The GALE ENCYCLOPEDIA of DIETS

A GUIDE TO HEALTH AND NUTRITION

SECOND EDITION

The GALE ENCYCLOPEDIA of DIETS

A GUIDE TO HEALTH AND NUTRITION

SECOND EDITION

VOLUME

A–L

KRISTIN KEY, EDITOR

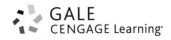

Detroit • New York • San Francisco • New Haven, Conn • Waterville, Maine • London

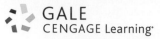
GALE
CENGAGE Learning·

Gale Encyclopedia of Diets, Second Edition

Project Editor: Kristin Key

Product Manager: Anne Marie Sumner

Editorial Support Services: Andrea Lopeman

Indexing Services: Laurie Andriot

Rights Acquisition and Management: Robyn Young

Composition: Evi Abou-El-Seoud

Manufacturing: Wendy Blurton

Imaging: John Watkins

Product Design: Kristine Julien

For product information and technology assistance, contact us at
Gale Customer Support, 1-800-877-4253.
For permission to use material from this text or product,
submit all requests online at **www.cengage.com/permissions.**
Further permissions questions can be emailed to
permissionrequest@cengage.com

While every effort has been made to ensure the reliability of the information presented in this publication, Gale, a part of Cengage Learning, does not guarantee the accuracy of the data contained herein. Gale accepts no payment for listing; and inclusion in the publication of any organization, agency, institution, publication, service, or individual does not imply endorsement of the editors or publisher. Errors brought to the attention of the publisher and verified to the satisfaction of the publisher will be corrected in future editions.

Library of Congress Cataloging-in-Publication Data

The Gale encyclopedia of diets : a guide to health and nutrition / Kristin Key, editor.– Second edition.
    2 volumes cm
   Includes bibliographical references and index.
   ISBN 978-1-4144-9884-3 (set) – ISBN 1-4144-9884-5 (set) – ISBN 978-1-4144-9885-0 (v. 1) – ISBN 1-4144-9885-3 (v. 1) – ISBN 978-1-4144-9886-7 (v.2) – ISBN 1-4144-9886-1 (v. 2) – ISBN 978-1-4144-9887-4 (ebk.) – ISBN 1-4144-9887-X (ebk.)
   1. Nutrition–Encyclopedias. 2. Diet–Encyclopedias. 3. Health–Encyclopedias. I. Key, Kristin, editor. II. Title: Encyclopedia of diets.
   RA784.G345 2013
   613.203--dc23   2012042115

Gale
27500 Drake Rd.
Farmington Hills, MI, 48331-3535

ISBN-13: 978-1-4144-9884-3 (set)   ISBN-10: 1-4144-9884-5 (set)
ISBN-13: 978-1-4144-9885-0 (vol. 1)   ISBN-10: 1-4144-9885-3 (vol. 1)
ISBN-13: 978-1-4144-9886-7 (vol. 2)   ISBN-10: 1-4144-9886-1 (vol. 2)

This title is also available as an e-book.
ISBN-13: 978-1-4144-9887-4 ISBN-10: 1-4144-9887-X
Contact your Gale, a part of Cengage Learning sales representative for ordering information.

Printed in China
1 2 3 4 5 6 7 17 16 15 14 13

CONTENTS

ALPHABETICAL LIST OF ENTRIES

PLEASE READ—IMPORTANT INFORMATION

The *Gale Encyclopedia of Diets: A Guide to Health and Nutrition* is a health reference product designed to inform and educate readers about a wide variety of diets, nutrition and dietary practices, and diseases and conditions associated with nutrition. Gale, Cengage Learning believes the product to be comprehensive, but not necessarily definitive. It is intended to supplement, not replace, consultation with a physician or other healthcare practitioner. While Gale, Cengage Learning has made substantial efforts to provide information that is accurate, comprehensive, and up-to-date, Gale, Cengage Learning makes no representations or warranties of any kind, including without limitation, warranties of merchantability or fitness for a particular purpose, nor does it guarantee the accuracy, comprehensiveness, or timeliness of the information contained in this product. Readers should be aware that the universe of medical knowledge is constantly growing and changing, and that differences of opinion exist among authorities. Readers are also advised to seek professional diagnosis and treatment for any medical condition, and to discuss information obtained from this book with their healthcare provider.

INTRODUCTION

The *Gale Encyclopedia of Diets: A Guide to Health and Nutrition* is a one-stop source for diet and nutrition information that covers popular and special diets, nutrition basics, and nutrition-related health conditions. It also addresses health and nutrition concerns across all age groups, from infants to seniors. The encyclopedia minimizes medical jargon, using language that any reader can understand while still providing thorough coverage of each topic. The *Gale Encyclopedia of Diets: A Guide to Health and Nutrition* does not endorse any one diet or lifestyle but aims to present readers with authoritative and balanced information.

SCOPE

Approximately 300 full-length articles are included in *The Gale Encyclopedia of Diets: A Guide to Health and Nutrition*. Entries follow a standardized format to provide information at a glance. Categories include:

Special and popular diets

- Definition
- Origins
- Description
- Function
- Benefits
- Precautions
- Risks
- Research and general acceptance

Nutrition basics

- Definition
- Purpose
- Description
- Recommended intake (for vitamins/minerals)

- Precautions
- Interactions
- Aftercare
- Complications
- Parental concerns

Diseases and conditions

- Definition
- Demographics
- Description
- Causes and symptoms
- Diagnosis
- Treatment
- Nutrition and dietary concerns
- Therapy
- Prognosis
- Prevention

Drugs and dietary supplements

- Definition
- Purpose
- Description
- Recommended dosage
- Precautions
- Side effects
- Interactions

INCLUSION CRITERIA

A preliminary list of diets and other nutrition topics was compiled from a wide variety of sources, including professional medical guides and textbooks as well as consumer guides and encyclopedias. An advisory board comprised of professionals in nutrition and medicine evaluated the topics and made suggestions for inclusion. The final selections were determined by Gale editors in conjunction with the advisory board.

ABOUT THE CONTRIBUTORS

The entries were written by experienced medical writers, including registered dietitians, nutritionists, healthcare practitioners and educators, pharmacists, researchers, and other professionals. The essays were reviewed by advisors to ensure that they are appropriate, up to date, and accurate.

HOW TO USE THIS BOOK

The Gale Encyclopedia of Diets: A Guide to Health and Nutrition has been designed with ready reference in mind:

- Straight **alphabetical arrangement** of topics allows users to locate information quickly.

- **Bold-faced terms** within entries direct the reader to related articles.

- Lists of **key terms** are provided where appropriate to define unfamiliar terms or concepts. A **glossary** of key terms is also included at the back of Volume 2.

- **Cross-references** placed throughout the *Encyclopedia* direct readers to primary entries from alternate names, drug brand names, and related topics.

- **Questions to Ask Your Doctor** sidebars provide sample questions that patients can ask their physicians.

- **Resources** at the end of every entry direct readers to additional sources of information on a topic.

- Valuable **contact information** for organizations and support groups is included with each entry and compiled in the back of Volume 2.

- A comprehensive **general index** allows users to easily find areas of interest.

GRAPHICS

The Gale Encyclopedia of Diets: A Guide to Health and Nutrition is enhanced with approximately 220 full-color images, including photographs, tables, and custom illustrations.

ADVISORY BOARD

A number of experts in health and nutrition have provided invaluable assistance in the formulation of this encyclopedia. Several of the advisors listed have also acted as contributing advisors, writing various articles related to their fields of expertise and experience.

CONTRIBUTORS

Margaret Alic, PhD
Science Writer
Eastsound, Washington

William Arthur Atkins
Science Writer
Atkins Research and Consulting
Pekin, Illinois

Jennifer Byrnes
Medical Writer
Lake Orion, Michigan

Stacy Chamberlin
Freelance Writer
New Albany, Ohio

William Connor
Oregon Health Sciences
    University
Portland, Oregon

Helen Davidson
Freelance Writer
Eugene, Oregon

Tish Davidson, AM
Medical Writer
Fremont, California

**Annette Dunne, BSc (Hons),
MSc, RD**
Freelance Dietitian
Cardiff, Wales, United
    Kingdom

Douglas Dupler, MA
Science Writer
Boulder, Colorado

Mohammed-Reza Forouzesh
California State University at
    Long Beach
Long Beach, California

Marie Fortin, MEd, RD
Family Health Nutritionist
Markham, Ontario, Canada

Marjorie Freedman
San Jose, California

Rebecca Frey, PhD
*Research and Administrative
Associate*
East Rock Institute
New Haven, Connecticut

Emil Ginter
Institute of Preventive and
    Clinical Medicine
Bratislava, Slovak Republic

Kirsten Herbes
University of Florida
Gainesville, Florida

Delores C. S. James
University of Florida
Gainesville, Florida

Warren B. Karp
The Medical College
    of Georgia
Augusta, Georgia

Monique Laberge, PhD
Research Associate
Department of Biochemistry
    and Biophysics
University of Pennsylvania
Philadelphia, Pennsylvania

Jens Levy
University of North Carolina
Chapel Hill, North Carolina

**Deborah Lycett, BSc (Hons), RD,
MBDA**
Freelance Dietitian
Worcester, England, United
    Kingdom

Emma Mills, RD
Registered Dietitian
Farnsfield, England, United
    Kingdom

Ranjita Misra
San Diego State University
San Diego, California

Braxton Mitchell
University of Maryland
Baltimore, Maryland

Susan Mitchell
Practicalories, Inc.
Winter Park, Florida

Laura Nelson
Texas A&M University
College Station, Texas

David E. Newton
Medical Writer
Ashland, Oregon

Debbie Nurmi, MS
*Medical Writer, Public Health
Researcher*
Atlanta, Georgia

**Melinda Granger Oberleitner, RN,
DNS**
*Acting Department Head and
Associate Professor*
Department of Nursing
University of Louisiana at Lafayette
Lafayette, Louisiana

Contributors

Teresa Odle
Medical Writer
Albuquerque, New Mexico

Lee Ann Paradise
Science Writer
Lubbock, Texas

Tracy Parker, Bsc (Hons), RD, HFI (ACSM)
Freelance Dietitian
London, England, United Kingdom

Gita Patel
Nutrition Consultant
Etna, New Hampshire

Megan Porter, RD, LD
Research Dietitian and Weight-Loss Instructor
Portland, Oregon

Thomas Prychitko
Research Scientist
Department of Nutrition and Food Science

Wayne State University
Detroit, Michigan

Sarah Schenker, SRD, PhD, RPHNutr
Nutrition Scientist
British Nutrition Institute
London, England, United Kingdom

Judith Sims, MS
Science Writer
Logan, Utah

Paulette Sinclair-Weir
University of North Carolina
Chapel Hill, North Carolina

Sara Stanner, MSc RPHNutr
Public Health Nutritionist
Welwyn, England, United Kingdom

Lisa A. Sutherland
University of North Carolina
Chapel Hill, North Carolina

Amy Sutton
Science Writer
Narvon, Pennsylvania

Liz Swain
Medical Writer
San Diego, California

Katherine Tucker
USDA/HNRCA at Tufts University
Boston, Massachusetts

Samuel Uretsky, PharmD
Pharmacist and Medical Writer
Wantagh, New York

Ruth Waibel
Elmont, New York

Ken Wells
Freelance Writer
Laguna Hills, California

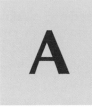

A

Abs diet

Definition

The Abs diet is a six-week plan that combines nutrition and exercise. It emphasizes 12 power foods that are the staples of the diet. It focuses on building muscle through strength training, aerobic exercises, and a dietary balance of proteins, **carbohydrates**, and fat. An updated version of the diet (the New Abs Diet) was released in 2010, and there is also a version targeted for women.

Origins

David Zinczenko, editor of *Men's Health*, developed the diet in 2004. He introduced it in the magazine and in his book *The Abs Diet: The Six-Week Plan to Flatten Your Stomach and Keep You Lean for Life*. Zinczenko says he grew up as an overweight child and by age 14 was 5 ft. 10 in. (1.8 m) tall and weighed 212 lb. (96 kg). He learned about fitness while in the U.S. Naval Reserve and nutrition from his tenure at *Men's Health*.

Despite its name, the diet does not specifically target abdominal fat. Exercise helps the body burn excess fat but it is not possible to target specific areas of fat, such as the abdomen. Diet and exercise help eliminate excess fat from all areas. If the bulk of a person's fat is around the belly, then that is where the greatest amount of fat-burning will occur. The Abs diet is designed to provide the necessary **vitamins**, **minerals**, and **fiber** for good health, while it promotes building muscle that helps increase the body's fat burning process.

Description

The Abs diet claims it will allow people to lose weight—primarily fat—while developing a leaner abdomen and increasing muscle tone, strength, general health, and sexual health. The diet has two components: exercise and nutrition. There are six general guidelines that are the basic principles of the diet. These are:

- eat six meals a day
- drink smoothies regularly
- know what to drink and what not to drink
- do not count calories
- eat anything for one meal a week
- focus on the Abs diet 12 power foods

The diet strongly recommends its followers eat six meals a day to help maintain what researchers call an energy balance. This is the number of **calories** burned in an hour versus the number of calories taken in. Georgia State University researchers found that when the hourly surplus or deficit of calories is 300–500 at any given time, the body is most susceptible to burning fat and building lean muscle mass. To stay within this range, Zinczenko recommends the following daily meal schedule: breakfast, mid-morning snack, lunch, mid-afternoon snack, dinner, and evening snack.

Another guideline is to drink smoothies regularly in place of a meal or snack. Smoothies are mixtures of low-fat milk and yogurt prepared in a blender with ingredients such as ice, **protein** powder, fruits, and peanut butter. Although there are no definitive studies, some researchers suggest that the **calcium** in the milk and yogurt helps to burn body fat and restricts the amount of fat produced by the body.

A third guideline details what to drink and not to drink. Drinking eight glasses of water daily is recommended. The benefits of 64 ounces of water are that it helps to alleviate hunger pangs, flushes waste products from the body, and delivers nutrients to muscles. Other acceptable drinks are low-fat milk, **green tea**, and no more than two glasses of diet soda a day. Alcohol is not recommended since it does not help to make a person feel full. It also decreases by one-third the body's ability to burn fat and makes the body store more of the fat from food. In addition, it decreases the production of testosterone and human growth hormone that help burn fat and increase muscle mass.

Although burning calories is required to lose fat, Zinczenko says calorie counting makes people lose focus and motivation. The foods allowed on the diet are energy-efficient and help curb feelings of hunger, according to Zinczenko.

People following the diet are allowed to cheat for one meal a week. The meal should include foods that the dieter misses most, including items high in carbohydrates and **fats**. This helps prevent feelings of burnout or frustration that are often experienced when dieting, at least in the early stages.

The last guideline is to focus on the 12 power foods of the diet to help meet core nutritional requirements. The 12 power foods are:

• almonds and other nuts (unsalted and unsmoked)
• beans (except refried and baked)
• green vegetables, including spinach, broccoli, Brussels sprouts, and asparagus
• non-fat or low-fat dairy products
• instant oatmeal (unsweetened and unflavored)
• eggs and egg substitute products
• lean meats, including turkey, chicken, fish, and beef
• peanut butter
• olive oil
• whole-grain breads and cereals
• whey protein powder
• berries

Other foods that can be eaten often include almond butter, apples, avocados, bananas, bean dips, brown rice, Canadian bacon, canola oil, cashew butter, citrus fruit and juices, edamame, fruit juices (sugar-free), garlic, hummus, lentils, mushrooms, melons, pasta (whole-wheat), peaches, peanut oil, peas, peppers (green, yellow, and orange), popcorn (fat-free), pretzels (whole-wheat), pumpkin seeds, sesame oil, shellfish, soup (broth-based), sunflower seeds, sweet potatoes, tomatoes, and yellow wax beans.

Exercise

Adequate exercise is as important as good nutrition in losing fat and flattening the stomach in the Abs diet. It includes strength training three times a week, abdominal exercises two or three days a week, and optional aerobic exercises two or three times a week. There are three basic principles to the exercise program: leave at least 48 hours between weight workouts of the same body part; do no exercises one day a week; and warm up for five minutes before exercising by jogging lightly, riding a stationary bike, jumping rope, or doing jumping jacks. There are three components of the plan that target different types of exercise:

• Strength training—Total-body workouts three days a week, with one workout placing extra emphasis on the leg muscles.
• Cardiovascular exercises—Do these twice a week in between strength training days. Activities include cycling, running, swimming, brisk walking, and stair climbing.
• Abdominal (ab) exercises—Do ab exercises two or three times a week, before strength training workouts.

GETTING STARTED. People who are not already exercising should do light strengthening exercises three days a week for the first two weeks. One sample routine is to alternate between three sets of 8–10 push-ups and three sets of 15–20 squats with no weights. Rest for one minute between sets. When it becomes easy to do 10 or more pushups and 20 or more squats, increase the number of pushups and add weights to the squats, using either a barbell or dumbbells. The weights routine should be followed by 30 minutes of brisk walking.

People who already exercise regularly should consider switching from their current workout routine to the Abs diet workout for at least the first few weeks, according to Zinczenko. For maximum results, it is best to change the workout routine every month to keep the body from adapting to a repetitious routine that can slow muscle development. The Abs diet suggests the basic workout be done on Mondays and Wednesdays, starting with one set of an ab exercise from each of the five categories of abdominal regions. Follow this with two circuits of one set of the core exercises in the order listed. On Tuesdays and Thursdays, do 20–30 minutes of cardiovascular exercise. On Friday, do the Monday and Wednesday workout, but replace the ab exercises with traveling lunges, 10–12 repetitions (reps), and step-ups, 10–12 reps each leg. Do two complete circuits.

ABDOMINAL EXERCISES. These exercises strengthen the abdominal muscles in five regions: upper abs, 12–15 reps; lower abs, 6–12 reps; obliques, 10 each side; transverse abdominis, 5–10 reps; and lower back, 12–15 reps. The following are exercises for each of the five abdominal regions. Upper abs: traditional crunch and modified raised-feet crunch; lower abs: figure-eight crunch and bent-leg knee raise; transverse abdominis: two-point bridge and Swiss ball pull-in; obliques: medicine ball torso rotation and two-handed wood chop; lower back: twisting back extension and Swiss ball Superman.

CORE EXERCISES. These are the basic exercises that promote muscle strength: squat, 10–12 reps; bench press, 10 reps; pulldown, 10 reps; military press, 10 reps; upright row, 10 reps; triceps pushdown, 10–12 reps; leg extension, 10–12 reps; biceps curl, 10 reps; and leg curl, 10–12 reps.

Function

The primary purpose of the Abs diet is to help people, especially men, develop a lean, flat, and hard stomach—referred to in fitness circles as a "six-pack"—and maintain a healthy weight and lifestyle. The diet is designed to promote a longer and healthier life by helping prevent **cancer**, heart disease, high blood pressure, diabetes, and other diseases. These diseases are more prevalent in overweight and obese people compared to people who maintain a normal or below normal weight. The diet is also designed to promote a healthier sex life in men since some of the causes of erectile dysfunction are **obesity**, heart disease, and diabetes.

Benefits

Excessive fat, especially around the belly, is a major risk factor for heart disease, high blood pressure, high LDL ("bad") cholesterol, diabetes, erectile dysfunction, and other diseases. By reducing or eliminating excess body fat, people can live healthier and longer lives. The health benefits increase when regular exercise is added. People on the Abs diet can expect to lose up to 12 lb. (5.4 kg) in the first two weeks followed by 5–8 lb. (2.3–3.6 kg) in the next two weeks, according to Juliette Kellow, a registered dietitian who reviews diets for Weight Loss Resources (http://www.weightlossresources.co.uk).

Most diets include cardiovascular (aerobic) exercise as part of a weight loss routine. Studies have shown that people who engage in aerobic exercise burn more calories than people who do strength training or weightlifting. However, additional research indicates that the fat-burning metabolic effects of aerobic exercise last 30–60 minutes, while the metabolic effects of strength training last up to 48 hours. Also, the Abs diet promotes increased muscle mass, which increases **metabolism** so that the body burns up to 50 calories per day for every pound of muscle. Adding 10 lb. (4.5 kg) of muscle can burn up to 500 extra calories each day.

Precautions

Overall, the Abs diet is healthy and poses no known dangers. Some of the items listed in the 12 power foods

---

---

can contain high amounts of **sodium**, such as canned and frozen vegetables, instant oatmeal, and peanut butter. People who want to limit salt intake or who have high blood pressure may want to avoid these foods. Since exercise is a main component of the diet, people with arthritis or back, knee, or other joint problems should discuss the diet with their physicians before starting exercise. People who are allergic to peanuts or nuts should avoid foods containing these products.

The diet does not address whether it is suitable for vegetarians or vegans. Menus in the book do not have meatless options. However, 8 of the 12 power foods do not contain meat or animal products. All of the protein required in the diet can be obtained by adding more beans and legumes and by replacing meat with **soy** protein sources, such as tofu or meat substitutes that are high in protein.

Risks

Since the diet includes a rigorous and regular exercise program, people with heart disease or other health problems should consult their physicians before going on the diet. Men with erectile dysfunction should discuss their condition with their physicians, urologists, or endocrinologists. Also, one of the 12 power foods is nuts, so people with peanut or other nut allergies should eliminate or modify the nut component of the diet.

Research and general acceptance

There is no specific research that proves the Abs diet delivers on what it promises: fat loss, muscle gain, increased sex drive, and six-pack abs. It is also unclear

QUESTIONS TO ASK YOUR DOCTOR

- Is the Abs diet a healthy weight-loss option for me?
- Do I have any physical or dietary restrictions that would prevent me from following this diet plan?
- If I have a nut allergy, what foods can I substitute for the recommended nut products?
- Is it safe for me to start an exercise program?

whether the diet will help people maintain a healthy weight once the initial weight is lost. The book contains many anecdotal stories of success, but there are no scientific studies that document the claims.

Zinczenko, along with fellow author Matt Goulding, also published a popular book called *Eat This, Not That!* There are a variety of titles in this series, which educate readers on making healthy food choices in restaurants, the supermarket, and at home.

Resources

BOOKS

Zinczenko, David. *The New Abs Diet for Women: The Six-Week Plan to Flatten Your Stomach and Keep You Lean for Life.* Emmaus, PA: Rodale, 2011.

Zinczenko, David, and Ted Spiker. *The Abs Diet Eat Right Every Time Guide.* Emmaus, PA: Rodale, 2005.

———. *The Abs Diet Get Fit Stay Fit Plan: The Exercise Program to Flatten Your Belly, Reshape Your Body, and Give You Abs for Life!* Emmaus, PA: Rodale, 2005.

———. *The Abs Diet 6-Minute Meals for 6-Pack Abs: More Than 150 Great-Tasting Recipes to Melt Away Fat!* Emmaus, PA: Rodale, 2006.

———. *The New Abs Diet: The Six-Week Plan to Flatten Your Stomach and Keep You Lean for Life.* Emmaus, PA: Rodale, 2010.

PERIODICALS

Aceto, Chris. "Build Muscle, Stay Lean! Open Up Our Nutritional Toolbox and Head to the Job Site: Your Kitchen Table. This State-of-the-Art Diet Plan Will Help You Add Muscle Without Gaining Fat." *Muscle & Fitness* (November 2006): 110–14.

———. "Protein & Carbs: Carbohydrates and Protein Have Been Misunderstood For Years. Here Are the Top 10 Myths That Plague Your Diet—And Your Physique." *Muscle & Fitness* (September 2005): 100–104.

Donnelly, Allan. "Critical Condition: Need to Get Ripped in a Hurry? Mark Dugdale's Fast-Track Nutritional Overhaul Will Help You Drop Body Fat in Five Easy Steps." *Flex* (October 2006): 216–20.

Horn, Beth. "M & F Blueprint: 6 Weeks to a Six-Pack; Build Awesome Abs With This Step-By-Step Training and Diet Program." *Muscle & Fitness* (May 2002): 142–45.

Zinczenko, David. "Abs Diet." *Men's Health* (Jul–Aug 2004): 154.

———. "Eat Right Every Time." *Men's Health* (Jan–Feb 2005): 130.

———. "7 Days to a 6-Pack." *Men's Health* (September 2004): 158.

WEBSITES

"The Abs Diet." http://www.absdiet.com (accessed August 7, 2012).

Truex, Leslie. "The Abs Diet." Livestrong.com. http://www.livestrong.com/article/488677-the-abs-diet (accessed August 7, 2012).

U.S. News & World Report. "The Abs Diet." http://health.usnews.com/best-diet/abs-diet (accessed August 16, 2012).

Zinczenko, David. "The 7-Day Abs Diet Meal Plan." Men's Health.com. http://www.menshealth.com/nutrition/abs-diet-weekly-meal-plan-recipes (accessed August 16, 2012).

ORGANIZATIONS

Academy of Nutrition and Dietetics, 120 South Riverside Plz., Ste. 2000, Chicago, IL 60606-6995, (312) 899-0040, (800) 877-1600, amacmunn@eatright.org, http://www.eatright.org.

Center for Nutrition Policy and Promotion, U.S. Department of Agriculture, 3101 Park Center Drive, 10th Fl., Alexandria, VA 22302, (703) 305-7600, Fax: (703) 305-3300, support@cnpp.usda.gov, http://www.cnpp.usda.gov.

Ken R. Wells
Stacey Chamberlin

Academy of Nutrition and Dietetics

Definition

The American Academy of Nutrition and Dietetics is the largest organization of registered dietitians in the world. With approximately 72,000 members in the United States, including the District of Columbia and Puerto Rico, the organization has an annual budget of $26 million. Formerly the American Dietetic Association (ADA), in January 2012 the association changed its name to the Academy of Nutrition and Dietetics and eschewed the use of any acronym for its name. Once the new name has become established, the organization will adopt the acronym AND; until then, it is to be known simply as "The Academy."

Origins

The Academy was founded by a group of women in Cleveland, Ohio, in 1917. Led by Lenna F. Cooper and first president Lulu C. Graves, the goal of the organization was to aid the government in food conservation and enhance the public's understanding of health and nutrition during a time of war.

Purpose

The Academy is committed to helping the public benefit from a healthy lifestyle, focusing on five critical health areas:

- obesity and overweight, with special emphasis on children
- healthy aging
- having a safe, sustainable, and nutritious food supply
- nutrigenetics and nutrigenomics
- integrative medicine, including supplements and alternative medicine

The Academy's mission is "leading the future of dietetics." Every March, the Academy sponsors National Nutrition Month, providing food and nutrition information to the public through numerous programs and services.

Description

Most of the Academy's members are registered dietitians (RDs), with a small percentage coming from dietetic technicians, registered (DTRs). Other members include clinical and community dietetics professionals, consultants, foodservice managers, educators, researchers, dietetic technicians, and students. Academy members are able to join focused dietetic practice groups within the Academy. These groups represent a wide range of practice areas and interests including public health; **sports nutrition**; medical nutrition therapy; diet counseling, cholesterol reduction; diabetes, heart, and kidney disease; **vegetarianism**; food service management in business, hospitals, restaurants, long-term care facilities, and education systems; education of other healthcare professionals; entrepreneurism; and scientific research.

Professionals choose to belong to the Academy to receive the membership benefits. The Academy provides continuing education opportunities, access to the Academy Evidence Analysis Library, subscription to the *Journal of the Academy of Nutrition and Dietetics*, and access to additional information and resources. Membership dues are paid annually and range from $110–$245.

RDs and DTRs

A registered dietitian is a professional who has met academic training requirements in the areas of food and nutrition. Some RDs hold additional certifications in specialized areas of practice, such as pediatric or **renal nutrition** and diabetes education. RDs must possess a bachelor's degree with course work approved by the Academy's Accreditation Council for Education in Nutrition and Dietetics. Coursework typically includes food and nutrition sciences, foodservice systems management, business, economics, computer science, sociology, biochemistry, physiology, microbiology, and chemistry. RDs must also complete an accredited, supervised, experiential practice program at a health-care facility, community agency, or foodservice corporation, and must pass a national examination administered by the Commission on Dietetic Registration. Continuing professional education is required to maintain registration.

Dietetic technicians, registered, must complete a two-year associate's degree in an approved dietetic technician program, have supervised practice experience, and pass a nationwide examination administered by the Academy to earn the DTR credential, and must complete continuing education courses throughout their careers.

Credentialing

The Academy is involved in the process of accrediting educational programs for RDs and DTRs. The development of an accreditation process was incorporated into the Academy to maintain the reputability of nutrition and dietetics education programs. RDs and DTRs must continue their education programs and meet certain eligibility requirements to keep their titles. The Academy is also affiliated with the Commission on Dietetic Registration, which oversees the registration of dietitians and diet technicians.

The Accreditation Council for Education in Nutrition and Dietetics (ACEND; formerly the Commission on Accreditation for Dietetics Education, CADE) is the Academy's accrediting agency for education programs that prepare dietetic students for careers as nutrition professionals. Recognized by the U.S. Department of Education and the Council for Higher Education Accreditation, ACEND is a reliable authority on the quality of nutrition and dietetics education programs. All dietetic programs that meet their standards are accredited through ACEND.

The Commission on Dietetic Registration

The Commission on Dietetic Registration (CDR) is the overseer of the professions of RD, DTR, board-certified specialist in renal nutrition (CSR), board-certified specialist in pediatric nutrition (CSP), board-certified specialist in sports dietetics (CSSD), board-certified specialist in gerontological nutrition (CSG), and board-certified specialist in oncology nutrition (CSO). Since the credentialing process began, more than 80,000 dietitians and dietetic technicians worldwide have taken the CDR exams.

The CDR consists of 11 members: 7 RDs, an RD specialist, and a DTR, who serve five-year terms; a newly credentialed RD, who serves for one year; a public representative, who serves for five years; and the chair and vice-chair, who each serve a one-year term. The CDR's certification programs are accredited by the National Commission for Certifying Agencies (NCCA), the accrediting arm of the Institute for Credentialing Excellence in Washington, DC.

Government and public policy

To help fulfill their mission, the Academy began an advocacy network based in Washington, DC. This government affairs office negotiates with state and federal legislators and agencies on public policy issues related to dietetics. Through their efforts, the Academy has influenced Medicare coverage of medical nutrition therapy, child nutrition, **obesity**, the Dietary Guidelines for Americans, and other health and nutrition concerns.

Academy of Nutrition and Dietetics Foundation (ANDF)

The ANDF was established in 1966 as a 501(c)(3) public charity and is the philanthropic arm of the Academy. It provides money for research, education, and public awareness programs. The Foundation's primary foci are funding of scholarships for nutrition and dietetic students, supporting food and nutrition research, providing leadership in promoting and achieving healthy weight for children, and helping to reduce the growing prevalence of **childhood obesity**. The ANDF's mission is to fund the future of the dietetics profession through research and education. ANDF is the largest grantor of scholarships in the nutrition and dietetic fields for graduate, undergraduate, and continuing education scholarships.

A 13-member board of directors that includes the president-elect, financial officer, and CEO of the Academy, as well as up to five public members, governs the Academy Foundation. It has an operating budget of over $7 million in endowed support for its causes and operations, donated by both individuals and industries. Approximately $1.4 million of the operating budget goes to fundraising and grantmaking activities.

Professional publications

The Academy publishes the *Journal of the Academy of Nutrition and Dietetics*. The peer-reviewed journal is written by and for dietetics professionals. The journal covers topics in nutritional science, medical nutrition therapy, public health nutrition, food science and biotechnology, foodservice systems, leadership and management, and dietetics education.

The Academy also promotes nutrition information for consumers through various media. Its website is filled with content such as news releases and consumer tips, including nutrition fact sheets, consumer FAQs, and a "Good Nutrition Reading List." The "Find a Registered Dietitian" feature allows consumers seeking the services of an RD to search for one in their area.

Relatively new to the Academy is a series of position statements that are regularly produced by the association. These position statements encompass multifaceted issues related to nutrition and are the official opinions of the Academy on issues that affect the nutritional and health status of the public. These statements are based on the latest scientific research available and are reviewed and updated on a regular basis.

Resources

WEBSITES

Academy of Nutrition and Dietetics. "Academy Position Papers." http://www.eatright.org/About/Content.aspx?id=6442460576 (accessed June 20, 2012).
———. "Accreditation Council for Education in Nutrition and Dietetics." http://www.eatright.org/ACEND/content.aspx?id=7877 (accessed June 20, 2012).
Commission on Dietetic Registration. http://www.cdrnet.org (accessed June 20, 2012).
Journal of the Academy of Nutrition and Dietetics. http://www.adajournal.org (accessed June 20, 2012).

ORGANIZATIONS

Academy of Nutrition and Dietetics, 120 South Riverside Plz., Ste. 2000, Chicago, IL 60606-6995, (312) 899-0040, (800) 877-1600, amacmunn@eatright.org, http://www.eatright.org.

Megan C.M. Porter, RD, LD
David Newton

Açaí berry

Definition

Açaí (pronounced ah-sah-EE) berry is the drupe, or fruit, of the açaí palm tree (*Euterpe oleracea*), a species of palm native to Central and South America. The name of the plant is the Portuguese form of its name in the Tupi language—a word that means "fruit that cries water." At one time the açaí palm was cultivated primarily for hearts of palm, a vegetable obtained from the inner core and growing bud of the tree. Since the early 2000s, however, the açaí palm has been cultivated primarily for its fruit while closely related species of palm are grown for hearts of palm.

Other names for açaí berry include Açaí Palm, Amazon Açaí Fruit, Assai, Assaí Palm, Baie de Palmier Pinot, Cabbage Palm, Chou Palmiste, and Palmier d'Açaí.

Purpose

Açaí berries are a traditional food for the indigenous tribes of the Amazon rainforest; the berries were also used by the tribespeople to treat diarrhea. In Canada and the United States, the berries are most often sold in health food stores or specialty supermarkets as frozen pulp or used in juices and juice products, smoothie mixes, jellies, ice cream, liqueurs, and similar fruit-flavored products. Açaí berries may be blended with other fruits or berries in these products or used as the sole flavoring.

Açaí berries are also used in the manufacture of **dietary supplements** that include liquid tonics, tablets, shake mixes, and snack bars. These products claim to produce health benefits ranging from weight loss and boosting of the immune system to diabetes management and increased virility in men. However, no scientific studies provide any proof of these claims.

There were four clinical trials of açaí berries registered with the National Institutes of Health (NIH) as of summer 2012: one study evaluated the effects of the berries when added to a high-antioxidant diet to slow the effects of aging; a second study concerned the effects of açaí in lowering risk factors for atherosclerosis; the third study was recruiting subjects for a study of the effectiveness of açaí in treating men with high levels of prostate-specific antigen; and the fourth study evaluated a high-fiber product that contained açaí berries as a treatment for **constipation**. Açaí berries have been used as an ingredient in some skin care products, as the plant oils contained in the berries appear to be beneficial in reducing inflammation and hyperpigmentation. Açaí has also been used in a pilot study as a possible treatment for **metabolic syndrome**, a condition that is often a precursor of type 2 diabetes, but the authors recommend further study to replicate their tentative findings.

Description

The açaí berry itself is a small, round, blackish-purple fruit about an inch in diameter that grows in branched clusters of 500–900 fruits under the fronds of the açaí palm, a slender species of palm tree that ranges from 45 to 90 feet in height. Its dark color is caused by anthocyanins, a class of flavonoids or plant pigments. The berries resemble grapes in size and general shape but contain much less pulp; the seed of the açaí berry comprises about 80% of the fruit. Açaí berries are not naturally sweet.

According to a 2006 study published in the *Journal of Agricultural and Food Chemistry*, a standardized freeze-dried powder made from the skin and pulp of açaí berries contains 533 **calories** per 100 grams (about 3.5 ounces dry weight), 52.2 g **carbohydrates**, 8.1 g **protein**, and 32.5 g total fat. The carbohydrate portion of the pulp included 44 grams of dietary **fiber** and little **sugar**. Of the fat content, 56.2% is oleic acid (the same fat found in olive oil), 24.1% is palmitic acid, and 12.5% linoleic acid. With regard to **vitamins** and **minerals**, the **vitamin C** content of the powder is very low, but the preparation does contain 260 mg of **calcium**, 4.4 mg of **iron**, and 1,002 units of **vitamin A**.

Brand names

The most common brands of açaí berry products sold in the United States and Canada are marketed by Sambazon and MonaVie. The latter company, which also markets its products in Australia, New Zealand,

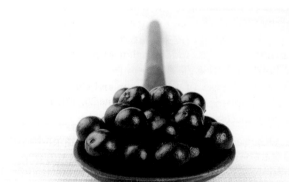

Açaí berries. (© Istockphoto.com/Brasil2)

Brazil, Hungary, Japan, Israel, Singapore, Austria, the United Kingdom, Mexico, Thailand, and Taiwan, has been subjected to enforcement actions by the U.S. Food and Drug Administration (FDA) in the United States for exaggerated health claims made about its products.

Sambazon primarily sells bottled juices, smoothie mixes, energy drinks, sorbet, and the freeze-dried powder. Its products include combinations of açaí berries and cranberries, pomegranates, and other fruits as well as pure açaí products. Although Sambazon describes açaí as a "superfood," it does not claim that its products will speed up weight loss, cure the common cold, or reverse the aging process.

As of 2012, neither the FDA nor any other government regulatory agency had evaluated açaí berries as a foodstuff. The **Academy of Nutrition and Dietetics** (formerly the American Dietetic Association) considers açaí to be as healthful as other fruits such as strawberries or blueberries, and safe to eat, but not as exceptional as it is made out to be in mass-market advertising.

Recommended dosage

There is no particular recommended dosage for açaí berry products used in so-called functional foods or nutraceuticals in combination with other ingredients, including other fruits or fruit flavorings. The Sambazon freeze-dried açaí berry supplement recommends adding one "scoop" (3 grams) to "your favorite smoothie, juice or milk." There is not enough scientific information to provide guidance on appropriate dosages of açaí as a dietary supplement.

Precautions

Açaí berries used in beverages, smoothies, and similar products appear to be safe for most people to eat; a toxicology report published in 2010 found nothing harmful in the fruit itself. Because the berries are acidic like most other fruits, consumers who have gastric **ulcers** or recurrent problems with **heartburn** should be careful not to ingest them together with NSAIDs like aspirin or ibuprofen. Until açaí dietary supplements have been evaluated for safety, they should not be used by children and pregnant or lactating women.

The chief danger for consumers of açaí berry products is the risk of false advertising claims, contaminated or mislabeled products, and credit card scams. As early as 2007, the FDA sent a registered letter to one of the executives of MonaVie, warning the company that its advertising of açaí as a fruit that can lower blood cholesterol levels, relieve the pain of arthritis, and relieve muscle pain was in effect to "establish the products as

KEY TERMS

Anthocyanins—A subgroup of flavonoids that cause the red, dark blue, or purple color of certain plants. Anthocyanins are responsible for the dark purplish color of açaí berries.

Antioxidant—Any molecule that inhibits the oxidation of other molecules. Antioxidant compounds in dietary supplements or cosmetics are claimed to benefit health and slow down the aging process.

Drupe—Any fruit that contains a soft, fleshy pulp (mesocarp) surrounded by an outer skin (exocarp) and containing a central inner stone or pit (endocarp) that contains the seed. Açaí berries are drupes.

Flavonoid—Any member of a large group of aromatic compounds that occur naturally in higher plants, mostly as plant pigments.

Functional food—A term used to describe a natural or processed food that contains biologically active compounds in sufficient amounts to benefit health.

Nutraceutical—A fortified food or dietary supplement that provides health benefits. Nutraceutical is often used as a synonym for functional food.

Rhabdomyolysis—A condition in which damaged skeletal muscle tissue breaks down and the breakdown products are released into the bloodstream.

Superfood—An unscientific term used largely in marketing to describe foods that have a high nutrient content or plant-derived compounds thought to be beneficial to health.

drugs" and violated the Federal Food, Drug, and Cosmetic Act. The company is largely responsible for the worldwide interest in açaí berries, which began with its aggressive marketing of the fruit in 2005. In addition to making unsupported claims about the health benefits of its products, MonaVie sells its tonics, dietary supplements, shake mixes, and energy drinks at inflated prices: one bottle of MonaVie Active (a fruit drink) is priced at $37, while a case of four bottles sells for $130. The dietary supplement, "designed to promote weight management success," is $65 for a one-month supply.

Other açaí berry products have been found by the FDA to be mislabeled. In one case, a man developed rhabdomyolysis (a muscle disorder) after taking a product labeled as an açaí berry dietary supplement. Chemical analysis revealed that the product did not contain any açaí. In an October 2011 case, the FDA issued a public warning about an açaí berry product,

Açaí Berry Soft Gel ABC, which contained sibutramine, a controlled substance removed from the market in 2010 for safety reasons. Sibutramine raises blood pressure and pulse rate and thus poses a risk to people with high blood pressure, heart disease, or a history of stroke. The FDA issued the statement "to inform the public of a growing trend of products marketed as dietary supplements or conventional foods with hidden drugs and chemicals."

Credit card scams involving açaí berry products first came to media attention in 2009, when the Center for Science in the Public Interest (CSPI) issued a warning about Web-based açaí scams. The scams promise consumers a "free" trial of açaí products provided the customer pays a $5.95 shipping and handling fee, for which a credit card number must be supplied. The company then continues to charge the customer each month for a shipment of the product, and customers who try to cancel the shipments have difficulty stopping the recurrent charges. The Better Business Bureau (BBB) has specifically given "F" ratings to such companies as FX Supplements, which markets Açaí Berry Maxx; Advanced Wellness Research, which sells Pure Açaí Berry Pro and AçaíBurn; and SFL Nutrition.

Some people believe that consuming açaí berries will negate the effects of an unhealthy diet. This is not true, and eating açaí berries or using açaí berry products does not replace the need to consume a wide variety of fruits and vegetables, many of which are cheaper than açaí.

Side effects

No serious side effects have been reported for açaí berry functional foods and flavored beverages. The case of rhabdomyolysis concerned a patient who had used a dietary supplement mislabeled as containing açaí when none was present in the product.

Interactions

Little information is available on interactions between açaí berries and other drugs. People taking pain medications or **cancer** drugs should check with their doctor before using açaí, however, as it may lower their effectiveness. It is a good idea for adults to check with their doctor before adding açaí products to their diet.

Resources

BOOKS

Qian, Michael C., and Agnes M. Rimando, eds. *Flavor and Health Benefits of Small Fruits*, sponsored by the ACS Division of Agricultural and Food Chemistry. Washington, DC: American Chemical Society, 2010.

Zoumbaris, Sharon, ed. *Encyclopedia of Wellness: From Açaí Berry to Yo-yo Dieting*. Santa Barbara, CA: Greenwood, 2012.

PERIODICALS

Elsayed, R.K., et al. "Rhabdomyolysis Associated with the Use of a Mislabeled 'Açaí Berry' Dietary Supplement." *American Journal of the Medical Sciences* 342 (December 2011): 535–38.

Fowler, J.F. Jr., et al. "Innovations in Natural Ingredients and Their Use in Skin Care." *Journal of Drugs in Dermatology* 9 (June 2010): suppl. 6: S72–S81.

Jensen, G.S., et al. "Pain Reduction and Improvement in Range of Motion after Daily Consumption of an Açaí (*Euterpe oleracea* Mart.) Pulp-fortified Polyphenolic-rich Fruit and Berry Juice Blend." *Journal of Medicinal Food* 14 (Jul–Aug 2011): 702–11.

Marcason, W. "What is the Açaí Berry and Are There Health Benefits?" *Journal of the American Dietetic Association* 109 (November 2009): 1968.

Schauss, A.G., et al. "Phytochemical and Nutrient Composition of the Freeze-Dried Amazonian Palm Berry *Euterpe oleraceae* mart. (Açaí)." *Journal of Agricultural and Food Chemistry* 54 (November 1, 2006): 8598–8603.

Schauss, A.G., et al. "Safety Evaluation of an Açaí-fortified Fruit and Berry Functional Juice Beverage (MonaVie Active®)." *Toxicology* 278 (November 28, 2010): 46–54.

Udani, J.K., et al. "Effects of Açaí (*Euterpe oleracea* Mart.) Berry Preparation on Metabolic Parameters in a Healthy Overweight Population: A Pilot Study." *Nutrition Journal* 10 (May 2011): 45. http://dx.doi.org/10.1186/1475-2891-10-45 (accessed September 19, 2012).

WEBSITES

Academy of Nutrition and Dietetics. "The Facts on Açaí." http://www.eatright.org/Public/content.aspx?id=10726 (accessed September 19, 2012).

Center for Science in the Public Interest (CSPI). "Consumers Warned of Web-Based Açaí Scams." http://www.cspinet.org/new/200903231_print.html (accessed September 19, 2012).

Mayo Clinic. "Açaí Berries: Do They Have Health Benefits?" http://www.mayoclinic.com/health/acai/AN01836 (accessed September 19, 2012).

National Center for Complementary and Alternative Medicine. "Açaí Berry." http://nccam.nih.gov/health/acai (accessed September 19, 2012).

U.S. Food and Drug Administration (FDA). "Public Notification: 'Açaí Berry Soft Gel ABC' Contains Undeclared Drug Ingredient," October 18, 2011. http://www.fda.gov/Drugs/ResourcesForYou/Consumers/BuyingUsing MedicineSafely/MedicationHealthFraud/ucm276098.htm (accessed September 12, 2012).

U.S. Food and Drug Administration (FDA) Enforcement Activities. "MonaVie Original," "MonaVie Active," "MonaVie Combo," and "MonaVie Gel." http://www.fda.gov/downloads/Drugs/GuidanceComplianceRegu latoryInformation/EnforcementActivitiesbyFDA/Cyber Letters/ucm056937.pdf (accessed September 12, 2012).

ORGANIZATIONS

Academy of Nutrition and Dietetics, 120 South Riverside Plz., Ste. 2000, Chicago, IL 60606-6995, (312) 899-0040, (800) 877-1600, amacmunn@eatright.org, http://www.eatright.org.

Center for Science in the Public Interest, 1220 L St. NW, Ste. 300, Washington, DC 20005, (202) 332-9110, Fax: (202) 265-4954, http://www.cspinet.org.

Center for Science in the Public Interest (Canada), Ste. 2701, CTTC Bldg., 1125 Colonel By Dr., Ottawa, Ontario, Canada K1S 5R1, (613) 244-7337, jefferyb@istar.ca, http://www.cspinet.org.

U.S. Food and Drug Administration, 10903 New Hampshire Ave., Silver Spring, MD 20993-0002, (888) INFO-FDA (463-6332), http://www.fda.gov.

Rebecca J. Frey, PhD

Acid reflux *see* **Gastroesophageal reflux disease (GERD)**

Acne diet

Definition

The acne diet—or, more accurately, the acne-free diet—is a way of eating that claims to improve or eliminate acne. There is some debate in the medical community about the impact of diet on acne; however, there is a body of evidence to support the idea that certain foods affect the skin.

By reviewing research from over 40 years, doctors such as dermatologist Dean Goodless have developed a set of recommendations regarding foods that may prevent acne. Goodless presents his recommendations

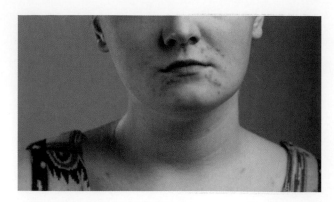

Teenage girl with acne. *(Melianiaka Kanstantsin/ Shutterstock.com)*

in his book *The Acne-Free Diet Plan.* He suggests eating a diet low in fat and high in **fiber** along with avoiding peanut products, fried foods, excessive salt, dairy products, foods high in refined sugars, and high-carbohydrate foods.

Origins

Most cultures had folk remedies to help clear the skin, but it was not until the later part of the twentieth century that serious scientific research began to confirm or disprove these folk tales and myths. One of the earliest studies about food and acne focused on chocolate, based on the belief that chocolate contributed to acne. (The study found that chocolate did not increase acne breakouts, and other studies since have confirmed this finding.) Other studies have investigated ethnic groups and communities where there is little or no incidence of acne, such as in the Pacific Islands and Africa. When the diets of these areas were compared to the typical Western diet, there were nutritionally significant differences: the ethnic groups with very low incidence of acne ate predominately plant-based diets that were low in fat and virtually **sugar** free, whereas the Western diets were heavy in meats, saturated fat, refined sugar, and processed foods. By studying these differences, doctors and researchers developed suggestions for dietary changes to improve or eliminate acne.

Description

Acne is caused when glands in the skin called sebaceous glands begin to form a sticky oil called sebum. These glands are stimulated by hormones that become active at puberty, which is why acne occurs most often in adolescence, when these hormones are produced in abundance. The oils formed by the sebaceous glands hold dead skin cells, preventing them from being sloughed off. As these cells die, they create the perfect

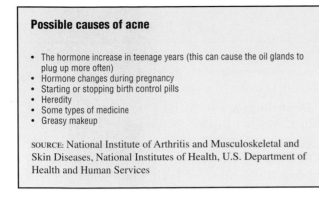

Possible causes of acne

- The hormone increase in teenage years (this can cause the oil glands to plug up more often)
- Hormone changes during pregnancy
- Starting or stopping birth control pills
- Heredity
- Some types of medicine
- Greasy makeup

SOURCE: National Institute of Arthritis and Musculoskeletal and Skin Diseases, National Institutes of Health, U.S. Department of Health and Human Services

(Table by GGS Information Services. © 2013 Cengage Learning.)

environment for bacteria to grow. When these bacteria, called acne vulgaris, become too plentiful, they will attempt to erupt from the skin, causing a pimple. Sometimes, when the bacteria grow, the body sends white blood cells to fight the infection. This natural reaction can cause large, painful cysts to form in the deeper layers of skin.

Opinions vary in the medical community as to whether or not diet plays a significant role in acne. Some dietary changes that have been proposed to help prevent acne breakouts include:

- Eat 20 to 30 grams of fiber every day. Fiber helps keep the colon clean and may remove toxins from the body before they reach the skin.
- Eat a low-fat diet. High fat consumption may elevate hormone levels in the body that cause blemishes on the skin.
- Avoid peanut products. Peanut products were found to cause acne flare ups in a study of 500 adolescents.
- Avoid fried foods.
- Limit salt intake, especially table salt or iodized salt. Many people with acne have elevated levels of iodine, found in table salt, in their bloodstream during acne flare-ups.
- Avoid dairy products such as milk, cheese, and ice cream.

Other **vitamins** and **minerals** proposed to affect acne include vitamins A, E, and B; **selenium**; **zinc**; **omega-3 fatty acids**; and **chromium**.

Carbohydrates

Many high-carbohydrate foods are believed to worsen acne, due to the spike in blood sugar caused by eating white sugar or refined carbs. This spike raises the level of **insulin** in the body, and elevated insulin levels may increase production of acne-causing hormones. However, some **carbohydrates**, such as those made with **whole grains**, digest more slowly than others, causing a gradual (as opposed to rapid) rise in blood sugar after eating. A system known as the glycemic index ranks carbohydrates and other foods according to the effect they have on blood sugar.

The glycemic index ranks foods based on a scale of 0–100. Foods with higher glycemic index ratings break down quickly and cause a sharp spike in blood sugar. When blood sugar rises quickly, the body produces a surge of insulin to lower the amount of glucose (sugar) in the blood. Insulin is a hormone that helps the body take glucose out of the bloodstream and put it into cells, where it can be used for energy or stored in fat. Foods with lower glycemic index ratings break down more slowly and cause a more gradual rise in blood sugar, meaning that less insulin will be needed.

Foods that have a high glycemic index rating include:

- white bread
- white rice
- white potatoes, depending on how they are cooked
- beer
- corn products and some products containing refined sugars

Foods with moderate glycemic index ratings include:

- whole grain breads and pastas
- brown rice
- sweet potatoes
- green peas
- many fruits (especially when eaten alone)
- yogurt

Low glycemic index foods may be enjoyed often without worsening acne. These include:

- rye grain
- nuts
- legumes such as black beans and lentils
- green vegetables
- apricots
- cherries

Foods that are high in fiber tend to have lower glycemic index numbers, because fiber takes longer to digest. Studies have shown that the presence of healthy **fats**, such as olive oil, can also slow digestion and keep blood sugar from rising too quickly.

Function

Eliminating certain foods from the diet and increasing the amount of specific vitamins and minerals may help reduce the amount of sebum produced and prevent acne breakouts. However, the interaction between diet and acne is not a simple cause-and-effect relationship—if an oily food is eaten, the oil does not travel to the skin or cause it to be oily. However, high levels of fat in the blood may effect the production of hormones such as testosterone, and higher levels of hormones may cause acne to worsen.

Benefits

Habits such as limiting **sodium**, processed foods, and saturated fats (found in fried foods) and increasing intake of whole grains, vegetables, and fiber are in line with federal dietary recommendations and support overall health. However, foods such as fruits and low-fat dairy products provide important nutrients like **calcium** and **vitamin C**, and eliminating entire food groups could potentially lead to vitamin or mineral deficiencies. People interested in the acne diet should consult with a physician or registered dietitian before starting the diet.

Precautions

Some acne diets suggest zinc or **vitamin A** supplementation. People should always consult with their physicians before taking any supplements or other drugs. Zinc supplements can cause stomach upset, and authors of acne diet plans recommend no more than 30 mg of zinc per day to avoid this.

Pregnant women or those who may become pregnant should not take vitamin A supplements or any medications containing vitamin A, as excessive amounts of vitamin A may cause birth defects.

Limiting the amount of dairy products in the diet may limit the amount of calcium consumed. A calcium supplement may be needed to ensure that daily dietary calcium requirements are met.

Dietary supplements could potentially interact with medications prescribed for acne. Some acne medications contain retinol, a form of vitamin A. Taking a vitamin A supplement with these prescriptions can cause a dangerous buildup of vitamin A in the body.

Risks

There are few risks associated with an acne diet. Most relate to taking dietary supplements. Zinc may prevent the body from absorbing enough **copper**. To avoid this,

---

KEY TERMS

Acne vulgaris—An inflammatory disease of the skin characterized by pimples and cysts that may cause scarring in severe cases.

Dermatologist—A doctor who specializes in the treatment of the skin.

Glycemic index—A scale for rating how quickly foods are converted to glucose or sugar by the body. It describes the impact on insulin levels of foods as they are digested.

Hormone—Substances in the body that regulate a process such as metabolism or growth.

Insulin—A hormone that regulates the conversion of food into glucose or sugar so it can be used by the body for energy.

Metabolism—The process by which food is converted into energy.

Sebaceous glands—Small glands in the skin, usually part of hair follicles, that produce sebum.

Sebum—The fatty substance secreted by sebaceous glands. It helps moisturize and protect skin and hair.

---

consumers should look for supplements that specifically state that they do not prevent copper absorption.

Vitamin A is a fat-soluble vitamin. That means that excess vitamin A is stored in the body rather than eliminated in the urine. Many acne prescriptions contain concentrated forms of vitamin A, but too much vitamin A can be toxic. Consult a doctor before taking vitamin A supplements.

Research and general acceptance

There is no consensus on whether or not diet plays a role in causing or preventing acne. Many dermatologists do not believe that diet has a significant effect on acne. Early studies about diet and acne focused on specific foods believed to trigger acne breakouts. Most of these studies found no evidence that individual foods cause acne.

Studies of the diets of ethnic groups that have a low incidence of acne form the basis of most of the acne diets. Studies of the diets of tribes in New Guinea, Paraguay, and the Bantu of South Africa, all of whom have little or no acne, found that they ate a primarily plant-based diet. Similar studies on populations in Japan and Korea support these findings.

A 2005 study of over 45,000 nurses claimed a link between the amount of dairy products consumed and severity of acne; women who reported consuming higher amounts of dairy products also reported more severe acne. However, of the women who drank at least two glasses of milk a day, only 8% experienced more severe breakouts.

The theory with the strongest support is that foods high on the glycemic index contribute to acne. Studies have shown that half of acne patients tested had abnormal glucose levels, and in another study, 80% of premenstrual women with acne had abnormal glucose **metabolism**. This data and others that show a high-carbohydrate diet increases the levels of testosterone in the blood have led to the recommendation of limiting consumption of refined carbohydrates as a means of treating acne.

Several studies have compared the results of zinc supplementation with oral antibiotic therapy to resolved acne and found zinc to be almost as effective as the antibiotic tetracycline.

Resources

BOOKS

Goodless, Dean R. *The Acne-Free Diet.* Celebration, FL: New Paradigm Dermatology, 2005.

Logan, Alan C., and Valori Treloar. *The Clear Skin Diet.* Nashville: Cumberland House, 2007.

Perricone, Nicholas. *The Acne Prescription: The Perricone Program for Clear and Healthy Skin at Every Age.* New York: HarperCollins, 2003.

PERIODICALS

Adebamowo, C.A., et al. "High School Dietary Intake and Teenage Acne." *Journal of the American Academy of Dermatology* 52, no. 2 (2005): 207–14.

Bae, Y.S., et al. "Innovative Uses for Zinc in Dermatology." *Dermatologic Clinics* 28, no. 3 (2010): 587–97.

Bowe, Whitney P., Smita S. Joshi, and Alan R. Shalita. "Diet and Acne." *Journal of the American Academy of Dermatology* 63, no. 1 (2010): 124–41.

Cordain, L., et al. "Acne Vulgaris: A Disease of Western Civilization." *Archives of Dermatology* 138, no. 12 (2002): 1584–90.

Davidovici, Batva B., and Ronni Wolf. "The Role of Diet in Acne: Facts and Controversies." *Clinics in Dermatology* 28, no. 1 (2010): 12–16.

Deplewski, D. and R. L. Rosenfield. "Growth Hormone and Insulin-like Growth Factors Have Different Effects on Sebaceous Cell Growth and Differentiation." *Endocrinology* 140, no. 9 (Sept 1999): 4089–94.

Smith, R.N., et al. "The Effect of a High-Protein, Low Glycemic-Load Diet Versus a Conventional, High Glycemic-Load Diet on Biochemical Parameters Associated with Acne Vulgaris: A Randomized, Investigator-Masked, Controlled Trial." *Journal of the American Academy of Dermatology* 57, no. 2 (2007): 247–56.

Veith, W.B., and N.B. Silverberg. "The Association of Acne Vulgaris with Diet." *Cutis* 88, no. 2 (2011): 84–91.

Williams, Hywel C., Robert P. Dellavalle, and Sarah Garner. "Acne Vulgaris." *The Lancet* 379, no. 9813 (2012): 361–72. http://dx.doi.org/10.1016/S0140-6736%2811%2960321-8 (accessed August 9, 2012).

WEBSITES

Bowers, Jan. "Diet and Acne: Role of Food Remains Controversial." American Academy of Dermatology Association. http://www.aad.org/dermatology-world/monthly-archives/2012/acne/diet-and-acne (accessed August 9, 2012).

University of Maryland Medical Center. "Acne." http://www.aad.org/dermatology-world/monthly-archives/2012/acne/diet-and-acne (accessed August 9, 2012).

Wilson, Bee. "Acne: Is Our Diet the Cause?" *The Telegraph* UK: Health, August 21, 2011. http://www.telegraph.co.uk/health/8701775/Acne-is-our-diet-the-cause.html (accessed August 9, 2012).

ORGANIZATIONS

American Academy of Dermatology, 930 E Woodfield Rd., Schaumburg, IL 60173, (847) 240-1280, (866) 503-SKIN (7546), Fax: (847) 240-1859, MRC@aad.org, http://www.aad.org.

Deborah L. Nurmi, MS

Acquired immunodeficiency syndrome (AIDS) diet *see* **AIDS/HIV diet and nutrition**

ADHD diet

Definition

Attention deficit **hyperactivity** disorder (ADHD) is defined as the combination of inattentive, hyperactive, and impulsive behaviors that are severe, developmentally inappropriate, and impair function at home and in

Behaviors associated with ADHD can be caused by other factors. It is best to consult a medical professional to rule out these possibilities. (Table by GGS Information Services. © 2013 Cengage Learning.)

school. Common features include mood swings, anxiety, impulsivity, hostility, poor concentration, and sleeping disorders, along with physical complaints such as headaches, migraines, and stomach upsets. Individuals with ADHD are also more likely to have been of low birth weight and to have allergies or autoimmune problems. Proportionally, more males than females are affected, with inattention tending to be a more female trait, and hyperactivity more common in males.

ADHD does persist into adulthood, although symptoms tend to diminish with time. The main focus of research and therapy relates to the problems of children with ADHD. Growing children are especially vulnerable to nutritional and environmental factors that influence brain development and function, which can have either a negative or positive impact. The symptoms of this difficult condition can also significantly compromise an individual's education, making them challenging to teach and consequently having a deleterious effect on their life-potential. The daily challenges of living with ADHD place a huge strain on families and can reduce overall quality of life for all involved.

Origins

In 1981, two British researchers, I. Colquhoun and S. Bunday, undertook a comprehensive survey of children with ADHD and discovered that many showed physical signs of essential fatty acid (EFA) deficiency, including excessive thirst, polyuria, and dry hair and skin. These authors were the first authorities to propose that fatty acid deficiency may be a factor in ADHD. Their groundbreaking work prompted more research studies and clinical trials designed to increase understanding of those nutritional factors involved in ADHD.

It has now been proposed that many developmental and psychiatric conditions—including ADHD, dyslexia, dyspraxia, autism, depression, and schizophrenia—may involve deficiencies of certain long-chain fatty acids, especially eicosapentaenoic acid (EPA) and docosahexaenoic acid (DHA). Both **iron** deficiency and **zinc** deficiency have also been associated with the development of ADHD.

Description

Dietary fats

Fats have a fundamental structural and functional role in the brain and central nervous system (CNS) and are a key factor in the development of ADHD. The two fatty acids that are thought to be especially important are EPA and DHA, not only because of their role in the brain and body, but because of the relative lack of them in many people's diets. EPA is the precursor of a complex group of substances, called eicosanoids, that perform numerous regulatory functions in the brain and body. DHA is a major building block of brain and neuronal membranes and has a profound influence on cell signaling. Both EPA and DHA are components of omega-3 fats and can be made from the omega-3 essential fatty acid, alpha linolenic acid (ALA). However, this conversion process can be problematic as genetic and environmental factors, including diet, can cause great variation in an individual's constitutional ability to convert ALA into EPA and DHA. Dietary factors known to adversely affect this conversion include low intake of ALA and high intake of **omega-6 fatty acids**, saturated fat, or hydrogenated fats, in addition to vitamin and mineral deficiencies, testosterone, and stress hormones. Unfortunately, many dietary surveys have revealed that a typical modern-day diet is rich in omega-6 fats, saturated fats, and hydrogenated fats and often low in omega-3 fats and micronutrients. Children with ADHD are often found to have iron and zinc deficiencies, and the fact that more boys than girls tend to be affected may be partly explained by the negative effect of testosterone on this conversion process.

In order to avoid a functional deficiency of these important fats, the diet should have a smaller ratio of the omega-6 essential fatty acid, linoleic acid (LA) to omega-3 essential fat (ALA), at an ideal ratio of no more than 5:1. The diet should also include adequate amounts of pre-formed EPA and DHA. The richest dietary sources of LA are certain vegetable and seed oils, including sunflower, safflower, soya, palm, peanut, and sesame, all of which should be eaten in adequate amounts along with oils that are rich in

ALA such as rapeseed (canola), **flaxseed** (linseed), and walnut oil. Olive oil is also recommended, despite having a quite low ALA content, as it is rich in beneficial monounsaturated fats. Looking at types of spreading fat available, many margarines have been specifically formulated to be rich in ALA, although some brands still contain harmful hydrogenated fats. Butter actually has a low LA content, and when mixed with equal quantities of rapeseed or olive oil, the saturated fat content is much reduced. Other sources of ALA include green, leafy vegetables such as rocket, watercress, and spinach, and fresh green herbs such as basil, coriander, mint, and parsley. Consequently, the food products of animals allowed to graze on open pasture will also be rich in ALA, and so organic, free-range, and outdoor-reared meat, milk, and eggs are the best choices.

When it comes to sources of EPA and DHA, fish and seafood are the best sources. Oily fish, such as salmon, trout, mackerel, sardines, herring, and anchovies, are especially rich in these fatty acids. Fresh tuna is classed as an oily fish, but the canning process causes a significant loss of fatty acids so tinned tuna has an EPA and DHA content comparable to white fish, such as cod, haddock, and plaice. Certain varieties of fish are more likely to contain large amounts of pollutants such as mercury and lead, which are known to be neurotoxic, and so it is prudent for people with ADHD, and all children under 16 years of age, to avoid eating shark, marlin, and swordfish. DHA can also be found in liver and egg yolks. These foods should be incorporated into the diet regularly, unless taking a nutritional supplement that contains **vitamin A**, in which case a person should not eat liver or foods containing liver such as pâté.

A general recommendation of a combined daily dose of 500 milligrams (0.5 grams) EPA and DHA is needed to avoid functional deficiency of these important fats, although individuals with ADHD may have an even higher requirement. This weekly total of 3,500 mg (3.5 g) is the equivalent of about three portions of salmon every week. In the United Kingdom, the recommended number of servings per week for girls and women of childbearing age is two, and for boys, men, and women past childbearing age is four. The relative amounts of EPA and DHA vary greatly between varieties of fish, with mackerel providing 2,700 mg (2.7 g) per average portion and haddock providing a much lower 170 mg (0.17 g) for a medium sized fillet. For many people, this variability in EPA and DHA intake is unlikely to have significant consequences as long as fish is regularly consumed, but for individuals with ADHD it may compromise brain function. For this reason, pure fish oil supplements that provide a daily standard dose of EPA and DHA are useful in addition to a diet containing fish and seafood. Increasing evidence from clinical trials has indeed shown that supplementation with EPA and DHA alleviate ADHD-related symptoms in some children. These supplements also have the advantage of being relatively safe and offering general health benefits, specifically in terms of cardiovascular protection. Although pure fish oil supplements may be beneficial in some individuals with ADHD, it is important to note that more research needs to be done to fully establish the durability of any treatment effects as well as optimal dosages and formulations.

Dietary antioxidants

If intakes of long-chain polyunsaturated fatty acids (PUFAs), such as EPA and DHA, increase, then so does the risk of lipid peroxidation by the action of harmful free radicals. Free radicals are unstable molecules that are created during normal bodily processes such as breathing and **metabolism**. The body is able to maintain a balance against the negative effects of free radicals in small amounts; however, they are also produced in response to stress or environmental toxins, such as smoking and pollution. PUFAs are highly susceptible to attacks from these reactive substances and need the protection of **antioxidants** to avoid damage. When free radical production is insufficiently countered by antioxidants, the resultant damage to the brain and body is termed "oxidative injury."

Dietary antioxidants include nutrients, such as **vitamin E** and **selenium**, as well as biologically active substances, such as flavonols, anthocyanins, and **carotenoids**, which are found in highly colored fruits and vegetables, nuts, teas, and red wines. Vitamin E is naturally found in PUFA-rich foods such as oils and nuts while selenium is found in fish, seafood, liver, egg, brazil nuts, mushrooms, and lentils. Eating the recommended daily minimum of five portions of fruit and/or vegetables should provide adequate amounts of complementary dietary antioxidants, especially if a wide range of colors and varieties are chosen.

Dietary iron

Iron deficiency has been associated with ADHD in children and tends to be worse even when compared with iron-deficient non-ADHD controls. Lower serum ferritin levels correlate with more severe ADHD symptoms and greater cognitive deficits.

Dietary sources of iron include red meat, fortified breakfast cereals, pulses, and dried apricots. These foods should feature regularly in the ADHD diet. Additional supplementary iron may be required in cases of proven iron deficiency.

Dietary zinc

Zinc has a range of important functions in the body, including the metabolism of neurotransmitters and fatty acids, with zinc deficiency possibly having an effect on the development of ADHD. Children with ADHD who have been treated with supplementary zinc have exhibited reduced hyperactive, impulsive, and impaired-socialization symptoms.

Foods known to be rich in zinc include seafood, liver, pine nuts, cashew nuts, and whole-grain cereals, and should be eaten regularly to help avoid deficiency.

Synthetic food additives

Certain synthetic food colorings, flavorings, and preservatives have been linked to increased hyperactivity in some ADHD and non-ADHD children. Many of these additives are unnecessary and are frequently used to sell poor-quality foods that are often marketed specifically toward children.

The following additives have been implicated in adverse reactions:

- tartrazine (E102)
- quinoline yellow (E104)
- yellow 2G (E107)
- sunset yellow (E110)
- azorubine (E122)
- amaranth (E123)
- ponceau 4R (E124)
- 128
- indigotine (E133)
- green S (E142)
- caramel (E150)
- brilliant black BN (E151)
- brown FK (E154)
- brown HT (E155)
- lithol rubine BK (E180)
- benzoic acid (E210)
- sodium benzoate (E211)
- sulfur dioxide (E220)
- sodium sulfite (E221)
- sodium hydrogen sulfite (E222)
- sodium metabisulfite (E223)
- potassium metabisulfite (E224)
- calcium sulfite (E226)
- calcium hydrogen sulfite (E227)
- potassium hydrogen sulfite (E228)
- vanillin

Function

The ADHD diet works by providing the right type and amount of fatty acids needed for the brain and CNS, as well as providing sufficient amounts of iron and zinc to avoid nutritional deficiencies that are known to be associated with worsening ADHD symptoms. Nutritional supplements should be taken upon the advice of a doctor or dietitian and in addition to a healthy, balanced diet. Dietary provision of antioxidants is needed to protect the long-chain fatty acids from breakdown, which would affect brain structure and compromise signaling within the brain and CNS. Finally, the ADHD diet excludes those synthetic **food additives** that have been identified as having the potential to adversely affect the behavior of ADHD and non-ADHD children alike.

Benefits

The key benefit of the ADHD diet is that it provides the correct types of foods needed to support the nutritional requirements of both the brain and body. It provides the nutrients needed to sustain good growth and development in children, as well as general health promotion for all, while excluding potential antagonistic additives. The diet supports other treatment strategies, including stimulant medication, and helps to improve the quality of life and educational possibilities of those individuals affected.

Precautions

Detailed, personalized advice should always be sought from a suitably qualified dietitian, especially when dealing with children. Any nutritional supplements should always be taken according to the manufacturer's instructions and at the prescribed dosage. If other medication is being taken, advice should be sought from a doctor.

Risks

It has been reported that fish oil supplements, when taken along with stimulant medication, can exacerbate hyperactive behavior in some individuals with ADHD. In these circumstances, the supplement should continue to be taken and the dosage of the medication should be altered accordingly under the supervision of a doctor.

Attention deficit hyperactivity disorder (ADHD)—A persistent pattern of inattention, hyperactivity, and/or impulsiveness; the pattern is more frequent and severe than is typically observed in people at a similar level of development.

Autism—Autism, or autistic spectrum disorder (ASD), is a serious developmental disorder, characterized by profound deficits in language, communication, and socialization, as well as resistance to learning.

Benzoic acid—A type of preservative used in processed foods known to cause food sensitivity in some individuals when consumed in the diet.

Carnitine—This is a naturally occurring substance, needed for the oxidation of fatty acids, a deficiency of which is known to have major adverse effects on the CNS.

Dietitian—A healthcare professional, qualified to a degree or post-graduate level, who advises individuals on diet and nutrition as part of a treatment strategy for particular medical conditions or for disease prevention.

Dyslexia—An inherent dysfunction affecting the language centers of the brain that results in difficulties with reading and writing.

Dyspraxia—A developmental disorder that affects coordination and movement.

Elimination diet—A diet consisting of a limited range of foods, classed as low risk in terms of causing food sensitivity or allergy.

Essential fatty acid—A type of fat that is necessary for the normal function of the brain and body and that the body is unable to produce itself, making it essential to be taken through the diet and/or supplements.

Ferritin—Iron is stored in the body, mainly in the liver, spleen, and bone marrow, as ferritin.

Functional deficiency—The depleted state of a particular nutrient that precipitates compromised function within the brain or body.

Hydrogenated fats—Also known as *trans* fats; a type of fat made by the process of hydrogenation, which turns liquid oils into solid fat. Biohydrogenation occurs in ruminant animals (e.g., cows), so small amounts of hydrogenated fats are found in butter, dairy foods, and meat, but these are accepted as being harmless. The commercial hydrogenation of oils produces large quantities of hydrogenated fats and has been implicated in the development of coronary heart disease and impaired cell signalling in the brain.

Lipid peroxidation—Refers to the chemical breakdown of fats.

Neurotoxic—A substance that has a specific toxic effect on the nervous system.

Oxidative injury—Damage that occurs to the cells and tissues of the brain and body by highly reactive substances known as free radicals.

Polyuria—An excessive production of urine.

Sodium benzoate—A type of preservative used in processed foods known to cause food sensitivity in some individuals when consumed in the diet.

Sulfur dioxide—A type of preservative used in processed foods known to cause food sensitivity in some individuals when consumed in the diet.

Sulphites—A type of preservative used in processed foods known to cause food sensitivity in some individuals when consumed in the diet.

Vanillin—A synthetic version of vanilla flavoring.

Fish oil supplements can also reduce blood clotting time and should not be used if anti-coagulant medication is already being taken.

There is no risk attached to the ADHD diet in terms of foods chosen and the diet can be safely followed by ADHD and non-ADHD individuals alike.

Research and general acceptance

Among the specialists working in this particular field, there is a general consensus that ADHD is a disorder that involves a functional deficiency of the long-chain fatty acids, EPA and DHA, that frequently co-exist with zinc and iron deficiencies. Among the wider community, there remains a great deal of skepticism about ADHD and the role that diet has in its development or management.

In terms of supplementation, insufficient data is available to formulate a standardized treatment strategy and it is unclear whether the micronutrient deficiencies are a cause of, or secondary to, ADHD. Other intervention studies have looked to carnitine supplementation and **elimination diets**, but their findings remain inconclusive.

QUESTIONS TO ASK YOUR DOCTOR

- What does the most recent research have to say about the connection between nutrition and ADHD?

- How can I find out what aspects of my child's diet may be contributing to his/her ADHD problems?

- What recommendations can you make for dietary changes that will reduce the ADHD symptoms evidenced by my child?

- Can you recommend a local resource to whom I can speak in more detail about recommended nutritional practices for my ADHD child?

Most researchers generally agree that there is still much to be learned about ADHD and how nutrients interact to either exacerbate or improve ADHD-related symptoms. More research is planned, and new findings may help improve the lives of all those affected by this debilitating condition.

Resources

BOOKS

Brown, Richard P., and Patricia L. Gerbarg. *Non-drug Treatments for ADHD: New Options for Kids, Adults, and Clinicians.* New York: W. W. Norton & Company, 2012.

Richardson, Alex. *They Are What You Feed Them.* London: HarperThorsons, 2006.

Simopoulos, Artemis, and Jo Robinson. *The Omega Diet.* New York: Harper Perennial, 1999.

Stevens, Laura. *12 Effective Ways to Help Your ADD/ADHD Child.* New York: Avery, 2000.

Stordy, Jacqueline and Malcolm Nicholl. *The LCP Solution.* New York: Ballantine Books, 2002.

PERIODICALS

Akhondzadeh, Shahin, Mohammad-Reza Mohammadi, and Mojgan Khademi. "Zinc Sulphate as an Adjunct to Methylphenidate for the Treatment of Attention Deficit Hyperactivity Disorder in Children: A Double-Blind and Randomised Trial." *BMC Psychiatry* 4, no. 9 (2004): 8–13.

Antalis, C. J., et al. "Omega 3 Fatty Acid Status in Attention-Deficit/Hyperactivity Disorder." *Prostaglandins, Leukotrienes, and Essential Fatty Acids* 75, nos. 4–5 (2006): 299–308.

Bilici, Mustafa, et al. "Double-Blind, Placebo-Controlled Study of Zinc Sulfate in the Treatment of Attention Deficit Hyperactivity Disorder." *Progress in Neuropsychopharmacology and Biological Psychiatry* 28, no. 1 (2004): 181–190.

Bourre, J. M. "Effects of Nutrients (in Food) on the Structure and Function of the Nervous System: Update on Dietary Requirements for Brain. Part 1: Micronutrients." *Journal of Nutrition, Health and Aging* 10, no. 5 (2006): 377–385.

———. "Effects of Nutrients (in Food) on the Structure and Function of the Nervous System: Update on Dietary Requirements for Brain. Part 2: Macronutrients." *Journal of Nutrition, Health and Aging* 10, no. 5 (2006): 386–399.

Brookes, Keeley J., et al. "Association of Fatty Acid Desaturase Genes with Attention Deficit/hyperactivity Disorder." *Biological Psychiatry* 60, no. 10 (2006): 1053–1061.

Colquhoun, Irene, and Sally Bunday. "A Lack of Essential Fatty Acids as a Possible Cause of Hyperactivity in Children." *Medical Hypotheses* 7, no. 5 (1981): 673–679.

Georgieff, Michael K. "Nutrition and the Developing Brain: Nutrient Priorities and Measurement." *American Journal of Clinical Nutrition* 85, no. 2 (2007): 614S–620S.

Hallahan, Brian, and Malcolm R. Garland. "Essential Fatty Acids and Their Role in the Treatment of Impulsivity Disorders." *Prostaglandins Leukotrienes and Essential Fatty Acids* 71, no. 4 (2004): 211–216.

Kanarek, R. B. "Artificial Food Dyes and Attention Deficit Hyperactivity Disorder." *Nutrition Reviews* 69, no. 7 (2011): 385–391. Available online at http://dx.doi.org/10.1111/j.1753-4887.2011.00385.x (accessed July 2, 2012).

Konofal, Eric, et al. "Iron-Deficiency in Children with Attention-Deficit/Hyperactivity Disorder." *Archives of Pediatric and Adolescent Medicine* 158, no. 12 (2004) 1113–1115.

Millichap, J. Gordon, and Michelle M. Yee. "The Diet Factor in Attention-Deficit/Hyperactivity Disorder." *Pediatrics* 129, no. 2 (2012): 330–337. Available online at http://dx.doi.org/10.1542/peds.2011-2199 (accessed July 2, 2012).

Richardson, Alex J. "Clinical Trials of Fatty Acid Treatment in ADHD, Dyslexia, Dyspraxia and the Autistic Spectrum." *Prostaglandins Leukotrienes and Essential Fatty Acids* 70, no. 4 (2004): 383–390.

———. "Long-Chain Polyunsaturated Fatty Acids in Childhood Developmental and Psychiatric Disorders." *Lipids* 39, no. 12 (2004): 1215–1222.

———. "Omega 3 Fatty Acids in ADHD and Related Neurodevelopmental Disorders." *International Review of Psychiatry* 18, no. 2 (2006): 155–172.

Schab, David W., and Nhi-Ha T. Trinh. "Do Artificial Food Colors Promote Hyperactivity in Children with Hyperactive Syndromes? A Meta-Analysis of Double-Blind, Placebo-Controlled Trials." *Journal of Developmental and Behavioural Pediatrics* 25, no. 6 (2004): 423–434.

Stevenson, Jim. "Dietary Influences on Cognitive Development and Behaviour in Children." *Proceedings of the Nutrition Society* 65 (2006): 361–365.

Virmani, Ashraf, Franco Gaetani, and Zbigniew Binienda. "Effects of Metabolic Modifiers Such as Carnitines,

Coenzyme Q10 and PUFAs against Different Forms of Neurotoxic Insults: Metabolic Inhibitors, MPTP and Methamphetamine." *Annals of the New York Academy of Science* 1053 (2008): 183–189.

WEBSITES

Huxsahl, John. "ADHD Diet: Do Food Additives Cause Hyperactivity?" MayoClinic.com. http://www.mayoclinic.com/health/adhd/AN01721 (accessed July 2, 2012).

NPR Staff. "Study: Diet May Help ADHD Kids More Than Drugs." *All Things Considered*, NPR.org. http://www.npr.org/2011/03/12/134456594/study-diet-may-help-adhd-kids-more-than-drugs (accessed July 2, 2012).

ORGANIZATIONS

Academy of Nutrition and Dietetics, 120 South Riverside Plz., Ste. 2000, Chicago, IL 60606-6995, (312) 899-0040, (800) 877-1600, http://www.eatright.org.

Children and Adults with Attention Deficit/Hyperactivity Disorder, 8181 Professional Pl., Ste. 150, Landover, MD 20785, (301) 306-7070, Fax: (301) 306-7090, (800) 233-4050, http://www.chadd.org.

Emma Mills, RD
David Newton

Calorie[1] requirements by age, gender, and activity level[2]

Age (years)	Sedentary	Moderately active	Active
Males			
2–3	1,000–1,200	1,000–1,400	1,000–1,400
4–8	1,200–1,400	1,400–1,600	1,600–2,000
9–13	1,600–2,000	1,800–2,200	2,000–2,600
14–18	2,000–2,400	2,400–2,800	2,800–3,200
Females			
2–3	1,000–1,200	1,000–1,400	1,000–1,400
4–8	1,200–1,400	1,400–1,600	1,400–1,800
9–13	1,400–1,600	1,600–2,000	1,800–2,200
14–18	1,800	2,000	2,400

[2]Sedentary refers to participating only in the light physical activity associated with day-to-day tasks. Moderately active refers to engaging in physical activity equivalent to walking about 1.5–3 miles per day at a 3–4 miles-per-hour (MPH) pace, in addition to everyday tasks. Active refers to daily physical activity equivalent to walking more than 3 miles per day at 3–4 MPH, in addition to routine tasks.

SOURCE: U.S. Department of Agriculture and U.S. Department of Health and Human Services, *Dietary Guidelines for Americans, 2010*, 7th ed., Washington, DC: U.S. Government Printing Office, December 2010.

(Table by PreMediaGlobal. © 2013 Cengage Learning.)

Adolescent nutrition

Definition

It is important for teenagers and adolescents to eat healthy foods to help them grow and develop normally, as well as to help prevent **obesity** and obesity-related diseases. Proper nutrition includes following **dietary guidelines** recommended by federal agencies and medical professionals to ensure that the specific nutritional needs of adolescents are met. The U.S. Department of Agriculture's (USDA) **MyPlate**, for example, offers age-specific information for children and adolescents. By following these and similar recommendations, parents can ensure that their children eat a well-balanced diet that supplies the **vitamins** and **calories** they need to stay healthy as they grow through puberty and into adulthood.

Purpose

Proper nutrition is essential for helping teens stay healthy and grow and develop properly. Eating right also helps teens participate better in both cognitive and athletic school activities. Studies have shown that children and teens who skip breakfast struggle with concentrating and do not perform as well in school, so it is important that teens eat three meals daily, starting with breakfast.

The nutritional status and health of children and adolescents in the United States has declined in recent years. In 2011, the U.S. Centers for Disease Control and Prevention reported that approximately one-third of children and adolescents aged 2 to 19 were considered overweight or obese. Of those children, approximately 17% were classified as obese. Other factors, such as poverty, can affect food intake and result in poor health and **malnutrition**.

Many adolescents consume more calories than they need but do not meet recommended daily intakes for a number of nutrients. Adequate intakes of vitamins and **minerals** are an important part of nutrition. Vitamins are required by the body in small amounts to regulate **metabolism** and to maintain normal growth and functioning. Minerals help make up the muscles, tissues, and bones and also support hormones, transport of oxygen, and enzyme systems. Of particular concern for children and adolescents is consuming adequate levels of **calcium**, potassium, **fiber**, **magnesium**, and **vitamin E**. Studies have shown that eating habits and nutrition in adolescence can impact not only adult weight but also other health issues later in life. For instance, not eating enough calcium as a teenager can increase a person's risk of developing osteoporosis as an older adult.

Some teens have health conditions that require special diets. Type 1 diabetes is diagnosed in as many as 15,000 children a year, according to the Juvenile Diabetes Research Foundation (JDRF). Treatment requires controlling both diet and lifestyle factors, which can be particularly difficult for busy teenagers. Increasing obesity rates have also correlated with a rise in type 2 diabetes among adolescents, which before had primarily been diagnosed in adults.

Description

Federal dietary guidelines for healthy eating are available for children age two and older. The U.S. Department of Agriculture (USDA) and the U.S. Department of Health and Human Services (HHS) produces the *Dietary Guidelines for Americans*, last revised in 2010. The guidelines are based on research and outline advice for choosing a nutritious diet and maintaining a healthy weight. The guidelines include key recommendations for children and adolescents and also address physical activity and **food safety**. In the 2010 revision, the USDA abandoned the former food pyramid approach to nutritional guidelines in favor of the new MyPlate approach to nutritional planning.

MyPlate

The food groups in the MyPlate recommendations for adolescents (ages 9–13) include:

- Grains. The guidelines recommend that girls and boys eat 5–6 ounces of grains each day, respectively. Sources include whole-grain bread, cereal, crackers, rice, or pasta. At least one-half of all grains consumed should be whole grains, which can be determined by looking for the word "whole" before the grain name on the list of ingredients.
- Vegetables. The USDA list includes dark green leafy vegetables, such as spinach and kale; red and orange vegetables, such as bell peppers and carrots; starchy vegetables, such as potatoes; and other vegetables, such as asparagus, avocado, eggplant, and turnips. Beans or peas may be counted as a vegetable serving once protein needs have been met. The recommendation is 2 cups daily for girls and 2.5 cups daily for boys.
- Fruits. Fresh, frozen, canned, or dried fruit are all acceptable fruit options. The USDA recommends limiting consumption of fruit juices due to added sugars, though 100% fruit juices are considered a fruit serving. Adolescents are encouraged to eat at least 1.5 cups per day.

- Protein. Protein options include low-fat or lean meats and poultry, fish, eggs, beans, peas, nuts, seeds, and soy. The daily recommendation for adolescents is 5 ounces.
- Dairy. The dairy group consists of all forms of milk, cheese, and yogurt (including soy), as well as milk-based desserts (such as puddings and frozen yogurt). The suggested daily amount for adolescents is 3 cups.

Fats and oils are not listed as a separate food group in the MyPlate diagram, but the USDA points out that they do provide essential nutrients and should be included in an individual's diet in limited quantities. Adolescents are allotted approximately 5 teaspoons per day.

Calcium

Calcium requirements are particularly important for teens, yet studies show that many adolescents fail to get the recommended daily allowance of calcium, which is 1,200–1,300 milligrams (mg) for teens aged 9–18. Calcium helps strengthen bones and teeth and also helps prevent osteoporosis, a condition characterized by a loss of bone density. Good sources of calcium include low-fat milk, cheese, and yogurt; calcium-fortified cereals; and low-fat pudding.

Iron

Iron requirements are very important for adolescent health and growth. Males need 8–11 mg of iron per day, depending on age. Females require more iron than males due to blood loss during menstruation; requirements range from 8 to 15 mg. The best sources of iron are found in the **protein** group (beef, poultry, fish, peanut butter). Other sources include iron-fortified **whole grains**, dark green leafy vegetables, and strawberries.

Fluid

Many adolescents do not realize the important role that fluids play in nutrition. It is important to stay hydrated and to limit consumption of high-sugar beverages and fruit juices. **Caffeine** from sodas and coffee drinks can interfere with sleep if consumed late at night, which can be a health and school performance issue. Adolescents should ensure that they drink an adequate amount of water; recommended intakes range from 2.4–3.3 L for males and 2.1–2.3 L for females. Teens who participate in sports especially need to remember to hydrate; some experts say an easy formula is one bottle (16 oz.) of fluid for every half hour of physical activity.

Physical activity

Teens who are very active and participate in organized sports will have different nutrition needs than other teenagers of the same age. They will require more fluids while exercising and may require more **carbohydrates**, which provide energy. Carbohydrates should come from whole grains and fruits and not from refined sugars. Some extra servings of lean protein may be helpful in building strong muscles, but eating too much of just one food group, rather than eating a balanced diet, is not recommended. According to the *Dietary Guidelines*, active teens aged 9–18 need between 2,000–3,200 calories per day for males and 1,800–2,400 for females.

Vegetarian diets

Some teenagers follow vegetarian diets. Some people may worry that a vegetarian diet is harmful for children and teens, but with proper planning, teenagers can meet nutritional requirements and achieve adequate growth with a vegetarian diet. Some people make the mistake of substituting meat with unhealthy choices, such as french fries and cheese pizza. An imbalanced diet can result in nutrient deficiencies, leading to side effects such as stunted growth, fragile bones, and stress fractures. Some vegetarian teens may need vitamin supplements to make up for some of the vitamins normally obtained in meats or meat products; a physician or registered dietitian (RD) can help determine the proper type and level of supplement(s) needed. Teenagers should not start taking **dietary supplements** without first consulting with their physician or RD.

Processed and prepared foods

At home, parents may choose snack and fast foods due to their convenience. Due to bigger portions and increased time spent in front of the television instead of being physically active, obesity in the United States is increasing. Adolescents are receiving and growing accustomed to less nutritional food choices. Highly processed foods often do not contain significant amounts of essential minerals and instead contain high amounts of fats and **sugar**, as well as **artificial preservatives** and other additives. Tips for parents looking to save time preparing meals include cooking meals on weekends and freezing them for busy weekdays and looking for cookbooks or online sources of quick and healthy recipes. To reduce fat in a teen's diet, parents and their teenage children can switch to low-fat or nonfat milk; remove skin from poultry or trim fat from red meat; reduce use of margarine and butter; use low-fat cooking methods such as baking, broiling, and steaming; and serve foods rich in fiber such as fruits, vegetables, and whole grains. Fresh salads can improve fiber in diet, as can adding

oat or wheat bran to baked foods. Milk, cheeses, tofu, and salmon are good sources of calcium. Fruit smoothies are healthy replacements for milk shakes.

School lunches

In recent years, a major emphasis has been placed on improving the nutritional value of lunch choices in schools. Schools generally offer balanced lunches, but many also offer snack bars or vending machines with sodas and snacks with high levels of sugar, fat, and **sodium**. Many teens choose these snacks over prepared **school lunches**. In addition, some schools may not offer physical education classes or the classes may not include enough activity to meet daily recommendations. Nutrition experts have worked with educators to present adolescents with healthier choices at school, to decrease or change the messages of food advertising, and to better educate students in the classroom about good nutritional choices.

Calories and weight management

Weight gain is caused by taking in more calories than are expended. By managing portions, eating a balanced diet from the food groups, limiting calories from high-sugar or high-fat foods, and participating in physical activity, adolescents can maintain a reasonable balance between calories in and calories out. Research has shown that subtracting just 100 calories a day from the diet can help manage weight, if needed—that could mean eliminating just one soda per day. Adults need to help teens understand that balanced eating and calorie management help manage weight, not unhealthy stretches of fasting or reliance on **fad diets**. Physical activity also helps manage weight. Encouraging participation in sports or spending time outside with family and friends instead of watching television, using the computer, or playing video games can also help manage weight safely.

Children and their parents are cautioned not to turn to fad diets for teenage weight problems. Many diets and diet products on the market have not been proven by clinical studies to be effective in the long term for adults, and so they certainly have not been proven safe or effective as a solution to weight problems in children and teens. Often, teenagers are more susceptible to claims made about diet plans. If weight is becoming a health issue, parents should encourage their teens to talk to a physician or RD to discuss safe weight-loss plans.

Eating disorders

Repeated fad dieting can be an important predictor of **eating disorders** among adolescents, especially teenage girls. Adolescents who worry too much about weight and appearance can develop social anxieties and eating disorders such as **anorexia nervosa** and **bulimia nervosa**. Anorexia usually occurs in teenage girls and young women who have a greater than normal fear of being fat. People with anorexia eat very little and obsess over the food they do eat. A teenager with anorexia might weigh every bit of food consumed, compulsively count all calories, or exercise to work off calories. The difference between anorexia and normal dieting is the serious compulsion with weight loss and the desire to go beyond being fit and trim to being as thin as possible, no matter the consequences. Warning signs for anorexia include dropping weight to about 20% below the normal range, claiming to "feel fat," exercising excessively, withdrawing from social activities, and finding excuses to avoid eating.

People with bulimia binge on food but then quickly purge by vomiting or taking laxatives. This behavior can be more difficult to spot than anorexia, because the teenager may be of average weight. Warning signs for bulimia include frequently going to the restroom immediately after meals, eating huge amounts of food without gaining weight, and using laxatives or diuretics.

Eating disorders lead to poor nutritional status and can affect growth and development for teenagers of both sexes. They rank as the third most common form of chronic illness in adolescents; according to the American Academy of Child and Adolescent Psychiatry, as many as 10% of young women in the United States have some type of eating disorder. If a child is diagnosed with an eating disorder, he or she should receive therapy to help treat both the disorder and the underlying causes. Nutritional therapy for teens with eating disorders is designed to correct possible malnutrition caused by the eating disorder. Refeeding must be carefully planned to avoid complications brought on by sudden increased calories and weight gain. The prescribed meal plan will gradually increase in calories as the teen's lean body mass increases.

Some adolescents with diabetes have been known to use doses of **insulin** below those recommended by their physicians to promote weight loss. This is a very dangerous practice. Teens with type 1 diabetes are encouraged to receive nutritional counseling upon diagnosis and schedule regular checkups with an RD. Teens with type 2 diabetes should also be taught how to control blood glucose levels.

Precautions

Like adults, adolescents need to understand that it is best to achieve recommended levels of nutrients

KEY TERMS

Anorexia nervosa—A serious eating disorder characterized by extreme weight loss, distorted body image, and fear of gaining weight.

Bulimia nervosa—An eating disorder in which an individual eats a large amount of food (binges) and then expels the food (purges) to maintain or lose weight.

Malnutrition—Any disorder of nutrition caused by insufficient or unbalanced diet that can result in impaired absorption or use of foods.

Puberty—The period of life in which boys' and girls' sexual organs begin to reach maturity and the ability to reproduce begins.

through consumption of foods instead of through vitamins and supplements. Use of supplements should be done only under the supervision of a professional medical provider who understands adolescent nutrition needs. Adolescents should understand that the best way to manage weight is through a balanced approach to eating fresh foods and through remaining physically active, not through fasting, use of drugs or supplements, or participation in fad diets.

Complications

Failing to eat a nutritious diet can cause growth and developmental problems in adolescents and long-term complications such as obesity or osteoporosis. Eating disorders can lead to serious complications in teens, including malnutrition, changes in heart function caused by starvation, stomach bleeding, and, in some cases, depression that may lead to suicide. Improper management of diabetes can lead to loss of consciousness and seizures, and in the longer term, eye disease, kidney and heart disease, or nerve damage.

Eating disorders

If a teen weighs less than 15% of the normal weight for his or her height, he or she may not have enough body fat to keep vital organs functioning. When a person is undernourished, the body slows down as if it is starving and blood pressure, pulse rate, and breathing slow. Girls with anorexia often stop having their menstrual cycles. People with anorexia can also experience lack of energy and concentration, as well as lightheadedness. They may become anemic, their bones can become brittle, and they can damage their heart, liver, and kidneys.

QUESTIONS TO ASK YOUR DOCTOR

- What special dietary provisions should we provide for my teenager, who is involved in active sports such as basketball and cross-country running?
- My child wants to follow a vegetarian diet. How can I make sure he/she is getting enough nutrients?
- How can I influence my child's school lunch programs to make sure that they provide adequate amounts of nutritious foods?
- What signs can I watch for to indicate that my children are not following a nutritious diet?

In the most severe cases, anorexia can result in malnutrition or even death.

The repeated vomiting behavior of bulimia causes constant stomach pain and can damage the stomach and kidneys. Acids from the stomach that come up into the mouth when vomiting can cause tooth decay. Teenage girls with bulimia may also stop having menstrual cycles. Constant vomiting may also cause the loss of too much potassium, which in severe cases can lead to heart problems and even death.

Parental concerns

Parents are up against the peer pressures and constant conflicting images that their children get from the media. Teens see unrealistic images of body types on television and in magazines but are also bombarded with advertisements for processed, convenient, and unhealthy foods. Magazines often feature articles about dieting and weight loss, which if followed obsessively can lead to unhealthy weight-control behaviors. Internet websites exist that provide advice to teens on how to accomplish and hide their eating disorders and products that help people with bulimia nervosa in their purging of foods.

Parents can help their teens navigate these messages by promoting healthy habits at home. Teens can be encouraged to snack on healthy foods, and parents can educate their teens about nutrition and the nutrients that are essential for them as they grow. Participating in sport and recreational activities, or at least supplementing television or computer use with activities like walking the family dog, can help instill long-lasting healthy habits and weight maintenance.

Resources

BOOKS

Pollan, Michael. *Food Rules: An Eater's Manual.* New York: Penguin Books, 2011.

Whitney, Eleanor Noss, and Sharon Rady Rolfes. *Understanding Nutrition.* Belmont, CA: Wadsworth, Cengage Learning, 2011.

PERIODICALS

American Academy of Child and Adolescent Psychiatry. "Teenagers with Eating Disorders." *Facts for Families* no. 2 (May 2008). http://aacap.org/cs/root/facts_for_families/teenagers_with_eating_disorders (accessed September 24, 2012).

Larson, N., and D. Neumark-Sztainer. "Adolescent Nutrition." *Pediatrics in Review* 30, no. 12 (2009): 494–496. http://dx.doi.org/10.1542/pir.30-12-494 (accessed March 5, 2012).

OTHER

U.S. Department of Agriculture. "Be a Healthy Role Model for Children." *10 Tips Nutrition Education Series*, DG Tip Sheet no. 12. Washington, DC: USDA Center for Nutrition Policy and Promotion, June 2011. http://www.choosemyplate.gov/food-groups/downloads/TenTips/DGTipsheet12BeAHealthyRoleModel.pdf (accessed November 6, 2012).

U.S. Department of Agriculture, U.S. Department of Health and Human Services. *Let's Eat for the Health of It.* Washington, DC: U.S. Department of Health and Human Services, June 2011. http://www.choosemyplate.gov/food-groups/downloads/MyPlate/DG2010Brochure.pdf (accessed March 5, 2012).

WEBSITES

Centers for Disease Control and Prevention. "Adolescent and School Health: Nutrition Facts." National Center for Chronic Disease Prevention and Health Promotion, Division of Adolescent and School Health. http://www.cdc.gov/healthyyouth/nutrition/facts.htm (accessed March 5, 2012).

———. "BMI Percentile Calculator for Children and Teens." http://apps.nccd.cdc.gov/dnpabmi (accessed September 24, 2012).

National Association of Anorexia Nervosa and Associated Disorders (ANAD). "Eating Disorders Statistics." http://www.anad.org/get-information/about-eating-disorders/eating-disorders-statistics (accessed September 24, 2012).

Nemours Foundation. "Eating Disorders." KidsHealth.org. http://kidshealth.org/parent/emotions/feelings/eating_disorders.html (accessed September 24, 2012).

Nutrition.gov. "For Tweens and Teens." http://www.nutrition.gov/nal_display/index.php?info_center=11&tax_level=3&tax_subject=395&topic_id=1688&level3_id=6570&level4_id=0&level5_id=0&placement_default=0 (accessed March 5, 2012).

U.S. Department of Agriculture. "Lifecycle Nutrition: Adolescence." National Agricultural Library. http://fnic.nal.usda.gov/nal_display/index.php?info_center=4&

tax_level = 2&tax_subject = 257&topic_id = 1354 (accessed March 5, 2012).

U.S. Department of Agriculture. "MyPlate." ChooseMy-Plate.gov. http://www.choosemyplate.gov/food-groups (accessed March 5, 2012).

ORGANIZATIONS

American Academy of Pediatrics (AAP), 141 Northwest Point Blvd., Elk Grove Village, IL 60007, (847) 434-4000, (800) 433-9016, Fax: (847) 434-8000, http://www.aap.org.

International Food Information Council Foundation, 1100 Connecticut Ave., NW Ste. 430, Washington, DC 20036, (202) 296-6540, info@foodinsight.org, http://www.foodinsight.org.

Juvenile Diabetes Research Foundation International, 26 Broadway, 14th Fl., New York, NY 10004, (800) 533-CURE (2873), Fax: (212) 785-9595, info@jdrf.org, http://www.jdrf.org.

National Eating Disorders Association, 165 West 46th St., New York, NY 10036, (212) 575-6200, (800) 931-2237, info@NationalEatingDisorders.org, http://www.nationaleatingdisorders.org.

U.S. Department of Agriculture, 1400 Independence Ave. SW, Washington, DC 20250, (202) 720-2791, http://www.usda.gov.

Teresa G. Odle
David Newton

Adult nutrition

Definition

Nutrition describes the processes by which the food a person eats is taken in and broken down into its chemical compounds, and nutrients that the body needs are absorbed. Good nutrition can help prevent disease and promote health. Adult nutrition refers to the specific nutritional needs of adults, which differ from those of children.

Purpose

For children, a healthy diet is important for normal growth and development. For adults, nutrition still promotes health and reduces the risk of disease. Studies have shown that the increasing rate of **obesity** in the United States and many other countries can be linked to both eating too much and making unhealthy food choices. A healthy diet can help prevent weight gain by increasing consumption of foods that are flavorful and filling, but that have a low calorie to volume ratio (known as a low energy density). Nutrition also plays a role in preventing diseases and helping individuals maintain good health. For example, poor nutrition can lead to high cholesterol levels, which are a risk factor for coronary artery disease and other

Calorie[1] requirements by age, gender, and activity level[2]

Age (years)	Male, sedentary	Male, moderately active	Male, active	Female, sedentary	Female, moderately active	Female, active
18	2,400	2,800	3,200	1,800	2,000	2,400
19–20	2,600	2,800	3,000	2,000	2,200	2,400
21–25	2,400	2,800	3,000	2,000	2,200	2,400
26–30	2,400	2,600	3,000	1,800	2,000	2,400
31–35	2,400	2,600	3,000	1,800	2,000	2,200
36–40	2,400	2,600	2,800	1,800	2,000	2,200
41–45	2,200	2,600	2,800	1,800	2,000	2,200
46–50	2,200	2,400	2,800	1,800	2,000	2,200
51–55	2,200	2,400	2,800	1,600	1,800	2,200
56–60	2,200	2,400	2,600	1,600	1,800	2,200
61–65	2,000	2,400	2,600	1,600	1,800	2,000
66–70	2,000	2,200	2,600	1,600	1,800	2,000
71–75	2,000	2,200	2,600	1,600	1,800	2,000
76+	2,000	2,200	2,400	1,600	1,800	2,000

[1]Calories determined using a 5'10", 154 lb. man and a 5'4", 126 lb. woman. Estimates for females do not include women who are pregnant or breastfeeding.
[2]Sedentary refers to participating only in the light physical activity associated with day-to-day tasks. Moderately active refers to engaging in physical activity equivalent to walking about 1.5–3 miles per day at a 3–4 miles-per-hour (MPH) pace, in addition to everyday tasks. Active refers to daily physical activity equivalent to walking more than 3 miles per day at 3–4 MPH, in addition to routine tasks.

SOURCE: U.S. Department of Agriculture and U.S. Department of Health and Human Services, *Dietary Guidelines for Americans, 2010*, 7th ed., Washington, DC: U.S. Government Printing Office, December 2010.

(Table by PreMediaGlobal. © 2013 Cengage Learning.)

vascular system problems. Lowering salt in the diet can help reduce blood pressure. Individuals with diabetes can improve their health by eating a healthy diet to control blood glucose levels. Poor nutrition has also been linked to an increased risk of many diseases, including osteoporosis, gout, and some types of **cancer**.

Special diets or nutritional therapies may be used to complement other treatments prescribed by a physician to treat some diseases and conditions. Examples include:

- High cholesterol. Eating a diet that is low in saturated fat, moderate in calories, and high in fiber can help keep blood cholesterol in check.

- High blood pressure. Reducing salt and saturated fat, as well as reducing overall weight (if overweight), helps lower blood pressure. Special diets have been developed to lower the risk of high blood pressure and heart disease.

- Diabetes. Good nutrition is critical for adults with type 2 diabetes. Dietary recommendations include controlling portion sizes, eating regular meals, and choosing whole-grain and other nutrient-rich foods.

- Iron deficiency anemia. Individuals with anemia need to get more iron from their diets and will be encouraged to eat foods such as red meat, legumes (e.g., beans, peas, lentils), and dark green leafy vegetables (e.g., spinach, kale).

Sometimes, people who are very ill need artificial nutrition to ensure they receive the proper nutrients. The nutrition may come in the form of special drinks that supplement their diets or may be provided through intravenous (IV) infusion in a hospital or other facility.

Nutrition is important throughout adults' lives. For younger adults, good nutrition provides the energy for active lives that may involve athletic pursuits and busy days filled with work and raising children. Good nutrition is especially important for pregnant women, as their dietary intake affects both their health and that of the developing baby. During middle age, proper nutrition helps prevent disease and weight gain that are more common when lives become more sedentary. As people reach their mature years, nutrition becomes especially critical to maintaining good health. It can also become more of a challenge, as many people in their later years find it difficult to eat a healthy, balanced diet due to medical conditions, medications, and social factors such as eating alone and difficulty cooking and shopping.

Description

On January 31, 2011, the United States Department of Agriculture (USDA) and the Department of Health and Human Services announced the 2010 Dietary Guidelines for Americans. The 2010 release was the seventh edition of the dietary guidelines. The new version of the guidelines was developed to help combat the increasing obesity problem in the United States, and focuses on providing recommendations that are easy for busy people to put into practice in their daily lives.

Some of the 2010 guidelines for adults:

- Enjoy your food, but eat less.
- Avoid oversized portions.
- Make half your plate fruits and vegetables.
- Drink water instead of sugary drinks.
- Switch to nonfat or low-fat milk.

The 2010 guidelines also include a variety of other recommendations. The two major themes of the recommendations are (1) Maintain calorie balance over time to achieve and sustain a healthy weight, and (2) Focus on consuming nutrient-dense foods and beverages. The full text of the recommendations, as well as a variety of interactive tools and other helpful nutrition information, can be found at http://www.dietaryguidelines.gov.

Basic food groups

The following are the basic food groups included in **MyPlate**, the food recommendations provided by the United States Department of Agriculture (USDA):

- Grains. The MyPlate dietary guidelines recommend consuming 3 to 3.5 ounces of grains each day, and making half of all grains consumed whole grains. Whole grains include whole-wheat flour, oatmeal, and brown rice.

- Fruits. The MyPlate dietary guidelines encourage individuals to make half their plate fruits and vegetables, for a total of 1.5 to 2 cups of fruits a day. Fruits include 100% fruit juices, and fresh, frozen, dried, canned, and other fruit preparations.

- Vegetables. The MyPlate dietary guidelines encourage individuals to make half their plate fruits and vegetables, for a total of about 2.5 to 3 cups of vegetables a day. Vegetables include vegetable juices, and fresh, frozen, dried, canned, mashed, and other vegetables, either raw or cooked.

- Dairy. The MyPlate dietary guidelines recommend 3 cups of dairy products per day for adults. The guidelines also recommend switching from full-fat dairy products to lower/reduced-fat or fat-free products.

- Protein. MyPlate recommends 5–6 ounces from this group each day, and that at least one serving per week be of fish or other seafood. Most Americans get enough protein, and should concentrate on selecting leaner, less processed food from this group.
- Oils. The MyPlate guidelines recommend no more than 5–6 teaspoons of oils per day. It is recommended that individuals replace fats in their diet that are solid at room temperature with oils, which are liquid at room temperature.

Recommendations for specific adult populations

Not every adult has the same nutritional needs. In addition to specific nutritional needs related to diseases or activity, the following recommendations apply to certain groups:

- People over age 50. Calcium supplementation and consumption of calcium-rich foods (e.g., low-fat milk) or calcium-fortified foods (e.g., calcium-fortified orange juice) is recommended.
- Women of childbearing age. If a woman may become pregnant, she should eat iron-rich foods and those that help absorb iron, such as foods rich in vitamin C. Women in their first trimester of pregnancy should consume adequate folic acid (usually as a doctor-prescribed supplement).
- Older adults, people with dark skin, and people not exposed to sufficient sunlight. These individuals should consume extra vitamin D from foods fortified with vitamin D and/or from supplements.

Getting adequate nutrients

Vitamins and **minerals** are substances present in food that do not provide energy (**calories**) but are required by the body in small amounts to regulate **metabolism** and to maintain normal growth and functioning. They play vital roles in building and maintaining muscles, tissues, and bones. They also are important to many life-supporting systems, such as hormones, transport of oxygen, and enzyme systems. Because different foods contain different nutrients, it is important to eat a diet that contains a variety of foods from each of the food groups. This helps ensure that the body gets enough of all the vitamins and minerals that it needs to function at its best. The actual amount of any nutrient a person needs, as well as the amount each individual gets from his or her diet, will vary. Many adults do not receive enough **calcium** from their diets, which can lead to osteoporosis later in life. Other nutrients of concern are potassium, **fiber**,

magnesium, and **vitamin E**. Some population groups also need more **vitamin B$_{12}$**, **iron**, folic acid, and **vitamin D**. These nutrients should come from food when possible (with the exception of vitamin D, which is also synthesized by sunlight), and from supplements if necessary.

Fluids

Many adults underestimate the role that fluids play in health. It is important to limit high-sugar beverages and fruit juices, even those that are 100% fruit. The high-sugar content of fruit beverages can contribute to weight gain and dental cavities if consumed too often. Alcoholic beverages are okay in moderation but contribute to **dehydration** and should be limited. The *Dietary Guidelines for Americans* recommend no more than one drink a day for women and two drinks a day for men. A drink is defined as 12 oz. of beer, 5 oz. of wine, or 1.5 oz. of liquor.

It is recommended that men consume about 3 liters (13 cups) of fluids each day, preferably water, and that women take in about 2.2 liters (9 cups) daily. Most people will get adequate **hydration** from normal thirst and drinking behavior, especially by consuming fluids with meals. Also, fluid in foods, such as water contained in fruits and vegetables, contributes to overall fluid requirements; food usually provides up to 20% of daily fluid needs. People with limited mobility, such as those in wheelchairs or who are bedridden, may not get enough fluids, especially in hot weather.

Nutrition for strength

Adults who are physically active and who strength train or pursue athletic activities will have different nutrition needs than typical adults of the same age. For example, they will require more fluids while exercising. In general, athletes and those who are very active also require more **carbohydrates** and calories in their diets than more sedentary individuals. Carbohydrates provide energy, but they should come mainly from **whole grains** and fruits.

Vegetarian diets

Vegetarians can achieve recommended nutrient intakes by carefully choosing foods from the basic food groups. They should pay careful attention to intake of **protein**, iron, and other vitamins, depending on the type of vegetarian diet they choose. Choosing a variety of foods including nuts, seeds, legumes, and **soy** products can help ensure good nutrition. Vegans may need to take vitamin supplements (e.g., vitamin B$_{12}$) to maintain adequate nutrition.

KEY TERMS

Cholesterol—A waxy substance made by the liver and also acquired through diet. High levels in the blood may increase the risk of cardiovascular disease.

Monounsaturated fats—Fats that contain one double or triple bond per molecule. Though these fats are still calorie dense, they can help lower blood cholesterol if used in place of saturated fats. Examples of foods rich in monounsaturated fats are canola oil and olive oil.

Osteoporosis—A condition found in older individuals in which bones decrease in density and become fragile and more likely to break. It can be caused by a lack of vitamin D and/or calcium in the diet.

Polyunsaturated fats—Fats that contain two or more double or triple bonds per molecule. Examples include fish, safflower, sunflower, corn, and soybean oils.

Processed and prepared foods

Americans frequently eat out and buy many foods at the grocery store that are highly processed. In general, fresh foods are healthier than those that are processed, and health care professionals generally agree that healthy diets are those that include many fresh foods and few highly processed ones. Highly processed foods often have a higher **sodium** content and can also contain more fat and **sugar**, as well as **artificial preservatives** and other additives. Many restaurants, including fast food restaurants, are trying to offer healthier selections, and healthy options are increasingly available in supermarkets. It is important for consumers to read nutrition labels on product packaging when making such decisions. Consumers may wish to check overall calorie, fat, sodium, sugar, fiber, protein, and other nutrient content, as well as the list of ingredients.

Calories and weight management

Weight management generally involves balancing energy, or the amount of calories eaten vs. the amount of calories used by the body. By watching portion sizes, eating a balanced diet from all the food groups, and reducing intake of high-sugar and high-fat foods and snacks, it is possible to balance energy intake (calories) and requirements. Regular physical activity is also important for achieving this balance. Research has shown that subtracting just 100 calories a day from the diet can help manage weight, and

eating 500 fewer calories a day can result in the loss of one to two pounds per week in weight. However, every individual, especially children and older adults, should consult a physician or dietitian before beginning a weight-loss plan.

Precautions

Though supplementation of nutrients sometimes is necessary, physicians and dietitians recommend that nutrients come from food, not from vitamins and supplements. High doses of vitamins and minerals from supplements can lead to serious health problems. It is important to consult a physician to ensure that supplements are being used at appropriate and safe levels and that they do not interfere with the actions of any prescribed medications the individual is taking. It also is best not to make significant changes to one's diet without the advice of a nutritional expert or health care professional. People who are chronically ill and women who are pregnant or **breastfeeding** should seek professional medical advice before beginning any new dietary regime.

Resources

BOOKS

Blake, Joan Salge. *Nutrition and You.* 2nd ed. San Francisco: Pearson Benjamin Cummings, 2012.

Iowa Dietetic Association, Andrea K. Maher, ed. *Simplified Diet Manual.* 11th ed. Chichester, West Sussex: Wiley-Blackwell, 2012.

Stephanie Maze, ed. *Healthy Foods From A to Z.* Sarasota, FL: Moonstone Press, 2012.

PERIODICALS

"A Healthy Diet and Physical Activity Help Reduce Your Cancer Risk." *CA: A Cancer Journal for Clinicians* 62, no. 1 (Jan–Feb 2012): 68–69.

Inzarty, M., et al. "Nutrition in the Age-Related Disablement Process." *Journal of Nutrition, Health, and Aging* 15, no. 8 (August 2011): 599–604.

"12 for 2012: Twelve Tips for Healthier Eating. It's Not About Individual Nutrients Anymore." *Harvard Women's Health Watch* 19, no. 5 (January 2012): 1–3.

OTHER

U.S. Department of Agriculture and U.S. Department of Health and Human Services. *Dietary Guidelines for Americans, 2010.* 7th ed. Washington, DC: U.S. Government Printing Office, December 2010. http://www.cnpp.usda.gov/Publications/DietaryGuidelines/2010/PolicyDoc/PolicyDoc.pdf (accessed July 9, 2012).

WEBSITES

ChooseMyPlate.gov. United States Department of Agriculture. http://www.choosemyplate.gov (accessed July 9, 2012).

Mayo Clinic staff. "Nutrition Basics." MayoClinic.com. http://www.mayoclinic.com/health/nutrition-and-healthy-eating/MY00431 (accessed July 9, 2012).

ORGANIZATIONS

Academy of Nutrition and Dietetics, 120 South Riverside Plz., Ste. 2000, Chicago, IL 60606-6995, (312) 899-0040, (800) 877-1600, amacmunn@eatright.org, http://www.eatright.org.

American Society for Nutrition, 9650 Rockville Pike, Bethesda, MD 20814, (301) 634-7050, Fax: (301) 634-7894, http://www.nutrition.org.

Office of Dietary Supplements, National Institutes of Health, 6100 Executive Blvd., Rm. 3B01, MSC 7517, Bethesda, MD 20892-7517, (301) 435-2920, Fax: (301) 480-1845, ods@nih.gov, http://ods.od.nih.gov.

Teresa Odle
Tish Davidson, AM

African American diet

Definition

There is no "African American diet" in the sense that African Americans follow a specific diet. However, African American culture has had a significant influence on American cuisine. Food associated with African American culture is diverse and flavorful. Despite cultural, political, economic, and racial struggles, African Americans have retained a strong sense of culture that is, in part, reflected in the food.

Origins

The roots of the diversity of African American cuisine may be traced back to 1619, when the first African slaves were sold in the New World. In a quest to build new cities in America, Europeans actively transported Africans and West Indians (people from the West Indies) to the new land. The West Indies (in the Caribbean Sea) was part of the slave route to America. Because the West Indians' skin color was similar to that of Africans, they were not treated any differently. As a result, some West Indian food traditions are similar to those of African Americans.

African American food has a distinctive culinary heritage with diverse flavors and includes traditions drawn from the African continent, the West Indies, and North America. In the southern United States, where the slave population was most dense, there is a cooking culture that remains true to the African American tradition. Commonly referred to as "soul food,"

southern cooking styles are considered to be based on African American recipes that have been passed down from generation to generation, just like other rituals. There is some controversy surrounding the term "soul food"—many civil rights advocates believe that using this word perpetuates a negative connection between African Americans and slavery. Other people, however, assert that the "soul" of the food refers loosely to the food's origins in Africa.

Description

Popular southern foods, such as the vegetable okra (brought to New Orleans by African slaves), are often attributed to the importation of goods from Africa, or by way of Africa, the West Indies, and the slave trade. Okra, which is the principal ingredient in the popular Creole stew referred to as gumbo, is believed to have spiritual and healthful properties. Rice and seafood (along with sausage or chicken) and filé (a sassafras powder inspired by the Choctaw Indians) are also key ingredients in gumbo. Other common foods that are rooted in African American culture include black-eyed peas, benne seeds (sesame), eggplant, sorghum (a grain that produces sweet syrup and different types of flour), watermelon, and peanuts.

In his 1962 essay "Soul Food," Amiri Baraka makes a clear distinction between southern cooking and soul food. To Baraka, soul food includes chitterlings (pronounced chitlins), pork chops, fried porgies, potlikker, turnips, watermelon, black-eyed peas, grits, hoppin' John, hushpuppies, okra, and pancakes. Southern food, on the other hand, includes only fried chicken, sweet potato pie, collard greens, and barbecue, according to Baraka. The idea of what soul food is differs greatly.

General dietary influences

There are many notable regional influences on cooking throughout the United States. Many regionally influenced cuisines emerged from the interactions of Native American, European, Caribbean, and African cultures. After emancipation, many slaves left the south and spread the influence of soul food to other parts of the United States. Barbecue is one example of African-influenced cuisine that is still widely popular throughout the United States. The Africans who came to colonial South Carolina from the West Indies brought with them what is today considered signature southern cookery, known as *barbacoa*, or barbecue. The original barbecue recipe's main ingredient was roasted pig, which was heavily seasoned in red pepper and vinegar. Because of regional differences in livestock availability, pork barbecue became popular in the eastern United States, while beef barbecue became popular in the west of the country.

Cajun and Creole cooking originated with the French and Spanish but were transformed by the influence of African cooks. African chefs brought with them specific skills in using various spices and introduced okra and other foodstuffs, such as crawfish, shrimp, oysters, crabs, and pecans, into both Cajun and Creole cuisine. Originally, Cajun meals were bland, and nearly all foods were boiled. Rice was used in Cajun dishes to stretch out meals to feed large families. Today, Cajun cooking tends to be spicier and more robust than Creole. Some popular Cajun dishes include pork-based sausages, jambalayas, gumbos, and coush-coush (a creamed corn dish). The symbol of Cajun cooking is perhaps crawfish, but until the 1960s crawfish were used mainly as bait.

More recently, the immigration of people from the Caribbean and South America has influenced African American cuisine in the south. New spices, ingredients, combinations, and cooking methods have produced popular dishes such as Jamaican jerk chicken, fried plantains, and bean dishes such as Puerto Rican *habichuelas* and Brazilian *feijoada*.

Holidays and traditions

African American meals are deeply rooted in traditions, holidays, and celebrations. For American slaves, after working long hours in the fields, the evening meal was a time for families to gather, reflect, tell stories, and visit with loved ones and friends. Today, the Sunday meal after church continues to serve as a prime gathering time for friends and family.

Kwanzaa, which means "first fruits of the harvest," is a holiday observed by more than 18 million people worldwide. Kwanzaa is an African American celebration that focuses on the traditional African values of family, community responsibility, commerce, and self-improvement. The Kwanzaa Feast, or Karamu, is traditionally held on December 31. This symbolizes the celebration that brings the community together to exchange and to give thanks for their accomplishments during the year. A typical menu includes a black-eyed peas dish, greens, sweet potato pudding, cornbread, fruit cobbler or compote dessert, and many other special family dishes.

Risks

There have been large changes in the overall quality of the diet of African Americans and in the United States in general since the 1960s. In 2010, according to the U.S. National Center for Health Statistics, rates of **obesity** in the United States were higher in African

KEY TERMS

Diabetes—A condition in which the body either does not make or cannot respond to the hormone insulin. As a result, the body cannot use glucose (sugar). There are two types: type 1 (juvenile onset) and type 2 (primarily adult onset).

Hypertension—High blood pressure.

Obesity—Defined as having a body mass index (BMI) of 30 or greater.

Americans than other ethnicities, especially in African American women (54%). Diets tend to be higher in fat and low in fruits, vegetables, and **whole grains**. Some factors in this shift include the greater market availability of packaged and processed foods; higher costs of fresh fruit, vegetables, and lean cuts of meat; prevalence of fried foods; and high use of **fats** in cooking.

African Americans tend to experience high rates of obesity, **hypertension**, type 2 diabetes, and heart disease, which are all partly associated with diet. Obesity and hypertension are major causes of heart disease, diabetes, kidney disease, and certain cancers. According to the U.S. Centers for Disease and Prevention (CDC), from 2005–2007, African Americans had the highest mortality rates for heart disease, stroke, and **cancer**, as well as overall. In the United States, the prevalence of high blood pressure in African Americans is among the highest in the world. Many U.S. government agencies have created national initiatives to improve the diet quality and the overall health of African Americans.

Resources

BOOKS

Foner, Eric, and Garraty, John A., eds. *The Reader's Companion to American History*. Boston: Houghton Mifflin, 1991.

Genovese, Eugene D. *Roll, Jordan, Roll: The World the Slaves Made*. New York: Vintage, 1974.

Harris, Jessica. *A Kwanzaa Keepsake: Celebrating the Holiday with New Traditions and Feasts*. New York: Simon & Schuster, 1995.

———. *Iron Pots and Wooden Spoons: Africa's Gift to the New World Cooking*. New York: Simon & Schuster, 1999.

Mitchell, William Frank. *African American Food Culture*. Westport, CT: Greenwood Press, 2009.

Wilson, Charles Reagan. *The New Encyclopedia of Southern Culture*. Chapel Hill: University of North Carolina Press, 2006.

Witt, Doris. *Black Hunger*. New York: Oxford University Press, 1999.

PERIODICALS

Dirks, R. T., and Duran, N. "African American Dietary Patterns at the Beginning of the 20th Century." *Journal of Nutrition* 131, no. 7 (2000): 1881–89.

Epstein, Dawn E., et al. "Determinants and Consequences of Adherence to the Dietary Approaches to Stop Hypertension Diet in African-American and White Adults with High Blood Pressure: Results from the ENCORE Trial." *Journal of the Academy of Nutrition and Dietetics* 112, no. 11 (November 2012). http://dx.doi.org/10.1016/j.jand.2012.07.007 (accessed September 20, 2012).

Kulkarni, Karmeen. "Food, Culture, and Diabetes in the United States." *Clinical Diabetes* 22, no. 4 (2004): 190–92. http://dx.doi.org/10.2337/diaclin.22.4.190 (accessed September 20, 2012).

OTHER

National Center for Health Statistics. *Health, United States, 2011: With Special Feature on Socioeconomic Status and Health.* Hyattsville, MD: 2012. http://www.cdc.gov/nchs/data/hus/hus11.pdf (accessed September 20, 2012).

Rastogi, Tallese D. Johnson, Elizabeth M. Hoeffel, and Malcolm P. Drewery, Jr. *The Black Population: 2010.* 2010 Census Briefs. Washington, DC: U.S. Census Bureau, 2011. http://www.census.gov/prod/cen2010/briefs/c2010br-06.pdf (accessed September 20, 2012).

WEBSITES

Centers for Disease Control and Prevention, Office of Minority Health & Health Equity (OMHHE). "Black or African American Populations." http://www.cdc.gov/minorityhealth/populations/REMP/black.html (accessed September 20, 2012).

Haederle, Michael. "Fighting Heart Disease, High Blood Pressure Among African Americans." *AARP Bulletin*, February 25, 2011. http://www.aarp.org/health/conditions-treatments/info-02-2011/african-americans-heart-disease-high-blood-pressure.html (accessed September 20, 2012).

MedlinePlus. "African-American Health." U.S. National Library of Medicine, National Institutes of Health. http://www.nlm.nih.gov/medlineplus/africanamerican health.html (accessed September 20, 2012).

Oldways. "African Heritage & Health." http://oldwayspt.org/programs/african-heritage-health (accessed September 20, 2012).

ORGANIZATIONS

Office of Minority Health & Health Equity (OMHHE), U.S. Centers for Disease Control and Prevention (CDC), Mail Stop K-77, 4770 Buford Hwy, Atlanta, GA 30341, (770) 488-8343, Fax: (770) 488-8140, OMHHE@cdc.gov, http://www.cdc.gov/minorityhealth/index.html.

M. Cristina F. Garces
Lisa A. Sutherland

African diet

Definition

The African diet is as rich and diverse as the geography and culture of the world's second-largest continent. Although fish is a mainstay of the African diet in coastal regions and near rivers and lakes, in many parts of Africa the diet is primarily vegetarian, with meat reserved for special occasions. For this reason, and because the human species evolved eating African foods and is therefore presumably well-adapted to those foods, a traditional African diet—sometimes called an African heritage diet—has been promoted as both a healthy alternative to Western diets, especially for black Americans, and as a path to weight loss.

Origins

The African diet evolved and adapted with the evolution of *Homo sapiens*. Some anthropologists believe that the selection pressure that led to bipedalism (walking on two legs) was an adaptation to changing environments that necessitated travel in search of tubers (underground plant stems) and other food sources. Africa's history includes some of humankind's earliest food production, with the Nile Valley being one of the most fertile centers of the ancient world. The Nile Valley has always been a rich source of fish, animal, and plant foods. In the drier African savannas, especially once the Saharan region became arid after 6000 BCE, nomadic tribes raised cattle, goats, and sheep as food sources. Crops that are less affected by extreme weather—cereals, such as wheat, barley, millet, and sorghum, and tubers such as yams—spread throughout the continent and remain important staples of the African diet today.

Much of the variety in the African diet results from the great differences in climate and terrain across the continent. Tribes and peoples migrated and traded in spices and foods, resulting in the mixing of cultures, traditions, and diets. European colonialism introduced a plethora of new foods, many of which were incorporated into traditional diets. In the modern era, globalization is transforming the African diet, just as aspects of African diets are reaching a worldwide population.

Description

Each region of Africa has its own distinct cuisine and staple foods. Among primary staples, cereal grains—mostly millet, sorghum, teff, and wheat—account for 46% of the energy supplied by the average African diet. Another 20% comes from roots and tubers, especially

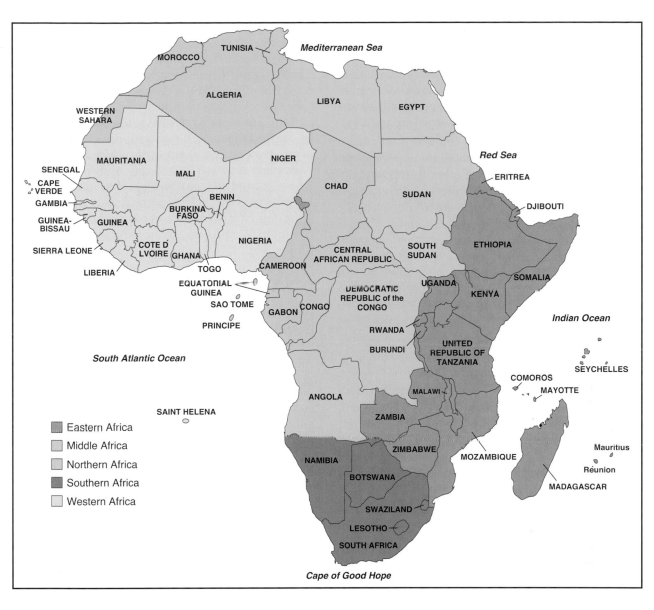

Map of Africa. *(Map by Electronic Illustrators Group. © 2013 Cengage Learning.)*

Legend:
- Eastern Africa
- Middle Africa
- Northern Africa
- Southern Africa
- Western Africa

yams. Roots and tubers account for about 40% of all food eaten by half of the population of sub-Saharan Africa. Although roots and tubers are high in **carbohydrates**, **calcium**, and **vitamin C**, they are low in **protein**. Other important African food crops include rice, sweet potatoes, leafy greens, okra (a vegetable native to African rainforests), beans, nuts and peanuts, oil palm, and coffee. Sauces and marinades made from herbs and spices, as well as fish, eggs, yogurt, and poultry, are also important components of traditional African diets, with minimal meat and sweets. Although meat is considered a staple in some parts of Africa, animal products supply only 7% of dietary energy in the average diet. Beef, goat, lamb, and sheep (mutton) are very expensive; however, many Africans consume bushmeat.

Throughout Africa, the midday meal is the main meal of the day. It is usually a combination of vegetables, legumes, and possibly meat. Depending on the region, stews, soups, or sauces made with vegetables are served over a porridge or mash made from a root vegetable (such as cassava) or a grain (such as millet, teff, rice, or corn). Variations on this basic meal reflect regional differences. In the traditional African diet, meat and fish are not the focus of a meal but are instead used to enhance the stew that accompanies the mash or porridge. The largest variety of ingredients is found in coastal areas and in the fertile highlands. Flavorings and spices vary with regional plants and local histories of trade with other regions.

Traditional African cooking methods include steaming food in leaf wrappers (banana or corn husks), boiling, frying in oil, grilling beside a fire, roasting in a fire, or baking in ashes. Africans have traditionally cooked outdoors or in a building separate from the living quarters. African kitchens commonly have a stew pot sitting on three stones arranged around a fire. Meals are normally eaten with the hands.

White South Africans, including Dutch descendants known as Afrikaners and other Europeans, and Asian Indians in Africa have diets similar to their countries of origin. In urban areas, however, the diets of black Africans are changing rapidly. There is an increasing dependence on meat, and poached bushmeat is decimating wildlife in many regions. Traditional African diets are also being rapidly replaced, especially in urban areas, by Western processed foods that typically contain high amounts of "empty" **calories**, meaning that they are void of or low in **vitamins** or **minerals**.

North Africa

The North African countries that border the Mediterranean Sea are predominantly Muslim. As a result, their diet reflects Islamic traditions. Islam does not permit the eating of pork or any animal that has not been butchered in accordance with the traditions of the faith. Like other regions of Africa, much of the North African diet is based on grains. However, cooking with olive oil, onions, and garlic is more common in North African countries. Notable spices include cumin, caraway, clove, and cinnamon. Flatbreads are a common staple and can accompany any meal, including breakfast, which is usually porridge prepared from millet or chickpea flour. Couscous (made from hard wheat) and millet are common staples for the main midday meal, often accompanied by a vegetable salad. *Tajine* is a main meal named for the conical clay pot in which it is prepared. Lamb is cooked in tajines, as well as on kabobs (roasted on a skewer). Vegetables include okra, meloukhia (spinach-like greens), and radishes. Common fruits are oranges, lemons, pears, and mandrakes. Legumes such as broad beans (fava beans), lentils, yellow peas, and black-eyed peas are also important staples. Mint tea and coffee are very popular beverages in North Africa. Alcoholic drinks are forbidden by Islamic tradition.

West Africa

There is considerable variation in staple foods across West Africa. Traditional West African meals are high in carbohydrates such as yam, rice, or plantain. Okra and fish soup is a traditional West African dish. Rice is predominant from Mauritania to Liberia and across to the Sahel, the region that traverses the continent between the Sahara and the southern savannas. Couscous is prevalent in the Sahara. Along the coast from Côte d'Ivoire (Ivory Coast) to Nigeria and Cameroon, root crops, primarily varieties of yam and cassava, are common. Cassava, imported from Brazil by the Portuguese, is boiled and then pounded into a nearly pure starch. Yam is the chief crop in West Africa and is served in a variety of dishes, including *amala* (pounded yam) and *egwansi* (melon) sauce. Millet is used for making porridge and beer. Palm oil is the stew base in Gambia and in southern and eastern regions of West Africa. In the Sahel, groundnut paste (peanut butter) is the main ingredient for stews. Other stews are based on okra, beans, sweet potato leaves, or cassava. Common vegetables include eggplant, cabbage, carrots, French beans, lettuce, onions, and cherry tomatoes. Stews in this region tend to be heavily spiced, often with chilies.

Plantain, a variety of banana, is abundant in more tropical regions of West Africa. Sweet plantains are normally fried, whereas hard plantains are boiled or pounded into *fufu*. Dates, bananas, guava, melons, passionfruit, figs, jackfruit, mangos, pineapples, cashews, and wild lemons and oranges are also common in West Africa.

Many West African households keep a few domestic animals, such as goats, sheep, cattle, or chickens, although their consumption is generally reserved for ceremonial and festive occasions. Bushmeat, including bush rat, antelope, and monkey, remains a major food source for rural West Africans, providing 20%–90% of their total animal dietary protein. Fish is a staple in coastal areas, and giant snails are eaten in various parts of West Africa. Pork is generally restricted to non-Muslim areas.

East Africa

Extensive trade with and migration to and from Arabic countries and South Asia have made East African food culture unique, particularly in the coastal areas. The main staples include potatoes, rice, *matake* (mashed plantains), and a maize meal that is cooked up into a thick porridge. Beans or a stew with meat, potatoes, or vegetables often accompany the porridge. Beef, goat, chicken, and sheep are the most common meats. Outside of Kenya and the horn of Africa, stews are less spicy, but the coastal areas of East Africa feature spicy, coconut-based stews.

Two herding tribes, the Maasai and Fulbe, have notably different diets. Meat is generally reserved for special occasions, but these tribes have traditionally depended on fresh and soured milk and butter as staples. This is unusual because most Africans consume little milk or other dairy products, primarily due to widespread lactose intolerance.

Diets in the horn of Africa, which includes Somalia and Ethiopia, are characterized by their spicy foods, prepared with chilies and garlic. The staple grain, teff, has a considerably higher **iron** and nutrient content than other African staple grains. A common traditional food is *injera*, a spongy flatbread that is eaten by tearing it and then using it to scoop up meat or stew.

Southern Africa

A greater variety of fruits and vegetables are available in the southern part of the continent, including bananas, pineapples, mangoes, avocados, tomatoes, carrots, onions, potatoes, and cabbage. Nevertheless, the southern African diet is heavily reliant on maize, and traditional southern African meals are generally centered around maize or rice stews. The most common dish made from cornmeal is called *mealie meal* or *pap*. Known as *nshima* or *nsima* farther north, it is usually covered with stew that includes boiled vegetables, such as cabbage, spinach, or turnips, or on special occasions, fish, beans, or chicken.

Risks

In many parts of Africa, traditional indigenous diets are often inadequate in essential vitamins, minerals, and protein. These deficiencies can cause or contribute to a variety of diseases. Micronutrient deficiencies are prevalent throughout much of Africa, particularly in **vitamin A**, **iodine**, and iron deficiencies, which can result in vision impairment, goiter (enlarged thyroid), and anemia, respectively. Deficiencies are most common in arid areas where the soil is either naturally poor or has been depleted through poor agricultural practices.

Food insecurity

Although depleted agricultural soils and a growing dependence on processed Western-type foods are problems throughout Africa, food insecurity—a lack of consistent and affordable staple food due to drought, floods, warfare, or other natural and man-made disasters—is a far greater (and growing) threat. Although the African continent has long suffered periodic famines, widespread famine has become increasingly frequent in recent decades. During the late twentieth century, the worsening HIV/AIDS

KEY TERMS

Anemia—Red blood cell deficiency.

Bushmeat—Meat of wild animals killed for subsistence.

Cassava—A tropical and subtropical shrub cultivated for its starchy tuberous root that is rich in carbohydrates but poor in protein; a major staple food throughout the developing world.

Couscous—A North African food made from semolina, the ground endosperm of hard durum wheat, and generally served in spicy stews.

Famine—An extreme and widespread food shortage.

Food insecurity—Occasional or consistent lack of access to a sufficient amount of safe and nutritious foods for supplying the dietary requirements necessary for a healthy, active life.

Lactose intolerance—The inability to digest lactose, the sugar in milk and other dairy products; common among Africans.

Sorghum—A food grain that is also cultivated for syrup, alcohol production, and animal fodder.

Staple—A food that is regularly consumed in such quantities that it constitutes a major portion of the diet and supplies the majority of a population's energy and nutritional requirements.

Teff—A cereal grain from North Africa.

---

epidemic threatened the food supply, as adults fell ill and died and agricultural production declined. Rural communities and women and children were the hardest hit. By the early twenty-first century, climate change was adversely affecting agricultural production in many parts of Africa. In particular, severe drought in the horn of Africa was causing widespread famine.

With its immense and growing population and depleting resources, maintaining healthy, well-balanced, and culturally appropriate diets presents immense challenges for the entire African continent. Preserving traditional food cultures and maintaining and improving agricultural land and practices are vitally important. Climate change has added a new dimension to feeding a continent where geography, politics, culture, and religion have affected the food supply and diet for centuries. Preserving the fertility of African land to feed the people of the continent is an important challenge for the entire world.

Resources

BOOKS

Ekunsanmi, Toye. *What Africans Eat: Traditional Foods and Food Traditions of West Africa.* Denver: Outskirts Press, 2010.

WEBSITES

"African Heritage Diet & Pyramid." Oldways. http://old-wayspt.org/resources/heritage-pyramids/african-diet-pyramid (accessed August 15, 2012).

Food and Agriculture Organization of the United Nations (FAO), Agriculture and Consumer Protection Department. "Staple Foods: What Do People Eat?" *Dimensions of Need—An Atlas of Food and Agriculture.* http://www.fao.org/docrep/u8480e/U8480E07.htm (accessed September 19, 2012).

Govindji, Azmina, and Shams Dharamshi. "Healthy Eating, West African Style." The Ismaili Nutrition Centre. http://www.theismaili.org/cms/997/Healthy-eating-West-African-style (accessed September 19, 2012).

ORGANIZATIONS

Build Africa, Vale House, Second Floor, Clarence Rd., Tunbridge Wells, UK Kent TN1 1HE, 44 0 1892 519619, hello@build-africa.org.uk, http://www.build-africa.org.

Food and Agricultural Organization of the United Nations, Viale delle Terme di Caracalla, Rome, Italy 00153, 3906 57051, Fax: 39 06 570 53152, FAO-HQ@fao.org, http://www.fao.org.

Oldways, 266 Beacon St., Boston, MA 02116, (617) 421-5500, Fax: (617) 421-5511, http://oldwayspt.org.

Jens Levy
M. Cristina F. Garces
Margaret Alic, PhD

Aging and nutrition *see* **Senior nutrition**

AIDS/HIV diet and nutrition

Definition

Human immunodeficiency virus (HIV) infection is a complex illness caused by a retrovirus, which is a single-strand virus that replicates by using reverse transcription to produce copies of DNA that become incorporated within the genome of the host cell. The HIV virus destroys a type of white blood cell known as CD4+ T lymphocyte, or T helper cell. These cells are important in maintaining the various functions of the human immune system. When the level of CD4+ T cells in the bloodstream falls, the patient loses the ability to fight off bacteria, viruses, and fungi that would not cause disease in a person with a strong immune system. Infections that occur in people with weakened immune systems are called opportunistic infections.

Acquired immunodeficiency syndrome (AIDS) is an advanced form of HIV infection in which the patient has developed opportunistic infections or certain types of **cancer** and/or the CD4+ T cell count has dropped below 200/mL. According to the Centers for Disease Control and Prevention (CDC), more than 1.1 million people in the United States were living with HIV/AIDS at the beginning of 2012, of whom about 20% were undiagnosed and unaware that they were infected. An estimated 33.4 million people around the world were infected with HIV as of 2012, with approximately 7,200 new infections every day. The disease causes nearly 2 million deaths worldwide each year, 95% of them in developing countries.

Nutritional issues are common in patients with HIV infection. Some problems with diet and nutrition are caused by HIV infection directly while others are related to opportunistic infections or medication side effects. Maintaining adequate food intake and balanced nutrition in patients with HIV infection is complicated not only by the many ways in which the disease can affect the body—including the fact that the virus mutates rapidly—but also by frequent updating of treatment strategies for AIDS, including nutritional therapy. As a result, nutritional care of patients with AIDS must be tailored to each person and reviewed carefully every few months. In 2010, the **Academy of Nutrition and Dietetics** issued a set of guidelines on the care of people with HIV infection that recommended appropriate nutritional care for individuals with HIV/AIDS. That publication is available on the Academy website.

Origins

AIDS is a relative newcomer to the list of major infectious diseases. According to the National Institutes of Health (NIH), researchers think that HIV originated in a species of chimpanzees native to west equatorial Africa and jumped the species barrier into humans through hunters' contact with the blood of infected chimpanzees—most likely somewhere in western Africa in the second half of the twentieth century. The earliest known case of HIV infection was found in a blood sample collected from a man in Kinshasa in the Congo in 1959.

The first cases of AIDS were not diagnosed in the United States until June 1981, when the CDC reported a cluster of five cases of an opportunistic lung infection among homosexual men in Los Angeles. In the first 15 years of the epidemic, there were no effective treatments for HIV infection (there is still no cure as of 2012). As a result, many patients turned to alternative dietary treatments to help them manage the nausea, weight loss, and other symptoms associated with the infection. Alternative food-related therapies that were used in this period included:

- Herbal compounds used in traditional Chinese medicine (TCM) for the treatment of fevers or energy deficiency, particularly medicines containing astragalus (*Astragalus membranaceus*).
- Western herbal preparations recommended by naturopaths, including goldenseal (*Hydrastis canadensis*), licorice (*Glycyrrhiza glabra*), osha root (*Ligusticum porteri*), and echinacea.
- Detoxification diets, including the Master Cleanser lemon juice diet.
- Juice fasts, often taken together with laxatives or colonics.
- Nutritional supplements, particularly blue-green algae, zinc, vitamin C, beta-carotene, and catechin (an antioxidant).
- Vegetarian and raw food diets.

Prior to 1996, nutritional management of AIDS patients focused largely on prevention of weight loss and wasting, sometimes called the "slim disease." After the introduction of highly active antiretroviral therapy (HAART) in 1996, however, nutritionists were confronted with a range of other dietary problems related either to the new drugs or to prolonged survival itself. HAART is not one drug but a combination of various antiretroviral agents given to patients to prevent the virus from replicating and to discourage mutations of the virus. The drugs must be taken in combination because no medication by itself is able to suppress HIV for very long. One early problem with HAART was the complicated dosing schedules of the different drugs prescribed for an individual patient. To encourage adherence to treatment schedules (which must be at least 98% complete to protect the patient from developing a strain of the virus resistant to HAART), some pharmaceutical companies developed fixed-dose combinations. A fixed-dose combination is a medication in which several antiretroviral drugs that are known to work well together are combined in a single pill.

Guidelines for offering antiretroviral treatment (ART) to patients were published in the late 1990s because the drugs have so many adverse effects (including hair loss, muscle cramps and pains, kidney or liver failure, insomnia, inflammation of the pancreas, dizziness and mental confusion, headache, nausea and vomiting, and numbness in hands or feet) that many patients were not compliant with dosage schedules and developed drug-resistant mutations of the HIV virus. Recommendations for ART have been revised several times by the U.S. Department of Health and Human Services. The most recent version of the guidelines was issued in October 2011, devoting 174 pages to every aspect of antiretroviral care for HIV patients, including laboratory testing for initial assessment of a patient's HIV status; treatment goals; therapy recommendations for patients without earlier treatment and with earlier treatment regimens; treatments that are not recommended; antiretroviral treatments in patients with other medical issues; limitations to safety and efficacy of various treatments; and preventing secondary infections of HIV. The primary recommendations for treatment standards for antiretroviral therapy as provided in the 2011 guidelines include:

- ART should be initiated in all patients with a history of an AIDS-defining illness or with a CD4+ count of under 350 cells/mm^3.
- ART is also recommended for patients with CD4+ counts between 350 and 500 cells/mm^3.
- A combination antiretroviral drug regimen is also recommended for pregnant women who do not meet criteria for treatment to prevent perinatal transmission.
- Patients initiating ART should be willing and able to commit to lifelong treatment and should understand the benefits and risks of therapy and the importance of adherence.
- Patients may choose to postpone therapy, and providers, on a case-by-case basis, may elect to defer therapy based on clinical and/or psychosocial factors.

It is this set of guidelines for ART that nutritionists currently work with when planning healthful diets for patients with HIV infection and AIDS.

Description

While there is no standard "HIV diet" or "AIDS diet" because patients' symptoms, medication regimens, and corresponding nutritional needs vary so widely, there are general practices followed by registered dietitians who work with doctors and other health care professionals to care for these patients.

Dietetics consultation and follow-up

Patients with HIV infection should consult a registered dietitian (RD) as soon as possible after diagnosis, because good nutrition is essential to maintaining a normal level of activity and self-care as well as supporting the patient's immune system. RDs use several screening questionnaires to evaluate patients for potential nutritional problems. On the patient's first visit, he or she may be given a quick nutrition screen or QNS to fill out. The QNS identifies such problems as unintentional weight loss, nausea, difficulty swallowing, and diarrhea. The dietitian then measures the patient's height, weight, skinfold thickness, and the circumference of the muscles on the patient's midarm. These last two measurements are needed in order to monitor changes in body fat distribution and muscle wasting that often accompany HIV infection.

The next step in the initial assessment involves the patient's completion of a food intake record (FIR). The patient is asked to record everything he or she eats or drinks in a 24-hour period, including snacks and alcoholic beverages. If possible, the patient will fill out two FIRs, one for a working day and one for a weekend day or holiday. The FIR allows the dietitian to evaluate the patient's usual eating habits, portion sizes, food preferences, and average calorie intake. It also establishes a baseline for the individual patient, so that loss of appetite later on or other nutritional problems can be detected as quickly as possible.

Follow-up visits to the dietitian are scheduled according to the degree of the patient's nutritional risk. One system originally developed by the American Dietetic Association (now the Academy of Nutrition and Dietetics) and the Los Angeles County Commission on HIV Health Services used the following timelines for HIV patients at nutritional risk:

- Low risk: The patient's weight is stable, with a balanced and adequate food intake; normal blood levels of cholesterol, triglycerides, and glucose; no evidence of kidney or liver disorders; regular physical exercise; and low levels of psychosocial stress. Low-risk patients are evaluated by the RD as needed, but at least once a year.
- Moderate risk: The patient is obese or suffers from changing patterns of body fat distribution; has high blood cholesterol levels or high blood pressure; has developed an eating disorder, nausea, vomiting, or diarrhea; has been recently diagnosed with type 2 diabetes or food allergies; is in recovery from substance abuse; or is under psychosocial stress. Moderate-risk patients should be seen by the RD within a month.
- High risk: The patient is pregnant; suffers from poorly controlled diabetes; has lost 10% of body weight over the previous 4–6 months; has lost 5% of body weight in the previous 4 weeks; has dental problems, involvement of the central nervous system, severe nausea or vomiting, severe pain on swallowing, or chronic diarrhea; has one or more opportunistic infections; or is under severe psychosocial stress. These patients should be seen by an RD within one week.

In addition to assessment of the patient's nutritional needs, RDs also evaluate his or her living situation and other issues that may affect receiving adequate nutrition.

Specific issues in nutritional care of HIV patients

NAUSEA, VOMITING, AND DIARRHEA. Nausea and vomiting are common symptoms of HIV infection as well as side effects of HAART. They can lead to long-term damage to the esophagus and dental problems as well as weight loss and inability to take needed medications. About 30% of patients develop nausea and vomiting within 1 to 4 weeks following infection as part of a condition called acute retroviral syndrome or ARS, which resembles influenza or mononucleosis. Most patients, however, develop nausea, vomiting, and diarrhea later on in the course of the disease as side effects of HAART or from opportunistic infections of the gastrointestinal system. Patients with HIV infection are highly susceptible to such diseases as **giardiasis**, cryptosporidiosis, listeriosis, *Campylobacter* infections, and *Salmonella* infections.

Treatment of nausea, vomiting, and diarrhea in patients with HIV infections may require a number of diagnostic tests and imaging studies as well as evaluation of the patient's medications in order to determine the cause(s) of the symptoms.

LIPODYSTROPHY. Lipodystrophy is the medical term for the redistribution of body fat that sometimes occurs in patients with HIV infection as a result of HAART, genetic factors, the length of time a person has been HIV-positive, and the severity of the disease. As of 2012, it was not completely understood why antiretroviral drugs and other factors have this effect. The patient may notice new deposits of fat at the back of the neck (sometimes called "buffalo humps") and around the abdomen. Conversely, fat may be lost under the skin of the face, resulting in sunken cheeks, or lost under the skin of the buttocks, arms, or legs. Lipodystrophy is not necessarily associated with weight loss.

Lipodystrophy may be accompanied by other changes in the patient's **metabolism**, particularly **insulin** resistance and higher levels of blood cholesterol and **triglycerides**. One recommendation registered dietitians often give to patients with lipodystrophy and metabolic changes is to follow a **Mediterranean diet**, which is high in fiber-rich **whole grains**, fruits, and vegetables and a high proportion of saturated **fats**. Another recommendation is to maintain regular physical exercise (particularly weight training), which has been shown to lower insulin resistance and decrease abdominal fat deposits.

WASTING. Wasting refers to rapid unintentional weight loss (usually defined as 5% of body weight over a period of 6 months) combined with changes in the composition of body tissue. Specifically, the patient is losing lean muscle tissue and replacing it with fat. The patient's outward appearance may not be a reliable guide to wasting, particularly if he or she also has lipodystrophy. Weight loss associated with wasting may result from nausea and vomiting related to opportunistic infections of the digestive tract as well as from reactions to medication.

Nutrition is the first line of defense against wasting. To help the patient maintain weight, nutritionists recommend raising the daily calorie intake from 17–20 **calories** per pound of body weight (a guideline used for patients whose weight has been stable) to 25 calories per pound. Patients with wasting syndrome may require as much as 3500 calories per day to maintain their weight. Nutrient ratios should be 15–20% **protein**, 50–60% **carbohydrates**, and 25% fats to protect the body's muscle tissue. Patients who need more calories or protein may benefit from adding supplements such as Ensure or Instant Breakfast to their daily diet. In addition, weight training or other forms of regular exercise help to maintain muscle tissue.

Other treatments for wasting include the use of appetite stimulants to increase food intake and hormonal treatments to build lean muscle tissue, particularly in male patients.

MEDICATION INTERACTIONS. Most medications used in HAART have the potential to cause nausea and vomiting. Some antiretroviral medications should be taken with food to minimize these side effects. Digestive disturbances are the single most common reason given by patients for discontinuing antiretroviral therapy. In some cases, switching to a different combination of drugs helps to relieve nausea, vomiting, or diarrhea.

Function

The function of nutritional education and dietary management in patients with HIV infection and AIDS is to maintain the patient's energy level and ability to carry out normal activities of daily life; lower the risk of opportunistic infections of the digestive system; support the immune system; and minimize the side effects of HAART on the patient's ability to eat and enjoy food.

Benefits

The benefits of good nutritional care for patients with HIV infection are prolonged survival, improved quality of life, and fewer or less severe side effects from medical treatment.

Precautions

Food safety issues

Food safety is an important concern for patients with HIV infection because their immune systems have difficulty fighting off food- or waterborne disease organisms. While most people can get **food poisoning** or parasitic infections of the digestive tract if they drink contaminated water or do not prepare food properly, patients with HIV infection can become severely ill due to their compromised immune systems. Foodborne illnesses are also much more difficult to treat in people with AIDS or HIV infection, and may lead to malabsorption syndrome, a condition in which the body cannot absorb and make use of needed nutrients in food. The CDC and NIH have brochures with detailed instructions for patients about safety issues in purchasing and preparing foods, particularly when traveling abroad. Basic safeguards include the following:

- Wash hands repeatedly in warm soapy water before and after preparing or eating food. Instant hand sanitizers should be used when away from home.
- Cook all meats, fish, and poultry to the well-done stage; do not eat sushi, raw oysters, or raw meat in any form.
- Do not use unpasteurized milk or dairy products.
- Do not eat raw, soft-boiled, or "wet" scrambled eggs, or Caesar salad made with raw egg in the dressing. Hard-boiled or hard-scrambled eggs are safe.
- Rinse all fruits and vegetables carefully in clean, safe water, and clean all cutting boards and knives that touch chicken and meat with soap and hot water before using these utensils with other food items.
- Keep all refrigerated foods below 40°F; check expiration dates on food packaging.
- Completely reheat leftovers before eating, and do not eat leftovers that have been stored in the refrigerator for longer than 3 days.
- Do not drink water that comes directly from lakes, streams, rivers, or springs, and ask for drinks without ice in restaurants.

HIV patients with special needs

Patients with special needs include those with limited food budgets or without access to a kitchen for preparing their own food.

Complementary and alternative (CAM) dietary treatments

In general, multivitamins, other **dietary supplements**, or herbal teas prepared by reliable manufacturers and approved by the patient's physician are useful

KEY TERMS

Acquired immune deficiency syndrome (AIDS)— HIV infection that has led to certain opportunistic infections, cancers, or a CD4+ T-lymphocyte (helper cell) blood cell count lower than 200/mL.

Acute retroviral syndrome (ARS)—A syndrome that develops in about 30% of HIV patients within a few weeks of infection. ARS is characterized by nausea, vomiting, fever, headache, general tiredness, and muscle cramps.

Carrier—A person who bears or carries a disease agent in or on their body and can transmit the disease to others, but is immune to the disease or has no symptoms of it.

Colonic—Sometimes called colonic hydrotherapy, a colonic is a procedure similar to an enema in which the patient's colon is irrigated (washed out) with large amounts of water. Some people undergoing a detoxification diet have one or more colonics to remove fecal matter remaining in the intestines during the diet; however, this procedure is discouraged by mainstream physicians because of its potential risks to health.

Dietitian—A healthcare professional who specializes in individual or group nutritional planning, public education in nutrition, or research in food science. To be licensed as a registered dietitian (RD) in the United States, a person must complete a bachelor's degree in a nutrition-related field and pass a state licensing examination. Dietitians are also called registered dietitians.

Highly active antiretroviral therapy (HAART)—The major form of pharmacological treatment for HIV since 1996. HAART is a combination of several different antiretroviral drugs selected for patients on an individual basis. It is not a cure for HIV infection but acts to slow the replication of the virus and discourage new mutations. HAART has a number of side effects that complicate maintaining good nutrition in HIV patients.

Lipodystrophy—The medical term for redistribution of body fat in response to HAART, insulin injections for diabetes, or rare hereditary disorders.

Malabsorption syndrome—A condition characterized by indigestion, bloating, diarrhea, loss of appetite, and weakness, caused by poor absorption of nutrients from food as a result of HIV infection itself, giardiasis or other opportunistic infections of the digestive tract, or certain surgical procedures involving the stomach or intestines.

Opportunistic infection—An infection caused by a normally harmless organism that causes disease when the host's immune system is weakened. Opportunistic infections are a major problem in the medical and nutritional care of HIV patients.

Retrovirus—A single-stranded virus that replicates by reverse transcription to produce DNA copies that are incorporated into the genome of infected cells. AIDS is caused by a retrovirus.

Wasting syndrome—A combination of weight loss and change in composition of body tissues that occurs in patients with HIV infection. Typically, the patient's body loses lean muscle tissue and replaces it with fat as well as losing weight overall.

---

complementary treatments for HIV patients. Traditional Chinese medicines made outside the United States, however, should be used with great caution as their purity cannot be guaranteed.

Patients interested in a vegetarian diet should consult their physician and nutritionist before starting one; raw-food vegetarian diets should be avoided because of the increased risk of contracting food-borne diseases. **Detoxification diets** and colonics are risky practices for HIV patients and should not be used.

Risks

There are no known risks to nutritional management of patients with HIV infection by qualified professionals working with the patient's physicians and nurses. There are few risks to the use of naturopathic dietary supplements or herbal formulas provided that the patient reports the use of alternative therapies to the medical care team and does not use them as substitutes for HAART or other mainstream medications.

Research and general acceptance

Research in the field of nutrition for HIV patients is ongoing and can be expected to produce revised guidelines for dietary management every few years for the foreseeable future. These changes will result as much from mutations in the disease organism as from discoveries of new drugs and other forms of treatment for HIV infection.

QUESTIONS TO ASK YOUR DOCTOR

- Can I continue to maintain my vegetarian diet now that I have been diagnosed with HIV disease?

- Can you recommend a specialist in nutrition with whom I can consult about a diet appropriate for my HIV status?

- Are there foods that are likely to interact with the drugs you have prescribed for my HIV status?

- Should I be concerned about drug interactions between my HIV medications and dietary supplements that I use?

Resources

BOOKS

Lehmann, Robert H. *Cooking for Life: A Guide to Nutrition and Food Safety for the HIV-positive Community.* New York: Dell Publishing, 1997.

Pibram, Vivian, ed. *Nutrition and HIV.* New York: Wiley-Blackwell, 2010.

Romeyn, Mary. *Nutrition and HIV: A New Model for Treatment,* 2nd ed. San Francisco: Jossey-Bass Publishers, 1998.

Watson, Ronald R. *Nutrition and AIDS.* 2nd ed. Boca Raton, FL: CRC Press, 2001.

PERIODICALS

Fields-Gardner, Cade. "Position of the American Dietetic Association: Nutrition Intervention and Human Immunodeficiency Virus Infection." *Journal of the American Dietetic Association* 104, no. 7 (2010): 1105–1119.

Grinspoon, Steven, and Kathleen Mulligan. "Weight Loss and Wasting in Patients Infected with Human Immunodeficiency Virus." *Clinical Infectious Diseases* 36, Suppl. 2 (2003): S69–S78.

Highleyman, Liz. "Managing Nausea, Vomiting, and Diarrhea." *Bulletin of Experimental Treatment for AIDS* (BETA) 15, no. 2 (2002): 29–39.

Lo, J. "Dyslipidemia and Lipid Management in HIV-infected Patients." *Current Opinion in Endocrinology, Diabetes, and Obesity* 18, no. 2 (2011): 144–47.

Mangili, A., et al. "Nutrition and HIV Infection: Review of Weight Loss and Wasting in the Era of Highly Active Antiretroviral Therapy from the Nutrition for Healthy Living Cohort." *Clinical Infectious Diseases* 42, 6 (2006): 836–842.

Mondy, Kristin, and Pablo Tebas. "Emerging Bone Problems in Patients Infected with Human Immunodeficiency Virus." *Clinical Infectious Diseases* 36, Suppl. 2 (2003): S101–S105.

Nerad, Judith, et al. "General Nutrition Management in Patients Infected with Human Immunodeficiency Virus." *Clinical Infectious Diseases* 36, Suppl. 2 (2003): S52–S62.

WEBSITES

Centers for Disease Control and Prevention (CDC), Division of HIV/AIDS Prevention. "Safe Food and Water." U.S. Department of Health and Human Services. http://www.cdc.gov/hiv/pubs/brochure/food.htm (accessed July 6, 2012).

"HIV and Nutrition." AVERT.org. http://www.avert.org/hiv-nutrition.htm (accessed July 6, 2012).

HIV InSite. "Diet and Nutrition." University of California, San Francisco (UCSF) Center for HIV Information. http://hivinsite.ucsf.edu/insite?page=pb-daily-diet (accessed July 10, 2012).

Tufts University School of Medicine, Public Health and Community Medicine, Nutrition/Infection Unit. "HIV Nutrition & Health." http://www.tufts.edu/med/nutrition-infection/hiv/health.html (accessed July 6, 2012).

U.S. Department of Agriculture, Food and Nutrition Information Center. "Diet and Disease: HIV/AIDS." http://fnic.nal.usda.gov/nal_display/index.php?info_center=4&tax_level=2&tax_subject=278&topic_id=1380 (accessed July 6, 2012).

U.S. Food and Drug Administration. "Integrating Nutrition Therapy into Medical Management of HIV." http://www.fda.gov/ForConsumers/ByAudience/ForPatientAdvocates/HIVandAIDSActivities/ucm125087.htm (accessed July 6, 2012).

ORGANIZATIONS

AIDS Education and Training Centers (AETC), National Resource Center, School of Nursing, University of Medicine and Dentistry of New Jersey, 65 Bergen St., 8th fl., Newark, NJ 07101, info@aidsetc.org, http://www.aidsetc.org.

Academy of Nutrition and Dietetics, 120 South Riverside Plz., Ste. 2000, Chicago, IL 60606-6995, (312) 899-0040, (800) 877-1600, amacmunn@eatright.org, http://www.eatright.org.

Centers for Disease Control and Prevention, 1600 Clifton Rd. NE, Atlanta, GA 30333, (800) CDC-INFO (232-4636), TTY: (888) 232-6348, cdcinfo@cdc.gov, http://www.cdc.gov.

University of California San Francisco (UCSF), Center for HIV Information, 4150 Clement St., Bldg 16, VAMC 111V - UCSF, San Francisco, CA 94121, (415) 379-5601, Fax: (415) 379-5547, chi@ucsf.edu, http://chi.ucsf.edu.

U.S. Food and Drug Administration, 10903 New Hampshire Ave., Silver Spring, MD 20993-0002, (888) INFO-FDA (463-6332), http://www.fda.gov.

Rebecca J. Frey, PhD

Alcohol consumption

Definition

Alcohol consumption is drinking beverages that contain ethyl alcohol, such as beer, wine, or distilled spirits such as gin, whiskey, or vodka.

Purpose

In earlier times, when subsistence agriculture was the norm, alcoholic beverages, usually beer or mead (fermented honey and water), provided a substantial percentage of **calories** in the diet. Today people drink alcohol to relax and socialize, to get high, or because they are physically addicted to it.

Description

Ethyl alcohol, or ethanol, is produced by yeast fermentation of the natural sugars in plants, such as grapes (wine), hops (beer), **sugar** cane (rum), agave (tequila), or rice (saki). The process of fermenting

Calories in alcohol

Beverage	Serving amount (ounce)	Average (calories)
Beer		
Regular	12	149
Light	12	110
Distilled (80 proof)		
Gin, rum, vodka, whisky, tequila	1.0	65
Brandy, cognac	1.0	65
Liqueurs (Drambuie, Cointreau, Kahlua)	1.5	188
Wine		
Red	4	80
Dry white	4	75
Sweet	4	105
Sherry	2	75
Port	2	90
Champagne	4	84
Vermouth, sweet	3	140
Vermouth, dry	3	105
Cocktails		
Martini	3.5	140
Manhattan	3.5	164
Daiquiri	4	122
Whiskey sour	3	122
Margarita cocktail	4	168
Coolers	6	150

SOURCE: National Institute on Alcohol Abuse and Alcoholism, National Institutes of Health, U.S. Department of Health and Human Services

(Table by GGS Information Services. © 2013 Cengage Learning.)

plants to produce alcohol is at least 10,000 years old and appears to have developed independently in many cultures.

Alcohol affects almost every system of the body. Research suggests that when alcohol is consumed in moderation, there are some health benefits and some health risks. Heavy use of alcohol has no health benefits and many health risks. The federal *Dietary Guidelines for Americans 2010* define moderate alcohol consumption as one drink per day for women and two drinks per day for men. This difference by gender is based on the fact that women tend to be smaller in body size than men and their bodies contain a lower percentage of water. An equivalent amount of alcohol in a woman's bloodstream will be more concentrated than in a man's. A "drink" according to these guidelines contains about 14 grams of alcohol and is defined as:

- 12 fluid ounces of regular beer
- 5 fluid ounces of wine
- 1.5 fluid ounces of 80 proof (40% alcohol) distilled spirits

Using this definition, one regular beer contains about 145 calories. One glass of red wine has 105 calories and white wine has about 100 calories. One shot of distilled spirits has about 95 calories plus any calories in the mixer used to make mixed drinks.

Benefits of moderate alcohol consumption

Evidence based on more than 100 studies shows that moderate alcohol consumption can help prevent heart attacks, sudden cardiac death, peripheral vascular disease, and strokes caused by blood clots (ischemic stroke). The risk of these diseases is reduced between 25–40% in both men and women. The reduction is seen in people who have no apparent heart disease, as well as those who are at high risk of heart disease because they have type 2 diabetes, high blood pressure (**hypertension**), angina (chest pain), or have already had one heart attack. Researchers suggest that this protective effect occurs because alcohol increases the amount of HDL, or "good" cholesterol, and also affects various proteins in ways that make blood clotting less likely.

In two other large studies, people who were moderate drinkers were also less likely to develop type 2 diabetes and **gallstones**. Gallstones are hard masses of cholesterol and **calcium** that form in the gallbladder. Finally, moderate drinking serves a social purpose that can provide psychological benefits.

Risks of moderate alcohol consumption

Moderate alcohol consumption also carries with it some risks. In women, even moderate drinking is associated with a modest increase in the risk of developing breast **cancer**. Consuming enough **folate** (folic acid), at least 600 mg daily, may help counteract this increased risk in women.

Women who are pregnant or **breastfeeding** should avoid alcohol completely, as even moderate consumption can affect the fetus. Alcohol consumption can also alter sleep patterns and interact with many medications. However, by far the greatest risk of moderate drinking is that for some people it will lead to heavy alcohol consumption, alcohol abuse, and alcohol dependency. Twin and family studies indicated that there is an inherited tendency for some individuals to develop alcohol abuse disorders.

Risks of heavy alcohol consumption

Heavy alcohol consumption is defined for men as consuming 15 or more alcoholic drinks per week and for women as consuming 8 or more drinks per week. Between moderate and heavy alcohol consumption is a gray area of potentially problematic drinking that includes binge drinking.

Binge drinking is heavy alcohol consumption that occurs intermittently. Bingeing for men means consuming five or more drinks in a period of about two hours. For women, it is consuming four or more drinks in the same time period. According to the U.S. Substance Abuse and Mental Health Services Administration (SAMHSA), in 2010 approximately 31% of males and 16% of females 12 and older binge drank in a given month, with 18-to-25-year-olds engaging in binge drinking the most (41%).

Heavy alcohol consumption leads to two alcohol abuse disorders that are recognized in the *Diagnostic and Statistical Manual for Mental Disorders Fourth Edition (DSM-IV-TR)* published by the American Psychiatric Association. The disorders are called alcohol dependence and alcohol abuse (alcoholism). Men are more likely to abuse alcohol than women because they usually begin drinking at an earlier age than women.

Alcohol dependence is diagnosed when one or more of the following occur within a 12-month period:

- failure to fulfill obligations at work, home, or school due to repeated alcohol use
- repeatedly performing hazardous activities, such as driving or operating machinery, while under the influence of alcohol
- experiencing legal problems caused by alcohol use
- continued alcohol use despite problems it causes in relationships.
- symptoms do not rise to the level of alcohol abuse

Alcohol abuse, or alcoholism, is diagnosed when three or more of the following occur within a 12-month period:

- tolerance to the effects of alcohol develops
- stopping drinking causes physical symptoms of withdrawal
- more alcohol is regularly drunk than is intended
- efforts to reduce alcohol consumption are unsuccessful
- getting alcohol, drinking, and recovering from drinking alcohol consumes a great deal of time
- work, social, and recreational activities are replaced by drinking or recovering from drinking
- alcohol use continues, despite its causing obvious physical and/or psychological problems

On any given day, about 7% of Americans, or more than 17 million people, are alcohol dependent or have alcoholism. Costs related to alcohol disorders are estimated to be more than $185 billion annually. Alcohol disorders are related to increased rates of motor vehicle deaths, homicides, suicides, and domestic violence. About 34% of Americans do not drink alcohol.

People with alcoholism generally do not eat healthy, balanced diets. An increasing problem in young women, particularly women with **body image** issues or **eating disorders**, is the deprivation of food to save calories for alcohol (to avoid weight gain). This is a dangerous practice. When 30% or more of an individual's calories come from alcohol, serious nutritional deficiencies develop. Not only do people with alcoholism fail to get the **protein**, **vitamins**, and **minerals** they need, but alcohol also interferes with the absorption of the nutrients they do eat. People who abuse alcohol develop **malnutrition** and deficiencies in essential amino acids, B-complex vitamins (especially vitamins B_1, B_2, and B_6), and **vitamin C**. They may develop either deficiencies or excesses of **vitamin A**. Along with nutritional deficiencies, the person with alcoholism often has liver damage. Cirrhosis, a disease in which the liver develops scar tissue and stops functioning, is the cause of death in about 32% of people with alcoholism worldwide. Alcoholism also substantially increases the chance of dying by violence, or developing esophageal cancer, mouth cancer, liver cancer, or breast cancer in women. Heavy drinking increases the risk of stroke and cardiovascular disease and can cause brain damage, loss of judgment, loss of motor skills, and memory loss.

Precautions

Some people should never drink alcohol. These include:

- children and adolescents under the age of 21
- women who are pregnant, breastfeeding, or who could become pregnant
- people who cannot control their drinking and keep it at the level of moderate consumption
- people who plan to drive, fly a plane, operate dangerous equipment, act as a lifeguard, or perform any activity that requires quick reactions, good judgment, and coordination
- people who are unable to control their aggression when they drink
- people taking certain medications (see below)
- people with liver or kidney damage
- people who are recovering from alcoholism

Interactions

Alcohol is a central nervous system depressant. More than 150 drugs interact with alcohol. Some of these interactions can be fatal, especially those that involve narcotic drugs that also depress the central nervous system. Categories of drugs that interact with alcohol include:

- narcotic drugs
- sleeping pills
- antidepressants
- anti-anxiety medications
- antihistamines

Aftercare

The best-known treatment for alcohol abuse disorders is the 12-step program of Alcoholics Anonymous. This program uses social support, rewards, and mentoring to change behavior. For it to succeed, the person with alcoholism must want to recover and must be willing to work at achieving sobriety. Relapses are common. Families of alcoholics may be helped by Al-Anon and teens by Alateen, whether or not their family member with alcoholism participates in Alcoholics Anonymous.

The United States Food and Drug Administration (FDA) approved three medications for the treatment of alcoholism. Disulfiram (Antabuse) makes the individual feel ill after drinking alcohol. Naltrexone (Depade, ReVia) acts on the brain to reduce the craving for alcohol. Acamprosate (Canpral) reduces withdrawal

---

KEY TERMS

B-complex vitamins—A group of water-soluble vitamins that often work together in the body. These include thiamin (B_1), riboflavin (B_2), niacin (B_3), pantothenic acid (B_5), pyridoxine (B_6), biotin (B_7 or vitamin H), folate/folic acid (B_9), and cobalamin (B_{12}).

Essential amino acid—An amino acid that is necessary for health but that cannot be made by the human body and must be acquired through diet.

Folic acid—Also called vitamin B_9, a stable synthetic form of folate that is found in dietary supplements and is added to fortified foods such as flour and cereal.

Mineral—An inorganic substance that is necessary in small quantities for the body to maintain good health. Examples include zinc, copper, and iron.

Peripheral vascular disease—A disease of blood vessels except those that supply blood to the heart.

Proof—A measure of alcohol. In the United States, one proof is equal to 0.5% alcohol content.

Tolerance—Adjustment of the body to a drug so that it takes more and more of the drug to produce the same physiological or psychological effect.

Type 2 diabetes—Sometimes called adult-onset diabetes, this disease prevents the body from properly using glucose (blood sugar).

Vitamin—A nutrient that the body needs in small amounts to remain healthy, but that the body cannot manufacture for itself and must acquire through diet.

---

symptoms. These medications are more effective with some people than others.

Complications

Complications of moderate and heavy alcohol abuse are listed above. In addition to physical complications, alcohol consumption can take an emotional and psychological toll on relationships and families, especially on children who have a parent with alcoholism.

Parental concerns

Alcohol consumption by adolescents substantially increases their risk of being in both fatal and nonfatal motor vehicle accidents. It also increases the chance of participating in risky sexual behavior, failing or dropping out of school, committing suicide, and

- What local resources can you recommend for assistance in dealing with my (or my family member's) drinking problems?
- What do you recommend as a way of gaining the potential benefits of drinking alcohol without encountering the possible risks associated with drinking?
- How much alcohol do I need to drink to achieve the health benefits?
- Can I drink alcohol if I am trying to become pregnant?

being a homicide victim. Children who begin to drink before age 15 are four times more likely to become alcohol dependent, according to the National Institute on Alcohol Abuse and Alcoholism.

Resources

BOOKS

Dasgupta, Amitava. *The Science of Drinking: How Alcohol Affects Your Body and Mind.* Lanham, MD: Rowman & Littlefield Publishers, 2011.

Watson, Ronald R. and Victor R. Preedy, eds. *Nutrition and Alcohol: Linking Nutrient Interactions and Dietary Intake.* Boca Raton, FL: CRC Press, 2004.

Wilson, Ted, and Norman J. Temple. *Beverages in Nutrition and Health.* Totowa, NJ: Humana Press, 2010. Reprint edition.

PERIODICALS

Nova, E., et al. "Potential Health Benefits of Moderate Alcohol Consumption: Current Perspectives in Research." *Proceedings of the Nutrition Society* 71, no. 2 (2012): 307–15.

Vasanthi, H.R., et al. "Health Benefits of Wine and Alcohol from Neuroprotection to Heart Health." *Frontiers in Bioscience* 4 (January 2012): 1505–12.

OTHER

Substance Abuse and Mental Health Services Administration (SAMHSA). *Results from the 2010 National Survey on Drug Use and Health: Summary of National Findings,* NSDUH Series H-41, HHS Publication No. (SMA) 11-4658. Rockville, MD: SAMHSA, 2011. http://www.oas.samhsa.gov/nsduhLatest.htm (accessed July 13, 2012).

WEBSITES

Centers for Disease Control and Prevention. "Alcohol and Public Health: Frequently Asked Questions." http://www.cdc.gov/alcohol/faqs.htm (accessed June 29, 2012).

Harvard School of Public Health. "Alcohol: Balancing Risks and Benefits." The Nutrition Source, Department of Nutrition, Harvard University. http://www.hsph.harvard.edu/nutritionsource/what-should-you-eat/alcohol-full-story/index.html (accessed July 3, 2012).

Higdon, Jane. "Alcoholic Beverages." Linus Pauling Institute, Oregon State University. http://lpi.oregonstate.edu/infocenter/foods/alcohol (accessed June 29, 2012).

———. "Folic Acid." Linus Pauling Institute, Oregon State University. http://lpi.oregonstate.edu/infocenter/vitamins/fa (accessed June 29, 2012).

Jennings, Ashley. "Drunkorexia: Alcohol Mixes With Eating Disorders." ABC News, October 21, 2010. http://abcnews.go.com/Health/drunkorexia-alcohol-mixes-eating-disorders/story?id=11936398 (accessed June 29, 2012).

Lieber, Charles S. "Relationships Between Nutrition, Alcohol Use, and Liver Disease." National Institute on Alcohol Abuse and Alcoholism. http://pubs.niaaa.nih.gov/publications/arh27-3/220-231.htm (accessed June 29, 2012).

MedlinePlus. "Alcohol." U.S. National Library of Medicine. http://www.nlm.nih.gov/medlineplus/alcohol.html (accessed June 29, 2012).

National Institute on Alcohol Abuse and Alcoholism (NIAAA). "Alcohol Calorie Counter." CollegeDrinking-Prevention.gov. http://www.collegedrinkingprevention.gov/CollegeStudents/calculator/alcoholcalc.aspx (accessed June 29, 2012).

———. "Alcohol & Health." http://www.niaaa.nih.gov/alcohol-health (accessed July 3, 2012).

Thompson, Warren. "Alcoholism." Medscape Reference. http://www.emedicine.com/med/topic98.htm (accessed June 29, 2012).

U.S. Department of Health and Human Services and the United States Department of Agriculture. "Dietary Guidelines for Americans." Health.gov. http://health.gov/dietaryguidelines/2010.asp (accessed June 29, 2012).

ORGANIZATIONS

Academy of Nutrition and Dietetics, 120 S Riverside Plaza, Ste. 2000, Chicago, IL 60606-6995, (312) 899-0040, (800) 877-1600, http://www.eatright.org.

Centers for Disease Control and Prevention, 1600 Clifton Rd NE, Atlanta, GA 30329, (404) 639-3534, (800) 232-4636, http://www.cdc.gov.

Linus Pauling Institute, 307 Linus Pauling Science Center, Corvallis, OR 97331, (541) 737-5075, Fax: (541) 737-5077, lpi@oregonstate.edu, http://lpi.oregeonstate.edu.

National Council on Alcoholism and Drug Dependence, Inc. (NCADD), 244 E 58th St., 4th Floor, New York, NY 10022, (212) 269-7797, Fax: (212) 269-7510, (800) 622-2255, http://www.ncadd.org.

National Institute on Alcohol Abuse and Alcoholism, 635 Fishers Ln., MSC 9304, Bethesda, MD 20892-9304, (301) 443-3860, niaaaweb-r@exchange.nih.gov, http://www.niaaa.nih.gov.

Tish Davidson, AM
David Newton

Algae *see* **Spirulina**
Alli *see* **Orlistat**
Alpha-tocophero *see* **Vitamin E**

American Diabetes Association

Description

Founded in 1940, the American Diabetes Association (ADA) is a leading 501(c)3 nonprofit health organization in the United States. It boasts more than 280,000 members and has a network of more than one million volunteers. The ADA serves 800 local groups within 53 state groups.

Origins

The ADA was created by a group of physicians and was originally intended to share information among doctors, researchers, and other healthcare professionals. As the organization made more and more contact with the public, advocating for the rights of people with diabetes and sponsoring programs such as children's camps, the group opened its membership to the public. The ADA has since created different divisions and programs aimed at increasing awareness and providing support. In 2009, the ADA started its Stop Diabetes campaign, an annual effort with the goal of bringing at least one million people into the fight against diabetes.

Purpose

The mission of the ADA is to prevent and cure diabetes and to improve the lives of all people affected by diabetes.

To fulfill their mission, the ADA promotes research, provides information, and advocates to find means of preventing and curing diabetes. The ADA uses different techniques to educate people at risk of or with diabetes so that they can improve their quality of life. The ADA also disseminates information to healthcare professionals and to family and caregivers of those with or at risk for diabetes. The organization is one of the largest advocates for the rights of people with diabetes.

Description

ADA members include but are not limited to physicians, nurses, dietitians, physical and occupational therapists, other health professionals, and any person affected by **diabetes mellitus**. The ADA offers membership to both consumers and health professionals who pay annual membership dues. Consumer membership is for people with diabetes, their families, and caregivers. Consumer members receive monthly issues of *Diabetes Forecast* magazine, discounts on ADA books and cookbooks, and access to a network of diabetes support and informational resources. Consumer membership dues are $28 annually.

Professional membership provides health professionals, research scientists, and diabetes educators with recent information in diabetes research and treatment options. As members, they receive benefits such as access to the ADA journal that is most relevant to their practice, registration discounts for ADA scientific sessions, and discounts on medical journals and books. Professional memberships can range from $50–$350 annually.

Education program recognition

To ensure quality education for people with diabetes, the ADA endorses the National Standards for Diabetes Self-Management Education Programs. The Standards are designed to endorse any health care setting offering diabetes education, from physicians' offices and HMOs to clinics and hospitals. All applicants must meet the National Standards before they are awarded the endorsement from the ADA.

The National Diabetes Advisory Board (NDAB) developed the National Standards for Diabetes Patient Education Programs. The ADA then endorsed the Standards in 1983 while participating in the nationwide pilot testing of the Standards and review criteria in 1984. The first edition of the Standards was published in *Diabetes Care* in 1984. In 1986, an application and review process was established through the ADA to determine whether an education program met the Standards. Then in 1987, the first programs to meet the Standards were recognized by the ADA.

The Standards are reviewed and revised about every five years. Such reviews involve a task force of representatives from the diabetes community compiled from the American Association of Diabetes Educators, American Diabetes Association, Academy of Nutrition and Dietetics, Centers for Disease Control and Prevention, Department of Veterans Affairs, Diabetes Research and Training Centers, Indian Health Service, Juvenile Diabetes Foundation, and National Certification Board for Diabetes Educators. The most recent version of the Standards was released in March 2007. It is now called the National Standards for Diabetes Self-Management Education and is endorsed by all organizations involved in its development.

Resources

The ADA supports a variety of tools to educate its members and the public.

Their National Call Center provides diabetes information and referral for callers nationwide through their toll-free 800 number. The Call Center responds to approximately 350,000 inquiries each year.

The ADA also supports a website that is available for anyone with Internet access with links to pertinent diabetes and diabetes prevention information, advocacy, membership information, and community and local events.

ADA research

Funds provided by ADARF support peer-reviewed basic and clinical diabetes research proposed to prevent, treat, and/or cure diabetes. Past research projects supported by the ADARF vary from microcellular research to educational and psychological issues related to diabetes.

All ADARF grants become part of the Diabetes Research database that is accessible to anyone with access to the ADA website. This database provides brief descriptions of each funded project, and gives brief summaries on the value the study findings may have for the field of diabetes research. Database contents are updated at least every six months.

Other methods ADA uses to distribute research findings are through Access: Diabetes Research, and the *Forefront Research* magazine. Both publications present summaries of diabetes research.

Publications

The ADA is the world's foremost publisher in the field of diabetes literature, including *Diabetes Forecast*, a monthly consumer magazine, and a range of publications and journals for research and health care professionals, such as *Diabetes*, *Diabetes Care*, *Diabetes*

Spectrum, *Clinical Diabetes*, and access to a comprehensive library of medical management guides.

Fund-raising activities

Each year, the ADA state chapters organize local events to increase awareness of diabetes within their communities, while at the same time helping to raise money for the ADA. The state chapters assist in organizing the ADA signature fund-raising events. The signature events that occur annually are America's Walk for Diabetes; Tour De Cure, a cycling event that takes place in over 70 cities nationwide; and School Walk for Diabetes, an educational, school-based program that promotes community service, school spirit, and healthy living to students. Another unique fund-raising campaign, Kiss-A-Pig, is a tribute to the pig for aiding in the discovery of the role of insulin for people with diabetes. It ends with the participant who raises the most money kissing the Kiss-A-Pig pig.

One of the goals of the ADA is to make the public aware of diabetes and the serious health effects it may have on a person. Throughout the year, the ADA sponsors events to educate the public about diabetes and diabetes prevention. Every November, the ADA sponsors American Diabetes Month, a month-long public awareness activity with the goal of raising awareness about serious and often preventable diabetes complications. A variety of events and educational activities are included in this awareness effort. The American Diabetes Alert is another program conducted annually on the fourth Tuesday in March to raise awareness about the seriousness of pre-diabetes and diabetes and its risk factors. The centerpiece of the Alert is a diabetes risk test, which is widely distributed and promoted through community activities and national and local media.

For professionals, the ADA provides educational and informative materials and programs through various media. Annually, they sponsor a Scientific Sessions diabetes conference, in addition to other medical and scientific programs. The ADA publishes and updates their medical care guidelines and recommendations for health professionals and also supports special interest groups.

Program services

The ethnic groups in the United States with the highest risk of developing type 2 diabetes are African Americans, Mexican Americans, Pima Indians, Asian Americans, and Pacific Islanders. The ADA reaches out to these communities through community campaigns.

THE DIABETES ASSISTANCE AND RESOURCES PROGRAM (DAR). DAR, which means, "to give" in Spanish, provides valuable information in English and Spanish to the Latino/Hispanic community. The goal of the DAR program is to increase awareness of the seriousness of diabetes and the importance of prevention and control.

DIABETES SUNDAY AND GET UP AND MOVE. The African American program's goal is to increase awareness about the seriousness of diabetes in the community and importance of early diagnosis and treatment. The program includes fun and informative church and community-based activities.

AWAKENING THE SPIRIT: PATHWAYS TO DIABETES PREVENTION AND CONTROL. This program is aimed at the Native American community, including American Indians, Alaska Natives, and Native Hawaiians. The program stresses the importance of choosing a healthy lifestyle for oneself and the generations that will follow.

Youth programs

The ADA is the largest provider of camps for children with diabetes in the world. Each year, more than 10,000 children benefit from camping programs provided through ADA funding.

The organization has developed a youth zone program that provides a web site especially for kids. It offers games, tips, links, and information to help kids manage their diabetes.

The ADA also provides information and resources for teens. It gives information on how diabetes may impact one's lifestyle. It gives resources and tools to help the teen understand diabetes and how it impacts the choices they make and their health.

Advocacy

Realizing a need for equality for those with diabetes, the AADA formed the Government Affairs & Advocacy program to help fulfill their mission of improving the lives of all those affected with diabetes. The main goals of this program are to:

• improve access to quality medical care for people with diabetes

• eliminate discrimination against people because of their diabetes

• ensure the federal government is adequately funding diabetes research and programs

ORGANIZATIONS

American Diabetes Association, 1701 North Beauregard St., Alexandria, VA 22311, (800) DIABETES (342-2383), askADA@diabetes.org, http://www.diabetes.org.

Megan C.M. Porter, RD, LD
David Newton

American Dietetic Association *see* **Academy of Nutrition and Dietetics**

American Heart Association No-Fad Diet

Definition

The *American Heart Association No-Fad Diet* is a book published by the American Heart Association (AHA) that focuses on planning weight loss rather than going on a diet in the traditional sense. The first edition of the book was published in 2005. The second edition, published in 2010, runs 450 pages and consists of three major parts: guidelines to losing weight and keeping it off, meal planning and recipes, and a "toolkit" of sample food diaries and other templates.

Origins

The first edition of the *American Heart Association No-Fad Diet* represented the AHA's first attempt to provide guidance for the general public about sensible weight loss. The organization had published a variety of low-fat, low-cholesterol, low-salt, and general "heart-healthy" cookbooks from 1973 onward, but had not yet produced a book on weight loss and weight maintenance. The 2005 edition was about 445 pages, about the same length as the second edition.

The AHA stated in the introduction to the first edition that its reason for publishing the *No-Fad Diet* was its concern about "the growing prevalence of **obesity** in the United States and around the world and the cardiovascular risks that come as a result...we have written this comprehensive weight-loss book...to provide a science-based, no-fad approach to losing weight for your better overall health and the accompanying decreased risk of heart disease, stroke, and diabetes."

Description

The *American Heart Association No-Fad Diet* is the product of an organization that is well respected by the medical community, as well as nutrition and

46

dietetics experts; it is not written by or associated with individual celebrities, bodybuilders, professional chefs, or alternative medical systems. The introduction to the second edition emphasizes the collective input and scientific agreement that underlies the book: "The American Heart Association recommendations reflect the opinions of many experts—physicians, registered dietitians, and specialists in physical activity and behavior modification. Our panel of scientists has reviewed the most current research and come to a consensus so you can cut through the confusion with confidence."

The subtitle of the book, *A Personal Plan for Healthy Weight Loss*, makes it clear that the book is the opposite of a one-size-fits all diet; in fact, the reader is expected to do considerable introspection, reflection, note-taking, mathematical calculation, and diary-keeping in the process of working out an individualized weight-loss regimen that will work over the long term.

Basic principles

The *No-Fad Diet* begins with a straightforward statement that there is nothing easy about losing weight and keeping it off, and that people seeking to lose weight must make a lifetime commitment to changing their present lifestyle. The authors of the *No-Fad Diet* attribute the current prevalence of obesity in developed countries to a combination of readily available, inexpensive food and high-calorie snacks combined with lower levels of exercise and physical activity. They note that the replacement of walking to work with commuting by automobile and the displacement of jobs that required physical activity with jobs requiring computer-based skills means that most people expend less energy while at the same time taking in more **calories**. The diet is based on balancing the number of calories taken in versus the number expended through physical activity.

Part I of the second edition of the *No-Fad Diet* consists of five chapters, the first three of which introduce the reader to the "three circles of success," summarized as "think smart," "eat well," and "move more." "Think smart" refers to the authors' theory that thoughts and beliefs are the primary obstacle to success in losing weight—that people either fail to analyze their current eating patterns, or instead rationalize them, or sometimes both. Readers are encouraged to take action, visualize success, root out negative thought patterns ("retrain your brain"), set definite and measurable goals, anticipate setbacks and plan in advance to deal with them, write everything down in a weight-loss diary, and be persistent ("practice makes perfect").

"Eat well" is about food choices and diet planning. The *No-Fad Diet* offers readers three different approaches to meal planning based on personal preference. The three strategies are identified as "switch and swap," the "75% solution," and menu plans devised by the AHA. The first strategy is based on substituting lower-calorie foods for high-calorie foods, such as having a piece of fruit instead of ice cream, or using a vinegar and tomato juice dressing on a salad instead of blue cheese. The second strategy uses portion control—a dieter can have his or her favorite foods but should eat less of them, such as eating one slice of pizza instead of two, a hamburger patty made from 4 ounces of meat rather than 6, and so on. The third approach, the set of AHA meal plans, is intended for dieters who feel more comfortable having a system to follow. The second edition of the book includes a questionnaire to help readers discover which approach is best suited to them.

Eating well also involves defining one's ideal weight and weight loss goals. The book includes a set of height and weight tables, a **body mass index** (BMI) table, and a calorie calculator to help readers determine whether they are in fact overweight/obese, how much weight they need to lose to attain their ideal weight, how many calories they presently expend in an average day, and how many fewer calories they should take in to lose weight. The reader is then instructed to keep a daily food diary of what they eat, when they eat it, the food's calorie content, and the reasons for eating it if other than to satisfy hunger (such as boredom, loneliness, etc.). The purpose of the diary is to help the dieter identify emotional triggers for overeating, as well as specific food **cravings**.

"Move more" is about increasing daily energy expenditure. Readers are expected to analyze their current level of physical activity, followed by setting a personal fitness goal and adding a minimum of 10 minutes of physical exercise each day. Similar to the three strategies for eating well, the *No-Fad Diet* offers three ways to become more active: the lifestyle approach, which consists of integrating fitness activities within the daily routine; the walking approach, which incorporates walking into a daily routine in 10-minute increments; and an organized activity strategy, which emphasizes exercise classes, team sports or group fitness activities, or scheduled workouts. Dieters are expected to record their activity in a log that includes the type of exercise, level of intensity, time involved, and, if applicable, the reason for failing to exercise. Dieters are also asked to assess their progress every six weeks.

Following through

Chapters four and five of the *No-Fad Diet* are concerned with weight maintenance and establishing healthy eating and exercise habits in one's family. Chapter four reminds the reader that the first two years following weight loss are the most difficult for maintaining that loss, and that dieters who do not regain the lost weight during those two years have a good chance of maintaining their lower weight permanently. Chapter five offers advice about teaching children healthy eating habits and encouraging them to be physically active.

Part II of the second edition contains menu plans and recipes for dieters who prefer that strategy. There are three sets of two-week plans, designed for 1200-, 1600-, and 2000-calorie daily intake levels. The meal plans are followed by 150 pages of recipes.

Part III of the second edition is a "toolkit" that contains templates for food and exercise diaries, as well as additional tips for maintaining weight loss.

Function

The function of the *No-Fad Diet* is to help individuals formulate a diet and exercise regimen that will allow them to lose weight slowly, maintain the weight loss, and make the changes a permanent part of their lifestyle. The *No-Fad Diet* is not intended to promote rapid weight loss and does not recommend any unusual or eccentric patterns of food consumption or nutritional composition.

Benefits

The benefits of the *No-Fad Diet* are its association with recognized authorities on nutrition, exercise, and preventive health care, and the soundness of its recommendations. Its outline of three different approaches to eating well reflects an understanding of the differences among human personalities and the need to take human psychology into account when introducing long-term lifestyle changes. The flexibility of the program in allowing food choices rather than imposing a rigid set of meal plans means that people with **food allergies**, chronic digestive problems, or other health issues as well as those having to cook for or eat with a family, can still benefit from the *No-Fad Diet*. Many readers will also like the book's advice on dining out, eating on social occasions, eating in fast-food restaurants, and similar situations.

Precautions

While the *No-Fad Diet* does not pose any health risks, it may not appeal to people who want to see rapid results from a weight-loss program. In addition, some readers may find the heavy emphasis on behavioral modification and psychological self-examination off-putting.

KEY TERMS

Behavior modification—Changing an individual's behavior through positive and negative responses to achieve a desired result, such as exercising regularly or sticking to a weight-loss diet.

Body mass index (BMI)—Measurement used to determine whether a person is at a healthy weight, underweight, overweight, or obese. BMI is calculated by dividing height squared (in inches) by weight (in pounds) and then multiplying that number by 703. The metric formula for BMI is the weight in kilograms divided by the square of height in meters.

The authors of the book note that while their recommendations about physical exercise are moderate and should not be difficult for most readers to implement, people with chronic medical conditions should consult their physicians before beginning an exercise program.

Criticisms of the *No-Fad Diet* surround the book's meal plans, which include foods known to contain *trans* fatty acids, despite the AHA's acknowledgement of **trans fats** as being associated with higher risk of heart disease, stroke, and type 2 diabetes. The AHA recommends obtaining less than 1% of daily calorie intake from *trans* **fats**, a limit that is not always followed in the meal plans.

Risks

The *No-Fad Diet* does not pose any obvious risks to adults who follow the book's recommendations in designing their own meal plans, exercise schedules, and weight-loss regimens. It is possible, however, that people with a history of **eating disorders** or obsessive-compulsive disorder (OCD) may find that the book's emphasis on keeping detailed records of exercise duration and intensity along with "everything you eat and drink," including habits, such as finishing another family member's uneaten food portion, could trigger an obsession with calorie counting or reduction that sometimes characterizes these disorders.

Research and general acceptance

The *American Heart Association No-Fad Diet* represents a summary or distillation of recent clinical research in nutrition and weight control rather than a specific diet. Given the book's insistence that weight loss and maintenance is a personal matter, it is difficult to see how a clinical study could be designed to

---

accommodate the variety of individual meal plans and exercise schedules that different dieters could adopt based on the three "circles of success." There are no clinical studies of the *No-Fad Diet* registered with the NIH, nor are there any studies of the diet reported in the medical literature. In addition, the book has not been reviewed to date by the **Academy of Nutrition and Dietetics**, again most likely because it reflects the general consensus of medical and nutrition professionals rather than an extreme or controversial point of view. Possibly for the same reason, the book has received infrequent reviews on popular diet websites.

Resources

BOOKS

American Heart Association. *American Heart Association No-Fad Diet: A Personal Plan for Healthy Weight Loss.* 2nd ed. New York: Clarkson Potter, 2011.

———. *The New American Heart Association Cookbook.* 8th ed. New York: Clarkson Potter, 2010.

WEBSITES

American Heart Association. "No-Fad Diet Tips." http://www.heart.org/HEARTORG/GettingHealthy/Weight Management/No-Fad-Diet-Tips_UCM_305838_Article. jsp (accessed September 13, 2012).

———. "Trans Fats." http://www.heart.org/HEARTORG/GettingHealthy/FatsAndOils/Fats101/Trans-Fats_UCM_301120_Article.jsp (accessed September 13, 2012).

———. "Welcome to the No-Fad Diet!" http://www.heart.org/HEARTORG/GettingHealthy/WeightManagement/Welcome-to-the-No-Fad-Diet_UCM_305835_SubHome Page.jsp# (accessed September 13, 2012).

EveryDiet.org. "No Fad Diet." http://www.everydiet.org/diet/no-fad-diet (accessed September 13, 2012).

Haynes, Fiona. "The No-Fad Diet: A Personal Plan for Healthy Weight Loss." About.com. http://lowfatcooking.about.com/od/lowfatcookingtools/fr/nofaddiet.htm (accessed September 13, 2012).

Morales, Tatiana. "Why 'No-Fad Diet' Really Works." CBS News, February 11, 2009. http://www.cbsnews.

com/2100-500165_162-705423.html (accessed September 13, 2012).

ORGANIZATIONS

Academy of Nutrition and Dietetics, 120 South Riverside Plz., Ste. 2000, Chicago, IL 60606-6995, (312) 899-0040, (800) 877-1600, amacmunn@eatright.org, http://www.eatright.org.

American Heart Association, 7272 Greenville Ave., Dallas, TX 75231, (800) 242-8721, http://www.americanheart.org.

Rebecca J. Frey, PhD

Anne Collins weight loss program

Definition

The Anne Collins weight loss program is a subscription-based weight-loss system available online. The system consists of nine separate diet plans. The system also includes advice regarding nutrition, exercise, and specific physical disorders; an on-line support community; and personal advice available through e-mail. However, Collins' credentials and background are not clear.

Origins

Anne Collins is an Irish nutritionist who says about herself, "I have been involved in the weight loss and fitness industry as a diet consultant, nutritionist, and personal adviser. I have written for many newspapers and magazines including a weekly weight loss and health column." She states that she first formulated her weight loss system in 1982.

Description

Overview

The Anne Collins system is available only through the author's website (http://www.anne-collins.com). Some parts of the website are available to the public, but most pages require an annual subscription; as of 2012, all diet plans were available for free for a limited time as the program underwent substantive updating. The release date of the new plan was unknown.

Included with the annual subscription fee is access to the following: all of the e-books for the nine specific diet plans, a community forum, updates to the existing diets and any new diet plans, advice about nutrition and exercise, shopping lists, advice and tips to stay motivated, and personal support either online or by telephone. The e-books average 55–60 pages in length and contain daily meal plans for a 28-day period, including options for snacks and fast foods. The motivational articles, nutrition information, and other sections of the website come to about 600 pages of material.

The Anne Collins weight loss program is not available in a print edition. In addition, neither the Library of Congress nor the British Library has a record of any book on nutrition or weight loss written by Anne Collins.

Specific diets

LOW-CARB DIET. The Low-Carb Diet is designed to be followed for 28 days, after which the dieter may repeat the 28-day cycle or switch to another Anne Collins plan. The four weeks are divided into two phases of 14 days each. Phase one supplies meal plans for three meals a day, averaging 30 g of **carbohydrates** per day. In phase two, the day's carbohydrate allotment is raised to 55 g per day. The diet plan includes a number of food substitutes, advice on eating in fast food restaurants, a shopping list, and a list of acceptable snack foods.

LOW GLYCEMIC DIET. The glycemic index (GI) is a measurement system for ranking the effects of dietary carbohydrates on blood sugar. The GI measures carbohydrates in individual foods on a gram-for-gram basis in regard to changes in blood glucose levels in the first two hours after a meal. The higher the index number, the more rapidly the carbohydrate breaks down in the digestive tract, releasing glucose into the bloodstream. A lower GI number is thought to relate to a longer feeling of fullness in the stomach, better control over **insulin** and blood sugar levels, and lower levels of blood lipids (**fats**).

Like the Anne Collins Low-Carb Diet, the Low Glycemic Diet has a 28-day cycle of meal plans and shopping lists, but is not divided into two phases. It is a lean-protein and low-GI carbohydrate diet intended to stabilize blood glucose levels during weight loss. The meal plans allow about 1,100 **calories** per day but may be adjusted upward to 2,000 calories for men (and for dieters who wish to lose weight more slowly) by adding calorie-controlled snacks.

10-MINUTE MEALS DIET. The "10-Minute Meals" Convenience Diet is geared for dieters who wish to lose weight rapidly but have little time to cook. The lunch menus provide fast food, brown-bag, and quick-cook options. Dinners provide fast food, quick-cook, and two-day meal options, which are dinners intended to last for two days.

Like the meal plans for the Low GI Diet, the meal plans for the 10-Minute Meals Diet allow about 1,100 calories per day, adjustable upward to 2,000 or 2,100 calories through snacks. After four weeks, the dieter can either repeat the 28-day cycle or choose another Anne Collins diet plan.

CHOLESTEROL-LOWERING DIET. This diet is intended for people who must lower blood cholesterol levels while losing weight and/or who wish to lose weight rapidly. The 28-day cycle of meal plans shows the total fat, saturated fat, and cholesterol content of every food item on the diet, as well as the calorie values. The diet allows about 1,200 calories per day, with an average content of 22 grams of total fat, 4 grams of saturated fat, and 120 milligrams of cholesterol. The meal plans are rich in dietary **fiber**, particularly soluble fiber, which has a number of important health benefits that include lowering blood cholesterol levels. The cholesterol and fat values of this diet plan fall within the guidelines recommended by the U.S. Food and Drug Administration (FDA). As with other Anne Collins diet plans, the calorie level can be adjusted upward for men and people who desire to lose weight more slowly.

The e-book that comes with this plan contains suggestions about and guidelines for exercise as a way to further lower blood cholesterol levels. The diet plan suggests that cholesterol levels should begin to fall within two to three weeks of beginning the diet. After four weeks, the dieter may repeat the cycle if blood cholesterol has not fallen to the desired level, or choose another diet in the program to continue losing weight.

14-DAY LOW-CALORIE BOOSTER DIET. This diet plan has only a 14-day rather than a 28-day cycle. It is intended for dieters with short-term weight-loss goals. The plan allows for six meals or snacks per day to promote rapid food **metabolism**. The meal plans include a number of quick-cook recipes and convenience food or fast-food options.

The basic diet plan allows about 1,000 calories a day to maximize weight loss but can be adjusted upward for men.

VEGETARIAN QUICK-START DIET. The Vegetarian Quick-Start Diet is a rapid weight-loss plan for committed vegetarians, people interested in a vegetarian lifestyle, or people trying to reduce their meat and poultry consumption. Technically, the diet is an ovo-lacto vegetarian plan, which means that it includes eggs and dairy products.

This diet plan is based on a 28-day cycle and allows about 1,250 calories per day, adjustable upward to about 2,000 calories for men. It contains about 90 recipes, advice about cooking **whole grains**, vegetarian fast-food options, and calorie counts for all menu items.

NO-NONSENSE BALANCED DIET. The No-Nonsense Balanced Diet is intended for dieters who want to lose weight rapidly but also want some flexibility in a diet plan. This diet also has a 28-day cycle, with meal plans averaging 1,100 calories per day. Flexibility includes home-cooked and convenience meal options for every lunch as well as every dinner.

As with the other Anne Collins plans, the calorie level can be adjusted upward for men. Sample menus from this diet include:

- Breakfast: 2 low-fat pancakes with 1 Tbsp. maple syrup, 2 slices Canadian bacon, one-half cup berries. Alternate menu: 1 cup fat-free yogurt, 2 Tbsp. wheat germ, 1 medium banana, 1 Tbsp. sesame seeds.

- Convenience option for lunch: Subway six-inch roasted chicken breast sandwich and 1 serving fruit. Home-cooked option: 1 cup low-fat ready-to-serve soup, 2 slices whole wheat bread spread with 2 Tbsp. fat-free mayonnaise and filled with chopped vegetables, 1 oz. fat-free cheese.

- Convenience meal option for dinner: Lean Cuisine angel hair pasta meal, 2 cups salad, 1 Tbsp. fat-free dressing, 2 graham crackers with 1 Tbsp. fat-free cream cheese, 1 serving fruit. Home recipe option: 1 oz. (dry weight) pasta or thin spaghetti, 3 oz. very lean ground beef, one-half cup sliced bell peppers, 1 chopped large tomato, 1 minced clove of garlic, one-half tsp. oregano, one-half tsp. Italian seasoning.

- Snacks: Select from list included with diet plan.

DIET FOR LIFE. The Diet For Life is essentially a slow weight-loss or maintenance-level diet plan that contains a 14-day starter set of meal plans. The meal plans are low in fat, moderate in **protein**, and high in carbohydrates. In addition to the usual calorie counts, this plan contains guidelines for lifelong sensible eating habits. It can be continued indefinitely, or the dieter may switch to another Anne Collins plan.

The basic calorie allowance in the Diet For Life is 1,300 calories per day, adjustable upward to 2,000 or 2,100 calories.

VEGETARIAN DIET FOR LIFE. The Vegetarian Diet For Life is similar to the general Diet For Life plan, with a 14-day set of starter menus, a large number of easy-to-prepare recipes, and advice about lifelong sensible eating habits. Like the Diet For Life, the Vegetarian Diet For Life plan is low in fat and moderate in protein. The menu plans provide about 1,250 calories per day but can be adjusted.

Function

The Anne Collins weight loss system is intended for weight loss. Most of the specific plans are intended for more rapid weight loss, but several are maintenance diets, including a maintenance diet for vegetarians. All of the specific plans can be tailored to allow higher calorie intakes for men or for dieters less concerned about losing weight rapidly.

Benefits

The system's website claims the following benefits for the nine diets:

- The dieter can lose weight.
- The system does not depend on appetite suppressants, dietary supplements, or other special products.
- There are no forbidden foods. The dieter can fit fast foods, chocolate, and other foods that are avoided on most diets into most of the specific diets.

One benefit mentioned by several reviewers of the Anne Collins system as a whole is its accommodation of vegetarians—at least ovo-lacto vegetarians. Of the nine diets, two are designed for vegetarians who use eggs and dairy products. Another benefit

QUESTIONS TO ASK YOUR DOCTOR

- Is this diet safe for me?
- Is this the best diet to meet my long-term weight-loss goals?
- Will I need to take a multivitamin or other supplement on this diet?
- How can I tell if I am getting the right nutrients?

noted by reviewers is the relatively low cost of the Anne Collins plans. The $19.97 subscription fee is roughly the same as the cost of most novels in e-book form, and subscribers may download all nine PDFs if they wish.

Many dieters seem to like the flexibility of the Anne Collins plans, in particular the option of using convenience foods and switching among the various plans to avoid monotony. Opinion is mixed, however, regarding the use of fast foods in the Collins plans. Some reviewers maintain that the fast-food options are a necessary adaptation to contemporary eating patterns, while others regard the fast-food choices as exposing dieters to a high degree of temptation to stray from the plan.

Precautions

Although none of the Anne Collins diet plans are very low-calorie diets (VLCDs), they still fall well below the calorie intakes recommended by the U.S. Department of Agriculture (USDA). People who exercise or lead an active lifestyle may need to consume more calories. It is always a good idea to consult with a physician before starting a new diet, especially for people who need to lose 30 pounds (13.6 kg) or more; are pregnant or nursing; are below the age of 18; or have a chronic disorder such as diabetes, kidney disease, or liver disease. People with type 2 diabetes should not substitute the Low-Glycemic Diet Plan for treatment and should not start the diet without consent from a doctor.

Risks

There do not appear to be any significant health risks associated with any of the nine plans for dieters who have been evaluated by a physician for any previously undiagnosed disorders.

Research and general acceptance

The Anne Collins system does not appear to have been used in any clinical trials reported in the medical literature. In addition, Collins' credentials as a nutritionist are not listed on her website, which makes it difficult to verify her qualifications as a weight loss expert. Existing feedback about this diet is informal, consisting solely of testimonials on the website itself and comments or reviews on various Internet diet websites and online chat groups. Alternate sources, such as the USDA's *Dietary Guidelines for Americans* and **MyPlate**, provide more widely accepted information on nutrition and healthy eating.

Resources

WEBSITES

ChooseMyPlate.gov. U.S. Department of Agriculture. http://www.choosemyplate.gov (accessed August 22, 2012).

U.S. Department of Agriculture. "Calories: How Many Can I Have?" ChooseMyPlate.gov. http://www.choosemyplate.gov/weight-management-calories/calories/empty-calories-amount.html (accessed August 22, 2012).

U.S. Department of Agriculture and U.S. Department of Health and Human Services. *Dietary Guidelines for Americans, 2010.* 7th ed. Washington, DC: U.S. Government Printing Office, December 2010. http://health.gov/dietaryguidelines (accessed August 22, 2012).

"Weight Loss with Anne Collins." http://www.annecollins.com (accessed August 22, 2012).

ORGANIZATIONS

U.S. Department of Agriculture, 1400 Independence Ave. SW, Washington, DC 20250, (202) 720-2791, http://www.usda.gov.

Rebecca J. Frey, PhD
Laura Jean Cataldo, RN, EdD

Anorexia nervosa

Definition

Anorexia nervosa is an eating disorder that involves self-imposed starvation. The individual is obsessed with becoming increasingly thinner and limits food intake to the point where health is compromised. Anorexia nervosa can be fatal.

Description

Anorexia is often thought of as a modern problem, but the English physician Richard Morton first described it in 1689. In the twenty-first century, anorexia nervosa is recognized as a psychiatric disorder in the *Diagnostic and Statistical Manual for Mental Disorders, Fourth Edition (DSM-IV-TR)* published by the American Psychiatric Association.

Individuals with anorexia are on an irrational, unrelenting quest to lose weight, and no matter how much they lose and how much their health is compromised, they want to lose more weight. Recognizing the development of anorexia can be difficult, but dieting is often a trigger. Warning signs for anorexia may include skipping meals, taking only tiny portions, being secretive about food, not wanting to eat in public, or sudden concerns about body image. The person may seem to always have an excuse for why he or she does not want to eat, such as not feeling hungry, feeling ill, having just eaten with someone else, or not liking the food served. The person may also begin to read food labels obsessively and know exactly how many **calories** and how much fat are in foods. Many people with anorexia practically eliminate fat and **sugar** from their diets. Some people may exercise compulsively to burn extra calories. These practices can have serious health consequences. At some point, the line between problem eating and an eating disorder is crossed.

Anorexia nervosa is diagnosed when most of the following conditions are present:

- an overriding obsession with food and thinness that controls activities and eating patterns every hour of every day
- weighing less than 85% of the average weight for his or her age and height group and willfully and intentionally refusing to maintain an appropriate body weight
- extreme fear of gaining weight or becoming fat, even when the individual is significantly underweight
- a distorted self-image that fuels a refusal to admit to being underweight, even when this is demonstrably true
- refusal to admit that being severely underweight is dangerous to health
- for women, three missed menstrual periods in a row after menstruation has been established

People with anorexia may spend a lot of time looking in the mirror, obsessing about clothing size, and practicing negative self-talk about their bodies. Some are secretive about eating and will avoid eating in front of other people. They may develop strange eating habits such as chewing their food and then spitting it out, or they may have rigid ideas about "good" and "bad" food. People with anorexia may hide their eating habits and their weight from friends, family, and healthcare providers. Many experience depression and anxiety disorders.

Demographics

Anorexia is a disorder of industrialized countries where food is abundant and the culture values a thin appearance. About 1% of Americans have anorexia, and females outnumber males 10:1. In men, the disorder is more often diagnosed in homosexuals than in heterosexuals. Some experts believe that number of people diagnosed with anorexia represents only the most severe cases, and that many more people have anorexic tendencies, but their symptoms do not rise to the level needed for a medical diagnosis.

Most people diagnosed with anorexia are white, and about three-quarters come from households at the middle income level or above. However, the number of blacks and Hispanics diagnosed with anorexia has increased. Competitive athletes of all races have an increased risk of developing anorexia nervosa, especially in sports where weight is tied to performance. Jockeys, wrestlers, figure skaters, cross-country runners, and gymnasts (especially female gymnasts) have higher than average rates of anorexia. People such as actors, models, cheerleaders, and dancers (especially ballet dancers) who are judged mainly on their appearance are also at high risk of developing the disorder.

Anorexia can occur to people as young as age 7. However, the disorder usually begins during adolescence. It is most likely to start at one of two times, either age 14 or 18. This corresponds with the age of transitioning into and out of high school. The younger the age at which anorexic behavior starts, the more difficult it is to cure. Preteens who develop anorexia often show signs of compulsive behavior and depression in addition to anorexia.

Causes and symptoms

Causes

Anorexia is a complex disorder that does not have a single cause. Research suggests that some people have a predisposition toward anorexia and that something triggers the behavior, which then becomes self-reinforcing. Hereditary (especially on the mother's side), biological, psychological, and social factors all appear to play a role.

- Heredity. Twin studies show that if one twin has anorexia nervosa, the other has a greater likelihood of developing the disorder. Having a close relative, usually a mother or a sister, with anorexia nervosa also increases the likelihood of other (usually female) family members developing the disorder. However, when compared to many other diseases, the inherited component of anorexia nervosa appears to be fairly small.

- Biological factors. There is some evidence that anorexia nervosa is linked to abnormal neurotransmitter activity in the part of the brain that controls pleasure and appetite. Neurotransmitters are also involved in other mental disorders such as depression. Research in this area is relatively new and the findings are unclear. People with anorexia tend to feel full sooner than other people. Some researchers believe that this is related to the fact that the stomach of people with anorexia tends to empty more slowly than normal; others think it may be related to the appetite control mechanism of the brain.

- Psychological factors. Certain personality types appear to be more vulnerable to developing anorexia nervosa. People with anorexia tend to be perfectionists who have unrealistic expectations about how they "should" look and perform. They tend to have a black-and-white, right-or-wrong, all-or-nothing way of seeing situations. Many people with anorexia lack a strong sense of identity and instead take their identity from pleasing others. Most have low self-worth. Many experience depression and anxiety disorders, although researchers do not know if this is a cause or a result of the eating disorder.

- Social factors. People with anorexia are more likely to come either from overprotective families or disordered families where there is a lot of conflict and inconsistency. Either way, the person feels a need to be in control of something, and that something becomes body weight. The family often has high and sometimes unrealistic and rigid expectations. Often something stressful or upsetting triggers the start of anorexic behaviors. This may be as simple as a family member teasing about the person's weight, nagging about eating junk food, commenting on how clothes fit, or comparing the person unfavorably to someone who is thin. Life events such as moving, starting a new school, breaking up with a boyfriend or girlfriend, or even entering puberty and feeling awkward about one's changing body can trigger anorexic behavior. Overlaying the family situation is the unrelenting media message that thin is "good" and fat is "bad."

Signs and symptoms

Anorexic behavior has physical and psychological consequences. These include:

- excessive weight loss; loss of muscle

- stunted growth and delayed sexual maturation in preteens

- gastrointestinal complications: liver damage, diarrhea, constipation, bloating, stomach pain
- cardiovascular complications: irregular heartbeat, low pulse rate, cardiac arrest
- urinary system complications: kidney damage, kidney failure, incontinence, urinary tract infections
- skeletal system complications: loss of bone mass, increased risk of fractures, teeth erosion by stomach acid from repeat vomiting
- reproductive system complications (women): missed menstrual periods, infertility
- reproductive system complications (men): loss of sex drive, infertility
- fatigue, irritation, headaches, depression, anxiety, impaired judgment and thinking
- fainting, seizures, low blood sugar
- chronically cold hands and feet
- weakened immune system, swollen glands, increased susceptibility to infections
- development of fine hair called lanugo on the shoulders, back, arms, and face; head hair loss; blotchy, dry skin
- potentially life-threatening electrolyte imbalances
- coma
- increased risk of self-mutilation (cutting)
- increased risk of suicide
- death

Diagnosis

Diagnosis is based on several factors including a patient history, physical examination, laboratory tests, and a mental status evaluation. A patient history is less helpful in diagnosing anorexia than in diagnosing many diseases because many people with anorexia lie repeatedly about how much they eat and their use of laxatives, enemas, and medications. The patient may, however, complain about related symptoms such as fatigue, headaches, dizziness, **constipation**, or frequent infections.

A physical examination begins with weight and blood pressure and then checks for potential symptoms. Based on the physical exam, the physician may order laboratory tests. In general, these tests will include a complete blood count (CBC), urinalysis, blood chemistries (to determine electrolyte levels), and liver function tests. The physician may also order an electrocardiogram to look for heart abnormalities.

Several different mental status evaluations can be used. In general, the physician will evaluate things such as whether the person is oriented in time and space, appearance, observable state of emotion (affect), attitude toward food and weight, delusional thinking, and thoughts of self-harm or suicide.

Treatment

Treatment choices depend on the degree to which anorexic behavior has resulted in physical damage and whether the person is a danger to him or herself. Medical treatment should be supplemented with psychiatric treatment (see Therapies below). Patients are frequently uncooperative and resist treatment, denying that their life may be endangered and insisting that the doctor only wants to "make them get fat."

Hospital impatient care is first geared toward correcting problems that present immediate medical crises, such as severe **malnutrition**, severe electrolyte imbalance, irregular heart beat, pulse below 45 beats per minute, or low body temperature. Patients are hospitalized if they are a high suicide risk, have severe clinical depression, or exhibit signs of an altered mental state. They may also need to be hospitalized to interrupt weight loss; stop the cycle of vomiting, exercising, and/or laxative abuse; treat substance disorders; or for additional medical evaluation.

Day treatment or partial hospitalization, where the patient goes every day to an extensive treatment program, provides structured mealtimes, nutrition education, intensive therapy, medical monitoring, and supervision. If day treatment fails, the patient may need to be hospitalized or enter a full-time residential treatment facility.

Anorexia nervosa is a chronic disease and relapses are common and to be expected. Outpatient treatment provides medical supervision, nutrition counseling, self-help strategies, and cognitive-behavioral therapy after the patient has reached some weight goals and shows stability.

Nutrition and dietary concerns

A nutrition consultant or dietitian is an essential part of the team needed to successfully treat anorexia. The first treatment concern is to get the individual medically stable by increasing calorie intake and balancing **electrolytes**. After that, nutritional therapy is needed to support the long process of recovery and stable weight gain. This is an intensive process involving nutrition education, meal planning, nutrition monitoring, and helping the patient develop a healthy relationship with food.

Therapy

Medical intervention helps alleviate the immediate physical problems associated with anorexia, but by itself, it rarely changes behavior. Psychotherapy plays a major role in helping the patient understand and recover from anorexia. Several different types of psychotherapy are used depending on the individual's situation. Generally, the goal of psychotherapy is to help the individual develop a healthy attitude toward their body and food. This may involve addressing the root causes of anorexic behavior as well as addressing the behavior itself.

Some types of psychotherapy that have been successful in treating anorexia include:

- Cognitive behavior therapy (CBT) is designed to change the individual's thoughts and feelings about his or her body and behaviors toward food, but it does not address why those thoughts or feelings exist. This therapy is relatively short-term.
- Psychodynamic therapy, also called psychoanalytic therapy, attempts to help the individual gain insight into the cause of the emotions that trigger their anorexic behavior. This therapy tends to be longer term that CBT.
- Interpersonal therapy is short-term therapy that helps the individual identify issues and problems in relationships. The individual may be asked to look back at his or her family history to try to recognize problem areas and work toward resolving them.
- Family and couples therapy is helpful in dealing with conflict or disorder that may be a factor in perpetuating anorexic behavior. Family therapy is especially useful in helping parents with a history of anorexia avoid passing their attitudes and behaviors on to their children.

Prognosis

Anorexia nervosa is difficult to treat successfully. Medical stabilization, nutrition therapy, continued medical monitoring, and substantial psychiatric treatment give a person with anorexia the best chance of recovery. Estimates suggest that between 20% and 30% of people in treatment drop out too soon and have major relapses. Even those who stay in treatment relapse occasionally. Treating anorexia is often a long, slow, frustrating process that can cost thousands of dollars. The earlier in life that the disorder starts and the longer the disorder continues untreated, the more difficult it is bring about recovery. Many individuals with anorexia are willfully uncooperative and do not want to recover.

About half of the people treated for anorexia nervosa recover completely and are able (sometimes with difficulty) to maintain a normal weight. Of the remaining 50%, between 6% and 20% die, usually of health complications related to starvation. About

KEY TERMS

Diuretic—A substance that removes water from the body by increasing urine production.

Electrolyte—Ions in the body that participate in metabolic reactions. The major human electrolytes are sodium (Na+), potassium (K+), calcium (Ca 2+), magnesium (Mg2+), chloride (Cl−), phosphate (HPO$_4$ 2−), bicarbonate (HCO$_3$−), and sulfate (SO$_4$ 2−).

Neurotransmitter—One of a group of chemicals secreted by a nerve cell (neuron) to carry a chemical message to another nerve cell, often as a way of transmitting a nerve impulse. Examples of neurotransmitters include acetylcholine, dopamine, serotonin, and norepinephrine.

20% remain dangerously underweight, and the rest remain thin.

Prevention

Research has found that a mother's attitude toward body weight and dieting may have a significant impact on her children's views. Some behaviors to try and help prevent anorexia nervosa from developing include:

- Parents should not obsess about their weight or appearance in front of their children.
- Do not tease children about their body shape or compare them to others.
- Make sure children know that they are loved and accepted.
- Try to eat meals together as a family whenever possible.
- Remind children that the models they see on television and in fashion magazines have extreme, not normal or healthy, bodies.
- Do not put children on a diet unless advised by a pediatrician.
- Block children from visiting pro-anorexia Websites. These are sites where people with anorexia give advice on extreme weight loss techniques and support each other's distorted body image.
- If a child is a competitive athlete, get to know the coach and the coach's attitude toward weight.

If parents suspect that their child has an eating disorder, they should not wait to intervene and get professional help. The sooner the disorder is recognized, the easier it is to treat.

Relapses happen to many people with anorexia. People who are recovering from anorexia can help prevent relapse by:

- never dieting; instead plan healthy meals
- staying in treatment
- monitoring negative self-talk; practicing positive self-talk
- spending time doing something enjoyable every day
- staying busy, but not overly busy; getting at least seven hours of sleep each night
- spending time each day with friends and family

Resources

BOOKS

Carleton, Pamela, and Deborah Ashin. *Take Charge of Your Child's Eating Disorder: A Physician's Step-By-Step Guide to Defeating Anorexia and Bulimia.* New York: Marlowe, 2007.

Heaton, Jeanne A., and Claudia J. Strauss. *Talking to Eating Disorders: Simple Ways to Support Someone Who Has Anorexia, Bulimia, Binge Eating or Body Image Issues.* New York: New American Library, 2005.

Herzog, David B., Debra L. Franko, and Patricia Cable. *Unlocking the Mysteries of Eating Disorders.* New York: McGraw-Hill, 2007.

Liu, Aimee. *Gaining: The Truth About Life After Eating Disorders.* New York: Warner Books, 2007.

Messinger, Lisa, and Merle Goldberg. *My Thin Excuse: Understanding, Recognizing, and Overcoming Eating Disorders.* Garden City Park, NY: Square One, 2006.

Rubin, Jerome S., ed. *Eating Disorders and Weight Loss Research.* Hauppauge, NY: Nova Science, 2006.

Walsh, B. Timothy. *If Your Adolescent Has an Eating Disorder: An Essential Resource for Parents.* New York: Oxford University Press, 2005.

PERIODICALS

Arcelus, Jon, et al. "Mortality Rates in Patients With Anorexia Nervosa and Other Eating Disorders: A Meta-Analysis of 36 Studies." *Archives of General Psychiatry* 68, no. 7 (2011): 724–31. http://dx.doi.org/10.1001/archgenpsychiatry.2011.74 (accessed November 14, 2011).

Genders, R., and K. Tchanturia. "Cognitive Remediation Therapy (CRT) for Anorexia in Group Format: A Pilot Study." *Eating and Weight Disorders* 15, no. 4 (2010): e234–39.

Hudson, James, et al. "The Prevalence and Correlates of Eating Disorders in the National Comorbidity Survey Replication." *Biological Psychiatry* 61, no. 3 (2007): 348–58.

Wilson, Jenny L., et al. "Surfing for Thinness: A Pilot Study of Pro-Eating Disorder Website Usage in Adolescents With Eating Disorders." *Pediatrics* 118, no. 6 (December 2006): e1635–43. http://dx.doi.org/10.1542/peds.2006-1133 (accessed October 2, 2012).

WEBSITES

American Academy of Family Physicians. "Anorexia nervosa." FamilyDoctor.org. http://familydoctor.org/familydoctor/en/diseases-conditions/eating-disorders.html (accessed October 2, 2012).

American Psychological Association. "Eating Disorders." http://www.apa.org/helpcenter/eating.aspx (accessed September 16, 2011).

Anorexia Nervosa and Related Eating Disorders (ANRED). "Table of Contents." http://www.anred.com/toc.html (accessed September 7, 2012).

Bernstein, Bettina E. "Eating Disorder: Anorexia." Medscape Reference. October 14, 2010. http://emedicine.medscape.com/article/912187-overview (accessed September 16, 2011).

MedlinePlus. "Eating Disorders." U.S. National Library of Medicine, National Institutes of Health. http://www.nlm.nih.gov/medlineplus/eatingdisorders.html (accessed September 16, 2011).

ORGANIZATIONS

American Academy of Child and Adolescent Psychiatry, 3615 Wisconsin Ave. NW, Washington, DC 20016-3007, (202) 966-7300, Fax: (202) 966-2891, http://aacap.org.

American Psychiatric Association, 1000 Wilson Blvd., Ste. 1825, Arlington, VA 22209-3901, (703) 907-7300, apa@psych.org, http://www.psych.org.

American Psychological Association, 750 1st St., NE, Washington, DC 20002-4242, (202) 336-5500, TTY: (202) 336-6123, (800) 374-2721, http://www.apa.org.

National Association of Anorexia Nervosa and Related Eating Disorders, PO Box 640, Naperville, IL 60566, (630) 577-1330, anadhelp@anad.org, http://www.anad.org.

National Eating Disorders Association, 165 W 46th St., New York, NY 10036, (212) 575-6200, (800) 931-2237, Fax: (212) 575-1650, info@NationalEatingDisorders.org, http://www.nationaleatingdisorders.org.

Tish Davidson, A.M.

Anti-aging diet

Definition

The anti-aging diet, also called the calorie-restriction diet, is one that restricts calorie intake by 30%–50% of the normal or recommended intake with the goal of increasing human lifespan by at least 30%. When combined with a healthy lifestyle, people on the diet tend to have improved health, providing they consume adequate **vitamins**, **minerals**, and other essential nutrients.

Origins

The idea that a calorie-restrictive diet can significantly increase lifespan has been around since the 1930s. In 1935, Cornell University food researchers Clive McCay and Leonard Maynard published their first in a series of studies in which laboratory rats were fed a diet that had one-third fewer **calories** than a control group of rats. The lower-calorie diet still contained adequate amounts of vitamins, minerals, **protein**, and other essential nutrients. This calorie-restrictive diet provided much less energy than researchers had previously thought rats needed to maintain growth and normal activities. The rats on the lower-calorie diet lived 30%–40% longer than the rats on a normal calorie diet. Since then, more than 2,000 studies have been carried out, mostly on animals, investigating the connection between **calorie restriction** and increased longevity.

A reduced-calorie diet was taken a step further by University of California, Los Angeles, pathologist Roy Walford, who studied the biology of aging. In 1986, he published *The 120-Year Diet* and a follow-up book in 2000, *Beyond the 120-Year Diet*, in which he argued that human longevity can be significantly increased by adhering to a strict diet that contains all the nutrients needed by humans, but with about one-third the calories. In 1994, he co-authored *The Anti-Aging Plan: Strategies and Recipes for Extending Your Healthy Years*. His anti-aging plan was based on his own research and that of other scientists, including his study of diet and aging conducted as chief physician of the Biosphere 2 project in Arizona in the early 1990s. Walford was one of eight people sealed in Biosphere 2 from 1991 to 1993 in an attempt to prove that an artificial closed ecological system could sustain human life. He also co-founded Calorie Restriction Society International in 1994. Walford died in 2004 at the age of 79 from complications of amyotrophic lateral sclerosis (ALS), also known as Lou Gehrig's disease (US) and motor neurone disease (UK).

Description

Anti-aging diets are regimes that reduce the number of calories consumed by 30%–50%, while allowing the necessary amounts of vitamins, minerals, and other nutrients the body needs to sustain itself and grow. Calorie restriction has been shown to increase the lifespan of various animals, including rats, fish, fruit flies, dogs, and monkeys, by 30%–50%. A few human studies have been done, but evidence of its impact on humans is very limited compared to results available from the animal studies. The completed studies suggest that calorie restriction may increase the maximum human lifespan by about 30%. The problem preventing scientists from offering substantive proof that humans can greatly increase their lifespan by restricting calories is that the current maximum human lifespan is 110–120 years and full compliance with the diet is difficult. A 30% increase would extend the human lifespan to 143–156 years. This is an exceptionally long time for a scientific study and requires involvement of several generations of scientists. Only several hundred people have ever been documented to live past age 110. The oldest person with confirmed documentation was Jeanne Louise Calmet (1875–1997) of France, who lived 122 years and 164 days.

Since 1980, dozens of books have been published offering specific calorie-reduction diets aimed at increasing lifespan. The most popular diets include the **Okinawa Diet**, Anti-Inflammatory Diet, Longevity Diet, **Blood Type Diet**, Anti-Aging Plan, and the 120-Year Diet. In the 2010s, other anti-aging diets emerged that were not entirely based on very low calorie intake. These include the Origin Diet (unprocessed food only, wild game), the RealAge diet (fruits, vegetables, **whole grains**, **soy**), the Eat Right, Live Longer diet (organic vegetarian), and the Age-Free **Zone Diet** (a high-protein, low-carbohydrate, calorie-restricted version of the Zone Diet).

Despite calorie restriction, maintaining a balanced intake of nutrients is essential for achieving any anti-aging effects. People who experience starvation or famine receive no longevity benefits since their low calorie intake contains inadequate nutrition. The calorie-restrictive diet is believed to most benefit people who start in their mid-20s, with the beneficial effects decreasing proportionately with the age one begins the diet.

Although there are variations among anti-aging diets, most reduced-calorie diets recommend a core set of foods. These include vegetables, fruits, fish, soy, low-fat or non-fat dairy products, nuts, avocados, and olive oil. The primary beverages recommended are water and green or black tea.

Guidelines on calorie reduction vary from diet to diet, ranging from a 10% reduction to a 50% reduction of normal intake. Roy L. Walford (1924–2004), author of several books on anti-aging diets, says a reasonable goal is to achieve a 10%–25% reduction in a person's normal weight based on age, height, and body frame. The Anti-Aging Plan diet recommends men of normal weight lose up to 18% of their weight in the first six months of the diet. For a six-foot male weighing 175 lb. (79.3 kg), that means a loss of about 31 lb. ((14 kg). For a small-framed woman who is five-foot, six-inches tall and weighs 120 lb. (54.4 kg), the plan recommends losing 10% of her weight in the first six months, a loss of 12 lb. (5.4 kg).

Walford's Anti-Aging Plan is a diet based on decades of animal experimentation. It consists of computer-generated food combinations and meal menus containing the United States Department of Agriculture's **dietary reference intakes** (formerly called recommended daily allowances) of vitamins and other essential nutrients using foods low in calories. On the diet, the maximum number of calories allowed is 1,800 per day. There are two methods for starting the diet: rapid orientation and gradual orientation.

The rapid orientation method allows people to eat low-calorie meals rich in nutrients. This is a radical change for most people and requires a good deal of willpower. All foods low in nutrients are eliminated from the diet. The nutritional value and calories in foods and meals is determined by a software program available for purchase from Calorie Restriction Society International.

The gradual orientation method allows people to adopt the diet over time. The first week, people eat a high-nutrient meal on one day. This increases by one meal a week until participants are eating one meal high in nutrients every day at the end of seven weeks. Other meals during the day consist of low-calorie, healthy foods, but there is no limit on the amount a person can eat. After two months, participants switch to eating low-calorie, high-nutrition foods for all meals. Dieters are advised to view this diet as a lifestyle change rather than a quick weight-loss program.

A sample one-day, low-calorie, high-nutrition menu developed by Walford is:

- Breakfast: One cup of orange juice, one poached egg, one slice of mixed whole-grain bread, and one cup of brewed coffee or tea.
- Lunch: One-half cup of low-fat cottage cheese mixed with one-half cup of non-fat yogurt and one tablespoon of toasted wheat germ, an apple, and one whole wheat English muffin.
- Dinner: Three ounces of roasted chicken breast without the skin, a baked potato, and one cup of steamed spinach.
- Snack: Five dates, an oat bran muffin, and one cup of low-fat milk.

The three meals and snack contain 1,472 calories, 92 g protein, 24 g fat, 234 g **carbohydrates**, 27 g **fiber**, and 310 g cholesterol.

Function

The goal of the anti-aging diet is to slow the aging process, thereby extending the human lifespan. Even though it is not a weight loss diet, people taking in significantly fewer calories than what is considered normal by registered dietitians are likely to lose weight. Exercise is not part of calorie reduction diets. Researchers suggest people gradually transition to a reduced calorie diet over one or two years since a sudden calorie reduction can be unhealthy and even shorten the lifespan.

There is no clear answer as to why severely reducing calorie intake results in a longer and healthier life. Researchers have various explanations, and many suggest it may be due to a combination of factors. One theory is that calorie restriction protects DNA from damage, increases the enzyme repair of damaged DNA, and reduces the potential for genes to be altered to become cancerous. Other calorie reduction (CR) theories suggest that:

- CR helps reduce the production of free radicals (unstable molecules that attack healthy, stable molecules). Damage caused by free radicals increases as people age.
- CR delays the age-related decline of the human immune system and improved immune function may slow aging.
- CR slows metabolism (the body's use of energy). Some scientists propose that the higher a person's metabolism, the faster they age.

Benefits

The primary benefits of the anti-aging diet are improved health and prevention or forestalling of diseases such as coronary artery disease, **cancer**, stroke, diabetes, osteoporosis, Alzheimer's, and Parkinson's disease. Studies show that most physiologic functions and mental abilities of animals on reduced calorie diets correspond to those of much younger animals. The diet also has demonstrated extension of the maximum lifespan for many of the life forms on which it has been tested.

Precautions

A reduced-calorie diet is not recommended for people under the age of 21 as it may impair physical growth. This impairment has been seen in research on young laboratory animals. In humans, mental development and physical changes to the brain occur in teenagers and people in their early 20s that may be negatively affected by a low-calorie diet.

Other individuals advised against starting a calorie-restricted diet include women who plan to become pregnant, women who are pregnant, and those who are **breastfeeding**. A low **body mass index** (BMI), which occurs with a low-calorie diet, is a risk factor in pregnancy and can result in dysfunctional ovaries and infertility. A low BMI increases the risk of premature birth and low birth weights in newborns. People with existing medical conditions or diseases should

---

KEY TERMS

Alzheimer's disease—A degenerative disorder that affects the brain, causing dementia and loss of memory usually late in life.

Antioxidant—Substance that inhibits the destructive effects of oxidation in the body.

Body mass index (BMI)—A scale that expresses a person's weight in relation to their height.

Calorie restriction—A (usually substantial) limit on the number of calories a person consumes.

Deoxyribonucleic acid (DNA)—A nucleic acid molecule in a twisted double strand, called a double helix, that is the major component of chromosomes. DNA carries genetic information and is the basis of life.

Free radicals—Highly reactive atoms or molecules that can damage DNA.

Osteoporosis—A disorder that causes bones to become porous, break easily, and heal slowly.

Parkinson's disease—An incurable nervous disorder marked by symptoms of trembling hands and a slow, shuffling walk.

Testosterone—A male sex hormone responsible for secondary sex characteristics.

---

be especially cautious and consult with their physician before starting.

It is imperative that participants ensure that they continue to consume adequate levels of essential nutrients. Nutritional supplements and other forms of nutritional help are likely to be needed.

Risks

The anti-aging diet is very restrictive, and dieters need to adhere strictly to diet plans to ensure that they are receiving required amounts of key nutrients. A wide range of risks, related to physical, mental, social, and lifestyle issues, is associated with such a low-calorie diet. They include:

- hunger, food cravings, and obsession with food
- loss of strength or stamina and loss of muscle mass, which can affect physical activities, such as sports
- decreased levels of testosterone, which can be compensated with testosterone supplementation
- rapid weight loss (more than two pounds a week), which can negatively impact health

QUESTIONS TO ASK YOUR DOCTOR

- Do I need to take any vitamin, mineral, or other nutritional supplements if I go on this diet?
- Will an anti-aging diet have any negative effects on my health?
- Is there another diet that would better allow me to reach the same goals as the anti-aging diet?
- How will restricting my calorie intake effect my metabolism and energy level?

- slower wound healing
- reduced bone mass, which increases the risk of fracture
- increased sensitivity to cold
- reduced energy reserves and fatigue
- menstrual irregularity
- headaches
- drastic appearance changes from loss of fat and muscle, causing people to look thin or anorexic

Social issues can arise over family meals, since not all family members may be on a reduced-calorie diet. Conflict related to the types of food served, the amount of food served, the number of meals in a day, and fasting may develop. Other social issues involve eating in restaurants, workplace food, parties, and holidays. The long-term psychological effects of a reduced-calorie diet are unknown. However, since a low-calorie diet represents a major change in a person's life, psychological problems can be expected, including, in some cases, **anorexia nervosa**, **binge eating**, and obsessive thoughts about food and eating.

Research and general acceptance

Animal studies generally support the idea that a calorie-restrictive diet with adequate intake of essential nutrients increases lifespan. Few studies have been done in humans. In some small studies, people consuming a calorie-restrictive diet (under 1,400 calories daily) for five or more years had better heart function and lower blood pressure than those who consumed a diet of more than 2,000 calories daily. It is not clear whether the benefits come only from calorie restriction or from the increased fruits, vegetables, and whole grains consumed on most of these diets.

Resources

BOOKS

D'Adamo, Peter, and Catherine Whitney. *Aging: Fighting It With the Blood Type Diet: The Individual Plan for Preventing and Treating Brain Decline, Cognitive Impairment, Hormonal Deficiency, and the Loss of Vitality Associated With Advancing Years.* New York: Berkley Trade, 2006.

Delaney, Brian M., and Lisa Walford. *The Longevity Diet.* New York: Marlowe & Company, 2005.

Gates, Donna and Lyndi Schrecengost. *The Baby Boomer Diet: Body Ecology's Guide to Growing Younger: Anti-Aging Wisdom for Every Generation.* Carlsbad, CA: Hay House 2011.

Goode, Thomas. *The Holistic Guide to Weight Loss, Anti-Aging, and Fat Prevention.* Tucson, AZ: Inspired Living International, LLC, 2005.

Walford, Roy L., and Lisa Walford. *The Anti-Aging Plan: The Nutrient-Rich, Low-Calorie Way of Eating for a Longer Life—The Only Diet Scientifically Proven to Extend Your Healthy Years.* New York: Marlowe & Company, 2005.

Willcox, Bradley J., and D. Craig Willcox. *The Okinawa Diet Plan: Get Leaner, Live Longer, and Never Feel Hungry.* New York: Clarkson Potter, 2004.

WEBSITES

EveryDiet.com. "The Longevity Diet." http://www.every diet.org/diet/longevity-diet (accessed June 24, 2012).

"50+: Live Better, Longer. Aging Well: Eating Right for Longevity." WebMD. http://www.webmd.com/healthy-aging/features/aging-well-eating-right-for-longevity (accessed June 24, 2012).

Scientific Psychic. "Calorie Restriction Diet." http://www.scientificpsychic.com/health/crondiet.html (accessed June 24, 2012).

Walford.com. "Getting Started On The Anti-Aging Diet." http://www.walford.com/aastart.htm (accessed June 24, 2012).

ORGANIZATIONS

American Aging Association, 25373 Tyndall Falls Dr., Olmsted Falls, OH 44138, (440) 793-6565, Fax: (440) 793-6598, americanaging@gmail.com, http://www.americanaging.org.

Calorie Restriction Society International, 187 Ocean Dr., Newport, NC 28570, (877) 481-4841, http://www.crsociety.org.

National Institute on Aging, Bldg. 31, Rm. 5C27, 31 Center Dr., MSC 2292, Bethesda, MD 20892, (800) 222-2225, TTY: (800) 222-4225, Fax: (301) 496-1072, http://www.nia.nih.gov.

Ken R. Wells
Tish Davidson, AM

Anti-inflammatory diets

Definition

Anti-inflammatory diets are used to prevent or treat inflammation, which is the body's immune reaction to an injury or an irritation. There are two types of inflammation: acute and chronic. Acute inflammation is the body's response to an injury like a wound, broken bone, or bee sting. It is a normal reaction and helps the body heal. Chronic inflammation, also known as low-grade or systemic inflammation, is the body's reaction to any irritation that it regards as a foreign substance. Possible irritants include germs, cigarette smoke, and excess weight. Chronic inflammation is associated with arthritis and chronic conditions such as **obesity**, heart disease, some cancers, and diabetes.

Foods like oily fish (which are rich in **omega-3 fatty acids**), fruits, and vegetables are part of an anti-inflammatory diet. Foods and nutrients thought to trigger chronic inflammation include red meat, full-fat dairy products, processed foods, and saturated and **trans fats**.

Origins

The discovery of the relationship between inflammation and chronic disease grew out of laboratory and clinical studies to develop therapies for pneumococcal pneumonia. In 1930, William S. Tillett and Thomas Francis Jr. discovered a new antigen of the bacteria *pneumococcus*. The substance was later identified as C-reactive **protein** (CRP). The body produces CRP in the liver in response to injury and infection. High levels of the protein signify acute general inflammation in the body. CRP tests are also used to monitor patients with inflammatory diseases like rheumatoid arthritis.

Chronic inflammation may be the continuation of acute inflammation or a low-grade form of inflammation caused by the body's mistaken reaction to a threat that does not exist. For example, fat cells can produce certain proteins that may trigger defensive mechanisms in the body. A number of organizations, including the Arthritis Foundation, recommend weight loss (if needed) to help reduce inflammation. Anti-inflammatory diets are based on the theory that certain foods provoke inflammatory responses.

Description

Inflammation is the localized immune reaction of body tissue to an injury, such as a cut or a fracture. It can also be a response to an irritation, such as bacteria, viral infection, trauma, cigarette smoke, chemicals, or heat. Inflammation is characterized by redness, swelling, heat, pain, and sometimes loss of function or mobility. The acute inflammation process starts with the dilation of the blood vessel, which results in increased blood flow to the affected area. The increased blood flow causes the heat and redness; the dilation produces the swelling. Pain is caused by the release of the messenger compounds that send white blood cells to kill the foreign substance.

Elements of inflammation

The cells produce different types of proteins called cytokines that serve in different functions in the body; they may be released into the bloodstream or into

Anti-inflammatory diet

Anti-inflammatory foods

Fruits	Fresh fruits, berries, blueberries, blackberries, and strawberries
Legumes and beans	Pinto, kidney, borlotti, mung, cannellini, adzuki, fava, and black beans; soybeans; chickpeas
Nuts and seeds	Walnuts, flax seeds, pumpkin seeds (raw, unsalted)
Oils	Expeller pressed canola oil; extra-virgin olive oil; rice bran, grape seed, evening primrose, and walnut oils
Poultry, lean	Grass fed and free of preservatives, sodium, nitrates, or coloring
Soy products	Soybeans, edamame, tofu, tempeh, soymilk, other products from soybeans
Spices and herbs	Use to replace salt, sugar, added saturated fats
Seafood and wild fish	Herring, mackerel, salmon, trout
Vegetables, fresh	Green leafy vegetables, brightly colored vegetables
Whole grains	Amaranth, barley, bulgur, wild rice, millet, oats, quinoa, rye, spelt, wheat berries, buckwheat, whole wheat

Pro-inflammatory foods

Dairy products, high fat	Butter, cream, sour cream, whole milk
Processed meats	Lunch meats, hot dogs, sausages
Red meats	Beef, lamb, pork
Refined grains	White bread; white rice; pasta (unless whole grain); chips; products made with white flour, such as cake, cookies, crackers, pretzels, doughnuts, bagels, muffins
Saturated fats	Meats, dairy products, eggs
Sugars, refined, and high sugar foods	Sodas, pastries, presweetened cereals, candy, white and brown sugar, confectioners sugar, corn syrup, processed corn fructose
Trans fats	Found in some meats, dairy products, cakes, cookies, crackers, pies, breads, margarines, fried potatoes, potato chips, corn chips, popcorn, shortenings, salad dressings

(Table by PreMediaGlobal. © 2013 Cengage Learning.)

tissue. The cytokines in the immune system are interferon, interleukins, and tumor necrosis factor-alpha (TNF-alpha). The cytokines act as messengers between cells and regulate inflammatory responses. Some cytokines are involved in acute inflammation, and others are involved in chronic inflammation.

Prostaglandins serve different functions in the body that include the activation of the inflammatory response. Prostaglandins are unsaturated carboxylic acids that are synthesized by the body from arachidonic acid, an omega-6 fatty acid. Leukotrienes are products of arachidonic acid **metabolism**. The body releases these chemicals in response to an allergen. Leukotrienes take place in leukocytes, which are white blood cells. During the inflammation process, leukocytes protect the body from threats such as viruses and bacteria.

Conditions associated with chronic inflammation

Chronic inflammation is related to conditions including obesity, **metabolic syndrome**, asthma, allergies, irritable bowel disease, **celiac disease** and other digestive system diseases, stress, and sleep disorders such as sleep apnea. According to the American Heart Association (AHA), inflammation has not been proven to cause heart disease, but it is a common symptom of heart disease and stroke. Risk factors for inflammation include smoking cigarettes, high blood pressure, and low-density lipoprotein (LDL) cholesterol, also known as "bad" cholesterol.

Traditional treatment

General medical treatments for inflammation include relaxation therapies, moderate exercise such as walking, weight maintenance or loss, and medications designed to reduce the inflammation and control pain. These medications may include ibuprofen or aspirin, nonsteroidal anti-inflammatory drugs (NSAIDs), or steroid medications. NSAIDs are widely used as the initial form of therapy. However, use of these medications may irritate the stomach and could cause other complications, including the risk of stomach bleeding for people who are 60 or older.

Preventive measures

Dietary recommendations for preventing some conditions associated with inflammation, including rheumatoid arthritis, obesity, diabetes, and stress, include eating a healthy diet, getting regular physical exercise, losing weight if necessary, and not smoking. Chronic inflammation is linked to excess weight and

obesity because fat cells create cytokines, the proteins that stimulate inflammation. Inflammation and obesity are also linked to high blood pressure and elevated levels of lipids such as **triglycerides** and cholesterol. Inflammation and being overweight or obese place a person at risk for conditions including heart disease, diabetes, stroke, and arthritis. Excess weight places stress on the body that includes pressure on joints such as the knees.

Nutrition and acute inflammation

Acute inflammation is caused by injuries such as wounds, bites, and bee stings. Treating severe injuries may involve a special diet. The Cleveland Clinic recommends that injured people eat a variety of foods from the five food groups to obtain the **calories**, proteins, and **minerals** needed for healing. The healing process for a severe wound requires an increase in calories. The Clinic also recommends consumption of "power foods," which include:

- two to three servings per day of protein, such as lean meats, fish, poultry, eggs, dairy products, lentils, nuts, and seeds
- one serving per day of vitamin A, found in spinach, orange and yellow vegetables, orange fruits, and fortified dairy products
- one serving per day of vitamin C, found in citrus fruits and juices, strawberries, tomatoes, peppers, potatoes, spinach, and cruciferous vegetables such as broccoli and cauliflower
- zinc, found in red meats, seafood, and fortified cereals

Nutrition and chronic inflammation

There is no one anti-inflammatory diet. Rather, there are several healthy eating plans and recommendations designed around foods believed to decrease inflammation, as well as foods to avoid. Many popular diets, such as the **Zone diet**, the **Perricone diet**, and Dr. Weil's diet, claim to help prevent and treat inflammation. Organizations such as Harvard Medical School and the Arthritis Foundation also offer anti-inflammatory diet recommendations.

GENERAL RECOMMENDATIONS. Many professional organizations offer recommendations on what foods reduce inflammation. Harvard Medical School's *Family Health Guide* attributes acute inflammation to "modern irritations like smoking, lack of exercise, high-fat and high-calorie meals, and highly processed foods." The guide contains recommendations about foods that either relieve or promote inflammation. Suggestions from the guide include:

- Avoid saturated fats and *trans* fats. Healthier sources of fats include olive oil and omega-3 fatty acids found in oily fish.
- Choose whole grains and avoid highly refined carbohydrates such as white bread, white rice, white potatoes, and soda, which raise blood sugar levels and promote production of cytokines.
- Increase intake of fruits and vegetables. Many contain antioxidants that help fight free radicals, molecules that damage cells and contribute to inflammation. Other sources of antioxidants include cocoa and dark chocolate, which have been found in some studies to help prevent inflammation.
- Eat more seeds and nuts. Nuts such as walnuts and almonds are thought to help relieve inflammation.
- Consume cocoa and chocolate because they slow the production of signaling molecules involved in inflammation. However, the guide advises choosing types low in sugar and fat.

The Arthritis Foundation website provides recommendations similar to those found in the Harvard guide, highlighting the need for omega-3 fatty acids in the diet as well as consumption of vegetables, fruits, nuts, and small amounts of dark chocolate.

MEDITERRANEAN DIETS. According to an article in the *Mayo Clinic Health Letter* by Brent Bauer, MD, there is limited evidence that anti-inflammation diets work directly to stop inflammation. However, foods recommended in anti-inflammatory diets are often typical of the Mediterranean style of eating and are generally good choices. Key components of Mediterranean diets include:

- generous amounts of fruits and vegetables
- healthy fats such as olive oil and canola oil
- regular consumption of fish
- small portions of nuts
- very little red meat
- red wine in moderation

POPULAR DIETS. Mainstream anti-inflammatory diets include the 2005 book *Healthy Aging: A Lifelong Guide to Your Physical and Spiritual Well-Being* by Andrew Weil, MD. Weil is the founder of the Arizona Center for Integrative Medicine at the University of Arizona and designed the diet to reduce the risks of age-related diseases and to optimize health. His diet recommendations are based on the glycemic load (GL), a measure of the effect of food on blood sugar. Low GL recommendations include consuming lean protein, healthy **fats**, and high quantities of **fiber** from fruits and vegetables. Weil advises people to swap meat and poultry for fish and vegetable proteins

---

KEY TERMS

Antioxidant—A chemical compound or substance that inhibits oxidation; for example, vitamin E, vitamin C, or beta-carotene.

Chronic disease—An illness or medical condition that lasts over a long period of time and sometimes causes a long-term change in the body.

Inflammation—Swelling, redness, heat, and pain produced in an area of the body as a reaction to injury or infection.

---

such as beans, **soy** foods, grains, and nuts. Foods to avoid or give up include fast food, processed foods, and products made with flour or high-fructose corn syrup.

Barry Sears, developer of the Zone diet, wrote about how that particular eating plan could be used to fight inflammation in his book *The Anti-Inflammation Zone: Reversing the Silent Epidemic That's Destroying Our Health.* Sears used the 40:30:30 framework of his Zone diet—40% of daily calories from **carbohydrates**, 30% from protein, and 30% from fat—to build an anti-inflammatory plan with an emphasis on fish, vegetables, berries, olive oil, almonds, avocados, and spices.

Function

Anti-inflammatory diets aim to reduce or prevent inflammation in the body. The foods recommended to reduce or relieve inflammation are frequently the same foods recommended to maintain health and to decrease the risk of developing chronic diseases. These foods include fish and other sources of omega-3 fatty acids. The body uses these fats to manufacture prostaglandins, chemicals that play an important role in reducing inflammation and promoting a healthy immune response. Nuts and seeds may also reduce inflammation but are high in fat, so intake should be limited.

Fish, including tuna, shellfish, and crab; Brazil nuts; and whole-wheat products are good sources of **selenium**, a trace mineral essential to health. Selenium is incorporated into proteins to make selenoproteins, which are important antioxidant enzymes. The antioxidant properties of selenoproteins include an important role in the cell's defense system. Selenium may be useful in preventing arthritis and other inflammatory conditions, according to *Arthritis Today*.

Flavonoids are a type of antioxidant thought to have anti-inflammatory effects. Flavonoids may help

QUESTIONS TO ASK YOUR DOCTOR

- Could an anti-inflammatory diet help me?
- Are there any foods I should avoid to decrease inflammation and my risk of chronic disease?
- Will losing weight help me to reduce my risks of inflammation and chronic disease?
- Are there any foods I could eat to decrease my dosage of anti-inflammatory medications?
- While my wound heals, how many calories should I consume each day?

to prevent arthritis and provide pain relief. Sources of flavonoids include fruits, such as blueberries, blackberries, strawberries, apples, and citrus fruits; dark chocolate; red wine; legumes; and vegetables such as broccoli, celery, thyme, hot peppers, onions, kale, and scallions. Diets high in legumes are also inversely related to plasma concentrations of CRP. Isoflavones are a subcategory of flavonoids that are found in soymilk and other soy foods such as soybeans, edamame, tofu, and tempeh.

Herbs and spices are also recommended in some anti-inflammatory diets because of their antioxidant properties. However, they would need to be consumed in large amounts to have any antioxidant effect. However, herbs and spices are useful as flavor replacements for less healthy recipe ingredients such as salt, sugar, and saturated fats.

Benefits

Diet and exercise help to maintain a healthy weight and to prevent inflammation and reduce the risk of developing chronic diseases. Furthermore, the combination of diet and exercise is usually accompanied by an elevation of energy and emotional health.

Precautions

People should consult with their doctors before beginning a new diet. Women who are pregnant or **breastfeeding** should also discuss the consumption of fish with their doctors, due to the risk of mercury contamination.

There is some support for the belief that **food sensitivities** or allergies to foods may be a trigger for inflammation. Often hard to detect with common blood tests, some people have seen alleviation of symptoms of chronic diseases, such as arthritis, when the aggravating foods are removed from their diet. Common allergic foods are milk and dairy, wheat, corn, eggs, beef, yeast, and soy.

Risks

In general, the recommendations provided by trusted organizations such as Harvard and the Mayo Clinic are in line with the federal guidelines for nutrition and provide no risks. However, people with diabetes or other chronic conditions should not change their diet without discussing it with their doctor. Also, anyone taking medication to treat a condition should not stop taking that medication without their physician's consent.

Research and general acceptance

The benefits of a healthy diet and regular physical activity are widely accepted; however, it is not as clear whether certain foods reduce or relieve the symptoms of chronic inflammation. The strongest evidence-based recommendations to reduce or prevent inflammation are for people to eat a healthy diet, lose weight if needed, and not smoke.

Whole grains and whole-grain foods have been shown in some studies to decrease inflammatory markers. However, other research, such as the WHOLEheart study in the United Kingdom, found no change in markers for the risk of cardiovascular disease when whole grain intake was significantly increased, according to the July 2010 issue of the *British Journal of Nutrition*. Inflammatory markers were among the measurements used in the 16-week study, which involved 316 people between the ages of 18 and 65.

Resources

BOOKS

Black, Jessica K. *The Anti-Inflammation Diet and Recipe Book: Protect Yourself and Your Family from Heart Disease, Arthritis, Diabetes, Allergies—and More.* Alameda, CA: Hunter House, 2006.

Challem, Jack. *The Inflammation Syndrome: Your Nutrition Plan for Great Health, Weight Loss, and Pain-Free Living.* 2nd ed. New York: Wiley, 2010.

Reinagel, Monica. *The Inflammation-Free Diet Plan.* New York: McGraw Hill, 2007.

Sears, Barry. *The Anti-Inflammation Zone: Reversing the Silent Epidemic That's Destroying Our Health.* New York: HarperCollins, 2005.

Weil, Andrew. *Healthy Aging: A Lifelong Guide to Your Physical and Spiritual Well-Being.* New York: Alfred A. Knopf, 2005.

PERIODICALS

Brownlee, Iain A., et al. "Markers of Cardiovascular Risk are Not Changed by Increased Whole-Grain Intake: The Wholeheart Study, a Randomised, Controlled Dietary Intervention." *British Journal of Nutrition* 104, no. 1 (July 2010): 125–34.

Dod, Harvinder, et al. "Effect of Intensive Lifestyle Changes on Endothelial Function and on Inflammatory Markers of Atherosclerosis." *The American Journal of Cardiology* 105, no. 3 (February 1, 2010): 362–67.

Feghali, Carol A., and Timothy M. Wright. "Cytokines in Acute and Chronic Inflammation." *Frontiers in Bioscience* (January 1, 1997). http://immuneweb.xxmu.edu.cn/ckine-infec.pdf (accessed September 20, 2012).

Greer, Ashley. "An Anti-Inflammatory Diet: The Next Frontier in Preventive Medicine." *JAPA: Official Journal of the American Academy of Physician Assistants* 25, no. 2 (2012): 38+. http://www.jaapa.com/an-anti-inflammatory-diet-the-next-frontier-in-preventive-medicine/article/224941 (accessed September 20, 2012).

Messier Stephen P., et al. "Weight Loss Reduces Knee-Joint Loads in Overweight and Obese Older Adults with Knee Osteoarthritis." *Arthritis & Rheumatism* 52, no. 7 (July 2005): 2026–32.

Sears, Barry, and Stacey Bell. "The Zone Diet: An Anti-Inflammatory, Low Glycemic-Load Diet." *Metabolic Syndrome and Related Disorders* 2, no. 1 (2004): 24–38.

WEBSITES

American Heart Association. "Inflammation and Heart Disease." http://www.heart.org/HEARTORG/Conditions/Inflammation-and-Heart-Disease_UCM_432150_Article.jsp (accessed September 20, 2012).

"Anti-Inflammatory Diet & Pyramid." DrWeil.com. http://www.drweil.com/drw/u/ART02012/anti-inflammatory-diet (accessed September 20, 2012).

Bauer, Brent. "Buzzed on Inflammation." *Mayo Clinic Health Letter* online edition, July 2008. http://healthletter.mayoclinic.com/editorial/editorial.cfm/i/163/t/Buzzed%20on%20inflammation (accessed September 20, 2012).

Breyer, Melissa. "Anti-Inflammatory Diet 101." Care 2 Make a Difference. http://www.care2.com/greenliving/anti-inflammatory-diet-101.html (accessed September 20, 2012).

Cleveland Clinic. "Nutrition Guidelines to Improve Wound Healing." http://my.clevelandclinic.org/healthy_living/nutrition/hic_nutrition_guidelines_to_improve_wound_healing.aspx (accessed September 20, 2012).

Drake, Victoria J. "Nutrition and Inflammation." Linus Pauling Institute, Oregon State University. http://lpi.oregonstate.edu/infocenter/inflammation.html (accessed September 20, 2012).

"Eat to Beat Joint Inflammation." *Arthritis Today.* http://www.arthritistoday.org/nutrition-and-weight-loss/healthy-eating/food-and-inflammation/eat-to-beat-inflammation.php (accessed September 20, 2012).

Harvard Medical School. "What You Eat Can Fuel or Cool Inflammation, A Key Driver of Heart Disease, Diabetes, and Other Chronic Conditions." *Harvard Medical School Family Health Guide.* http://www.health.harvard.edu/fhg/updates/What-you-eat-can-fuel-or-cool-inflammation-a-key-driver-of-heart-disease-diabetes-and-other-chronic-conditions.shtml (accessed September 20, 2012).

Higdon, Jane, and Victoria J. Drake. "Flavonoids." Linus Pauling Institute, Oregon State University. http://lpi.oregonstate.edu/infocenter/phytochemicals/flavonoids (accessed September 20, 2012).

"Nutrient-Rich Foods That Can Be Medicine." *Arthritis Today.* http://www.arthritistoday.org/conditions/rheumatoid-arthritis/nutrition-and-ra/foods-as-medicine.php (accessed September 20, 2012).

Reinagel, Monica. "The Anti-Inflammatory Diet." Epicurious.com. http://www.epicurious.com/articlesguides/healthy/news/diet_antiinflammatory (accessed September 20, 2012).

Rockefeller University Hospital. "C-Reactive Protein: From Pneumococcal Pneumonia to Cardiovascular Disease Risk." http://centennial.rucares.org/index.php?page=C-Reactive_Protein (accessed September 20, 2012).

Sandon, Lona. "Food and Inflammation." Academy of Nutrition and Dietetics. http://www.eatright.org/media/blog.aspx?id=4294968470&blogid=269 (accessed September 20, 2012).

U.S. Office of Dietary Supplements. "What is Selenium?" National Institutes of Health. http://ods.od.nih.gov/factsheets/Selenium-HealthProfessional (accessed September 20, 2012).

ORGANIZATIONS

Academy of Nutrition and Dietetics, 120 South Riverside Plz., Ste. 2000, Chicago, IL 60606-6995, (312) 899-0040, (800) 877-1600, amacmunn@eatright.org, http://www.eatright.org.

Arthritis Foundation, PO Box 7669, Atlanta, GA 30357-0669, (800) 283-7800, http://www.arthritis.org.

Megan C. M. Porter, RD, LD
David Newton
Liz Swain

Antioxidants

Definition

Antioxidants are substances that prevent oxygen molecules from interacting with other molecules in a process called oxidation. In the body, antioxidants combine with potentially damaging molecules called free radicals to prevent the free radicals from causing damage to cell membranes, DNA, and proteins in the cell. Common antioxidants important to human health are **vitamins** A, C, E; beta-carotene; and **selenium**. By some estimates, up to 10% of North Americans and Europeans were taking at least one antioxidant dietary supplement in 2012.

Purpose

The role of antioxidants in the body is complex and not completely understood. Antioxidants combine with free radicals so that the free radicals cannot react with, or oxidize, other molecules. In this way, antioxidants help slow or prevent damage to cells. Antioxidant enzymes present in the body also work to prevent oxidation. Damage caused by free radicals is thought to cause or contribute to cardiovascular disease, **cancer**, Alzheimer's disease, age-related changes in vision, and other signs of aging. However, no direct cause-and-effect relationship between antioxidant intake and disease prevention has been proven. Antioxidants unrelated to those of importance in the body have commercial uses in the preservation of processed food and in many industrial processes.

Description

Oxygen is essential to many reactions that occur within cells. Free radicals form mainly as a result of normal cellular **metabolism** involving oxygen. They can also form in abnormally large amounts when the body is exposed to radiation, ultraviolet (UV) light, and toxins such as cigarette smoke or certain chemicals.

The common feature of free radicals is that their molecular structure contains an unpaired electron. Free radical molecules with an unpaired electron are unstable and have a strong tendency to react with other molecules by "stealing" an electron from them to form a more stable electron pair. This reaction is called oxidation (even when it happens with molecules other than oxygen). In the body, free radicals cause damage when they react with deoxyribonucleic acid (DNA), proteins, and lipids (**fats**). Antioxidants are molecules that react with free radicals in ways that neutralize them so they are no longer able to "steal" electrons and cause damage.

Some important human antioxidants must be acquired through diet, while others can be made by the body. **Vitamin C** (ascorbic acid), **vitamin E** (alpha-tocopherol), **vitamin A** (retinol), and beta-carotene are the most important antioxidants obtained from food sources. Flavonoids found in tea, chocolate, grapes, berries, onions, and wine also appear to have antioxidant activity, although their role in health is unclear. Selenium is sometimes classified as an antioxidant due to its activities in the body, but strictly, it is not.

Selenium is a mineral that must be acquired through diet. Plants grown in geographic locations with selenium-rich soil provide a rich source of this mineral. Brazil nuts and fish (e.g., tuna, halibut, sardines, salmon) are considered the best sources of selenium. Shellfish, meat, poultry, eggs, mushrooms, and grains (wheat, barley, rice, oats) also contain selenium, although the amounts in plant-based foods depend on the concentration of selenium in the soil in which they were grown. Selenium is necessary in the formation of the enzymes involved in antioxidant reactions. Glutathione and coenzyme Q (ubiquinone) are the most important antioxidants produced by the body.

Antioxidants and disease

When free radicals build up faster than antioxidants can neutralize them, the body develops a condition called oxidative stress. Oxidative stress reduces the body's ability to deal with damage to cells and is thought to play a role in the development of chronic diseases such as cardiovascular disease, cancer, and Alzheimer's disease. Researchers know that a diet high in fruits and vegetables containing antioxidants promotes health and decreases the risk of developing some chronic diseases such as atherosclerosis (hardening of the arteries). In the early 2000s, **dietary supplements** containing antioxidants were popularized as a way to reduce oxidative stress; prevent health problems such as cancer, stroke, heart attack, and dementia; and live longer. Research has since shown that although there are relationships between antioxidant levels and health, antioxidant dietary supplements are not adept at preventing age-related diseases. In fact, some evidence now suggests that high intakes of antioxidants may actually have harmful effects in promoting the development of cancers and preventing the prophylactic effects of certain cholesterol-reducing medications.

One problem in determining whether there is a cause-and-effect relationship between oxidative stress and disease is that it is often unclear whether oxidative stress causes a disease or if the disease brings about oxidative stress. Also, everyone develops oxidative stress as they age, but not everyone develops the same diseases. The interactions among an individual's diet, environment, genetic make-up, and health are complex and still not well understood. Antioxidants remain of great interest to researchers seeking ways to prevent and cure chronic disease. Many clinical trials are underway to determine safety and effectiveness of different antioxidants, both alone and in combination with other drugs and supplements.

CARDIOVASCULAR DISEASE. The strongest link between antioxidant levels and health is related to the development of cardiovascular disease. Low-density lipoprotein cholesterol (LDL or "bad" cholesterol) appears to react with free radicals. This changes the LDL cholesterol in a way that allows it to accumulate in cells lining the blood vessels. These cholesterol-loaded cells are precursors to the development of plaque, hard deposits that line blood vessels and cause cardiovascular disease, heart attack, and stroke.

High dietary intakes and blood levels of antioxidant nutrients (e.g., beta-carotene) have been associated with lower risk of cardiovascular disease. This led researchers to hypothesize that increasing the amount of antioxidants in the blood by taking supplements would decrease the number of free radicals available to interact with LDL cholesterol, lowering the risk of developing cardiovascular disease. However, studies have found this not to be the case. A paper published in the *Journal of the American Medical Association* in 2007 analyzed 68 trials of antioxidant supplements, involving about 232,600 patients, and found that antioxidant supplements did not prolong life. In fact, when only rigorous, well-controlled studies were analyzed, the risk of dying increased 5%. This analysis is quite controversial, with some experts questioning the analytical methods used. However, the American Heart Association and similar organizations in other countries continue to advocate cardiovascular disease prevention through dietary consumption of antioxidants—in fruits, vegetables, **whole grains**, and nuts—instead of antioxidant supplements.

CANCER. In some laboratory cell cultures and animal studies, antioxidants have appeared to slow the development of cancer. The results have been mixed, however, in studies where humans took antioxidant dietary supplements. A large study of 29,000 men showed that when a beta-carotene dietary supplement was taken by men who smoked, they developed lung cancer at a rate 18% higher and died at a rate 8% higher than men who did not receive the supplement. Another study that gave men dietary supplements of beta-carotene and vitamin A was stopped when researchers found that the men receiving the beta-carotene had a 46% greater chance of dying from lung cancer than those who did not receive the supplement. Other large studies have shown either no or only slight protective effects against cancer. The position of the American Cancer Society, the National Cancer Institute, and several international health organizations is that antioxidants should come from a healthy diet high in fruits and vegetables and low in fat and not from dietary supplements.

AGE-RELATED VISION IMPAIRMENT. Cataracts and age-related macular degeneration are two types of vision impairment common in older individuals. Cataracts

develop because of changes in the **protein** in the lens of the eye. These changes cause the lens to become cloudy and limit vision. The changes may be due to damage by free radicals. Age-related macular degeneration is an irreversible disease of the retina that causes blindness. Two carotenoid antioxidants, zeaxanthin and lutein, are found in the retina and are essential to vision. However, study participants who took antioxidant supplements over several years did not have a reduced risk of developing these diseases.

ALZHEIMER'S DISEASE. Antioxidants have been associated with slowing the progression of memory loss and other cognitive disorders, including Alzheimer's disease, but results have been inconclusive. A 1997 study sponsored by the National Institute on Aging found that high doses of vitamin E prolonged the ability of participants to carry out activities of daily life when facing cognitive

QUESTIONS TO ASK YOUR DOCTOR

- Are there any circumstances in which you would recommend that I begin to take antioxidant dietary supplements?

- What specific foods would you recommend to ensure that I obtain an adequate level of antioxidants in my daily diet?

- What does the most recent research have to say about the effectiveness of antioxidants in preventing heart disease? Cancer?

- Is there really any harm in my taking antioxidant dietary supplements if I really want to do so? If so, what is the risk?

decline. However, subsequent studies have found conflicting evidence, and too much vitamin E may cause adverse side effects, including an increased risk of death. Vitamin E is sometimes prescribed to patients with Alzheimer's disease but should only be taken under close physician supervision. Again, the best sources of antioxidants are whole foods and not supplements.

Flavonoids found in berries, which are a class of antioxidants, have been linked to positive cognitive function, including delayed memory loss and lowered risk of Parkinson's disease, but a cause-and-effect relationship has not been established, and further research is needed.

Precautions

The mixed results obtained in human studies of antioxidant supplements suggests that all antioxidants should come from foods and not from dietary supplements. There is also little information on the safety of antioxidant supplements in children and women who are pregnant or **breastfeeding**.

The amount of antioxidant in a supplement often is many times greater than that acquired by eating fruits and vegetables. Some antioxidants (e.g., vitamin A in the form of retinol) can build up to potentially dangerous levels in the body. In the case of supplementation, more is not necessarily better. Consult a physician before taking any antioxidant supplements.

Interactions

The interaction among various antioxidants, enzymes, coenzymes, drugs, and herbal and dietary supplements is complex and not completely understood. Specific antioxidants may have known interactions with other substances, and any supplements should be discussed with a physician.

Complications

Antioxidants acquired by eating fruits and vegetables promote health. No complications are expected from antioxidants in food. Antioxidant dietary supplements may interact with other substances or increase the levels of antioxidants in the body in ways that cause undesirable side effects. Consult a physician prior to taking an antioxidant supplement.

Parental concerns

Parents should encourage their children to eat a healthy and varied diet high in fruits, vegetables, and whole grains. There is no need to give children antioxidant dietary supplements. The safety of these supplements in children has not been studied.

Resources

BOOKS

DeCava, Judith A. *The Real Truth about Vitamins and Antioxidants*. 2nd ed. Fort Collins, CO: Selene River Press, 2006.

Frei, Balz, ed. *Natural Antioxidants in Human Health and Disease*. San Diego: Academic Press, 2006.

Panglossi, Harold V., ed. *Antioxidants: New Research*. New York: Nova Science Publishers, 2006.

Paur, I., et al. "Antioxidants in Herbs and Spices: Roles in Oxidative Stress and Redox Signaling." In *Herbal Medicine: Biomolecular and Clinical Aspects*, 2nd ed., edited by Iris F.F. Benzie and Sissi Watchel-Galor. Boca Raton, FL: CRC Press, 2011.

Wildman, Robert E. C., ed. *Handbook of Nutraceuticals and Functional Foods*. 2nd ed. Boca Raton, FL: CRC/Taylor &Francis, 2007.

PERIODICALS

Bjelakovic, G., et al. "Antioxidant Supplements for Prevention of Mortality in Healthy Participants and Patients with Various Diseases." *Cochrane Database of Systematic Reviews* 3, art no. CD007176 (March 12, 2012). http://dx.doi.org/10.1002/14651858.CD007176.pub2 (accessed June 12, 2012).

Bjelakovic, G., et al. "Mortality in Randomized Trials of Antioxidant Supplements for Primary and Secondary Prevention: Systematic Review and Meta-Analysis." *Journal of the American Medical Association* 297, no. 8 (2007): 842–57.

Feng-Jiao, Li, Liang Shen, and Hong-Fang Ji. "Dietary Intakes of Vitamin E, Vitamin C, and ß-Carotene, and Risk of Alzheimer's Disease: A Meta-Analysis." *Journal of Alzheimer's Disease* 31, no. 2 (2012).

Halliwell, B. "Free Radicals and Antioxidants: Updating a Personal View." *Nutrition Reviews* 70, no. 5 (2012): 257–65.

http://dx.doi.org/10.1111/j.1753-4887.2012.00476.x (accessed June 12, 2012).

Piero, Dolara, Elisabetta Bigagli, and Andrew Collins. "Antioxidant Vitamins and Mineral Supplementation, Life Span Expansion, and Cancer Incidence: A Critical Commentary." *European Journal of Nutrition* (2012): e-pub ahead of print. http://www.springerlink.com/content/l3m8913643721808 (accessed June 12, 2012).

WEBSITES

Alzheimer's Association. "Medications for Memory Loss." http://www.alz.org/alzheimers_disease_standard_pre scriptions.asp (accessed June 12, 2012).

Consumer Reports on Health. "Vitamins, Supplements: New Evidence Shows They Can't Compete with Mother Nature," March 2010. ConsumerReports.org. http://www.consumerreports.org/cro/2012/05/vitamins-supplements/index.htm (accessed June 12, 2012).

Dillner, Luisa. "Should I Take Antioxidant Supplements?" *Dr. Dillner's Health Dilemmas* (blog), *The Guardian*, August 8, 2011. http://www.guardian.co.uk/lifeandstyle/2011/aug/08/should-i-take-antioxidant-supplements (accessed June 12, 2012).

HealthDay News. "Eating Berries Might Help Preserve Your Memory." MedlinePlus. http://www.nlm.nih.gov/medline plus/news/fullstory_124533.html (accessed June 12, 2012).

International Food Information Council Foundation. "Functional Foods Fact Sheet: Antioxidants." FoodInsight.org. http://www.foodinsight.org/Resources/Detail.aspx?topic=Functional_Foods_Fact_Sheet_Antioxidants (accessed June 12, 2012).

MedlinePlus. "Antioxidants." U.S. National Library of Medicine, National Institutes of Health. http://www.nlm.nih.gov/medlineplus/antioxidants.html (accessed June 12, 2012).

National Cancer Institute. "Antioxidants and Cancer Prevention: Fact Sheet." http://www.cancer.gov/cancertopics/factsheet/prevention/antioxidants (accessed June 12, 2012).

ORGANIZATIONS

Academy of Nutrition and Dietetics, 120 South Riverside Plz., Ste. 2000, Chicago, IL 60606-6995, (312) 899-0040, (800) 877-1600, amacmunn@eatright.org, http://www.eatright.org.

American Heart Association, 7272 Greenville Ave., Dallas, TX 75231, (800) 242-8721, http://www.americanheart.org.

National Cancer Institute, 6116 Executive Blvd., Ste. 300, Bethesda, MD 20892-8322, (800) 4-CANCER (422-6237), http://www.cancer.gov.

Office of Dietary Supplements, National Institutes of Health, 6100 Executive Blvd., Rm. 3B01, MSC 7517, Bethesda, MD 20892-7517, (301) 435-2920, Fax: (301) 480-1845, ods@nih.gov, http://ods.od.nih.gov.

Tish Davidson, AM
David Newton

Antiscorbutic vitamin *see* **Vitamin C**

Arthritis diet

Definition

Arthritis is the general medical term for the inflammation of a joint or a disorder characterized by such inflammation. There are a number of different kinds of arthritis, and therefore there is no "arthritis diet" as such that has been proposed as a treatment for all of these different joint disorders. Dietary therapies for osteoarthritis (OA) and rheumatoid arthritis (RA), the two most common forms of arthritis, fall into three major categories. The first is a mainstream management strategy that focuses on weight reduction and well-balanced diets as a way to relieve stress on damaged joints and slow the progression of arthritis. The second has **dietary supplements** of various types that have been evaluated in clinical trials and have been found to benefit at least some patients. A third category uses alternative medical approaches that rely on

Differences between osteoarthritis and rheumatoid arthritis

	Osteoarthritis	Rheumatoid arthritis
Risk factors		
Age related	✔	
Family history	✔	✔
Overuse of joints	✔	
Excessive weight	✔	
Physical effects		
Affects joints	✔	✔
Autoimmune disease		✔
Bony spurs	✔	✔
Enlarged or malformed joints	✔	✔
Treatment options		
Weight management	✔	
Glucocorticoids		✔
Nonsteroidal anti-inflammatory drugs	✔	✔
Methotrexate		✔
Disease-modifying antirheumatic drugs		✔
Pain management		
Support groups	✔	✔
Exercise	✔	✔
Joint splitting	✔	✔
Physical therapy	✔	✔
Passive exercise	✔	✔
Joint replacement	✔	✔
Hot and cold therapy	✔	✔
Massage therapy	✔	✔
Acupuncture	✔	✔
Psychological approaches (relaxation, visualization)	✔	✔
Tai chi	✔	✔
Low-stress yoga	✔	✔

(Table by PreMediaGlobal. © 2013 Cengage Learning.)

dietary adjustments (including **elimination diets**) and/ or traditional herbal remedies to treat arthritis.

Osteoarthritis vs. rheumatoid arthritis

It is necessary to understand the differences between OA and RA in order to understand both mainstream and alternative approaches to these disorders. Osteoarthritis (OA) is the more common of the two in the North American population, particularly among middle-aged and older adults. OA is also the most common joint disorder worldwide. In 2012, it was estimated to affect about 27 million adults in the United States and to account for at least $86 billion in health care costs each year. It is also the single most common condition for which people seek help from complementary and alternative medical (CAM) treatments.

The rate of OA increases in older age groups; about 80%–90% of people over the age of 65 show some evidence of OA when they are X-rayed. Only about half of these older adults, however, are affected severely enough to develop noticeable symptoms. By age 80, 100% of individuals show some signs of OA. OA usually does not completely disable people; most patients can manage its symptoms by watching their weight, staying active, avoiding overuse of affected joints, and taking over-the-counter or prescription pain relievers. OA most commonly affects the weight-bearing joints in the hips, knees, and spine, although some people first notice its symptoms in their fingers or neck. It is often unilateral, which means that it affects the joints on only one side of the body. The symptoms of OA vary considerably in severity from person to person.

OA results from progressive damage to the cartilage that cushions the joints, especially joints involving the long bones. As cartilage deteriorates, fluid accumulates in the joints, bony overgrowths develop, and the muscles and tendons may weaken, leading to stiffness on arising, pain, swelling, and restricted movement. OA is gradual in onset, often taking years to develop before the person notices pain or a limited range of motion in the joint. OA is most likely to be diagnosed in people over the age of 50, although younger adults are occasionally affected. OA affects more men than women under age 45; while more women than men are affected in the age group over 55.

OA is not simply caused by the aging process. It is thought to result from a combination of factors, including traumatic damage to joints from accidents or sports injuries, repetitive use of the joint, **obesity**, and heredity. In an effort to clarify the role of heredity, British scientists in 2010 began a two-year study involving 14,000 people to determine what gene mutations are linked to OA. Race does not appear to be a factor. Some risk factors for OA include osteoporosis and **vitamin D** deficiency.

Rheumatoid arthritis (RA), by contrast, is most likely to be diagnosed in adults between the ages of 30 and 50, two-thirds of whom are women. RA affects about 1% of adults worldwide. Race appears to be a factor. RA is much more common among Native Americans (5%–6%) and rare among blacks of Caribbean origin. There is a hereditary component to RA; people with relatives who have RA are more likely to develop the disease.

Unlike OA, which is caused by degeneration of a body tissue, RA is an autoimmune disorder in which the body's immune system attacks some of its own tissues. RA often develops suddenly and may affect other organ systems, not just the joints. RA is more debilitating than OA; 30% of patients with RA will become permanently disabled within two to three years of diagnosis if they are not treated. In addition, patients with RA have a higher risk of heart attacks and strokes. RA differs from OA, too, in that the joints it most commonly affects are the fingers, wrists, knuckles, elbows, and shoulders. RA is typically a bilateral disorder, which means that both sides of the body are affected. In addition, people with RA often feel sick, feverish, or generally unwell, while those with OA usually feel normal, except for the stiffness or discomfort in the affected joints.

Origins

The role of diet and nutrition in both OA and RA has been studied since the 1930s, but there is little agreement, as of 2012, regarding the details of dietary therapy for these disorders. One clear finding that has emerged from decades of research is the importance of weight reduction or maintenance in the treatment of patients with OA. Another agreed upon finding is the need for nutritional balance and healthy eating patterns in the treatment of either form of arthritis. Findings regarding the use of dietary supplements and complementary and alternative medicine (CAM) therapies will be discussed in more detail below.

Various elimination diets have been proposed since the 1960s as treatments for OA. The best known of these is the Dong diet, introduced by Dr. Collin Dong in a book published in 1975. This diet is based on traditional Chinese beliefs about the effects of certain foods on increasing the pain of arthritis. The Dong diet requires the patient to eliminate all fruits, red meat, alcohol, dairy products, herbs, and all foods containing

KEY TERMS

Arthritis—A general term for the inflammation of a joint or a condition characterized by joint inflammation.

Ayurveda—The traditional system of natural medicine that originated in India around 3500 BC. Its name is Sanskrit for "science of long life." Some people have tried Ayurvedic medicines and dietary recommendations in the treatment of arthritis.

Chondroitin sulfate—A compound found naturally in the body that is part of a large protein molecule (proteoglycan) helping cartilage to retain its elasticity. Chondroitin sulfate derived from animal or shark cartilage can be taken as a dietary supplement by people with OA.

Dietary supplement—A product, such as a vitamin, mineral, herb, amino acid, or enzyme, that is intended to be consumed in addition to an individual's diet with the expectation that it will improve health.

Disease-modifying antirheumatic drugs (DMARDs)—A class of prescription medications given to patients with rheumatoid arthritis that suppress the immune system and slow the progression of RA.

Elimination diet—A diet in which the patient excludes a specific food (or group of foods) for a period of time in order to determine whether the food is responsible for symptoms of an allergy or other disorder. Elimination diets are also known as food challenge diets.

Glucosamine—A type of amino sugar that is thought to help in the formation and repair of cartilage. It can be extracted from crab or shrimp shells and used as a dietary supplement by people with OA.

Naturopathy—A system of disease treatment that emphasizes natural means of health care, such as water, natural foods, dietary adjustments, massage and manipulation, and electrotherapy, rather than conventional drugs and surgery. Naturopaths (practitioners

of naturopathy) often recommend dietary therapy in the treatment of arthritis.

Nonsteroidal anti-inflammatory drugs (NSAIDs)—A class of drugs commonly given to treat the inflammation and pain associated with both RA and OA. NSAIDs work by blocking prostaglandins, which are hormone-like compounds that cause pain, fever, muscle cramps, and inflammation. Some NSAIDs are prescription drugs while others are available in over-the-counter (OTC) formulations.

Placebo—A pill or liquid given during the study of a drug or dietary supplement that contains no medication or active ingredient. Usually study participants do not know if they are receiving a pill containing the drug or an identical-appearing placebo.

Osteoarthritis (OA)—The most common form of arthritis, characterized by erosion of the cartilage layer that lies between the bones in weight-bearing joints. OA is also known as degenerative joint disease or DJD.

Rheumatoid arthritis (RA)—An autoimmune disorder that can affect organ systems as well as the joints. It is much less common than OA but is potentially much more serious.

Rheumatologist—A physician, usually a pediatrician or internist, who has additional specialized training in the diagnosis and treatment of diseases that affect the bones, muscles, and joints.

Turmeric—A perennial herb of the ginger family used as a coloring agent as well as a spice in food preparation. It is used in some traditional Ayurvedic medicines for the relief of joint pain and inflammation.

Vegan—A vegetarian who excludes all animal products from the diet, including those that can be obtained without killing the animal. Vegans are also known as strict vegetarians. Some people believe that a vegan diet is helpful in managing arthritis.

---

additives or preservatives. There is, however, no clinical evidence as of 2012 that this diet is effective.

Another type of elimination diet, still recommended by naturopaths and some vegetarians, is called the nightshade elimination diet. It takes its name from a group of plants belonging to the family Solanaceae. There are over 1,700 plants in this category, including various herbs, potatoes, tomatoes, bell peppers, and eggplants as well as nightshade

itself, a poisonous plant also known as belladonna. The nightshade elimination diet began in the 1960s when a researcher in horticulture at Rutgers University noticed that his joint pain increased after eating vegetables belonging to the nightshade family. He eventually published a book recommending the elimination of vegetables and herbs in the nightshade family from the diet. However, there is no clinical evidence that people with OA will benefit from avoiding these foods, and nightshade vegetables may even help reduce arthritis symptoms.

Description

Osteoarthritis

WEIGHT REDUCTION. The major dietary recommendation approved by mainstream physicians for patients with OA is keeping one's weight at a healthy level. The reason is that OA primarily affects the weight-bearing joints of the body, and even a few pounds of extra weight can increase the pressure on damaged joints when the person moves or uses the joint. It is estimated that a force of three to six times the weight of the body is exerted across the knee joint when a person walks or runs; thus being only 10 pounds overweight increases the forces on the knee by 30 to 60 pounds with each step. Conversely, even a modest amount of weight reduction lowers the pain level in people with OA affecting the knee or foot joints. Obesity is a definite risk factor for developing OA; data from the National Institutes of Health (NIH) indicate that obese women are four times as likely to develop OA as non-obese women, while for obese men the risk is five times as great.

Although some doctors recommend trying a vegetarian or vegan diet as a safe approach to weight loss for patients with OA, most will approve any nutritionally sound calorie-reduction diet that works well for the individual patient.

It is important to note that weight reduction is not recommended for patients with RA who are at a healthy weight. Excessive weight loss, especially if caused by avoiding lots of foods or adopting fasting diets, may worsen RA symptoms. Too low of a body weight in people with RA may even cause faster destruction of joints than in people who are slightly overweight. Eating a healthy diet to avoid nutritional deficiencies is key.

DIETARY SUPPLEMENTS. Some dietary supplements that are commonly recommended for managing the discomfort of OA and/or slowing the rate of cartilage deterioration include:

- Chondroitin sulfate. Chondroitin sulfate is a compound found naturally as part of a large protein in the body that imparts elasticity to cartilage. The supplemental form is derived from animal or shark cartilage. A commonly recommended daily dose is 1200 mg (1.2 grams).
- Glucosamine. Glucosamine is a form of amino sugar that is thought to support the formation and repair of cartilage. It can be extracted from crab, shrimp, or lobster shells. A commonly recommended daily dose is 1500 mg (1.5 grams). Dietary supplements that combine chondroitin sulfate and glucosamine can be obtained over the counter in most pharmacies or health food stores.
- Botanical preparations. Some naturopaths recommend extracts of yucca, devil's claw, hawthorn berries, blueberries, and cherries. These extracts are thought to reduce inflammation in the joints and enhance the formation of cartilage. Powdered ginger has also been used to treat joint pain associated with OA.
- Vitamin therapy. Some doctors recommend increasing one's daily intake of vitamins C, E, A, and B$_6$, which are required to maintain cartilage structure.
- Avocado soybean unsaponifiables (ASU). ASU is a compound of the fractions of avocado oil and soybean oil that are left over from the process of making soap. It contains one-part avocado oil to two-parts soybean oil. ASU was first developed in France, where it is available by prescription only under the name Piasclédine, and has been used as a treatment for OA in the 1990s. It appears to work by reducing inflammation and helping cartilage to repair itself. ASU can be purchased in the United States as an over-the-counter dietary supplement. A common recommended daily dose is 300 mg (0.3 grams).

CAM DIETARY THERAPIES. Two alternative medical systems use dietary changes and herbal medicine to treat OA. The first is Ayurveda, the traditional medical system of India. Practitioners of Ayurveda regard OA as caused by an imbalance among the three *doshas*, or subtle energies, in the human body. This imbalance produces toxic by-products during digestion, known as *ama*, which lodge in the joints of the body instead of being eliminated through the colon. To remove these toxins from the joints, the digestive fire, or *agni*, must be increased. The Ayurvedic practitioner typically recommends adding such spices such as turmeric, cayenne pepper, and ginger to food, and undergoing a three- to five-day detoxification diet followed by a cleansing enema to purify the body.

Traditional Chinese medicine (TCM) treats OA with various compounds containing **ephedra** (a substance now banned in the United States and Canada), cinnamon, aconite, and coix. This combination herbal medicine has been used for at least 1,200 years in TCM, and is known as *Du Huo Ji Sheng Wan*, or Joint Strength. Most Westerners who try TCM for relief of OA, however, seem to find acupuncture more helpful as an alternative therapy than Chinese herbal medicines.

Rheumatoid arthritis

DIETARY ALTERATIONS. There is some indication that patients with RA benefit from cutting back on red meat consumption or switching entirely to a vegetarian or vegan diet.

Another dietary adjustment that appears to benefit some people with RA is switching from cooking oils that are high in **omega-6 fatty acids** (which increase inflammation) to oils that are high in **omega-3 fatty acids** (which reduce inflammation). This second group includes olive oil, canola oil, and **flaxseed** oil.

DIETARY SUPPLEMENTS. The most common dietary supplements recommended for patients with RA are as follows:

• Fish oils. The oils from cold-water fish have been reported to reduce inflammation and relieve joint pain in some patients with RA. A common recommended daily dose is 1 to 2 teaspoons. Consuming oily fish (e.g., salmon, trout, sardines) also may help reduce risk of heart disease, which is higher in people with arthritis.

• Plant oils. Studies suggest that plant oils that are high in gamma-linolenic acid (GLA) reduce inflammation in the joints. These plant oils include evening primrose oil, borage oil, and black currant oil. A common recommended daily dose is 200 to 300 mg (0.2–0.3 grams).

• Green tea. Drinking four cups of green tea per day is thought to benefit RA patients by reducing inflammation in the joints.

CAM DIETARY THERAPIES. Ayurvedic medicine recommends a compound of ginger, turmeric, boswellia, and ashwaganda to relieve the pain and fever associated with RA.

Traditional Chinese medicine (TCM) uses such plants as hare's ear (*Bupleurum falcatum*) and thunder god vine (*Tripterygium wilfordii*) to reduce fever and joint pain in patients with RA.

Function

Osteoarthritis

The function of dietary treatment for OA is to lower (or maintain) the individual's weight to a healthy level in order to minimize stress on damaged weight-bearing joints; to maintain the structure and composition of the cartilage in the joints; to protect the general health of tissues by including bioflavonoids and **antioxidants** in the diet; and by conducting food challenges, when appropriate, to determine whether specific foods are affecting the individual's symptoms.

Rheumatoid arthritis

Dietary treatment of RA is primarily used in addition to pharmaceutical treatment, as the disease cannot be managed by nutritional changes alone. Patients with RA must take a combination of medications, usually a combination of disease-modifying anti-rheumatic drugs (DMARDs) and nonsteroidal anti-inflammatory drugs (NSAIDs), to control pain, inflammation, and slow the progression of the disease. A well-balanced and healthful diet, however, can help to offset the depression that often accompanies RA and enable patients to maintain a normal schedule of activities. It also helps to prevent nutritional deficiencies in these patients that may be caused by the use of prescription drugs to control the disease. For instance, the steroids used to treat RA reduce the level of **calcium** absorption in the body, which may increase the risk of osteoporosis.

Benefits

Osteoarthritis

The benefits of weight reduction in overweight individuals with OA are a noticeable reduction in discomfort and improved range of motion in the affected joints. The benefits of dietary supplements vary from patient to patient depending on the specific joints affected and the degree of erosion of the joint cartilage.

Rheumatoid arthritis

The benefits of dietary adjustments or dietary supplements for RA vary considerably from patient to patient. Maintenance of a balanced diet, however, is valuable in preventing the nutritional deficiencies that sometimes occur in patients with RA as side effects of high dosages of DMARDs and NSAIDs. **Vitamin B_6** deficiencies have been associated with the development of RA, and vitamin B_6 supplementation may help reduce inflammation levels; patients should talk to their physicians before taking any supplements.

Precautions

Some general precautions for all people with arthritis:

• Before beginning any form of dietary treatment for joint pain, consult a physician to obtain an accurate diagnosis of the type of arthritis that is causing the pain. When RA is suspected, it is vital to get systemic treatment as soon as possible to minimize long-term damage to health.

- Consult a physician before taking any dietary supplements, as certain over-the-counter (nonprescription) and prescription medications can interact with these compounds. Chondroitin sulfate, for example, may increase bleeding time in some people, particularly if it is taken together with aspirin.
- Purchase dietary supplements only from well-established companies that can be held accountable for the quality of their products.
- Do not stop taking any medications currently prescribed by a doctor without consulting him or her.
- If maintaining a primarily vegetarian diet, be aware of the potential for iron deficiency.

People with either form of arthritis who are more than 30 pounds (13.6 kg) overweight, are pregnant, nursing, under age 18, or diagnosed with type 2 diabetes, kidney disorders, or liver disorders should consult a physician before attempting a weight-reduction program.

Osteoarthritis

People with diabetes should monitor blood sugar levels more frequently if they are taking **glucosamine**, because it is an amino sugar. Similarly, individuals who are taking blood thinners should have their blood clotting time checked periodically if they are taking chondroitin sulfate.

Rheumatoid arthritis

Plant oils containing gamma linolenic acid (GLA) have been reported to cause intestinal gas, bloating, diarrhea, and nausea in some people. In addition, these oils may interact with other prescription medications, particularly blood thinners. Some borage seed oil preparations contain ingredients known pyrrolizidine alkaloids, or PAs, that can harm the liver or worsen liver disease. Only forms of borage oil that are certified to be PA-free should be used. Evening primrose oil may interact with a group of tranquilizers used in the treatment of schizophrenia known as phenothiazines. This group of drugs includes chlorpromazine and prochlorperazine.

Fish oil may affect the rate of blood clotting and cause nausea or a fishy odor of the breath in some people. Some fish oil supplements may also contain overly high levels of **vitamin A**. In addition, patients who take fish oil supplements must usually take them for several months before they experience any benefits.

QUESTIONS TO ASK YOUR DOCTOR

- Would you recommend glucosamine and chondroitin supplements for mild OA?
- Have any of your other patients benefited from taking ASU or other dietary supplements for arthritis?
- What is your opinion of elimination diets as treatment for arthritis?
- Would you recommend a vegetarian diet for patients with OA as well as patients with RA?
- How can I reduce my risk of cardiovascular disease?

Risks

Osteoarthritis

Most dietary supplements for OA appear to be safe when purchased from reputable manufacturers and used as directed. Glucosamine and chondroitin sulfate have been reported to cause intestinal gas or mild diarrhea in some people. ASU causes nausea and skin rashes in some people.

Cost may be a consideration for some people, as these supplements are not usually covered by health insurance.

Rheumatoid arthritis

Chinese thunder god vine is reported to weaken bone structure and increase the risk of osteoporosis in patients with RA. Fish oils with high levels of vitamin A have been reported to cause vitamin A toxicity in some people.

Research and general acceptance

Osteoarthritis

Weight loss is universally accepted by medical practitioners as a positive way to decrease joint pain and improve the general health of people with OA.

No mainstream clinical studies have found that patients with OA benefit from elimination diets. With regard to dietary supplements, findings are mixed. A large study of glucosamine and chondroitin sulfate supplements, the Glucosamine/chondroitin Arthritis Intervention Trial (GAIT), done under the sponsorship of the National Center for Complementary and Alternative Medicine (NCCAM), reported in 2008 that a combination of these two supplements appeared to be beneficial to a small subgroup of patients with moderate to severe pain from OA. In individuals with only mild discomfort, the glucosamine/chondroitin supplement produced no greater pain relief than a placebo.

A 2009 study reviewed 35 studies of herbal medicines used to treat OA. The authors concluded that it is likely that ASU is beneficial, but that a large, well-designed study is needed to clarify the benefits. The same study reported that it is likely that a Chinese herbal remedy known as SKI 306X reduces pain from OA. SKI 306X is a combination of three herbs, *Clematis mandshurica*, *Trichosanthes kirilowii* and *Prunella vulgaris*.

Some clinical studies carried out in India report that an Ayurvedic compound that combines ginger, turmeric, and **zinc** reduced pain in patients with OA of the knees even when other aspects of Ayurvedic practice were not followed.

Rheumatoid arthritis

NCCAM has noted in a recent review of alternative treatments of RA that few high-quality human studies of these treatments have been published as of 2012. Several studies indicate that vegetarian or vegan diets and the **Mediterranean diet** can benefit patients with RA. According to NCCAM, fish oil supplements look promising, but more studies need to be done. They have been reported to reduce the risk of heart attacks in patients with RA as well as reduce joint pain and inflammation. **Green tea** has reduced joint swelling in mice with RA, but as of 2012, it had not been tested on human subjects. A study conducted at the University of Arizona reported in 2006 that turmeric by itself inhibits the destruction of joint tissue in rats with RA as well as reduces joint inflammation, but as of 2012, turmeric supplements had not been used in clinical trials with human subjects with RA.

Resources

BOOKS

Black, Jessica. *The Anti-Inflammation Diet and Recipe Book: Protect Yourself and Your Family from Heart Disease, Arthritis, Diabetes, Allergies—and More.* Alameda, CA: Hunter House, 2006.

Cannon, Christopher P. and Elizabeth Vierck. *The Complete Idiot's Guide to the Anti-Inflammation Diet.* Indianapolis, IN: Alpha Books, 2006.

Challem, Jack. *The Inflammation Syndrome: Your Nutrition Plan for Great Health, Weight Loss, and Pain-Free Living.* Hoboken, NJ: John Wiley & Sons, 2010.

WEBSITES

Betsch, Mara. "6 Dietary Changes That May Help Ease Rheumatoid Arthritis Pain." Health.com. http://www.health.com/health/gallery/0,,20387825,00.html (accessed June 23, 2012).

Linder, Larry. "Arthritis Food Myths." *Arthritis Today.* http://www.arthritistoday.org/nutrition-and-weight-loss/healthy-eating/food-and-inflammation/food-myths-arthritis.php (accessed July 23, 2012).

Mayo Clinic staff. "Osteoarthritis." MayoClinic.com http://www.mayoclinic.com/health/osteoarthritis/DS00019 (accessed June 23, 2012).

National Center for Complementary and Alternative Medicine. "Green Tea May Help Protect Against Rheumatoid Arthritis." http://nccam.nih.gov/research/results/spotlight/120808.htm (accessed July 23, 2012).

Physicians Committee for Responsible Medicine. "Foods and Arthritis." http://www.pcrm.org/health/health-topics/foods-and-arthritis (accessed July 23, 2012).

University of Maryland Medical Center. "Vitamin B_6 (Pyridoxine)." http://www.umm.edu/altmed/articles/vitamin-b6-000337.htm (accessed June 23, 2012).

ORGANIZATIONS

American Association of Naturopathic Physicians, 818 18th St. NW, Ste. 250, Washington, DC 20006, (202) 237-8150, (866) 538-2267, Fax: (202) 237-8152, member services@naturopathic.org, http://www.naturopathic.org.

Arthritis Foundation, PO Box 7669, Atlanta, GA 30357-0669, (800) 283-7800, http://www.arthritis.org.

National Center for Complementary and Alternative Medicine Clearinghouse, PO Box 7923, Gaithersburg, MD 20898, (888) 644-6226, Fax: (866) 464-3616, info@nccam.nih.gov, http://nccam.nih.gov.

National Institute of Arthritis and Musculoskeletal and Skin Diseases (NIAMS) Information Clearinghouse, 1 AMS Circle, Bethesda, MD 20892-3675, (301) 495-4484, (877) 226-4267, TTY: (301) 565-2966, Fax: (301) 718-6366, NIAMSinfo@mail.nih.gov, http://www.niams.nih.gov.

National Institute of Ayurvedic Medicine (NIAM), 584 Milltown Rd., Brewster, NY 10509, (845) 278-8700, http://niam.com.

Rebecca J. Frey, PhD
Tish Davidson, AM

Artificial preservatives

Definition

Artificial preservatives are a group of chemical substances added to food or to certain medications to slow or prevent spoilage, discoloration, or contamination by bacteria and other disease organisms. Most

Artificial preservatives

Antimicrobial agents	Antioxidants	Chelating agent
Benzoates. Inhibits the growth of molds, yeasts, and bacteria in acidic drinks and liquids, including fruit juice, vinegar, sparkling drinks, and soft drinks.	**Sulfites.** Prevents oxidation and inhibits the growth of yeasts and fungi in beer and wines, and preserves meats, dried potato products, and dried fruits.	**Disodium ethylenediaminetetraacetic acid (EDTA).** Delays spoilage (used in food processing).
Sodium benzoate. Used as an antimicrobial agent in foods with a pH below 3.6, including salad dressings, carbonated drinks, fruit juices, and Oriental food sauces such as soy sauce and duck sauce.	**Vitamin E.** Slows oxidation of fresh-cut fruits and vegetables, used to fortify breakfast cereals and pet foods.	**Polyphosphates.** Used as an anti-browning agent in dips and washes for fresh-peeled fruits and vegetables.
Sorbates. Prevents the growth of molds, yeasts, and fungi in foods or beverages.	**Vitamin C.** Prevents browning of fresh-cut apples, peaches, and other fruits.	**Citric acid.** Used as a flavoring agent and antioxidant in foods.
Propionates. Inhibits the growth of mold in baked goods.	**Butylated hydroxyanisole (BHA).** Prevents oxidation in butter, lard, meats, baked goods, beer, vegetable oils, potato chips and other snack foods, nuts and nut products, and dry mixes for beverages and desserts.	
Nitrites. Prevents the growth of bacteria, particularly *Clostridium botulinum* (bacterium responsible for botulism), in meat or smoked fish.	**Butylated hydroxytoluene (BHT).** Used in fats, oils, shortening, and similar products.	

(Table by PreMediaGlobal. © 2013 Cengage Learning.)

preservatives are categorized by the United States government as **food additives**.

Purpose

The use of artificial preservatives is an extension of centuries-old methods of food preservation, some of which involved adding naturally occurring chemicals to food. To keep food from spoiling before it could be eaten, early humans found ways to dry it or, in colder climates, freeze it. Drying or dehydrating foods, a process known as desiccation, worked well with fruits, herbs, some meats, and some vegetables. Another method for preserving fruit was **sugar** preservation, which involved cooking the fruit in a high concentration of sugar that discouraged the growth of bacteria. In terms of natural chemicals, vinegar, ethanol (beverage alcohol), olive oil, and salt have been used for centuries to preserve foods by pickling. Meats and some types of fish were preserved by smoking and curing, which draws moisture from the meat without cooking it. Smoking introduces **antioxidants** into meat or fish, while some spices used to flavor foods, such as curries and hot chilies, contain antimicrobial compounds.

As technology advanced, artificial preservatives were designed with the same goal as the earlier methods—to prevent food from spoiling or discoloring. Spoilage usually involves one of two processes: contamination by microorganisms or oxidation. The primary causes of contamination are bacteria, molds, fungi, and yeasts. Oxidation is the scientific name for the process that takes place in some foods when they combine with the oxygen in the atmosphere in the presence of heat, light, or certain metals. Oxidized foods typically turn brown, develop black spots, or acquire a bad or "off" smell. Cooking oils; oily foods like potato chips, sausage, or nuts; or buttery spreads that develop an unpleasant taste or smell are said to have gone rancid. Some **minerals** in food—particularly **iron** and copper—can speed up the process of food spoilage through oxidation. Preservatives that are added to food to prevent oxidation related to these minerals are called chelating agents.

Some antimicrobial preservatives are added to medications to prevent the growth of bacteria. Most of these preparations are topical, which means that they are intended for use on the outside of the body, such as the skin, the eyes, or the ears. Eye drops formulated to relieve dry eyes are the most common topical medications that may contain artificial preservatives, but some asthma drugs also contain benzoates or other antimicrobials. Sulfites (sometimes spelled sulphites) are added to asthma inhalers, injectable epinephrine, and some other medications to prevent browning of the solution.

Description

Most artificial preservatives are categorized by the federal government as food additives, which are defined by the Federal Food, Drug, and Cosmetic Act (FD&C) of 1938 as "any substance, the intended use of which results directly or indirectly, in its becoming a component or otherwise affecting the characteristics of food." A subcategory of food preservatives are classified as "generally recognized as safe" (GRAS), which means that the government accepts the current scientific consensus on their safety, based on either their use prior to 1958 or well-known scientific information.

Government regulations of artificial preservatives

In order to gain FDA approval, producers of artificial preservatives must submit an application to show:

- that the amount of the preservative that will be consumed is a safe amount
- that the preservative will not have a harmful cumulative effect in the diet
- whether or not the preservative is carcinogenic or has other toxic effects in humans or animals
- that the preservative does not change the appearance of the food

There are three major groups of artificial food preservatives: antimicrobial agents, antioxidants, and chelating agents.

Antimicrobial agents

Antimicrobial preservatives are added to food to destroy bacteria or to inhibit the growth of mold on foods.

BENZOATES. Benzoates are salts of benzoic acid, a weak acid that was at one time derived from benzoin resin, a gum obtained from the bark of trees native to Thailand and Indonesia. The benzoates used as food preservatives are potassium benzoate and sodium benzoate.

Potassium benzoate works best in products with a low pH (below 4.5). A substance's pH value is a measure of its acidity or alkalinity. Solutions with a pH below 7 are considered acidic, and those above 7 are alkaline. Potassium benzoate is used to inhibit the growth of molds, yeasts, and bacteria in some processed foods and beverages, including fruit juice and sparkling drinks. Potassium benzoate is used most commonly in soft drinks. It is listed on some products as being used to "protect taste" and "preserve freshness." When potassium benzoate is dissolved into liquid, it breaks down into sodium benzoate and the electrolyte potassium.

Sodium benzoate can be produced commercially by reacting sodium hydroxide with benzoic acid. It is used as an antimicrobial agent in foods with a pH below 3.6, such as salad dressings, carbonated drinks, fruit juices, and Asian food sauces such as **soy** sauce and duck sauce.

It is also used in some mouthwashes. Sodium benzoate occurs naturally in cranberries, prunes, greengage plums, cloves, cinnamon, and apples. Although the FDA limits the concentration of sodium benzoate as a preservative to 0.1%, organically grown cranberries and prunes may contain higher levels.

When sodium benzoate is added to beverages that contain **vitamin C** (ascorbic acid), the combination could produce small amounts of benzene, a chemical known to cause leukemia and other cancers at high levels of exposure. Though the amounts present in foods and beverages are very small, the FDA has worked with manufacturers to keep levels below 5 parts per billion (ppb), the acceptable amount established by the U.S. Environmental Protection Agency (EPA) for benzene in drinking water.

SORBATES. The sorbates are a group of antimicrobial food preservatives comprising sorbic acid and its three mineral salts: potassium sorbate, **calcium** sorbate, and sodium sorbate. The name of the group comes from the botanical name of the rowan tree, *Sorbus aucuparia*, because sorbic acid was first isolated from unripe rowan berries. In general, food manufacturers prefer the three salts of sorbic acid to the acid itself because they are easier to dissolve in water.

The sorbates are used to prevent the growth of molds, yeasts, and fungi in foods or beverages with a pH below 6.5. They are generally used at concentrations of 0.025%–0.10%. Potassium sorbate, which is made by reacting sorbic acid with potassium hydroxide, is a mild preservative. It is often used to stabilize wine as well as to prevent the growth of molds in cheese, yogurt, dry fruit, jelly, syrup, and baked goods such as cake. Allergic reactions to the sorbates are uncommon and limited to minor skin rashes or itching.

PROPIONATES. Propionates are salts of propionic acid. The three propionates most commonly used as food preservatives are calcium propionate, sodium propionate, and potassium propionate. They are used to inhibit the growth of mold in baked goods such as bread, cakes, pies, and rolls. The propionates are often used instead of benzoates in bakery products because they do not require an acidic environment to be effective. Calcium propionate is also added to animal feed to prevent milk fever in cows.

NITRITES. Nitrites are salts of nitrous acid that were used more often in the past for curing meat than they are now. The most commonly used nitrite in food preservation is sodium nitrite. When added to meat or smoked fish, it prevents the growth of bacteria, particularly *Clostridium botulinum*, the bacterium responsible for botulism, a potentially deadly disease. Sodium nitrite also turns meat an appealing dark red color when it interacts with myoglobin, the primary oxygen-carrying pigment in muscle tissue.

Nitrites are being gradually phased out of food processing for two reasons. The first reason is that they are toxic in large amounts; a lethal dose of nitrites for a human is 22 mg per kg of body weight. The second reason is that nitrites in meat can react with the breakdown products of amino acids in the acidic environment of the human stomach to form nitrosamines, substances that are known to be carcinogenic. For a manufacturer to be permitted to use sodium nitrite to prevent the growth of *C. botulinum* in smoked fish or meat, the manufacturer must show that the maximum amount of nitrite in the food will be no more than 200 parts per million (ppm). Sodium ascorbate, a salt of ascorbic acid (vitamin C), is often added to foods containing nitrites to inhibit or prevent the formation of nitrosamines.

It is highly unlikely that a person would consume a lethal amount of nitrites through food, but according to the American Cancer Society, studies have linked eating large amounts of processed meats, which contain nitrites, with an increased risk of colorectal cancer.

Antioxidants

Antioxidants are preservatives added to oils and fatty foods to prevent them from becoming rancid.

SULFITES. The sulfites are a group of compounds containing charged molecules of sulfur compounded with oxygen. There are five used as preservatives: sodium sulfite, sodium bisulfite, sodium metabisulfite, potassium bisulfite, and potassium metabisulfite. They are applied to foods as dips or sprays. Sodium metabisulfite and potassium metabisulfite are commonly used to stabilize wine or beer. When added to these fluids, the sulfite compounds release sulfur dioxide gas, which prevents oxidation and also inhibits the growth of yeasts and fungi. Sodium sulfite is used to preserve meats, dried potato products, and dried fruits.

Sulfites have been used for centuries as food preservatives since they occur naturally in almost all wines. Of all the groups of food preservatives, however, sulfites are the most likely to produce hypersensitivity reactions. People with asthma or allergies to aspirin are at an elevated risk for this type of reaction. A severe systemic reaction known as anaphylaxis or anaphylactic shock may be fatal and requires immediate treatment at an emergency room. Anaphylaxis is characterized by hives, difficulty breathing, and cardiovascular collapse.

VITAMIN E. Vitamin E (tocopherol) is a fat-soluble vitamin that occurs as a natural antioxidant in many foods, particularly vegetable oils, **whole grains**, nuts, wheat germ, and green leafy vegetables. It may be added to fresh-cut fruits and vegetables to slow oxidation. It is also used to fortify some breakfast cereals and pet foods.

VITAMIN C. Vitamin C (ascorbic acid) also occurs naturally in many fruits and vegetables, particularly citrus fruits. It is a water-soluble vitamin. The salts of ascorbic acid—sodium ascorbate, calcium ascorbate, and potassium ascorbate—are also water-soluble and are often added to fresh-cut apples, peaches, and other fruits to prevent browning. These three compounds are not fat soluble and cannot be used to prevent **fats** from going rancid. To protect fats or oils from oxidation, a fat-soluble ester of ascorbic acid, known as ascorbyl palmitate, must be used.

BUTYLATED HYDROXYANISOLE (BHA). BHA, which is a white or slightly yellow waxy solid in its pure form, is widely used in the food industry to prevent oxidation in butter, lard, meats, baked goods, beer, vegetable oils, potato chips and other snack foods, nuts and nut products, dry mixes for beverages and desserts, and many other foods. BHA is also used in cosmetics, particularly lipsticks and eye shadows. It is effective as an antioxidant because oxygen reacts preferentially with it rather than with the fats or oils containing it, thereby protecting them from spoilage. Although the FDA considers BHA a GRAS substance when its content is no greater than 0.02% of the total fat content of the product by weight (200 ppm), the National Toxicology Program (NTP) of the Department of Health and Human Services (HHS) listed it in 2011 as "reasonably anticipated to be a human carcinogen" on the basis of experimental findings in animals. The NTP stated that the maximum content of BHA in various foods that it sampled ranged from 2 to 1,000 ppm.

BUTYLATED HYDROXYTOLUENE (BHT). BHT is similar to BHA in its structure and uses as an antioxidant, although it is ordinarily a white powder rather than a waxy substance at room temperature. BHT is often added to packaging materials as well as directly to fats, oils, shortening, and similar products. The FDA first approved it as a food preservative in 1954. BHT has been banned in Japan, Romania, Sweden, and Australia but not in the United States. Although the use of BHT is controversial, it has not been shown conclusively to be carcinogenic.

Chelating agents

Chelating agents work by binding or sequestering metal ions, usually iron or **copper**, in certain foods in

KEY TERMS

Anaphylaxis—A severe and potentially fatal systemic allergic reaction characterized by itching, hives, fainting, and respiratory symptoms. Sulfites may trigger anaphylaxis in a small number of people who are unusually sensitive to them.

Antimicrobial—A type of food preservative that works by preventing the growth of bacteria, fungi, molds, or yeast in foods.

Antioxidant—A type of food preservative that prevents rancidity in oils and fatty foods.

Botulism—A potentially deadly disease characterized by respiratory and musculoskeletal paralysis caused by a bacterium called *Clostridium botulinum*.

Carcinogen—A substance or other agent that causes cancer. Some artificial preservatives have been banned in the United States on the grounds that they may be carcinogens or produce carcinogenic substances when added to food.

Chelating agent—A type of food preservative that works by binding (or sequestering) metal ions (usually iron or copper) in certain foods in order to prevent the metals from oxidizing and speeding up spoilage.

Food additive—Defined by the Federal Food, Drug, and Cosmetic Act (FD&C) of 1938 as "any substance, the intended use of which results directly or indirectly, in its becoming a component or otherwise affecting the characteristics of food." Food additives include flavoring and coloring agents as well as artificial preservatives.

Nitrosamine—Any of various organic compounds produced by the interaction of nitrites in food with the breakdown products of amino acids. Nitrosamines are also found in tobacco smoke. Some nitrosamines are powerful carcinogens.

Oxidation—In food chemistry, the process that takes place in some foods when they combine with the oxygen in the atmosphere in the presence of heat, light, or such metals as iron or copper.

pH—A measure of the acidity or alkalinity of a solution. Solutions with a pH below 7 are considered acidic while those above 7 are alkaline. A pH of exactly 7 (pure water) is neutral.

Rancid—Spoiled; having a bad smell or taste.

order to prevent the metals from oxidizing and speeding up spoilage.

DISODIUM ETHYLENEDIAMINETETRAACETIC ACID (EDTA). EDTA is used in food processing to bind **manganese**, cobalt, iron, or copper ions in order to slow spoilage in foods such as salad dressing, margarine, soft drinks, and canned shellfish. It is sometimes added to eye drops to reinforce the action of other preservatives. It is also used in dentistry to wash out the teeth during root canal procedures and in medicine to treat mercury or lead poisoning. EDTA is added to soft drinks containing both ascorbic acid (vitamin C) and sodium benzoate to prevent the formation of benzene.

POLYPHOSPHATES. Polyphosphates are chelating agents with limited solubility in cold water that are used in low concentrations (0.5%–2%) as anti-browning agents in dips and washes for fresh-peeled fruits and vegetables. They are also used to soften water and to remove mineral deposits from beverage production equipment. Polyphosphates are considered nontoxic.

CITRIC ACID. Citric acid, which is found naturally in citrus fruits, can be used not only as a flavoring agent and antioxidant in foods, but also as a chelating agent in soaps and detergents. By chelating the

minerals that are present in hard water, citric acid allows the cleaning agents to produce foam without the need for added water softeners. Allergic reactions to citric acid are rare; it is regarded as a safe food additive by all major international food regulatory organizations as well as by the FDA, because excess citric acid is easily metabolized by the body and excreted.

Precautions

The categorization of a preservative is never permanent; it may change as new information about the preservative's safety is reported and analyzed. Certain preservatives that were once considered safe—most notably sulfites and nitrites—have since been banned or greatly restricted in their permissible uses. Information about the current status of more than 3,000 substances (including coloring and flavoring agents as well as preservatives) that the FDA has either approved as food additives or listed or affirmed as GRAS may be obtained from the U.S. Food and Drug Administration's EAFUS (Everything Added to Food in the United States) database, available online: http://www.accessdata.fda.gov/scripts/fcn/fcnNavigation.cfm?rpt=eafusListing&displayAll=true.

Some people may wish to avoid eating meat containing nitrites such as bacon, sausage, and ham. Although no studies have proven that nitrites cause cancer, people concerned about the effects of nitrites or nitrates should consult with their doctor. Studies have indicated a link between consuming large amounts of processed meat and an increased risk of colorectal cancer, but it is not known whether nitrites are the cause or if other factors contribute to the risk. Nitrosamines, however, are known carcinogens, and may be produced when nitrites are combined with other substances, especially **protein**.

Some hypersensitivity reactions to food preservatives occur in relation to food eaten at restaurants. Restaurant foods are most likely to be the culprit when the person has a reaction to a specific dish served in a restaurant but not to that same food when made at home. People who already know that they are sensitive to sulfites may need to ask about specific dishes at a restaurant ahead of time to inquire whether they are made from foods containing high levels of sulfites.

Complications

Allergic reactions to artificial preservatives (or coloring or flavoring additives) in food may involve the skin (flushing, itching, or rashes), the digestive system (nausea, vomiting, or diarrhea), the respiratory system (wheezing, cough, or runny nose), or the muscles (cramping or aching sensations). Some doctors think that reactions to food additives are underdiagnosed because they are not often suspected; most maintain, however, that hypersensitivity to food additives involves at most 1% of the adult population and perhaps 2% of children.

The food preservatives most likely to cause allergic reactions are the sulfites and the benzoates. Prior to 1986, sulfites were commonly added to fresh produce in supermarkets and on restaurant salad bars to prevent browning. Reports of sensitivity reactions, however, led the FDA to ban the use of sulfites on fresh produce, especially lettuce put out on salad bars. The FDA requires all foods containing more than 10 ppm of sulfites to declare sulfites on the label. Foods containing less than 10 ppm of sulfites have not been shown to cause allergic symptoms, even in people who are hypersensitive to sulfites.

Testing for sulfite allergy should be done only by a physician who has been trained in this procedure and has some experience in using it. The test involves administering increasing amounts of sulfites by mouth to the patient while the doctor monitors the patient's lung function and other vital signs such as blood pressure and pulse rate. A sudden and

significant drop in lung function indicates that the patient is sensitive to sulfites.

People allergic to high levels of sulfites should avoid anything containing or garnished with bottled (non-frozen) lemon or lime juice, wine, molasses, grape juices, pickled cocktail onions, dried potatoes, wine vinegar, gravies or sauces, Maraschino cherries, fruit toppings, and sauerkraut. People who are sensitive to moderate or low levels of sulfites should also avoid fresh mushrooms, canned clams, avocado dip or guacamole, pickles and relishes, maple syrup, corn syrup, fresh shrimp, apple cider, and cider vinegar.

Sodium benzoate has been reported to cause skin rashes or facial swelling in some people when used as a preservative in acidic foods and beverages, and to worsen asthma attacks in some patients taking asthma medications. Reactions to benzoates, however, are a very low percentage of **food allergies**; one team of physicians in Italy rated reactions to benzoates as no more than 2% of all allergic responses to foods or drugs.

Consumers who are concerned about a specific artificial preservative in their food can check for its presence by reading the labels of processed foods, which are required by law to state the ingredients in order by weight from the greatest amount to the least. Those who wish to cut down on their intake of preservatives in general could try growing their own produce, or purchasing fresh fruits and vegetables only from local farmers during the growing season.

To report allergic reactions to preservatives or other food additives, consumers should contact the FDA's consumer complaint coordinator for their region. Contact information is available on the FDA website: http://www.fda.gov/safety/reportaproblem/consumercomplaintcoordinators/default.htm. If the problem concerns food eaten in or purchased from a restaurant, however, the incident should be reported to the local or state health department.

Parental concerns

In general, food preservatives are no more likely to cause allergic reactions in children than either coloring agents or flavoring agents, which are the other major categories of food additives. Some people develop hives, itching, or nasal congestion when exposed to one particular type of yellow food coloring, FD&C 5, known as tartrazine.

Resources

BOOKS

Institute of Medicine (IOM). *Dietary Reference Intakes for Water, Potassium, Sodium, Chloride, and Sulfate.* Washington, DC: The National Academies Press, 2006.

Russell, N. J., and G. W. Gould. *Food Preservatives.* 2nd ed. New York: Kluwer Academic/Plenum Publishers, 2003.

PERIODICALS

"Benzoate Contained in Some Antiasthmatic Drugs." *International Journal of Immunopathology and Pharmacology* 17 (May–Aug 2004): 225–26.

Wilson, B.G., and S.L. Bahna. "Adverse Reactions to Food Additives." *Annals of Allergy, Asthma and Immunology* 95 (December 2005): 499–507.

OTHER

National Toxicology Program (NTP). *Report on Carcinogens.* 12th edition. Washington, DC: U.S. Department of Health and Human Services, 2011. http://ntp.niehs.nih.gov/?objectid = 03C9AF75-E1BF-FF40-DBA9EC 0928DF8B15 (accessed August 21, 2012).

WEBSITES

American Cancer Society. "Food Additives, Safety, and Organic Foods." http://www.cancer.org/Healthy/Eat HealthyGetActive/ACSGuidelinesonNutritionPhysical ActivityforCancerPrevention/acs-guidelines-on-nutrition-and-physical-activity-for-cancer-prevention-food-additives (accessed August 21, 2012).

Center for Science in the Public Interest (CSPI). "Chemical Cuisine: Learn about Food Additives." http://www.cspinet.org/reports/chemcuisine.htm?&LS-2659 (accessed August 21, 2012).

Epley, Richard J., Paul B. Addis and Joseph J. Warthesen. "Nitrite in Meat." University of Minnesota Extension. http://www.extension.umn.edu/distribution/nutrition/DJ0974.html (accessed August 21, 2012).

Hardin, Ashley. "Myth or Fact: Hot Dogs Cause Cancer." DukeHealth.org. http://www.dukehealth.org/health_library/health_articles/myth-or-fact-hot-dogs-cause-cancer (accessed August 21, 2012).

International Food Information Council (IFIC) and U.S. Food and Drug Administration (FDA). *Food Ingredients & Colors.* http://www.fda.gov/food/foodingredientspack aging/ucm094211.htm (accessed August 14, 2012).

U.S. Department of Agriculture Food Safety and Inspection Service (FSIS). "Food Labeling: Additives in Meat and Poultry Products." http://www.fsis.usda.gov/Factsheets/Additives_in_Meat_&_Poultry_Products/index.asp (accessed August 14, 2012).

U.S. Food and Drug Administration (FDA). "Everything Added to Food in the United States (EAFUS)." (updated November 14, 2011). FDA.gov. http://www.accessdata.fda.gov/scripts/fcn/fcnNavigation. cfm?rpt = eafusListing&displayAll = true (accessed August 15, 2012).

U.S. Food and Drug Administration (FDA). "Guidance for Industry: Frequently Asked Questions about GRAS." http://www.fda.gov/Food/GuidanceComplianceRegu latoryInformation/GuidanceDocuments/FoodIngre dientsandPackaging/ucm061846.htm (accessed August 15, 2012)

U.S. Food and Drug Administration (FDA). "Questions and Answers on the Occurrence of Benzene in Soft Drinks and Other Beverages." http://www.fda.gov/Food/Food Safety/FoodContaminantsAdulteration/Chemical Contaminants/Benzene/ucm055131.htm (accessed August 14, 2012).

ORGANIZATIONS

Center for Science in the Public Interest, 1220 L St. NW, Ste. 300, Washington, DC 20005, (202) 332-9110, Fax: (202) 265-4954, http://www.cspinet.org.

Institute of Food Technologists (IFT), 525 W. Van Buren, Ste. 1000, Chicago, IL 60607, (312) 782-8424, (800) 438-3663, Fax: (312) 782-8348, info@ift.org, http://www.ift.org.

U.S. Food and Drug Administration, 10903 New Hampshire Ave., Silver Spring, MD 20993-0002, (888) INFO-FDA (463-6332), http://www.fda.gov.

Rebecca J. Frey, PhD
Liz Swain

Artificial sweeteners

Definition

Artificial sweeteners, which are also called **sugar** substitutes, alternative sweeteners, or non-sugar sweeteners, are substances used to replace sugar in foods and beverages. They can be divided into two large groups: nutritive sweeteners, which add some energy value **(calories)** to food; and nonnutritive sweeteners, which are also called high-intensity sweeteners because they are used in very small quantities and add no energy value to food. Nutritive sweeteners include the natural sugars—sucrose (table sugar; a compound of glucose

Artificial sweeteners

Sweetener	Times sweeter than sugar	Calories	Brand name(s)
aspartame	200	4 kcal/g	Nutrasweet and Equal
saccharin	200–700	0	Sweet'N Low, Twin, and Necta Sweet
acesulfame-K (potassium)	200	0	Sunett and Sweet One
neotame	7,000–13,000	0	Neotame
sucralose	600	0	Splenda

SOURCE: Food and Drug Administration, U.S. Department of Health and Human Services

(Table by GGS Information Services. © 2013 Cengage Learning.)

and fructose), fructose (found in fruit as well as table sugar), and galactose (milk sugar)—as well as the polyols, which are a group of carbohydrate compounds that are not sugars but provide about half the calories of the natural sugars. The polyols are sometimes called sugar replacers, sugar-free sweeteners, sugar alcohols, or novel sugars. Polyols occur naturally in plants but can also be produced commercially. They include such compounds as sorbitol, mannitol, xylitol, and hydrogenated starch hydrolysates.

Nonnutritive sweeteners are synthetic compounds that range between 160 and 13,000 times as sweet as sucrose, which is the standard for the measurement of sweetness. There are five nonnutritive sweeteners approved by the Food and Drug Administration (FDA) for use in the United States. They are saccharin, aspartame, acesulfame potassium (or acesulfame-K), sucralose, and neotame. There are other nonnutritive sweeteners that have been approved for use elsewhere in the world by the Scientific Committee on Food (SCF) of the European Commission, the Joint Expert Committee of Food Additions (JECFA) of the United Nations Food and Agricultural Organization, and the World Health Organization (WHO) but have not been approved by the FDA. These substances are alitame, cyclamate, neohesperidine dihydrochalcone, stevia, and thaumatin. All of these will be described in further detail below.

The FDA uses two categories to classify both nutritive and nonnutritive sweeteners for regulatory purposes. Some are classified as *food additives*, which is a term that was introduced by the Federal Food, Drug, and Cosmetic (FD&C) Act of 1938. This legislation was passed by Congress in response to a mass poisoning tragedy that took the lives of over a hundred people in 1937. A company in Tennessee that manufactured an antibacterial drug known as sulfanilamide, which had been used safely in powdered or pill form to treat childhood infections, dissolved the sulfanilamide in diethylene glycol—related to the active ingredient in automobile antifreeze—in order to market it as a liquid medicine. Diethylene glycol is highly toxic to human beings and household pets, causing painful death from kidney failure. In 1937 there was no requirement for medications to be tested for toxicity before being placed on the market. The FD&C Act of 1938 thus included a legal definition of a food additive as "any substance, the intended use of which results directly or indirectly, in its becoming a component or otherwise affecting the characteristics of food."

The FDA asks the following questions in evaluating a proposed new sweetener as a food additive:

- How is the sweetener made?
- What are its properties when it is added to foods or beverages?
- How much of the sweetener will be digested or otherwise absorbed by the body?
- Are certain groups of people likely to be more susceptible than others to the additive?
- Does the sweetener have any known toxic effects, including hereditary disorders or cancer?

Other sweeteners are classified as *generally regarded as safe* or GRAS, and are not defined for legal purposes as **food additives**. The GRAS category was created in 1958 when the FD&C Act was modified by the passage of the Food Additives Amendment. A sweetener, whether nutritive or nonnutritive, can be given GRAS status on the basis of "experience based on common use in food" or a scientific consensus represented by published studies. Sorbitol and a few other polyols have GRAS status along with the natural sugars. Most artificial sweeteners, however, are considered food additives by the FDA.

Purpose

Artificial sweeteners are used in food products for several reasons: to lower the calorie content of soda pop and other sweetened drinks and foods as part of weight reduction and weight maintenance diets; to assist patients with diabetes in controlling blood sugar levels more effectively; and to lower the risk of tooth decay (e.g., in chewing gum). They are also added as excipients (inert substances used to make drugs easier to take in tablet or liquid form) to some prescription medications to disguise unpleasant tastes because they do not react with the active drug ingredients as natural sugars sometimes do. Sorbitol and mannitol are commonly added to toothpaste, mouthwash, breath mints, cough drops, cough syrups, sugarless gum, over-the-counter liquid

KEY TERMS

Acceptable daily intake level (ADI)—The level of a substance that a person can consume every day over a lifetime without risk. The ADIs for artificial sweeteners are very conservative measurements.

Carcinogen—A substance or other agent that causes cancer. Some artificial sweeteners have been banned in the United States and elsewhere on the grounds that they may be carcinogens.

Excipient—An inert substance, such as certain gums or starches, used to make drugs easier to take by allowing them to be formulated into tablets or liquids. Some artificial sweeteners are used as excipients.

Food additive—Defined by the Federal Food, Drug, and Cosmetic Act (FD&C) of 1938 as "any substance, the intended use of which results directly or indirectly, in its becoming a component or otherwise affecting the characteristics of food."

Fructose—A simple sugar that occurs naturally in sucrose and fruit. It can be added in combination with sucrose in the form of high-fructose corn syrup (HFCS) to sweeten foods because it is sweeter than sucrose. Large amounts of fructose can cause diarrhea in infants and young children.

Generally recognized as safe (GRAS)—A phrase used by the federal government to refer to exceptions to the FD&C Act of 1938 as modified by the Food Additives Amendment of 1958. Sweeteners that have a scientific consensus on their safety, based on either their use prior to 1958 or to well-known scientific information, may be given GRAS status.

Gulf war syndrome (GWS)—A disorder characterized by a wide range of symptoms, including skin rashes, migraine headaches, chronic fatigue, arthritis, and muscle cramps, possibly related to military service in the Persian Gulf war of 1991. GWS was briefly attributed to the troops' high consumption of beverages containing aspartame, but this explanation has been discredited.

High-intensity sweetener—Another term for nonnutritive sweetener, used because these substances add sweetness to food with very little volume.

Nonnutritive sweetener—Any sweetener that offers little or no energy value when added to food.

Nutritive sweetener—Any sweetener that adds some energy value to food.

Phenylketonuria (PKU)—A rare inherited metabolic disorder resulting in accumulation of phenylalanine, an amino acid, in the body. It can lead to intellectual disability and seizures. People with PKU should not use products containing the artificial sweetener aspartame because it is broken down into phenylalanine (and other products) during digestion.

Sucrose—The natural sweetener commonly used as table sugar; sucrose is a compound of two simple sugars, glucose and fructose. It is used as the standard for measuring the sweetening power of high-intensity artificial sweeteners.

---

antacids, and similar personal oral care products to add bulk to the product's texture as well as minimize the risk of tooth decay.

In addition to adding a sweet flavor, artificial sweeteners are also used in the manufacture of baked goods, beverages, syrups, and other food products to improve texture, add bulk, retard spoilage, or as part of a fermentation process. The polyols in particular are used to retard spoilage because they do not support the growth of mold or bacteria to the same extent as natural sugars.

Description

Nonnutritive sweeteners approved by the FDA

There are seven nonnutritive sweeteners approved by the FDA for use in the United States:

- Acesulfame potassium (acesulfame-K). Acesulfame potassium is a high-intensity nonnutritive sweetener that is about 200 times sweeter than sucrose; 95% of it is excreted from the body unchanged. It was discovered by a German company, Hoechst AG, in 1967. It was first approved by the FDA for use in nonalcoholic beverages in 1998 and for general use in 2003. In addition to its usefulness in reducing the calorie content of foods, in diabetic diets, and in preventing tooth decay, acesulfame potassium remains stable at the high temperatures used for cooking and baking, has a long shelf life, does not leave any bitter aftertaste, and combines well with other sweeteners. It is sold under the brand names ACK, Sunett, Sweet & Safe, and Sweet One.

- Aspartame. Aspartame, which is also about 200 times sweeter than sugar, was discovered in 1965 by a researcher at Searle Laboratories working on anti-ulcer medications. It is unusual among nonnutritive sweeteners in that it is completely broken down during digestion into its basic components—the amino acids aspartic acid and phenylalanine plus a small amount of methanol. Aspartame was approved by the FDA for tabletop use in 1981 and for use in carbonated beverages in 1983. As of the early 2000s, the United States used 75% of the aspartame produced in the world, with 70% of this amount consumed in diet beverages. Aspartame is the nonnutritive sweetener that has received the greatest amount of negative attention in the mass media because of a rumor that it caused Gulf War syndrome (GWS) in veterans of the Persian Gulf conflict of 1991, and because of a study done in Europe in 2005 that linked aspartame to two types of cancer (leukemia and lymphomas) in female laboratory rats. In response to the 2005 European study, the National Cancer Institute (NCI) conducted a study of half a million people in the United States in 2006 and found no connection between cancer rates and aspartame consumption. The details of this study can be found in a fact sheet available on the NCI website. Another study conducted by the National Toxicology Program (NTP) of the National Institute of Environmental Health Sciences (NIEHS) of aspartame as a possible carcinogen found no evidence that the sweetener causes cancer in humans. Aspartame is sold under the brand names NutraSweet, Equal, and Sugar Twin (blue box). Although it is considered safe for consumption in the United States, it is under review by the European Food Safety Authority.

- Neotame. Neotame is similar chemically to aspartame but is between 7,000 and 13,000 times sweeter than sugar. In July 2002, neotame was approved as a general-purpose sweetener by the FDA. Neotame is partially absorbed in the small intestine, the remainder excreted in urine and feces. It is not concentrated in any body organs and has not been identified as a cancer risk. Like acesulfame potassium, neotame has a clean taste with no bitter aftertaste, combines well with other sweeteners, and is stable when used in cooking and baking. It is also used to enhance the flavors of fruit and other ingredients in food. Neotame is manufactured in the United States by the NutraSweet Company of Mount Prospect, Illinois, but does not have a commercial or brand name.

- Saccharin. Saccharin is the oldest nonnutritive sweetener, having been discovered in 1879 by a chemist working at Johns Hopkins University. It is about 200 to 700 times as sweet as sugar. It was used extensively during World Wars I and II, when sugar was rationed in the United States as well as in Europe. It is still the least expensive high-intensity sweetener used around the world—about 65 million pounds (29 million kg) per year in the late 1990s. Saccharin passes through the body essentially unchanged. It was so widely used in the United States that it was considered a GRAS substance when the Food Additives Amendment was passed in 1958, but it lost that status when studies performed on laboratory rats in the 1970s indicated that it might cause bladder cancer. At that point Congress mandated that all foods containing saccharin must carry a warning label that they might be hazardous to health. Later studies indicated that the bladder tumors in rats are caused by a mechanism that does not operate in humans, and that there is no evidence that saccharin is unsafe for humans. In 2000 the NTP took saccharin off its list of carcinogens and the saccharin-warning label was removed from food. Details of the controversy over saccharin and cancer can be found on the NCI website. Saccharin is presently sold under the trade names of Sweet 'N Low, Sweet Twin, and Necta Sweet.

- Sucralose. Sucralose is unusual in that it is the only nonnutritive sweetener made from sugar, but it is about 600 times as sweet as table sugar. Sucralose is manufactured from sugar by substituting three chlorine atoms for three hydroxyl groups in the sugar molecule. Only about 11% of sucralose is absorbed during digestion; the remainder is excreted unchanged. The FDA approved sucralose in 1998 as a tabletop sweetener and in 1999 as a general-purpose sweetener. The acceptable daily intake (ADI) for sucralose is 5 mg per kilogram of body weight per day. Like acesulfame potassium, sucralose is highly heat-stable and works well in foods that must be baked or cooked. Sucralose is sold under the trade name Splenda for table use.

- Stevia. Stevia is a sweetener derived from a shrub native to South America. The FDA has designated certain refined preparations of stevia as GRAS, although the plant itself or plant extracts are not approved.

- Luo han guo fruit extract, or monk fruit; sold under the brand name Nectresse.

Nonnutritive sweeteners not approved for use in the United States

- Alitame. Alitame is a compound of aspartic acid, D-alanine, and an amide; it is 2,000 times sweeter than sugar. In 1986 it was reviewed by the FDA, which found the application to be deficient. As of 2012, alitame was approved for use only in Australia, New Zealand, Mexico, and China.

• Cyclamate. Cyclamate, which is about 30 times sweeter than sugar, was used as a nonnutritive sweetener in the United States until 1969, when it was shown to cause cancer in laboratory rats when combined with saccharin. Although cyclamate by itself was found by the National Academy of Sciences not to be a carcinogen in 1985 and is approved for use in over 50 countries, it has not been reinstated by the FDA for use in the United States.

• Neohesperidine dihydrochalcone. Neohesperidine dihydrochalcone is a compound that is about 1,500 times sweeter than sugar and adds a slight licorice flavor to foods and beverages. The FDA considers neohesperidine GRAS as a flavoring but not as a sweetener.

• Thaumatin. Thaumatin is an intensely sweet mixture of proteins that also acts as a flavor enhancer. The FDA has given thaumatin GRAS status as a flavor adjunct but had not approved it as a sweetener as of 2012.

Precautions

Artificial sweeteners are generally regarded as safe when used appropriately. The official position of the Academy of Nutrition and Dietetics is that nutritive and nonnutritive sweeteners are safe as long as they are consumed in moderation and a person's overall diet follows the current federation recommendations for nutrition.

The Institute of Medicine (IOM) maintains measurements of acceptable daily intake (ADI) levels for artificial sweeteners approved for use in the United States. The ADI is a regulatory definition that is often misunderstood. It is a very conservative estimate of the amount of a sweetener that can be safely consumed on a daily basis over the course of a person's lifetime. The ADI is *not* intended to be used as a specific point at which safe use ends and health risks begin, as occasional use of an artificial sweetener over the ADI is not of concern. To use aspartame as an example, its ADI is 50 mg per kilogram of body weight per day. An adult weighing 150 pounds (68 kg) would have to drink 20 12-ounce containers of diet soft drink containing aspartame, eat 42 servings of gelatin, or use 97 packets of tabletop sweetener to reach the ADI.

Some specific artificial sweeteners must be used cautiously by certain groups of people:

• Polyols: Some polyols—most commonly mannitol and sorbitol—have a laxative effect in some people if they are consumed in large amounts (more than 50 g/day of sorbitol or 20 g/day of mannitol). People with diabetes may wish to limit their consumption of products containing polyols or increase their use

gradually until they see how their bodies react to these sweeteners.

• Aspartame: Because aspartame is broken down in the body to the amino acid phenylalanine, foods or beverages containing aspartame should not be used by people with phenylketonuria (PKU), a rare inherited disease that causes phenylalanine to accumulate in the body. The FDA requires all products containing aspartame sold in the United States to be labeled with the following warning: "Phenylketonurics: Contains Phenylalanine." Although the breakdown products of neotame also include phenylalanine, the amount is so small that it does not affect people with PKU.

Interactions

There are no known interactions with prescription drugs caused by the use of nutritive or nonnutritive sweeteners. As was noted above, some nonnutritive sweeteners are considered useful excipients for medications precisely because they are chemically inert.

Parental concerns

There have been concerns expressed about the use of artificial sweeteners by children because children consume more sweeteners, both nutritive and nonnutritive, per pound of body weight on a daily basis than adults. The use of fruit juice and other sweet beverages by children has greatly increased since the 1980s; however, studies indicate that even children who drink large amounts of diet soda and other beverages usually remain well below the ADI levels for aspartame and other nonnutritive sweeteners. The chief risk to children's digestive health is fructose, which is found in such popular children's drinks as apple juice. Fructose is incompletely digested by children below the age of 18 months and may cause diarrhea in older children. Children diagnosed with nonspecific diarrhea may benefit from being given smaller amounts of fruit juice to drink.

During the early 1990s, some researchers identified a possible connection between high levels of aspartame consumption and attention-deficit **hyperactivity** disorder (ADHD) in children. Two studies published in 1994 in *Pediatrics* and the *New England Journal of Medicine* respectively, however, found no connection between aspartame and ADHD, even when the children were given 10 times the normal daily amount of aspartame. Aspartame and other nonnutritive sweeteners, however, may have an additive effect on nerve cell development when they are combined with food colorings. This possibility was suggested by a 2006 study of laboratory mice in the

United Kingdom, but the implications for humans are far from clear.

High intake of sweeteners added to food is of greatest concern during adolescence. As people age, they generally lower their intake of calories from added sugars. Fewer than 10% of adults over age 50 derive more than 25% of their daily calories from sugars, which is the maximal intake value established by the IOM. Nearly a third of adolescent females exceed this level, however, with almost a third of the extra sugar intake coming from carbonated beverages sweetened with high-fructose corn syrup. Although the rise in **obesity** in children and adolescents is a complex problem that cannot be attributed to a single factor, preliminary studies suggest that nonnutritive sweeteners may be useful in reducing adolescents' consumption of drinks sweetened with HFCS.

Resources

BOOKS

Nabors, Lyn O'Brien, ed. *Alternative Sweeteners*. 3rd ed. New York: M. Dekker, 2001.

Peña, Carolyn Thomas de la. *Empty Pleasures: The Story of Artificial Sweeteners from Saccharin to Splenda*. Chapel Hill: University of North Carolina Press, 2010.

PERIODICALS

Lau, K., et al. "Synergistic Interactions between Commonly Used Food Additives in a Developmental Neurotoxicity Test." *Toxicological Sciences* 90 (March 2006): 178–87.

Shaywitz, B.A., et al. "Aspartame, Behavior, and Cognitive Function in Children with Attention Deficit Disorder." *Pediatrics* 93 (January 1994): 70–75.

Wax, Paul M. "Elixirs, Diluents, and the Passage of the 1938 Federal Food, Drug, and Cosmetic Act." *Annals of Internal Medicine* 122 (March 15, 1995): 456–461. http://www.annals.org/cgi/content/full/122/6/456 (accessed October 2, 2012).

Whitehouse, C.R., J. Boullata, and L.A. McCauley. "The Potential Toxicity of Artificial Sweeteners." *AAOHN (American Association of Occupational Health Nurses) Journal* 56, no. 6 (2008): 251–59.

Wolraich, M.L., et al. "Effects of Diets High in Sucrose or Aspartame on the Behavior and Cognitive Performance of Children." *New England Journal of Medicine* 330 (February 3, 1994): 301–7.

Yang, Q. "Gain Weight by 'Going Diet?' Artificial Sweeteners and the Neurobiology of Sugar Cravings: Neuroscience 2010." *Yale Journal of Biology and Medicine* 83, no. 2 (2010): 101–8.

WEBSITES

Mayo Clinic staff. "Artificial Sweeteners: Understanding These and Other Sugar Substitutes." MayoClinic.com. http://www.mayoclinic.com/health/artificial-sweeteners/MY00073 (accessed September 28, 2012).

National Cancer Institute. "Artificial Sweeteners and Cancer: Questions and Answers." http://www.cancer.gov/cancertopics/factsheet/Risk/artificial-sweeteners (accessed October 2, 2012).

U.S. Food and Drug Administration. "Generally Recognized as Safe (GRAS)." http://www.fda.gov/Food/FoodIngredientsPackaging/GenerallyRecognizedas SafeGRAS/default.htm (accessed October 2, 2012).

ORGANIZATIONS

Academy of Nutrition and Dietetics, 120 South Riverside Plz., Ste. 2000, Chicago, IL 60606-6995, (312) 899-0040, (800) 877-1600, amacmunn@eatright.org, http://www.eatright.org.

Dietitians of Canada, 480 University Ave., Ste. 604, Toronto, Ontario, Canada M5G 1V2, (416) 596-0857, Fax: (416) 596-0603, centralinfo@dietitians.ca, http://www.dietitians.ca.

National Cancer Institute, 6116 Executive Blvd., Ste. 300, Bethesda, MD 20892-8322, (800) 4-CANCER (422-6237), http://www.cancer.gov.

U.S. Food and Drug Administration, 10903 New Hampshire Ave., Silver Spring, MD 20993-0002, (888) INFO-FDA (463-6332), http://www.fda.gov.

Rebecca J. Frey, PhD

Ascorbic acid *see* **Vitamin C**

Asian diet

Definition

The traditional Asian diet, based on plant foods such as vegetables, beans, legumes, fruits, nuts, and vegetable oils, has been followed across the continent for thousands of years. Although specific diets vary among different countries and regions, they have many components in common. Rice and/or noodles are staples. Although fish and/or seafood are common where available, meat is rarely a main course but may be used in dishes for accent and flavor.

Description

Approximately 60% of the world's population lives in Asia, and more than 43 countries follow some form of Asian diet. Food is an important part of daily life across Asia, and meals are an essential component of family relationships. Although varying religious practices and traditions dictate the types of foods eaten in specific Asian diets, and each country and region has distinct ingredients and cooking styles, there are many common elements. The Asian diet is based on fresh plant foods served raw, steamed, stir-fried, or deep-fried. Fish and

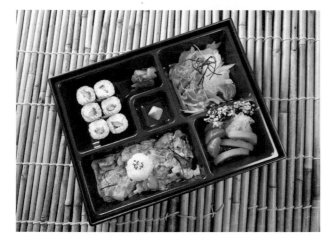

The bento box is a very popular lunch in Japan. *(Fanfo/Shutterstock.com)*

seafood are common in island nations and along coastlines, but meat is relatively rare. The Asian diet generally focuses on balance, with an ideal daily energy (calorie) content of about 1,200–1,400 **calories**.

Asian food pyramid

Like other healthy diets, the Asian diet can be represented by a food pyramid. The organization Oldways, in conjunction with the Cornell-China-Oxford Project on Nutrition, Health, and Environment and the Harvard School of Public Health, developed the Asian diet pyramid, based on the traditional Asian diet, as a model for healthy eating.

The base of the Asian food pyramid consists of daily rice, millet, corn, barley, other **whole grains**, noodles, and breads. Rice is an important part of almost every meal across most of Asia, although its preparation and uses vary. Rice also has religious significance, having saved many lives in times of famine. Rice is used as a main ingredient in candy and cakes and is fermented for wines, Japanese sake, and beer. Noodles may be made from rice, buckwheat (soba), wheat (somen and udon), or other grains. Breads take the form of dumplings, chapatis, roti, mantou, and naan.

The second tier of the pyramid consists of daily vegetables, fruits, legumes, seeds, and nuts. The last three serve as the primary **protein** sources in Asian diets. Soybeans, the seeds of a member of the pea family, have been integral to the traditional Asian diet for thousands of years. Soybeans are cooked or made into products including tofu, miso, tempeh, **soy** sauce, flour, and milk. Soybeans are high in protein and healthy isoflavones. Chickpeas (garbanzo beans) are also important. They are a good source of

carbohydrates; dietary **fiber**; high-quality protein, meaning they contain almost all of the essential amino acids; and several **vitamins** and **minerals**, especially potassium. Chickpeas are low in fat but contain important unsaturated fatty acids such as linoleic and oleic acids. Chickpea oil contains important sterols. Other beans include adzuki, edamame, lentils, and mung. Nuts and seeds include almonds, cashews, hazelnuts, lentils, peanuts, and sesame seeds. Common vegetables and tubers include bamboo shoots, bean sprouts, bok choy (cabbage), broccoli, carrots, chilies, daikon (radish), eggplant, leeks, lemongrass, lettuce, lotus root, peppers, kale, mushrooms, mustard greens, scallions, seaweed, snow peas, spinach, sweet potatoes, taro root, turnips, water chestnuts, and yams. Common fruits include lemons, kumquats, limes, apricots, bananas, cherries, coconut, dragon fruit, dates, grapes, kiwi, longan, lychee, mandarins, mangoes, melons, mangosteen, milk fruit, oranges, papaya, pears, pineapple, rambutan, and tangerines.

The other tiers of the Asian food pyramid are, in ascending order:

- daily vegetable oils, with highly saturated fats for cooking in very small amounts
- optional daily fish or shellfish—including abalone, clams, cockles, crab, eel, king fish, mussels, octopus, oysters, roe, scallops, sea bass, shrimp, squid, tuna, whelk, and yellowtail—or dairy such as cheese (paneer), butter (ghee), and yogurt (chaas, lassi)
- weekly eggs and poultry (chicken, quail, and duck)
- monthly sweets, such as Chinese mooncakes, Indian rice pudding, Japanese sugared sweet potatoes, or Thai mango-coconut pudding
- meat monthly or more frequently in very small portions, usually pork or beef

Common Asian herbs and spices include amchoor, asafoetida, basil in Thai food, cardamom, chilies, cloves, coriander, curry leaves, fennel, fenugreek, garlic, ginger, **ginseng**, lime leaves, masala, mint, parsley, pepper, scallion, star anise, and tumeric. Tea is widely consumed throughout Asia.

East Asia

China, the world's most populous country, has many regional cuisines. Although rice is a staple throughout most of China, in some regions noodles are the main staple. Chinese food is generally prepared by mincing and cooking in a wok with a small amount of oil. The traditional southern Chinese diet features more rice and vegetables, with moderate amounts of seafood, pork, and poultry. The northern Chinese diet

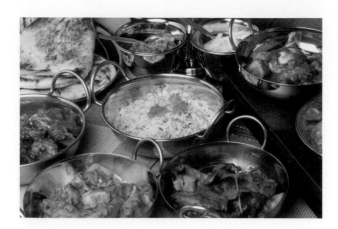

Traditional Indian foods, including curry, Naan bread, and rice. *(Joe Gough/Shutterstock.com)*

uses more refined wheat products and potatoes. Shanghai is known for its hot and spicy chili pepper flavorings and distinctive red-colored meats. The Cantonese and Chao Zhao regions are associated with flavorful meat and vegetable combinations. In the Beijing, Mandarin, and Shandong regions, noodles and steamed dumplings, rather than rice, form the foundation of most meals.

As an island nation with extensive coastline, Japan cuisine features fish and fish-based ingredients. Rice and soy products are staples. Vegetables are sliced and salted. Sushi, meats with teriyaki sauce, and tempura—lightly battered and fried meats, fish, and shellfish—are common. The Japanese diet features onions, ginger, soy sauce, and black pepper, which are all rich in phytochemicals. Mirin is fermented rice used as a **sugar** substitute that contains B vitamins and **probiotics**.

The Korean diet is comprised of a blend of Chinese and Japanese influences with its own distinct flavors, including soy sauces, garlic, ginger, chilies, pine nuts, and sesame seeds, among other spices. Traditional Korean meals include meats and seafood. Most meals include a vegetable dish called gimchi made of grated vegetables pickled with garlic, chili, and ginger.

South and Southeast Asia

South Asian or Indian cuisine is the only type of Asian diet that regularly includes dairy products, primarily in the form of lassi, ghee, and cheese (paneer), as well as milk. Rice is a staple, and dairy products, legumes, and nuts are the major protein sources. Hindi, the predominant religion in India, holds cows sacred and forbids the consumption of beef. Curry is a ubiquitous dish, commonly prepared with vegetable

oil, turmeric, black pepper, chili pepper, cumin, onion, garlic, and coriander, all of which are high in phytochemicals. Saffron, cardamom, ginger, tamarind, mustard, and aniseed are also common spices. The cuisines of other Southern Asian countries, including Pakistan, Bangladesh, and Sri Lanka, have been influenced by Indian cooking.

Southeast Asian countries—Vietnam, Thailand, Cambodia, Laos, Burma, Indonesia, Malaysia, Singapore, and the Philippines—all have unique cuisines that tend to be ancient fusions of East and South Asian diets. Rice and vegetables are the foundation of Vietnamese cooking, with meat and fish used sparingly. Fish sauces called *nuoc mam* are the primary source of flavoring. Fruits such as bananas, mangoes, papayas, coconut, and pineapple are an important part of each meal.

Malaysia and Singapore share a spicy cuisine that incorporates Chinese, Indian, and Muslim influences. Rice and Chinese noodles are eaten daily. Traditional foods include meat kebabs called satays that are served with a spicy peanut sauce. Curry is added to meat and marinades. Desserts made from coconut milk, green noodles, sugar syrup, and sweet beans are local favorites.

Filipino cuisine is a unique blend of Japanese, Chinese, Islamic, Spanish, and American influences. The typical day includes three main meals and a light afternoon snack. Rice and noodles are served with most meals, along with vegetables such as broccoli, bitter melon, mung bean, bean sprouts, and okra. Unlike in other parts of Asia, meat is very important in the Philippines. Meats consumed include pork, beef, and chicken, as well as water buffalo in rural provinces.

Function

The Asian diet is nutritionally balanced and provides ample phytochemicals and micronutrients, with fewer calories and less saturated fat than the typical Western diet. Spices, herbs, fermented vegetables, sprouts, and healthy **fats** make the Asian diet highly flavorful. Vegetables, broths, and spices provide satiety with fewer calories.

Benefits

The traditional plant-based Asian diet is considered to be very healthy. It is high in fresh fruits and vegetables and fiber and low in fat and calories. The traditional Asian diet is also high in vitamins, minerals, **antioxidants**, and other micronutrients. Antioxidants help to prevent oxidative damage to the cells of the body from free radicals. Free radicals are the byproducts of normal metabolic functions as well as environmental toxins that are ingested and inhaled. Antioxidants may reduce the risk of certain forms of **cancer** and heart disease. Saturated fats, which contribute to chronic illnesses, including **obesity, coronary heart disease**, and cancer, are almost completely absent from the Asian diet. Asians following a traditional diet are among the healthiest and longest-lived peoples, with lower rates of many illnesses common in the Western world, such as type 2 diabetes, heart disease, **hypertension**, cancer, and obesity. Death rates from cardiovascular disease in Japan are less than half the rates in the United States. Residents of Okinawa, off the Japanese coast, are one of the longest-lived populations on earth. An increase in Western-style diets in Asia has correlated with increases in heart disease, cancer, and obesity rates across the continent.

Precautions

Growing children may require more fat and pregnant women may require more calories than are provided by a traditional Asian diet. Furthermore, dairy products, which are a good source of **calcium**, are rare or absent in the traditional Asian diet. Modern versions of the traditional Asian diet generally include moderate amounts of low- or reduced-fat dairy products. Pregnant or **breastfeeding** women and growing children may require calcium supplements. Weight-bearing exercise strengthens bones and may help compensate for lower calcium intake.

Risks

Low calcium can contribute to osteoporosis, a weakening of the bones, especially in postmenopausal women. Nevertheless, there are lower rates of bone fractures from osteoporosis, as well as lower rates of breast cancer and cardiovascular disease, among Asian women compared with Western women. This has generally been attributed to the high soy content of the Asian diet, although scientific evidence for this claim is lacking.

Many Asian restaurants in Western countries have adopted Western tastes, altering the authentic meals by adding high amounts of fat and **sodium** to foods. Likewise, many people in Asia have adopted Western diets, resulting in an increase in chronic health problems that are traditionally more common in the West. Throughout Asia, overweight and obesity are becoming significant problems, as many people turn to fast food instead of home-cooked meals and sedentary work and lifestyles replace manual labor.

KEY TERMS

Antioxidant—Substances, including many phytonutrients, that prevent or reduce cellular damage from reactive oxygen species such as free radicals.

Body mass index (BMI)—A measure of body fat; the ratio of weight in kilograms to the square of height in meters.

Isoflavones—Various phytonutrients with antioxidant and estrogenic activities; found especially in soy.

Micronutrients—Nutrients, such as vitamins, that are required in minute amounts for growth and health.

Obesity—Excessive weight due to accumulation of fat; usually defined as a body mass index of 30 or above or body weight greater than 30% above normal on standard height-weight tables.

Osteoporosis—A disease characterized by low bone mass and structural deterioration of bone tissue, leading to bone fragility.

Overweight—A body mass index between 25 and 30.

Phytochemicals—Phytonutrients; micronutrients from plants, especially whole grains.

Probiotic—Foods or supplements containing beneficial live bacteria such as lactobacilli.

Saturated fat—Hydrogenated fat; fat molecules that contain only single bonds, especially animal fats.

Staple—A food that is regularly consumed in such quantities that it constitutes a major portion of the diet and supplies the majority of a population's energy and nutritional requirements.

Type 2 diabetes—A disease that prevents the proper utilization of glucose (sugar); sometimes called adult-onset diabetes, although it is increasingly being diagnosed in children.

Research and general acceptance

Research supports the health benefits of the traditional Asian diet, which is comprised primarily of fruits, vegetables, and fish; is high in fiber and micronutrients; and is low in fat. Such a diet can lower blood fat and cholesterol levels and blood pressure and help prevent cardiovascular disease. Studies also have identified specific health benefits for various foods that are common in the Asian diet, including soybeans, viscous vegetables such as Japanese yams and okra, red mold rice (a fermented product), and **green tea**.

A recent study found that increased consumption of hamburgers, fried chicken, pizza, and other American-style fast food among Southeast Asians greatly increased their risk of death from heart disease. A study of Chinese-Singaporeans found that those who ate fast food twice per week were 56% more likely to die of heart disease and 27% more likely to develop type 2 diabetes. Those who ate fast food four times per week were 80% more likely to die of heart disease. Research suggests that Asians may be at increased risk for cardiovascular disease at a lower **body mass index** (BMI) and waist circumference than those that are considered risk factors for Westerners.

Resources

BOOKS

Jacob, Anna, and Ng Hooi Lin. *Fit Not Fat: An Asian Diet Plan*. Singapore: Marshall Cavendish Cuisine, 2011.

Phyo, Ani. *Ani's Raw Food Asia: Easy East-West Fusion Recipes*. Cambridge, MA: Da Capo Lifelong Books, 2011.

Reader's Digest Association. *Low-Fat, No-Fat Asian Cooking: 150 Simple, Delicious Recipes for a Healthier You*. White Plains, NY: Reader's Digest, 2011.

Russell, Laura Byrne. *The Gluten-Free Asian Kitchen: Recipes for Noodles, Dumplings, Sauces, and More*. Berkeley, CA: Celestial Arts, 2011.

Simonds, Nina. *A Spoonful of Ginger: Irresistible, Health-Giving Recipes from Asian Kitchens*. New York: Alfred A. Knopf, 2011.

Trang, Corinne. *Asian Flavors Diabetes Cookbook: Simple, Fresh Meals Perfect for Every Day*. Alexandria, VA: American Diabetes Association, 2012.

Wang, Yuan, Warren Sheir, and Mika Ono. *Ancient Wisdom, Modern Kitchen: Recipes from the East for Health, Healing and Long Life*. Cambridge, MA: Da Capo Lifelong, 2010.

PERIODICALS

Li, Y., et al. "Dietary Patterns Are Associated with Stroke in Chinese Adults." *Journal of Nutrition* 141, no. 10 (October 2011): 1834–39.

"No Bone or Menopause Benefits from Soy." *Tufts University Health & Nutrition Letter* 29, no. 9 (November 2011): 6.

Taniguchi-Fukatsu, A., et al. "Natto and Viscous Vegetables in Japanese-Style Breakfast Improved Insulin Sensitivity, Lipid Metabolism and Oxidative Stress in Overweight Subjects with Impaired Glucose Tolerance." *British Journal of Nutrition* 107, no. 8 (April 2012): 1184–91.

Yang, H. Y., et al. "Beneficial Effects of Catechin-Rich Green Tea and Inulin on the Body Composition of Overweight Adults." *British Journal of Nutrition* 107, no. 5 (March 2012): 749–54.

WEBSITES

"Asian Diet & Pyramid." Oldways. http://oldwayspt.org/resources/heritage-pyramids/asian-diet-pyramid (accessed August 26, 2012).

Mayo Clinic staff. "Pyramid or Plate? Explore These Healthy Diet Options." MayoClinic.com. http://www.mayoclinic.com/health/healthy-diet/NU00190/NSECTIONGROUP = 2 (accessed August 26, 2012).

National Center for Complementary and Alternative Medicine. "Soy." National Institutes of Health. http://nccam.nih.gov/health/soy/ataglance.htm (accessed August 26, 2012).

ORGANIZATIONS

American Heart Association, 7272 Greenville Ave., Dallas, TX 75231, (800) AHA-USA-1 (242-8721), http://www.heart.org.

Oldways, 266 Beacon St., Boston, MA, USA 02116, (617) 421-5500, Fax: (617) 421-5511, http://oldwayspt.org.

Deborah L. Nurmi, MS
Margaret Alic, PhD

Aspartame *see* **Artificial sweeteners**

Atkins diet

Definition

The Atkins diet, also known as the Atkins Nutritional Approach, is a high-protein, high-fat, very low-carbohydrate regimen. It emphasizes meat, cheese, eggs, and oils while severely limiting foods such as bread, pasta, fruit, and **sugar**. It is a form of ketogenic diet.

Origins

Robert C. Atkins, a cardiologist and internist, developed the Atkins diet in the early 1970s. The original premise for developing the diet came about because of Atkins' frustration with the increasing rates of American **obesity** and chronic diseases such as type 2 diabetes. The diet first came to public attention in 1972 with the publication of *Dr. Atkins' Diet Revolution*. It quickly became a bestseller, but unlike most other **fad diets**, it remained very popular until about 2004.

Before his death in 2003, Atkins authored many books, including cookbooks and many books promoting variations on his diet. After his death, the popularity of the diet declined substantially. In 2005, Atkins' company, Atkins Nutritionals, filed for Chapter 11 bankruptcy. Until 2005, the company had concentrated on providing diet information through the sale of its books. When the company emerged from bankruptcy in 2006, it had a new business strategy that focused on providing low-carbohydrate foods (mostly

---

Phases of the Atkins diet

Induction—At least two weeks
No more than 20 net carbohydrates per day (with 12–15 grams from low-carb vegetables)
Liberal amounts of protein, including meats, fish, poultry, and eggs, as well as healthy fats
Fatty condiments (mayonnaise, sour cream, olive oil, butter) are allowed in unlimited quantities
Weight loss during the induction phase may be significant

Ongoing weight loss—Begin after two weeks
Slow introduction of foods with carbohydrates that are considered nutrient dense (nuts, berries, seeds)
In week one, eat 25 grams of carbohydrates per day
In week two, 30 grams of carbohydrates are allowed
The addition of five grams per week continues until weight loss stalls, then drop back to the previous gram level

Pre-maintenance goal—Begin when within 5–10 pounds of weight-loss goal
Gradually increase carbohydrate intake by 10 grams per week until weight loss stops, then drop back to the previous carbohydrate gram level
Level weight loss to less than one pound per week
Add in some fruits, whole grains, and starchy vegetables

Lifetime maintenance—Begin one month after weight-loss goal is achieved
May be able to consume from 75 to 120 grams of carbohydrates a day, depending on age, gender, and activity level
Maintaining weight goal is more likely if carbohydrate intake remains at the level discovered in pre-maintenance

SOURCE: Atkins diet official website, http://www.atkins.com/Home.aspx.

(Table by PreMediaGlobal. © 2013 Cengage Learning.)

shakes and bars) that conform to the Atkins diet. In 2011, Atkins Nutritionals began a refocused advertising campaign aimed at individuals who wanted quick weight loss of up to 15 pounds (6.8 kg) in two weeks. This quick weight-loss continued to be the focus of the Atkins Nutritionals website as of 2012.

Description

The Atkins diet has been one of the most popular fad diets in the United States. It started a "low-carb revolution," leading to the development of low-carbohydrate choices in grocery stores and restaurants. The regimen is a very-low-carbohydrate, or ketogenic diet, characterized by initial rapid weight loss, usually due to water loss. Drastically reducing carbohydrate intake causes liver and muscle glycogen loss, which has a strong but temporary diuretic effect. Long-term weight loss is said to occur because a very low carbohydrate intake causes the body to burn stored fat for energy.

The Atkins diet consists of four phases that participants are expected to progress through to achieve and maintain weight loss. Throughout these phases, the dieter is encouraged to drink at least eight 8-ounce glasses of water daily to avoid **dehydration** and **constipation**, to take a good multivitamin supplement, and to exercise to speed weight loss.

Induction

The four-phase diet starts with a two-week induction program designed to rebalance an individual's **metabolism**. This is by far the most restrictive of the four phases. Unlimited amounts of fat and **protein** are allowed but carbohydrate intake is restricted to 15–20 grams per day. Foods allowed include butter, oil, mayonnaise, sour cream, guacamole, meat, poultry, fish, eggs, cheese, and cream. The Atkins theory is that high-fat foods enhance the flavor of meals, making the Atkins diet easier to maintain. The daily amount of **carbohydrates** allowed equals about three cups of salad vegetables, such as lettuce, cucumbers, and celery. Dieters are said to feel hungry for the first 48 hours as their bodies adjust to the abrupt reduction in carbohydrates.

Atkins Nutritionals claims that the induction phase can make people feel revitalized, since carbohydrates can cause blood sugar spikes that lead to fatigue and other symptoms. The diet also claims that the induction phase will help dieters see the benefits of fat burning and strengthen their immune systems. Weight loss during this phase often is often substantial and quick, which can motivate the dieter to continue.

Ongoing weight loss

The second phase of the Atkins diet moves into ongoing weight loss. It involves the slow introduction of foods containing carbohydrates that are also considered nutrient dense and allows 15–40 grams of carbohydrates per day. Most of the carbohydrates come from vegetables. Atkins dieters still eat a high proportion of proteins and fat, but they gradually add more carbohydrates into the diet. The purpose of the phase is to continue to burn fat while controlling appetite and **cravings**. This phase also introduces the dieter to a broader range of foods and helps determine the dieter's threshold level of carbohydrate consumption (the maximum amount that still promotes weight loss). It is the intention of this phase to deliberately slow weight loss.

If weight loss continues, carbohydrate intake is gradually increased each week. In week one, the dieter can increase carbohydrate intake to 25 grams per day. In week two, if weight loss continues, 30 grams of carbohydrates are allowed. This process of allowing an additional 5 grams of carbohydrates per day continues on a weekly basis until weight loss stalls, then the dieter drops back to the previous gram level.

Typical tolerance levels range anywhere from 30 grams to 90 grams of carbohydrates per day. The more a dieter exercises, the more carbohydrates he or she can consume and still lose weight. The Atkins diet recommends choosing first from vegetables that are low in carbohydrates, then from other sources that are fresh foods high in nutrients and **fiber**. Examples of low-carbohydrate vegetables are lettuce, raw celery, and cucumbers. Nutrient-rich carbohydrates include green beans, Brazil nuts, avocados, berries, and **whole grains**.

Pre-maintenance

The Atkins diet considers the third phase as practice for lifetime maintenance of the individual's goal weight and "healthy eating habits." When the dieter is within 5–10 lb. (2.3–4.5 kg) of the goal weight, carbohydrate intake gradually is increased by 10 grams per day each week until weight is gained. Then the dieter drops back to the previous carbohydrate gram level. The purpose is to level weight loss to less than one pound per week. The dieter should continue at this rate until the goal weight is reached and for one month past that time. The goal is to achieve a level at which weight is neither gained nor lost and to internalize habits that become part of a permanent lifestyle.

Examples of vegetables that contain about 10 grams of carbohydrates are 3/4 cup of carrots, 1/2 c. of acorn squash, 1 c. of beets, and 1/4 c. of white potatoes. Legumes and fruit are the next preferred food groups for adding 10 grams daily. One-half apple contains 10 grams of carbohydrates, as does 1/3 c. of kidney beans.

Lifetime maintenance

This final phase of the Atkins diet occurs when the dieter's goal weight is reached. Although an adult may be able to consume 90–120 grams of carbohydrates daily, depending on age, gender, and activity level, maintaining the goal weight is more likely if carbohydrate intake remains at the level discovered in pre-maintenance, generally in the range of 40–60 grams of carbohydrates per day. The key, according to Atkins, is never letting weight vary by more than three to five pounds before making corrections.

Eco-Atkins

Though Atkins himself did not believe his high-carbohydrate diet was suitable for vegetarians or vegans, a vegan alternative, dubbed "Eco-Atkins," has been developed for dieters who do not eat meat or animal products. The protein in the diet comes primarily from **soy**, gluten (a protein found in wheat), and nuts. Small-scale studies saw slight reductions in dieters' LDL (low density lipoprotein, or "bad") cholesterol levels, as well as weight loss. The Atkins website warns that vegan dieters will have trouble with the induction phase of the Atkins program and should start in one of the other three phases. The studies were done on dieters who skipped right to the lifetime maintenance part of the plan, without ever following phases one, two, or three.

Function

Atkins and his followers believe that the traditional approach to weight loss of counting **calories** and cutting fat does not work. They believe that carbohydrates contribute to rising rates of obesity and obesity-related diseases. Through several updates of the Atkins diet, the same basic premise has held with minor revisions. The function of the diet is to enjoy eating while severely limiting carbohydrates. The Atkins diet makes some distinctions between trans **fats** and other fats. A more clear distinction is also made between carbohydrates in general and sugar in particular. The Atkins diet emphasizes that protein builds energy, repairs muscles and bones, and boosts the metabolism.

Benefits

The primary benefit of the diet is initial rapid and substantial weight loss. When carbohydrate intake is severely restricted, the body burns more fat stored in the body. There are no limits on the amount of calories or quantities of foods allowed while on the diet, so there is little hunger between meals. According to Atkins, the diet can alleviate symptoms of conditions such as fatigue, irritability, headaches, depression, and some types of joint and muscle pain.

Research also suggests that a high-fat, low-carbohydrate diet similar to the Atkins diet may help certain individuals with epilepsy avoid seizures. Research regarding the effects of diet on epilepsy is ongoing. Clinical trials are underway to determine the safety and effectiveness of a modified Atkins diet on epilepsy. A list of current clinical trials recruiting patients can be found at http://www.clinicaltrials.gov. There is no fee to participate in a clinical trial.

Precautions

The average carbohydrate intake recommended by the Atkins diet is well below the average level generally recommended by other experts and federal **dietary**

guidelines. The U.S. Department of Agriculture suggests eating six (1 oz.) servings each day (on average), and the Institute of Medicine, which determines the recommended daily intake values of **vitamins** and **minerals**, advises obtaining 45%–65% of daily calories from carbs. Studies have shown that even though people lose weight on the Atkins plan, they do not necessarily keep the weight off in the long term because the diet does not teach sustainable lifestyle changes.

Like many fad diets, the Atkins plan produces and promotes many food products associated with its diet plan. As of 2012, these products included bars, shakes, candy, pasta, and a baking mix. So although the plan argues against processed foods and snacking, the company heavily promotes the use of its nutritional products to support weight loss or maintenance.

Due to the diet's restrictive nature, adherence to the Atkins diet can result in vitamin and mineral deficiencies. In his books, Atkins recommends a wide range of nutritional supplements, including a multivitamin. Among his recommendations, Atkins suggests the following daily dosages: 300–600 micrograms (mcg) of **chromium** picolinate, 100–400 milligrams (mg) of pantetheine, 200 mcg of **selenium**, and 450–675 mcg of **biotin**.

Risks

According to Atkins, this diet causes no adverse side effects. Many health care professionals disagree. Some of the complications reported as resulting from the diet include ketosis, dehydration, electrolyte loss, **calcium** depletion, weakness, nausea, headaches, and kidney problems. There is also significant concern that since the diet is high in animal fats it could lead to increased levels of cholesterol and an increased risk of heart disease.

People with diabetes who are taking **insulin** are at risk of becoming hypoglycemic if they do not eat appropriate quantities of carbohydrates. Also, individuals who exercise regularly may experience low energy levels and muscle fatigue from low carbohydrate intake.

Followers of the Atkins diet have reported muscle cramps, diarrhea, general weakness, and rashes more frequently than people on low-fat diets. Others have reported bad breath, headache, and fatigue. Constipation is also a risk due to the limited intake of fruits and vegetables, which contain dietary fiber. The Academy of Nutrition and Dietetics warns that any diet that severely limits one food group should viewed very cautiously by dieters.

KEY TERMS

Biotin—A B-complex vitamin, found naturally in yeast, liver, and egg yolks.

Diuretic—A substance that removes water from the body by increasing urine production.

Electrolyte—Salts and minerals that ionize in body fluids. The major human electrolytes are sodium (Na^+), potassium (K^+), calcium ($Ca\ 2+$), magnesium ($Mg2+$), chloride ($Cl-$), phosphate ($HPO4\ 2-$), bicarbonate ($HCO3-$), and sulfate ($SO4\ 2-$). Electrolytes control the fluid balance of the body and are important in muscle contraction, energy generation, and almost all major biochemical reactions in the body.

Gluten—An elastic protein found in wheat and some other grains that gives cohesiveness to bread dough.

Ketoacidosis—An imbalance in the makeup of body fluids caused by the increased production of ketone bodies. Ketones are caused by fat breakdown.

LDL cholesterol—Low-density lipoprotein containing a high proportion of cholesterol that is associated with the development of heart disease.

High-protein diets may have adverse effects on bone health. A high protein intake causes increased calcium excretion in urine, and low calcium can lead to decreased bone health and risk of fractures. However, recent studies have found that while more calcium is lost, high protein intake may increase calcium absorption, helping to counteract the effects. In addition, although studies comparing low-fat diets with low-carb diets have not found differences in kidney function in obese patients, physicians have warned that high-protein diets may cause permanent loss of kidney function in anyone with kidney dysfunction.

Research & general acceptance

The Atkins diet has been hotly debated by lay people and the medical community alike. Although many studies have been carried out, the results often seem to be contradictory. In general, research has supported the idea that although short-term weight loss is often successfully achieved using the Atkins diet, long-term health may be put at risk. A study published in the March 2007 volume of the *Journal of the American Medical Association* found that weight loss achieved by women on the Atkins diet was higher

QUESTIONS TO ASK YOUR DOCTOR

- What aspects of the Atkins diet do you feel are appropriate for weight loss?

- How often would I need to be seen by a physician or registered dietitian while following the Atkins diet?

- Is this diet appropriate for my whole family?

- Would you recommend I take a vitamin or supplement while on this diet?

- Are there any possible negative side effects of the diet I should watch out for?

than that achieved by women on the Zone, Ornish, or LEARN diets. This would seem to indicate that the Atkins diet might be an effective approach to weight loss that is likely to lead to improved health in the longer term. However, a study published in the April 2007 volume of the *Journal of Internal Medicine* followed a group of more than 40,000 Swedish women for 12 years. The study found that those who followed a low-carbohydrate, high-fat diet were much more likely to have cardiovascular problems, and were at a higher risk of mortality. This type of back-and-forth between evidence supporting the Atkins diet and evidence warning of its risks makes it very controversial.

Although opinion from the general medical community remains mixed on the Atkins diet, it is not generally recommended. A number of leading medical and health organizations, including the American Medical Association, Academy of Nutrition and Dietetics, American Heart Association, and the American Cancer Association advise against the diet in most cases. The Atkins diet calls for eating a mix of foods drastically different than the dietary intakes recommended by the U.S. Department of Agriculture and the National Institutes of Health.

Controversy even surrounded Atkins' death in 2003. Although he died when he slipped on the ice outside his office in February 2003, he spent eight days in a coma before dying, and a copy of the medical examiner's report showed that his weight upon death was 258 pounds. Critics of Atkins' diet said that this was considered obese for a man who was six feet tall. His allies said that most of the pounds were gained in Atkins' time in a coma because of fluid retention. Even while Atkins was alive, he had reported problems with his heart, though these purportedly stemmed from an

enlarged heart caused by a viral infection, not from his diet.

Resources

BOOKS

Atkins, Robert C. *Atkins for Life: The Complete Controlled Carb Program for Permanent Weight Loss and Good Health.* New York: St. Martin's Press, 2003.

Haekes, Corinna, et al., Eds. *Trade, Food, Diet, and Health: Perspectives and Policy Opinions.* Ames, IA: Blackwell, 2010.

Heimowitz, Colette. *The New Atkins for You Cookbook: 200 Simple and Delicious Low-Carb Recipes in 30 Minutes or Less.* New York: Simon & Schuster, 2011.

Phinney, Stephen D., Jeff S. Volek, and Eric C. Westman. *The New Atkins for a New You: The Ultimate Diet for Shedding Weight and Feeling Great Forever.* New York: Simon & Schuster, 2010.

PERIODICALS

Fung, Teresa T., et al. "Low-Carbohydrate Diets, Dietary Approaches to Stop Hypertension-Style Diets, and the Risk of Postmenopausal Breast Cancer." *American Journal of Epidemiology* (September 15, 2011) 174, no. 6: 652–60.

Jenkins, David J.A., et al. "The Effect of a Plant-Based Low-Carbohydrate ('Eco-Atkins') Diet on Body Weight and Blood Lipid Concentrations in Hyperlipidemic Subjects." *Archives of Internal Medicine* 169, no. 11 (2009): 1046–54. http://dx.doi.org/10.1001/archinternmed.2009. 115 (accessed July 8, 2012).

Kerstetter, Jane E., Kimberly O. O'Brien, and Karl L. Insogna. "High Protein Diets, Calcium Economy, and Bone Health." *Topics in Clinical Nutrition* 19, no. 1 (2004): 57–70.

Knight, Christine. "Most People Are Simply Not Designed to Eat Pasta: Evolution Explanations for Obesity in the Low-Carbohydrate Diet Movement." *Public Understanding of Science* (September 2011) 20, no. 5: 706–19.

Lagiou, P., et al. "Low Carbohydrate-High Protein Diet and Mortality in a Cohort of Swedish Women." *Journal of Internal Medicine* 261, no. 4 (2007): 366–74. http://dx. doi.org/10.1111/j.1365-2796.2007.01774.x (accessed July 8, 2012).

Neal, E. G. and J. H. Cross. "Efficacy of Dietary Treatment for Epilepsy." *Journal of Human Nutrition and Diet* 23, no. 2 (2010): 113–19.

Surdykowski, Anna K. "Optimizing Bone Health in Older Adults: The Importance of Dietary Protein." *Aging Health* 6, no. 3 (2010): 345–57. http://dx.doi.org/ 10.2217/ahe.10.16 (accessed July 8, 2012).

WEBSITES

Atkins official website. http://www.atkins.com (accessed November 6, 2012).

Dietary Guidelines Advisory Committee. *Report of the Dietary Guidelines Advisory Committee on the Dietary Guidelines for Americans, 2010, to the Secretary of Agriculture and the Secretary of Health and Human Services.*

Washington, DC: U.S. Department of Agriculture, Agricultural Research Service, 2010. See esp. "Section 5: Carbohydrates." http://www.cnpp.usda.gov/DGAs2010-DGACReport.htm (accessed June 13, 2012).

Gardner, Amanda. "'Eco-Atkins' Diet Sheds More Than Pounds." ABC News, June 8, 2009. http://abcnews.go.com/Health/Healthday/story?id=7788145 (accessed July 8, 2012).

Hellmich, Nanci. "Digesting the Facts on the 'New Atkins' Low-Carb Diet." USA TODAY, March 2, 2010. http://www.usatoday.com/news/health/weightloss/2010-03-03-atkins03_ST_N.htm (accessed July 8, 2012).

U.S. Department of Agriculture. "How Many Grain Foods Are Needed Daily?" ChooseMyPlate.gov. http://www.choosemyplate.gov/food-groups/grains_amount_table.html (accessed July 8, 2012).

ORGANIZATIONS

Academy of Nutrition and Dietetics, 120 South Riverside Plz., Ste. 2000, Chicago, IL 60606-6995, (312) 899-0040, (800) 877-1600, amacmunn@eatright.org, http://www.eatright.org.

Teresa Odle
Tish Davidson, AM

Attention deficit hyperactivity disorder diet *see* **ADHD diet**

Autism spectrum disorders *see* **Casein-free diet**

B

Bariatric surgery

Definition

Bariatric surgery is a surgical weight-loss procedure that reduces or bypasses the stomach or small intestine so that severely overweight people can achieve significant and permanent weight loss.

Purpose

Bariatric surgery is performed only on severely overweight people who are more than twice their ideal weight. This level of **obesity** is often referred to as morbid obesity since it can result in many serious, and potentially deadly, health problems, including **hypertension**, Type 2 **diabetes mellitus** (non-insulin dependent diabetes), increased risk for coronary disease, increased unexplained heart attack, **hyperlipidemia**, and a higher prevalence of colon, prostate, endometrial, and, possibly, breast **cancer**. This surgery is performed on people whose risk of complications of surgery is outweighed by the need to lose weight to prevent health complications, and for whom supervised weight-loss and exercise programs have repeatedly failed. Obesity surgery, however, does not make people thin. Most people lose about 60% of their excess weight through this treatment. Changes in diet and exercise are required to maintain a normal weight.

The theory behind obesity surgery is that if the volume the stomach holds is reduced and the entrance into the intestine is made smaller to slow stomach emptying, or part of the small intestine is bypassed or shortened, people will not be able to consume and/or absorb as many **calories**. With obesity surgery the volume of food the stomach can hold is reduced from about 4 cups to about 1/2 cup.

Insurers may consider obesity surgery elective surgery and not cover it under their policies. Documentation of the necessity for surgery and approval from the insurer should be sought before this operation is performed.

Precautions

Obesity surgery should not be performed on people who are less than twice their ideal weight. It also is not appropriate for people who have substance addictions or who have psychological disorders. Other considerations in choosing candidates for obesity surgery include the general health of the person and his or her willingness to comply with follow-up treatment.

Description

Obesity surgery is usually performed in a hospital by a surgeon who has experience with obesity surgery or at a center that specializes in the procedure. General anesthesia is used, and the operation takes 2–3 hours. The hospital stay lasts about one week.

Three procedures are currently used for obesity surgery:

- Gastric bypass surgery. Probably the most common type of obesity surgery, gastric bypass surgery has been performed in the United States for about 35 years. In this procedure, the volume of the stomach is reduced by four rows of stainless steel staples that separate the main body of the stomach from a small, newly created pouch. The pouch is attached at one end to the esophagus. At the other end is a very small opening into the small intestine. Food flows through this pouch, bypassing the main portion of the stomach and emptying slowly into the small intestine where it is absorbed.

- Vertical banding gastroplasty. In this procedure, an artificial pouch is created using staples in a different section of the stomach. Plastic mesh is sutured into part of the pouch to prevent it from dilating. In both surgeries, food enters the small intestine farther along than it would enter if exiting the stomach normally. This reduces the time available for

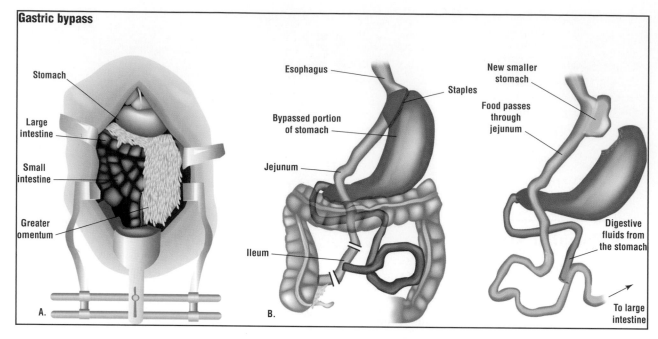

Gastric bypass

A. Stomach / Large intestine / Small intestine / Greater omentum

B. Esophagus / Bypassed portion of stomach / Jejunum / Ileum / Staples / New smaller stomach / Food passes through jejunum / Digestive fluids from the stomach / To large intestine

In this Roux-en-Y gastric bypass, the stomach is separated into two sections. Food is bypassed from the larger stomach to the smaller stomach. *(Illustration by PreMediaGlobal. © 2013 Cengage Learning.)*

absorption of nutrients. The procedure is normally done laparoscopically, meaning that the surgeon makes one or more small incisions in the abdomen and inserts the necessary tools and instruments through the tiny holes. The surgeon can then view the patient's organs via an inserted camera that displays pictures on a monitor. This method makes for a faster and easier recovery than a large incision.

• Jejunoileal bypass. Now a rarely performed procedure, jejunoileal bypass involves shortening the small intestine. Because of the high occurrence of serious complications involving chronic diarrhea and liver disease, it has largely been abandoned for the other, safer procedures.

Preparation

After patients are carefully selected as appropriate for obesity surgery, they receive standard preoperative blood and urine tests and meet with an anesthesiologist to discuss how their health may affect the administration of anesthesia. Pre-surgery counseling is done to help patients anticipate what to expect after the operation.

Aftercare

Immediately after the operation, most patients are restricted to a liquid diet for 2–3 weeks; however, some may remain on it for up to 12 weeks. Patients then move on to a diet of pureed food for about a month, and after about two months most can tolerate solid food. High-fat food is restricted because it is hard to digest and causes diarrhea. Patients are expected to work on changing their eating and exercise habits to assist in weight loss. Most people eat 3–4 small meals a day once they return to solid food. Eating too quickly or too much after obesity surgery can cause nausea and vomiting as well as intestinal "dumping," a condition in which undigested food is shunted too quickly into the small intestine, causing pain, diarrhea, weakness, and dizziness.

Risks

As in any abdominal surgery, there is always a risk of excessive bleeding, infection, and allergic reaction to anesthesia. Specific risks associated with obesity surgery include leaking or stretching of the pouch and loosening of the gastric staples. Although the average death rate associated with this procedure is less than one percent, the rate varies from center to center, ranging from 0%–4%. Long-term failure rates can reach 50%, sometimes making additional surgery necessary. Other complications of obesity surgery include an intolerance to foods high in **fats**, lactose intolerance, bouts of vomiting and diarrhea, and intestinal discomfort.

Studies on the risks of these surgeries continue. A 2003 report showed that gastric bypass surgery risk increases with age, weight, and male gender. Patients age 55 and older experienced more complications than younger patients, and male patients had more life-threatening complications than female patients, particularly those who were more severely obese.

Normal results

Many people lose about 60% of the weight they need to reach their ideal weight through obesity surgery. However, surgery is not a magic weight-loss operation, and success also depends on the patient's willingness to exercise and eat low-calorie foods. A 2003 report showed that super-obese patients had a lower success rate with laparoscopic vertical banding gastroplasty than those considered morbidly obese. However, the overall success rate was nearly 77% of patients carrying less than 50% excess weight four years after the procedure.

Resources

BOOKS

Cook, Colleen. *The Success Habits of Weight-Loss Surgery Patients.* 2nd ed. Salt Lake City, UT: Bariatric Support Centers Int., 2003.

Deitel, M., et al., eds. *Handbook of Obesity Surgery.* Toronto: FD-Communications Inc., 2010.

Levine, Patt. *Eating Well After Weight Loss Surgery: Over 140 Delicious Low-Fat High-Protein Recipes to Enjoy the Weeks, Months and Years After Surgery.* New York: Marlowe & Co., 2004.

PERIODICALS

Colquitt, J. L., J. Picot, E. Loveman, and A. J. Clegg. "Surgery for Obesity." *Cochrane Database of Systematic Reviews* 2, art no. CD003641 (2009).

Available online at http://dx.doi.org/10.1002/14651858.CD003641.pub3 (accessed September 19, 2012).

Guilherme, M., et al. "Better Weight Loss, Resolution of Diabetes, and Quality of Life for Laparoscopic Gastric Bypass vs Banding: Results of a 2-Cohort Pair-Matched Study." *Archives of Surgery* 146, no. 2 (2011): 149–55.

Laurenius, A., et al. "Changes in Eating Behaviour and Meal Pattern Following Roux-en-Y Gastric Bypass." *International Journal of Obesity* 36 (March 2012): 348–355.

Sjöström, Lars, et al. "Effects of Bariatric Surgery on Mortality in Swedish Obese Subjects." *New England Journal of Medicine* 357 (August 2007): 741–52.

WEBSITES

"Bariatric Surgery 101." Consumer Guide to Bariatric Surgery. http://www.yourbariatricsurgeryguide.com/intro (accessed September 19, 2012).

Mayo Clinic staff. "Gastric Bypass Surgery." MayoClinic.com. http://www.mayoclinic.com/health/gastric-bypass/MY00825 (accessed September 19, 2012).

National Institute of Diabetes, Digestive and Kidney Diseases. "Bariatric Surgery for Severe Obesity." Weight-Control Information Network. http://win.niddk.nih.gov/publications/gastric.htm (accessed September 19, 2012).

ORGANIZATIONS

American Society of Bariatric Physicians, 2821 S. Parker Rd., Ste. 625, Aurora, CO 80014, (303) 770-2526, Fax: (303) 779-4834, http://asbp.org.

American Society for Metabolic and Bariatric Surgery, 100 SW 75th St., Ste. 201, Gainesville, FL 32607, (352) 331-4900, Fax: (352) 331-4975, info@asmbs.org, http://asmbs.org.

Tish Davidson, AM
Stacey Chamberlin

Bernstein diet

Definition

The Bernstein diet is a low-carbohydrate, high-fat diet for people with diabetes. It goes against the conventional high-carbohydrate, low-fat **diabetic diet** recommended by much of the medical community.

Origins

The diet was developed by endocrinologist Richard K. Bernstein, who has type 1 diabetes. It was first published in his 1997 book *Dr. Bernstein's Diabetes Solution: A Complete Guide to Achieving Normal Blood Sugars.* The diet is intended for people with diabetes and **insulin** resistance syndrome. Diabetes is a disease in which the body does not produce or properly use insulin. Insulin is a hormone that is needed to convert **sugar**, starches, and other food into energy. Insulin resistance often goes along with other health problems, including diabetes, high cholesterol, high blood pressure, and heart attack. When a person has many of these conditions together, it is referred to as insulin resistance syndrome.

Bernstein was diagnosed with diabetes in 1946 at the age of 12 and was put on a low-fat, high-carbohydrate diet. He remained on this diet until 1969. During this time, he experienced frequent bouts of hypoglycemia (excessively low blood sugar) along with headaches and fatigue, which he said was caused by the large doses of insulin he was taking to help regulate his blood sugar levels. He blamed this cycle of hypoglycemia followed by insulin injections on his diet. Doctors typically recommend a high-carbohydrate diet for people with diabetes because it raises blood sugar. Bernstein, an engineer, began adjusting his insulin regimen and diet to see how it affected his condition. Within one year, Bernstein said he had nearly constant normal blood sugar levels, and his health improved considerably. He spent the next few years trying to convince others that his methods were effective, but his attempts failed. In 1979, Bernstein quit his engineering job and entered medical school. In 1983, he opened his own medical practice in New York. After that, he began formulating his diet plan, which became the focus of his 1997 book. Bernstein went on to publish several more books, the most recent being *Dr. Bernstein's Diabetes Solution: The Complete Guide to Achieving Normal Blood Sugars*, 4th edition, published in 2011.

Description

The Bernstein diet is designed as a medical diet rather than a diet for weight loss, although people can lose weight on it. It is similar in many respects to other high-fat/low-carb diets, such as the **Atkins diet**. Both diets stress foods that are high in **fats** and **protein** and low in **carbohydrates**. This formula is controversial in weight loss and health circles, and the Bernstein diet as a treatment for diabetes is especially controversial in the medical community.

The Bernstein diet does not recommend a specific ratio of the three main food groups: proteins, fats, and carbohydrates. Instead, Bernstein advocates an individualized approach to diet. He recommends that people with diabetes test their blood sugar levels at least five to eight times a day to learn how different foods affect them.

Bernstein has three basic rules for developing meal plans that normalize blood sugar levels. They are:

- Eliminate all foods from the diet that contain simple sugars, which are fast-acting carbohydrates. These foods include table sugar, most starchy foods such as breads and pasta, grains, and potatoes.
- Limit total carbohydrate intake to an amount that will work with insulin, either injected or produced naturally by the body. This will avoid a post-meal blood sugar increase.
- Stop eating when there is no longer a feeling of hunger.

Bernstein advises people with diabetes to avoid hidden dangers in foods, especially sugar-free foods, that can cause blood sugar levels to rise too much and too rapidly. Food labels should be carefully checked for foods containing carob, honey, saccharose, corn syrup, lactose, sorbitol, dextrin, levulose, sorghum, dextrose, maltodextrin, treacle, dulcitol, maltose, turbinado, fructose, mannitol, xylitol, glucose, mannose, xylose, and molasses, which are all forms of sugars.

The Bernstein diet recommends avoiding eating breakfast cereals, snack foods (candy, cookies, cakes, potato and tortilla chips, popcorn, and pretzels), protein bars, milk and cottage cheese (except for **soy** milk), fruits and fruit juices, certain vegetables (beans, beets, carrots, corn, potatoes, tomatoes and tomato products), and canned and packaged soups.

Foods that are allowed on the Bernstein diet include meat, fish and seafood, poultry, eggs, tofu, soy meat substitutes, cheese, butter, margarine, cream, yogurt, soymilk, soy flour, and bran crackers. Other food items allowed include toasted nori (seaweed), **artificial sweeteners** (Equal, Sweet'n Low, NutraSweet, and Splenda), No-Cal brand syrups, Da Vinci Gourmet brand syrups, flavor extracts, herbs and spices, low-carbohydrate salad dressings, nuts, and sugar-free gelatin and puddings.

Bernstein admits that his diet is somewhat restrictive and that people will still have **cravings** for sweets and bakery items, but believes that the benefits of the diet (such as improved health) help override these urges.

Function

The main function of the Bernstein diet is to help people with diabetes to maintain constant, normal blood sugar levels throughout the day. Maintaining control of blood sugar levels can help avoid long-term complications of diabetes, including neuropathy of the feet, amputation, cataracts and blindness, heart disease, erectile dysfunction, glaucoma, **ulcers** of the feet, high blood pressure, and high cholesterol. Since the diet is similar to the Atkins diet in that it emphasizes low-carbohydrate foods, people who are overweight or obese may lose weight on the Bernstein diet.

Benefits

The primary benefits of the Bernstein diet come from being able to maintain constant, normal blood sugar levels. In the long-term, this can help reduce the number of diabetes-related complications. These complications include heart disease, high blood pressure, eye problems, serious conditions affecting the feet that sometimes lead to amputation, gastroparesis (a condition in which the stomach requires significantly longer than its normal time to empty), kidney disease, and fatigue. The importance of maintaining constant, normal blood sugar levels (by checking the levels at least five to eight times a day with home glucose monitors and then adjusting insulin levels accordingly) was proven by the Diabetes Control and Complications Trial, a study of people with diabetes from 1983–1993, the most comprehensive large-scale diabetes study ever conducted. The study found that for people who intensely controlled their blood sugar levels, the risk for eye disease was reduced by 76 percent, nerve disease by 60 percent, and kidney disease by 50 percent. The diet can also help people who are overweight or obese to lose weight.

Precautions

The Bernstein diet goes against the recommendations of major medical organizations such as the American Medical Association, **Academy of Nutrition and Dietetics**, and **American Diabetes Association** (ADA). According to an article published in *Diabetes Forecast*, most people with diabetes obtain about 40%–45% of their daily **calories** from carbohydrates, which is in line with ADA recommendations. People with diabetes should not start the Bernstein diet without first discussing it with their doctor or a specialist in diabetes, called

---

KEY TERMS

Carbohydrate—A nutrient that the body uses as an energy source.

Diabetes—A condition in which the body either does not make or cannot respond to the hormone insulin. As a result, the body cannot use glucose (sugar). There are two types: type 1 (juvenile onset) and type 2 (primarily adult onset).

Endocrinologist—A medical specialist who treats diseases of the endocrine (glands) system, including diabetes.

Hypoglycemia—Abnormally low blood sugar levels.

Insulin—A hormone that regulates the level of glucose (sugar) in the blood.

Insulin resistance syndrome—A medical condition in which insulin fails to function normally in regulating blood glucose (sugar) levels.

Ketoacidosis—A condition caused by low insulin levels where the amount of sugar and ketones in the blood is high.

---

an endocrinologist. They may also wish to consult a diabetic dietitian or nutritionist.

People with diabetes should never use a diet as a substitute for medication without first talking to their doctor. They should not stop taking any prescribed medications without their physician's approval.

Risks

People with type 1 diabetes who take insulin are at a high risk of hypoglycemia (abnormally low blood sugar levels) and ketoacidosis (dangerously high blood sugar levels) if they remove too much carbohydrate from their diet. It is also important for people with diabetes to eat enough calories, which can be difficult when removing food sources. Following a low-carbohydrate diet requires proper planning and should not be attempted without consulting a physician or dietitian.

Critics of the Bernstein diet say that it contains too much fat and is not nutritionally balanced. The high fat intake may be especially be an issue for people with type 2 diabetes who are trying to lose weight. They also say it is difficult for many people to maintain a low-carb diet over the long-term.

Research and general acceptance

Among the critics of the Bernstein diabetic diet are the ADA, Academy of Nutrition and Dietetics,

QUESTIONS TO ASK YOUR DOCTOR

- Is it safe for me to go on the Bernstein diet?
- Are there any other diets you would recommend to help control my diabetes?
- How often should I check my blood sugar levels throughout the day?
- Will losing weight help my diabetes?

American Medical Association, American Heart Association, United States Department of Agriculture, and the Physicians Committee for Responsible Medicine. They state that high-fat, low-carbohydrate diets tend to be lower in **fiber**, **calcium**, fruits, and vegetables, and higher in cholesterol, fat, and saturated fat. However, since 2002, a number of scientific studies that compared high- and low-carbohydrate diets concluded that low-carbohydrate diets reduced blood sugars and risk factors for heart disease. Many practicing endocrinologists endorse the Bernstein diet and other low-carbohydrate diets for their patients. They point out that the ADA has traditionally been slow to adopt new developments in diabetes monitoring and treatment; for example, the ADA did not endorse patient blood glucose monitors until 1983, about ten years after they were developed. Still, further research is needed on the effectiveness of low-carbohydrate diets in treating diabetes.

People with type 2 diabetes may be able to improve control of their blood sugar levels, lose weight, and lower cholesterol levels significantly with a low-carbohydrate diet, such as the Bernstein diet, than with diets that restrict calorie intake, according to two studies presented in 2006 at the ADA annual scientific sessions. One of the studies, conducted by Duke University researchers, was funded by the Robert C. Atkins Foundation; Atkins authored a number of books on his own low-carbohydrate diet.

Resources

BOOKS

Bernstein, Richard K. *The Diabetes Diet: Dr. Bernstein's Low-Carbohydrate Solution*. New York: Little, Brown and Company, 2005.

———. *Dr. Bernstein's Diabetes Solution: The Complete Guide to Achieving Normal Blood Sugars*. Rev. ed. New York: Little, Brown and Company, 2011.

PERIODICALS

American Diabetes Association. "Nutrition Principles and Recommendations in Diabetes." *Diabetes Care* (January 2004): S36–S46.

Evans, Jeff. "Low-Carb Diet Trumps Caloric Restriction in Type 2 Diabetes." *Family Practice News* (October 15, 2006): 21.

Govindji, Azmina. "The Role of Carbohydrates in a Healthy Diet." *Nursing Standard* (September 27, 2006): 56–64.

Kirk, J.K., et al. "Restricted-Carbohydrate Diets in Patients with Type 2 Diabetes: A Meta-Analysis." *Journal of the American Dietetic Association* 108, no. 1 (2008): 91–100.

Morrison, Katharine. "Low Carbohydrate Diets For Diabetes Control." *British Journal of General Practice* 55, no. 520 (2005): 884.

Neithercott, Tracey. "Are Carbs the Enemy?" *Diabetes Forecast* (March 2011). http://forecast.diabetes.org/carbs-enemy (accessed September 20, 2012).

Vaughan, Lisa. "Dietary Guidelines for the Management of Diabetes." *Nursing Standard* (July 13, 2005): 56–64.

WEBSITES

American Diabetes Association. "Carbohydrates." http://www.diabetes.org/food-and-fitness/food/what-can-i-eat/carbohydrates.html (accessed September 20, 2012).

Davidson, Nancy Klobassa, and Peggy Moreland. "Dr. Bernstein Diet and Beyond." MayoClinic.com, *Living with Diabetes* (blog), July 8, 2011. http://www.mayoclinic.com/health/dr-bernstein-diet/MY01817 (accessed September 20, 2012).

ORGANIZATIONS

American Diabetes Association, 1701 North Beauregard St., Alexandria, VA 22311, (800) DIABETES (342-2383), askADA@diabetes.org, http://www.diabetes.org.

National Diabetes Education Program, One Diabetes Way, Bethesda, MD 20814-9692, (301) 496-3583, http://www.ndep.nih.gov.

National Diabetes Information Clearinghouse, 1 Information Way, Bethesda, MD 20892-3560, (800) 860-8747, TTY: (866) 569-1162, Fax: (703) 738-4929, ndic@info.niddk.nih.gov, http://diabetes.niddk.nih.gov.

Ken R. Wells

Best Life diet *see* **Bob Greene's diet**

Beta-carotene *see* **Carotenoids**

Beverly Hills Diet

Definition

The Beverly Hills Diet is a fad diet created by Judy Mazel (1943–2007). Mazel believed that weight loss could be achieved by eating foods in the proper combinations and in the correct order. Her diet is strongly opposed by mainstream medical organizations, including the American Medical Association.

Origins

Judy Mazel claimed to be an overweight child who struggled with her weight for 20 years. She was told by a doctor that she was "destined to always be fat." Six months after this pronouncement, she went skiing and broke her leg. While she was recuperating, she read a book on nutrition that a friend had given her. From this she developed her ideas about how the body works and how to lose weight and stay thin.

Mazel reported that she used her new theories to lose 72 lb. (29 kg) without ever regaining the weight. In 1981, she published her diet in *The Beverly Hills Diet*. The original book reportedly sold more than one million copies, and in 1996 Mazel published a revised and updated version called *The New Beverly Hills Diet*. Mazel also wrote a cookbook designed to go with the diet as well as *The New Beverly Hills Diet Skinny Little Companion*, a slim volume designed to provide inspiration and tips to help dieters through their first 35 days on the diet.

Mazel died at age 63 due to complications from peripheral vascular disease.

Description

The Beverly Hills Diet is based on the idea that the order and combinations in which foods are eaten causes weight gain. Mazel claimed that eating foods in the wrong order could stop some foods from being digested, causing fat build-up. The diet divides foods into four groups: **carbohydrates**, proteins, fruits, and **fats**. Fruit, even different types of fruit, must always be eaten alone. If a different type of food is eaten, such as a **protein**, the dieter must wait until the next day to eat fruit again.

On the Beverly Hills Diet, protein and carbohydrates cannot be eaten together. Most dairy products fall under the protein group for purposes of categorization. This means that dieters can drink milk with protein meals but not with carbohydrate meals. Fat is allowed to be eaten with either group but may not be eaten with fruit.

The order throughout the day in which food is eaten is very important on the Beverly Hills Diet. Each day, fruit should be eaten first. After fruit, the carbohydrate group can be eaten, then protein. Once a dieter has changed food groups, he or she cannot eat from the previous groups again until the next day.

Dieters must wait two hours between eating foods from different food groups.

Dieters cannot consume diet sodas or anything with **artificial sweeteners**, although alcohol is not restricted. The diet categorizes most alcoholic drinks, such as beer, vodka, and rum, as carbohydrates, and says they must only be consumed with carbohydrates. Wine is categorized as a fruit, and unlike the rules for eating other fruits, wine does not have to be consumed alone but can be drunk with another fruit. Mazel says that champagne is a neutral food and can be drunk with anything.

The diet provides readers with a 35-day plan. Every day, dieters are told what foods are allowed and in what order they must be eaten. Most foods do not have a quantity limit. Instead, dieters may consume as much of a given food as desired until they move on to the next food. Dieters must eat the foods in the order listed and cannot go back or make substitutions. The diet is very restrictive, with most days allowing no more than two or three types of foods.

For example, on the first day of the diet, dieters are instructed to eat pineapple, corn on the cob, and a salad made of lettuce, tomatoes, and onions with Mazel dressing. (Mazel dressing is a recipe included in the book that shows up frequently throughout the diet.) This means that dieters may eat as much pineapple as desired in the morning, but once they begin eating corn on the cob, they cannot go back and eat more pineapple. Once the salad is eaten, both corn on the cob and pineapple are no longer allowed. Dieters are instructed to wait between changing foods to ensure proper digestion.

Some days on the New Beverly Hills diet, only one type of food is permitted during the entire day. Day three of the diet allows the dieter only to consume grapes. On other days, the dieter is only allowed to eat watermelon. Although these rules are extremely restrictive, they are not as restrictive as original Beverly Hills Diet—on that diet, dieters were only allowed to eat fruit for the first 10 days, and animal protein was not allowed until the 19th day. The New Beverly Hills Diet includes vegetables and carbohydrates occasionally during the first week and lamb chops and shrimp on the 6th day.

Function

The Beverly Hills Diet promises dieters that they will lose up to 25 lb. (11.5 kg) in 35 days. The Beverly Hills Diet is intended to be a lifestyle, and dieters are expected to continue to follow the rules of the diet after the 35 days of meal plans are finished. The diet does not provide exercise recommendations.

Benefits

Although there are benefits to losing weight, the Beverly Hills diet is very restrictive and is not recommended. A healthy rate of weight loss is 1–2 lb. per week. It may also be difficult to consume enough **calories** while on this diet. Very low-calorie diets, which are diets below 800 calories per day, are usually medically supervised. Following such a restrictive diet for an extended period of time could result in nutritional deficiencies.

Precautions

The New Beverly Hills Diet's website, while no longer active, cautioned that women who are pregnant or **breastfeeding** and people with diabetes, **ulcers**, spastic colon, or various forms of irritable bowel disease should not follow this diet. The website also cautioned that anyone with a serious illness or chronic disease should only begin this diet under medical supervision.

Even dieters who do not have a serious illness should consult a doctor or other medical professional if considering this diet. It limits important sources of nutrients and is not recommended. A physician or registered dietitian will be able to suggest alternative and healthy diets.

Risks

This diet requires that dieters eat only a small variety of foods each day, and on some days, only

one type of food is allowed. No protein is allowed until the sixth day of the diet and it is not included regularly after that. This means that it will be extremely hard for dieters to get the **vitamins**, **minerals**, and nutrients that are needed each day for good health. No vitamin or supplement can replace eating a healthy, balanced diet.

The excessive consumption of fruit and the limited consumption of other foods may cause diarrhea, which can lead to severe **dehydration** and **malnutrition**. People considering this diet are advised against it and should talk to a medical professional about safe options for losing weight.

Research and general acceptance

There is no scientific evidence to support Mazel's claims. In 1981, after the original Beverly Hills Diet book debuted, the *Journal of the American Medical Association* published an article stressing the dangers of the diet. It called the diet "the latest, and perhaps worst, entry in the diet-fad derby" and said that the diet could cause severe enough diarrhea to cause fever, muscle weakness, and, in the most severe cases, extreme drops in blood pressure that could lead to death. The article told physicians to discourage their patients from trying this diet.

People interested in the Beverly Hills Diet are strongly encouraged to meet with a registered dietitian or physician to discuss alternative options for weight loss. The Beverly Hills Diet is highly restrictive and is both impractical and potentially dangerous in the long term. Federal sources such as the U.S. Department of Agriculture's (USDA) *Dietary Guidelines for Americans* and **MyPlate** (ChooseMyPlate.gov) provide consumers with credible information on a well-rounded diet.

Resources

BOOKS

Mazel, Judy, and Susan Shultz. *The Beverly Hills Diet*. New York: Macmillan, 1981.

——. *The Beverly Hills Style.* New York: Stein and Day, 1985.

——. *The New Beverly Hills Diet.* Deerfield Beach, FL: Health Communications, 1996.

PERIODICALS

Mirkin, G.B., and R.N. Shore. "The Beverly Hills Diet. Dangers of the Newest Weight Loss Fad." *The Journal of the American Medical Association* (Nov. 1981): 2235–37.

WEBSITES

ChooseMyPlate.gov. U.S. Department of Agriculture. http://www.choosemyplate.gov (accessed August 22, 2012).

U.S. Department of Agriculture and U.S. Department of Health and Human Services. *Dietary Guidelines for Americans, 2010.* 7th ed. Washington, DC: U.S. Government Printing Office, December 2010. http://health.gov/dietaryguidelines (accessed August 22, 2012).

ORGANIZATIONS

Academy of Nutrition and Dietetics, 120 South Riverside Plz., Ste. 2000, Chicago, IL 60606-6995, (312) 899-0040, (800) 877-1600, amacmunn@eatright.org, http://www.eatright.org.

U.S. Department of Agriculture, 1400 Independence Ave. SW, Washington, DC 20250, (202) 720-2791, http://www.usda.gov.

Tish Davidson, AM
Laura Jean Cataldo, RN, EdD

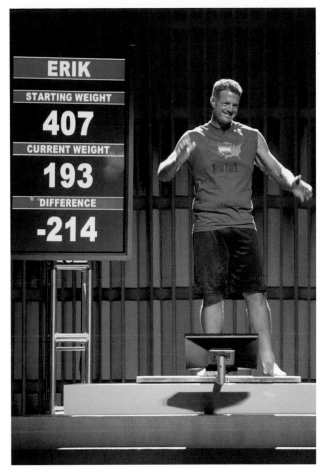

Contestant during a weigh-in on the television show *The Biggest Loser.* *(NBC-TV/THE KOBAL COLLECTION/HASTON, CHRIS)*

Biggest Loser diet

Definition

The Biggest Loser diet is a diet and exercise plan based on the NBC television show of the same name. It emphasizes healthy eating and regular exercise.

Origins

The Biggest Loser diet is based on the NBC television program *The Biggest Loser*, which began airing in 2004. By 2012, the show was in its 14th season (two seasons per year began airing in 2008). On the television show, morbidly obese individuals compete to see who can lose the most weight by the end of the series, often losing more than 100 pounds (45 kg) each. The winner receives a prize of $250,000.

The Biggest Loser became extremely popular very quickly, with millions of viewers tuning into each episode. While the show began in the United States, it has since been syndicated in more than 20 other countries, including India, Germany, and Sweden.

On the television show, series contestants eat a closely monitored diet and engage in hours of high-intensity exercise and strength training. They also learn strategies to help them continue to improve and support their new lifestyle after they leave the show.

The first Biggest Loser diet book, *The Biggest Loser: The Weight Loss Program to Transform Your Body, Health, and Life*, was published in 2005. Since then, more than 14 additional Biggest Loser books have been released, including *Biggest Loser 30-Day Jump Start*, and a wide variety of cookbooks.

The Biggest Loser diet program was developed by the experts that worked on the television show, along with Michael Dansinger, MD, an **obesity** specialist from Tufts University; Cheryl Forberg, RD, a chef and registered dietitian; and two trainers from the show, Bob Harper and Jillian Michaels.

Description

The Biggest Loser diet is a 12-week diet and exercise program designed to help individuals begin to lose weight, get in shape, and eat nutritious foods. It combines both food and exercise recommendations, along with motivation, advice, and success stories to help encourage dieters.

Food

Before beginning the Biggest Loser diet, the dieter must determine the daily calorie level that is right for him or her. The diet suggests that an individual multiply his or her current weight by seven to get the correct number of daily **calories**. For example, a 200-pound (91 kg) individual should aim for 1,400 calories per day.

The core of the Biggest Loser food program is the Biggest Loser 4-3-2-1 pyramid. This pyramid represents the amount of food that should be eaten each day: four servings of fruits and vegetables, three servings of lean proteins, two servings of healthy **whole grains**, and one serving of a treat such as sweets or alcohol.

The Biggest Loser diet provides a variety of recipes and sample menus for different target calorie levels. Aside from this, however, it is up to the dieter to monitor his or her calorie intake. Using suggested rules of thumb for correct portion sizes can be helpful for individuals who do not want to spend time counting every calorie. The diet emphasizes eating smaller meals, containing filling and fresh foods, more frequently to help combat hunger and **cravings**.

Exercise

Regular exercise is a core part of the Biggest Loser diet. The diet's message is that good health cannot exist without both a healthy, well-balanced diet and regular aerobic and strength training exercises. The Biggest Loser diet provides both extensive aerobic and strength training routines, and more are available from additional DVDs, books, and the Biggest Loser website. At the beginning of the diet, 30 minutes of exercise daily is required. This amount is increased to 60 minutes daily after a few weeks. It is important to note that contestants on the Biggest Loser television show perform well over this amount of exercise. The contestants are closely monitored, and the intense levels of exercise on the show are not recommended for the average person.

Additional content

The Biggest Loser diet has a wide variety of additional content available to dieters willing to pay for it.

There are many DVDs, CDs, pieces of fitness equipment, sportswear, and even video games for dieters who want additional motivation and encouragement. There is also the Biggest Loser Club website, where for a monthly fee individuals can access exclusive content such as additional recipes, meal plans, food and weight trackers, and message boards. The website also provides "Buddy Challenges" where dieters can compete against each other to lose weight.

Function

The Biggest Loser diet functions by providing dieters with guidelines for healthy eating that include fruits, vegetables, whole grains, and lean sources of **protein**. It is a calorie-limited diet, which when combined with the exercises suggested by the plan helps to produce steady weight loss. The emphasis on eating frequent, small meals full of fresh, wholesome ingredients was designed so that dieters do not feel hungry or deprived, helping them stay on the plan successfully. The Biggest Loser diet can easily be modified to help dieters maintain their weight loss once they have reached their goal weight.

Benefits

There are a wide variety of benefits to weight loss, regular exercise, and eating a healthy and well-balanced diet. Maintaining a healthy weight can help reduce the risk of cardiovascular disease, type 2 diabetes, some types of cancers, and possibly Alzheimer's disease. Eating a wide variety of fruits, vegetables, and whole grains can help maintain a healthy weight and reduce cholesterol and blood pressure levels. Getting regular exercise can also improve mood, flexibility, and cognitive function.

Precautions

Before beginning a new diet or exercise program, individuals should always consult with a doctor or other medical professional. Beginning an intense exercise regime after a period of inactivity can increase the risk of muscle strains and sprains, stroke, heart attack, and even sudden death. The contestants on *The Biggest Loser* are closely monitored by medical professionals during the show. Individuals at home should not exercise to the extremes that the contestants do without medical supervision and should not expect weight loss to occur as quickly as it does for contestants participating in the television show.

Risks

The risks to following the Biggest Loser diet are relatively low. The recommended food plan is similar to what is generally recommended for good health and is designed to provide a variety of **vitamins** and **minerals** each day. Dieters should be sure to eat the recommended number of calories each day for their weight, and not eat less in an attempt to lose weight more quickly. Eating fewer calories than recommended can cause dieters to eliminate vital nutrients and vitamins needed for good health. There are always some risks to exercise, including muscle sprains and strains. To reduce these risks, dieters should be sure to take the time to warm up before and cool down after each workout.

Research and general acceptance

The Biggest Loser diet has not been scientifically studied for its safety or effectiveness. However, it provides guidelines for daily eating that are generally considered healthy for most adults. Its emphasis on fruits and vegetables, whole grains, and lean proteins is similar to what is recommended in the U.S. Department of Agriculture's *Dietary Guidelines for Americans.* Many registered dietitians and other health professionals who have reviewed the diet find it to be a reasonable diet for most healthy adults, although some recommend taking a vitamin or dietary supplement while following the diet.

The U.S. Centers for Disease Control and Prevention recommends that all adults get 2 hours and 30 minutes of moderate-intensity aerobic exercise or 1 hour and 15 minutes of vigorous-intensity aerobic activity each week, along with strength-training exercises on at least two days weekly. Following the

---

QUESTIONS TO ASK YOUR DOCTOR

- Do I have any medical conditions that would make it unsafe for me to try this diet?
- Can you recommend a weight loss support group in this area?
- Does my insurance cover a visit with a registered dietitian? If so, can you refer me to one?
- How many calories per day should I aim for if I want to lose weight at a healthy pace?
- Are there any signs or symptoms that I should be aware of that could indicate a problem while on this diet?

---

exercise suggestions of the Biggest Loser diet would exceed these recommendations.

Resources

BOOKS

Alexander, Devin. *The Biggest Loser Quick and Easy Cookbook.* New York: Macmillan, 2011.

Forberg, Cheryl, Melissa Roberson, and Lisa Wheeler. *The Biggest Loser: 6 Weeks to a Healthier You.* Emmaus, PA: Rodale, 2010.

Gandy, Joan, Angela Madden, and Michelle Holdsworth, eds. *Oxford Handbook of Nutrition and Dietetics.* 2nd ed. New York: Oxford University Press, 2012.

PERIODICALS

Neve, Melinda J., Clare E. Collins, and Phillip P. Morgan. "Dropout, Nonusage Attrition, and Pretreatment Predictors of Nonusage Attrition in a Commercial Web-Based Weight Loss Program." *Journal of Medical Internet Research* 12, no. 4 (2010): e69.

OTHER

U.S. Department of Agriculture and U.S. Department of Health and Human Services. *Dietary Guidelines for Americans, 2010.* 7th ed. Washington, DC: U.S. Government Printing Office, December 2010. http://health.gov/dietaryguidelines (accessed August 22, 2012).

WEBSITES

"Biggest Loser Diet." US News and World Report: Health. http://health.usnews.com/best-diet/biggest-loser-diet (accessed August 22, 2012).

Mayo Clinic staff. "Weight Loss: Choosing a Diet That's Right for You." MayoClinic.com. http://www.mayoclinic.com/health/weight-loss/NU00616 (accessed August 22, 2012).

Zelman, Kathleen M. "'The Biggest Loser' Diet." WebMD.com. http://www.webmd.com/diet/features/biggest-loser-diet (accessed August 22, 2012).

ORGANIZATIONS

Academy of Nutrition and Dietetics, 120 South Riverside Plz., Ste. 2000, Chicago, IL 60606-6995, (312) 899-0040, (800) 877-1600, amacmunn@eatright.org, http://www.eatright.org.

The Biggest Loser Club, (800) 914-9367, customer_service@biggestloserclub.com, http://www.biggestloserclub.com.

Center for Nutrition Policy and Promotion, U.S. Department of Agriculture, 3101 Park Center Drive, 10th Fl., Alexandria, VA 22302, (703) 305-7600, Fax: (703) 305-3300, support@cnpp.usda.gov, http://www.cnpp.usda.gov.

Tish Davidson, AM

Binge eating

Definition

Binge eating is an abnormal eating pattern characterized by the consumption of a large amount of food within a limited time period, such as one or two hours. A pattern of frequent overeating is classified as binge eating disorder (BED), a serious eating disorder also known as compulsive overeating.

Demographics

Binge eating disorder is the most commonly diagnosed eating disorder, affecting 3.5% of women and 2% of men at some point in their adult lives. Although it often begins in late adolescence or early twenties, BED is also common during middle age. As many as one-half of people attending weight-loss clinics are considered to have BED. Although BED affects blacks and whites equally, little research has been done on binge eating in other racial or ethnic groups.

Data from a 2011 study conducted by the U.S. National Institute of Mental Health showed that the lifetime prevalence of binge eating disorder in teens is 1.6% (approximately 300,000 teens). The study was based on interviews with more than 10,000 adolescents aged 13 to 18 years. The study data also showed that rates of binge eating disorder, as well as **bulimia nervosa**, have approximately doubled since 1990, while the rates of **anorexia nervosa** have remained fairly stable. More girls were affected by binge eating disorder than boys, and approximately 15% of any teens with binge eating disorder had attempted suicide.

Description

Although most people overeat on occasion, BED is a pattern of frequent overeating, which is different from continuous snacking and often occurs in the absence of hunger. Although the duration of a binge may vary significantly, binge eating is characterized by an inability to stop eating during each episode and a general feeling of being out of control. A binge typically ends only when all of the desirable binge foods have been consumed or when the person feels too full to continue. Binge eaters generally eat very fast and alone—usually out of embarrassment—and suffer strong negative feelings such as guilt, shame, or depression following the binge.

The American Psychiatric Association recognizes BED as an eating disorder, and it has been proposed to be included in the *Diagnostic and Statistical Manual of Mental Disorders*, the diagnostic guide used by professionals in the field of mental health.

Some experts believe that binge eating should be classified as an obesity-related behavior. However, not all binge eaters are obese, and not all obese people are binge eaters. Further, binge eaters are far more likely to report significant mood problems, especially depression, and greater dissatisfaction with their weight and shape, as compared to people with **obesity**.

Other experts believe that binge eating is a subtype of bulimia. Bulimia is characterized by episodes of binge eating followed by self-induced purging through vomiting; abuse of laxatives, diuretics, or enemas; fasting; or compulsive exercise. Although people with BED often attempt to diet between binges, they do not purge the extra **calories**. They also do not exhibit anorexic or self-starving behaviors, which may occur in people with bulimia.

Risk factors

Risk factors for binge eating are similar to risk factors for other **eating disorders**. These include:

- a family history of eating disorders
- frequent dieting, especially rigorous dieting or weight cycling
- preoccupation with weight and body image
- impulsiveness or poor impulse control
- low self-esteem and negative self-talk
- difficulty expressing feelings appropriately and managing anger
- a history of sexual abuse
- depression, which can be both a risk factor for binge eating or a result of binge eating

Causes and symptoms

Like other eating disorders, BED has multiple causes. Some people appear to be genetically predisposed to binge eating. Researchers believe that this may be related to abnormalities in the brain neurotransmitters that help regulate appetite. Episodes of binge eating may occur in response to strong negative emotions, such as depression or anxiety, or to less defined feelings of stress or tension. People who binge eat are far more likely than others to describe themselves as experiencing personal and work problems and as being hypersensitive to the opinions of others. Like with bulimia, people with BED are more likely than others to be diagnosed with major depression, substance-related disorders, and personality disorders. Binge eating is often triggered by stress—sometimes the stress is caused by very restrictive diets, but often the stress is caused by social and cultural factors, such as family conflicts or dysfunctional relationships. Pressure felt from cultural and media messages that promote being thin as desirable can also result in binge eating, which may be used as a coping mechanism. Some patients report that their binges are related to the ingestion of certain "trigger foods," usually **carbohydrates**.

Whatever the cause, binge eating appears to temporarily alleviate uncomfortable or painful feelings. When binge eating, patients typically describe themselves as "numb" or "spaced out." The relief is short-lived, leading to repeated episodes. The out-of-control eating is a frightening experience for most people, and they usually report feeling embarrassed and ashamed about their bingeing. In the aftermath of a binge, many people experience overwhelming feelings of guilt, self-disgust, anxiety, or depression. They may vow never to binge again but are unable to prevent it.

Symptoms of binge eating can be difficult to detect. The eating often occurs in private, and the eater tends to be secretive about food. Specific symptoms of binge eating include:

- feeling out of control and unable to stop eating
- continuing to eat despite feeling full or even painfully uncomfortable
- eating abnormally large amounts of food at one sitting, sometimes as many as 3,000–10,000 calories in a short period
- eating abnormally fast
- eating alone or in secret
- hoarding food and hiding empty food containers
- constant dieting without weight loss
- obsessive concern with weight
- depression
- anxiety
- substance abuse

Diagnosis

Binge eating can be hard for healthcare providers to diagnose. People with BED often go out of their way to hide how much they eat. They may, for example, buy snack food at the grocery store and eat it in the car before they go home, or they may buy food in secret and hide it so that people close to them will not know they are bingeing. Normally, healthcare professionals begin diagnosis with a family and personal history. However, patients may not reveal their true eating habits.

If a patient (or family member) does tell their doctor about their eating behaviors, the physician will conduct a physical examination and usually order standard laboratory tests such as a complete blood count (CBC), urinalysis, and blood tests to check the level of cholesterol, **triglycerides**, and **electrolytes**. Additional tests, such as a thyroid function test, may be ordered to rule out other disorders. If the individual is obese, tests may be done check for obesity-related diseases such as diabetes, cardiovascular disease, and sleep apnea.

Several different evaluations can be used to examine the patient's mental state. A doctor or mental health professional will assess the individual's thoughts and feelings about themselves, their body, their relationships with others, and their risk for self-harm. These tests are usually administered in an office setting.

Treatment

BED is usually treated most effectively by a combination of psychotherapy and group therapy. However, physicians are more likely to concentrate on weight-control issues, using drugs, diet, and nutrition counseling to reduce the health risks of obesity-related diseases. Although nutrition counseling and meal planning may help control weight, they do not address the impulse to binge eat. Psychologists are more likely to treat behavior and thought patterns that cause abnormal eating, since obesity may be easier to treat once bingeing behavior is controlled.

There are no drugs specifically approved by the U.S. Food and Drug Administration (FDA) for treating binge eating. However, the FDA has approved antidepressants called selective serotonin reuptake inhibitors (SSRIs), such as fluoxetine (Prozac) and sertraline (Zoloft), for the treatment of bulimia, which involves binge-eating behavior. These medications increase serotonin levels in the brain and are thought to affect the body's sense of fullness. SSRIs may be prescribed for BED, regardless of whether there are signs of depression. Tricyclic antidepressants (TCAs) and appetite suppressants may be prescribed for BED, but their use is rare. The anticonvulsant topiramate (Topamax), which is normally used to control seizures, has been found to reduce binge-eating episodes, but this drug can have serious side effects.

Although weight-loss programs are helpful for some people with BED, they generally are not recommended until after BED treatment, since low-calorie diets can trigger binge eating. Weight-loss programs generally do not address binge-eating triggers to the same extent as psychotherapy. Weight loss should be medically supervised.

Self-help programs, including books and manuals, videos, and support groups, can be helpful for treating BED. A 2010 study of patients with at least one binge-eating episode per week found that 64% of patients who attended eight therapy sessions utilizing a six-step self-help program were binge free after one year. This compared with 45% of patients who were given only basic healthy eating information and informed of available services.

Self-help programs are cost-effective as well. In another 2010 study of 123 patients with binge eating disorder, a guided self-help program was significantly more cost effective than simply providing patients with options for treatment. The cost to society in terms of binge-free days and workplace productivity was significantly reduced in the intervention group, with a savings of more than $26,000 per quality-adjusted life year.

Nutrition and dietary concerns

People with binge eating disorder understand that their eating pattern is abnormal and unhealthy. Nutrition counseling and meal planning can help bring weight under control, but they do not address the inability to control the impulse to binge. Nutrition counseling needs to be part of a broader treatment program that includes psychotherapy and possibly drug therapy.

Therapy

Several types of psychotherapy may be effective for treating BED. Cognitive-behavioral therapy (CBT) is a relatively short-term therapy designed to confront and change thoughts and feelings about one's body and behaviors toward food. It does not address the origins of those thoughts and feelings, but rather explores self-control strategies and the development of skills for coping with emotional distress. Interpersonal therapy is short-term therapy to help identify and resolve specific relationship issues and problems and has been shown to

be successful in the treatment of BED. Dialectical behavior therapy (DBT) utilizes structured private and group sessions for reducing behaviors that interfere with quality of life, finding alternate solutions to current problem situations, and learning to regulate emotions. Family therapy is helpful for treating children who binge eat. It teaches strategies for reducing conflict, disorder, and stress that can trigger binge eating. Regardless of the type of therapy used, in order for it to be effective, the individual must truly want to stop binge eating.

Prognosis

There is no clear prognosis for binge eating disorder, though overall rates of recovery are higher for

BED than for bulimia. Since stress often triggers bingeing, relapses are most likely to occur in response to stressful life events. Some individuals find that simply seeking help improves their control over binge eating. For example, some studies have found that receiving a placebo is as effective as receiving medication, although this is one reason why some parts of the medical community refuse to accept binge eating as a genuine disorder. Many studies are underway to test different approaches to treating binge eating. Individuals interested in participating in a clinical trial at no cost can find a list of studies currently enrolling volunteers at http://www.clinicaltrials.gov.

Prevention

Binge eating is difficult to prevent, since its causes are unclear, and it can be difficult to detect. Prevention strategies include:

- eating small meals every three or four hours to avoid hunger
- tracking food intake
- avoiding eating alone
- avoiding using food for comfort in times of stress
- monitoring negative self-talk and practicing positive self-talk
- spending time doing something enjoyable every day
- staying busy without becoming frantic or stressed
- being aware of situations that invite bingeing and looking for ways to avoid or defuse such situations
- avoiding extreme diets

- teaching children to have healthy attitudes toward their weight, appearance, and diet
- avoiding comparisons or teasing about body size and shape
- loving and accepting family members for who they are
- being alert for signs of low self-esteem, anxiety, depression, and drug or alcohol abuse, and seeking help if signs appear

Resources

BOOKS

Agras, W. Stewart. *Overcoming Eating Disorders: A Cognitive-Behavioral Therapy Approach for Bulimia Nervosa and Binge-Eating Disorder*. 2nd ed. New York: Oxford University Press, 2008.

Bulik, Cynthia M. *Crave: Why You Binge Eat and How to Stop*. New York: Walker, 2009.

Favor, Lesli J. *Food as Foe: Nutrition and Eating Disorders*. New York: Marshall Cavendish Benchmark, 2008.

Heaton, Jeanne A. and Claudia J. Strauss. *Talking to Eating Disorders: Simple Ways to Support Someone Who Has Anorexia, Bulimia, Binge Eating or Body Image Issues*. New York: New American Library, 2005.

Herzog, David B., Debra L. Franko, and Patricia Cable. *Unlocking the Mysteries of Eating Disorders*. New York: McGraw-Hill, 2007.

Munsch, Simone and Christoph Beglinger, eds. *Obesity and Binge Eating Disorder*. New York: Karger, 2005.

Rubin, Jerome S., ed. *Eating Disorders and Weight Loss Research*. Hauppauge, NY: Nova Science Publishers, 2006.

Saxen, Ron. *The Good Eater: The True Story of One Man's Struggle With Binge Eating Disorder*. Oakland, CA: New Harbinger Publications, 2007.

Silverstein, Alvin, Virginia B. Silverstein, and Laura Silverstein Nunn. *The Eating Disorders Update: Understanding Anorexia, Bulimia, and Binge Eating*. Berkeley Heights, NJ: Enslow, 2009.

Walsh, B. Timothy. *If Your Adolescent Has an Eating Disorder: An Essential Resource for Parents*. New York: Oxford University Press, 2005.

Watson, Stephanie. *Binge Eating*. New York: Rosen Pub. Group, 2007.

PERIODICALS

Arikian, A., et al. "Establishing Thresholds for Unusually Large Binge Eating Episodes." *International Journal of Eating Disorders* 45, no. 2 (2012): 222–26. http://dx.doi.org/10.1002/eat.20930 (accessed June 25, 2012).

Hellmich, Nanci. "Treating Binge Eating Need Not Be Extensive or Expensive Study: 64% Stopped with Six-Step Plan." *USA Today* (April 6, 2010): D4. http://www.usatoday.com/news/health/2010-04-06-bingeeating05_ST_N.htm (accessed June 25, 2012).

Lynch, Frances, et al. "Cost-Effectiveness of Guided Self-Help Treatment for Recurrent Binge Eating." *Journal of Consulting and Clinical Psychology* 78, no. 3 (June 2010): 322–33.

Mond, Jonathan M., Carol B. Peterson, and Phillipa J. Hay. "Prior Use of Extreme Weight-Control Behaviors in a Community Sample of Women with Binge Eating Disorder or Subthreshold Binge Eating Disorder: A Descriptive Study." *International Journal of Eating Disorders* 43, no. 5 (July 2010): 440–46.

Moon, Kenneth T. "Comparison of Psychological Treatments for Binge Eating Disorder." *American Family Physician* 82, no. 5 (September 1, 2010): 534.

Roberto, Christina A., et al. "Binge Eating, Purging, or Both: Eating Disorder Psychopathology Findings from an Internet Community Survey." *International Journal of Eating Disorders* 43, no. 8 (December 2010): 724–31.

Treasure, Janet, Angélica M. Claudino, and Nancy Zucker. "Eating Disorders." *Lancet* 375, no. 9714 (February 13–19, 2010): 583–93.

WEBSITES

Doheny, Kathleen. "Study: Eating Disorders in Teens Are Common." WebMD. March 7, 2011. http://www.webmd.com/mental-health/anorexia-nervosa/news/20110307/study-eating-disorders-in-teens-are-common (accessed June 25, 2012).

Mayo Clinic staff. "Binge-Eating Disorder." MayoClinic.com. October 9, 2010. http://www.mayoclinic.com/health/binge-eating-disorder/DS00608 (accessed June 25, 2012).

MedlinePlus. "Eating Disorders." U.S. National Library of Medicine, National Institutes of Health. http://www.nlm.nih.gov/medlineplus/eatingdisorders.html (accessed June 25, 2012).

Nemours Foundation. "Binge Eating Disorder." KidsHealth.org. http://www.kidshealth.org/parent/emotions/behavior/binge_eating.html (accessed June 25, 2012).

Weight-Control Information Network. "Binge Eating Disorder." National Institute of Diabetes and Digestive and Kidney Diseases (NIDDK). http://win.niddk.nih.gov/publications/binge.htm (accessed June 25, 2012).

ORGANIZATIONS

American Psychological Association, 750 1st St. NE, Washington, DC 20002-4242, (202) 336-5500, (800) 374-2721, http://www.apa.org.

National Association of Anorexia Nervosa and Associated Disorders, PO Box 640, Naperville, IL 60566, (630) 577-1330, anadhelp@anad.org, http://www.anad.org.

National Eating Disorders Association, 165 W 46th St., New York, NY 10036, (212) 575-6200, (800) 931-2237, Fax: (212) 575-1650, info@NationalEatingDisorders.org, http://www.nationaleatingdisorders.org.

Overeaters Anonymous, PO Box 44020, Rio Rancho, NM 87174-4020, (505) 891-2664, Fax: (505) 891-4320, http://www.oa.org.

Weight-control Information Network, 1 WIN Way, Bethesda, MD 20892-3665, (202) 828-1025, (877) 946-4627, Fax: (202) 828-1028, win@info.niddk.nih.gov, http://win.niddk.nih.gov/index.htm.

Tish Davidson, AM
Margaret Alic, PhD
Heidi Splete

Bioengineered foods

Definition

Bioengineered foods are foods that have had a gene from a different species of plant or other organism introduced to produce desired characteristics or traits. Bioengineered foods are also referred to as

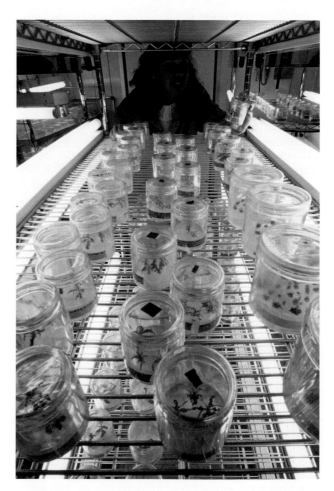

A technician checks on plants in a lab. Each dish holds tiny peach or apple trees grown from lab-cultured cells that have been given new genes. *(Scott Bauer/U.S. Department of Agriculture (USDA))*

genetically modified organisms (GMOs) or living modified organisms (LMOs).

Purpose

The general purpose of bioengineering is to create plants or animals that are in some way superior to a current breed of plant or animal in existence. For example, some genetically engineered plants are modified to resist specific insects or diseases. This means that those plants are more likely to grow large and to stay healthy. Because most farming uses pesticides or insecticides to protect plants, plants that are bioengineered to be pest resistant allow farmers to use less of these chemicals. This change is positive for the environment, as well as possibly less costly for the farmer, and can often provide cheaper products for the consumer.

In addition to producing heartier crops, some bioengineering is done to improve the taste of crops. Other bioengineering is done to introduce traits that will help the crops get to the consumer in better condition or have a longer period of freshness. In 1994, the first bioengineered food to be introduced to the consumer market in the United States was the Flavr Savr tomato. This tomato was bioengineered to ripen more slowly and to remain on the vine longer so that it would be available to consumers later in the year than other tomatoes. However, it remained on the market for only three years because it proved not to be economically viable.

Bioengineering can also be used to increase crop yields, the nutrient content of foods, or to add **vitamins** that are not usually found in a certain food. A variety of rice, sometimes referred to as "golden rice," that includes beta-carotene has been developed. Beta-carotene is a provitamin to **vitamin A**, which means that the body can use it to produce vitamin A. Rice is a staple of the diet of many people around the world, and because rice does not normally contain vitamin A, many people in Asia are vitamin A deficient. This deficiency is believed to have resulted in blindness in a quarter of a million children in southeast Asia alone. If the new strain of rice that contains beta-carotene is introduced to this area, it has the potential to reduce or even eliminate vitamin A deficiency and significantly reduce childhood blindness.

Description

All living organisms have deoxyribonucleic acid (DNA) in their cells. DNA is the chemical compound that carries all of the information needed to produce

and sustain life in an organism. DNA is made up of strands of nucleic acids that are grouped to form individual genes. Each gene contains the information needed to synthesize a particular **protein**. Synthesized proteins are responsible for individual characteristics, such as hair and eye color in humans.

When scientists genetically engineer a plant, they take a gene from another plant or organism such as a bacterium and insert it into the original plant or trade it for a gene in the original plant. This trading of genes is called transposition.

Scientists did not learn how to insert and transpose genes successfully until the 1980s. However, long before this, people had been trying to create better, heartier plants and animals through selective breeding. For hundreds of years farmers had selected and bred animals based on characteristics that they wanted the offspring to have. Farmers might decide to breed a cow that gave a higher quantity of milk than other cows in the hopes of producing more cows that gave an above-average quantity of milk. Farmers also planted the seeds of plants that had desirable characteristics, hoping to produce more plants with those same traits.

Although many people were engaged in trying to make new and better plants and animals for many years, it was not until the work of Gregor Mendel in the nineteenth century that people began to understand how traits were passed from one generation to the next. Mendel did research on pea plants and discovered that traits were passed from one generation to the next in a way that could be predicated. Peas had a much simpler inheritance pattern than most organisms, so even with this knowledge it was very difficult for scientists to produce plants with the exact traits they wanted. Plants with the desired trait had to be cross bred, and then plants from the resulting generation that had the desired traits had to be selected and cross bred again and again. It takes many generations of plants to produce offspring that regularly have the desired trait.

Today, scientists do not have to cross breed plants repeatedly to get a new variety of plant that has the traits or characteristics they desire. Instead, they search for a gene in another plant that will produce the desired characteristic and insert it into the DNA of the original plant. Often two or three different genes are inserted, sometimes each from different plants or animals. Plants that have had this done are considered bioengineered. As of 2011, 94% of all soybeans grown in the United States, 90% of all cotton, and 88% of all corn had been genetically engineered. In addition, about two-thirds of all processed foods contained some form of bioengineered crop.

Bioengineered foods are regulated and monitored in the United States by three different government agencies: the U.S. Food and Drug Administration (FDA), the U.S. Department of Agriculture (USDA), and the Environmental Protection Agency (EPA). The FDA is responsible for the regulation and labeling of the bioengineered foods, the USDA oversees the safety and completeness of test fields used by bioengineering companies to test their new plants, and the EPA regulates any bioengineered plants that contain pesticide-related genes.

Before companies can put a genetically engineered food on the market, they need to prove that it is safe for consumers. The FDA requires that companies prove that the bioengineered food is just as safe and nutritious as the non-bioengineered equivalent. This process includes providing information for the FDA to review about the kinds of proteins synthesized by the new gene or genes, nutritional content, toxicology reports, and other information.

In the United States, labeling of bioengineered foods is voluntary and is left to the discretion of the company. The European Union has strict labeling laws for food and animal feed containing bioengineered components in EU member states. The EU laws require that any food or animal feed product containing a proportion of bioengineered product greater than 0.9% must be labeled. This can include statements such as "genetically modified" or "made from genetically modified [the name of the ingredient]" on the package. On foods that are not packaged, the EU requires a sign displaying this information to be placed near the item for sale, such as on a counter or a supermarket shelf.

Precautions

There is a small chance that some people might have an unexpected allergic reaction to proteins synthesized by plants that have been genetically modified. This is unlikely, however, as the FDA regulates bioengineered foods and requires tests for safety and the presence of known allergens before the food is allowed on the market.

Interactions

There are no expected interactions between bioengineered foods and any other foods, medicines, or products.

Complications

There are no complications expected from consuming bioengineered foods.

Parental concerns

Some parents might be concerned that allergens that could affect their child might be introduced into unexpected plant species. Ninety percent of **food allergies** in the United States are to milk, eggs, fish, shellfish, nuts, wheat, and legumes (including peanuts and soybeans). The FDA ensures that each bioengineered food is tested to ensure that none of the common proteins that cause reactions to these foods can be sold to consumers. They also test for additional, less common proteins that have been known to cause allergic reactions.

Resources

BOOKS

Bodiguel, Luc, and Cardwell, Michael, eds. *The Regulation of Genetically Modified Organisms: Comparative Approaches.* New York: Oxford University Press, 2010.

Forman, Lillian E. *Genetically Modified Foods.* Edina, MN: ABDO, 2010.

Healey, Justin, ed. *Genetically Modified Food and Crops.* Thirroul, Australia: Spinney Press, 2010.

Heldman, Dennis R., Matthew B. Wheeler, and Dallas G. Hoover, eds. *Encyclopedia of Biotechnology in Agriculture and Food.* Boca Raton, FL: CRC Press, 2011.

Miller, Debra A. *Genetically Engineered Food.* Detroit: Greenhaven Press, 2011.

PERIODICALS

Gamarra, Luis Fernando Rimachi, Jorge Enrique Alacantara, and Rodomiro Ortiz. "Controversy Over GM Maize in Peru." *Nature* 470, no. 7332 (February 3, 2011): 39.

McHughen, Alan, and Robert Wagner. "Popular Misconceptions: Agricultural Biotechnology." *New Biotechnology* 27, no. 6 (2010): 724–28.

Stone, R. "Activists Go on Warpath Against Transgenic Crops—And Scientists." *Science* 331, no. 6020 (February 25, 2011): 1000–1001.

WEBSITES

University of Maryland Medical Center. "Genetically Engineered Foods." http://www.umm.edu/ency/article/002432.htm (accessed September 28, 2012).

ORGANIZATIONS

U.S. Department of Agriculture, 1400 Independence Ave. SW, Washington, DC 20250, (202) 720-2791, http://www.usda.gov.

U.S. Food and Drug Administration, 10903 New Hampshire Ave., Silver Spring, MD 20993-0002, (888) INFO-FDA (463-6332), http://www.fda.gov.

World Health Organization, Avenue Appia 20, 1211 Geneva 27, Switzerland, +4122791-2111, Fax: +4122791-3111, info@who.int, http://www.who.int.

Tish Davidson, MA
David Newton

Biotin

Definition

Biotin, also known as vitamin H or vitamin B₇, belongs to the group of B-complex water-soluble **vitamins**. The body produces only a small amount of biotin, so most of the biotin we need must come from food. Biotin is involved in the conversion of **carbohydrates**, **fats**, and **protein** into usable energy for the body.

Purpose

Biotin joins with protein enzymes to regulate the breakdown of foods in the body and convert them to energy. Some researchers believe that biotin also plays a role in the duplication and "reading" (replication and transcription) of deoxyribonucleic acid (DNA).

Makers of dietary supplements promote biotin to treat brittle fingernails, dry skin, and hair loss. It is sold as a dietary supplement in capsules or tablets, either alone, in a multivitamin, or combined with brewer's yeast. Biotin is also added to cosmetics and skin creams. In animal studies, biotin has improved the condition of horse hooves, but no controlled studies have shown the same effect on human fingernails. Biotin deficiency does cause hair loss, but there is no proof that supplemental biotin prevents hair loss.

Description

Biotin is one of the less familiar B vitamins. It was discovered in the 1930s by researchers experimenting with different diets for chickens and rats, and later it was discovered to be essential to human health. Bacteria, yeasts, mold, algae, and some plants make biotin. The large intestine (colon) in humans contains some bacteria that synthesize biotin. Researchers believe that a portion of this biotin is absorbed into the bloodstream, but they are uncertain how much or how available it is to the body.

Biotin is essential to life. It combines with four different enzymes that control different metabolic reactions related to energy production and the building of new molecules from simple nutrients. Biotin helps the body:

- form glucose from fats and amino acids (but not from carbohydrates)
- build fatty acids
- synthesize leucine, an amino acid necessary for health
- metabolize amino acids, cholesterol, and some fatty acids

Some researchers believe that biotin binds to proteins called histones, which open up chromosomes so that their DNA becomes accessible and can be copied. If this is true, biotin could play a role in gene expression.

Normal biotin requirements

The Institute of Medicine (IOM) of the National Academy of Sciences has developed values called **dietary reference intakes (DRIs)** for vitamins and **minerals**. The **DRIs** consist of three sets of numbers: recommended dietary allowance (RDA), adequate intake (AI), and tolerable upper intake level (UL). RDAs define the average daily amount of the nutrient

Biotin	
Age	Adequate intake (mcg/day)
Children 0–6 mos.	5
Children 7–12 mos.	6
Children 1–3 yrs.	8
Children 4–8 yrs.	12
Children 9–13 yrs.	20
Children 14–18 yrs.	25
Adults 19≤ yrs.	30
Pregnant women	30
Breastfeeding women	35

mcg = microgram

SOURCE: U.S. Department of Agriculture, National Agricultural Library, Food and Nutrition Information Center.

(Table by PreMediaGlobal. © 2013 Cengage Learning.)

needed to meet the health needs of 97%–98% of the population. AIs are estimates set when there is not enough information to determine an RDA. The UL is the average maximum amount that can be taken daily without risking negative side effects. DRIs are calculated for children, adults, and pregnant and **breastfeeding** women.

The IOM has not set RDA values for biotin because of incomplete scientific information. Instead, there are AI levels for all age groups. AI levels for biotin are measured by weight (micrograms or mcg). No UL levels have been set due to a lack of data.

The AIs for biotin for healthy individuals are:

• infants 0–6 months: 5 mcg
• infants 7–12 months: 6 mcg
• children 1–3 years: 8 mcg
• children 4–8 years: 12 mcg
• children 9–13 years: 20 mcg
• children 14–18 years: 25 mcg
• adults 19 and older: 30 mcg
• pregnant women: 30 mcg
• breastfeeding women: 35 mcg

Sources of biotin

Biotin is found in small quantities in many foods. Bacteria in the large intestine also make biotin. Unlike some vitamins, biotin is recycled and reused by the body, meaning that daily intake does not need to be high. Only small amounts of biotin are lost in urine. Biotin in food is stable and minimally affected by heat, light, or air.

The approximate biotin content in some common foods is:

• bread, whole wheat, 1 slice: 6 mcg
• cauliflower, raw, 1/2 cup: 2 mcg
• chicken, cooked, 3 ounces: 3 mcg
• egg, 1 cooked: 25 mcg
• liver, cooked, 3 ounces: 27 mcg
• pork, cooked, 3 ounces: 2 mcg
• salmon, cooked, 3 ounces: 4 mcg
• swiss chard, cooked, 1/2 cup: 5.2 mcg

Biotin deficiency

Biotin deficiency is very rare worldwide. Only a few conditions are known to cause biotin deficiency. Two rare inherited genetic disorders cause the body to need excessive amounts of biotin. These disorders are treated with high-dose biotin supplements. Prolonged (months or years) consumption of raw egg whites can also cause a deficiency. A protein in raw egg whites binds biotin and makes it unavailable to the body. Cooking the egg releases the biotin. Receiving all nutrition through intravenous feeding (total parenteral nutrition or TPN) for an extended period may also lead to a shortage of biotin in the body.

Symptoms of biotin deficiency include skin and hair problems, such as a red, scaly rash on the face, increased susceptibility to fungal infections, brittle hair, and hair loss. Individuals may also develop seizures, problems with coordination, and muscle cramps. Biotin deficiency has not been known to cause death. These symptoms have many other causes that should be considered first, however, because biotin deficiency is so rare.

Precautions

In many species, pregnant animals who are biotin deficient give birth to offspring with birth defects at a higher rate than animals who have adequate levels of biotin. The same effect has not been seen in humans, but blood levels of biotin tend to drop in pregnant women, causing concern among researchers that pregnant women may develop marginal biotin deficiencies with no visible symptoms. **Dietary supplements** of biotin are not routinely recommended for women who are pregnant, but these women should make a special effort to obtain the adequate intake of 30 mcg biotin daily through diet. Pregnant and breastfeeding women should not take a biotin dietary supplement unless directed by their healthcare provider.

Interactions

Biotin is known to interact with a few drugs and dietary supplements:

• Antibiotics taken over a long period may reduce the amount of bacteria in the large intestine that synthesize biotin.
• Long-term use of drugs to prevent seizures—such as phenytoin (Dilantin), primidone (Mysoline), carbamazepine (Tegretol), phenobarbital (Solfoton), and possibly valproic acid—cause a reduction in the blood level of biotin.
• High doses of pantothenic acid may decrease the amount of biotin absorbed from the large intestine.

Complications

No complications are expected from biotin. Even when large doses are taken for long periods, there are no reported side effects.

KEY TERMS

B-complex vitamins—A group of water-soluble vitamins that often work together in the body. These include thiamin (B_1), riboflavin (B_2), niacin (B_3), pantothenic acid (B_5), pyridoxine (B_6), biotin (B_7 or vitamin H), folate/folic acid (B_9), and cobalamin (B_{12}).

Dietary supplement—Any product, such as a vitamin, mineral, herb, amino acid, or enzyme, intended to be consumed in addition to an individual's diet with the expectation that it will improve health.

Enzyme—A protein that changes the rate of a chemical reaction within the body without being depleted in the reaction.

Fatty acids—Complex molecules found in fats and oils. Essential fatty acids are fatty acids that the body needs but cannot synthesize. They are made by plants and must be obtained through diet.

Glucose—A simple sugar resulting from the breakdown of carbohydrates. Glucose circulates in the blood and is the main source of energy for the body.

Vitamin—A nutrient the body needs in small amounts to remain healthy but that the body cannot manufacture for itself and must acquire through diet.

Water-soluble vitamin—A vitamin that dissolves in water and can be removed from the body in urine.

Parental concerns

Biotin deficiency is rare, so as long as children are eating a well-balanced diet, parents should have almost no concern about their children's biotin needs being met.

Resources

BOOKS

Berkson, Burt, and Arthur J. Berkson. *Basic Health Publications User's Guide to the B-complex Vitamins.* Laguna Beach, CA: Basic Health Publications, 2006.

Gaby, Alan R., ed. *A–Z Guide to Drug-Herb-Vitamin Interactions: Improve Your Health and Avoid Side Effects When Using Common Medications and Natural Supplements Together.* 2nd ed., rev. New York: Three Rivers Press, 2006.

Lieberman, Shari, and Nancy Bruning. *The Real Vitamin and Mineral Book: The Definitive Guide to Designing Your Personal Supplement Program.* 4th ed. New York: Avery, 2007.

Rucker, Robert B., ed. *Handbook of Vitamins.* Boca Raton, FL: Taylor & Francis, 2007.

PERIODICALS

Mock, Donald M. "Marginal Biotin Deficiency Is Common in Normal Human Pregnancy and Is Highly Teratogenic in Mice." *Journal of Nutrition* 139, no. 1 (2009): 154–57. http://dx.crossref.org/10.3945%2Fjn.108.095273 (accessed August 9, 2012).

WEBSITES

Higdon, Jane, and Victoria Drake. "Biotin." Linus Pauling Institute, Oregon State University. http://lpi.oregonstate.edu/infocenter/vitamins/biotin (accessed August 9, 2012).

MedlinePlus. "Biotin." U.S. National Library of Medicine, National Institutes of Health. http://www.nlm.nih.gov/medlineplus/druginfo/natural/313.html (accessed August 9, 2012).

University of Maryland Medical Center. "Vitamin H (Biotin)." http://www.umm.edu/altmed/articles/vitamin-h-000342.htm (accessed August 9, 2012).

ORGANIZATIONS

Academy of Nutrition and Dietetics, 120 South Riverside Plz., Ste. 2000, Chicago, IL 60606-6995, (312) 899-0040, (800) 877-1600, amacmunn@eatright.org, http://www.eatright.org.

Food and Nutrition Information Center, National Agricultural Library, 10301 Baltimore Ave., Rm. 105, Beltsville, MD 20705, (301) 504-5414, Fax: (301) 504-6409, fnic@ars.usda.gov, http://fnic.nal.usda.gov.

Institute of Medicine, National Academy of Sciences, 500 Fifth St. NW, Washington, DC 20001, (202) 334-2352, iomwww@nas.edu, http://www.iom.edu.

Tish Davidson, AM

Blood type diet

Definition

The Blood Type diet is a fad diet that claims that an individual's blood type (A, B, AB, or O) can affect diet and health. In his 1996 book, *Eat Right for Your Blood Type*, naturopathic doctor Peter D'Adamo presents the idea that an individual's blood type determines which foods are healthy for that person and which are not. The book describes the anthropological origins of each of the four blood types and explains why each blood type develops specific antibodies against certain foods.

Purported benefits of the Blood Type diet

Blood type O
Weight loss
Prevents blood clotting disorder and inflammatory diseases, including arthritis, hypothyroidism, ulcers, and asthma

Blood type A
Weight loss
Reduced risk of heart disease, cancer, anemia, liver and gallbladder disorders, and type I diabetes

Blood type B
Weight loss
Reduction of the risk of type I diabetes, chronic fatigue syndrome, and autoimmune disorders such as Lou Gehrig's disease, lupus, and multiple sclerosis

Blood type AB
Weight loss
Reduction in the risk of developing heart disease, cancer, or anemia

(Table by GGS Information Services. © 2013 Cengage Learning.)

Origins

In 1901, Dr. Karl Landsteiner discovered that there were four types of human blood. He named them A, B, AB, and O. He received the Nobel Prize in Physiology or Medicine in 1930 for that discovery and research that made it safer to do blood transfusions. Before Landsteiner's discovery about blood types, transfusions could be fatal because mixing blood from two people could lead to blood clumping, known as agglutination. Landsteiner discovered that blood clumping was an immunological reaction that occurred when the recipient of the blood transfusion had antibodies against the donor blood.

D'Adamo's father, James, also a naturopathic physician, noticed that different diets worked better with some patients than others. In Peter D'Adamo's 1994 book, *One Man's Food—Is Someone Else's Poison*, he attributed this difference to the differences in blood type. Peter D'Adamo continued his father's research by studying the agglutination process that occurred between specific blood types and certain foods. He maintained that it was the result of the evolution of the unique blood types. As of July 2012, he served as academic dean for the Institute for Human Individuality, an institution with the goal of fostering education and research in **nutrigenomics** and epigenetics.

The evolution of blood types

Anthropologists have traced the origins of each blood type. The earliest human blood type was type O. Since these people were ancient hunter-gatherers and ate a diet dominated by meat, blood type O individuals developed antibodies against the lectins found in agricultural foods such as wheat and other grains. D'Adamo suggested that individuals with type O blood should eat a diet more similar to their ancient ancestors—that is, a diet with more meats and fewer grains.

The next blood type to evolve was type A. As the environmental conditions changed, humans began to grow food rather than hunt it. The diet shifted from predominantly meat to plant-based. As the diet changed and the blood type A evolved, antibodies for lectins in meat were formed. According to D'Adamo, individuals with blood type A have antibodies against many lectins found in meat and will benefit from a largely vegetarian or plant-based diet.

The next blood type to emerge was type B. As ancient peoples migrated and adapted to further climate change, blood type B evolved. Their diet included meats, plants, and dairy products. D'Adamo claimed this was the reason individuals with blood type B developed fewer antibodies against lectins found in meat and grain. He also maintained this was why people with blood type B were more tolerant of milk products than other blood types.

The final blood type to evolve was type AB. It remains a rare blood type, with fewer than 5% of the world's population having type AB blood. Type AB evolved when the A and B blood types intermingled. D'Adamo described this blood type as a complex blood type with many strengths and many contradictions.

Description

The Blood Type diet includes extensive lists of foods that are beneficial for each blood type. The food lists also include foods that each blood type should avoid and foods that are neutral or benign. D'Adamo reports that following this diet will not only improve health but will help individuals achieve an ideal weight.

The Blood Type diet

The Blood Type diet divides all foods into 16 food groups:

- Meats—beef, poultry, and pork
- Seafood—fish and shellfish
- Dairy and eggs—milk, yogurt, ice cream, cheese, and eggs
- Oils and fats—all oils such as peanut oil, linseed oil, and sesame oil
- Nuts and seeds—all nuts or seeds
- Beans and legumes—all beans and peas
- Cereals—oats such as barley, cream of wheat, corn flakes, and puffed rice

- Breads and muffins—all baked goods including loaf breads and crackers
- Grains and pasta—this includes all flour, buckwheat, noodles, and spaghetti
- Vegetables—all vegetables, olives, peppers, and avocado
- Fruit—fresh, dried, and canned fruits
- Juices and fluids—all fruit juices, fresh and from concentrate
- Spices—all spices fresh and dried, syrups, miso, soy sauce, and other sauces that are not dairy based
- Condiments—mayonnaise, mustard, ketchup, jellies and jams, pickles, pickle relish, and salad dressing
- Herbal teas—all herbal teas
- Miscellaneous beverages—coffee, black tea, green tea, seltzer waters, colas, wine, beer, and liquor

Within each of the 16 food groups, there are foods that promote weight gain, foods that support weight loss, beneficial foods, neutral foods, and foods to avoid. The diet is unique and individual for each blood type. For example, chicken is considered neutral for individuals with blood type O and blood type A. However, it is on the foods-to-avoid list for individuals with blood type B and blood type AB.

In addition to specific and detailed **dietary guidelines**, *Eat Right for Your Blood Type* also includes advice for each blood type concerning the impact of stress on the body and strategies for coping with stress. D'Adamo outlined the best supplements for each blood type and addressed the best form of exercise for individuals of each blood type.

GenoType diet

D'Adamo presented another approach to dieting in the 2007 book, *The GenoType Diet: Change Your Genetic Destiny to Live the Longest, Fullest and Healthiest Life Possible*. The book divides people into six genetic categories (GenoTypes). Similar to the Blood Type diet, each GenoType category has an eating plan of foods to emphasize, foods to limit or avoid, and neutral foods.

Blood type is one of the criteria used to determine a person's GenoType. According to D'Adamo, the six GenoTypes are:

- hunter (tall, thin, intense)
- gatherer (full figured)
- teacher (strong, stable)
- explorer (muscular, adventurous, problem solver)
- warrior (long, lean)
- nomad (sensitive, vulnerable)

There is a food list for each GenoType. Foods in the book are categorized as "superfoods to emphasize" and "toxins to limit or avoid." Superfoods that provide additional benefits are marked with a diamond. Food in the Toxins list with a black dot may be added to the diet in moderate amounts three to six months after the person has been on the diet. Neutral foods, or those that do not have nutritional benefits for that GenoType, are the remaining foods that are not on either list. D'Adamo also makes recommendations for supplements, stress reduction, and exercise.

Function

The Blood Type diet was built on the fact that all foods have lectins, or proteins that can interact with antibodies in blood. D'Adamo believes that when a specific food's lectin reacts with a specific blood type (A, B, AB, or O), it can cause agglutination to occur. In agglutination, the lectins cause the blood to become sticky, and D'Adamo asserts that these sticky blood cells can lead to medical conditions including **obesity**, impaired digestion, kidney and liver problems, headache, and diabetes. The Blood Type diet claims to reverse this process by eliminating the foods that cause agglutination. The GenoType diet is based on a similar premise, with diet activating "good" genes and shutting down "bad" genes. However, all of D'Adamo's claims are speculative and are not supported by scientific evidence.

Benefits

D'Adamo claims that people who follow his diets will lose weight and reduce their risk of developing certain diseases. There is no proof behind these claims and they are not supported by the scientific community; however, critics do agree that certain aspects of the diets, such as limiting the amount of saturated fat and highly processed "junk" foods, will benefit most people.

Precautions

The Blood Type and GenoType diets are considered **fad diets** and are not generally supported in the scientific and medical communities. People should consult with their physician before beginning any weight loss plan, including the Blood Type or GenoType diet. This is especially true for pregnant and **breastfeeding** women. These diets restrict many healthful foods, including certain fruits, vegetables, and proteins. These foods are considered to be part of traditionally accepted dietary recommendations, such as the *2010 Dietary Guidelines for Americans* issued by the U.S. Department of Agriculture (USDA) and the Department of Health and Human Services (HHS). Other foods that the guidelines caution about limiting (such as **fats**) are acceptable in larger quantities on the Blood Type and GenoType diets.

Risks

People with certain conditions, such as diabetes, **hypertension**, heart disease, or **food allergies**, may be at higher risk of adverse side effects if following the Blood Type and GenoType diets. People with these and other conditions should never change their diets without first discussing the changes with their physician. People taking prescribed medications should also not stop taking medications unless approved by their doctor.

Research and general acceptance

While many followers of the Blood Type diet reported improved health and weight loss, the Blood Type diet has drawn some criticism, primarily that there is virtually no data to support the plans. There have been no well-designed, well-controlled studies to validate the diet claims, and critics assert that if agglutination was as widespread and common as D'Adamo claims, thousands of people would die each year from organ failure caused by this process. No such evidence has been presented or found in reviews of the literature. Similar criticisms have also been made of the GenoType diet.

Although it is recognized that there is a relationship between genetics and obesity, the workings of this relationship are not yet fully understood. According to the U.S. Centers for Disease and

QUESTIONS TO ASK YOUR DOCTOR

- Is this diet appropriate for me?
- Are there any special precautions I should follow?
- What are the potential health risks if I follow this diet?
- Will I need any dietary supplements if I adopt this diet?
- Am I healthy enough for the exercises recommended for my GenoType?

Prevention (CDC), the best course of prevention for people genetically predisposed to gaining weight is a combination of a healthy diet, physical activity, and, if needed, medication. Pharmaceutical companies have begun using genetic approaches (pharmacogenomics) to develop new drug strategies to treat obesity, according to the CDC.

Resources

BOOKS

D'Adamo, Peter, with Allan Richards. *One Man's Food—Is Someone Else's Poison*. Toronto, Ontario, Canada: Health Thru Herbs (1994).

D'Adamo, Peter J., and Catherine Whitney. *Cook Right 4 Your Blood Type: The Practical Kitchen Companion to Eat Right 4 Your Blood Type*. Berkeley, CA: Berkeley Trade, 2000.

———. *The Eat Right 4 Your Blood Type Encyclopedia*. New York: G. P. Putnam and Sons, Riverhead Books, 2002.

———. *Eat Right 4 Your Type: The Individualized Diet Solution to Staying Healthy, Living Longer, and Achieving your Ideal Weight*. New York: G. P. Putnam and Sons, 1996.

———. *The GenoType Diet: Change Your Genetic Destiny to Live the Longest, Fullest and Healthiest Life Possible*. New York: Broadway Books, 2007.

———. *Live Right 4 Your Blood Type*. New York: Putnam Adult, 2000.

Nomi, Toshitaka, and Alexander Besher. *You Are Your Blood Type*. New York: St. Martin's Press, 1983.

PERIODICALS

Boblett, Michael. "What is the Genotype Diet?" *The Huffington Post* (blog), January 25, 2011. http://www.huffingtonpost.com/michael-boblett/what-is-the-genotype-diet_b_813812.html (accessed September 11, 2012).

Dorsey-Straff, Nicole. "*The GenoType Diet* Review." ThatsFit.com. http://www.thatsfit.com/2010/10/04/the-genotype-diet-review (accessed September 11, 2012).

Frazier Roberts, J.A. "Some Associations between Blood Types and Disease." *British Medical Bulletin* 15 (1959): 129–133.

Freed, D.L.F. "Dietary Lectins and Disease." *Food Allergy and Intolerance* (1987): 375–400.

———. "Lectins." *British Medical Journal* 290 (1985): 585–586.

Wyman, L.C. and W.C. Boyd. "Human Blood Groups and Anthropology." *American Anthropologist* 37 (1953): 181.

WEBSITES

"Blood Groups, Blood Typing, and Blood Transfusions." Nobelprize.org. http://www.nobelprize.org/educational/medicine/landsteiner/readmore.html (accessed September 11, 2012).

"Eat Right For Your Type." http://www.dadamo.com (accessed September 18, 2012).

"The GenoType Diet." GenotypeDiet.com. http://www.genotypediet.com (accessed September 11, 2012).

"The GenoType Diet or The Blood Type Diet: Which is Best For You?" http://www.dadamo.com/which_diet_is_right.htm (accessed September 11, 2012).

"Obesity and Genetics: What We Know, What We Don't Know and What It Means." U.S. Centers for Disease Control and Prevention. CDC.com. http://www.cdc.gov/genomics/resources/diseases/obesity/obesknow.htm (accessed September 11, 2012).

ORGANIZATIONS

Institute for Human Individuality, 213 Danbury Rd., Wilton, CT 06897, (203) 761-6701, ifhi@dadamo.com, http://www.dadamo.com/ifhi.

Deborah L. Nurmi, MS
Liz Swain

Blue-green algae *see* **Spirulina**
BMI *see* **Body mass index**

Bob Greene's diet

Definition

Bob Greene is a personal trainer and the creator of several diet and fitness programs, including *Get with the Program! (GWTP!)* and *The Best Life Diet*. Both programs are moderate and nutritionally balanced weight loss regimens combined with an exercise program and psychological introspection.

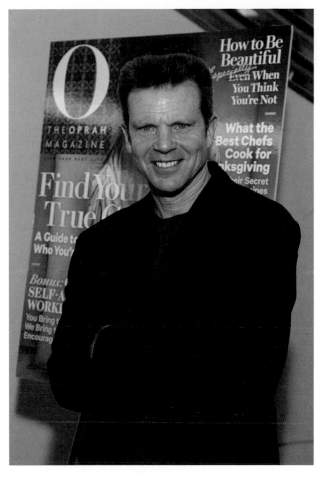

Bob Greene. *(Ben Rose/WireImage/Getty Images)*

Origins

Greene holds educational and professional credentials in physical education and exercise physiology. He maintains that his interest in health and fitness began as early as seven, when he was told that the reason his great-grandmother was bedridden was because of her excess weight. He noticed that many of his other relatives were overweight and began to read articles about food and nutrition in the daily newspaper. After high school, Greene majored in physical education at the University of Delaware and completed a master's degree in exercise physiology at the University of Arizona. He worked as the director of exercise physiology for a medical management company and as the manager and trainer of the fitness staff at a health spa in Telluride, Colorado.

Both GWTP! and the Best Life program were preceded by Greene's first book, *Make the Connection: 10 Steps to a Better Body—And a Better Life*, which he co-authored with talk show host Oprah Winfrey and published in 1996. He met Winfrey while working at the spa in Telluride, later moving to Chicago to set up a training practice and make regular appearances on her television show.

Description

Get with the Program!

GWTP! is a four-phase program that focuses on the user's slow and gradual development of new eating and exercise habits. Dieters proceed through the phases of the program at their own pace. GWTP! emphasizes the importance of organization in personal weight loss.

PHASE 1. Phase 1 centers on truth, commitment, and self-control. The theory behind this phase is that an individual will make healthier lifestyle choices if they care about their well-being. The program offers participants a contract they can use to make a commitment to themselves for a healthier lifestyle. The participant is encouraged to post it where it can be seen every day as a reminder of commitment. Physical exercise in this phase consists of flexibility, stretching, and range-of-motion exercises. Phase 1 should be completed in one to three weeks. Completion of the phase 1 checklist signifies preparation for the next phase.

PHASE 2. GWTP! asserts that many dieters make the mistake of trying to cut back on **calories** too quickly rather than increasing their level of physical activity. Phase 2 introduces participants to a physical fitness program that increases their body's **metabolism** rate. Certain types of exercise produce an effect known as the "after-burn," when the body burns calories at a higher rate for several hours after an exercise session, in addition to calories burned during the workout. Exercise also helps reinforce the commitment to healthy eating because physical changes usually present fairly rapidly. Cardiovascular workouts average 50–75 minutes per week in this phase. After one to three months, participants should be ready for Phase 3.

PHASE 3. The primary component of phase 3 is recognizing emotional eating habits. The focus on this behavior is a distinctive feature of Greene's overall approach to health and fitness. A participant needs to understand the distinction between physical hunger and eating for such emotional reasons as boredom, loneliness, job-related stress, or general anxiety. In order to learn how to tell the difference, participants are asked to choose a specific day and delay their normal meal times for several hours so that they can experience real physical hunger. (People with diabetes or other medical conditions should consult their physicians before undertaking this step.) After reestablishing an awareness of physical hunger, participants are advised to keep journals to record when events or other stimuli (television advertising, eating out, the smell of food from a nearby restaurant, stress, etc.) trigger episodes of emotional eating. Readers are encouraged to use behavior modification to alter these habits, such as substituting other activities—such as reading, taking a class, working on a hobby or craft, or going for a walk—for eating. Exercise during phase three is increased to 100–125 minutes per week. Phase 3 typically lasts one to three months.

PHASE 4. Phase 4 focuses on enhancing the changes in activity level and conscious food choices made in the first three phases. The exercise program is scaled up to include weight training. A checklist verifies that the participant met the major program goals. No specific time line is provided for this phase since it leads to a lifetime of weight management using the tools acquired throughout the program.

GWTP! stresses many of the same themes in all four phases. Participants are continuously encouraged to increase their activity level, drink more water, become aware of what triggers their hunger, and eat sensibly. Guidelines for exercise are provided at each phase. Information about nutrition and making healthy food selections is also provided. Greene believes that many people overeat because they eat haphazardly, without any meal planning, and that this lack of structure is conducive to poor nutrition and exercise habits. He recommends a schedule of three meals and two snacks a day, with a cutoff point for stopping food consumption two hours before bedtime.

The Best Life diet

PHASE 1. The chief objective in the Best Life diet is to establish a regular pattern of exercise and eating. Phase 1 begins with an initial weigh-in followed by an increase in physical activity. Participants are allowed three meals plus one or two snacks daily, but no alcohol and no eating for a minimum of two hours before bedtime. If the overall weight loss has been a pound or more per week and the daily objectives outlined in the plan are met consistently, the participant may move on to Phase 2 at the end of four weeks or continue in this phase until their goals are met.

PHASE 2. Phase 2 emphasizes significant and consistent weight loss through controlling hunger and implementing changes in eating patterns. The participant is expected to explore the physical and emotional reasons for hunger and to rate their hunger using a ten-point scale (one being very hungry and ten being very full). Participants are also expected to eat smaller food portions and remove six foods from their diet that lack nutritional value or are problem foods. Physical activity may be increased. Weight is checked every week for four weeks. When participants are within 20 lb. (9 kg) of their goal weight and the weight loss has stopped, it is time to begin phase 3.

PHASE 3. This is the lifetime maintenance phase. The objective is to continue improving the quality of the participant's diet for good health and long-term weight maintenance. The participant is asked to weigh themselves a minimum of once a month but no more than once a week. Additional nutritious foods should replace less wholesome foods on shopping lists and menus. Physical activity remains a focus, and levels should be increased as the participant improves their fitness.

SAMPLE MENUS. Week 1, Day 1:

- Breakfast: Skim milk, pear muffin, 1 fresh apple
- Snack: Low-fat yogurt
- Lunch: Walnut cannellini wrap + chopped green salad
- High-calcium snack: Whole-grain crackers with reduced-fat cheddar cheese
- Dinner: Pasta with chicken or shrimp + mixed green salad
- "Anytime treat": 1 oz. piece of dark chocolate

Week 1, Day 2:

- Breakfast: Best Life Kashi Go Lean Mix with pecans and skim milk + one half grapefruit
- Snack: Iced vanilla soy latte with graham cracker
- Lunch: Nut butter and pear whole-wheat sandwich + carrot sticks
- High-calcium snack: Maple-nut yogurt
- Dinner: Lemon and herb grilled trout + corn + sautéed sugar peas with ginger
- "Anytime treat": Low-fat ice cream

Online programs

As of 2012, the Best Life diet also included an online program featuring weight loss plans, recipes, tracking tools, and community support. The paid program cost less than $6 per month, according to the website. GWTP! was still available in book form. The books for both diet plans are roughly 300 pages long and contain recipes, meal plans, and suggestions for reexamining and making changes in one's food choices. An updated version of the Best Life diet was published in 2009 and includes Oprah's personal meal plans in addition to the Best Life menus. Two additional books can be used with GWTP!: *Get with the Program! Guide to Good Eating* (2003), containing supplementary recipes and menu plans, and *Get with*

KEY TERMS

After-burn—The increased rate of body metabolism that lasts for several hours after a session of vigorous exercise.

Emotional eating—Term for eating to alter mood or relieve stress, boredom, or loneliness.

Ovo-lacto vegetarian—A vegetarian who consumes eggs and dairy products as well as plant-based foods.

Personal trainer—An individual specializing in diet and exercise who works with clients on an individual basis.

Pesce/pollo vegetarian—A vegetarian who avoids the use of red meat but will include fish (*pesce* in Italian) or chicken (*pollo* in Italian) in the diet.

---

the Program! Guide to Fast Food and Family Restaurants (2003), covering over 75 restaurants.

Function

Greene's diet plans aim to restructure participants' present eating and exercise habits, with changes phased in gradually at their own pace. The plans require a committed intention to lose weight based on a willingness to look honestly at personal patterns of food consumption, including emotional as well as physical reasons for eating.

Benefits

One of the benefits of the diet programs is their common sense approach to the necessity of personal commitment to change as well as the lifestyle modifications necessary to lose weight and keep it off. Many users find the plans' emphasis on introspection and emotional honesty helpful in breaking the psychological patterns that cause them to regain the pounds after a period of successful weight loss.

The flexibility of food choices built into the program makes it easier for participants with **food allergies** or those who must cook for or share meals with a family to use this plan. The foods Greene recommends are moderate in cost, and vegetarians also find it easy to adjust for an ovo-lacto vegetarian or pesce/pollo vegetarian diet.

Precautions

Dieters who select the individualized programs offered on Greene's websites should check with their

---

primary care physicians to verify that the dietary changes and physical exercises suggested for them are appropriate. People with diabetes or other medical conditions may not be able to forgo eating at scheduled intervals.

Risks

Greene's diet plan does not pose any risks to health for users who have consulted with their healthcare providers prior to starting the plan.

Research and general acceptance

Most references to Greene's diets are in popular print media—daily newspapers and monthly women's magazines with wide circulations—rather than medical or nutritional journals. Although Greene does not publicize his associations with celebrities, his websites as well as newspaper and magazine articles always emphasize that he is Oprah Winfrey's personal trainer. Crediting Winfrey as the co-author of his first book is generally regarded as the key to Greene's rapid success in the late 1990s.

There are no published reports on clinical trials of Bob Greene's diet plan. Reviews of the diet plan by registered dietitians are generally favorable; they typically describe it as a simple program that establishes the groundwork for a lifetime of healthy living. The programs are easy to follow and include **dietary guidelines** aligned with those recommended by the U.S. Department of Agriculture (USDA). Greene is realistic about the difficulty of long-term weight loss and up front about the commitment required to make long-term changes.

On the other hand, some registered dietitians point out that Greene's diets require a greater time commitment for journaling and exercise than most people can manage on a regular basis. The program is not designed for rapid weight loss.

Resources

BOOKS

Greene, Bob W. *The Best Life Diet.* New York: Simon & Schuster, 2006.

———. *The Best Life Diet.* Rev. and upd. New York: Simon & Schuster, 2009.

———. *Get with the Program!: Getting Real about Your Health, Weight, and Emotional Well-Being.* New York: Simon & Schuster, 2002.

———. *The Get with the Program! Guide to Fast Food and Family Restaurants.* New York: Simon & Schuster, 2004.

———. *The Get with the Program! Guide to Good Eating.* New York: Simon & Schuster, 2003.

Greene, Bob W., and Oprah Winfrey. *Make the Connection: Ten Steps to a Better Body—and a Better Life.* New York: Hyperion, 1996.

PERIODICALS

Baldacci, Leslie. "Oprah's Trainer Asks What Candy Means." *Chicago Sun-Times* (November 21, 2006): 44.

Eller, Daryn. "Food to Go: Have It Your Way; When It Comes to Restaurant Eating, Bob Greene Says the Choice Is Yours." *Muscle & Fitness/Hers* (December 2003): 54.

WEBSITES

"Best Life Diet." Everydiet.org. http://www.everydiet.org/diet/best-life-diet (accessed November 6, 2012).

Best Life diet official website. http://www.thebestlife.com (accessed August 10, 2012).

Moore, Marissa. "The Best Life Diet, Revised and Updated (Book Review)." Academy of Nutrition and Dietetics. http://www.eatright.org/Media/content.aspx?id=10410 (accessed August 10, 2012).

ORGANIZATIONS

Academy of Nutrition and Dietetics, 120 South Riverside Plz., Ste. 2000, Chicago, IL 60606-6995, (312) 899-0040, (800) 877-1600, amacmunn@eatright.org, http://www.eatright.org.

Rebecca J. Frey, PhD

Body for Life diet

Definition

Body for Life is a 12-week diet and rigorous exercise program designed by former competitive bodybuilder Bill Phillips. The program promises those who follow it faithfully that after 12 weeks they will not only have lost about 25 lb. (10 kg) if they are overweight, but they will have a new shape and a more muscular body.

Origins

Bill Phillips, the originator of the Body for Life program, is a former bodybuilder and was the founder of EAS, a dietary supplement manufacturer. In Body for Life, he has taken some of the principles of body-building and incorporated them into a motivational program that is easily understandable to the general public. In 1996, when Phillips still owned EAS (he has since sold the company), he began the "EAS Grand Spokesperson Challenge." The following year he changed its name to the Body for Life Challenge. This is a self-improvement competition based on the Body for Life program.

The Body for Life program became widely known with the publication of *Body for Life: 12 Weeks to Mental and Physical Strength* in 1999. Other books, videos, and a website have followed. Phillips claims that in a decade more than 2 million people have successfully changed their bodies and their lives through the Body for Life program.

Description

Body for Life is both a diet and a rigorous exercise program served up with a big helping of motivational psychology. The diet part of the plan is relatively simple and offers some benefits over other plans in that it does not require calorie counting or careful measuring of food.

Diet

For 12 weeks, people on the Body for Life diet eat five or six small meals a day. The meals consist of a portion of lean, protein-rich food and a portion of unrefined or whole-grain **carbohydrates**. In addition, at least two meals daily must include a vegetable portion, and the diet should be supplemented by one tablespoon daily of oil high in monounsaturated **fats**. A portion is defined as being equal to the size and thickness of the dieter's hand (**protein**) or fist (carbohydrates and vegetables). Dieters estimate portion size rather than measuring.

Approved proteins include lean poultry, most fish and seafood, egg whites, low-fat cottage cheese, and, unlike many diets, lean beef and ham. For vegetarians, approved proteins include tempeh, **soy**, textured vegetable protein, and seitan. Vegetarians will have a hard time meeting the protein requirements of this diet. Vegans will most likely not be able to do so.

Approved carbohydrates include baked potato, sweet potato, both brown and white rice, pasta, whole wheat bread, whole wheat tortillas, dried beans, oatmeal, and **whole grains** such as quinoa. Also included in the approved carbohydrates list are apples, melon, strawberries, oranges, and corn. This is a much less restrictive list of carbohydrates than appears in many diets.

Approved vegetables include lettuce, tomato, carrots, broccoli, cauliflower, asparagus, spinach, mushrooms, zucchini, peas, bell peppers, celery, and onions. All are to be served as plain vegetables without sauce. The daily oil allotment can come from salad dressing.

The fats requirement of this diet can be met with unsaturated oils such as canola, olive, safflower, or **flaxseed**, but also through eating salmon three times a week or with avocados, natural peanut butter, or a handful of nuts or seeds daily.

In addition to allowed foods, the dieter is required to drink 10 or more glasses of water daily. The diet is to be followed rigorously for six days. On the seventh day, the dieter can eat anything he or she wants. Overall, this diet allows a larger diversity of foods than many diets, but it is a high-protein, low-fat diet with about half the **calories** consumed coming from protein and very few from fats. Generally, dietitians recommend a diet that is about 55% carbohydrates, with emphasis on whole-grain carbohydrates; 15%–20% protein; and no more than 30% fat. The diet recommends unsaturated fats and restricts sweets, junk food, and empty calories that add few nutrients. One criticism of the diet is that Phillips repeatedly recommends **dietary supplements** made by his former company.

Exercise

The exercise portion of Body for Life is more complicated than the food portion. It consists of a two-week block of exercises. Forty-five minute weight-training exercises for either the upper or lower body alternate with a minimum of 20-minute aerobic exercises with every seventh day as a day of rest.

Exercises are to be done at specific levels of exertion using a 10-point rating scale developed by the American College of Sports Medicine. This scale allows the level of difficulty to be personalized to the individual. Most exercises consist of multiple repetitions beginning around level 5 (hard, but with plenty of energy to continue). They move on to a completely flat effort at level 10, where the individual is putting out the maximal effort possible. These exercises are intended to be difficult. Phillips believes that short bursts of maximal exercise burn more calories than longer exercise periods at lower intensities. One drawback is that these exercises are best done in a gym with equipment and a supervised environment because of their intensity.

Motivation

Bill Phillips uses strong motivational techniques to help people succeed in the Body for Life Program. The program asks the dieter to determine his or her reasons for wanting to change and then set a goal for that change. Phillips then applies the psychology of competition by encouraging people to become involved in the Body for Life Challenge. This is a contest to see which dieter can improve his or her body the most using the program. Prizes in 2007 were substantial. The grand prize was $50,000, a home gym, and a $5,000 gift certificate for EAS supplement products. Eight category champions received $20,000, a home gym, and a $2,500 gift certificate for EAS products. The official Body for Life website offers inspiring stories, pictures of former champions, and plenty of tips and information on how to succeed.

Function

The theory behind the Body for Life diet is that eating many small meals high in protein during the day helps keep **insulin** levels steady and boosts **metabolism** so that the body burns calories at a higher rate. Insulin is a hormone that regulates blood glucose (sugar) levels in the body. When blood glucose is too high, cells store the extra glucose as glycogen or fat. In addition, Phillips says that protein suppresses energy and is essential for building muscle mass. The goal of the Body for Life plan is not just to lose weight, but to develop a sculpted body.

Benefits

With increased exercise; a low-fat, high-protein diet; and reduced portion sizes, Body for Life does help people lose weight rapidly. People do gain muscle and strength through exercise. The main drawback to achieving these benefits is the rigorousness of the program and the difficulty people have staying on it. Eating five or six times a day and finding time to exercise daily requires a major lifestyle change. The committed will see benefits, but this program is definitely not for everyone.

Precautions

Because of the high level of exercise involved in this program, dieters should talk to their doctor about whether their physical condition will allow them to participate. This is probably not a good program for people with heart or respiratory problems. Children and teens who are still growing and pregnant women also are unlikely candidates for this program. People with kidney disease should discuss the diet aspect of the program with their doctor since their kidneys may not be able to handle a high-protein diet. Anecdotally, the program appears to be most successful with out-

---

KEY TERMS

Dietary supplement—A product, such as a vitamin, mineral, herb, amino acid, or enzyme, that is intended to be consumed in addition to an individual's diet with the expectation that it will improve health.

Glycogen—A compound made when the level of glucose (sugar) in the blood is too high. Glycogen is stored in the liver and muscles for release when blood glucose levels are too low.

Hormone—A chemical messenger that is produced by one type of cell and travels through the bloodstream to change the metabolism of a different type of cell.

Insulin—A hormone made by the pancreas that controls blood glucose (sugar) levels by moving excess glucose into muscle, liver, and other cells for storage.

Pancreas—A gland near the liver and stomach that secretes digestive fluid into the intestine and the hormones insulin and glucagon into the bloodstream.

Quinoa—A high-protein grain native to South America (pronounced keen-wah).

---

of-shape athletes who want to lose weight and get back in shape.

Risks

People who are not used to the level of exercise required by Body for Life are at high risk for developing injuries as a result of the exercise component of the program. In addition, many **obesity** experts feel that rapid weight loss—that is, loss of more than 1–1.5 lb. (0.5–7 kg) per week—increases the chance of **weight cycling** or putting the weight back on once the dieter begins eating a regular diet. Weight cycling is thought to have some harmful cardiovascular effects.

Research and general acceptance

No scholarly research has been done on Body for Life. However, bodybuilders have used the diet and exercise principles behind the program for many years. Some registered dietitians (RDs) support the idea of eating many small meals during the day and using only unsaturated fats. They tend to dislike the high-protein content of the diet. The aspect criticized most strongly, however, is the need for dietary supplements in this program Body for Life unabashedly pushes dieters to use EAS supplements. Many RDs feel that a healthy diet should not require protein shakes and other supplements beyond perhaps a multivitamin for certain dieters.

Resources

BOOKS

Peeke, Pamela. *Body-for-Life for Women: A Woman's Plan for Physical and Mental Transformation.* Emmaus, PA: Rodale, 2005.

Phillips, Bill. *Body for Life: 12 Weeks to Mental and Physical Strength.* New York: HarperCollins, 1999.

———. *Eating for Life: Your Guide to Great Health, Fat Loss and Increased Energy!* Golden, CO: High Point Media, 2003.

———. *Transformation; How to Change Everything.* Carlsbad, CA: Hay House, Inc., 2007.

WEBSITES

"Body for Life (Eating for Life)." EveryDiet.org. http://www.everydiet.org/diet/body-for-life (accessed September 25, 2012).

Body-for-LIFE offical website. http://bodyforlife.com (accessed September 25, 2012).

Callahan, Maureen. "Body-for-Life." Health.com. http://www.health.com/health/article/0,,20410208,00.html (accessed September 25, 2012).

Tish Davidson, AM

Body image

Definition

Body image is a mental opinion or description that individuals have of their own physical appearance. It is a subjective concept, based on comparisons to socially constructed standards or ideals. A person's body image can range from very negative to very positive. Depending on age and other factors, the degree of concern with body image can also vary widely among individuals.

Individuals who have a poor body image perceive their body as unattractive to others, whereas those with a positive body image view their body as acceptable to others. Their views do not necessarily reflect their actual appearance or how others perceive them, though outside judgments may skew personal perceptions.

Origins

Scientists have found that body image is first formed as an infant during contact (or lack thereof) with people such as parents and family members. Personal contact in the form of hugs, kisses, and other forms of affection can help develop an early positive body image, whereas the absence of such contact can have the opposite effect, forming an early negative body image.

Body image is then generally developed through comparison, as people compare themselves to others based on physical traits and characteristics. Within the field of psychoanalysis, a person's body image is often measured by asking a person to rate parts of his/her current body (such as face, stomach, and buttocks) with respect to a series of pictures representing an ideal body image. The difference in rating between a person's current body image and a perceived idea body image is generally considered the amount a person is dissatisfied with his or her body.

Description

Body image, especially among young people going through puberty, can become a problem, especially if there is excessive concern placed on appearance. For example, parents who are overly concerned with their children's weight and appearance may cause their children to develop negative views of their body. Similarly, parents who are preoccupied with their own weight and appearance can indirectly teach their children to be critical of their bodies. A person's peers or colleagues can exert pressure, urging each other to attain a certain ideal figure or criticizing individuals who somehow do not measure up to their expectations. Media depictions of models and actors and popular discussion of celebrities in terms of their physical appearance may contribute to beliefs about the "ideal" body type. Body image is also closely associated with self-esteem, which is defined as the amount of value or personal worth individuals subjectively feel they have.

Older children and young adults tend to be more concerned about how other people view them than other age groups, so they are usually much more sensitive regarding body image and vulnerable to external pressures. This can affect their self-esteem as their body goes through dramatic changes from adolescence to adulthood during puberty. Boys may be overly concerned with height when seeing girls of their same age growing faster. Girls may be sensitive about their height, weight, or other noticeable changes happening within their bodies.

Statistically, according to the National Eating Disorders Association, 91% of young college women report having been on at least one diet. Seventy percent of young college men report being unhappy with their body image—with 32% of all college men stating that they have been on one or more diets. Other studies show similar percentages in older children and young adults, which help to support the contention that young people are very concerned with body image— a body image where the ideal is to be very slim.

Differences among men and women

Concern with body image is generally more important to women than it is to men. Women are usually more critical of their overall body and individual parts of their body than men. However, the gap between the two genders has been narrowing over recent years as men become more concerned with their body image.

Poor body image often relates to a feeling of being overweight, especially with women. Men, on the other hand, desire more muscle mass when considering their body image. A desire to be more masculine can parallel an interest in obtaining additional muscle mass and more definition in current muscles.

Generally, a poor body image can lead to constant and fad dieting, **obesity**, and eating disorders, along with low self-esteem, depression, anxiety, and overall emotional distress. However, for the most part, people with good exercise habits, positive personal and sexual experiences, and excellent emotional and mental states have better and more accurate perceptions of their body image than people without those characteristics and experiences. These people also have fewer problems associated with poor body image.

Causes of negative body image

Body image can be affected by outside influences. Media sources, such as television, the Internet, and magazines, often portray people closer to a supposed "ideal" body type than the average body type in order

KEY TERMS

Anorexia nervosa—A mental eating disorder that features an extreme fear and obsession of becoming overweight, which leads to extreme forms of dieting that can result in sickness and sometimes even death.

Binge eating disorder—A mental eating disorder that features the consumption of large amounts of food in short periods of time.

Body dysmorphic disorder (BDD)—A mental disorder that features a distorted or disturbed body image. People with BDD are very critical of their physical body and body image even though no defect is easily visible.

Bulimia nervosa—A mental eating disorder that is characterized by periods of overeating followed with periods of undereating.

Narcissism—Excessive admiration of oneself.

Psychoanalysis—A psychological theory that concerns the mental functions of humans both on the conscious and unconscious levels.

Puberty—A stage of physiological maturity that marks the start of being capable of sexual reproduction, causing physical changes in the body.

Subjective—Based on feelings and opinions.

to sell their products and services. Consequently, people can be overly influenced by such depictions of the "perfect" body. The average U.S. citizen is exposed to potentially thousands of advertising messages each day, and studies of network television commercials have shown that attractiveness is a desirable trait that advertisers regularly use to convince viewers to purchase their products.

Family life can also affect a person's perception of their body image. Parents that criticize their children in the way they look, talk, or act may have a negative effect on the development of self-esteem in their offspring, and young people may also be adversely affected by the comments of classmates and peers. Children and adolescents often try to pressure their peers to conform to what is currently popular in clothing styles, language, and other characteristics, and not meeting these expectations can negatively affect body image.

Precautions

Exaggerated and distorted concerns with body image have been linked in medical studies with decreases in self-esteem and increases in dieting and eating disorders, including **anorexia nervosa**, **binge eating** disorder, and **bulimia nervosa**. Bulimia is an eating disorder marked by episodes of binge eating followed by one or more behaviors to control weight, most commonly self-induced vomiting, laxative abuse, fasting, or excessive exercise. The disorder is rare in children under age 14. It is estimated to occur in 1%–3% of high school and college-aged women in the United States.

People with extreme body image problems may have body dysmorphic disorder (BDD), which involves a distorted body image without any eating disorders. Body dysmorphic disorder was recognized as a psychiatric disorder in 1997, although its symptoms have been exhibited in patients for more than 100 years. The disorder involves obsession and complete preoccupation with an imagined or mild physical flaw. It is known to occur in 1%–2% of Americans, but it is thought to be underdiagnosed because it often occurs in conjunction with other psychiatric disorders such as major depression and obsessive-compulsive disorder. Excessive preoccupation with body image and an obsession with positive body image has also been associated with narcissism, a personality disorder marked by self-admiration or an overestimation regarding the attractiveness of one's appearance.

If taken to the extreme, the behaviors that accompany these psychological disorders can be life-threatening. Body image disorders are often accompanied by additional psychological problems such as depression or anxiety and even thoughts of suicide. For some individuals, body image eventually becomes an all-consuming preoccupation.

Complications

If poor body image is not addressed, it could develop into a more serious problem. Feelings of depression, anxiety, or isolation may occur. Some people turn to alcohol or drugs to offset those negative feelings, while others turn away from their regular activities and their usual friends, becoming withdrawn and showing lack of interest in previously enjoyed situations.

Sometimes, people can recover from such feelings by focusing on their good qualities, accepting things that cannot be changed, and realistically working on things that could be improved. In some cases, outside help is needed in the form of a guidance counselor, parent, coach, religious leader, or someone else that is trusted and accepting of personal feelings. Crisis hotlines are also available to help with such problems.

> ## QUESTIONS TO ASK YOUR DOCTOR
>
> - What are the indications that my child may have a problem with body image?
> - What treatment options do you recommend?
> - What physical symptoms or behaviors are important enough that I should seek immediate treatment?

Parental concerns

Parents should be concerned if their children have excessive concerns about their appearance and looks. All children will be concerned with some aspect of their body; this is normal and is not a medical problem. However, an obsession with body and appearance is not normal and may be indicative of BDD or another disorder. Parents should consult with their family doctor about any concerns for the health and well-being of their children.

Resources

BOOKS

Kilpatrick, Haley., and Whitney Joiner. *The Drama Years: Real Girls Talk About Surviving Middle School—Bullies, Brands, Body Image, and More*. New York: Free Press, 2012.

Knoblich, Gunther, et al. eds. *Human Body Perception from the Inside Out*. Oxford, UK: Oxford University Press, 2006.

Moore, Karen. *True Images Devotional: 90 Daily Devotions for Teen Girls*. Grand Rapids, MI: Zondervan, 2012.

Robertson, Cathie. *Safety, Nutrition and Health in Early Education*. 4th ed. Florence, KY: Wadsworth Publishing, 2009.

Smith, Rita. *Self-Image and Eating Disorders*. New York: Rosen Pub Group, 2012.

Wilhelm, Sabine. *Feeling Good About the Way You Look: A Program for Overcoming Body Image Problems*. New York: Guilford Press, 2006.

WEBSITES

Brown University Health Education. "Body Image." http://brown.edu/Student_Services/Health_Services/Health_Education/nutrition_&_eating_concerns/body_image.php (accessed August 22, 2012).

MedlinePlus. "Anorexia Nervosa." U.S. National Library of Medicine, National Institutes of Health. http://www.nlm.nih.gov/medlineplus/ency/article/000362.htm (accessed August 22, 2012).

———. "Bulimia." U.S. National Library of Medicine, National Institutes of Health. http://www.nlm.nih.gov/

medlineplus/ency/article/000341.htm (accessed August 22, 2012).

Nemours Foundation. "Body Image and Self-Esteem." KidsHealth.org. http://kidshealth.org/teen/your_mind/body_image/body_image.html (accessed August 22, 2012).

U.S. Department of Health and Human Services, Office on Women's Health. "Body Image." Womenshealth.gov. http://www.womenshealth.gov/body-image (accessed August 22, 2012).

ORGANIZATIONS

Association of Body Image and Disordered Eating, UCD Counseling & Psychological Services, Davis, CA 95616, http://abide.ucdavis.edu.

National Association of Anorexia Nervosa & Associated Disorders, 800 E Diehl Rd. #160, Naperville, IL 60563, (630) 577-1333, (630) 577-1330 (helpline), anadhelp@anad.org, http://www.anad.org.

National Eating Disorders Association, 165 West 46th St., New York, NY 10036, (212) 575-6200, (800) 931-2237, info@NationalEatingDisorders.org, http://www.nationaleatingdisorders.org.

William Arthur Atkins
Laura Jean Cataldo, RN, EdD

Body mass index

Definition

Body mass index (BMI), also called the Quetelet Index, is a calculation used to determine an individual's amount of body fat.

Purpose

The BMI gives healthcare professionals a consistent way of assessing their patients' weight and an objective way of discussing it with them. It is also useful in suggesting the degree to which the patient may be at risk for obesity-related diseases.

Description

BMI is a statistical calculation intended as an assessment tool. It can be applied to groups of people to determine trends or it can be applied to individuals. When applied to individuals, it is only one of several assessments used to determine health risks related to being underweight, overweight, or obese.

The history of BMI

The formula used to calculate BMI was developed more than one hundred years ago by Belgian mathematician and scientist Lambert Adolphe Quetelet (1796-1874). Quetelet, who called his calculation the Quetelet Index of Obesity, was one of the first statisticians to apply the concept of a regular bell-shaped statistical distribution to physical and behavioral features of humans. He believed that by careful measurement and statistical analysis, the general characteristics of populations could be mathematically determined. Mathematically describing the traits of a population led him to the concept of the hypothetical "average man" against which other individuals could be measured. In his quest to describe the weight to height relationship in the average man, he developed the formula for calculating the body mass index.

Calculating BMI requires two measurements: weight and height. To calculate BMI using metric units, weight in kilograms (kg) is divided by the height squared measured in meters (m). To calculate BMI in imperial units, weight in pounds (lb.) is divided by height squared in inches (in.) and then multiplied by 703. This calculation produces a number that is the individual's BMI. This number, when compared to the statistical distribution of BMIs for adults ages 20–29, indicates whether the individual is underweight, average weight, overweight, or obese. The 20–29 age group was

Body mass index (BMI) calculation and meaning

Body mass index is determined by a person's weight and height:

Pounds/inches		Kilograms/meters	BMI	Weight status
$\frac{weight\ (lb) \times 703}{[height\ (in)]^2}$	(or)	$\frac{weight\ (kg)}{[height\ (m)]^2}$	Below 18.5	Underweight
			18.5–24.9	Normal
			25.0–29.9	Overweight
			30.0 and above	Obese

(Table by PreMediaGlobal. © 2013 Cengage Learning.)

chosen as the standard because it represents fully developed adults at the point in their lives when they statistically have the least amount of body fat. The formula for calculating the BMI of children is the same as for adults, but the resulting number is interpreted differently.

Although the formula for calculating BMI was developed in the mid-1800s, it was not commonly used in the United States before the mid-1980s. Until then, fatness or thinness was determined by tables that set an ideal weight or weight range for each height. Heights were measured in one-inch intervals, and the ideal weight range was calculated separately for men and women. The information used to develop these ideal weight-for-height tables came from several decades of data compiled by life insurance companies. These tables determined the probability of death as it related to height and weight and were used by the companies to set life insurance rates. The data excluded anyone with a chronic disease or anyone who, for whatever health reason, could not obtain life insurance.

Interest in using the BMI in the United States increased in the early 1980s when researchers became concerned that Americans were rapidly becoming obese. In 1984, the national percentage of overweight individuals was reported in a major assessment of the nation's health. Men having a BMI of 28 or greater were considered overweight. This BMI number was chosen to define overweight because 85% of American men ages 20–29 fell below it. A different calculation, not BMI, was used for women in the report.

In 1985, the term overweight was redefined as a BMI equal to or greater than 27.8 for men and equal to or greater than 27.3 for women. No BMI was selected to define underweight individuals. This definition of overweight was used in reports on obesity until 1998. In 1998, the United States National Institutes of Health revised its weight definitions to bring them in line with the definitions used by the World Health Organization. Overnight, 30 million Americans went from being classified as normal weight to being classified as overweight. Overweight is now defined for both men and women as a BMI of 25–29.9. At the same time, an underweight classification was added, as was the classification of obese for individuals with a BMI greater than or equal to 30.

Interpreting BMI calculations for adults

All adults age 20 and older are evaluated on the same BMI scale as follows:

- BMI below 18.5: Underweight
- BMI 18.5–24.9: Normal weight
- BMI 25.0–29.9: Overweight
- BMI 30 and above: Obese

Some researchers consider a BMI of 17 or below an indication of serious, health-threatening malnourishment. In developed countries, a BMI this low in the absence of disease is often an indication of **anorexia nervosa**. At the other end of the scale, a BMI of 40 or greater indicates morbid obesity that carries a very high risk of developing obesity-related diseases such as stroke, heart attack, and type 2 diabetes.

Interpreting BMI calculations for children and teens

The formula for calculating the BMI of children ages 2–20 is the same as the formula used in calculating adult BMIs, but the results are interpreted differently. Interpretation of BMI for children takes into consideration that the amount of body fat changes as children grow and that the amount of body fat is different in boys and girls of the same age and weight.

Instead of assigning a child to a specific weight category based on their BMI, a child's BMI is compared to other children of the same age and sex. Children are then assigned a percentile based on their BMI. The percentile provides a comparison between their weight and that of other children the same age and gender. For example, if a girl is in the 75th percentile for her age group, 75 of every 100 children who are her age weigh less than she does and 25 of every 100 weigh more than she does. The weight categories for children are:

- Below the 5th percentile: Underweight
- 5th percentile to less than the 85th percentile: Healthy weight
- 85th percentile to less than the 95th percentile: At risk of overweight
- 95th percentile and above: Overweight

Application of BMI information

The BMI was originally designed to observe groups of people. It is still used to spot trends, such as increasing weight in a particular age group over time. It is also a valuable tool for comparing body mass among different ethnic or cultural groups, and can indicate to what degree populations are undernourished or overnourished.

When applied to individuals, the BMI is not a diagnostic tool. Although there is an established link between BMI and the prevalence of certain diseases such as type 2 diabetes, some cancers, and cardiovascular disease, BMI alone is not intended to predict the likelihood of an individual developing these diseases. The National Heart, Lung, and Blood Institute recommends that the following measures be used to assess the impact of weight on health:

- BMI
- waist circumference (an alternate measure of body fat)
- risk factors for disease associated with obesity (e.g., high blood pressure, high LDL or "bad" cholesterol)
- low HDL or "good" cholesterol
- high blood glucose (sugar)
- high triglycerides
- family history of cardiovascular disease
- low physical activity level
- cigarette smoking

Precautions

BMI is very accurate when defining characteristics of populations, but less accurate when applied to individuals. However, because it is inexpensive and easy to determine, BMI is widely used. Calculating BMI requires a scale, a measuring rod, and the ability to do simple arithmetic or use a calculator. Potential limitations of BMI when applied to individuals are:

- BMI does not distinguish between fat and muscle. BMI tends to overestimate the degree of "fatness" among elite athletes in sports such as football, weightlifting, and bodybuilding. Since muscle weighs more than fat, many athletes who develop heavily muscled bodies are classified as overweight, even though they have a low percentage of body fat and are in top physical condition.
- BMI tends to underestimate the degree of fatness in the elderly, as muscle and bone mass is lost and replaced by fat, for the same reason it overestimates fatness in athletes.
- BMI makes no distinction between body types. People with large frames (big boned) are held to the same standards as people with small frames.
- BMI weight classes have absolute cut-offs, while in many cases health risks change gradually along with changing BMIs. A person with a BMI of 24.9 is classified as normal weight, while one with a BMI of 25.1 is overweight. In reality, their health risks may be quite similar.
- BMI does not take into consideration diseases or drugs that may cause significant water retention.
- BMI makes no distinction between genders, races, or ethnicities. Two people with the same BMI may have different health risks because of their gender or genetic heritage.

BMI is a comparative index and does not measure the amount of body fat directly. Other methods do give a direct measure of body fat, but these methods generally are expensive and require specialized equipment and training to be performed accurately. Among them are measurement of skin fold thickness, underwater (hydrostatic) weighing, bioelectrical impedance, and dual-energy x-ray absorptiometry (DXA). Combining BMI, waist circumference, family health history, and lifestyle analysis gives healthcare providers enough information to analyze health risks related to weight at minimal cost to the patient.

Parental concerns

Childhood obesity is an increasing concern. Research shows that overweight children are more likely to become obese adults than normal weight children. Excess weight in childhood is also linked to early development of type 2 diabetes, cardiovascular disease, and early onset of certain cancers. In addition, overweight or severely underweight children often pay a heavy social and emotional price as objects of scorn or teasing.

Both the American Academy of Pediatrics (AAP) and the United States Centers for Disease Control and Prevention (CDC) recommend that the BMI of children over age two be reviewed at regular intervals during pediatric visits. Parents of children whose BMI falls above the 85th percentile (at risk of being overweight and overweight categories) should seek information from their healthcare provider about health risks related to a high BMI and guidance on how to moderate their child's weight. Strenuous dieting is rarely advised for growing children, but healthcare providers can give guidance on improving the child's diet, such as eliminating empty **calories** (such as those found in soda and candy) and increasing the child's activity level in order to burn more calories and improve fitness.

Resources

WEBSITES

American Heart Association. "Body Mass Index (BMI Calculator)." http://www.heart.org/HEARTORG/GettingHealthy/WeightManagement/BodyMassIndex/Body-Mass-Index-BMI-Calculator_UCM_307849_Article.jsp (accessed October 2, 2012).

Centers for Disease Control and Prevention. "Body Mass Index." http://www.cdc.gov/healthyweight/assessing/bmi (accessed October 2, 2012).

National Heart, Lung, and Blood Institute. "Calculate Your Body Mass Index." National Institutes of Health. http://nhlbisupport.com/bmi (accessed October 2, 2012).

ORGANIZATIONS

Centers for Disease Control and Prevention, 1600 Clifton Rd. NE, Atlanta, GA 30333, (800) CDC-INFO (232-4636), TTY: (888) 232-6348, cdcinfo@cdc.gov, http://www.cdc.gov.

National Heart, Lung, and Blood Institute, PO Box 30105, Bethesda, MD 20824-0105, (301) 592-8573, TTY: (240) 629-3255, Fax: (240) 629-3246, nhlbiinfo@nhlbi.nih.gov, http://www.nhlbi.nih.gov.

Weight-Control Information Network (WIN), 1 WIN Way, Bethesda, MD 20892-3665, (202) 828-1025, (877) 946-4627, Fax: (202) 828-1028, win@http://win.niddk.nih.gov, http://win.niddk.nih.gov.

Tish Davidson, A.M.

Bodybuilding diet

Definition

The bodybuilding diet is designed to build muscle and reduce body fat. It emphasizes foods high in **protein** and complex **carbohydrates**, such as whole grain bread, pasta, and cereal. There are many variations of the bodybuilding diet but an essential component remains the same throughout: a regular strength-building exercise program.

Origins

Many scholars believe bodybuilding diets began with the ancient Greeks, whose gods, like Hercules and Apollo, were often portrayed as quite muscular. This influenced ancient Greek society to emulate the concept of a perfect physique. The same desire for physical perfection is found in ancient Rome and Egypt. The modern era of bodybuilding began in the late 1800s in England; German strongman Eugen Sandow is credited with being the first professional bodybuilder of the modern era. He was a featured attraction at the 1893 World Columbian Exposition in Chicago for his feats of strength. He opened a chain of 20 weight training studios in England and published a magazine that included tips on diet. Sandow's own diet was high in **calories**, protein, carbohydrates, and **fats**.

Description

A bodybuilding diet generally contains 2,500–5,500 calories per day for men and 1,500–3,000 calories daily for women, depending on the types and levels of exercise. The diet's ratio of protein, carbohydrates, and fat can differ. Some programs recommend 40% carbohydrates, 40% protein, and 20% fats. Others suggest a ratio of 40% protein, 30% carbohydrates, and 30% fat. There are many variations of this diet where the calorie intake and ratios are different. Most bodybuilding diets include nutritional supplements as well as protein powders. The focus of bodybuilding has shifted away from an emphasis on health toward an emphasis on appearance at all costs. To achieve a bigger, better body, many bodybuilders have placed a huge emphasis on nutritional and other types of supplements, including the illegal use of steroids.

All diets require an exercise routine of three to seven days a week, usually with weightlifting and cardiovascular exercises. The body burns up to 50 calories per day for every pound of muscle. So adding 10 pounds of muscle can burn up to 500 extra calories each day. The exact diet and exercise routine can vary greatly and can be confusing, especially to people new to bodybuilding. When it comes to either diet or exercise, no two people follow the same routine.

Basic nutrition of bodybuilding

The three main components of a bodybuilding diet are the three **macronutrients**: carbohydrates, protein, and fat.

CARBOHYDRATES. Carbohydrates are the main source of energy for the body. They are especially important in aerobic exercise and high-volume weight training, including aiding in muscle recovery. Eating carbohydrates causes the pancreas to release the hormone **insulin**, which helps regulate blood glucose (sugar) levels. Insulin takes carbohydrates and stores them as fat in muscle, or in the liver as glycogen. Insulin also takes amino acids from protein and stores them in muscle cells that aid in recovery and repair following strength-building exercise. All carbohydrates are broken down into glucose by the body and released into the blood; the speed at which this process

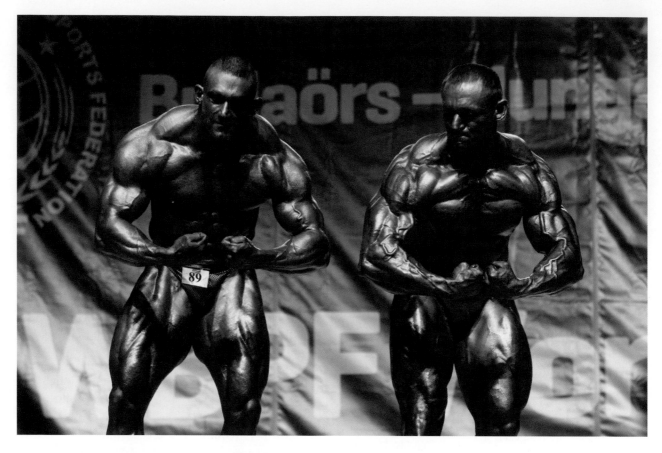

Two contestants in the WBPF Bodybuilding World Cup in 2012. *(Istvan Csak/Shutterstock.com)*

occurs varies depending on the type of carbohydrate and the presence of fat and protein in the stomach. This rate of absorption is a critical factor in maintaining energy levels, reducing body fat, and maintaining overall health.

Carbohydrates are often referred to as either simple or complex. A bodybuilding diet contains both simple and complex carbohydrates. Complex carbohydrates have a chemical structure composed of three or more sugars. They provide energy that is sustained over time. Simple carbohydrates have a chemical structure composed of one or two sugars and provide quick but short-lasting energy. A bodybuilding diet contains mostly complex carbohydrates eaten throughout the day. Simple carbohydrates are eaten immediately after working out to aid in faster recuperation and repair of muscles. Complex carbohydrates are found in whole-grain bread, pasta, cereal, beans, and most vegetables. Simple carbohydrates are found in fruit and sugary foods such as candy, juice, and sport drinks.

There are two other ways bodybuilding diets classify carbohydrates besides the simple and complex

designations: glycemic index (GI) and glycemic load. The GI measures the quality rather than the quantity of carbohydrates found in food. Quality refers to how quickly blood sugar levels are raised following eating. The standard for GI is white bread, which is assigned an index value of 100. Other foods are compared to the standard to arrive at their ratings. The higher the GI number, the faster blood sugar increases when that particular food is consumed. A high GI is 70 and greater, a medium GI is 56–69, and a low GI value is 55 or less. The GI is not a straightforward formula when it comes to reducing blood sugar levels. Various factors affect the GI value of a specific food, such as how the food is prepared (boiled, baked, sautéed, or fried, for example) and what other foods are consumed with it. Foods that are readily broken down and absorbed by the body are typically high on the GI. Foods that are digested slower, such as those high in **fiber**, have a lower GI value.

In 1997, epidemiologist and nutritionist Walter Willett of the Harvard School of Public Health developed the glycemic load as a more useful way of rating carbohydrates compared to the glycemic index. The glycemic load factors in the amount of a food eaten whereas the glycemic index does not. The glycemic load of a particular food or meal is determined by multiplying the amount of net carbohydrates in a serving by the glycemic index and dividing that number by 100. Net carbohydrates are determined by taking the amount of total carbohydrates and subtracting the amount of dietary fiber. For example, popcorn has a glycemic index of 72, which is considered high, but a serving of two cups has 10 net carbs for a glycemic load of seven, which is considered low.

PROTEIN. Muscle is composed primarily of protein and water. Protein builds muscle mass but not all protein consumed in the diet goes directly to muscle. Adequate consumption of protein helps preserve muscle tissue and enhance recovery from strenuous weight-bearing workouts. Since weight-bearing exercises cause significant damage to muscle tissue, the subsequent repair and growth of muscle requires a recovery period of at least 24 hours. If an inadequate amount of protein is consumed, muscle mass will suffer along with a decrease in **metabolism**. Most bodybuilding diets recommend 1–1.5 grams of protein per day for each pound of lean body mass (body weight minus body fat). Daily consumption of more than 3 grams per kilogram of body mass can lead to serious health problems, especially kidney damage. Protein is found in lean meat, poultry, fish, eggs, tofu, and **soy** products.

FATS. Fat in a diet is needed to maintain a healthy metabolism. There are four types of fat: saturated, trans, polyunsaturated, and monounsaturated. Saturated and trans fats are limited because high consumption is a risk factor for heart disease, **obesity**, high cholesterol, diabetes, and some cancers. Sources of saturated and trans fats are butter, whole milk products, fried foods, shortening, and coconut, palm, and other tropical oils. Meat with visible fat is also a source of saturated fat. Monounsaturated and polyunsaturated fats are good fats because they lower the risks of heart disease, diabetes, high cholesterol, and obesity. These fats are derived from avocados; most nuts; fish; flax; and olive, canola, peanut, safflower, corn, sunflower, soybean, and cottonseed oils.

Two other important factors in the bodybuilding diet are water and the number and timing of meals. Bodybuilding diets suggest drinking at least eight eight-ounce glasses of water a day. In addition, bodybuilders drink about a quarter cup of water every fifteen minutes during their workout. Water helps control appetite and drinking cold water increases metabolism.

The number and content of meals is important, as is the timing and quality of foods, especially just before

and just after workouts. An efficient way to burn fat is to elevate the body's metabolism. The process of digesting meals burns calories in itself, so a concept of this diet is to eat more frequently to make the process more efficient. Most bodybuilding diets recommend consuming six to eight smaller meals a day, starting with breakfast. Carbohydrates are important right after a workout because the body's supply of glycogen

---

KEY TERMS

Amino acids—A group of organic acids that are constituents of protein.

Carbohydrate—A nutrient that the body uses as an energy source. A carbohydrate provides 4 calories of energy per gram.

Cardiovascular—Pertaining to the heart and blood vessels.

Cholesterol—A solid compound found in blood and a number of foods, including eggs and fats.

Epidemiologist—A scientist or medical specialist who studies the origins and spread of diseases in populations.

Glycemic index (GI)—A method of ranking carbohydrates based on how they affect blood glucose levels.

Glycemic load (GL)—A more precise ranking of how an amount of a particular food affects blood glucose levels. The glycemic index (GI) is part of the equation for determining ranking.

Glycogen—A compound stored in the liver and muscles that is easily converted to glucose as an energy source.

Insulin—A hormone that regulates the level of glucose (sugar) in the blood.

Monounsaturated fat—A type of fat found in vegetable oils such as olive, peanut, and canola.

Pancreas—A digestive gland of the endocrine system that regulates several hormones, including insulin.

Polyunsaturated fat—A type of fat found in some vegetable oils, such as sunflower, safflower, and corn.

Saturated fat—A type of fat generally found in meat products with visible fat and dairy products.

Trans fat—A type of fat generally found in butter, whole milk products, fried foods, shortening, and coconut, palm, and other tropical oils.

(a compound easily converted to glucose for energy) is depleted. Many bodybuilding nutritionists recommend that the post-workout meal contain twice the calories, protein, and carbohydrates as the other meals of the day. The pre-workout meal contains foods high in carbohydrates since they improve exercise performance and enhance muscle recovery.

Function

The purpose of the bodybuilding diet is to gain muscle mass and lose fat. It is not a weight loss diet and most people will likely gain weight. Nutrition provides the body, especially muscles, with the raw materials needed for energy, recuperation, growth, and strength.

Benefits

The benefits of the bodybuilding diet are health and appearance. The bodybuilding diet promotes increased muscle mass, which increases metabolism.

Precautions

When monitored by a health professional, the bodybuilding diet can be a healthy method for increasing strength and body mass. Caution should be used in regard to nutritional supplements, especially protein powders. Excess protein intake is known to cause serious health problems such as kidney damage and **dehydration**. Bodybuilders should discuss any supplements with their doctor, and steroids, such as human growth hormone and testosterone, should only be used for medical reasons and with a doctor's prescription. Since exercise is a main component of the diet, people with arthritis or back, knee, or other joint problems should discuss the fitness regimen with their physicians before starting exercise. Making major changes to a person's diet should be done in small incremental steps so the body can adapt to the changes. A sudden reduction or increase in calories can cause the body to store or hoard fat.

Risks

The rigorous and regular exercise component of this diet is a risk to people with heart disease or certain other health problems. Individuals with these conditions should consult their physician before starting the diet. A bodybuilding diet is not recommended for women who are pregnant or nursing.

QUESTIONS TO ASK YOUR DOCTOR

- Is it safe for me to start a bodybuilding diet?
- Do I need to take dietary supplements?
- What are the health risks involved with this diet?
- Is it safe for me to start a weightlifting program?

Research and general acceptance

The bodybuilding diet is generally accepted by the medical and bodybuilding communities as being safe and effective in helping increase muscle mass and decrease fat. There is no general acceptance on the exact ratio of protein, carbohydrates, and fats.

Protein is considered the basic nutrient in repairing muscle that is broken down during weightlifting and for muscle maintenance and growth. The recommended dietary allowance (RDA) per day for protein is 0.8 g/kg. However, research shows that a greater amount of protein is needed for weightlifters. Depending on a person's level of activity, the amount of protein needed for a bodybuilder is greater than the RDA, but not more than 1.5–2 g/kg. Research indicates that muscles double the rate of protein synthesis following exercise and that it remains elevated for at least 24 hours.

The amount of carbohydrates in a bodybuilder's diet can range from 40%–60%, but such levels are not necessarily effective. An inadequate consumption of carbohydrates can have a negative effect on exercise performance and duration. Other studies have shown that the dominant factor in weight loss is a reduction of calorie intake. There has been a great deal of research on bodybuilding nutrition from the 1980s forward.

Resources

BOOKS

Campbell, Adam, and Jeff Volek. *The Men's Health TNT Diet: The Explosive New Plan to Blast Fat, Build Muscle, and Get Healthy in 12 Weeks.* Emmaus, PA: Rodale Books, 2007.

Cordain, Loren, and Joe Friel. *The Paleo Diet for Athletes: A Nutritional Formula for Peak Athletic Performance.* Emmaus, PA: Rodale Books, 2005.

Hofmekler, Ori. *Maximum Muscle: Minimum Fat.* St. Paul, MN: Dragon Door Publications, 2003.

Kleiner, Susan, and Maggie Greenwood-Robinson. *Power Eating.* Champaign, IL: Human Kinetics Publishers, 2006.

Larson-Meyer, D. Enette. *Vegetarian Sports Nutrition.* Champaign, IL: Human Kinetics Publishers, 2006.

Schuler, Lou, et al. *The Testosterone Advantage Plan: Lose Weight, Gain Muscle, Boost Energy.* New York: Fireside, 2002.

Sepe, Frank. *TRUTH Body Solutions: Truthful Nutritional Strategies for a Better Body and a Better Life.* Carlsbad, CA: Hay House, 2006.

PERIODICALS

Aceto, Chris. "Know the Score! Cheat Foods, When Properly Refereed, Can Help Boost Your Muscular Gains." *Flex* (August 2005): 94–99.

Karimian, J., and P.S. Esfahani. "Supplement Consumption in Body Builder Athletes." *Journal of Research in Medical Sciences* 16, no. 10 (2011): 1347–53.

Elliott, Tabatha. "Cholesterol for Muscle." *Muscle & Fitness* (October 2005): 245–46.

Slater, G., and S.M. Phillips. "Nutrition Guidelines for Strength Sports: Sprinting, Weightlifting, Throwing Events, and Bodybuilding." *Journal of Sports Sciences* 29, supp. no. 1 (2011): S67–77.

Stoppani, Jim. "Food Fixes: Want To Improve Your Results and Make Faster Gains? Here's a Guide You Can Use to Upgrade Your Bodybuilding Diet, One Meal At a Time." *Flex* (March 2007): 154–58.

Wuebben, Joe, et al. "The Bodybuilding Foods: From the Basics for Building Muscle to On-The-Go, Gotta-Eat-Now Fast Foods, Here are 111 Superfoods Every Bodybuilder Must Have in His Eating Arsenal." *Joe Weider's Muscle & Fitness* (March 2007): 142–50.

WEBSITES

Academy of Nutrition and Dietetics. "Strength Building and Muscle Mass." http://www.eatright.org/Public/content.aspx?id=11633 (accessed September 26, 2012).

ORGANIZATIONS

American College of Sports Medicine, 401 West Michigan St., Indianapolis, IN 46202-3233, (317) 637-9200, Fax. (317) 634-7817, http://www.acsm.org.

American Council on Exercise, 4851 Paramount Dr., San Diego, CA 92123, (888) 825-3636, support@acefitness.org, http://www.acefitness.org.

American Society for Nutrition, 9650 Rockville Pike, Bethesda, MD 20814, (301) 634-7050, Fax: (301) 634-7894, http://www.nutrition.org.

Sports, Cardiovascular, and Wellness Nutritionists, 1520 Kensington Rd., Ste. 202, Oak Brook, IL 60523, (800) 249-7288, Fax: (866) 381-7288, scandpg@gmail.com, http://www.scandpg.org.

Ken R. Wells

Brazilian diet *see* **South American diet**

Breastfeeding

Definition

Breastfeeding is the practice of feeding an infant milk through the mother's breast. According to La Leche League International (LLLI), human milk is "a living fluid that protects babies from disease and actively contributes to the development of every system in [a] baby's body." Breastfeeding stimulates babies' immune systems and protects against diarrhea and infection.

Purpose

Breast milk is the ideal food for an infant. It contains appropriate amounts of all the nutrients a baby needs to grow and stay healthy:

- Fats: Breast milk contains omega-3 fatty acids essential for the growth and development of the brain and nerve tissue. The amount of fat a baby receives depends on the length of the feeding. The milk at the beginning of the feeding is called the foremilk. It is the low-fat milk. The hind milk that comes at the end of the feeding contains higher concentrations of fat. Therefore, the longer the baby nurses the higher the fat content.

- Proteins: The whey proteins found in breast milk are easier to digest than formula. Taurine, an amino acid that is important in the development of brain tissue, is found in breast milk but not in cow's milk.

- Sugars: Breast milk contains lactose, a milk sugar that provides energy. Breast milk contains 20%–30% more lactose than cow's milk.

Global breastfeeding rates: percentage of infants younger than 6 mos. who are breastfed exclusively, by region, 2006–2010

Eastern and Southern Africa	49%
South Asia	45%
Latin America and Caribbean	42%
Middle East and North Africa	34%
East Asia and Pacific	30%
West and Central Africa	29%
Central Eastern Europe	24%
United States	16%

SOURCE: UNICEF, "Current Status: Breastfeeding," http://www.childinfo.org/breastfeeding_status.html, and U.S. Centers for Disease Control and Prevention, "Breastfeeding Report Card—United States, 2012," http://www.cdc.gov/breastfeeding/data/reportcard.htm.

(Table by PreMediaGlobal. © 2013 Cengage Learning.)

- Vitamins and minerals: Breast milk provides the most balanced source of vitamins and minerals for an infant.
- Immune system boosters: White blood cells and immunoglobulins are responsible for fighting and destroying infection.

The content of breast milk varies from feeding to feeding, at different times of day, and as the baby grows, often adjusting to exactly what is needed by the baby.

Description

The mother's body prepares for breastfeeding while she is pregnant. The fatty tissue of the breast is replaced by glandular tissue that is necessary to produce milk. When baby suckles the breast, the hormone oxytocin is released. This causes the muscle cells of the breast to squeeze milk from the milk ducts to the nipple.

Origins

Throughout time, millions of mothers have breastfed their babies. During ancient times, mothers breastfed their babies for 12-18 months, or until the mother's menstrual cycle returned.

For thousands of years, breastfeeding was the only source of nutrition for the first part of a baby's life. Before the invention of formula, few alternatives were available. If a mother could not breastfeed, a wet nurse was found or the baby was fed animal milk or "pap," a mixture of flour, rice, and water. In the early 1900s, most babies in America were still breastfed, and over half of them were breastfed for one year or longer. However, as more women entered the workforce and supplemental methods of feeding were introduced, breastfeeding rates in America decreased. According to a survey from Ross Labs, by 1971 only 24.7% of American babies were breastfed at birth, and of these babies, only 5.4% of them were still breastfed at six months.

Demographics

In 1982, the United States experienced a resurgence in breastfeeding and rates have continued to increase. The National Immunization Survey conducted by the Centers for Disease Control and Prevention (CDC) in 2005 revealed that 72% of American babies were breastfed at birth and 39% were still breastfed at six months.

The developing world has experienced a decline in breastfeeding rates as well due to urbanization, social change, and the promotion of formula. Mothers who choose to feed their babies formula often encounter unsafe hygienic conditions in which to prepare the bottles, or they cannot afford to purchase the fuel needed to heat the water. Two of the major causes of infant mortality in developing countries are diarrhea and acute respiratory infections. Both are conditions that breastfeeding can protect against.

The World Health Organization (WHO) and the United Nations Children Fund (UNICEF) are two organizations working together to bring about a change in the global breastfeeding culture. In 2002, they developed "The Global Strategy for Infant and Young Child Feeding," which recommends that all babies are exclusively breastfed for the first six months of life with continued breastfeeding up to two years or beyond. Exclusive breastfeeding means that breast milk is the child's only food source of nutrition for the first six months of life and that no other solids or liquids, such as formula or water, are introduced at this time, with the exception of liquid **vitamins** or medicines. Despite this recommendation, only one-third of all babies in the developing world were exclusively breastfed for six months in 2004. The highest rates of exclusive breastfeeding were in the East Asia/Pacific region (43%) and the lowest rates were in the Western/Central Africa region (20%), according to WHO.

During the first week of August, the organizations promote World Breastfeeding Week, celebrated in more than 170 countries "to encourage breastfeeding and improve the health of babies around the world." The event has been sponsored by WHO and UNICEF since 1990. Additional information about World Breastfeeding Week may be found on their website at http://worldbreastfeedingweek.org.

As of February 2012, the WHO reported that less than 40% of infants under six months of age were exclusively breastfed. Studies show that breastfeeding helps prevent **malnutrition** and can save the lives of about one million children. This organization promotes breastfeeding as the best source of nourishment for infants and young children, thus helping to ensure child health and survival.

Benefits for baby

There are a plethora of benefits for the breastfeeding baby, including:

- increased immunity due to antibodies not found in formula that help to protect the baby from bacteria and viruses
- lower incidence of ear infections and respiratory infections

- higher blood levels of the omega-3 fatty acid docosahexaenoic acid (DHA), which helps support brain health and function
- improved digestion and reduced constipation
- decreased risk of diarrhea, pneumonia, urinary tract infections, and certain types of spinal meningitis
- decrease in food allergies and eczema
- lower incidence of overweight
- reduced risk of type 1 and type 2 diabetes, celiac disease, cancer, rheumatoid arthritis, multiple sclerosis, liver disease, and acute appendicitis
- lower risk of sudden infant death syndrome (SIDS)
- reduced risk of breast cancer (in daughters who have been nursed)
- promotes development of jaw and facial structure
- promotes bonding between mother and child

Benefits for mother

Breastfeeding women also enjoy many benefits:

- reduced risk of breast, ovarian, and uterine cancers
- faster postpartum recovery—breastfeeding burns extra calories to help moms lose pregnancy weight and nursing helps the uterus shrink back to its normal size
- improved relaxation due to release of oxytocin when breastfeeding, a hormone that induces a calm, content feeling
- protection from osteoporosis
- saves money
- reduces environmental impact (since there are no bottles to wash or cans to dispose of)

Precautions

Breastfeeding requires lots of energy, and breastfeeding women need to make sure that they are taking in enough **calories** and consuming a healthy diet. The ideal diet of a breastfeeding woman is comprised of healthy and nutritious foods from the five basic food groups (dairy, **whole grains**, fruits, vegetables, and **protein**). The main concentration (50%–55%) should be made up of carbohydrate foods, such as pastas, grains, and fruits. Healthy **fats**, such as fatty fish and avocados, should be 30%, and proteins should equal 15%–20%. Breastfeeding women should make sure to eat foods that contain lots of **calcium**, such as dairy products, broccoli, and beans. They should also make sure they eat plenty of iron-rich foods such as lean red meat, fish, and poultry.

In order to compensate for the energy they expend breastfeeding their babies, breastfeeding women should add 300–500 extra nutritious calories to their diet each day and drink extra fluids. Breastfeeding mothers should also continue to take prenatal vitamins.

Complications

Every substance that a breastfeeding mother puts into her body has the potential to pass to her baby through her breast milk. This includes food, medicine, alcohol, and cigarettes.

- Foods such as dairy products, caffeine, grains and nuts, gassy foods, and spicy foods may cause the baby to fuss if the food upsets the baby's stomach. If this occurs, the mother should eliminate the suspect food from her diet for 10–14 days to see if the trouble stops.
- Any medication taken while breastfeeding should be approved by a doctor.
- The high estrogen type of birth control pills may decrease a breastfeeding mother's milk supply and are not recommended. A progestin-only pill, such as the "mini-pill," is the least likely to cause milk supply issues.
- Infants have a hard time detoxifying from the alcohol that passes through their mother's breast milk to them. It is recommended to limit alcohol consumption while breastfeeding.
- Cigarettes contain toxins that can pass through to the baby and are not recommended for breastfeeding women.

When breastfeeding is not an option

Although breastfeeding is the optimal way to feed an infant, sometimes it is not possible or feasible. A small percentage of women have conditions that prevent breast milk production, such as insufficient development of milk production glands, and cannot breastfeed. Women with HIV are advised against

QUESTIONS TO ASK YOUR
DOCTOR

- Is it safe for me to breastfeed my baby?
- What are the risks and benefits of breastfeeding?
- What are some alternate options for nutritional sources if I decide not to breastfeed?
- Will any of the medications I am taking pose a risk or preclude me from choosing to breastfeed my baby?
- Can you recommend any organizations that will provide me with additional information about breastfeeding?

breastfeeding as the virus may be passed to their babies. Women who are newly diagnosed with infectious tuberculosis should not breastfeed unless they are on medication. Babies with galactosemia, a rare genetic disorder where the infant cannot metabolize the **sugar** in breast milk, cannot breastfeed.

Resources

BOOKS

La Leche League International. *The Womanly Art of Breastfeeding*. 8th ed. London, UK: Pinter & Martin, 2010.

Meek, Joan Younger, and Winnie Yu. *American Academy of Pediatrics New Mother's Guide to Breastfeeding*. New York: Bantam Books, 2011.

Sears, William, et al. *The Baby Book: Everything You Need to Know About Your Baby from Birth to Age Two*. Boston, MA: Little, Brown and Company, 2013.

PERIODICALS

Faucher, M.A. "An Updated Scientific Review of the Benefits of Breastfeeding with Additional Resources for Use in Everyday Practice." *Journal of Midwifery & Women's Health*. 57, no. 4 (2012): 422–23.

Hunsberger, Monica, et al. "Infant Feeding Practices and Prevalence of Obesity in Eight European Countries— the IDEFICS Study." *Public Health Nutrition* (September 2012): e-pub ahead of print. http://dx.doi.org/10.1017/S1368980012003850 (accessed September 13, 2012).

Kramer, M.S., and R. Kakuma. "Optimal Duration of Exclusive Breastfeeding." *Cochrane Database of Systematic Reviews* 8, art no. CD003517 (August 15, 2012). http://dx.doi.org/10.1002/14651858. CD003517.pub2 (accessed September 13, 2012).

Young, J., et al. "Responding to Evidence: Breastfeed Baby If You Can—The Sixth Public Health Recommendation to Reduce the Risk of Sudden and Unexpected Death in Infancy." *Breastfeeding Review* 20, no. 1 (2012): 7–15.

WEBSITES

Office on Women's Health. "Breastfeeding." WomensHealth.gov. http://www.womenshealth.gov/ breastfeeding (accessed September 13, 2012).

ORGANIZATIONS

American Academy of Pediatrics, 141 NW Point Blvd., Elk Grove Village, IL 60007, (847) 434-4000, http:// www.aap.org.

Centers for Disease Control and Prevention, 1600 Clifton Rd., Atlanta, GA 30333, (800) 311-3435, http:// www.cdc.gov.

La Leche League International, 957 N. Plum Grove Rd., Schaumburg, IL 60173, (800) LA-LECHE (525-3243), http://www.lalecheleague.org.

United Nations Children Fund, 3 United Nations Plaza, New York, NY 10017, (212) 686-5522, http://www.unicef.org.

World Health Organization, Department of Maternal, Newborn, Child and Adolescent Health, Ave. Appia 20, CH-1211, Geneva 27, Switzerland, +0041(22) 791 21 11, http://www.who.int/maternal_child_adolescent/ about/en/index.html.

Jennifer L. Byrnes
Laura Jean Cataldo, RN, EdD

British diet *see* **Northern European diet**
British Heart Foundation diet *see* **3-day diet**

Bulimia nervosa

Definition

Bulimia nervosa is an eating disorder that involves repeated **binge eating** followed by purging the body of **calories** to avoid gaining weight. The person who has bulimia has an irrational fear of gaining weight and a distorted **body image**. Bulimia nervosa can have potentially fatal health consequences.

Description

Bulimia is an eating disorder whose main feature is eating an unreasonably large amount of food in a short time, then following this binge by purging the body of calories. Purging is most often done by self-induced vomiting, but it can also be done by laxative, enema, or diuretic abuse. Alternately, some people with bulimia do not purge but use extreme exercising and post-binge fasting to burn calories. This can lead to serious injury. Non-purging bulimia is sometimes

Effects of bulimia on the body

Blood	Anemia
Body fluids	Dehydration
	Low potassium, magnesium, and
	sodium
Brain	Anxiety
	Depression
	Dizziness
	Fear of gaining weight
	Low self-esteem
	Shame
Cheeks	Soreness
	Swelling
Heart	Heart failure
	Heart muscle weakened
	Irregular heart beat
	Low pulse and blood pressure
Intestines	Abdominal cramping
	Bloating
	Constipation
	Diarrhea
	Irregular bowel movements
Hormones	Irregular or absent period
Mouth	Cavities
	Gum disease
	Teeth sensitive to hot and cold food
	Tooth enamel erosion
Muscles	Fatigue
Skin	Abrasion of knuckles
	Dry skin
Stomach	Delayed emptying
	Pain
	Rupture
	Ulcers
Throat and esophagus	Blood in vomit
	Soreness and irritation
	Tears and ruptures

SOURCE: National Women's Health Information Center, Office on Women's Health, U.S. Department of Health and Human Services

(Table by GGS Information Services. © 2013 Cengage Learning.)

called exercise bulimia. Bulimia nervosa is officially recognized as a psychiatric disorder in the *Diagnostic and Statistical Manual for Mental Disorders, Fourth Edition-Text Revision (DSM-IV-TR)*, published by the American Psychiatric Association.

Bulimia nervosa is diagnosed when most of the following conditions are present:

• Repeated episodes of binge eating followed by behavior to compensate for the binge (e.g., purging, fasting, over-exercising). Binge eating is defined as eating a significantly larger amount of food in a limited time than most people typically would eat.

• Binge/purge episodes occur at least twice a week for a period of three or more months.

• The individual feels unable to control or stop an eating binge once it starts and will continue to eat even if uncomfortably full.

• The individual is overly concerned about body weight and shape and puts unreasonable emphasis on physical appearance when evaluating his or her self-worth.

• Bingeing and purging does not occur exclusively during periods of anorexia nervosa.

Many people with bulimia will consume 3,000–10,000 calories in an hour. For example, they will start out intending to eat one slice of cake and end up eating the entire cake. One distinguishing aspect of bulimia is how out of control people with bulimia feel when they are eating. They will eat and eat, continuing even when they feel full and become uncomfortable.

Most people with bulimia recognize that their behavior is not normal; they simply cannot control it. They usually feel ashamed and guilty over their binge/purge habits. As a result, they frequently become secretive about their eating and purging. They may, for example, eat at night after the family has gone to bed or buy food at the grocery store and eat it in the car before going home. Many people with bulimia choose high-fat, high-sugar foods that are easy to eat and easy to regurgitate. They become adept at inducing vomiting, usually by sticking a finger down their throat and triggering the gag reflex. After a while, they can vomit at will. Repeated purging has serious physical and emotional consequences.

Many individuals with bulimia are of normal weight, and a fair number of men who become bulimic were overweight as children. This makes it difficult for family and friends to recognize when someone is suffering from this disorder. People with bulimia may lie about induced vomiting and laxative abuse, although they may complain of symptoms related to their binge/purge cycles and seek medical help for those problems. People with bulimia tend to be more impulsive than people with other **eating disorders**. Lack of impulse control often leads to risky sexual behavior, anger management problems, and alcohol and drug abuse.

A subset of people with bulimia also have **anorexia nervosa**. Anorexia nervosa is an eating disorder that involves self-imposed starvation. These people often purge after eating only a small or a normal-sized portion of food. Some studies have shown that up to 60% of people with bulimia have a history of anorexia nervosa.

Dieting is usually the trigger that starts a person down the road to bulimia. The future bulimic is very concerned about weight gain and appearance, and may constantly be on a diet. She (most people with bulimia are female) may begin by going on a rigorous low-calorie diet. Unable to stick with the diet, she then eats voraciously, far more than she needs to satisfy her hunger, feels guilty about eating, and then exercises or purges to get rid of the unwanted calories. At first this may happen only occasionally, but gradually these sessions of bingeing and purging become routine and start to intrude on the person's friendships, daily activities, and health. Eventually these practices have serious physical and emotional consequences that need to be addressed by healthcare professionals.

Demographics

Bulimia nervosa is primarily a disorder of industrialized countries where food is abundant and the culture values a thin appearance. Internationally, the rate of bulimia has been increasing since the 1950s. Bulimia is the most common eating disorder in the United States. Overall, about 3% of Americans have bulimia. Of these, 85%–90% are female. The rate is highest among adolescents and college women, averaging 5%–6%. In men, the disorder is more often diagnosed in homosexuals than in heterosexuals. Some experts believe that the number of people diagnosed with bulimia represents only the most severe cases and that many more people have bulimic tendencies, but are successful in hiding their symptoms. In one study, 40% of college women reported isolated incidents of bingeing and purging.

Bulimia affects people from all racial, ethnic, and socioeconomic groups. The disorder usually begins later in life than anorexia nervosa. Most people begin bingeing and purging in their late teens through their twenties. Men tend to start at an older age than women. About 5% of people with bulimia begin the behavior after age 25. Bulimia is uncommon in children under age 14.

Competitive athletes have an increased risk of developing bulimia nervosa, especially in sports where weight is tied to performance and where a low percentage of body fat is highly desirable. Jockeys, wrestlers, bodybuilders, figure skaters, cross-country runners, and gymnasts have higher than average rates of bulimia. People such as actors, models, cheerleaders, and dancers who are judged mainly on their appearance are also at high risk of developing the disorder. This same group of people is also at higher risk for developing anorexia nervosa. Some people are primarily anorexic and severely restrict their calorie intake while also purging the small amounts they do eat. Others move back and forth between anorexic and bulimic behaviors.

A 2007 report from the National Institute of Mental Health (NIMH) noted that approximately 16% of individuals with bulimia nervosa received treatment for a 12 month period of time, and 43% of individuals with this disorder were receiving lifetime treatment.

Causes and symptoms

Bulimia nervosa is a complex disorder that does not have a single cause. Research suggests that some people have a predisposition toward bulimia and that something triggers the behavior, which then becomes self-reinforcing. Hereditary, biological, psychological, and social factors all appear to play a role.

Causes

- Heredity. Twin studies suggest that there is an inherited component to bulimia nervosa, but that it is small. Having a close relative, usually a mother or a sister, with bulimia slightly increases the likelihood of other (usually female) family members developing the disorder. However, when compared to other inherited diseases or even to anorexia nervosa, the genetic contribution to developing this disorder appears less important than many other factors. Family history of depression, alcoholism, and obesity also increase the risk of developing bulimia.

- Biological factors. There is some evidence that bulimia is linked to low levels of serotonin in the brain. Serotonin is a neurotransmitter. One of its functions is to help regulate the feeling of fullness or satiety that tells a person to stop eating. Neurotransmitters are also involved in other mental disorders, such as depression, that often occur with bulimia. Other research suggests that people with bulimia may have abnormal levels of leptin, a protein that helps regulate weight by telling the body to take in less food. Research in this area is relatively new, and the findings are still unclear.

- Psychological factors. Certain personality types appear to be more vulnerable to developing bulimia. People with bulimia tend to have poor impulse control. They are aware that their behavior is abnormal. After a binge/purge session, they may feel ashamed and vow never to repeat the cycle, but the next time they wish to eat and purge, they are unable to control the impulse. Major depression, obsessive-compulsive disorder, and anxiety disorders are more common among individuals who are bulimic.

- Social factors. The families of people who develop bulimia are more likely to have members who have problems with alcoholism, depression, and obesity. These families also tend to have a high level of open conflict and disordered, unpredictable lives. Often something stressful or upsetting triggers the urge to diet stringently and then begin binge/purge behaviors. This may be as simple as a family member teasing about the person's weight, nagging about eating junk food, commenting on how clothes fit, or comparing the person unfavorably to someone who is thin. Life events such as moving, starting a new school, and breaking up with a boyfriend or girlfriend can also trigger binge/purge behavior. Overlaying the family situation is the false but unrelenting media message that thin is "good" and fat is "bad."

Signs and symptoms

Binge/purge cycles have physical consequences, including:

- teeth damaged from repeated exposure to stomach acid from vomiting; eroded tooth enamel
- swollen salivary glands; sores in mouth and throat
- dehydration
- sores or calluses on knuckles or hands from using them to induce vomiting
- electrolyte imbalances revealed by laboratory tests
- dry skin
- fatigue
- irregular or absent menstrual cycles in women
- weight, heart rate, and blood pressure may be normal

Diagnosis

Diagnosis is based on several factors, including a patient history, physical examination, the results of laboratory tests, and a mental status evaluation. A patient history is less helpful in diagnosing bulimia than in diagnosing many diseases because many people with bulimia lie about their bingeing and purging and their use of laxatives, enemas, and medications. The patient may, however, complain about related symptoms such as fatigue or feeling bloated. Many people with bulimia are likely to express extreme concern about their weight during the examination.

A physical examination begins with weight and blood pressure and moves through the body looking for the signs listed above. Based on the physical exam and patient history, the physician may order laboratory tests. In general, these tests will include a complete blood count (CBC), urinalysis, and blood chemistries (to determine electrolyte levels). People suspected of extreme exercising may need to have x rays to look for damage to bones, such as stress fractures.

Several different evaluations can be used to examine a person's mental state. A doctor or mental health professional will assess the individual's thoughts and feelings about themselves, their body, their relationships with others, and their risk for self-harm.

Treatment

Treatment choices depend on the degree to which the bulimic behavior has resulted in physical damage and whether the person is a danger to him or herself. Hospital inpatient care may be needed to correct severe electrolyte imbalances that result from repeated vomiting and laxative abuse. Electrolyte imbalances can result in heart irregularities and other potentially fatal complications. Most people with bulimia do not require hospitalization. The rate of hospitalization is much lower than that for people with anorexia nervosa because many people with bulimia maintain a normal weight.

Day treatment or partial hospitalization, where the patient goes every day to an extensive treatment program, provides structured mealtimes, nutrition education, intensive therapy, medical monitoring, and supervision. If day treatment fails, the patient may need to be hospitalized or enter a full-time residential treatment facility.

Outpatient treatment provides medical supervision, nutrition counseling, self-help strategies, and psychotherapy. Self-help groups receive mixed reviews from healthcare professionals who work with people with bulimia. Some groups offer constructive support in stopping the binge/purge cycle, while others tend to reinforce the behavior.

Drug therapy helps many people with bulimia. Selective serotonin reuptake inhibitors (SSRIs) such as fluoxetine (Prozac) and sertraline (Zoloft) have been approved by the United States Food and Drug Administration (FDA) for treatment of bulimia. These medications increase serotonin levels in the brain and are thought to affect the body's sense of fullness. They are used whether or not the patient shows signs of depression. Drug treatment should always be supplemented with psychotherapy.

Other drugs are being explored for use in the treatment of bulimia. Individuals with bulimia interested in entering a clinical trial at no cost can find a list and description of clinical trials currently enrolling volunteers at http://www.clinicaltrials.gov.

Nutrition and dietary concerns

A dietitian is part of the team needed to successfully treat bulimia. These professionals usually perform a dietary review along with nutritional counseling so that the recovering bulimic can plan healthy meals and develop a healthy relationship with food.

Therapy

Medical intervention helps alleviate the immediate physical problems associated with bulimia. Medication can help the person with bulimia break the binge/purge cycle. However, drug therapy alone rarely produces recovery. Psychotherapy plays a major role in helping the individual with bulimia recover from the disorder. Several different types of psychotherapy are used depending on the individual's situation. Generally, the goal of psychotherapy is to help the individual change his or her behavior and develop a healthy attitude toward their body and food.

Some types of psychotherapy have been successful in treating people with bulimia:

- Cognitive behavior therapy (CBT) is designed to confront and then change the individual's thoughts and feelings about his or her body and behaviors toward food, but it does not address why those thoughts or feelings exist. Strategies to maintain self-control may be explored. This therapy is relatively short-term. CBT is often the therapy of choice for people with bulimia, and it is often successful at least in the short term.

- Interpersonal therapy is short-term therapy that helps the individual identify specific issues and problems in relationships. The individual may be asked to look back at his or her family history to try to recognize problem areas and work toward resolving them. Interpersonal therapy has about the same rate of success in people with bulimia as CBT.

- Family and/or couples therapy is helpful in dealing with conflict or disorder that may be a factor in triggering binge/purge behavior at home.

- Supportive-expressive therapy or group therapy may be helpful in addition to other types of therapy.

Prognosis

The long-term outlook for recovery from bulimia is mixed. About half of all people with bulimia show improvement in controlling their behavior after short-term interpersonal or cognitive behavioral therapy with nutritional counseling and drug therapy. However, after three years, only about one-third are still doing well. Relapses are common, and binge/purge episodes and bulimic behavior often comes and goes for many years. Stress seems to be a major trigger for relapse.

The sooner treatment is sought, the better the chances of recovery. Without professional intervention, recovery is unlikely. Untreated bulimia can lead to death from causes such as rupture of the stomach or esophagus. Associated problems such as substance abuse, depression, anxiety disorders, and poor impulse control also contribute to the death rate.

KEY TERMS

Diuretic—A substance that removes water from the body by increasing urine production.

Electrolyte—Ions in the body that participate in metabolic reactions. The major human electrolytes are sodium (Na+), potassium (K+), calcium (Ca 2+), magnesium (Mg2+), chloride (Cl−), phosphate (HPO$_4$ 2−), bicarbonate (HCO$_3$−), and sulfate (SO$_4$ 2−).

Neurotransmitter—One of a group of chemicals secreted by a nerve cell (neuron) to carry a chemical message to another nerve cell, often as a way of transmitting a nerve impulse. Examples of neurotransmitters include acetylcholine, dopamine, serotonin, and norepinephrine.

Obsessive-compulsive disorder—A psychiatric disorder in which a person is unable to control the desire to repeat the same action over and over.

Prevention

Some behaviors to try to help prevent bulimia nervosa from developing include:

- Parents should not obsess about their weight or appearance in front of their children.

- Do not tease children about their body shape or compare them to others.

- Make sure children know that they are loved and accepted.

- Try to eat meals together as a family whenever possible.

- Remind children that the models they see on television and in fashion magazines have extreme, not normal or healthy, bodies.

- Do not put children on a diet unless advised by a pediatrician.

- Block children from visiting pro-bulimia websites. These are sites where people with bulimia give advice on techniques and support each other's distorted body image.

- If a child is a competitive athlete, get to know the coach and the coach's attitude toward weight.

QUESTIONS TO ASK YOUR DOCTOR

- What are the indications that my loved one may suffer from an eating disorder?
- What are the indications that my child may have a problem with their perception of body image?
- Should we see a specialist? If so, what kind of specialist should I contact?
- What treatment options do you recommend?
- What dietary changes, if any, would you recommend for my child?
- What physical symptoms or behaviors are important enough that I should seek immediate treatment?

If parents suspect that their child has an eating disorder, they should not wait to intervene and get professional help. The sooner the disorder is recognized, the easier it is to treat.

Relapses happen to many people with bulimia. People who are recovering from bulimia can help prevent themselves from relapsing by doing the following:

- never dieting and planning healthy meals instead
- eating with other people and not alone
- staying in treatment and keeping therapy appointments
- monitoring negative and practicing positive self-talk
- spending time doing something enjoyable every day
- getting at least seven hours of sleep each night
- spending time each day with family and friends

Resources

BOOKS

Carleton, Pamela, and Deborah Ashin. *Take Charge of Your Child's Eating Disorder: A Physician's Step-By-Step Guide to Defeating Anorexia and Bulimia.* New York: Marlowe & Co., 2007.

Hall, Lindsey. *Bulimia: A Guide to Recovery.* Carlsbad, CA: Gurze Books, 2011.

Kilpatrick, Haley., and Whitney Joiner. *The Drama Years: Real Girls Talk About Surviving Middle School—Bullies, Brands, Body Image, and More.* New York: Free Press, 2012.

Knoblich, Gunther, et al, eds. *Human Body Perception from the Inside Out.* Oxford, UK: Oxford University Press, 2006.

Kolodny, Nancy J. *The Beginner's Guide to Eating Disorders Recovery.* Carlsbad, CA: Gurze Books, 2012.

Liu, Aimee. *Restoring Our Bodies, Reclaiming Our Lives: Guidance and Reflections on Recovery from Eating Disorders.* Boston: Trumpeter, 2011.

Messinger, Lisa, and Merle Goldberg. *My Thin Excuse: Understanding, Recognizing, and Overcoming Eating Disorders.* Garden City Park, NY: Square One Publishers, 2006.

Poppink, Joanna. *Healing Your Hungry Heart: Recovering from Your Eating Disorder.* San Francisco: Conari Press, 2011.

Smith, Rita. *Self-Image and Eating Disorders.* New York: Rosen, 2012.

Zweig, Rene D., and Robert L. Leahy. *Treatment Plans and Interventions for Bulimia and Binge-Eating Disorder.* New York: The Guilford Press, 2011.

PERIODICALS

McElroy, S.L., et al. "Current Pharmacotherapy Options for Bulimia Nervosa and Binge Eating Disorder." *Expert Opinion on Pharmacotherapy* 13, no. 14 (2012): 2015–26.

Moreno-Domínguez, S., et al. "Impact of Fasting on Food Craving, Mood and Consumption in Bulimia Nervosa and Healthy Women Participants." *European Eating Disorders Review* (July 5, 2012): e-pub ahead of print. http://dx.doi.org/10.1002/erv.2187 (accessed September 24, 2012).

Wilson, Jenny L., et al. "Surfing for Thinness: A Pilot Study of Pro-Eating Disorder Web Site Usage in Adolescents With Eating Disorders." *Pediatrics* 118, no. 6 (December 2006): e1635–43. http://dx.doi.org/ 10.1542/ peds.2006-1133 (accessed September 24, 2012).

WEBSITES

Anorexia Nervosa and Related Eating Disorders (ANRED). "Table of Contents." http://www.anred.com/toc.html (accessed September 24, 2012).

Mayo Clinic staff. "Bulimia Nervosa." MayoClinic.com. http://www.mayoclinic.com/health/bulimia/DS00607 (accessed September 24, 2012).

MedlinePlus. "Eating Disorders." U.S. National Library of Medicine, National Institutes of Health. http:// www.nlm.nih.gov/medlineplus/eatingdisorders.html (accessed September 24, 2012).

National Association of Anorexia Nervosa and Associated Disorders. "Eating Disorders Statistics." http:// www.anad.org/get-information/about-eating-disorders/eating-disorders-statistics (accessed September 24, 2012).

National Institute of Mental Health. "Eating Disorders Among Adults—Bulimia Nervosa." National Institutes of Health. http://www.nimh.nih.gov/statistics/ 1EAT_ADULT_RBUL.shtml (accessed September 24, 2012).

ORGANIZATIONS

Association of Body Image and Disordered Eating, UCD Counseling & Psychological Services, Davis, CA 95616, http://abide.ucdavis.edu.

National Association of Anorexia Nervosa & Associated Disorders, 800 E Diehl Rd. #160, Naperville, IL 60563, (630) 577-1333, (630) 577-1330 (helpline), anadhelp@anad.org, http://www.anad.org.

National Eating Disorders Association, 165 West 46th St., New York, NY 10036, (212) 575-6200, (800) 931-2237, info@NationalEatingDisorders.org, http://www.nationaleatingdisorders.org.

National Institute of Mental Health, 6001 Executive Blvd., Bethesda, MD 20892, (301) 443-4513, TTY: (866) 415-8051, (866) 615-6464, nimhinfo@nih.gov, http://www.nimh.nih.gov.

Tish Davidson, AM
Laura Jean Cataldo, RN, EdD

C

Cabbage soup diet

Definition

The cabbage soup diet is a quick weight-loss program intended to be followed for seven days. The centerpiece of the diet is a recipe for cabbage soup, which the dieter may consume in unlimited quantities. In addition to the cabbage soup, there are certain other foods that the dieter must eat on specific days during the week. There are several versions of the diet, most of which promise a 10–17 lb. (4.5–7.7 kg) weight loss after one week.

The cabbage soup diet has a number of other names, including the TWA Stewardess Diet, Model's Diet, Dolly Parton Diet, Military Cabbage Soup Diet, Mayo Clinic Diet, Sacred Heart Hospital Diet, Miami Heart Institute Diet, Spokane Diet, Fat-Burning Diet, T. J.'s Miracle Soup Diet, and the Skinny.

Origins

The cabbage soup diet may be the oldest fad diet still in use; it seems to resurface with a new name every 10 to 15 years. It has been described by some historians of popular culture as a good example of an urban legend—a type of modern folklore passed from person to person via word of mouth, photocopies, or e-mail. Urban legends are often stories or anecdotes, but some can be called "widely accepted misinformation."

No one seems to know when the cabbage soup diet was first formulated or the identity of its originator. According to the Academy of Nutrition and Dietetics' (formerly the American Dietetic Association) timeline of **fad diets**, the cabbage soup diet originated around 1950. After the 1950s, the cabbage soup diet was revived in the early 1980s not only as the Dolly Parton Diet but also as the Trans World Airlines (TWA) Stewardess Diet and the Model's Diet. It acquired these names because of the belief that celebrities, models, and flight attendants had to meet rigorous periodic weight check-ins in order to keep their jobs. The cabbage soup diet was passed around from person to person in the form of photocopies during this period. It was claimed that the dieter would lose 10–17 lb. during the first week, either because cabbage supposedly has no **calories** at all or because it contains a "miracle fat-burning" compound.

The cabbage soup diet reappeared again in the mid-1990s, when fax machines and the Internet made it easy for people to transmit copies of the diet to friends and workplace colleagues. The diet was also published in magazines such as *Cosmopolitan* and *Gentlemen's Quarterly* (now *GQ*) in 1995. The diet was attributed to health associations as well as the cardiology departments of several hospitals and medical centers in this period. These institutions supposedly gave the diet to overweight patients preparing for heart surgery to help them to lose weight quickly before their operations. Thus, the diet acquired such names as the Sacred Heart diet or the Spokane diet (from the names of hospitals in Brussels, Belgium; Montreal, Quebec; and Spokane, Washington), the American Heart Association Diet, the Mayo Clinic Diet, and the Miami Heart Institute Diet. However, these institutions have no official affiliation with the diet.

Description

The cabbage soup diet features very specific menus for each day of the diet, plus an unlimited amount of cabbage soup. There is no restriction on the amount of cabbage soup that can be eaten to help prevent hunger. The diet is intended to be followed for seven days. At least four glasses of water should be consumed each day, in addition to the required foods. The cabbage soup meal plan is as follows:

- Day one: Eat only the cabbage soup and unlimited fruit (except bananas). Cantaloupe and watermelon are recommended. Permissible drinks are water, black coffee, cranberry juice, or unsweetened tea.

- Day two: No fruit. Raw or cooked vegetables can be eaten in unlimited quantity along with the soup, except for corn, peas, and beans. A baked potato with butter can be eaten at dinnertime.
- Day three: Unlimited fruit or vegetables, but no baked potato.
- Day four: Eat at least three and as many as eight bananas, and drink an unlimited amount of skim milk. Day Four is supposed to curb a desire for sweets.
- Day five: Eat 10–20 oz. of beef and up to six fresh tomatoes (or one can of stewed tomatoes). Cabbage soup must be eaten for at least one meal. Drink 6–8 glasses of water to flush acids from the body. Baked or broiled chicken (without the skin) or fish may be substituted for beef at one meal.
- Day six: Eat cabbage soup at least once during the day; otherwise, an unlimited amount of beef and vegetables can be consumed, but no baked potato.
- Day seven: Eat an unlimited amount of brown rice and vegetables and drink an unlimited amount of unsweetened fruit juice. Cabbage soup must be eaten at least once during the day. No bread, alcohol, or carbonated beverages (including diet soda) are allowed.

Cabbage soup recipes

Most versions of the cabbage soup diet begin with a recipe for the soup. One change that has evolved since the diet first appeared in the 1950s is the cooking instructions; the earliest versions of the diet recommended cooking the soup for an hour, which would destroy most of the nutrients in the cabbage and other ingredients. Recent soup recipes recommend letting the soup simmer no more than 10 to 15 minutes after being brought to a boil.

STANDARD RECIPE.

- 6 large green onions
- 2 green peppers
- 1 or 2 cans diced tomatoes
- 1 bunch of celery
- 1 envelope of dry onion soup mix
- 1 or 2 bouillon cubes (some versions specify low-sodium vegetable flavor) if desired
- 1 large head of cabbage
- 1 8 oz. can of vegetable juice (optional)

MILITARY DIET RECIPE.

- 2 13-ounce cans of chicken broth
- 1 large bunch of celery
- 2 bunches of spring onions

- 1 large head of cabbage
- 1 large can of whole tomatoes
- 3 large bell peppers
- Salt and pepper to taste

GREEN CABBAGE SOUP RECIPE.

- One-half of a green cabbage, chopped
- 3 large onions, diced
- 1 large green pepper, sliced
- 1 cup fresh mushrooms, washed and sliced
- 1 or 2 cups washed fresh spinach leaves
- 1 can of diced tomatoes
- 1 envelope of dry onion soup mix
- 3 vegetable-flavored bouillon cubes
- 8 to 12 cups of water
- oregano, cilantro, garlic powder, basil, pepper, and/or parsley to taste

Function

The cabbage soup diet is intended only for short-term weight loss. It is very restrictive and is not in line with federal dietary recommendations. Safe and healthy weight loss is considered to be 1–2 lb. (0.45–0.9) per week. Most of the weight lost on the cabbage soup diet is water weight and will likely return after dieters revert back to previous eating habits.

Benefits

Due to the limited number of daily calories consumed on the cabbage soup diet, following it may result in weight loss. Some people like the fact that the diet offers a break from junk food or fast food and does not require any unusual or expensive ingredients, complex recipes, or appetite suppressants. However, it is not a realistic way of eating and is not intended for long-term maintenance. People interested in the cabbage soup diet should meet with a physician or registered dietitian to discuss healthier and more long-term weight-loss methods.

Precautions

Though not nutritionally sound, the cabbage soup diet poses no serious danger to adults in good health who follow it for no more than seven days. However, this does not mean that it is a recommended or safe diet. The cabbage soup diet does not include an adequate balance of nutrients and is too low in calories for long-term use. Claims that the diet can be used indefinitely or repeated within three days of completing the first cycle should be ignored as they are not safe. Frequent use could lead to **weight cycling**, which has been shown to be detrimental to health.

The diet should not be used by anyone without first consulting a doctor or registered dietitian, and it should not be used by individuals with type 2 diabetes, **eating disorders**, or other disorders requiring special diets.

Risks

Side effects from the diet may include dizziness, light-headedness, and flatulence (intestinal gas). The latter may be a social risk due to embarrassment related to passing gas in public. Common versions of the soup recipe are high in salt. Dieters who must restrict their **sodium** intake should discuss variations with their physician.

Research and general acceptance

The American Heart Association (AHA) and the hospitals whose names have been associated with the cabbage soup diet have issued formal disclaimers warning the public that they do not endorse this diet. The Hôpital du Sacré-Coeur de Montréal stated in a press release that the diet is contrary to healthy feeding patterns and even presents potential dangers to good health. The Sacred Heart Medical Center (SHMC) in Spokane requests that people do not affiliate the diet with their hospital as they do not consider it a safe or healthy method of weight loss. A SHMC disclaimer states, "This diet did not originate at SHMC and it is not endorsed by the dietitians or the staff of our cardiac rehabilitation program. One of our major concerns about this diet plan is it emphasizes the consumption of fruits and vegetables while excluding the consumption of meat or fish, cereal grains, and milk products on most days. Any diet that focuses on only certain food groups will be low or deficient in essential nutrients and, therefore, lead to poor nutritional status long-term. Our experience with any low-calorie diets, like this one, is that they do not lead to permanent weight loss. Once individuals start eating in a more normal pattern, the weight is regained. A very important factor in obtaining a healthy weight is to evaluate your physical activity and other lifestyle concerns. This is most appropriately done by consulting with a registered dietitian."

Scientific evidence is not available to support claims that cabbage has unique detoxifying, fat-burning, immunoprotective, antidepressant, or anticancer properties. Claims regarding the possibility of losing 17 pounds by the end of one week on this diet are exaggerated. In addition, there is no indication that any government has ever sponsored clinical trials of cabbage soup, whether in pill form or fully constituted.

Resources

BOOKS

Danbrot, Margaret. *The New Cabbage Soup Diet*. Rev. ed. New York: St. Martin's Press, 2004.

Scales, Mary Josephine. *Diets in a Nutshell: A Definitive Guide on Diets from A to Z*. Clifton, VA: Apex Publishers, 2005.

WEBSITES

Academy of Nutrition and Dietetics. "Fad Diet Timeline." http://www.eatright.org/nnm/games/timeline/index.html (accessed August 10, 2012).

"The 'Miracle Soup Diet.'" Providence Health and Services, Spokane. http://www2.providence.org/spokane/facilities/sacred-heart-medical-center/services/food-and-nutrition/Pages/soup-diet.aspx (accessed August 10, 2012).

Zeratsky, Katherine. "What is the Cabbage Soup Diet, and Can It Help Me Lose Weight?" Mayo Clinic. http://www.mayoclinic.com/health/cabbage-soup-diet/AN02134 (accessed August 14, 2012).

ORGANIZATIONS

Academy of Nutrition and Dietetics, 120 South Riverside Plz., Ste. 2000, Chicago, IL 60606-6995, (312) 899-0040, (800) 877-1600, amacmunn@eatright.org, http://www.eatright.org.

Dietitians of Canada, 480 University Ave., Ste. 604, Toronto, Ontario, Canada M5G 1V2, (416) 596-0857, Fax: (416) 596-0603, centralinfo@dietitians.ca, http://www.dietitians.ca.

Rebecca J. Frey, PhD

Caffeine

Definition

Caffeine is a mild alkaloid stimulant made by some plants. It is found in coffee beans, tea leaves, and cocoa beans; added to soft drinks, energy drinks, and energy bars; and sold in capsules and tablets as a dietary supplement.

Purpose

Caffeine is a mild stimulant. It is used to temporarily relieve fatigue and increase mental alertness. Caffeine is added to some antihistamine drugs to help counteract the sleepiness they may cause. It is also added to over-the-counter headache remedies (e.g., Excedrin) and migraine headache drugs to enhance their painkilling effects. Under medical supervision, citrated caffeine (a prescription drug) is used to treat breathing problems in premature infants.

Description

Caffeine, from the Italian word cafée, meaning coffee, is naturally made by about 60 plants. The most familiar of these are coffee leaves and beans, tea leaves, kola nuts, yerba mate, guarana berries, and cacao (the source of chocolate). In plants, caffeine is a pesticide. Insects eating plants that contain caffeine become disabled or die.

Humans have eaten plants containing caffeine for thousands of years; first chewing the seeds and leaves, and later boiling them and drinking the resulting liquid. Coffee, a major source of caffeine, was introduced to Europe from the Middle East in the seventeenth century and rapidly became a popular drink. Coffee houses began appearing in London in the mid-1600s. A German chemist purified caffeine in 1819. Today, besides being found naturally in coffee, tea, and chocolate, it is added to soft drinks, energy drinks and bars, headache remedies, and is sold as a dietary supplement to improve mental and physical functioning.

Caffeine has no nutritional value, but it has these effects on the body:

- increases heart rate
- temporarily increases blood pressure
- relaxes smooth muscle cells in the airways
- releases fatty acids and glycerol in the body for energy use
- easily crosses the blood-brain barrier and changes the level of neurotransmitters in the brain
- passes into breast milk

It used to be believed that caffeine acted as a diuretic, which is any substance that increases urine output. Research has since found that these effects are very mild, and that the diuretic effect is seen only when caffeine is consumed in large doses (500 to 600 milligrams [mg], or up to seven cups of coffee per day). This means that moderate consumption of coffee and other caffeinated beverages does not cause **dehydration**.

Caffeine is absorbed in the stomach. Its effects are noticeable in about 15 minutes and usually last several hours. However, there is a huge variation among people both in their sensitivity to caffeine and in how long it stays in their bodies. Although the average time it takes half a dose of caffeine to be eliminated from the body is three to four hours, this time may extend to six hours in women taking oral contraceptives, and be much longer in pregnant women and in people with liver damage.

Many well-designed, well-documented studies show that caffeine makes people more alert, improves short-term memory, enhances the ability to concentrate, increases the individual's capacity for physical work, and speeds up reaction time. In habitual caffeine drinkers, caffeine achieves this by preventing the detrimental effects of withdrawal. It does not boost functioning to above normal levels. All of these effects are

Approximate amounts of caffeine in popular products		
	Size	Amount of caffeine
Sprite, Fanta, 7 UP	12 oz (355 mL)	0 mg
Tea, decaffeinated	8 oz (240 mL)	1–4 mg
Coffee, decaffeinated, brewed	8 oz (240 mL)	2–12 mg
Hershey's Milk Chocolate	1.55 oz (43 g)	9 mg
Tea, green, brewed	8 oz (240 mL)	15 mg
Barq's Root Beer	12 oz (355 mL)	23 mg
Hershey's Special Dark Chocolate	1.45 oz (41 g)	31 mg
Coca-Cola Classic	12 oz (355 mL)	35 mg
Pepsi	12 oz (355 mL)	36–38 mg
Tea, black, brewed	8 oz (240 mL)	40–120 mg
Sunkist Orange, regular or diet	12 oz (355 mL)	41 mg
Dr Pepper	12 oz (355 mL)	42–44 mg
Diet Coke	12 oz (355 mL)	47 mg
Mountain Dew	12 oz (355 mL)	54 mg
Coffee, espresso	1 oz (30 mL)	58–75 mg
Excedrin® extra-strength headache	1 tablet	65 mg
Red Bull energy drink	8.3 oz (245 mL)	76 mg
SoBe No Fear energy drink	8 oz (240 mL)	83 mg
Coffee, brewed	8 oz (240 mL)	95–200 mg
5-hour ENERGY® drink	2 oz (59 mL)	138 mg
Monster Energy drink	16 oz (473 mL)	160 mg
NO-DOZ® maximum-strength caffeine	1 tablet	200 mg

(Table by PreMediaGlobal. © 2013 Cengage Learning.)

temporary. Caffeine does not replace the need for rest or sleep.

Caffeine is on the U.S. Food and Drug Administration's (FDA) list of foods generally recognized as safe (GRAS). In moderate amounts, caffeine does not appear to be harmful to humans, although it is poisonous to dogs, horses, and some birds. "Moderate" generally means consumption in the range of 300–400 mg or 3–4 cups of coffee daily. Caffeine has not been shown to cause birth defects and is considered safe in reasonable amounts during pregnancy. The March of Dimes Foundation recommends that pregnant women limit their caffeine intake to 200 mg per day, roughly the amount in one 12-ounce cup of coffee. Women experiencing difficulty becoming pregnant may wish to completely eliminate caffeine from their diet.

By law, caffeine must be listed as an ingredient on food labels, but the amount of caffeine per serving is not required to be disclosed. Since caffeine is added to so many products, it is difficult to measure the amount of caffeine in an individual's diet. Caffeine content of coffees and teas varies depending on where the plants were grown and how the beverages are prepared.

Benefits

Research is conflicting, but there seem to be some benefits to regular caffeine consumption. A 2012 study published in the *Journal of Alzheimer's Disease* found that drinking roughly three cups of coffee per day could help prevent or delay the onset of Alzheimer's disease. Other studies have linked similar amounts of caffeine consumption to improved memory and long-term cognition. A study of more than 50,000 women, published in the September 2011 issue of the *Archives of Internal Medicine*, found that women who drank at least four cups of coffee per day had a significantly lower rate (0.2%) of depression than women drinking fewer than one cup per week or even one cup per day (1.3% and 1.8%, respectively). Other benefits associated with moderate-to-high caffeine consumption include decreased risk of skin **cancer** (three cups per day), improved athletic performance (1–5 cups), and longer life expectancy (six cups).

Tea is another good source of caffeine. Though most caffeinated teas have less caffeine per cup than coffee, drinking tea is associated with myriad benefits, due to tea's antioxidant properties.

Precautions

People vary in their sensitivity to caffeine based on their weight, age, medications they may be taking, personal biology, and habitual intake. Individuals

---

KEY TERMS

Alkaloid—An organic compound found in plants; chemically it is a base and usually contains at least one nitrogen atom.

Blood-brain barrier—A specialized, semi-permeable layer of cells around the blood vessels in the brain that controls which substances can leave the circulatory system and enter the brain.

Diuretic—A substance that removes water from the body by increasing urine production.

Neurotransmitter—One of a group of chemicals secreted by a nerve cell (neuron) to carry a chemical message to another nerve cell, often as a way of transmitting a nerve impulse. Examples of neurotransmitters include acetylcholine, dopamine, serotonin, and norepinephrine.

Tolerance—Adjustment of the body to a drug so that it takes more and more to produce the same physiological or psychological effect, or adjustment to a drug so that side effects are diminished.

---

should be alert to how much caffeine they consume during a day and how it makes them feel, then adjust their intake accordingly. All of caffeine's effects are temporary, and a "crash" is likely to occur after a dose of caffeine wears off.

Caffeine stays in the system of pregnant women and people with liver damage longer than normal. These people should closely monitor their caffeine intake.

Caffeine passes into breast milk and although it may have no effect on the **breastfeeding** woman, it may make the infant restless, irritable, and less likely to sleep. Recommendations for breastfeeding women vary from one to three cups of coffee per day; if the infant seems to react to the caffeine, the mother should reduce her intake.

Athletes should be aware that the International Olympic Committee tests for caffeine levels over 12 mg/mL of urine. This level could be reached by drinking four large cups of coffee.

Caffeine has increasingly been added to alcoholic beverages. The FDA views this practice as unsafe and in 2010 ordered several manufacturers of caffeinated alcoholic beverages to cease production. Some beverages are still available, but the effects of combining caffeine and alcohol have not been sufficiently tested, and the full extent of possible adverse effects is not yet known.

Interactions

Caffeine appears to enhance the effectiveness of over-the-counter headache and migraine remedies. Some of these medications contain a mixture of caffeine and painkiller. People with a high sensitivity to caffeine or those trying to reduce or monitor their intake (e.g., pregnant women) should read the labels carefully.

People taking diuretic medication (water pills) may see increased urine output because caffeine is a weak diuretic.

Complications

Although caffeine in moderate amounts poses no major health risks, the body quickly develops tolerance to the effects of caffeine, along with a mild physical and psychological dependency. For example, tolerance to caffeine-related sleep disruption disappears in about a week among people who drink 3–4 cups of coffee daily. The amount of caffeine it takes to reach this state is highly variable.

Discontinuing caffeine among regular users can cause withdrawal symptoms. These can include headaches (very common), irritability, nausea, fatigue, sleepiness, inability to concentrate, and mild depression. Caffeine withdrawal symptoms begin 12–24 hours after caffeine is stopped. Withdrawal symptoms peak at around 48 hours, and can last up to five days. Tapering caffeine use, for example cutting down on caffeine by the equivalent of half a cup of coffee (about 50 mg) a day, minimizes or eliminates withdrawal symptoms.

People who consume more than 500 mg of caffeine a day—equivalent to about five cups of coffee—may develop a condition called caffeinism, though the threshold varies among individuals. Caffeinism produces unpleasant sensations, some of which are similar to withdrawal symptoms. Symptoms of caffeine overuse include restlessness, irritability, nervousness, anxiety, muscle twitching, headaches, inability to fall asleep, and a racing heart. Severe overuse of caffeine can cause a number of related disorders, including:

- Caffeine intoxication—usually the result of taking caffeine pills (e.g., NoDoz), this condition causes mental changes, rambling thoughts and speech, irregular heartbeat, and other symptoms associated with overuse. In severe cases death can result from ventricular fibrillation (unsynchronized contractions of the ventricle of the heart).
- Caffeine-induced anxiety disorder—severe anxiety that interferes with daily social interactions and occurs after caffeine intoxication or heavy long-term use of caffeine.

- Caffeine-induced sleep disorder—an inability to sleep that is so great it requires medical/psychiatric attention and occurs after prolonged caffeine consumption.
- Non-specific caffeine-induced disorder—disorders not listed that are attributable to either acute or long-term caffeine consumption.

Parental concerns

Children get most of their caffeine from soft drinks. Parents should choose soft drinks that contain little or no caffeine or replace soft drinks with water, fruit juice, or low-fat milk. Adolescents are increasingly using energy drinks and energy bars containing caffeine. In addition, adolescence is the time when many people start drinking coffee. Parents should educate their children about the effects of caffeine and encourage them to monitor their caffeine consumption from all sources.

Accidental overdose from caffeine pills can be fatal. Caffeine tablets, like all drugs, should be kept out of reach of children. Children who accidentally eat caffeine pills need immediate medical attention from a physician.

Resources

BOOKS

Klosterman, Lorrie. *The Facts About Caffeine.* New York: Marshall Cavendish Benchmark, 2006.

Smith, Barry D., Uma Gupta, and B. S. Gupta, eds. *Caffeine and Activation Theory: Effects on Health and Behavior.* Boca Raton, FL: CRC Press, 2007.

Weinberg, Bennett Alan, and Bonnie K. Bealer. *The World of Caffeine: The Science and Culture of the World's Most Popular Drug.* New York: Routledge, 2001.

PERIODICALS

Freedman, Neal, et al. "Association of Coffee Drinking with Total and Cause-Specific Mortality." *New England Journal of Medicine* 336 (May 17, 2012): 1891–1904.

Loomans, Eva M., et al. "Caffeine Intake During Pregnancy and Risk of Problem Behavior in 5- to 6-Year-Old Children." *Pediatrics* (July 9, 2012): e-pub ahead of print. http://dx.doi.org/10.1542/peds.2011-3361 (accessed August 8, 2012).

Lucas, Michel, et al. "Coffee, Caffeine, and Risk of Depression Among Women." *Archives of Internal Medicine* 171, no. 17 (2012): 1571–78. http://dx.doi.org/10.1001/archinternmed.2011.393 (accessed August 8, 2012).

Persad, Leeana Aarthi Bagwath. "Energy Drinks and the Neurophysiological Impact of Caffeine." *Frontiers in Neuroscience* 5, no. 116 (October 21, 2011). http://dx.doi.org/10.3389/fnins.2011.00116 (accessed August 8, 2012).

Song, Fengju, Abrar A. Qureshi, and Jiali Han. "Increased Caffeine Intake Is Associated with Reduced Risk of Basal Cell Carcinoma of the Skin." *Cancer Research* 72, no. 13 (2012): 3282–89. http://dx.doi.org/10.1158/0008-5472.CAN-11-3511 (accessed August 8, 2012).

WEBSITES

BabyCenter. "Caffeine and the Nursing Mom." http://www.babycenter.com/0_caffeine-and-the-nursing-mom_4488.bc (accessed August 8, 2012).

International Food Information Council Foundation. "Fact Sheet: Caffeine and Performance." FoodInsight.org. http://www.foodinsight.org/Resources/Detail.aspx?topic=Fact_Sheet_Caffeine_and_Performance (accessed August 8, 2012).

March of Dimes Foundation. "Eating and Nutrition: Caffeine in Pregnancy." http://www.marchofdimes.com/pregnancy/nutrition_caffeine.html (accessed August 8, 2012).

Mayo Clinic staff. "Caffeine: How Much is Too Much?" MayoClinic.com. http://www.mayoclinic.com/health/caffeine/NU00600 (accessed August 8, 2012).

———. "Caffeine Content for Coffee, Tea, Soda, and More." MayoClinic.com http://www.mayoclinic.com/health/caffeine/AN01211 (accessed August 8, 2012).

MedlinePlus. "Caffeine in the Diet." U.S. National Library of Medicine, National Institutes of Health. http://www.nlm.nih.gov/medlineplus/ency/article/002445.htm (accessed August 8, 2012).

Nemours Foundation. "Caffeine and Your Child." KidsHealth.org. http://kidshealth.org/parent/growth/feeding/child_caffeine.html (accessed August 8, 2012).

U.S. Food and Drug Administration. "Serious Concerns Over Alcoholic Beverages with Added Caffeine." http://www.fda.gov/ForConsumers/ConsumerUpdates/ucm233987.htm (accessed August 8, 2012).

Zeratsky, Katherine. "Caffeine: Is it Dehydrating or Not?" Mayo Clinic. http://www.mayoclinic.com/health/caffeinated-drinks/AN01661 (accessed August 8, 2012).

ORGANIZATIONS

International Food Information Council Foundation, 1100 Connecticut Ave. NW, Ste. 430, Washington, DC 20036, (202) 296-6540, info@foodinsight.org, http://www.foodinsight.org.

U.S. Food and Drug Administration, 10903 New Hampshire Ave., Silver Spring, MD 20993-0002, (888) INFO-FDA (463-6332), http://www.fda.gov.

Tish Davidson, AM

Calcium

Definition

Calcium (chemical symbol: Ca) is the most abundant mineral in the body. About 99% of calcium in the body is in bones and teeth. The remaining 1% is in blood and soft tissue. Calcium in body fluids is an electrolyte with a charge of $2+$. Humans must meet their need for calcium through diet.

Calcium

Age	Recommended dietary allowance (mg)	Tolerable upper intake level (mg)
Children 0–6 mos.	200 (AI)	1,000
Children 7–12 mos.	260 (AI)	1,500
Children 1–3 yrs.	700	2,500
Children 4–8 yrs.	1,000	2,500
Children 9–13 yrs.	1,300	3,000
Adolescents 14–18 yrs.	1,300	3,000
Adults 19–50 yrs.	1,000	2,500
Adults, male, 51–70 yrs.	1,000	2,000
Adults, female, 51–70 yrs.	1,200	2,000
Adults 71+ yrs.	1,200	2,000
Pregnant women 18≥ yrs.	1,300	3,000
Pregnant women 19≤ yrs.	1,000	2,500
Breastfeeding women 18≥ yrs.	1,300	3,000
Breastfeeding women 19≤ yrs.	1,000	2,500

AI = Adequate intake
mg = milligram

SOURCE: Office of Dietary Supplements, "Dietary Supplement Fact Sheet: Calcium," U.S. National Institutes of Health.

(Table by PreMediaGlobal. © 2013 Cengage Learning.)

Purpose

Calcium is essential for:

- building and maintaining strong bones and teeth
- muscle contraction
- blood vessel contraction and relaxation
- nerve impulse transmission
- regulating fluid balance in the body

Description

Most calcium in the body is stored in bones and teeth. Here it combines with phosphate to form strong, stable crystals. The remaining 1% is dissolved in body fluids and much of it occurs in the form of positively charged calcium ions, Ca^{2+}. In the body, these electrically charged particles are called **electrolytes**. Calcium and other electrolytes are not distributed evenly throughout the body. Dissolved calcium is found mainly in the fluid outside cells (extracellular fluid). Metabolic events cause the movement of calcium across cell membranes resulting in muscle contraction, nerve impulse transmission, and various chemical reactions. The cell then uses energy to restore the balance of calcium between the inside and outside of the cell membrane, so that the event can be repeated.

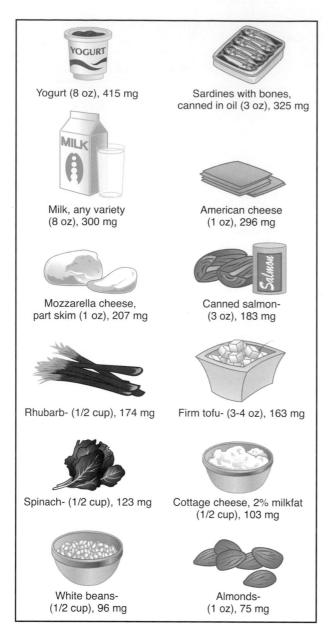

Yogurt (8 oz), 415 mg

Sardines with bones, canned in oil (3 oz), 325 mg

Milk, any variety (8 oz), 300 mg

American cheese (1 oz), 296 mg

Mozzarella cheese, part skim (1 oz), 207 mg

Canned salmon- (3 oz), 183 mg

Rhubarb- (1/2 cup), 174 mg

Firm tofu- (3-4 oz), 163 mg

Spinach- (1/2 cup), 123 mg

Cottage cheese, 2% milkfat (1/2 cup), 103 mg

White beans- (1/2 cup), 96 mg

Almonds- (1 oz), 75 mg

Sources of calcium. *(Illustration by Electronic Illustrators Group. © 2013 Cengage Learning.)*

To remain healthy, the amount of calcium dissolved in body fluids must stay within a very narrow range. Bone acts like a calcium bank. It is constantly being broken down by cells called osteoclasts and built up again by cells called osteoblasts. This process is called bone remodeling, and it continues throughout an individual's life. When excess calcium is present in the blood, osteoblasts deposit calcium into bones. When too little calcium is in the blood, osteoblasts dissolve calcium from bones and move it into the blood. This process is controlled by parathyroid hormones (PTH) secreted by the parathyroid glands. The parathyroid glands are extremely sensitive to the level of calcium in the blood, and in a healthy individual they are able to maintain the concentration of calcium ions within very close limits.

Normal calcium requirements

The United States Institute of Medicine (IOM) of the National Academy of Sciences has developed values called **dietary reference intakes (DRIs)** for many **vitamins** and **minerals**. The **DRIs** consist of three sets of numbers. The recommended dietary allowance (RDA) defines the average daily amount of a nutrient needed to meet the health needs of 97%–98% of the population. The adequate intake (AI) is an estimate set when there is not enough information to determine an RDA. The tolerable upper intake level (UL) is the average maximum amount that can be taken daily without risking negative side effects. The DRIs are calculated for children, adult men, adult women, pregnant women, and lactating women. The Food and Nutrition Board (FNB) of the IOM regularly reviews and, as necessary, revises the recommended RDAs, AIs, and ULs for all categories of men and women, boys and girls.

The current RDAs for calcium, as established by the FNB, are as follows:

- children 0–6 months: 200 mg (AI)
- children 7–12 months: 260 mg (AI)
- children 1–3 years: 700 mg
- children 4–8 years: 1,000 mg
- adolescents 9–18 years: 1,300 mg
- males 19–70 years: 1,000 mg
- females 19–50 years: 1,000 mg
- females 51 and older: 1,200 mg
- males 71 and older: 1,200 mg
- pregnant and lactating women 18 years and younger: 1,300 mg
- pregnant and lactating women over age 18: 1,000 mg

The U.S. RDAs tend to be higher than international recommended values. For example, the requirement for adults in the United Kingdom is 700 mg per day. Recommended dietary intakes in Australia are similar for adults but less for children (500 mg for children aged 1–3, 700 mg for children 4–8, and 1,000 mg for children 9–11).

Sources of calcium

In the United States, dairy products—milk, yogurt, and cheese—are the main sources of dietary calcium. Low-fat dairy products, such as skim milk or reduced-fat cheese, contain about the same amount of calcium as whole milk products. Other sources of calcium include canned fish with bones, dark green leafy vegetables, and tofu made with calcium sulfate. Other types of tofu do not contain significant amounts of calcium. Processed foods such as orange juice, breakfast cereal, instant breakfast drinks, and bread are often fortified with calcium. This fact will be indicated on the label.

The following list gives the approximate calcium content for some common foods:

- bok choy, 1/2 cup cooked: 61 mg
- bread, whole wheat, 1 slice: 20 mg
- breakfast cereal, fortified, 1 cup: 100–1,000 mg
- cheddar cheese, 1.5 ounces: 305 mg
- milk, any type, 1 cup (8 ounces): 300 mg
- mozzarella cheese, 1.5 ounces: 370 mg
- orange juice, fortified, 6 ounces: 200–260 mg
- pinto or red beans, cooked, 1/2 cup: 43 mg
- salmon with bones, canned, 3 ounces: 181 mg
- sardines with bones, canned in oil, 3 ounces: 324 mg
- spinach, cooked, 1/2 cup: 120 mg
- tofu, firm, made with calcium sulfate, 1/2 cup: 204 mg
- white beans, cooked, 1/2 cup: 113 mg
- yogurt, plain, 8 ounces: 415 mg
- yogurt, with fruit, 8 ounces: 245–380 mg

It is important to note that although a food may contain a significant amount of calcium, there is a difference between the total calcium content of a food and the amount that is available to the body (bioavailability). Other components present in foods may inhibit the body's access to those foods' calcium supplies. For example, oxalic acid, which is present in spinach, limits the absorption of calcium. So, although spinach is relatively high in calcium, not all of that calcium is absorbed by the body. Kale, on the other hand, contains less calcium than spinach but its calcium content is more easily absorbed in the body.

Although experts recommend that people meet as many of their vitamin and mineral needs as possible through diet, it is difficult for many people to get enough calcium from food alone. This is especially true for vegans, who eat no dairy products, adolescent girls who are very calorie conscious and tend to avoid milk and replace it with diet sodas, and people with lactose intolerance who cannot easily digest dairy products. Pregnant women and older individuals may also have a hard time eating enough to meet their calcium needs. People who do not get enough calcium through diet can benefit from taking a dietary supplement containing calcium.

Calcium supplements are available over-the-counter. The most common supplements supply calcium in the form of calcium carbonate or calcium citrate. Calcium carbonate is usually the most economical calcium supplement. People who are taking medications to reduce stomach acid may absorb calcium citrate more easily. Some supplements combine calcium and **vitamin D** because vitamin D helps the body absorb calcium. No calcium supplement contains enough calcium to meet the entire daily adequate intake, because the pill would be too large to swallow. In addition, the body absorbs calcium best in doses of 500 mg or less. People who need more than 500 mg of supplemental calcium should divide the dose in half to be taken in the morning and evening.

Calcium deficiency

Calcium deficiency, called hypocalcemia, can occur because of inadequate calcium intake, excess calcium excretion by the kidneys (usually caused by kidney damage), the inability to adequately absorb calcium, or interactions between calcium and some prescription drugs. People at highest risk of calcium deficiency are teenagers, women past the age of menopause, individuals who are lactose intolerant, vegans, and people with kidney (renal) damage.

Calcium deficiency rarely shows up in blood tests because calcium is withdrawn from the bones to maintain blood levels of calcium. The bones then become less dense, weaker, and more likely to break. This condition is called osteoporosis, and it is most noticeable in the elderly, who have a high rate of broken bones resulting from falls. Osteoporosis is a part of aging, but eating a healthy diet high in calcium, getting adequate vitamin D, and doing weight-bearing exercises regularly can delay its onset. Severe calcium deficiency is usually caused by a medical condition rather than inadequate calcium intake. It causes symptoms such as muscle cramps, tingling in the fingers, lethargy, convulsions, and heart rhythm abnormalities, and may even result in death. These symptoms can also be caused by many other diseases.

Calcium excess

Calcium excess is called hypercalcemia. It usually results from poor kidney function (renal failure) or from a malignant **cancer** tumor. It can also be caused by very large supplemental doses of vitamin D. Very rarely is hypercalcemia caused by too much calcium from food or **dietary supplements**. High levels of calcium interfere with the absorption of other minerals such as **iron, zinc, magnesium,** and phosphorous. People with hypercalcemia usually have multiple medical problems and are under the supervision of a physician.

Precautions

People of all ages, races, and genders need to be alert to getting enough calcium in their diet. Building strong, dense bones begins in childhood and adolescence, even though the results cannot be seen until old age. People who are at an especially high risk of low dietary calcium intake should investigate taking a calcium supplement.

Interactions

Absorption of calcium is affected by several conditions.

• Age. Infants absorb as much as 60% of the calcium in their digestive system. This decreases to 15–20% in adulthood, and even less in old age.

• Pregnancy. Pregnancy increases the efficiency of calcium absorption in the intestines to meet the demands of fetal development.

• Amount of calcium consumed. The more calcium consumed at one time, the less efficient absorption becomes. Calcium from supplements should be spaced out during the day for maximum absorption.

• Vitamin D. The presence of vitamin D improves calcium absorption. Vitamin D deficiency can worsen calcium deficiency.

• Plant products. Phytic acid, found in beans, and oxalic acid, found in spinach and leafy greens, decrease the amount of calcium absorbed from those foods but do not affect the absorption of calcium from other foods present at the same time in the intestines. Fiber also reduces calcium absorption.

Prescription medications can also affect or be affected by the absorption of calcium. These include:

• digoxin

• fluoroquinolones

• levothyroxine

• tetracycline antibiotics

• anticonvulsants

• thiazide-type diuretics

• glucocorticoids

• mineral oil

• stimulant laxatives

• antacids

People taking these drugs should check with their healthcare provider or pharmacist about potential adjustments in their medications or calcium intake.

QUESTIONS TO ASK YOUR DOCTOR

• Are my children receiving adequate amounts of calcium in their regular diets, or should they be taking supplements?

• Are there specific kinds of calcium supplements that you recommend?

• If our family is receiving inadequate amounts of calcium in our diets, what symptoms should we expect to see developing?

Complications

Some studies have found an increased risk of heart attack in people taking calcium supplements. An 11-year study published in the June 2012 issue of the journal *Heart* saw an 86% increase in heart attack risk among a group of almost 24,000 German adults. Previous studies done on post-menopausal women taking calcium supplements, with or without vitamin D supplementation, have found similar results. Calcium and vitamin D supplements are often recommended to older women to reduce the risk of osteoporosis and bone fractures, which increases with age and after menopause. The U.S. Preventive Services Task Force, an independent group that works in cooperation with the Agency for Healthcare Research and Quality, recommended in mid-2012 that older adults not take such supplements, due to a lack of supporting evidence. Although further research is needed, it is always advisable to obtain the majority of nutrients from foods and not supplements.

Calcium supplements may cause gas, nausea, and abdominal discomfort. Taking the supplement with meals, taking smaller doses spread out over the day, or changing the type of supplement usually solves this problem.

Parental concerns

Building strong bones starts in childhood, and parents should be aware of how much calcium their child needs compared to how much he or she is getting. As children get older they tend to replace milk in their diet with juice, bottled water, and especially carbonated soft drinks. This practice leads to large calcium deficiencies during adolescence. Parents should monitor their child's diet and encourage them to take calcium supplements if they cannot induce their adolescents to eat more dairy products and other calcium-rich food.

Resources

BOOKS

Fragakis, Allison. *The Health Professional's Guide to Popular Dietary Supplements.* Chicago: American Dietetic Association, 2003.

Gaby, Alan R., ed. *A–Z Guide to Drug-Herb-Vitamin Interactions Revised and Expanded 2nd Edition: Improve Your Health and Avoid Side Effects When Using Common Medications and Natural Supplements Together.* New York: Three Rivers Press, 2006.

Lieberman, Shari and Nancy Bruning. *The Real Vitamin and Mineral Book: The Definitive Guide to Designing Your Personal Supplement Program.* 4th ed. New York: Avery, 2007.

Pressman, Alan H. and Sheila Buff. *The Complete Idiot's Guide to Vitamins and Minerals.* 3rd ed. Indianapolis, IN: Alpha Books, 2007.

Rockwell, Sally. *Calcium Rich & Dairy Free: How to Get Calcium Without the Cow.* Pomeroy, WA: Health Research Books, 2005.

Weaver, Connie M., and Robert Proulx Heaney. *Calcium in Human Health.* Totowa, NJ: Humana Press, 2010. Reprint of 2006 edition.

PERIODICALS

Bolland, Mark J., et al. "Calcium Supplements with or without Vitamin D and Risk of Cardiovascular Events: Reanalysis of the Women's Health Initiative Limited Access Dataset and Meta-Analysis." *British Medical Journal* 342 (April 19, 2011): d2040. http://dx.doi.org/10.1136/bmj.d2040 (accessed June 21, 2012).

Kuanrong, Li., et al. "Associations of Dietary Calcium Intake and Calcium Supplementation with Myocardial Infarction and Stroke Risk and Overall Cardiovascular Mortality in the Heidelberg Cohort of the European Prospective Investigation into Cancer and Nutrition Study (EPIC-Heidelberg)." *Heart* 98, no. 12 (2012): 920–25. http://dx.doi.org/10.1136/heartjnl-2011-301345 (accessed June 21, 2012).

Reid, Ian R., and Mark J. Bolland. "Calcium Supplements: Bad for the Heart?" *Heart* 98, no. 12 (2012): 895–96. http://dx.doi.org/10.1136/heartjnl-2012-301904 (accessed June 21, 2012).

WEBSITES

"Calcium in Diet." *New York Times*, Health Guide. http://health.nytimes.com/health/guides/nutrition/calcium-in-diet/overview.html (accessed June 21, 2012).

Centers for Disease Control and Prevention. "Calcium and Bone Health." http://www.cdc.gov/nutrition/everyone/basics/vitamins/calcium.html (accessed June 21, 2012).

Harvard School of Public Health. "Calcium and Milk: What's Best for Your Bones and Health?" *The Nutrition Source*, Department of Nutrition, Harvard University. http://www.hsph.harvard.edu/nutritionsource/what-should-you-eat/calcium-full-story/index.html (accessed June 21, 2012).

MedlinePlus. "Calcium." U.S. National Library of Medicine. http://www.nlm.nih.gov/medlineplus/calcium.html (accessed June 21, 2012).

Moisse, Katie. "Calcium Supplements Linked to Increased Heart Attack Risk in Post-Menopausal Women: Study." ABC News, April 20, 2011. abcnews.go.com/Health/HeartHealth/calcium-supplements-linked-increased-heart-attack-risk-post/story?id=13411283 (accessed June 21, 2012).

Office of Dietary Supplements. "Dietary Supplement Fact Sheet: Calcium." U.S. National Institutes of Health. http://ods.od.nih.gov/factsheets/Calcium-QuickFacts (accessed June 21, 2012).

ORGANIZATIONS

Academy of Nutrition and Dietetics, 120 South Riverside Plz., Ste. 2000, Chicago, IL 60606-6995, (312) 899-0040, (800) 877-1600, amacmunn@eatright.org, http://www.eatright.org.

International Food Information Council Foundation, 1100 Connecticut Ave. NW, Ste. 430, Washington, DC 20036, (202) 296-6540, info@foodinsight.org, http://www.foodinsight.org.

NIH Osteoporosis and Related Bone Diseases National Resource Center, 2 AMS Circle, Bethesda, MD 20892-3676, (202) 223-0344, TTY: (202) 466-4315, (800) 624-BONE (2663), Fax: (202) 293-2356, NIHBoneInfo@mail.nih.gov, http://www.bones.nih.gov.

Office of Dietary Supplements, National Institutes of Health, 6100 Executive Blvd., Rm. 3B01, MSC 7517, Bethesda, MD 20892-7517, (301) 435-2920, Fax: (301) 480-1845, ods@nih.gov, http://ods.od.nih.gov.

Tish Davidson, AM
David Newton

Calorie restriction

Definition

Calorie restriction is a reduction in energy intake (food consumption). This may be involuntary, due to reasons such as an inadequate food supply, or voluntary, such as in individuals seeking to lose weight or people with the eating disorder **anorexia nervosa**. Extreme calorie restriction can result in **malnutrition** or a deficiency of one or more nutrients.

Purpose

The human body requires an adequate amount of energy or **calories** to enable us to grow, perform daily activities, produce hormones, and to minimize the risk of nutrition-related complications. Calorie requirements for individuals vary from one individual to the next and

- decreased libido
- decreased enjoyment in previously enjoyed activities

Parental concerns

Children who have an insufficient energy intake over prolonged periods of time may not reach expected growth rates. Furthermore, they may lose weight and ultimately experience stunted growth and develop nutrition-related complications. Parents should ensure that a physician monitors growth rates regularly.

Resources

BOOKS

Garrow, J.S., W.P.T. James, and A. Ralph. *Human Nutrition and Dietetics.* 10th ed. Churchill Livingstone, 2000.

Keys, A., J. Brozek, et al. *The Biology of Human Starvation.* Oxford: University of Minnesota Press, 1950.

Thomas, Briony, and Jacki Bishop. *Manual of Dietetic Practice.* 4th ed. Blackwell Science Ltd., 2007.

PERIODICALS

Ingram, D.K., et al. "Calorie Restriction Mimetics: An Emerging Research Field." *Aging Cell* 5, no. 2 (April 2006): 97–108.

Kemnitz, J.W. "Calorie Restriction and Aging in Nonhuman Primates." *Institute of Laboratory Animal Resources Journal* 52, no. 1 (2011): 66–77.

Mattison, Julie A. "Impact of Caloric Restriction on Health and Survival in Rhesus Monkeys from the NIA Study." *Nature* (August 2012): e-pub ahead of print. http://dx.doi.org/10.1038/nature11432 (accessed September 7, 2012).

Redman, Leanne, Corby Martin, Donald Williamson, and Eric Ravussin. "Effect of Caloric Restriction in Non-Obese Humans on Physiological, Psychological, and Behavioral Outcomes." *Physiology & Behavior* 94, no. 5 (August 2008): 643–48.

Rochon, James, et al. "Design and Conduct of the CAL-ERIE Study: Comprehensive Assessment of the Long-term Effects of Reducing Intake of Energy." *Journals of Gerontology: Biological Sciences* 66A, no. 1 (2011): 97–108. http://dx.doi.org/10.1093/gerona/glq168 (accessed August 28, 2012).

Speakerman, J.R., and S.E. Mitchell. "Caloric Restriction." *Molecular Aspects of Medicine* 32, no. 3 (June 2011): 159–221.

Williamson, D.A., et al. "Is Caloric Restriction Associated with Development of Eating-Disorder Symptoms? Results from the CALERIE Trial." *Health Psychology* 27, suppl. 1 (January 2008): S32–42.

WEBSITES

"Comprehensive Assessment of Long-Term Effects of Reducing Intake of Energy (CALERIE) Home Page." Duke University. http://calerie.dcri.duke.edu/index.html (accessed September 7, 2012).

Gertner, Jon. "The Calorie-Restriction Experiment." *New York Times Magazine*, October 7, 2009.

Lund, Jim. "Dismissing the Nonsense Calorie Restriction/Eating Disorder Link." March 14, 2008. *Fight Aging.* http://www.fightaging.org/archives/2008/03/dismissing-the-nonsense-calorie-restriction-eating-disorder-link.php (accessed September 7, 2012).

National Institute on Aging. "Topics of Interest: Calorie Restriction." U.S. National Institutes of Health. http://www.nia.nih.gov/newsroom/topics/calorie-restriction (accessed September 7, 2012).

ORGANIZATIONS

CR Society International, 187 Ocean Dr., Newport, NC 28570, (252) 241-3079, (877) 511-2702, http://www.calorierestriction.org.

Annette Laura Dunne, BSc (Hons) MSc RD
Stacey Chamberlin

Calories

Definition

The term calorie refers to a unit of energy. It can be further divided into two terms: small calorie and large calorie. A small calorie (or the gram calorie [cal]) is defined as a unit of energy that is equivalent to the amount of heat needed to increase the temperature of one gram (g) of water (H_2O) by one degree of Celsius (C).

As a unit of food energy, the large calorie (or the kilogram calorie [kilocalorie or Cal]) is the amount of energy needed to increase the temperature of one kilogram (kg) of water by one degree of Celsius. French chemist and physicist Nicolas Clément (1779–1842) became the first known person to define and utilize the calorie as a unit of heat in 1824. The definition for kilocalorie as a unit of energy has since been replaced with the unit of joule (J) by the International System of Units

KEY TERMS

Celsius—A scale and unit of measurement for temperature, where the freezing point of water is 0°C and the boiling point of water is 100°C.

Energy—The ability of a physical system to do work on other physical systems.

Gram—A metric unit of mass.

Joule—The International System of Units (SI) unit of energy.

Kilogram—The International System of Units (SI) unit of mass, where one such unit is equal to one thousand grams.

(SI), but it is still used as a measure of food energy. When people in the United States refer to "calories" in a diet or with food, they are really talking about kilocalories.

Purpose

Calories are needed to sustain life. Food provides energy in the form of calories—when a person eats food, the calories are either converted to physical energy and burned off by the body or are stored in the body as fat. All people have a base rate at which their bodies burn calories, called the basal metabolic rate. This is the number of calories burned by the body while at rest. Exercise or other movement burns more calories and increases the total number of calories burned in a day. Excess calories that are not expended by the body as energy are instead stored as fat within the body. A person's caloric intake may vary from day to day, but eating more food than the body can turn into energy for an extended period of time can result in weight gain.

Description

Everyone consumes calories, but people eat different foods every day. Some foods, because of the various essential nutrients they contain, possess more calories than others (by mass). **Macronutrients** such as **carbohydrates**, **fats**, **fiber**, and proteins all contain calories and release energy to the body, but they do so in varying amounts. Fats release a large amount of energy, about 9 kilocalories per gram (38 kJ/g). Carbohydrates and proteins release a bit less, at about 4 kilocalories per gram (17 kJ/g). In addition, alcohol is a source of calories, with about 7 kilocalories per gram (30 kJ/g). Two foods may have the same mass, but if one food is high in fat and the other is high in **protein**, the high-fat food will have more calories.

Calories and weight maintenance

Calories are burned (expended) during exercise or physical activity. Even moving a finger to change channels on the television burns a tiny bit of calories within the body. The amount of calories expended depends on the length and type of exercise, though it varies from person to person. For instance, according to the National Heart, Lung, and Blood Institute, for a 175-pound (79 kg) man and a 140-pound (63.5 kg) women performing light activity (such as daily housework, playing a round of golf, or working in an office), the number of calories expended in one hour is about 300 calories and 240 calories, respectively. For moderate activities such as bicycling, dancing, and walking briskly, men burn about 460 calories per hour, while women expend around 370 calories. Strenuous activities, such as playing football, swimming, or jogging, burn even more calories.

Regardless of where dietary calories come from, they are either converted to physical energy (as when people perform physical exercises) or are stored in the body as fat. If exercises and physical activities do not convert all of the calories consumed in one day, then the remaining calories (not consumed) are stored as fat in the body. These stored calories remain until they are used up another day with either additional physical activity or a caloric deficit. If more calories are consumed than are expended, a person gains weight. On the other hand, if fewer calories are consumed, a person loses weight. If the same number of calories are consumed as are expended in any particular day, the person remains at the same weight. For example, if 3,500 calories are burned in one day from playing basketball, walking, doing yard work, and all the other daily activities, and 3,000 are consumed as food in the form of calories, then 500 calories have been taken from fat and burned by the body for energy to the muscles and other life processes. If this happens for one week (seven days), then 3,500 calories of fat have been eliminated from the body and the person has lost about one pound. Conversely, if 3,500 calories are eaten and only 3,000 are burned, that person will gain one pound. When it comes to weight loss and maintenance, it all comes down to calories consumed (intake) versus calories expended (output).

To maintain a healthy lifestyle, the U.S. Department of Health and Human Services (HHS) recommends a minimum of 2.5 hours per week of moderate aerobic activity (such as walking or swimming) or 1.25 hour per week of vigorous aerobic activity (such as running). In addition, the HHS recommends that strength-training exercises (anaerobic exercises such as lifting weights) should be performed at least twice per week. This amount of physical exercise will make it more likely that a person maintains a healthy weight and fit lifestyle.

QUESTIONS TO ASK YOUR DOCTOR

- Why can't I lose weight?
- How can I find out how many calories I should eat each day?

Calorie tracking

People trying to alter their weight can track their calories by "counting them," or measuring the number of calories in foods against a daily calorie balance. Many free online calorie counters are available on the Web. The U.S. Department of Agriculture's (USDA) SuperTracker, released in December 2011, is a free calorie-tracking tool that also accounts for physical activity (calorie expenditure). The Super-Tracker MyPlan program will also assign users daily calorie balances based on weight loss goals and help them make meal plans to meet these goals.

Complications

Eating too many calories on a daily basis increases the risk of becoming overweight or excessively overweight (obese). However, not eating enough calories puts a person at risk of nutrient deficiencies, which can lead to undernutrition and **malnutrition**. Consuming too much of a specific nutrient, by way of foods or supplements, can also cause problems.

Undernutrition and malnutrition are more common than overnutrition in developing countries. The opposite is true in developed countries, such as the United States and Australia, two countries with highest percentages of obese citizens. Medical conditions may also cause caloric complications, whether as the result of eating too much or too little.

Older people are more apt to eat less calories and nutrients than younger people. Some older people in the United States live on less than 1,000 calories each day. Such a small caloric intake of food is not adequate to maintain healthy nutrient levels.

Parental concerns

Infants, children, and adolescents are often at increased risk from undernutrition because of their need for extra calories and nutrients as they grow rapidly into adulthood.

Resources

BOOKS

Dubé, Laurette, et al., eds. *Obesity Prevention: The Role of Brain and Society on Individual Behavior*. Amsterdam: Elsevier, 2010.

Karasu, Sylvia R., and T. Byram Karasu. *The Gravity of Weight: A Clinical Guide to Weight Loss and Maintenance*. Washington, DC: American Psychiatric, 2010.

The Mayo Clinic Diet: Eat Well, Enjoy Life, Lose Weight. Intercourse, PA: Good Books, 2010.

Roth, Ruth A. *Nutrition & Diet Therapy*. Clifton Park, NY: Delmar Cengage Learning, 2011.

Rust, Rosanne. *The Calorie Counter for Dummies*. Hoboken, NJ: Wiley, 2010.

Smith, Ian K. *Eat: The Effortless Weight Loss Solution*. New York: St. Martin's Press, 2011.

WEBSITES

"Calories Burned During Fitness Activities." MedicineNet.com. http://www.medicinenet.com/script/main/art.asp?articlekey=10289 (accessed June 7, 2011).

Mayo Clinic staff. "Counting Calories: Get Back to Weight-Loss Basics." MayoClinic.com. http://www.mayoclinic.com/health/calories/WT00011 (accessed June 7, 2012).

Merck. "Undernutrition." Merck Manual Home Health Handbook. http://www.merckmanuals.com/home/sec12/ch153/ch153a.html (accessed June 7, 2012).

U.S. Department of Agriculture. "ChooseMyPlate.gov." http://www.choosemyplate.gov (accessed June 8, 2011).

———. "SuperTracker." https://www.choosemyplate.gov/SuperTracker (accessed June 5, 2012).

U.S. Department of Agriculture and U.S. Department of Health and Human Services. *Dietary Guidelines for Americans, 2010*. 7th ed. Washington, DC: U.S. Government Printing Office, December 2010. http://health.gov/dietaryguidelines (accessed September 27, 2012).

ORGANIZATIONS

Academy of Nutrition and Dietetics, 120 South Riverside Plz., Ste. 2000, Chicago, IL 60606-6995, (312) 899-0040, (800) 877-1600, amacmunn@eatright.org, http://www.eatright.org.

U.S. Department of Agriculture, 1400 Independence Ave. SW, Washington, DC 20250, (202) 720-2791, http://www.usda.gov.

Weight-Control Information Network (WIN), 1 WIN Way, Bethesda, MD 20892-3665, (202) 828-1025, (877) 946-4627, Fax: (202) 828-1028, win@http://win.niddk.nih.gov, http://win.niddk.nih.gov.

William A. Atkins, BB, BS, MBA

Cambridge diet

Definition

The Cambridge diet is a commercial very low-calorie diet (VLCD). The diet was first used only in weight-loss clinics in the United Kingdom. In the early 1980s, the products associated with the diet (powder mix, meal bars, and liquid meals) started selling commercially in the United States and the United Kingdom. Formulations of the Cambridge diet in the United Kingdom differ from those that sold in the United States. In both the United Kingdom and North America, the Cambridge products are available only from distributors; they cannot be purchased over the counter at pharmacies or supermarkets.

Origins

United Kingdom and Western Europe

A scientist at Cambridge University in England, Alan Howard, initiated the research that eventually lead to the development of the Cambridge diet in the 1960s. Howard became interested in **obesity** as an increasingly common nutritional problem. He worked together with Ian McLean-Baird, a physician at the West Middlesex Hospital, to create a formula diet food that would allow people to lose weight rapidly without losing lean muscle tissue, create a mild ketosis (a condition in which the body begins to use fat rather than **carbohydrates** as a source of energy), and contain enough **vitamins**, **minerals**, and micronutrients to maintain health. Howard and McLean-Baird also organized the first national symposium on obesity in the United Kingdom, which was held in 1968.

The formula that satisfied the researchers' goals was successful in helping people in hospital obesity clinics lose weight, but was not particularly appetizing. The researchers collaborated with food technologists to improve the flavor of the formula. After further testing with clinic patients, the Cambridge diet was marketed commercially in the United Kingdom in 1984, four years after it was available in the United States. In 1985, the Cambridge diet became available in Germany, France, and the Scandinavian countries, and in 1990 in Poland and Eastern Europe. The British company, Cambridge Manufacturing Company Limited (CMC), which manufactures the diet products associated with the Cambridge Health and Weight Plan, was owned by the Howard Foundation between 1982 and 2005. The Howard Foundation is a charitable trust established by Alan Howard to offer scholarships to international students and to fund research in obesity and nutrition. In 2005 the Cambridge Manufacturing Company was sold to its three senior managers and became Cambridge Nutritional Foods Limited.

The present Cambridge diet products available in the United Kingdom are sachets (packets) of powder, Mix-a-Mousse granules, liquid meals, and meal bars.

Cambridge diet

British version—4 stages

Preparation
Reduce food intake gradually over a week or 10 days before beginning the diet

Losing weight (Sole Source program)
Women shorter than 5' 8": three servings of Cambridge diet products daily and no other food
Women taller than 5' 8" and men: four servings of Cambridge diet products daily and no other food
Coffee, tea, and tap and bottled water allowed
Drink at least 2 quarts of fluid per day
415 to 554 calories per day

Stabilization
After 4 weeks on the Sole Source program, add a meal of 3 oz. of lean white fish or poultry, cottage cheese, and a portion of green or white vegetables to the basic Cambridge meals
Total of 790 calories per day
Return, if necessary, to the Sole Source regimen for further rapid weight loss
Other options allow 1,000 or 1,200 calories per day for more gradual weight loss or to accommodate lifestyles

Weight maintenance
Begins at an intake of 1,500 calories per day

American version—5 programs

Regular
Designed for a weight loss of 2–5 pounds per week
820 calories per day: 3 servings of Cambridge Food for Life formula plus one 400-calorie conventional meal
A minimum of 8–10 glasses (8oz.) of water daily
Tea and coffee allowed, but not as substitutes for the water
Continue on the program until weight loss goal achieved

Fast start
For rapid and safe weight loss
Regimen is similar to the British Sole Source program
Do not remain on the program longer than 2 weeks at a time
Return to the Regular Program and contact a physician if experiencing headaches, nausea, or vomiting

Physician-monitored
Recommended for weight loss of 30 pounds or more, or for persons under doctor's care for other medical conditions
Essentially the British Sole Source program, with the added provision that the dieter switch to the Regular Program when 10 to 15 pounds from weight goal

Maintenance
Essentially the use of the Cambridge's Food for Life nutrition formula as a foundation, adding conventional foods while determining caloric level to maintain body weight

Lifetime nutrition
Use Cambridge diet products as meal substitutes for one or two meals a day, or as healthy snacks

(Table by GGS Information Services. © 2013 Cengage Learning.)

The sachets are intended to be mixed with a half-pint of water (hot or cold) to produce a shake or soup. The sachets, which provide about 138 **calories**, are sold in boxes of 21 servings, which is a week's supply. There are 12 different flavors, including banana, mixed fruit, and chicken mushroom. The dieter may also purchase Mix-a-Mousse granules that add 20 calories to the powdered formula, but give it a thicker texture. The liquid formula is available in a ready-to-drink version packaged as Tetra Briks—sealed cartons with straws. Tetra Briks come in banana or chocolate flavor. There are four flavors of chocolate-covered meal bars (caramel, chocolate, orange, and toffee), one of which can be consumed each day.

Each sachet or liquid formula contains enough nutrients to be used as a complete meal. The meal bars can replace a meal as well, but have extra carbohydrates and should only be eaten once a day. The Cambridge diet products can be consumed exclusively as meal replacements or used in conjunction with regular food (e.g., sachet for breakfast, Tetra Brik for lunch, and normal dinner).

United States

Rights to the original Cambridge diet formula—a powder to be mixed in a blender with water or diet soft drinks—in the United States were obtained by Cambridge Direct Sales in 1979. After working to improve the formula's flavor, the diet was placed on the market in 1980. It was initially quite popular. The original version of the Cambridge diet is sometimes known as the "Original 330 Formula" in the company's promotional literature because Dr. Howard's first rapid weight-loss program called for a total daily consumption of only 330 calories, provided by three servings of the original powder formula (110 calories per serving). The nutrient ratio of the original formula is 10–11 g of **protein** per serving, 15 g of carbohydrates (derived primarily from fructose or fruit **sugar**), and 1 g of fat.

In 1984 Cambridge Direct Sales hired Dr. Robert Nesheim to develop Cambridge Food for Life products. Like the Original 330 Formula, Food for Life is a powder that comes in a can to be reconstituted with conventional foods. Food for Life is available in a super oats cereal version and includes flavor choices such as tomato, potato, mushroom, chicken soup, vanilla, chocolate, strawberry, and eggnog. Nesheim was specifically asked to meet guidelines for nutrition supplements established by the U.S. Food and Drug Administration (FDA). The company states that Nesheim "increased the protein and carbohydrate content for an extra margin of safety when used as the sole source of nutrition." Food for Life contains 140 calories per serving, 13–15 g of protein, 18 g of carbohydrates, and 1 g of fat.

The American company introduced a Cambridge nutrition bar in 1983, but was unsuccessful as the product had a short shelf life and lacked flavor appeal. Dr. Nesheim tripled the shelf life of the nutrition bars and improved their taste. Each bar contains 170 calories, with 10 g of protein, 19–22 g of carbohydrates, and a low fat content.

Description

British version

The British version of the Cambridge diet cannot be used without the supervision of an official counselor, who "provide[s] a personal screening, advisory, monitoring and support service." The counselors are trained and accredited by the company, and must follow a code of conduct in their dealings with customers. According to the company, most counselors are people who have successfully used the Cambridge diet themselves.

The British version of the Cambridge diet is for adults over the age of 16 and has four stages:

- Preparation: The dieter is asked to reduce food intake gradually over a week to 10 days before beginning the diet.
- Losing weight: This initial step is called the "Sole Source" program and gives the dieter between 415 and 554 calories per day. Dieters are advised not to remain on the Sole Source program for longer than four weeks at a time. They are required to obtain a signed certificate from their doctor before they can begin the Sole Source program. Female dieters shorter than 5 ft. 8 in. take three servings of Cambridge diet products per day and eliminate other food; women taller than 5 ft. 8 in. and men are allowed four servings. Allowable beverages include coffee, tea, and tap or bottled water; forbidden beverages include alcoholic drinks, coffee or tea with milk added, fruit juices, and any drink containing sugar. The dieter is advised to drink at least two quarts of fluid per day.
- Stabilization: After four weeks on the Sole Source program, the dieter can add a meal of three ounces of lean white fish or poultry, cottage cheese, and a portion of green or white vegetables to the basic Cambridge meals for a total of 790 calories per day. The dieter can then return to the Sole Source regimen for further rapid weight loss. There are other options allowing the dieter 1,000-1,200 calories per day that are better suited for gradual weight loss.
- Weight maintenance: Begins at an intake of 1,500 calories per day.

American version

The American version of the Cambridge diet is divided into five separate programs:

- Regular: Designed for a weight loss of 2–5 lb. per week, the Regular Program provides 820 calories per day: three servings of Cambridge Food for Life formula, plus one 400 calorie conventional meal. The dieter is advised to drink a minimum of 8–10 eight-ounce glasses of water each day. Tea and coffee are allowed, but not as substitutes for the water. There is no stipulation that the Regular program is limited to four weeks.

- Fast Start: Similar to the British Sole Source program, the Fast Start program is to be followed no longer than two weeks at a time. The dieter is advised to return to the Regular Program and contact a physician if they experience headaches, nausea, or vomiting.

- Physician-Monitored: Recommended for people who need to lose 30 lb. or more, or who are under a doctor's care for other medical conditions. It is essentially the British Sole Source program with the added provision that the dieter should switch to the Regular Program when he or she is 10–15 lb. from their goal weight.

- Maintenance: Uses the Food for Life nutrition formula as a foundation, while adding conventional foods until a caloric intake is determined to maintain an ideal weight.

- Lifetime Nutrition: The Food for Life company recommends using the Cambridge diet products as meal substitutes for one or two meals a day, or as snacks indefinitely. This maintenance program is not endorsed by any government agency.

Function

The Cambridge diet claims to be a flexible plan that can be used as a VLCD for rapid initial weight loss and then modified to serve as a maintenance diet.

Benefits

The Cambridge diet offers a rapid initial weight loss that compensates (for some dieters) the low calorie intake and other food restrictions. The American version also offers a peer support network and a self-instruction program based on cognitive behavioral therapy (CBT) called Control for Life.

Precautions

People under a physician's care for high blood pressure, kidney or liver disease, or diabetes, or who need to lose more than 30 lb. should consult their physician before starting the Cambridge diet or any

---

KEY TERMS

Body mass index (BMI)—The ratio between a person's weight and the square of their height. A BMI over 25 is considered overweight; below 18.5 is considered underweight.

Cholelithiasis—The medical term for gallstones. People on a VLCD have an increased risk of developing gallstones from an increase of cholesterol content in the bile produced by the liver.

Cognitive behavioral therapy (CBT)—An approach to psychotherapy based on modifying the patient's day-to-day thoughts and behaviors, with the aim of changing long-standing emotional patterns. Some people consider CBT a useful or even necessary tool in maintaining long-term weight reduction.

Ketosis—An abnormal increase in the number of ketone bodies in the body, produced when the liver breaks down fat into fatty acids and ketone bodies. Ketosis is a common side effect of low-carbohydrate diets or VLCDs. If continued for a long period of time, ketosis can cause serious damage to the kidneys and liver.

Very low-calorie diet (VLCD)—A term used by registered dietitians to classify weight reduction diets that allow around 800 calories or fewer a day.

VLCD. The Cambridge diet should not be used by adolescents under the age of 16, and should only be used with caution by elderly people, pregnant women, or nursing women.

Risks

VLCDs in general should not be attempted without consulting a physician, and the Cambridge diet is no exception. The diet is not suitable for people whose work or athletic training requires high levels of physical activity. One physical risk from this diet, as from other VLCDs, is an increased likelihood of developing cholelithiasis, or **gallstones**.

There is also some financial risk to using the Cambridge diet. Although the American website states that the Physician-Monitored version is less expensive than VLCD hospital programs, all forms of the Cambridge diet cost $95–100 for a 15-day supply of the Original 330 Formula or $85–89 for a 15-day supply of the Food for Life formula. A case of six cans of the Original 330 Formula, supplying a total of 126 servings, is about $160. Although the cost per meal is

One-third of all cancer deaths are due to a poor adult diet. High-fat diets have been associated with development of cancers of the colon and rectum, prostate, endometrium, and breast cancer in women. Consumption of meat, particularly red meat, has been associated with increased risk for cancer of the colon and prostate. Additionally, a high-calorie diet and low levels of physical activity can lead to **obesity**, which increases risk for cancer at various sites including the breast, colon and rectum, prostate, kidney, and endometrium.

Causes and symptoms

There are numerous risk factors and causes of cancer. Among them are advancing age, gender, and family medical history. Some risk factors depend on the type of cancer. In some cases, a person may have more than one risk factor for the disease. Another person may be diagnosed with cancer and have no apparent risk factor. Genetic causes cannot be controlled by an individual, but people who know they are at risk because a close relative had a particular cancer should follow all recommendations for screening and prevention.

Cancer is a progressive disease that evolves through several stages. Each stage can produce a number of symptoms. Unfortunately, many types of cancer do not display any obvious symptoms or cause pain until the disease has progressed to an advanced stage. Early signs of cancer may be subtle and may be easily mistaken for signs of other less-dangerous diseases and conditions. In addition, some of the more commonly diagnosed cancers may not have any early signs or symptoms associated with their development.

Despite the fact that there are many different types of cancers with very different symptoms, the ACS has established the following symptoms as possible warning signs of cancer:

- feeling weak or very tired
- a lump or thickening in the breast or any other part of the body
- a new mole or changes in an existing mole
- changes to bowel or bladder habits
- hoarseness or a cough that will not go away
- a sore that does not heal
- difficulty swallowing or persistent indigestion
- unexplained weight loss or weight gain
- unusual discharge or bleeding

Diagnosis

Generally, the earlier cancer is found, the better in terms of outcome. Screening and early detection methods are available for many types of cancer. For example, a screening mammography helps detect breast cancer before symptoms occur. A Pap test screens for cervical cancer. Several tests, such as a colonoscopy, are recommended for people of certain ages or with certain risk factors to screen for colon and rectal cancer. It is important to follow the guidelines of organizations such as the ACS concerning recommended screening for cancers.

Physicians use a combination of family and medical history, screening examination results, laboratory examinations, imaging examinations, and other procedures to diagnose cancer. Family and medical history are important to look for hereditary links to many cancers. Medical history helps to determine if a person may have behaviors, such as smoking, that increase the risk for many cancers.

Laboratory examinations may test a person's blood, urine, or other fluids. These tests often are conducted to search for levels of substances called tumor markers. Laboratory tests alone cannot diagnose cancer, but can help lead a physician toward or away from a suspected diagnosis.

X rays may be the first type of imaging performed. Mammography is a form of x ray; it is the screening and diagnostic examination used to detect breast cancer. Chest x rays may be used to detect lung cancer. Other types of x rays may be used in cancer diagnosis.

Computed tomography (CT) scanning is another form of imaging. Because the use of the computer can generate finer, cross-sectional detail in combination with x rays, CT scans are often used to image a particular area. A CT colonography can screen for polyps and other lesions in the large intestine, much like a colonoscopy. But CT is noninvasive, meaning it does not penetrate the skin or enter the body. CT may involve the use of a contrast medium that is injected to help make certain fluids or tissues more visible on the image for the radiologist.

Nuclear medicine or radionuclide scans involve injection of a small amount of a radiopharmaceutical into a vein. The agent flows through the bloodstream and collects in certain areas or organs. When a special camera is used to take images, the agent shows "hot spots," which the radiologist will use to interpret the results. Often, nuclear medicine scans will be used to check for the spread of cancer to bone, but they also have other uses. Most of the radiopharmaceutical is eliminated from the body in urine or stool and the rest disappears through natural loss of radioactivity over time. Negative reactions to the agent are rare.

Ultrasound is an imaging examination that does not use radiation. Instead, high-frequency sound waves are used to produce images. Ultrasounds are often used to follow up on suspicious mammogram findings. Ultrasound images show fluids and soft tissues very well and often help radiologists determine if a mass is most likely a benign cyst or a malignant (cancerous) solid mass. Other common areas that ultrasound is used to image when diagnosing cancer are the thyroid, the abdomen, the pelvic area (ovaries, uterus), and the prostate.

Magnetic resonance imaging (MRI) also does not require the use of radiation. Instead, a strong magnetic field and radio waves provide clear and detailed pictures through a computer display. MRI has proven to be the most sensitive examination for brain tumors. MRI has also become increasingly useful in breast cancer imaging in recent years, as well as for many other suspected cancers.

Positron emission tomography, or PET scanning, is a nuclear medicine procedure that acquires images based on detection of radiation, as in a radionuclide scan, but through emission of positrons. Positrons are tiny particles emitted from a radioactive substance administered to the patient. Cancer cells sometimes show up as areas of high activity. In recent years, physicians have been able to combine these images with CT images, fusing them with one another to show superb detail of the anatomy from CT scans along with the functional details gained from PET. These images improve diagnosis, staging, and tracking of treatment progress for cancer patients.

In most cases, at least for cancers that are solid tumors, a biopsy is the only definite method for confirming a cancer diagnosis. Before many of the imaging methods discussed above were developed, a biopsy could be performed only through surgery, in which a small sample of the tissue is cut out and sent to a laboratory for evaluation by a pathologist. Today, these samples can be extracted using small needles. The physician can be guided to the site of the suspected cancer by use of ultrasound, CT, MRI, or other imaging methods. The biopsy method is often called fine needle aspiration biopsy or core needle biopsy. Biopsies also may be performed during surgery, particularly to verify and stage cancer when a mass is removed as part of treatment. Removal and biopsy of the entire tumor is called excisional biopsy, while removal of only a portion of the tumor is called incisional biopsy.

Advances in molecular biology and in understanding of the genetic basis of cancer have resulted in the development of several tests designed to assess an individual's risk for developing certain types of cancer. Genetic testing examines specific genes that have been linked to particular cancers, including cancers of the breast, ovary, and colon.

Treatment

Planning treatment for cancer first involves staging of the cancer. Once the physician has gathered the information needed to determine the cancer's stage, the physician will communicate with the patient about treatment options. Common modalities utilized in the treatment of cancer include chemotherapy, radiation therapy, surgery, immunotherapy and biologic or targeted therapies. A cancer patient may receive one or all of these treatments or a combination of them in any order. The particular use and details of each treatment depend on the type of cancer, the stage, and many other factors specific to each patient.

Staging

Cancer staging determines the extent to which cancer has spread in the body. The cancer's stage at diagnosis is based on the size of the original tumor, whether the cancer has spread to the lymph nodes, and whether the cancer has spread to organs of the body that are distant from the original site. Each cancer has its own staging system using letters and numbers. For example, in the TNM Classification System, the T in this cancer staging method describes the original tumor and the N stands for whether the cancer has spread to nearby lymph nodes. The M stands for metastases, or distant spread of the cancer. Numbers are assigned along with letters. Stage I cancers are the least advanced and have the best outlook for survival. Stage IV is the most advanced level.

Chemotherapy

Cancer can spread, even early in the cancer's development. Chemotherapy, referred to as systemic therapy, uses cancer-killing drugs that are given to the patient via various methods, most often by mouth or by intravenous injection. The drugs travel through the bloodstream to try to kill cancer cells throughout the body, not just at the original tumor site. Usually, the drugs are given in cycles and treatment can last six months or longer depending on the specific treatment protocol. Chemotherapy may cause side effects, including fatigue, nausea, and increased susceptibility to colds and infections due to the damage caused to blood cells and other rapidly dividing cells by some chemotherapy agents.

When chemotherapy is used prior to surgery, this form of therapy is known as primary or neoadjuvant chemotherapy. The purpose of administering chemotherapy prior to surgery is to reduce the size or bulk of the tumor. The more common use of chemotherapy is as adjuvant therapy, when chemotherapy is administered after surgery or radiation therapy to destroy any remaining cancer cells and to help prevent recurrence of the cancer.

Radiation therapy

Also called radiotherapy or radiation treatment, radiation therapy usually is used to shrink or control the growth of a tumor. The radiation destroys the cancer cells' ability to reproduce and the body naturally gets rid of the cells. In the past, radiation was available only from external beam radiation therapy, a process in which x-ray beams are directed toward the tumor from a machine outside the patient's body. But patients also may receive brachytherapy, a procedure in which radioactive sources, such as seeds, needles, or wires, are placed inside the body at the tumor site. Radiation therapy techniques have improved dramatically in recent years. Using computers and 3-D imaging, radiation oncologists and radiation therapists can precisely target the tumor area, sparing healthy tissues. Newer techniques even take into account natural movements such as breathing to better target the cancer cells. Radiation can produce some side effects, such as skin changes. Most of the effects are short term, although there are some effects that may last for a year or longer after treatment.

Surgery

When a surgeon removes cancerous tissue, he or she often removes a little bit of the tissue (margins) around the tumor. This step is taken to ensure that all of the cancer cells were removed, to help minimize the chance of recurrence. Surgery may require a hospital stay and recovery time, depending on the type and extent of the surgery. The belief that surgery for cancer leads to spreading of the disease is untrue.

Immunotherapy

Immunotherapy is the use of treatments that promote or support the body's immune system response to cancer. Examples of immunotherapy agents include interleukin, interferon, and colony-stimulating factors. The side effects of immunotherapy are variable but include flu-like symptoms, weakness, loss of appetite, and skin rash. These symptoms typically subside once treatment is completed.

Targeted therapies

There has been tremendous growth in the development of targeted therapies used in the treatment of cancer. Targeted therapies are drugs or other substances that are designed specifically to work at the cellular level by blocking the actions of specific molecules in or on the cancer cell. Many targeted therapies focus on blocking the actions of specific proteins that signal cancer cells to proliferate and grow. Examples of targeted therapies are monoclonal antibodies and small-molecule drugs. Because the action of the drug or substance is targeted to a specific site on or in the cancer cell, normal cells in the same area are less likely to be harmed, thereby potentially reducing side effects. In addition, the action of the targeted agent is more likely to be effective in damaging or killing the cancer cell.

Nutrition and dietary concerns

Numerous factors impact an individual's food and nutrient selection, including economic and educational status, dietary customs and habits, seasonal availability of foods, as well as food and nutritional practices based on cultural or religious values.

Nutritional intake and diet are the focus of many current studies examining the role of foods and **dietary supplements** in the prevention of cancer. In addition, research is being conducted to examine the optimal nutritional supportive care approaches for patients diagnosed with cancer during and after the treatment process.

Nutrition and cancer prevention

Thirty to forty percent of human cancers may be prevented by changes in food and nutrient consumption. Results of current research related to nutrition and cancer prevention suggest a strong role for **antioxidants** in decreasing or preventing DNA damage at the cellular level, which can lead to cancer. Beta-carotene, lycopene, **selenium**, and **vitamins** A, C, and E are nutrients recognized for their strong antioxidant properties.

In 2006, the ACS recommended that Americans maintain a healthy weight throughout life, adopt a physically active lifestyle as adults and children, and consume a healthy diet with an emphasis on plant sources. The physical activity suggestions include at least 30 minutes of moderate to vigorous physical activity for adults five or more days a week, with 45 to 60 minutes of activity preferred. Children and adolescents should engage in at least 60 minutes of activity at least five days a week.

The ACS recommends choosing food and beverages that help to achieve and maintain a healthy weight. The society also recommends eating nine or more servings of a variety of fruits and vegetables per day. **Whole grains** should replace processed grains and the recommendations say to limit consumption of processed and red meats. Scientific evidence shows that populations with diets rich in vegetables and fruits but low in animal fat, meat, and **calories** have a reduced risk of some common cancers.

Nutrition during cancer treatment

Assessment of nutritional deficiencies in patients newly diagnosed with cancer is critical. Deficiencies may lead to suboptimal response to treatment, which can result in diminished prospects for survival. Current recommendations include initiation of a nutritional assessment on newly diagnosed cancer patients within 48 hours after admission or diagnosis, when cancer treatment is started, or when the patient experiences a weight loss of 2%–5% of body weight. Components of the nutritional assessment include assessment of current weight and recent changes to body weight, evaluation of nutrient consumption, as well as physical examination and examination of the results of laboratory tests such as serum albumin, prealbumin, and **vitamin D** levels. In addition, evaluation of symptoms related to the cancer or cancer treatment that impact nutritional intake should be conducted as part of the nutritional assessment. Patients with certain types of cancers, such as cancers of the head and neck areas or cancers of the gastrointestinal tract, are at particularly high risk for the development of nutritional deficiencies due to the cancer or from treatment side effects.

Many cancer treatments can cause loss of appetite, and chemotherapy may cause nausea or changes in taste. Radiation can also affect appetite, depending on the location of the tumor and treatment. Other nutritional needs for cancer patients arise because of a tendency to lose weight and muscle mass. When cancer is diagnosed, patients may be encouraged to consume high-protein and high-calorie diets for a period of time to help maintain muscle mass and weight.

During treatment, dietitians, nurses, and other clinicians may recommend dietary strategies to help minimize side effects. If patients are having trouble chewing or difficulty swallowing, thick liquids such as milkshakes may be suggested. Other semi-solid foods such as mashed potatoes may be helpful until swallowing or chewing ability improves. Other patients may have pain, nausea, vomiting, or diarrhea. Eating a

KEY TERMS

Benign—Mild, does not threaten health or life. When referring to a tumor, it generally means noncancerous.

Cancer—A disease caused by uncontrolled growth of the body's cells.

Cancer staging—A surgical procedure to remove a lymph node and examine the cells for cancer. It determines the extent of the cancer and how far it has spread.

Chemotherapy—A cancer treatment that uses synthetic drugs to destroy the tumor either by inhibiting the growth of the cancerous cells or by killing the cancer cells.

Malignant—Unfavorable, tending to produce deterioration or death. For a tumor, it generally means cancerous.

Radiopharmaceutical—A drug that is radioactive. It is used for diagnosing or treating diseases.

meal of cold foods before treatment may ease nausea. Eating small meals several times a day and choosing bland foods are some suggestions caregivers will offer patients to deal with nausea caused by cancer treatment. Diarrhea can be treated by eating broth, soups, sports drinks, or bananas and avoiding greasy foods. Loss of appetite can be overcome by eating small snacks that contain plenty of calories and **protein**, and eating foods with odors that are appealing, as well as by trying new foods. Sometimes, cancer treatment alters the taste of foods. Rinsing the mouth before eating, using plastic utensils if foods taste metallic, and adding spices to foods may help ease the symptoms.

After cancer treatment, it is important to resume healthy eating habits, following the recommendations of the American Cancer Society to maintain a healthy weight, be as physically active as possible, and eat a balanced diet that leans toward whole grains and plant-based foods instead of red meats and processed foods.

Therapy

Some cancer patients will require nutrition therapy provided and monitored by an interdisciplinary team to restore nutrients and remain nourished, particularly if they experience **malnutrition** because of their cancer or cancer treatment. Nutrition therapy may consist of enteral nutrition, also known as tube

QUESTIONS TO ASK YOUR DOCTOR

- Can you recommend a specialist in cancer nutrition to advise our family about meal planning during our loved one's cancer treatments?
- What is your opinion about foods that may or may not provide additional protection against the development of cancers?
- Are there specific foods that I should include in my diet or eliminate from my diet for the type of cancer with which I have been diagnosed?

feeding. Enteral nutrition is food given in liquid form directly through a tube that is inserted into the stomach or small intestine. Parenteral nutrition is delivered into the bloodstream through a thin tube, or catheter, inserted into a vein. Eating by mouth always is preferred to these methods, and patients are encouraged to eat as soon as they can following these nutrition therapies.

Vitamin D deficiency may be corrected with high-dose supplementation until optimal levels of 50 ng/mL are reached.

Prognosis

Most cancers are curable if detected and treated in their early stages. The prognosis for a person with cancer is affected by many factors, especially the type of cancer and stage of the cancer, the extent to which it has metastasized, and its aggressiveness. In addition, a person's age, general health status, and the effectiveness of the treatments prescribed are important factors.

To help predict the outcome of cancer and the likelihood of recovery from the disease, five-year survival rates are used. In the United States, as of 2012, the five-year survival rate for all cancers combined was 67% for people diagnosed between 2001 and 2007. This means that 67% of people with cancer are expected to be alive at least five years after they are diagnosed. These people may be free of cancer, or they may be undergoing treatment. This is an increase of almost 50% compared to the five-year survival rate for people who were diagnosed with cancer between 1975 and 1977.

It is important to note that while this statistic can give some information about the average survival of people with cancer in a given population, it cannot be used to predict the course of cancer for an individual. No two people are genetically the same, and the survival rate can vary dramatically depending on cancer type and stage at diagnosis. The five-year survival rate does not account for differences in detection methods, types of treatments, individual response to treatment, additional illnesses, and the personal behavior of the individual.

Prevention

In addition to following the American Cancer Society guidelines concerning diet, nutrition, and activity, it is important to follow recommendations from the ACS, family physicians, and other credible health sources regarding behaviors that might lead to cancer. Examples of these behaviors include tobacco use and exposure to ultraviolet rays (sunshine) without protection. Anyone who has a first-degree relative with cancer should speak with their physician about their risk for the same type of cancer and participate in screening as recommended. In cancer, early detection is essential to treatment and a good prognosis.

Resources

BOOKS

American Cancer Society's Healthy Eating Cookbook. 3rd ed. Atlanta, GA: American Cancer Society, 2005.

DeVita, V. T., Jr., T. S. Lawrence, & S. A. Rosenberg. *DeVita, Hellman, and Rosenberg's Cancer Principles and Practice of Oncology.* 9th ed. Philadelphia: Lippincott, Williams, and Wilkins, 2011.

Good for You! Reducing Your Risk of Developing Cancer. Atlanta, GA: American Cancer Society, 2002.

Katzin, Carolyn. *The Cancer Nutrition Center Handbook: An Essential Guide for Cancer Patients and Their Families.* Los Angeles: Carolyn Katzin, 2011.

Wilkes, G. M. *Targeted Cancer Therapy: A Handbook for Nurses.* Sudbury, MA: Jones and Bartlett Publishers, 2011.

Yarbro, C. H., D. Wujcik, and B. H. Gobel. *Cancer Nursing: Principles and Practice.* 7th ed. Sudbury, MA: Jones and Bartlett Publishers, 2011.

PERIODICALS

Ardilio, S. "Calculating Nutrition Needs for a Patient with Head and Neck Cancer." *Clinical Journal of Oncology Nursing* 15, no. 5 (2011): 457–59.

Brown, C. H., S. M. Baidas, J. J. Hajdenberg, et al. "Lifestyle Interventions in the Prevention and Treatment of Cancer." *American Journal of Lifestyle Medicine* 3, no. 5 (2009): 337–48.

Davidson, W., et al. "Malnutrition and Chemotherapy-induced Nausea and Vomiting: Implications for Practice." *Oncology Nursing Forum* 39, no. 4 (2012): E340–E345.

Gotay, C. C. "Cancer Prevention: Major Initiatives and Looking into the Future." *Expert Review of Pharmacoeconomics & Outcomes Research* 10, no. 2 (2010): 143–54.

Granda-Cameron, C., et al. "An Interdisciplinary Approach to Manage Cancer Cachexia." *Clinical Journal of Oncology Nursing* 14, no. 1 (2010): 72–81.

Katzmarzyk, P. T., B. A. Reeder, S. Elliott, et al. "Body Mass Index and Risk of Cardiovascular Disease, Cancer and All-Cause Mortality." *Canadian Journal of Public Health* 103, no. 2 (2012): 147–51.

Klement, R. J., and Kammerer, U. "Is There a Role for Carbohydrate Restriction in the Treatment and Prevention of Cancer?" *Nutrition & Metabolism* 8, no. 75 (2011).

Lee, K. W., A. M. Bode, and Z. Dong. "Molecular Targets of Phytochemicals for Cancer Prevention." *National Review of Cancer* 11, no. 3 (2011): 211–18.

Mannion, C., et al. "Components of an Anticancer Diet: Dietary Recommendations, Restrictions and Supplements of the Bill Henderson Protocol." *Nutrients* 3, no. 1 (2011): 1–26.

Mitchell, D. "The Relationship Between Vitamin D and Cancer." *Clinical Journal of Oncology Nursing* 15, no. 5 (2011): 557–60.

Moreland, S. S. "Nutrition Screening and Counseling in Adults with Lung Cancer: A Systematic Review of the Evidence." *Clinical Journal of Oncology Nursing* 14, no. 5 (2010): 609–14.

Ralph, J., et al. "Diet Assessment Methods: A Guide for Oncology Nurses." *Clinical Journal of Oncology Nursing* 15, no. 6 (2011): E114–E121.

WEBSITES

American Cancer Society. "Complementary and Alternative Medicine: Diet and Nutrition." http://www.cancer.org/Treatment/TreatmentsandSideEffects/ComplementaryandAlternativeMedicine/DietandNutrition/index (accessed September 15, 2012).

———.*Facts and Figures 2012*. http://www.cancer.org (accessed September 15, 2012).

MedlinePlus. "Diet: Cancer Treatment." U.S. National Library of Medicine. http://www.nlm.nih.gov/medlineplus/ency/article/002439.htm (accessed September 15, 2012).

National Cancer Institute. "Eating Hints: Before, During, and After Cancer Treatment." U.S. Department of Health and Human Serivces, National Institutes of Health. http://www.cancer.gov/cancertopics/coping/eatinghints/page1/AllPages (accessed September 15, 2012).

ORGANIZATIONS

American Academy of Dermatology, PO Box 4014, Schaumburg, IL 60168, (866) 503-SKIN (7546), http://www.aad.org.

American Brain Tumor Association, 8550 W. Bryn Mawr Ave., Chicago, IL 60631, (773) 577-8750, (800) 886-2282, http://www.abta.org.

American Cancer Society, 250 Williams St. NW, Atlanta, GA 30303, http://www.cancer.org.

American Lung Association, 1301 Pennsylvania Avenue NW, Ste. 800, Washington, DC 20004, (202) 785-3355, http://www.lung.org.

American Society of Clinical Oncology, 2318 Mill Rd., Ste. 800, Alexandria, VA 22314, (571) 483-1300, http://www.asco.org.

American Urological Association, 1000 Corporate Blvd., Linthicum, MD 21090, (866) 746-4282, http://www.auanet.org.

Brain Tumor Foundation for Children, Inc., 6065 Roswell Road NE, Ste. 525, Atlanta, GA 30328, (404) 252-4107, http://www.braintumorkids.org.

Breastcancer.org, 7 East Lancaster Ave., 3rd Fl., Ardmore, PA 19003, http://www.breastcancer.org.

Colon Cancer Alliance, 1025 Vermont Ave. NW, Ste. 1066, Washington, DC 20005, (877) 422-2030, http://www.ccalliance.org.

Leukemia and Lymphoma Society, 1311 Mamaroneck Ave., Ste. 310, White Plains, NY 10605, (914) 949-5213, http://www.lls.org.

Lung Cancer Alliance, 888 16th St. NW, Ste. 150, Washington, DC 20006, (202) 463-2080, http://www.lungcanceralliance.org.

Lung Cancer Foundation of America, 15 S. Franklin St., New Ulm, NM 56073, (507) 354-1361, http://www.lcfamerica.org.

Melanoma Research Foundation, 1411 K St., NW, Ste. 500, Washington, DC 20005, (800) 673-1290, http://www.melanoma.org.

National Brain Tumor Foundation, 22 Battery St., Ste. 612, San Francisco, CA 94111-5520, (415) 834-9970, (800) 770-8287, http://www.braintumor.org.

National Cancer Institute, 6116 Executive Blvd., Ste. 300, Bethesda, MD 20892-8322, (800) 422-6237, http://www.cancer.gov.

National Children's Leukemia Foundation, 7316 Ave. U, Brooklyn, NY 11234, (800) 448-3467, http://www.leukemiafoundation.org.

National Comprehensive Cancer Network, 275 Commerce Dr., Ste. 300, Fort Washington, PA 19034, (215) 690-0300, http://www.nccn.org.

Oncology Nursing Society, 125 Enterprise Dr., Pittsburgh, PA 25275, (866) 257-4667, http://www.ons.org.

Prostate Cancer Foundation, 1250 Fourth St., Santa Monica, CA 90401, (800) 757-2873, http://www.pcf.org.

Skin Cancer Foundation, 149 Madison Ave., Ste. 901, New York, NY 10016, (212) 725-5176, http://www.skincancer.org.

Support for People with Oral and Head and Neck Cancer, PO Box 53, Locust Valley, NY 11560-0053, (800) 377-0928, http://www.spohnc.org.

Susan G. Komen for the Cure, 5005 LBJ Freeway, Ste. 250, Dallas, TX 75244, (877) 465-6636, ww5.komen.org.

The Oral Cancer Foundation, 3419 Via Lido, #205, Newport Beach, CA 92663, (949) 646-8000, http://oralcancerfoundation.org.

United Ostomy Associations of America, PO Box 512, Northfield, MN 55057-0512, (800) 826-0826, http://www.ostomy.org.

Us Too Prostate Cancer Education and Support, 5003 Fairview Ave., Downers Grove, IL 60515, (800) 808-7866, http://www.ustoo.org.

Teresa G. Odle
David Newton
Melinda Granger Oberleitner, RN, DNS

Cancer diet

Definition

The phrase *cancer diet* can be used to refer to several different approaches to the associations between **cancer** and nutrition. Some people think of a cancer diet as a preventive approach to cancer or a way to lower the risk of cancer by avoiding foods associated with specific types of cancer. *Cancer diet* may also refer to the special diets or nutritional therapy prescribed for cancer patients to prevent them from developing **malnutrition** as a side effect of their cancer therapy. Finally, *cancer diet* is sometimes used to refer to complementary and alternative (CAM) approaches to cancer that involve the use of special diets and nutritional supplements. The best-known of these are the **macrobiotic diet**, a largely vegetarian diet that originated in Japan; and the Gonzalez regimen, an alternative therapy for pancreatic cancer. The Gonzalez regimen includes a special diet, nutritional supplements, pancreatic enzymes in capsule form, and coffee enemas.

Purpose

The purpose of preventive cancer diets is to lower an individual's risk of cancer, particularly cancers of the digestive system. The purpose of nutritional therapy for cancer is to minimize loss of appetite, tissue wasting, and other symptoms of the disease or side effects of treatment; to help the patient tolerate cancer treatment; to protect the functioning of his or her immune system; and to maintain or improve the patient's quality of life. The purpose of the Gonzalez regimen and other CAM dietary therapies for cancer is to treat the disease itself rather than its symptoms or the side effects of mainstream cancer therapies.

Demographics

The World Health Organization (WHO) estimates that more than 30% of cancers can be prevented, and that the primary risk factors for cancer include tobacco use (the primary risk factor), alcohol use, unhealthy diet, and lack of physical activity. **Obesity** and/or a lack of physical activity have been linked specifically to up to 30% of colon, premenopausal breast, uterine, esophageal, and renal cell cancers. Further, diet has been associated with cancers of the mouth, esophagus, stomach, intestines, rectum, prostate, breast, kidney, liver, and pancreas. Obesity may also contribute to higher mortality rates in cancer patients.

According to the American Cancer Society (ACS), cancer accounts for 7.6 million deaths worldwide each year, or 13% of the global total. In 2008, 12.7 million people around the world were living with cancer; this figure is expected to jump to 21.4 million by 2030. More than half of all new cancers occur in developing countries. The greatest single risk factor for cancers related to diet is not race or sex but socio-economic status (SES); cancer risk factors are highest and survival rates are lowest in groups with the least education.

Description

Diet as a cancer preventive

Dietary changes as a preventive measure for lowering an individual's risk of cancer are sometimes called an anticancer diet, although this term does not have a precise definition. Most recommendations for lowering the risk of cancer through changes in eating habits include the following:

- Eat less total fat and avoid hydrogenated fats—the type of fats often used to prepare fast foods.
- Choose foods that are high in fiber, such as wheat bran, kidney beans, garbanzo beans, navy beans, whole wheat, whole grains, legumes, whole-grain bread, and prunes.
- Eat large amounts of fresh fruits and vegetables, particularly the cruciferous vegetables (broccoli, cabbage, Brussels sprouts, mustard greens, kale, and cauliflower).
- Switch from red meat to fish; if possible, move from a meat-based to a vegetarian diet.
- Use olive oil rather than oils containing saturated fats when cooking.
- Choose foods that are high in calcium.
- Drink less alcohol.

The ACS offers similar nutritional preventive guidelines, emphasizing the importance of choosing **whole grains** over processed, limiting consumption of red meat, eating a variety of fresh produce, limiting alcohol, and engaging in regular physical activity.

There has been research on the link between **antioxidants** and cancer prevention, but results are yet to be conclusive. The ACS promotes obtaining antioxidants from whole foods, such as berries, plums, and artichokes, over **dietary supplements**.

One mainstream approach to diet that is often recommended as a way to lower cancer risk is the **Mediterranean diet**. The Mediterranean diet is better described as a nutritional model or pattern of food consumption rather than a diet in the usual sense of the word. There is more than one Mediterranean diet, if the phrase is understood to refer to the traditional foods and eating patterns found in the countries bordering the Mediterranean Sea. In general, however, Mediterranean diets have five major characteristics:

- high levels of fruits and vegetables, breads and other cereals, potatoes, beans, nuts, and seeds
- olive oil as the principal or only source of fat in the diet
- low to moderate amounts of dairy products, fish, and poultry, little red meat
- eggs used no more than four times weekly
- wine consumed in moderate amounts—two glasses per day for men, one glass for women

These characteristics are in line with most of the recommendations of so-called anticancer diets.

It is important to remember, however, that diet is not the only risk factor for certain types of cancer. Occupation, environmental factors, and heredity also influence a given individual's risk of developing cancer, and changing the diet does not guarantee that a person will never develop cancer.

Nutritional therapy for cancer

Nutritional therapy for cancer patients is intended to help them maintain normal energy levels and avoid malnutrition. Appetite, taste, smell, and the ability to eat enough food or absorb the nutrients from food may be affected by the symptoms of the disease itself or by the side effects of treatment. Cancer patients frequently experience such symptoms as loss of appetite, nausea and vomiting, **constipation**, diarrhea, sore mouth, trouble swallowing, and depression. The most common nutritional problems in cancer patients are failure to eat enough high-protein foods and failure to take in enough overall **calories**.

The most common cause of malnutrition in cancer patients is anorexia, or loss of appetite. It may appear together with cachexia, a wasting syndrome in which the person loses weight, muscle, and fat tissue. Cachexia is not the same as starvation. A healthy person's body can adjust to starvation by slowing down its use of nutrients, but the body cannot adjust in this fashion in cancer patients with cachexia.

Nutrition therapy for cancer patients may be very different from standard guidelines for healthful eating. It is tailored to each patient's individual nutritional needs, response to cancer treatment, and personal food preferences. Patients who cannot take foods by mouth may require enteral nutrition (tube feeding) or parenteral nutrition (nutrients infused directly into the bloodstream through a catheter). Those who can take foods by mouth may need to change their eating habits by having several small meals a day rather than one large one; by taking medications for such problems as nausea, vomiting, constipation, or diarrhea; by drinking extra fluids to cope with such problems as dry mouth or changes in the sense of taste; and by adding as many high-protein, high-calorie foods to the diet as possible. Good choices include cheese and crackers, puddings, muffins, nutritional supplements, milk shakes, yogurt, ice cream, and chocolate.

CAM dietary therapies

Some CAM dietary therapies are promoted as cancer treatments. However, it is important to note that there is little scientific evidence to support these therapies. Patients should never take it upon themselves to replace any prescribed treatments with CAM therapies without first consulting with their physicians.

GONZALEZ REGIMEN. The Gonzalez regimen is an alternative dietary therapy for pancreatic cancer developed by Nicholas Gonzalez, a physician in New York City. It is a complex combination of dietary changes, various nutritional supplements, and detoxification procedures.

- Diet. In general, the diet in the Gonzalez regimen requires the patient to consume mostly organic foods, and avoid such synthetic and refined foods as white flour and white sugar. The diet is, however, tailored to each patient. There are ten basic diets with 90 variations, ranging from nearly vegetarian diets to diets high in meat and fat.
- Supplements. These may include vitamins, minerals, trace elements, antioxidants, animal glandular concentrates, and other food concentrates. Like the diet, the combination of supplements is also customized for the individual patient.
- Proteolytic enzymes made from the pancreas of a pig. The basic theory underlying the Gonzalez regimen is that toxins from processed foods and environmental sources are responsible for cancers in humans, and that the pancreas is the organ primarily responsible for detoxifying the body. Gonzalez maintains that

these pancreatic enzymes, taken in capsule form, enter the bloodstream and help the body eliminate and destroy malignant cells, waste material, and abnormal proteins that are toxic to the body. Overall, a cancer patient on the Gonzalez regimen will take between 150 and 175 capsules per day of nutrient supplements and pancreatic enzymes.

• Coffee enemas, taken twice daily. Gonzalez maintains that these enemas serve to detoxify the body by improving liver function and stimulate the gallbladder to empty, thereby speeding up the elimination of toxins and waste products.

MACROBIOTIC DIET. The macrobiotic diet is a diet based on the heavy consumption of whole grains, vegetables, **soy** products, seaweed, beans and bean products, mild flavorings, fruit, fish, nuts, and seeds. All products used should be locally grown whenever possible and processed as little as possible. The specific foods are selected according to the time of year; the climate; and the person's sex, age, activity level, and overall health status. The macrobiotic diet developed in Japan from traditional folk medicine. It was given the name "macrobiotic" in the 1950s by George Ohsawa (1893–1966) and brought to the West in the late 1950s.

The macrobiotic diet was first touted as a cure for cancer by one of Ohsawa's disciples, Michio Kushi (1926–). Kushi wrote a book about the macrobiotic diet as a cancer preventive and treatment, titled *The Cancer Prevention Diet: The Macrobiotic Approach to Preventing and Relieving Cancer*, and first published in 1993. The website of the Kushi Institute includes personal testimonials from people who maintain that their cancers, ranging from uterine and pancreatic cancers to leukemia and brain tumors, were cured by following the macrobiotic diet.

Precautions

People wishing to learn more about lowering their individual risk of cancer by changing their diet should consult their primary care physician. Sources like the American Cancer Society (ACS), the National Cancer Institute (NCI), the World Health Organization (WHO), and the World Cancer Research Fund (WCRF) also provide up-to-date information about the relationships between cancer and nutrition. Patients being treated with nutritional therapy as part of their cancer treatment should follow the recommendations of their doctors and dietitians. People considering CAM therapies for cancer should find out as much as they can about these approaches and talk to their primary care doctor before using them. Most experts advise that CAM therapies should not be used as substitutes for mainstream cancer treatments.

Risks

There are no known risks to eating a healthful diet in order to reduce the risk of cancer nor in following the nutritional recommendations of the treatment team if being treated for cancer.

Gonzalez notes that patients on his dietary regimen frequently experience muscle aches and pains, low-grade fevers, skin rashes, and other flu-like symptoms. He attributes these to the body's reaction to detoxification. Other reported side effects include bloating, gassiness, and indigestion.

The primary risk of following the macrobiotic diet is using it as a therapy for cancer instead of mainstream cancer treatment. Other people who have used it as a preventive diet to lower their risk of cancer have developed mild forms of malnutrition by failing to supplement the diet with **vitamin D** and **vitamin B$_{12}$**, which are not available in sufficient amounts in the foods that are the mainstays of the macrobiotic diet.

Health care team roles

Dietary changes as a cancer preventive for individual patients should be overseen and monitored by a primary care physician and a dietitian. Dietary therapy for cancer patients is usually designed and modified by a treatment team that includes a dietitian as well as doctors and nurses.

Patients with pancreatic cancer who are interested in the Gonzalez regimen should first consult their present treatment team for their advice and suggestions. Similarly, patients already diagnosed with cancer should consult their treatment team before using a macrobiotic diet as cancer therapy. The ACS "strongly urges individuals with cancer not to use a dietary program as an exclusive or primary means of treatment."

Research & general acceptance

The World Health Organization (WHO) has summarized recent findings about the relationship between lifestyle and dietary factors and cancer as follows:

• Convincing evidence for lowering cancer risk: Regular physical activity.

• Convincing evidence for increasing cancer risk: Overweight and obesity.

• Probable evidence for lowering cancer risk: High consumption of fresh fruits and vegetables.

• Probable evidence for increasing cancer risk: Excessive alcohol consumption; salted and preserved meats; highly cooked rather than rare or raw meats;

KEY TERMS

Aflatoxins—A group of naturally occurring toxins produced by fungi of the genus *Aspergillus*.

Cachexia—Unintentional loss of body weight and muscle mass, and weakness that may occur in patients with cancer, AIDS, or other chronic diseases.

Enteral nutrition—The medical term for tube feeding.

Gonzalez regimen—An alternative therapy for pancreatic cancer that includes a special diet, nutritional supplements, pancreatic enzymes, and coffee enemas.

Macrobiotic diet—A diet based primarily on whole grains, vegetables, and beans, and avoiding refined or processed foods. It is sometimes recommended by practitioners of alternative medicine as a preventive for cancer.

Parenteral nutrition—Providing a person with necessary nutrients through intravenous feeding.

fermented fish; very hot (temperature) drinks and food; and aflatoxins (toxins produced by fungi sometimes found in peanuts, grains, and tree nuts).

- Possible or insufficient evidence for lowering cancer risk: Plant fiber, soya, fish, omega-3 fatty acids, carotenoids, vitamins B_2, B_6, folate, B_{12}, C, D, E, calcium, zinc, selenium, and non-nutrient plant constituents.

- Possible or insufficient evidence for increasing cancer risk: Animal fats, heterocyclic amines (chemicals found in well-cooked meat), polycyclic aromatic hydrocarbons, and nitrosamines.

Evidence for CAM dietary therapies for cancer is considerably lower than that for preventive dietary modifications. The NCI's summary of the Gonzalez regimen states that "Existing clinical data concerning the effectiveness of the Gonzalez regimen as a treatment for cancer are limited and inconclusive," primarily because of the small size of the subject groups and the lack of a control group. In August 2009, a group of researchers in New York and Boston reported that patients following the Gonzalez regimen survived only a third as long as those receiving conventional chemotherapy and had a lower quality of life.

The macrobiotic diet is generally considered ineffective as a treatment for cancer. The ACS states, "After studying the literature and other available information, the American Cancer Society has found no evidence that a macrobiotic diet is useful as a cure for cancer in humans." The wife and daughter of Michio Kushi both died of cancer (as did two physicians who claimed to have cured themselves of cancer by following the macrobiotic diet), and Kushi himself had a cancerous tumor removed from his intestines in 2004.

Clinical trials investigating the link between diet and cancer are ongoing. Individuals interested in participating in clinical trials may find a list online at ClinicalTrials.gov.

See also Diet and disease prevention.

Resources

BOOKS

Gonzalez, Nicholas J. *One Man Alone: An Investigation of Nutrition, Cancer, and William Donald Kelley.* New York: New Spring Press, 2009.

Katz, David L. *Nutrition in Clinical Practice: A Comprehensive, Evidence-Based Manual for the Practitioner*, 2nd ed. Philadelphia: Lippincott Williams and Wilkins, 2008.

Keane, Maureen, and Daniella Chace. *What to Eat If You Have Cancer: Healing Foods That Boost Your Immune System*, updated 2nd ed. New York: McGraw-Hill, 2007.

Kushi, Michio, and Alex Jack. *The Cancer Prevention Diet: The Macrobiotic Approach to Preventing and Relieving Cancer*, revised and updated. New York: St. Martin's Press, 2009.

Oncology Nutrition Dietetic Practice Group. *Clinical Guide to Oncology Nutrition*, 2nd ed. Chicago, IL: American Dietetic Association, 2006.

PERIODICALS

Balbuena, L., and A.G. Casson. "Physical Activity, Obesity and Risk for Esophageal Adenocarcinoma." *Future Oncology* 5 (September 2009): 1051–63.

Bosetti, C., et al. "Diet and Cancer in Mediterranean Countries: Carbohydrates and Fats." *Public Health Nutrition* 12 (September 2009): 1595–1600.

Chabot, J.A., et al. "Pancreatic Proteolytic Enzyme Therapy Compared With Gemcitabine-Based Chemotherapy for the Treatment of Pancreatic Cancer." *Journal of Clinical Oncology*, April 2010.

Davis, C.D., and J.A. Milner. "Gastrointestinal Microflora, Food Components and Colon Cancer Prevention." *Journal of Nutritional Biochemistry* 20 (October 2009): 743–52.

Divisi, D., et al. "Diet and Cancer." *Acta Bio-Medica* 77 (August 2006): 118–23.

Holman, Dawn M., and Mary C. White. "Dietary Behaviors Related to Cancer Prevention among Pre-Adolescents and Adolescents: The Gap between Recommendations and Reality." *Nutrition Journal* 10 (June 2011): 60.

Holmes, S. "A Difficult Clinical Problem: Diagnosis, Impact and Clinical Management of Cachexia in Palliative Care." *International Journal of Palliative Nursing* 15 (July 2009): 320–326.

La Vecchia, C. "Association between Mediterranean Dietary Patterns and Cancer Risk." *Nutrition Reviews* 67 (May 2009), Suppl. 1, S126–S129.

Mosby, T.T., et al. "Nutritional Assessment of Children with Cancer." *Journal of Pediatric Oncology Nursing* 26 (July-August 2009): 186–97.

Rezash, V. "Can a Macrobiotic Diet Cure Cancer?" *Clinical Journal of Oncology Nursing* 12 (October 2008): 807–08.

Weitzman, S. "Complementary and Alternative (CAM) Dietary Therapies for Cancer." *Pediatric Blood and Cancer* 50 (February 2008): 494–97.

Zheng, W., and S.A. Lee. "Well-done Meat Intake, Heterocyclic Amine Exposure, and Cancer Risk." *Nutrition and Cancer* 61 (April 2009): 437–46.

OTHER

American Cancer Society (ACS). *Cancer Facts & Figures.* Atlanta: ACS, 2012. http://www.cancer.org/Research/CancerFactsFigures/CancerFactsFigures/cancer-facts-figures-2012 (accessed September 15, 2012).

WEBSITES

American Cancer Society (ACS). "ACS Guidelines on Nutrition and Physical Activity for Cancer Prevention." http://www.cancer.org/Healthy/EatHealthyGetActive/ACSGuidelinesonNutritionPhysicalActivityforCancerPrevention/index (accessed September 15, 2011).

National Cancer Institute. "Chemicals in Meat Cooked at High Temperatures and Cancer Risk." http://www.cancer.gov/cancertopics/factsheet/Risk/heterocyclic-amines (accessed September 15, 2012).

———. "Energy Balance: Weight and Obesity, Physical Activity, Diet." http://www.cancer.gov/cancertopics/prevention/energybalance (accessed September 15, 2011).

———. "Gonzalez Regimen." http://www.cancer.gov/cancertopics/pdq/cam/gonzalez/healthprofessional/allpages (accessed September 15, 2012).

———. "Nutrition in Cancer Care." http://www.cancer.gov/cancertopics/pdq/supportivecare/nutrition/patient/allpages (accessed September 15, 2012).

———. "What You Need to Know about Cancer: Risk Factors." http://www.cancer.gov/cancertopics/wyntk/overview/page4 (accessed September 15, 2012).

World Health Organization (WHO). "Cancer: Diet and Physical Activity's Impact." http://www.who.int/dietphysicalactivity/en (accessed September 15, 2012).

ORGANIZATIONS

Academy of Nutrition and Dietetics, 120 South Riverside Plz., Ste. 2000, Chicago, IL 60606-6995, (312) 899-0040, (800) 877-1600, amacmunn@eatright.org, http://www.eatright.org.

American Cancer Society, 250 Williams Street NW, Atlanta, GA 30303, (800) 227-2345, http://www.cancer.org.

Kushi Institute, 198 Leland Rd., Becket, MA 01223, (413) 623-5741, (800) 975-8744, Fax: (413) 623-8827, http://www.kushiinstitute.org.

National Cancer Institute, 6116 Executive Blvd., Ste. 300, Bethesda, MD 20892-8322, (800) 422-6237, cancergovstaff@mail.nih.gov, http://www.cancer.gov.

National Center for Complementary and Alternative Medicine (NCCAM), 9000 Rockville Pike, Bethesda, MD 20892, info@nccam.nih.gov, http://nccam.nih.gov.

World Health Organization (WHO), Avenue Appia 20, 1211 Geneva 27, Switzerland, 41 22 791 21 11, info@who.int, http://www.who.int/en.

Rebecca J. Frey, PhD

Cancer-fighting foods

Definition

Research on the link between foods and **cancer** tends to focus on two components: phytochemicals and **antioxidants**. Phytochemicals are plant-based substances that are believed to have positive effects on human health. Antioxidants are molecules that prevent free radicals (oxidizing molecules) from damaging cells. The goal of current research is to determine precisely how and why these substances—found primarily in fruits and vegetables—can prevent or stop the development of malignant cells. When animals are given vegetables and fruits before being exposed to carcinogens (cancer-causing agents), they are less likely to develop cancer. Although additional experimental data needs to be collected in

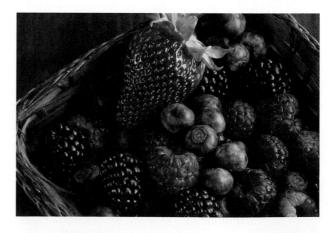

Berries are featured on the American Institute for Cancer Research's list of cancer-fighting foods. *(Minerva Studio/Shutterstock.com)*

humans, there is evidence that consumption of fruits and vegetables may play an important role in preventing cancer.

Purpose

Phytochemicals are chemicals that occur naturally in plants. Several hundred types of phytochemicals have been identified, but many more likely remain to be identified. Some examples include indoles in cabbage or cauliflower, saponins in peas and beans, genstain in soybeans, and isoflavones in **soy** milk and tofu. Over the past 20 years, nutrition scientists have consistently found that individuals who eat greater amounts of vegetables and fruits have lower rates of cancer. It has been only recently that the mechanisms by which phytochemicals assist the body in resisting cancer have begun to be understood. The phytochemicals present in fruits and vegetables protect the body by stunting the growth of malignant cells. It is not yet known how many phytochemicals exist and how they work, but the World Health Organization concluded that people who ate at least 400 grams of fruits and vegetables every day had a significantly lower risk of various cancers. This determination led many countries, including the United States and the United Kingdom, to campaign for increased produce intake, such as the U.K.'s 5 A DAY campaign. It is recommended that individuals mix and match their five servings a day of fruits and vegetables with seven or more starchy or protein-rich plant foods such as grains, peas and beans, and potatoes.

Supplements containing **vitamins** and **minerals** can help an individual gain some of the benefits of these substances. However, vitamin and mineral supplements are not a total replacement for real food. This is because vitamin and mineral supplements, although very beneficial, do not supply the thousands of phytochemicals that might be present in fruits and vegetables, according to the Cleveland Clinic Foundation in Ohio. For example, eating a sweet potato with its skin, which is a great source of both beta carotene and **fiber**, provides at least 5,000 phytochemicals that are not present in a beta-carotene supplement. That's an extremely important difference. Isolating a few compounds in a pill will not provide the hundreds of protective benefits that plant foods provide. The best advice is to obtain phytochemicals by eating a good variety of plant foods every day. Whether fruits and vegetables are consumed in raw or cooked form does not really matter with regard to phytochemical content. Even canned, frozen, and juiced fruits and vegetables pack a phytochemical punch. However, raw or steamed vegetables provide the best nutrient value.

The antioxidants found in fruits, vegetables, and other plant-based foods fight free radicals, which are compounds in the body that attack and destroy cell membranes. The uncontrolled activity of free radicals is believed to cause many cancers. Examples of antioxidants include **carotenoids**, such as beta-carotene, lycopene, and vitamins C and E.

The carotenoids, in particular, which give fruits and vegetables their bright yellow, orange, and red colors, are now gaining recognition for their nutritional worth. Numerous studies have extolled the virtues of lycopene (the carotenoid that makes tomatoes red) in preventing prostate cancer. One such study at Harvard University found that men who include tomato products in their meals twice a week could reduce their risk of developing prostate cancer by one-third compared with men who do not consume tomatoes.

Other lycopene-rich foods, such as watermelon, red grapefruit, and guava, are now piquing the interest of researchers. Watermelon not only yields more lycopene per serving (15 mg in 1 1/2 cups) than raw tomatoes (11 mg per 1 1/2 cups), but it's also a rich source of vitamins A and C.

Whether antioxidants can reduce the incidence of cancer is still uncertain at this point because of the lack of sufficient studies. However, research data obtained thus far indicates that antioxidants do appear to provide health benefits.

The National Cancer Institute estimates that roughly one-third of all cancer deaths may be diet-related. Scientists have recently estimated that approximately 30% to 40% of all cancers could be averted if people ate more fruits, vegetables, and plant-based foods and minimized high-fat, high-calorie edibles that have scant nutritional value. Food can have both positive and negative effects. In the past, researchers had linked fat consumption with the development of cancers, but they currently believe that eating fruits, vegetables, and grains may be more important in preventing the disease than not eating fat. Many of the common foods found in grocery stores or organic markets contain cancer-fighting properties, from the antioxidants that neutralize the damage caused by free radicals to the powerful phytochemicals that scientists are just beginning to explore. There isn't a single element in a particular food that does all the work. The best thing to do is eat a variety of foods.

Description

There are a number of foods that are thought to have the ability to help stave off cancer, and some may even help inhibit cancer cell growth or reduce tumor size. These foods have been determined to be the best cancer fighters based on the nutrients they contain.

AVOCADOS. Avocados are rich in glutathione, a powerful antioxidant that attacks free radicals in the body by blocking intestinal absorption of certain **fats**. They also supply even more potassium than bananas and are a good source of **vitamin E**. Scientists believe that avocados may also be useful in treating viral hepatitis (a cause of liver cancer), as well as other sources of liver damage. A 2007 study sponsored by Ohio State University and published in the journal *Seminars in Cancer Biology* found supportive evidence that the phytochemicals in avocados may help prevent oral cancer.

BEANS. Beans contain a number of phytochemicals, which have been shown to prevent or slow genetic damage to cells. While this makes beans beneficial for helping to reduce the risk of many types of cancer, specific research has suggested they are especially potent in preventing prostate cancer. As an added bonus, the high fiber content of beans has been connected with a lower risk of digestive cancers.

BERRIES. The two most widely studied cancer-fighting compounds in berries are ellagic acid (richest in strawberries and raspberries) and anthocyanosides (richest in blueberries). Ellagic acid is believed to help prevent skin, bladder, lung, and breast cancers, both by acting as an antioxidant and by slowing the reproduction of cancer cells. The anthocyanosides in blueberries are currently the most powerful antioxidants known to scientists and are beneficial in the prevention of all types of cancer. Raspberries contain many vitamins, minerals, plant compounds, and antioxidants known as anthocyanins that may protect against cancer. According to a 2001 study reported by *Cancer Research*, rats fed diets of 5% to 10% black raspberries saw the number of esophageal tumors decrease by 43% to 62%. A diet containing 5% black raspberries was actually more effective than a diet containing 10% black raspberries. Research using strawberries in 2011 supported the connection between berry intake and decreased risk of esophageal cancer. A study reported in the journal *Nutrition and Cancer* in May 2002 showed that black raspberries may also help thwart colon cancer. Black raspberries are rich in antioxidants and are thought to have even more cancer-preventing properties than blueberries and strawberries.

CARROTS. Carrots contain a plentiful amount of beta-carotene, which may help reduce a wide range of cancers including lung, mouth, throat, stomach, intestine, bladder, prostate, and breast. Some research indicates that beta-carotene may actually cause cancer, but this study has not confirmed that eating carrots,

unless in very large quantities (e.g., 2 to 3 kilos a day), can cause cancer. In fact, a substance called falcarinol that is found in carrots has been found to reduce the risk of cancer, according to researchers at the Danish Institute of Agricultural Sciences (DIAS). It has been demonstrated that isolated cancer cells grow more slowly when exposed to falcarinol. This substance is a polyacetylene.

CHILI PEPPERS. Chili peppers and jalapenos contain a chemical, capsaicin, which may neutralize certain cancer-causing substances called nitrosamines and may help prevent cancers such as stomach cancer.

CRUCIFEROUS VEGETABLES. All cruciferous vegetables (members of the Brassicaceae, or Cruciferae family), including cabbage and cauliflower, are rich in a variety of compounds that have been shown to slow cancer growth and development in a number of laboratory studies. These vegetables contain a chemical component called indole-3-carbinol that can combat breast cancer by converting a cancer-promoting estrogen into a more protective variety. Other larger human studies have shown that cruciferous vegetables can help to reduce the risk of lung and bladder cancers. The antioxidants lutein and zeaxanthin, which are present in cruciferous vegetables, may help decrease the risk of prostate and other cancers.

Broccoli, which is also a cruciferous vegetable, contains the phytochemical sulforaphane, a product of glucoraphanin, that is believed to aid in preventing some types of cancer, such as stomach, colon and rectal cancer. Sulforaphane induces the production of certain enzymes that can deactivate free radicals and carcinogens. The enzymes have been shown to inhibit the growth of tumors in laboratory animals. Studies by the U.S. Department of Agriculture of 71 types of broccoli plants found a 30-fold difference in the amounts of glucoraphanin. It appears that the more bitter the broccoli is, the more glucoraphanin it has. Broccoli sprouts have been developed under the trade name BroccoSprouts that have a consistent level of sulforaphane that is as much as 20 times higher than the levels found in mature heads of broccoli.

DARK GREEN LEAFY VEGETABLES. Leafy-green vegetables, such as romaine lettuce, mustard greens, chicory, and Swiss chard, are rich sources of antioxidants called carotenoids. These compounds scavenge dangerous free radicals from the body before they can promote cancer growth. The vegetables are also rich in **folate**, a vitamin shown to reduce the risk of lung and breast cancer.

FIGS. Figs contain a derivative of benzaldehyde. It has been reported by investigators at the Institute of

Physical and Chemical Research in Tokyo that benzaldehyde is highly effective at shrinking tumors, although further experiments need to be conducted. In addition, the U.S. Department of Agriculture says that figs, which contain vitamins A and C, and **calcium**, **magnesium** and potassium, may curtail appetite and improve weight-loss efforts. Fig juice is also a potent bacteria killer in test-tube studies.

FLAX. Flax contains lignans, which may have an antioxidant effect and block or suppress cancerous changes. Flax is also high in **omega-3 fatty acids**, which are thought to protect against colon cancer and heart disease. **Flaxseed** in the form of oil and meal contains phytoestrogens believed to reduce the risk of breast, skin, and lung cancer. Research on the potency of flaxseed as an anti-cancer food is still ongoing. A specialized diet called the Budwig diet, which has been used by some cancer patients, uses the combination of flaxseed oil and cottage cheese. When these two foods are consumed simultaneously, it is said that they increase the levels of substances called phosphatides and lipoproteins in the blood. Dr. Johanna Budwig, the creator of the diet, claims that the diet is both preventative and curative in regard to cancer.

GARLIC. Garlic has immune-enhancing allium compounds (diallyl sulfides) that appear to increase the activity of immune cells that fight cancer and indirectly help break down cancer causing substances. These substances also help block carcinogens from entering cells and slow tumor development. Diallyl sulfide, a component of garlic oil, has also been shown to render carcinogens in the liver inactive. Studies have linked garlic, as well as onions, leeks, and chives to lower risk of a variety of cancers including stomach, colon, lung, and skin cancer. Dr. Lenore Arab, professor of epidemiology and nutrition at the University of North Carolina at Chapel Hill Schools of Public Health and Medicine and colleagues analyzed a number of studies and reported their findings in the October 2000 issue of the *American Journal of Clinical Nutrition*. According to the report, individuals who consume raw or cooked garlic regularly face about half the risk of stomach cancer and two-thirds the risk of colorectal cancer as individuals who eat little or none. Their studies did not show that garlic supplements had the same effect. It is believed garlic may help prevent stomach cancer because it has anti-bacterial effects against a bacterium, *Helicobacter pylori*, found in the stomach and known to promote cancer there.

GRAPEFRUITS. Like oranges and other citrus fruits, grapefruits contain monoterpenes, which are believed to help prevent cancer by sweeping carcinogens out of the body. Some studies show that grapefruit may inhibit the proliferation of breast-cancer cells in vitro. Grapefruits also contain **vitamin C**, beta-carotene, and folic acid.

GRAPES. Red and purple grapes in particular are a rich source of resveratrol, a potent antioxidant and anti-inflammatory agent, which inhibits the enzymes that can stimulate cancer-cell growth and suppress immune response. Resveratrol is thought to work by preventing cell damage before it begins. Grapes also contain ellagic acid, a compound that blocks enzymes that are necessary for cancer cell growth. Ellagic acid also appears to help slow the growth of tumors. Red grapes also contain bioflavonoids, which are powerful antioxidants that work as cancer preventives.

KALE. Considered a cruciferous vegetable, kale contains indoles, which are a nitrogen compound that may help stop the conversion of certain lesions to cancerous cells in estrogen-sensitive tissues. In addition, isothiocyanates, phytochemicals found in kale, are thought to suppress tumor growth and block cancer-causing substances from reaching their targets.

LICORICE ROOT. Licorice root has a chemical, glycyrrhizin, that blocks a component of testosterone and therefore may help prevent the growth of prostate cancer. However, excessive amounts can lead to elevated blood pressure.

MUSHROOMS. There are a number of mushrooms that appear to help the body fight cancer and build the immune system. They include shiitake, maitake, reishi, *Agaricus blazei* Murill, and *Coriolus versicolor*. The active ingredients in medicinal mushrooms are polysaccharides called beta-glucans. These beta-glucans are powerful compounds that help in building immunity. Examples of beta-glucans include lentinan and a unique beta-glucan called D-fraction, that is found in the maitake mushroom. This D-fraction is believed to be responsible for the many health benefits of maitake. These mushrooms also have a **protein** called lectin, which attacks cancerous cells and prevents them from multiplying. They also contain thioproline. These mushrooms can stimulate the production of interferon in the body. Extracts from mushrooms have been successfully tested in recent years in Japan as an adjunct to chemotherapy.

NUTS. Many nuts contain the antioxidants quercetin and campferol that may suppress the growth of cancers. Brazil nuts contain 80 micrograms of **selenium**, which is important for those with prostate cancer.

ORANGES AND LEMONS. Oranges and lemons both contain limonene, which stimulates cancer-killing immune cells like lymphocytes that may also function in breaking down cancer-causing substances.

PAPAYAS. They have vitamin C, which is an antioxidant and may also reduce absorption of cancer-causing nitrosamines from the soil or processed foods. Papaya contains folacin (also known as folic acid), which has been shown to minimize cervical dysplasia and certain cancers.

RED WINE. Red wine has polyphenols that may protect against various types of cancer. Polyphenols are potent antioxidants, compounds that help neutralize disease-causing free radicals. Also, researchers at the University of North Carolina's Medical School in Chapel Hill found the compound resveratrol, which is present in grape skins. It appears that resveratrol inhibits cell proliferation and can help prevent cancer. However, the findings didn't extend to heavy imbibers, so wine should be used in moderation. In addition, alcohol can be toxic to the liver and to the nervous system, and many wines have sulfites, which may be harmful to your health.

ROSEMARY. Rosemary may help increase the activity of detoxification enzymes. An extract of rosemary, termed carnosol, has inhibited the development of both breast and skin tumors in animals. No comparable studies have as yet been conducted on humans. Rosemary can be used as a seasoning and it can also be consumed as a tea.

SEAWEED AND OTHER SEA VEGETABLES. Sea vegetables contain beta-carotene, protein, **vitamin B₁₂**, fiber, and chlorophyll, as well as chlorophylones, which are important fatty acids that may help combat breast cancer. Many sea vegetables also have high concentrations of the minerals potassium, calcium, magnesium, **iron**, and **iodine**.

SOY PRODUCTS. Soy products like tofu contain several types of phytoestrogens which are weak, non-steroidal estrogens that resemble some of the body's natural hormones. These compounds could help prevent both breast and prostate cancer by blocking and suppressing cancerous changes. There are a number of isoflavones in soy products, but research has shown that genistein is the most potent inhibitor of the growth and spread of cancerous cells. It appears to lower breast cancer risk by inhibiting the growth of epithelial cells and new blood vessels that tumors require to flourish, and is being scrutinized as a potential anticancer drug. However, there are some precautions to consider when adding soy to the diet. Eating up to four or five ounces of tofu or other soy products a day is probably fine, but research is being done to see if loading up on soy could cause hormone imbalances that stimulate cancer growth. As a precaution, women who have breast cancer or are at high risk should talk

---

KEY TERMS

Antioxidant—A molecule that prevents oxidation. In the body antioxidants attach to other molecules called free radicals and prevent the free radicals from causing damage to cell walls, DNA, and other parts of the cell.

Carcinogen—A cancer-causing substance.

Carotenoids—Fat-soluble plant pigments, some of which are important to human health.

Free radical—An unstable, highly reactive molecule that occurs naturally as a result of cellular metabolism, but can be increased by environmental toxins, ultraviolet rays, and nuclear radiation. Free radicals damage cellular DNA and are thought to play a role in aging, cancer, and other diseases. Free radicals can be neutralized by antioxidants.

Phytochemical—A nonnutritive bioactive plant substance, such as a flavonoid or carotenoid, considered to have a beneficial effect on human health.

---

to their doctors before taking pure isoflavone powder and pills, which are extracted from soy.

SWEET POTATOES. Sweet potatoes contain many anticancer properties, including beta-carotene, which may protect DNA in the cell nucleus from cancer-causing chemicals outside the nuclear membrane.

TEAS. Green tea and black tea contain certain antioxidants known as polyphenols (catechins) which appear to prevent cancer cells from dividing. Green tea is best, followed by black tea (herbal teas do not show this benefit). According to a report in the July 2001 issue of the *Journal of Cellular Biochemistry*, the polyphenols that are abundant in green tea, red wine, and olive oil may protect against various types of cancer. Study findings have suggested that dry green tea leaves, which are about 40% polyphenols by weight, may also reduce the risk of cancer of the stomach, lung, colon, rectum, liver, and pancreas.

TOMATOES. Tomatoes contain lycopene, an antioxidant that attacks roaming oxygen molecules, known as free radicals, which are suspected of triggering cancer. Lycopene appears to be more easily absorbed if the tomatoes are eaten in processed form—either as tomato sauce, paste, or juice. It appears that the hotter the weather, the more lycopene tomatoes produce. Lycopene has been shown to be especially potent in combating prostate cancer and may also protect against breast, lung, stomach, and pancreatic cancer. Scientists in Israel have shown that lycopene can kill mouth cancer cells. An increased intake of lycopene has already been linked to a reduced risk of breast, prostate, pancreas, and colorectal cancer. Recent studies indicate that for proper absorption, the body also needs some oil along with lycopene. Tomatoes also have vitamin C, an antioxidant that can prevent cellular damage that leads to cancer. Watermelons, carrots, and red peppers also contain these substances, but in lesser quantities. It is concentrated by cooking tomatoes.

TUMERIC. Tumeric is a member of the ginger family and is believed to have medicinal properties. Tumeric appears to inhibit the production of the inflammation-related enzyme cyclo-oxygenase 2 (COX-2), which reaches abnormally high levels in certain inflammatory diseases and cancers, especially bowel and colon cancer. A pharmaceutical company (Phytopharm in the United Kingdom) hopes to introduce a natural product, P54, that contains certain volatile oils, which greatly increase the potency of the turmeric spice.

WHOLE GRAINS. **Whole grains** contain a variety of anticancer compounds, including fiber, antioxidants, and phytoestrogens. When eaten as part of a balanced diet, whole grains can help decrease the risk of developing most types of cancer.

AICR superfoods

The American Institute of Cancer Research (AICR) maintains a list of foods thought to fight cancer. The list is constantly updated based on high-quality research and provides references to recent studies. As of 2012, the list included:

- apples
- beans
- berries (açaí, blueberries, cranberries, blackberries, raspberries, strawberries)
- broccoli and other cruciferous vegetables
- dark green leafy vegetables (spinach, kale)

- flaxseed
- garlic
- grapes and grape juice
- green tea
- legumes (dry beans, peas, lentils)
- soy
- tomatoes
- whole grains
- winter squash

Expected to be added soon were:

- carrots
- cherries
- chili peppers
- citrus fruits (oranges, lemons, grapefruit)
- melons
- mushrooms
- nuts
- onions
- papayas
- pomegranates
- sweet potatoes

Precautions

A considerable amount of information and knowledge has been accumulated regarding cancer-fighting foods. No single food or food substance alone can protect an individual against cancer, but the right combination of plant-based foods in the diet can greatly increase the chances of avoiding cancer. Evidence is mounting that the minerals, vitamins, antioxidants, and phytochemicals in many plant foods interact to provide extra cancer protection by working synergistically in the body. For this reason, many nutrition scientists recommend that at least two-thirds of a person's diet should consist of vegetables, fruits, whole grains, and beans.

High intakes of individual vitamins can carry specific risks in certain people—for example, high levels of beta-carotene may increase the risk of lung cancer in smokers.

Parental concerns

Children can greatly benefit from a diet rich in cancer-fighting foods. The healthy diet will promote a lifetime of good health as well as encourage proper growth. However, vitamin supplementation is not recommended outside of a physician's or registered dietitian's care as children have different vitamin requirements and the level of doses appropriate for an adult may not be the same for a child.

Resources

BOOKS

Béliveau, Richard, and Denis Gingras. *Foods That Fight Cancer: Preventing Cancer Through Diet*. London: Dorling Kindersley, 2007.

Greenwood-Robinson, Maggie. *Foods That Combat Cancer: The Nutritional Way to Wellness*. New York: Avon Books, HarperCollins, 2003.

Kushi, Michio. *The Cancer Prevention Diet, Revised and Updated Edition: The Macrobiotic Approach to Preventing and Relieving Cancer*. New York: St. Martin's Press, 2009.

Quillin, Patrick, and Noreen Quillin. *Beating Cancer with Nutrition*. 4th ed. Tulsa, OK: Nutrition Times Press, 2007.

Varona, Verne. *Nature's Cancer-Fighting Foods*. New York: Penguin Putnam Inc., 2001.

PERIODICALS

Ding, Haiming, et al. "Chemopreventive Characteristics of Avocado Fruit." *Seminars in Cancer Biology* 17, no. 5 (2007): 386–94. http://dx.doi.org/10.1016/j.semcancer.2007.04.003 (accessed August 14, 2012).

Gonzalez, C. A., and E. Riboli. "Diet and Cancer Prevention: Contributions from the European Prospective Investigation into Cancer and Nutrition (EPIC) Study." *European Journal of Cancer* 46, no. 14 (2010): 2555–2562.

OTHER

World Cancer Research Fund (WCRF) and American Institute for Cancer Research (AICR). *Food, Nutrition, Physical Activity, and the Prevention of Cancer: a Global Perspective*. Washington, DC: AICR, 2007. http://www.dietandcancerreport.org/cancer_resource_center/downloads/Second_Expert_Report_full.pdf (accessed August 14, 2012).

WEBSITES

American Institute for Cancer Research. "AICR's Foods That Fight Cancer." http://www.aicr.org/foods-that-fight-cancer (accessed August 9, 2012).

Carollo, Kim. "Could Cancer Prevention Someday Be As Easy As Eating Strawberries?" ABC News, April 6, 2011. http://abcnews.go.com/Health/strawberries-prevent-esophageal-cancer/story?id=13308917 (accessed August 14, 2012).

National Health Service in England (NHS). "5 A DAY." http://www.nhs.uk/Livewell/5ADAY/Pages/5ADAYhome.aspx (accessed August 14, 2012).

Paul, Maya W., and Melinda Smith. "The Anti-Cancer Diet: Cancer Prevention Nutrition Tips and Cancer-Fighting Foods." Helpguide.org. http://www.helpguide.org/life/healthy_diet_cancer_prevention.htm (accessed August 9, 2012).

ORGANIZATIONS

American Cancer Society, 250 Williams St. NW, Atlanta, GA 30303, (800) 227-2345, http://www.cancer.org.

American Institute for Cancer Research, 1759 R Street NW, Washington, DC 20009, (800) 843-8114, aicrweb@aicr.org, http://www.aicr.org.

The Cancer Cure Foundation, PO Box 3782, Westlake Village, CA 91359, (800) 282-2873, webmaster@cancure.org, http://www.cancure.org/home.htm.

National Cancer Institute, 6116 Executive Blvd., Ste. 300, Bethesda, MD 20892-8322, (800) 4-CANCER (422-6237), http://www.cancer.gov.

Thomas Prychitko
David Newton

Carbohydrate addict's diet

Definition

The carbohydrate addict's diet is an eating plan that emphasizes foods low in **carbohydrates** (carbs). It is based on the theory that some people develop unmanageable **cravings** for high-carb foods due to the pancreas producing too much of the hormone **insulin**, and that regular consumption of these foods leads to weight gain.

Origins

American research scientists Rachael Heller and Richard Heller developed the carbohydrate addict's diet in the early 1990s after they lost a combined 200 lb. (75 kg) on the diet. Both Hellers are professors and researchers specializing in biomedical sciences. They outlined their method in their first book, *The Carbohydrate Addict's Diet*, published in 1991. They have since expanded upon the diet in subsequent books and several updates of the original book. The term "carbohydrate addiction" was coined in 1963 by Robert Kemp, a biochemist at Yale University.

Description

The carbohydrate addict's diet is based on the theory that balancing insulin levels in the body will lead to reduced insulin resistance and less cravings for foods high in carbohydrates. The diet has two steps: reduce the amount of high-carbohydrate foods consumed and regulate insulin levels by using **dietary supplements**. Although the Hellers recommend an exercise program with the diet, there is not a major emphasis on exercise. The Hellers define carbohydrate addiction as a compelling hunger, craving, or desire for foods high in carbohydrates, or an escalating and recurring need for starchy foods, snack foods, junk foods, and sweets.

These foods include breads, bagels, cakes, cereals, chocolate, cookies, crackers, pastry, fruit and fruit juices, ice cream, potato chips, pasta, potatoes, pretzels, rice, pies, popcorn, and sugar-sweetened beverages. The Hellers also advocate avoiding **sugar** substitutes (Equal, NutraSweet, Splenda), which they believe causes the body to release insulin and to store fat.

The Hellers claim that carbohydrate addiction is caused by an overproduction of insulin when foods high in carbohydrates are eaten. The insulin tells the body to take in more food and once the food is eaten, the insulin signals the body to store the extra food energy as fat, according to the Hellers. When too much insulin is released after eating, it is called postprandial reactive hyperinsulinemia. Over time, some people with this condition develop insulin resistance, where cells in tissue stop responding to insulin. Normally, insulin helps the body process glucose, or sugar. In insulin resistance, the body continues to produce insulin but is unable to use the glucose (sugar) properly. Insulin resistance often occurs with other health problems, including diabetes, high cholesterol, high **triglycerides**, high blood pressure, and cardiovascular disease. Insulin resistance syndrome is the occurrence of more than one of these diseases together.

There is no medical test that indicates carbohydrate addiction, so the Hellers developed a self-administered quiz to determine if a person is a carbohydrate addict. The quiz, which is available in their books and on their Website, asks ten "yes" or "no" questions, such as "Is it hard to stop eating starches, snack foods, junk food, or sweets?" Scoring of the quiz is based on the number of "yes" answers. A score of 0–2 indicates no carbohydrate addiction, a score of 3–4 suggests a mild carbohydrate addiction, a score of 5–7 suggests a moderate addiction, and a score of 8–10 indicates severe addiction.

The carbohydrate addict's diet begins with the entry plan, which allows two complementary meals and one reward meal each day for the first week. In subsequent weeks, the diet is adjusted depending on a person's weight loss goal and amount of weight lost in the previous week. The diet also allows for a snack and salads. The complementary meal is composed of one serving of meat and two cups of low-carb vegetables or two cups of salad. There is an extensive list of meats and vegetables to choose from. The reward meal can be as large as the person wants but it must be composed of equal portions of **protein**, low-carb vegetables, and high-carb foods (including dessert). The reward meal must be eaten in an hour. A snack is the same as a complementary meal but half the size. The diet allows for an unlimited amount of water, diet drinks, and unsweetened coffee and tea.

KEY TERMS

Carbohydrates—A nutrient that the body uses as an energy source. A carbohydrate provides 4 calories of energy per gram.

Cardiovascular—Pertaining to the heart and blood vessels.

Cholesterol—A waxy substance made by the liver and also acquired through diet. High levels in the blood may increase the risk of cardiovascular disease.

Endocrinologist—A medical specialist who treats diseases of the endocrine (glands) system, including diabetes.

Insulin—A hormone that regulates the level of glucose (sugar) in the blood.

Pancreas—A digestive gland of the endocrine system that regulates and produces several hormones, including insulin.

Post-prandial reactive hyperinsulinemia—A condition resulting from excess insulin production after eating.

The Hellers claim that few people need to eat breakfast, which goes against the advice of all major medical and dietetic organizations. Skipping breakfast is not widely recommended by registered dietitians.

The Hellers offer two different carbohydrate addict's diets for children and teenagers. Both are outlined in the Hellers' book *Carbohydrate-Addicted Kids*. On the step-by-step carbohydrate addict's diet, children go at a slower pace, and are offered additional food incentives besides the rewards meal. The jump-start carbohydrate addict's diet is designed for older children and teens. It offers foods high in **fiber** and protein for meals and snacks. Like the adult diet, it provides a reward meal in which dieters can eat anything they want, provided it is equal portions of protein, low-carb vegetables, and high-carb foods. The book also provides information on meals for special occasions, such as birthdays, holidays, vacations, and other celebrations. The diets for adolescents also have a vegetarian component.

Function

The premise of the carbohydrate addict's diet is to correct the excess release of insulin, which occurs following consumption of foods high in carbohydrates. The Hellers claim that this triggers an intense and recurring craving for more carbohydrate-rich foods. The diet is designed to correct the underlying cause of the cravings.

Benefits

The primary benefit of the carbohydrate addict's diet is the control of cravings and weight loss. The diet is less strict than other low-carb diets, such as the **Atkins diet**, since it allows for one meal a day with three equal portions of foods high in carbohydrates, high in protein, and low in carbohydrates. The carbohydrate addict's diet is suitable for vegetarians (though not vegans) since it allows for low-fat cheeses, egg whites, egg substitutes, and tofu.

Precautions

Like any strict diet, the carbohydrate addict's diet should be undertaken with the supervision of a doctor. People with diabetes should consult an endocrinologist, who may recommend discussing the diet with a registered dietitian. Children and adolescents should not follow the carbohydrate addict's diet unless recommended by a physician.

Risks

Critics of the diet claim that it contains too much fat, is not nutritionally balanced, and is not a long-term solution for losing weight and keeping it off. It may be difficult for people to maintain a low-carb diet over the long-term. The diet is not recommended for women who are pregnant or nursing. Individuals who have a history of stroke, diabetes, heart disease, high cholesterol, or kidney stones should talk to their doctor before starting a low-carb diet.

Research and general acceptance

There is mixed acceptance of the carbohydrate addict's diet and low-carb diets in general by the medical community and dietitians. Some studies have shown that low-carb diets can be effective in controlling blood sugar levels in people with diabetes and in helping people lose weight. Other studies have contradicted these findings. Most professional organizations, including the U.S. federal dietary recommendations, do not support low-carb diets.

A 2003 study by researchers at the University of Pennsylvania School of Medicine found that a low-carb diet produced a greater weight loss than a conventional low-calorie, **low-fat diet** after six months. However, after one year, the two diets produced similar weight loss results. A 2004 study by the same medical center found that both a low-carb and a more conventional diet produced similar weight loss results after one year but that a low-carb diet improved the health of people with atherogenic dyslipidemia, a cholesterol disorder characterized by the elevation of triglycerides and a decrease in "good cholesterol" high-density lipoprotein (HDL) levels in the blood. This lipid disorder is associated with an increased risk of developing cardiovascular disease. Individuals participating in the study also had better control of blood sugar levels.

Resources

BOOKS

Heller, Richard F., and Rachael F. Heller. *The Carbohydrate Addict's Carbohydrate Counter.* New York: Signet, 2000.
———. *The Carbohydrate Addict's Diet.* New York: Vermilion, 2000.
———. *The Carbohydrate Addict's Healthy Heart Program: Break Your Carbo-Insulin Connection to Heart Disease.* New York: Ballantine Books, 2000.
———. *The Carbohydrate Addict's LifeSpan Program.* New York: Signet, 2001.
———. *The Carbohydrate Addict's No Cravings Cookbook.* New York: NAL Trade, 2006.
———. *The Carbohydrate Addict's 7-Day Plan: Start Fresh On Your Low-Carb Diet!* New York: Signet, 2004.
———. *Carbohydrate-Addicted Kids: Help Your Child or Teen Break Free of Junk Food and Sugar Cravings—For Life!* New York: Harper Paperback, 1998.

PERIODICALS

Baron, Melissa. "Fighting Obesity: Part 1: Review of Popular Low-Carb Diets." *Health Care Food & Nutrition Focus* (October 2004): 5.
Belden, Heidi. "Sticks and Kidney Stones; As Low-Carb, High-Protein Diets Grow in Popularity, the Risk of Developing Kidney Stones Rises As Well." *Drug Topics* (September 13, 2004): 36.
Bell, John R. "Jury Out on Value of Low-Carb Diets." *Family Practice News* (March 15, 2006): 20.

Chernikoff, Lisa. "Low-Carb Mania: A University of Michigan Expert Explains Why Low-Carb Diets are Not the Best Choice." *American Fitness* (May–June 2004): 45–48.

Last, Allen R., and Stephen A. Wilson. "Low-Carbohydrate Diets." *American Family Physician* (June 1, 2006): 1942–48.

Marks, Jennifer B. "The Weighty Issue of Low-Carb Diets, or Is the Carbohydrate the Enemy?" *Clinical Diabetes* (Fall 2004): 155–56.

Martin, C.K., et al. "Change in Food Cravings, Food Preferences, and Appetite During a Low-Carbohydrate and Low-Fat Diet." *Obesity* 19, no. 10 (2011): 1963–70. http://dx.doi.org/10.1038/oby.2011.62 (accessed September 20, 2012).

Shaughnessy, Allen F. "Low-Carb Diets Are Equal to Low-Fat Diets for Weight Loss." *American Family Physician* (June 1, 2006): 2020.

Sullivan, Michele G. "Teens Lose More Weight With Less Effort on Low-Carb Diets vs. Low-Fat Diets." *Family Practice News* (June 15, 2004): 64.

ORGANIZATIONS

Academy of Nutrition and Dietetics, 120 South Riverside Plz., Ste. 2000, Chicago, IL 60606-6995, (312) 899-0040, (800) 877-1600, amacmunn@eatright.org, http://www.eatright.org.

American Society for Nutrition, 9650 Rockville Pike, Bethesda, MD 20814, (301) 634-7050, Fax: (301) 634-7894, http://www.nutrition.org.

Ken R. Wells

Carbohydrates	
Refined and processed carbohydrates	**Whole grain and high-fiber carbohydrates**
White bread	100% whole wheat bread
White rice	Oatmeal
White potatoes	Brown rice
Pasta	Whole wheat pasta
Sugary cereals	Whole grain crackers
Cinnamon toast	Popcorn
Sweets	Cornmeal
Jellies	Hulled barley
Candy	Whole wheat bulgur
Soft drinks	Bran cereals
Sugars	Rye wafer crackers
Fruit drinks (fruitades and fruit punch)	English muffins
Cakes, cookies and pies	Dry beans and peas
Dairy desserts	Navy beans
Ice cream	Kidney beans
Sweetened yogurt	Split peas
Sweetened milk	Lentils
	White beans
	Pinto beans
	Green peas
	Soybeans
	Whole fruits, fresh, frozen or canned
	Vegetables
	Low-fat milk

(Table by GGS Information Services. © 2013 Cengage Learning.)

Carbohydrates

Definition

Carbohydrates are compounds that consist of carbon, hydrogen, and oxygen, linked together by energy-containing bonds. There are two types of carbohydrates: complex and simple. The complex carbohydrates, such as starch and **fiber**, are classified as polysaccharides. Simple carbohydrates are known as sugars and they are classified as either monosaccharides (one **sugar** molecule) or disaccharides (two sugar molecules). All carbohydrates are made from these simple sugars. The term "complex" depends on the molecular structure—if the carbohydrate is composed of more than two simple sugars forming a straight or branched chain of monosaccharides, it is considered complex.

Purpose

The primary role of carbohydrates in human nutrition is to supply the body with the energy needed to sustain life. Glucose is the body's primary source of energy, and glycogen is the stored form of glucose. In the human body, every cell depends on glucose for its fuel to some extent, with the cells of the brain and nervous system depending primarily on glucose as their energy source. For cells to function properly, the body must maintain blood glucose at high enough levels to support the cells. If glucose levels become too low, the body feels dizzy and weak; if levels are too high, a person may feel tired, confused, and have difficulty breathing. Blood glucose levels that are too low or too high may result in death if left untreated.

Description

Carbohydrates are one of the three major food groups, along with proteins and **fats**. They are essential to human life and health. Carbohydrates provide four **calories** per gram (g) and come almost exclusively from fruits, vegetables, legumes, and grains. Milk is the only animal-based product that contains a significant amount of carbohydrate. Simple carbohydrates include the single sugars, or monosaccharides, and the double sugars, or disaccharides. The monosaccharides include glucose, fructose, and galactose. Disaccharides include lactose, which is made of glucose and galactose; maltose, made of two glucose units; and sucrose, made of glucose and fructose. Glucose is the only sugar that can be absorbed in the mouth. Once in the small intestine, monosaccharides can be absorbed directly into the bloodstream, but disaccharides need to be broken down into their monosaccharide components before they can be absorbed.

When food is eaten, the digestion of carbohydrates begins in the mouth, where an enzyme in saliva (amylase) breaks down the starch molecules into shorter polysaccharides and the disaccharide maltose. The food then moves into the stomach, where it mixes with the stomach's acid and other juices and digestion of carbohydrates stops. The majority of carbohydrate digestion occurs in the small intestine. Starch is further broken down into glucose chains and disaccharides by pancreatic amylase. Cells lining the small intestine secrete the enzymes maltase, sucrase, and lactase, which further split these disaccharides and polysaccharides into monosaccharides. The cells lining the small intestine can absorb these monosaccharides, which are then taken to the liver. The liver converts fructose and galactose to glucose. If there is an excess of fructose or galactose, it may also be converted to fat. Lastly, the glucose is transported to the body's cells by the circulatory system, where it can be used for energy.

When there is an excess of glucose, the muscle and liver cells often convert it to glycogen, which is the form in which glucose is stored in the body. The muscles store two-thirds of the body's glycogen solely for their own use, and the liver stores the other one-third, which can be used by the brain or other organs when needed. When blood glucose levels decline, the body breaks down some of its glycogen stores and uses the glucose for energy. If blood glucose (sugar) levels are too high, the excess glucose is taken to the liver where it is converted into glycogen or fat and stored for future use.

Fiber

Fiber is the general term used to describe the non-starchy polysaccharides cellulose, hemicelluloses, pectins, gums, and mucilages in plant foods. It is also a term used for the nonpolysaccharides lignins, cutins, and tannins. They are usually categorized as either water insoluble, cellulose, hemicelluloses, or lignin. Gums, pectin, some hemicelluloses, and mucilages are called water soluble. Even though these compounds cannot be digested by human digestive enzymes, some are further broken down by the gut bacteria to short-chain fatty acids that yield a small portion of energy when metabolized and serve several important functions in human health. Insoluble fibers are found in high concentrations in wheat, cereals, and vegetables,

and their main function in human physiology is to assist in the movement of waste through the intestines and to increase fecal weight. They also bind with bile acids, which reduces fat and cholesterol absorption. Soluble fiber helps decrease low-density lipoprotein (LDL) cholesterol levels, also called "bad" cholesterol, and delays the stomach emptying, promoting satiety. It can be found in barley, fruit, legumes, and oats.

Fiber is an extremely important part of the diet. It aids in weight control by displacing calorie-dense fats. Fiber also absorbs water and slows the movement of food through the digestive tract, promoting a feeling of fullness. It improves large intestine function and health and may help prevent colon **cancer** and lower blood cholesterol levels. It also helps to reduce the glycemic response (how fast foods are turned into glucose). Too much fiber, however, may result in abdominal discomfort and lower nutrient availability.

Recommended intake

The Institute of Medicine of the National Academy of Sciences has established ranges for the percentage of calories in the diet that should come from carbohydrates. The acceptable macronutrient distribution ranges (AMDR) take into account both chronic disease risk reduction and required intake of essential nutrients. For carbohydrates, the AMDR is 45%–65% of daily caloric need for people older than age one, though percentages can vary depending on age, general health, certain diseases and conditions, and activity level. Of this intake, it is further recommended that half or more of grains consumed come from **whole grains**. The Adequate Intake (AI) level for fiber is 14 g per 1,000 calories, or about 25 g per day for women and 38 g per day for men. The U.S. Department of Agriculture's (USDA) *Dietary Guidelines for Americans* suggests that half of a person's plate be filled with fruits and vegetables at each meal and recommends consuming legumes in place of red meat on occasion. According to the American Heart Association guidelines, the recommended sugar intake for adult women is 5 teaspoons (20 g) of sugar per day; for adult men, 9 teaspoons (36 g) per day; and for children, 3 teaspoons (12 g) a day.

Precautions

A common concern among consumers is that high intake of carbohydrates will cause weight gain. Consuming too much of any particular food can cause an increase in weight, but eating a balanced diet with plenty of fruits, vegetables, and grains will help support weight management. Many of the carbohydrates

KEY TERMS

Dietary fiber—Also known as roughage or bulk. Insoluble fiber moves through the digestive system almost undigested and gives bulk to stools. Soluble fiber dissolves in water and helps keep stools soft.

Glucose—A simple sugar that results from the breakdown of carbohydrates. Glucose circulates in the blood and is the main source of energy for the body.

Glycogen—The storage form of glucose found in the liver and muscles.

Starch—A naturally abundant nutrient carbohydrate found in seeds, fruits, tubers, and roots.

consumed in the United States are made with high amounts of fat, **sodium**, and added sugars, which can promote weight gain. High-fructose corn syrup (HFCS) in particular is used in many foods in the United States. HFCS was first developed in the mid-1960s and, because of its unique physical and functional properties, was widely embraced by food formulators. The use of HFCS increased rapidly over the next 30 years, primarily used as a replacement for sucrose (table sugar). Since 1999, use of HFCS has declined somewhat due to noted adverse health concerns associated with its intake. Studies have shown that adults who consumed 25% of their daily calories as fructose or HFCS beverages (a percentage within current government guidelines) for two weeks experienced increases in serum levels of cholesterol and **triglycerides** (fatty acids in the blood). Other negative health claims associated with a high intake of fructose and/or HFCS include raised serum uric acid levels; increased risk of developing gout, dementia, cardiovascular disease, and high blood pressure; and accumulation of central fat storage. Smaller studies have also shown that it may play a role in the development of non-alcoholic fatty liver disease. Fructose is not only to blame—studies have also shown some of these same effects, such as central fat storage and increased blood pressure, with high intakes of other sugars. Regardless of form, when sugar displaces other nutrient dense foods and/or adds extra calories, usually through sweetened beverages, it has been shown to be a determinant of **obesity** and predicts the risk of developing cardiometabolic disease.

Interactions

Some people lack the enzyme lactase, which is required to break down the disaccharide lactose into glucose and galactose. This is termed lactose intolerance. People with lactose intolerance cannot consume dairy products, or else they will experience uncomfortable side effects such as bloating, abdominal discomfort, and diarrhea.

People on a **high-fiber diet** may lose **minerals** that become bound to phytic acid, which comes from husks of legumes, grains, and seeds and binds to **zinc**, **iron**, **calcium**, **magnesium**, and **copper**. These minerals then get excreted from the body unused, which could have health consequences, though this is not common in people consuming a well-balanced diet.

Complications

When carbohydrate intake is low, there is insufficient glucose production, which then causes the body to use its storage of fat and **protein** for energy. This ultimately prevents the body's protein from performing its more important functions, such as maintaining the body's immune system. Without carbohydrates, the body may go into a state of ketosis, in which byproducts of fat (called ketones) break down and accumulate in the blood. This causes a shift in the acid-base balance of the blood, which can be dangerous if left untreated.

Parental concerns

Parents can consult with a pediatrician, physician, registered dietitian (RD), or endocrinologist if they suspect that their child suffers from low or high blood sugar levels or if they have questions about **children's diets**. Parents should try to limit their child's consumption of added sugars, especially from sugared beverages, and refined grains. They should not attempt to place their child on a diet without consulting with a healthcare professional.

Resources

BOOKS

Collins, P. M. *Dictionary of Carbohydrates*. Boca Raton, FL: Chapman & Hall, 2005.

Eliasson, Ann-Charlotte. *Carbohydrates in Food*. 2nd ed. Boca Raton, FL: CRC Press, 2006.

Warshaw, Hope S., and Karen M. Bolderman. *Practical Carbohydrate Counting*. Alexandria, VA: American Diabetes Association, 2007.

Wrolstad, Ronald E. *Food Carbohydrate Chemistry*. Hoboken, NJ: Wiley-Blackwell, 2012.

PERIODICALS

"Continuing Carb Controversy: Are Carbohydrates the Culprits in Diabetes and Obesity?" *Food & Fitness Advisor* (July 2006): 3.

Govindji, Azmina. "Sugar-Sweetened Beverages and Risk of Obesity and Type 2 Diabetes: Epidemiologic Evidence." *Nursing Standard* 21, no. 3 (2006): 56–64.

Lattimer, James M., and Mark D. Haub. "Effects of Dietary Fiber and Its Components on Metabolic Health." *Nutrients* 2, no. 12 (2010): 1266–89. http://dx.doi.org/10.3390/nu2121266 (accessed September 21, 2012).

Lin, W.T, et al. "Effects on Uric Acid, Body Mass Index and Blood Pressure in Adolescents of [sic] Consuming Beverages Sweetened with High-Fructose Corn Syrup." *International Journal of Obesity* (August 14, 2012): e-pub ahead of print. http://dx.doi.org/10.1038/ijo.2012.121 (accessed September 21, 2012).

Moon, Mary Ann. "High-Carb, Low-Glycemic Index Diet Cuts Weight, Cardiac Risk." *Family Practice News* 36, no. 17 (2006): 15.

WEBSITES

Centers for Disease Control and Prevention. "Carbohydrates." http://www.cdc.gov/nutrition/everyone/basics/carbs.html (accessed September 21, 2012).

Harvard School of Public Health. "Carbohydrates: Good Carbs Guide the Way." The Nutrition Source, Department of Nutrition, Harvard University. http://www.hsph.harvard.edu/nutritionsource/what-should-you-eat/carbohydrates-full-story/index.html (accessed September 21, 2012).

MedlinePlus. "Carbohydrates." U.S. National Library of Medicine, National Institutes of Health. http://www.nlm.nih.gov/medlineplus/carbohydrates.html (accessed September 21, 2012).

ORGANIZATIONS

Academy of Nutrition and Dietetics, 120 South Riverside Plz., Ste. 2000, Chicago, IL 60606-6995, (312) 899-0040, (800) 877-1600, amacmunn@eatright.org, http://www.eatright.org.

Food and Nutrition Information Center, National Agricultural Library, 10301 Baltimore Ave., Rm. 105, Beltsville, MD 20705, (301) 504-5414, Fax: (301) 504-6409, fnic@ars.usda.gov, http://fnic.nal.usda.gov.

U.S. Department of Agriculture, 1400 Independence Ave. SW, Washington, DC 20250, (202) 720-2791, http://www.usda.gov.

Ken R. Wells
David Newton

Popular dishes of selected Caribbean islands

Island	Special dishes
Antigua, Montserrat, Nevis	Fish soup, pepper pot soup (any available fish, meat, chicken, and vegetables cooked in fermented cassava juice), saltfish with avocado and eggplant
Barbados	Flying fish, jug-jug (mashed stew of pigeon peas, usually served at Christmas) Black pudding (a type of sausage made by combining cooked rice mixed with fresh pig's blood; seasoned with salt, pepper, and other condiments; placed in thoroughly cleaned pieces of pig's intestine; and tied on both ends and boiled in seasoned water)
Belize	Rice and chicken, tamales, conch fritters, refried beans and iswa (fresh corn tortillas)
Dominica	Tannia (coco, a starch tuber soup), mountain chicken (frog's legs)
Grenada	Callaloo (soup with green vegetables), Lambi souse (conch marinated in lime juice, hot pepper, onion), oil-down (a highly seasoned dish of coconut milk and salted fish)
Guyana	Mellagee (one-pot stew of pickled meat/fish and coconut milk with tubers and vegetables), rice treat (rice with shrimp, vegetables, and pineapple)
Jamaica	Saltfish and ackee (a fruit commonly used as a vegetable, boiled and then sautéed in oil), escoveitched fish (fried fish marinated in vinegar, spices, and seasoning), roasted breadfruit, asham or brown George (parched dried corn that is finely beaten in a mortar, sifted, and mixed with sugar)
St. Vincent and the Grenadines	Stewed shark
British Virgin Islands	Fish chowder, conch salad, saltfish and rice
Trinidad and Tobago	Pelau (rice with meat, fish, peas, vegetables), pakoras, kachouri, palouri (fried vegetable fritters)
Guadeloupe and Martinique	Mechoui (spit-roasted sheep), pate en pot (finely chopped sheep and lamb parts cooked into a thick, highly seasoned stew)

(Table by PreMediaGlobal. © 2013 Cengage Learning.)

Caribbean Islander diet

Definition

The Caribbean Islander diet refers to the culinary traditions of the Caribbean Islands, which include Anguilla, Antigua and Barbuda, Aruba, the Bahamas, Barbados, the British Virgin Islands, the Cayman Islands, Cuba, Dominica, the Dominican Republic, Grenada, Guadeloupe, Haiti, Honduras, Jamaica, Martinique, Montserrat, Netherlands Antilles, Saint Barthélemy, Saint Kitts and Nevis, Saint Lucia, Saint Martin, Saint Vincent and the Grenadines, Trinidad and Tobago, Turks and Caicos Islands, and the U.S. Virgin Islands, as well as many more small islands.

Origins

Travel advertisements for the Caribbean Islands portray long stretches of sun-drenched beaches and swaying palm trees, with people dancing to jazz, calypso, reggae, or meringue music. Indeed, the beauty, warmth, and lush landscapes had Christopher Columbus in awe in 1492 when he came upon these tropical islands, stretching approximately 2,600 miles between Florida and Venezuela.

European settlement

The Arawaks and Caribs, the first natives of the islands, were not treated kindly as the Spanish, French, Dutch, and British conquered the islands at different periods, all but wiping out the native populations. Today, only a few aboriginals remain in the Caribbean. The European settlers soon realized that sugarcane was a profitable crop that could be exported to the European market. However, there was a shortage of European farmers, and slaves were brought from Africa to work on the **sugar** plantations. The slave trade started in 1698. European settlers fought to keep their territories and hoped for great wealth, while actively pursuing the sugar and slave trades.

Two things changed the situation on the islands. In 1756, missionaries from Germany (Moravian Protestants) came to the islands, though the landowners were opposed to their presence, fearing that any education of the slaves could lead to a revolution. At about the same time, a German scientist by the name of Margraf discovered that sugar could be produced from beets, and many European countries began to produce their own sugar.

In 1772, after many revolts and uprisings, the Europeans began to free their slaves. The sugar plantations still needed laborers, however, and indentured workers were brought from China and India to work in the fields. Sugar cane and its by-products, molasses and rum, brought great prosperity to the settlers. However, not wanting to depend solely on sugar, they began to grow yams, maize, cloves, nutmeg, cinnamon, coconuts, and pineapples on a very large scale. Coffee also began to flourish. Many of the islands had wild pigs and cattle on them, and spiced, smoked meat became part of the diet. Today, jerk meat is a specialty.

Description

Foods of the Islands

The foods of the Caribbean are marked by a wide variety of fruits, vegetables, meats, grains, and spices, all of which contribute to the area's unique cuisine.

Foods of Creole, Chinese, African, Indian, Hispanic, and European origin blend harmoniously to produce mouth-watering dishes.

FRUITS AND VEGETABLES. There are many fruits and vegetables found in the various Caribbean Islands, and because many of them have been exported to North America and Europe, people in other countries have become familiar with them. This exotic array of fruits and vegetables in vibrant colors forms the heart of island cooking.

Chayote, also called Christophene or Cho-cho, is a firm pear-shaped squash used in soups and stews. The Chinese vegetable bokchoy (or pakchoy) has become widely used on the islands. Plantains, which resemble bananas, are roasted, sautéed, fried, and added to stews and soups. The breadfruit grows profusely and is either boiled or baked, sliced, and eaten hot, or ground into flour. Breadfruit blossoms make a very good preserve.

Yucca, also known as cassava or manioc, is a slender tuber with bark-like skin and a very starchy flesh that must be cooked and served like a potato, or it can be made into cassava bread. Mangoes can be picked from trees and eaten by peeling the skin and slicing the flesh off the large pit. They are used in salads, desserts, frozen drinks, and salsa. Papaya, which has a cantaloupe-like flavor, contains the enzyme papain, which aids in digestion. To be eaten, the black seeds must be removed and the flesh scooped out.

The soursop is a large, oval, dark-green fruit with a thick skin that is soft to the touch when it ripens. The fruit has a creamy flesh with a sweet, tart flavor. Its rich custard-like flavor can be made into a sherbet, ice cream, or refreshing drink.

SPICES AND CONDIMENTS. Many foods of the Caribbean are highly spiced. The Scotch bonnet, a colorful pepper with a hot aroma, is widely used in soups, salads, sauces, and marinades. Some other important spices are annatto, curry, pimento, cinnamon, and ginger. Annatto seeds are often steeped in oil and used to flavor soups, stews, and fish dishes. Curry powder is made from a variety of freshly grounded spices. Curry dishes and hot sauces, which are used regularly in cooking, were brought to the islands by Indian settlers.

Pimento, also known as allspice, is used in pickles, marinades, soups, and stews and is an important ingredient in jerking, a method of cooking meat and poultry over an open fire. To bring out the flavor of meat and chicken, they are marinated in a mixture of scallions, garlic, thyme, onion, lemon juice, and salt. The spices and the method of slow cooking over a fire give jerk meat its distinctive flavor.

PROTEIN. Although fish, conch (a pink shellfish), goat meat, pork, and beef are used throughout the Caribbean, legumes make up a fair percentage of the region's **protein** intake. Kidney and lima beans, chickpeas, lentils, black-eyed peas, and other legumes are used in soups, stews, and rice dishes. Accra fritters, made from soaked black-eyed peas that are mashed, seasoned with pepper, and then fried, is a dish of West African origin similar to the Middle Eastern falafel. Sancocho is a hearty Caribbean stew made with vegetables, tubers, and meats.

COOKING METHODS. A "cook-up" dish is one made with whatever ingredients an individual has on hand, and presents an opportunity to be creative. Such a dish will often include rice, vegetables, and possibly meat. By adding coconut milk, this could turn into an enticing coconut-scented pilaf. Burning sugar to color stews is another technique used in island cooking. This process begins by heating oil, then adding sugar, and stirring until the sugar becomes an amber color.

The roti is a griddle-baked flour wrapping that is filled with curried meat, chicken, or potatoes. Coucou, or fungi, is a cornmeal mush that is served with meat, poultry, fish, or vegetable dishes.

BEVERAGES AND DESSERTS. A variety of fruit beverages are often served in the Caribbean. Beverages include **green tea** and "bush tea," served sweetened with sugar or honey and with or without milk. Bush tea is an infusion of tropical shrubs, grasses, and leaves that has a number of medicinal uses. People drink it as a remedy for gas, the common cold, asthma, high blood pressure, fever, and other ailments. Sweetened commercial drinks made from carrot, beet, guava, tamarind, and other fruits and vegetables are also popular.

A number of fermented drinks are also popular. *Garapina* is made from pineapple peelings, while *mauby* is made from the bark of the mauby tree. Grated ginger is used to produce ginger beer. *Horlicks* is a malted milk made with barley.

Fruit is eaten anytime of the day but is not considered a dessert unless prepared in a fruit salad or some other form. Coconut and banana form the basis for many desserts. A sweet pudding that goes by many names (e.g., duckunoo, blue drawers, pain me, paimee, and konkee) is made from grated banana, plantain, or sweet potato, which is then sugared, spiced, mixed with coconut milk or grated coconut, wrapped in banana leaves, and boiled in spiced water. A prepared sweet pone (pudding) cake or pie is a popular dessert. Black fruitcake, made from dried fruits soaked in wine, is popular at Christmas time, and is also used for weddings and other celebrations.

Health issues

In the Caribbean region, nutrition-related chronic diseases are common, threatening the well-being of the people of the islands. In the 1950s, the governments of the Caribbean were concerned about the **malnutrition** that permeated the region. They were able to meet the protein and calorie needs by making meat, **fats**, oils, and refined sugar more readily available. The health and nutrition initiatives introduced helped curb the malnutrition, but new and related health and nutrition problems began to emerge.

The health administrators of the Caribbean region are concerned with the rise of iron-deficiency anemia in pregnant women and school-aged children due to inadequate **iron** intake and poor absorption in the body. The increased incidence of diabetes, **hypertension**, **coronary heart disease**, **cancer**, and **obesity**, especially in people aged 35 and older, is thought to be directly linked to the existing lifestyle and dietary practices of the islanders.

The Caribbean Islands have seen a proliferation of fast-food restaurants, and the increased consumption of meals high in fat, sugar, and salt has contributed to the increase in chronic diseases. In addition, there has been a reduction in the amount of cereals, grains, fruits, vegetables, tubers, and legumes that are eaten. The popularity of fast foods among the youth has led the government to focus on improving nutrition in the schools. Also contributing to the health problems is the dependency on costly imported processed foods that can do the body harm. Overconsumption of imported foods high in fat and **sodium** has led to a deterioration of the health status of people throughout the region, with an increase in health problems such as obesity, diabetes, hypertension, cardiovascular disease, and cancer.

Nutrition programs

Due to insufficient resources and less than adequate planning, school-feeding programs on most of the islands exhibit many shortcomings. However, on the island of Dominica, where a self-help initiative involving the parents was introduced, the eating habits of school-aged children improved and the parents and communities adopted many of the program's menus and preparation methods. As a result, school attendance increased and the attention span of the children in class improved.

School nutrition programs need constant monitoring to improve the nutritional status of the children involved. Furthermore, a good nutrition promotion campaign must be designed to educate and promote a healthy lifestyle for the population at large.

The Caribbean region has the tremendous task of putting in place appropriate policies, plans, and programs to address the changing health and disease patterns of the region's people. This effort is made more difficult because of the socioeconomic, political, and cultural differences among the Caribbean countries. The various countries must not only examine the food availability and how it is consumed, but they must also assess and evaluate the quality of the food and the nutrition intake of those most at risk.

The Caribbean Food and Nutrition Institute (CFNI), established in 1967, aims to improve the food and nutrition status in member countries, which include Anguilla, Antigua, Bahamas, Barbados, Belize, the British Virgin Islands, Cayman Islands, Dominica, Grenada, Guyana, Jamaica, Montserrat, St. Christopher-Nevis, St. Lucia, St. Vincent, Suriname, Trinidad and Tobago, and Turks and Caicos Islands.

The governments of the Caribbean have come together under an initiative called Caribbean Cooperation in Health. They hope to work closely together through five types of activities: service, education training, providing information, coordination, and research. The food goals of each country must be analyzed, with care and attention paid to the agricultural policies and economic opportunities in each specific country.

Desiring a longer and richer quality of life, many governments of the Caribbean Islands have introduced programs to combat chronic diseases and promote a more physically active lifestyle. For example, in Grenada, a campaign to "grow what you eat and eat what you grow" demonstrates a move to increase consumption of local foods.

Adequate nutrition cannot be achieved without the consumption of sufficient foods containing a wide array of nutrients. Poor health status, whether as a result of insufficient food intake, overconsumption, or nutrition imbalance, threatens longevity and increases health care costs. The challenge is to improve the availability of nutritious foods and the eating habits of the varied population.

Resources

BOOKS

Campbell, Versada. *Caribbean Foodways.* Kingston, Jamaica: Caribbean Food and Nutrition Institute, 1988.

Houston, Lynn Marie. *Food Culture in the Caribbean.* Westport, CT: Greenwood Press, 2005.

Kittler, Pamela Goyan, Kathryn P. Sucher, and Marcia Nelms. *Food and Culture.* 6th edition. Belmont, CA: Wadsworth, Cengage Learning, 2011.

Sheridan, Richard B. *Sugar and Slavery.* Baltimore: Johns Hopkins University Press, 1974.

Stein-Barer, Thelma. *You Eat What You Are: People, Culture, and Food Tradition.* 2nd edition. Toronto: Firefly, 1999.

WEBSITES

"Caribbean Community in Health." http://www.caricom. org/jsp/community_organs/health/health_main_ page.jsp (accessed September 20, 2012).

ORGANIZATIONS

Caribbean Food & Nutrition Institute, University of the West Indies Campus Mona, PO Box 140, Kingston 7, Jamaica, (876) 927-1927, Fax: (876) 927-2657, e-mail@cfni.paho.org, http://new.paho.org/cfni.

Pan American Health Organization, 525 23rd St. NW, Washington, DC 20037, (202) 974-3000, Fax: (202) 974-3663, http://new.paho.org/index.php.

Paulette Sinclair-Weir

Carotenoids

Definition

Carotenoids are fat-soluble plant pigments, some of which are important to human health. The most common carotenoids in the diet of North Americans are alpha-carotene, beta-carotene, beta-cryptoxanthin, lutein, zeaxanthin, and lycopene.

Purpose

The role carotenoids play in human health is not well understood. Carotenoids are **antioxidants** that react with free radicals. Molecules, called free radicals, form during normal cell **metabolism** and with exposure to ultraviolet light or to toxins, such as cigarette smoke. Free radicals cause damage by reacting with **fats** and proteins in cell membranes and genetic material. This process is called oxidation. Antioxidants are compounds that attach themselves to free radicals so that it is impossible for the free radical to react with, or oxidize, other molecules. In this way, antioxidants may protect cells from damage. Although carotenoids have antioxidant activity in the laboratory, it is not clear how much they function as antioxidants in the body. Claims that carotenoids can protect against

Carotenoids

Carotenoid	Food sources
Alpha-carotene	Carrots Collard greens Peas Plantains Pumpkin Tangerines Tomatoes, raw Winter squash
Beta-carotene	Broccoli Cantaloupe Carrot juice Carrots Dandelion greens Kale Pumpkin Spinach Turnip greens Sweet potatoes Winter squash
Beta-cryptoxanthin	Carrots Corn, yellow Nectarines Orange juice Oranges Papaya Pumpkin Red bell peppers Tangerines Watermelon
Lutein and zeaxanthin	Broccoli Brussels sprouts Collard greens Corn, yellow Dandelion greens Kale Mustard greens Peas Pumpkin Spinach Summer squash Turnip greens Winter squash
Lycopene	Baked beans, canned Catsup Grapefruit, pink Marinara sauce Sweet red peppers Tomato juice Tomato paste and puree Tomato soup Tomatoes, raw Vegetable juice cocktail Watermelon

(Table by GGS Information Services. © 2013 Cengage Learning.)

cancer and cardiovascular disease are primarily based on their antioxidant properties.

One subgroup of carotenoids—which includes alpha-carotene, beta-carotene, and beta-cryptoxanthin— is converted into **vitamin A** (retinol) by the body. Vitamin A is important for maintaining good vision, a healthy immune system, and strong bones. Vitamin A also helps

turn on and off certain genes (gene expression) during cell division and differentiation. The degree to which this group of carotenoids is converted into vitamin A appears to depend on whether or not the body is getting enough vitamin A in other forms. Only 10% of all carotenoids can be converted into vitamin A.

Description

Carotenoids are highly colored red, orange, and yellow pigments found in many vegetables. The German chemist Heinrich Wilhelm Ferdinand Wackenroder isolated the first carotenoid in 1826 from carrots and named it beta-carotene. Since then, more than 600 carotenoids have been identified in plants, algae, fungi, and bacteria. Carotenoids must be dissolved in a small amount of fat to be absorbed from the intestine. **Dietary supplements** of carotenoids contain oil, which makes them more readily available to the body than carotenoids in food. Carotenoids in vegetables are best absorbed if they are cooked in oil or eaten in a meal that contains at least some fat. (A very tiny amount of fat is adequate.)

The United States Institute of Medicine (IOM) of the National Academy of Sciences develops values called **Dietary Reference Intakes (DRIs)** for **vitamins** and **minerals**. The **DRIs** define the amount of a nutrient a person needs to consume daily and the largest daily amount from food or dietary supplements that can be taken without harm. The IOM has not developed any DRIs for carotenoids because not enough scientific information is available, and because no diseases have been identified as being caused by inadequate intake of carotenoids. The IOM, the American Cancer Society, and the American Heart Association all recommend that people get all their antioxidants, including carotenoids, from a diet high in fruits, vegetables, and **whole grains** rather than from dietary supplements.

Health claims for carotenoids

Many health claims for carotenoids are based on laboratory and animal studies. Results from human studies are often inconsistent and confusing. One difficulty in evaluating these studies comes from the variety of ways in which they are conducted. When increased carotenoid intake comes from eating foods high in carotenoids, it is hard to separate the effects of the carotenoids from the effects of other vitamins and minerals in the food. When a dietary supplement is given to increase the level of a specific carotenoid, the outcomes often differ from those that occur in a diet of carotenoid-rich vegetables. In addition, the fact that some carotenoids are converted into vitamin A blurs the line between their effects and that of vitamin A from other sources. More controlled research needs to be done on these compounds. Many clinical trials are underway to determine safety and effectiveness of different carotenoids, both alone and in combination with other drugs and supplements.

BETA-CAROTENE. Beta-carotene is a yellow-orange provitamin A carotenoid. A provitamin is a substance that is converted into a vitamin in the body of an organism. Good sources of beta-carotene include carrots, sweet potatoes, winter squash, pumpkins, spinach, kale, and broccoli. When vitamin A stores are low, the body can convert beta-carotene into vitamin A to prevent symptoms of vitamin A deficiency. It takes 12 micrograms (mcg) of beta-carotene to make 1 mcg of retinol, the active form of vitamin A. Therefore, vitamin A deficiency is usually more effectively treated by eating more foods high in vitamin A and/or taking a vitamin A supplement than by increasing beta-carotene intake.

The only use for beta-carotene dietary supplements, proven in well-controlled clinical trials, is to treat a rare genetic disorder called erythropoietic protoporphyria, also called porphyria. This disorder causes the skin to be painfully sensitive to sunlight and causes the development of **gallstones** and problems with liver function. Symptoms are sometimes relieved by giving beta-carotene supplements under the supervision of a physician.

A diet high in vegetables rich in beta-carotene appears to reduce the risk of developing certain cancers. However, in a large study of 29,000 Finnish men (the Alpha-Tocopherol, Beta-Carotene Cancer Prevention [ATBC] Trial), when a beta-carotene dietary supplement was taken by men who smoked, they developed lung cancer at a rate of 18% higher and died at a rate of 8% higher than men who did not take the supplement. The study was halted in 1994, but side effects continued into the 2000s. A similar U.S. study (Carotene and Retinol Efficacy Trial [CARET]) that gave men dietary supplements of beta-carotene and vitamin A was also stopped when researchers found the men receiving the beta-carotene had a 46% greater chance of dying from lung cancer than those who did not take it. The official position of the IOM is that "beta-carotene supplements are not advisable for the general population."

ALPHA-CAROTENE. Alpha-carotene is the lesser-known cousin of beta-carotene. It also is a provitamin A carotenoid, but it takes 24 mcg of alpha-carotene to make 1 mcg of retinol. Good sources of alpha-carotene include pumpkins, carrots, winter squash, collard greens, raw tomatoes, tangerines, and peas. Less research has been done on alpha-carotene than beta-carotene, but it is not recommended as a dietary supplement.

KEY TERMS

Antioxidant—A molecule that prevents oxidation. In the body antioxidants attach to other molecules called free radicals and prevent the free radicals from causing damage to cell walls, DNA, and other parts of the cell.

Cell differentiation—The process by which stem cells develop into different types of specialized cells such as skin, heart, muscle, and blood cells.

Dietary supplement—A product, such as a vitamin, mineral, herb, amino acid, or enzyme, intended to be consumed in addition to an individual's diet with the expectation that it will improve health.

Provitamin—A substance the body can convert into a vitamin.

Retina—The layer of light-sensitive cells on the back of the eyeball that function in converting light into nerve impulses.

BETA-CRYPTOXANTHIN. Beta-cryptoxanthin is also a provitamin A carotenoid. It takes 24 mcg of beta-cryptoxanthin to make 1 mcg of retinol. Good sources of beta-cryptoxanthin include pumpkins, red bell peppers, papayas, tangerines, nectarines, oranges and orange juice, carrots, yellow corn, and watermelons.

LUTEIN AND ZEAXANTHIN. Lutein and zeaxanthin do not have vitamin A activity. They are the only carotenoids found in the human eye. It has been proposed, but not proven, that they may help slow the development of cataracts. Cataracts are changes in the lens of the eye that result in clouding and vision loss. These carotenoids are also found in the retina. They absorb light in the blue wavelength range. Some researchers theorize that they can help slow or prevent age-related breakdown of the retina (age-related macular degeneration), a common cause of vision loss in the elderly. Good sources of lutein and zeaxanthin include spinach, kale, turnips, collard and mustard greens, summer squash, peas, broccoli, Brussels sprouts, and yellow corn.

LYCOPENE. Lycopene is the carotenoid that gives tomatoes, watermelons, and guavas their reddish color. In the American diet, almost all dietary lycopene comes from tomato products.

The relationship between dietary intake of lycopene and the risk of men developing prostate cancer is of great interest to researchers. Results have been conflicting. A large study of 58,000 Dutch men found no relationship between the two, but a 2004 analysis of 21 observational studies examining the relationship between dietary lycopene intake and prostate cancer found that men with the highest dietary intake of lycopene were slightly less likely to develop prostate cancer. Studies conducted in 2007 on almost 30,000 found results similar to the original 1990s Dutch study, with no significant relationship. Research continues into the 2010s.

Precautions

The relationship between lung cancer and beta-carotene strongly suggests that all carotenoids should be obtained through diet and not through dietary supplements. There is also no information on the safety of carotenoid dietary supplements in children or women who are either pregnant or **breastfeeding**.

Interactions

Interactions of specific carotenoids with drugs, herbs, and dietary supplements have not been well studied. In general, cholesterol-lowering drugs, the weight-loss drug **orlistat** (Xenical or Alli), and mineral oil reduce the absorption of carotenoids from the intestine, but it is not known whether this has an effect on health.

Complications

There are no identified complications from carotenoid deficiency.

Beta-carotene supplements of 30 mg per day or more or excessive consumption of carrots and other beta-carotene rich food can cause the skin to become yellow, a condition called carotenodermia. Carotenodermia is not associated with any health problems and disappears when beta-carotene intake is reduced.

Lycopene supplements, or excessive intake of tomatoes and tomato products, can cause the skin to turn orange, a condition called lycopenodermia. This condition disappears when lycopene intake is reduced.

No recommendations have been set about the maximum daily intake of carotenoids from diet, but dietary supplements of carotenoids are not recommended by the IOM, the American Heart Association, or the American Cancer Society.

Parental concerns

Parents should encourage their children to eat a healthy and varied diet high in fruits, vegetables, and whole grains. There is no need to give children dietary supplements of carotenoids. The safety of these supplements in children has not been studied.

Resources

BOOKS

Gaby, Alan R., ed. *A–Z Guide to Drug-Herb-Vitamin Interactions.* 2nd ed. New York: Three Rivers Press, 2006.

Krinsky, Norman, Susan T. Mayne, and Helmut Sies, eds. *Carotenoids in Health and Disease.* New York: Marcel Dekker, 2004.

Lieberman, Shari, and Nancy Bruning. *The Real Vitamin and Mineral Book: The Definitive Guide to Designing Your Personal Supplement Program.* 4th ed. New York: Avery, 2007.

Rucker, Robert B., ed. *Handbook of Vitamins.* Boca Raton, FL: Taylor & Francis, 2007.

Yamaguchi, Masayoshi. *Carotenoids: Properties, Effects, and Diseases.* Hauppauge, NY: Nova Science Publishers, 2011.

PERIODICALS

Kushi, Lawrence H., et al. "American Cancer Society Guidelines on Nutrition and Physical Activity for Cancer Prevention." *CA: Cancer Journal for Clinicians* 56, no. 5 (2006): 254–281.

Redlich, C.A., et al. "Effect of Supplementation with Beta-Carotene and Vitamin A on Lung Nutrient Levels." *Cancer Epidemiology, Biomarkers & Prevention* 7, no. 3 (1998): 211–14.

Satia, Jessie A., et al. "Long-Term Use of ß-Carotene, Retinol, Lycopene, and Lutein Supplements and Lung Cancer Risk: Results from the VITamins and Lifestyle (VITAL) Study." *American Journal of Epidemiology* 169, no. 7 (2009): 815–28. http://dx.doi.org/10.1093/aje/kwn409 (accessed June 14, 2012).

Voutilainen, Sari, et al. "Carotenoids and Cardiovascular Health." *American Journal of Clinical Nutrition* 83, no. 6 (2006): 1265–1271.

WEBSITES

American Cancer Society. "Lycopene." http://www.cancer.org/Treatment/TreatmentsandSideEffects/ComplementaryandAlternativeMedicine/DietandNutrition/lycopene (accessed June 15, 2012).

Higdon, Jane, and Victoria Drake. "Carotenoids." Linus Pauling Institute, Oregon State University. http://lpi.oregonstate.edu/infocenter/phytochemicals/carotenoids (accessed June 14, 2012).

MedlinePlus. "Beta-carotene." U.S. National Library of Medicine, National Institutes of Health. http://www.nlm.nih.gov/medlineplus/druginfo/natural/patient-betacarotene.html (accessed June 14, 2012).

National Cancer Institute. "Alpha-Tocopherol, Beta-Carotene Cancer Prevention (ATBC) Trial." U.S. National Institutes of Health. http://www.cancer.gov/newscenter/qa/2003/atbcfollowupqa (accessed June 14, 2012).

Office of Dietary Supplements. "Dietary Supplement Fact Sheet: Vitamin A and Carotenoids." U.S. National Institutes of Health. http://ods.od.nih.gov/factsheets/VitaminA (accessed June 14, 2012).

ORGANIZATIONS

Academy of Nutrition and Dietetics, 120 South Riverside Plz., Ste. 2000, Chicago, IL 60606-6995, (312) 899-0040, (800) 877-1600, amacmunn@eatright.org, http://www.eatright.org.

American Cancer Society, 250 Williams St. NW, Atlanta, GA 30303, (800) 227-2345, http://www.cancer.org.

American Heart Association, 7272 Greenville Ave., Dallas, TX 75231, (800) 242-8721, http://www.americanheart.org.

Office of Dietary Supplements, National Institutes of Health, 6100 Executive Blvd., Rm. 3B01, MSC 7517, Bethesda, MD 20892-7517, (301) 435-2920, Fax: (301) 480-1845, ods@nih.gov, http://ods.od.nih.gov.

Tish Davidson, AM
David Newton

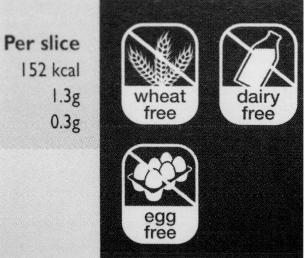

Dairy-free foods are free of casein, a protein found in milk. (© Tim Gainey/Alamy)

Casein-free diet

Definition

The casein-free diet is a diet that has been tried since the early 1990s as a treatment for autism. Casein is a **protein** that accounts for 80% of the protein in cow milk and cheese and is similar in its molecular structure to gluten, a protein found in wheat, barley, and other grains. If the diet excludes foods containing gluten as well as dairy products, it is called the gluten-free, casein-free (GFCF) diet. If **soy** products are also excluded, the diet is called the GFCFSF (gluten-free, casein-free, soy-free) diet. The American Academy of Pediatrics considers the GFCF diet an alternative therapy for autism rather than a mainstream medical treatment.

Origins

The basic idea that some psychiatric and developmental disorders can be treated with dietary interventions dates back to the 1960s, when some researchers noted that certain societies in the South Pacific had lower than average rates of schizophrenia as well as diets that were almost completely free of grain and dairy products. The researchers theorized that schizophrenia might be caused by a genetic mutation that prevents patients from completely digesting gluten and casein, and that elevated levels of peptides in the blood might be responsible for the bizarre behavior associated with schizophrenia.

This theory was not applied to autism until the early 1990s, when Kalle Reichelt, a physician-researcher in Norway, noted that urine samples from children with autism often contained higher-than-normal levels of peptides. Reichelt theorized that peptides from incomplete digestion of gluten and casein not only enter the bloodstream from the small intestine in these children, but also act like opioids on the brain and affect the development of the growing brain. Reichelt has since published several papers maintaining that the GFCF diet is an effective treatment for autism.

Description

The GFCF diet is essentially an elimination diet that works by excluding all foods containing gluten and casein. Parents are usually also warned against substituting soy products as substitutes for milk or cheese. The basic theory underlying the GFCF diet is that children with autism cannot digest such proteins as casein and gluten completely, and that this incomplete digestion results in the formation of peptide molecules that enter the bloodstream from the lumen of the small intestine—either because the child is lacking an enzyme necessary to complete digestion, or because the child's intestine is abnormally permeable and allows the peptides to enter the bloodstream in unusually large quantities. This latter hypothesis is sometimes called the "leaky gut" theory.

The GFCF diet requires parents to exclude all foods and personal care products made from or containing gluten and casein from the child's diet.

- Gluten is found in wheat, rye, triticale, barley, and oats. The basic foods containing gluten include bread, cereal, pasta, cake, donuts, flour, some alcohol, bouillon, and some vinegar and sauce thickeners. Prepackaged food mixes almost always contain gluten, as do flavored instant coffees and teas.
- Gluten is also found in some lip balms, lotions, medicines, and vitamin tablets.
- Casein is found in the milk of all mammals, including human breast milk as well as the milk of cows, goats, sheep, buffalo, and yaks. Common foods containing casein include ice cream, sour cream, yogurt, butter, luncheon meats, hot dogs, and cheese.

Most websites about the GFCF diet contain links to companies that make gluten- and casein-free substitutes for such popular foods as breakfast cereals, pasta, pizza, and ice cream, while others include lists of ingredients that can be substituted for flour, milk, butter, etc., in ordinary recipes.

Parents are usually advised to try the GFCF diet for at least three full months before determining whether or not it is helping their child.

Autism incidence and treatment

It is difficult to estimate how many families may be using the GFCF diet. According to the American Academy of Pediatrics (AAP) and the U.S. Centers for Disease Control and Prevention, approximately 1 in 88 children have an autism spectrum disorder. Opinions vary, however, on the best way to manage the symptoms of autism. The AAP classifies the two major types of treatment approaches as psychosocial (e.g., cognitive behavioral therapy) and medical. Medical approaches include both psychotropic medications and some complementary and alternative medicine (CAM) treatments. The AAP further subdivides CAM approaches into nonbiological treatments (craniosacral manipulation, auditory integration training, music therapy, and behavioral optometry) and biological treatments (vitamin supplements, **detoxification diets**, and chelation therapy, as well as the elimination diet).

GFCF diet preparation

Most parents who have tried the GFCF diet recommend introducing it in stages, to prevent the child from becoming emotionally upset by the sudden loss of favorite foods and to give the child's digestive system time to adjust to the removal of gluten and casein from the diet. It is commonly recommended to begin the diet during the summer or a lengthy school holiday when the child is at home most of the time. Each week or two, certain foods should be eliminated from the diet:

- Weeks 1–2: All milk products, including yogurt, sour cream, ice cream, and cheese, are removed from the diet and are not replaced by soy products. The child is given calcium supplements.
- Weeks 3–4: All products containing gluten are removed.
- Weeks 5–6: Anything else in the diet containing soy is removed.
- Weeks 7–8: The contents of the diet are rechecked and the child's toothpaste, shampoo, lip balm, and other personal care products are replaced if necessary.
- Weeks 9–10: Carbohydrates and sugars in the diet are assessed to ensure that they are within appropriate levels. Processed foods, even GFCF foods, may be high in sugar.

Function

The goal of the GFCF diet is to manage the symptoms of autism, especially the repetitive behavior and communication problems characteristic of the disorder; to improve the child's social interactions with others; and to improve the child's chances of eventual functional independence. The GFCF diet is used almost exclusively in treating preschool or school-age children with autism, but it is occasionally used to treat adults.

Benefits

Supporters of the GFCF diet maintain that it brings about "dramatic and remarkable improvements, not just in [children with autism's] level of functioning, but in their sleeping patterns, anxiety levels, and comfort levels." However, most proponents of the diet are careful to note that the degree of improvement depends on the child's age, basic gastrointestinal health, and the child's position on the spectrum of autistic disorders. The diet has not been touted as a cure for autism, but only as a way to manage symptoms of the disorder.

There appears to be some disagreement regarding the proportion of children with autism that are helped by the diet. Some websites about the diet state that about a third of children with autism show improvement on the GFCF diet, but estimates range up to 91%. Children who benefit from the GFCF diet will need to remain on it for the remainder of their lives to continue its effects.

Precautions

Parents considering the GFCF diet as a treatment for a child with autism should consult a registered dietitian (RD), as well as their pediatrician and possibly a psychologist or psychiatrist experienced in managing autism spectrum disorders.

There are several precautions that families considering the GFCF diet should keep in mind:

• Although the GFCF diet is less expensive than some other treatments for autism, it can add substantially to the cost of a family's groceries, particularly if special foods designed as substitutes for grain or dairy products are purchased.

• It may be difficult to balance the child's diet against the rest of the family's food, and measures may need to be taken to ensure that the child cannot access the rest of the family's foods (such as keeping food locked in a pantry).

• Special occasions and social get-togethers where an array of foods will be served may be hard for the child, especially if they do not understand why he or she cannot eat what everyone else is eating.

• The child may feel upset about being deprived of some favorite foods.

• Parents or caregivers will need to read food labels with extreme care. Many foods that may not appear to contain gluten or casein may in fact be prepared with coatings, flavorings, or other ingredients containing these substances.

It will be up to caregivers to make sure that the child remains on the diet. Parents will need to monitor the child's response to the diet and report it to the child's doctor periodically.

Risks

The GFCF diet is not known to pose any risks to a child's physical health as long as parents work with a pediatrician or RD to ensure that the child is still receiving enough **vitamins** and nutrients. However, the loss of foods that are favorites of many children—such as pizza, potato chips and other snack foods, chocolate, and ice cream—can lead to tantrums, food stealing, and other behavioral problems. It may help the child adjust to the diet if other family members do not eat any of the eliminated foods in front of the child. Parents may wish to explain the diet to other relatives and to the child's teachers, as well.

Research & general acceptance

Opinion is divided on the efficacy of the GFCF diet as a treatment for autism. The primary difficulty is the lack of solid evidence that the diet is effective. There have been few large studies of the GFCF diet in mainstream medical literature. Still, some mainstream physicians maintain that the diet is not likely to harm the child, is less expensive than medications, and may help some children.

To some extent the lack of consensus about the diet is rooted in a deeper problem, namely ongoing disagreement on the causes of autism. While many children with autism do have gastrointestinal disorders, there is not yet any evidence of gastrointestinal

QUESTIONS TO ASK YOUR DOCTOR

- What is your opinion of the GFCF diet?
- Do you know any families who have tried it?
- Do you think my child would benefit from a GFCF diet?
- Can you refer me to a registered dietitian?

factors specific to children with autism, and not all children with autism experience adverse gastrointestinal symptoms. Information on ongoing clinical trials is available at the U.S. National Institutes of Health–sponsored website ClinicalTrials.gov.

It should also be noted that the book-length guides and cookbooks related to the GFCF diet are written by parents rather than medical specialists. While this fact does not diminish their value as resources for those who wish to try the diet, it does reflect the lack of consensus among doctors about the effectiveness of the diet as a treatment for autism.

Resources

BOOKS

Compart, Pamela J. and Dana Laake. *The Kid-Friendly ADHD and Autism Cookbook: The Ultimate Guide to the Gluten-Free, Casein-Free Diet*, 2nd ed. Beverly, MA: Fair Winds, 2009.

Le Breton, Marilyn. *Diet Intervention and Autism: Implementing the Gluten-Free and Casein-Free Diet for Autistic Children and Adults: A Practical Guide for Parents*. Philadelphia: Jessica Kingsley, 2001.

Lord, Susan. *Getting Your Kid on a Gluten-Free Casein-Free Diet*. Philadelphia: Jessica Kingsley, 2009.

Oller, John W., and Stephen D. Oller. *Autism: The Diagnosis, Treatment & Etiology of the Undeniable Epidemic*. Sudbury, MA: Jones and Bartlett, 2010.

PERIODICALS

Autism Research Institute. "Parent Ratings of Behavioral Effects of Biomedical Interventions." *ARI Publication* 34 (March 2009). http://www.autism.com/pdf/providers/ParentRatings2009.pdf (accessed June 6, 2012).

Christison, G. W., and K. Ivany. "Elimination Diets in Autism Spectrum Disorders: Any Wheat amidst the Chaff?" *Journal of Developmental and Behavioral Pediatrics* 27 (April 2006): Suppl. 2, S162–S171.

Elder, J. H. "The Gluten-Free, Casein-Free Diet in Autism: An Overview with Clinical Implications." *Nutrition in Clinical Practice* 23 (December 2008–January 2009): 583–88.

Erickson, C. A., et al. "Gastrointestinal Factors in Autistic Disorder: A Critical Review." *Journal of Autism and Developmental Disorders* 35 (December 2005): 713–27.

Harrington, J. W., et al. "Parental Perceptions and Use of Complementary and Alternative Medicine Practices for Children with Autistic Spectrum Disorders in Private Practice." *Journal of Developmental and Behavioral Pediatrics* 27 (April 2006): Suppl. 2, S156–S161.

Myers, Scott M., and Chris P. Johnson. "Management of Children with Autism Spectrum Disorders." *Pediatrics* 120, no. 5 (November 2007; reaffirmed September 2010): 1162–82. http://dx.doi.org/10.1542/peds.2007-2362 (accessed September 14, 2012).

Pennesi, C. M., and L. C. Klein. "Effectiveness of the Gluten-Free, Casein-Free Diet for Children Diagnosed with Autism Spectrum Disorder: Based On Parental Report." *Nutritional Neuroscience* 15, no. 2 (2012): 85–91.

Reichelt, K. L., and A. M. Knivsberg. "The Possibility and Probability of a Gut-to-Brain Connection in Autism." *Annals of Clinical Psychiatry* 21 (Oct–Dec 2009): 205–11.

Whiteley, P., et al. "The ScanBrit Randomised, Controlled, Single-Blind Study of a Gluten- and Casein-Free Dietary Intervention for Children with Autism Spectrum Disorders." *Nutritional Neuroscience* 13, no. 2 (2010): 87–100.

WEBSITES

Autism Research Institute (ARI). "Tips for Implementing Special Diets." http://www.autism.com/index.php/treating_diets (accessed September 14, 2012).

Centers for Disease Control and Prevention. "Autism Spectrum Disorders." http://www.cdc.gov/ncbddd/autism/index.html (accessed September 14, 2012).

GFCF Diet Support Group. "Support Groups in the United States." http://www.gfcfdiet.com/communitybulletinboard.htm (accessed September 14, 2012).

National Institute of Neurological Disorders and Stroke. "Autism Fact Sheet." http://www.ninds.nih.gov/disorders/autism/detail_autism.htm (accessed September 14, 2012).

Talk About Curing Autism (TACA). "Going GFCFSF in 10 Weeks!" http://gfcf-diet.talkaboutcuringautism.org/gfcf-in-10-weeks.htm (accessed September 14, 2012).

ORGANIZATIONS

American Academy of Pediatrics (AAP), 141 Northwest Point Blvd., Elk Grove Village, IL 60007, (847) 434-4000, (800) 433-9016, Fax: (847) 434-8000, http://www.aap.org.

Autism Research Institute (ARI), 4182 Adams Ave., San Diego, CA 92116, (866) 366-3361, Fax: (619) 563-6840, http://www.autism.com.

Talk About Curing Autism (TACA), 2222 Martin St., Ste. 140, Irvine, CA 92612, (949) 640-4401, Fax: (949) 640-4424, http://www.tacanow.org.

Rebecca J. Frey, PhD

Caveman diet *see* **Paleo diet**

Celiac disease

Definition

Celiac disease—also known as sprue, celiac sprue, non-tropical sprue, and gluten-sensitive enteropathy—is a lifelong autoimmune disease in which the body's reaction to gluten causes damage to the intestines that results in poor absorption of nutrients.

Description

Absorption of most nutrients occurs in the small intestine. The intestine is lined with microscopic, hair-like projections called villi, and it is through these villi that nutrients are absorbed. Villi project into the intestine and provide an increased surface area for absorption. Damage to the villi results in inadequate absorption, especially of **vitamins**, **minerals**, and **fats**.

Celiac disease is an autoimmune disease. Whenever immune system cells in the body sense the presence of foreign material, they produce proteins called antibodies that act to disable the foreign material. In an autoimmune disease, the body treats some of its own cells as foreign and attacks them. Celiac disease is also classified as a malabsorption disease because the cells that are damaged by the body's immune system are cells of the villi lining the small intestine. When these cells are damaged, the villi flatten out, decreasing the surface area available for absorption. Nutrients are not properly absorbed, and vitamin and mineral deficiencies often develop.

The symptoms of celiac disease were described as early as 1888, but it was not until the 1950s that physicians began to understand what caused the disease. A Dutch pediatrician, W. K. Dicke, was the first person to make the connection between the consumption of foods containing wheat and symptoms of celiac disease. Today, researchers know that the problem substance is gluten, a **protein** found in wheat, rye, barley, and any products made from these grains such as flour, bread, and pasta. The role of oats and oat products in celiac disease remains controversial.

Demographics

Celiac disease is most common among people of Northern European ancestry and is uncommon to rare among people of African or Asian ancestry. Initially, celiac disease was thought to be uncommon in the United States, but recent improvements in genetic testing and disease awareness have changed that picture. Experts now believe that in areas of the world settled primarily by Europeans, including the United States, about 1 in every 133 people has celiac disease; prevalence

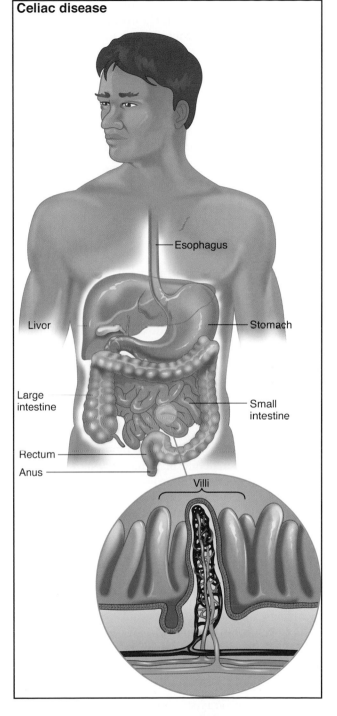

Celiac disease

Esophagus

Liver

Stomach

Large intestine

Small intestine

Rectum

Anus

Villi

When people with celiac disease eat foods or use products containing gluten, their immune system responds by damaging or destroying villi in the intestine. Villi allows nutrients from food to be absorbed into the bloodstream; without healthy villi, a person becomes malnourished, regardless of the quantity of food eaten. *(Illustration by Electronic Illustrators Group. © 2013 Cengage Learning.)*

for non-Hispanic whites in the United States is thought to be closer to 1 in 100 (1%). The disease has an inherited component, and the rate increases to 1 of every 22 people who are blood relatives of a parent, sibling, or child with the disease. In about 70% of identical twins, if one has celiac disease, the other also has it. Celiac disease is also more common among people with other genetically related autoimmune diseases, such as systemic lupus erythematosus, type 1 diabetes (juvenile diabetes), rheumatoid arthritis, and autoimmune thyroid disease.

People of any age can be diagnosed with celiac disease. However, there are two common peaks for diagnosis, one between 8–15 months (which is shortly after infants usually begin eating wheat products) and another between 30–40 years in adults.

Causes and symptoms

Researchers have traced the genetic component of celiac disease to a cluster of genes on chromosome six. Multiple genes are involved, which may account for the variation in symptoms and inheritability of the disease. Often, symptoms of the disease develop after a serious infection, physical trauma, pregnancy, or surgery. Researchers do not know why stress on the body appears to trigger symptoms.

Symptoms of celiac disease are varied. Some people have the disease (as diagnosed by samples that show damage to the small intestine), but they show no symptoms. Others go along for years with annoying or intermittent symptoms, and some, especially children, show severe symptoms of **malnutrition** that stunt growth despite eating a healthy diet. Symptoms are similar to those of other, more common, **digestive diseases**. Often, celiac disease is initially misdiagnosed.

Common symptoms of celiac disease fall into two categories, those primarily related to the immediate problems of digesting food and those that result mainly from long-term deficiencies in vitamins and minerals. Symptoms primarily related to immediate difficulties in digestion include:

- chronic diarrhea
- foul-smelling grayish stools, resulting from the inability to properly digest fats
- gas, abdominal bloating
- abdominal cramps
- weight loss

Other symptoms that develop because of vitamin and mineral deficiencies can include:

- iron deficiency anemia (low red blood cell count)
- joint pain, muscle pain, muscle cramps

- osteoporosis (inadequate calcium absorption)
- tingling in the legs from nerve damage
- seizures
- bleeding disorders (inadequate vitamin K)
- missed menstrual periods
- infertility (in women), frequent miscarriages
- failure to thrive in infants
- delayed mental and physical growth in children

Other symptoms include:

- fatigue
- irritability and behavioral changes, especially in children
- pale sores inside the mouth
- dermatitis herpetiformis (an itchy skin rash that usually appears on the trunk, buttocks, neck, and scalp)

Diagnosis

Celiac disease can be difficult to diagnose because its symptoms are similar to those of so many other diseases. Often, it is initially misdiagnosed as **irritable bowel syndrome** or **Crohn's disease**. Stool examination, blood tests, and lactose (milk **sugar**) tolerance tests are often done when the patient first complains of symptoms, but there are two definitive tests for celiac disease.

The immune system of people with celiac disease produces higher than normal levels of certain antibodies. Blood tests can detect abnormal levels of these antibodies. If blood tests are positive, a small bowel endoscopy with biopsies is done. Endoscopies are usually performed in a doctor's office or an outpatient clinic while the patient is under light sedation. In this procedure, the physician inserts a tube, called an endoscope, down the patient's throat, through the patient's stomach, and into the upper part of the small intestine. A tiny camera at the end of the endoscope allows the doctor to see if there is damage to villi. During this procedure, the doctor also removes small tissue samples (biopsies) from the intestinal lining in order to look for cell damage under the microscope. Presence of a specific type of damage is a positive diagnosis for celiac disease.

Treatment

There is no cure for celiac disease. The only treatment is life-long avoidance of any foods that contain gluten. This means not eating foods that contain wheat, rye, and barley, such as bread or baked goods, pizza, spaghetti, and many processed foods that use flour as a thickening agent.

When individuals fail to improve on a **gluten-free diet**, it is sometimes because they are unintentionally consuming sources of hidden gluten. A few people on truly gluten-free diets do not improve. They can be treated with corticosteroid drugs to reduce inflammation, but this does not heal the intestine. Clinical trials concerning treatment of celiac disease are underway. Patients interested in participating in a clinical trial at no cost can find a list of trials currently enrolling volunteers at http://www.clinicaltrials.gov.

Nutrition and dietary concerns

Individuals newly diagnosed with celiac disease may find it helpful to meet with a nutritionist or dietitian to aid with meal planning. Two issues need to be addressed. First, determining what is safe to eat, and second, learning how to get the right balance of nutrients in a gluten-free diet. Complicating matters, damage to the intestines may make some people lactose intolerant, so that they either cannot eat or must limit dairy products in their diet.

Many cookbooks are available to help people on a gluten-free diet. Home cooks must learn to substitute ingredients, such as cornstarch and rice flour, for wheat flour in their foods. An increasing number of gluten-free foods are available commercially. However, these often cost more than their gluten-containing counterparts. Foods people with celiac disease can safely eat include:

- plain fruits and vegetables
- plain meat that has not been breaded, coated, or mixed with fillers
- potatoes
- rice (all types)
- cornmeal, cornstarch, and products made of corn, such as corn tortillas
- tapioca
- buckwheat
- dried beans and peas
- nuts
- quinoa
- amaranth
- arrowroot

Other foods must be avoided. Individuals with celiac disease must also avoid cross-contamination with these foods. For example, they should not cut gluten-free bread using a knife that has cut regular wheat bread unless the knife has been thoroughly washed. Even small amounts of gluten can cause damage to the intestine. Some of the foods people with celiac disease must avoid are:

- wheat flours, including durum flour, enriched flour, graham flour, semolina flour, and white flour

---

KEY TERMS

Antibodies—Proteins that provoke the immune system to attack particular substances. In celiac disease, the immune system makes antibodies to a component of gluten.

Gluten—A protein found in wheat, rye, barley, and oats.

Villi—Tiny, finger-like projections that enable the small intestine to absorb nutrients from food.

- wheat germ, wheat starch, wheat bran, cracked wheat
- products made with the above mentioned wheat products such as pasta, bread, cakes, cookies
- barley, barley flour, and products made with barley
- rye, rye flour, and products made with rye
- triticale and other wheat hybrids

Learning how to read food labels is very important to people who must avoid gluten. However, this may become easier in the future. In January 2007, the United States Food and Drug Administration (FDA) published preliminary regulations for foods that could be labeled "gluten free." Labeling will be voluntary. As of early 2012, the FDA had still not implemented the new gluten labeling rules. Once those rules are implemented, shoppers who must avoid gluten should find it easier to find products they can safely eat. Meanwhile, people with celiac disease must be alert to "hidden" sources of gluten that often serve as binders or thickeners in commercially prepared foods. Some of these non-obvious sources of gluten that may appear on food labels are listed below.

- starch (type unspecified)
- modified food starch
- hydrolyzed vegetable protein (HVP)
- hydrolyzed plant protein (HPP)
- texturized vegetable protein (TVP)
- binders
- fillers
- extenders
- excipients (ingredients used in medications that do not have medicinal value, such as coatings of tablets. Consult a pharmacist or physician before taking drugs, vitamins, etc.)
- malt

Some brands of commercially prepared french fries, potato chips, hot dogs, meatballs, gravy mixes, soups,

QUESTIONS TO ASK YOUR DOCTOR

- Can you recommend a registered dietitian who can help our family develop a safe, gluten-free diet?
- Is it possible for someone with celiac disease to go off his or her diet once in a while without damage to bodily systems?
- How can I be sure that my child stays on the diet and does not stray from the diet when out with friends?

soy sauce, and candy contain these hidden sources of gluten. Others are gluten-free. A nutritionist and dietitian can help people with celiac disease learn to read labels accurately to distinguish that foods are safe for them.

Therapy

Switching to a gluten-free diet requires major lifestyle changes. It can be especially hard on children and teens who want to be able to go out with their friends and eat pizza and fast food. Many people find Internet support groups are helpful in making the transition to a gluten-free diet.

Prognosis

The intestines of people with celiac disease who go on a gluten-free diet heal. In children, the healing usually takes 3–6 months. In adults, healing can take 2 years. The intestinal villi remain intact and function properly so long as the diet remains free of gluten, but the disease is never cured.

People who are not diagnosed, or who do not stay on a gluten-free diet, face increased chances of developing **cancer** of the intestine. They may also develop osteoporosis because of poor **calcium** absorption. Other vitamin and mineral deficiencies may contribute to a multitude of health problems. Untreated pregnant women have higher than normal rates of miscarriage and babies born with birth defects, especially neural tube defects, which arise from inadequate amounts of folic acid. Untreated children may have stunted mental and physical growth.

Prevention

Celiac disease is a genetic autoimmune disorder that cannot be prevented. Once diagnosed, the only way to prevent symptoms and complications is to follow a strictly gluten-free diet.

Resources

BOOKS

Green, Peter H.R., and Rory Jones. *Celiac Disease: A Hidden Epidemic.* Rev. upd. ed. New York: HarperCollins, 2010.

Hauser, Stephen C. *Mayo Clinic on Digestive Health.* Rochester, MN: Mayo Clinic, 2011.

Washburn, Donna, and Heather Butt. *The Best Gluten-Free Family Cookbook.* West Toronto, ON: Robert Rose, 2005.

PERIODICALS

Rubio-Tapia, Alberto, et al. "The Prevalence of Celiac Disease in the United States." *American Journal of Gastroenterology* (July 31, 2012): e-pub ahead of print. http://dx.doi.org/10.1038/ajg.2012.219 (accessed August 15, 2012).

WEBSITES

Mayo Clinic staff. "Celiac Disease." MayoClinic.com. http://www.mayoclinic.com/health/celiac-disease/DS00319 (accessed June 23, 2012).

MedlinePlus. "Celiac Disease." U.S. National Library of Medicine. http://www.nlm.nih.gov/medlineplus/celiacdisease.html (accessed June 23, 2012).

National Digestive Diseases Information Clearinghouse. "Celiac Disease." National Institute of Diabetes and Digestive and Kidney Diseases (NIDDK). http://digestive.niddk.nih.gov/ddiseases/pubs/celiac (accessed June 23, 2012).

Neumors Foundation. "Celiac Disease." TeensHealth.org. http://teenshealth.org/teen/diseases_conditions/digestive/celiac.html (accessed June 23, 2012).

Picco, Michael F. "Celiac Disease Diet: How Do I Get Enough Grains?" http://www.mayoclinic.com/health/celiac-disease/AN00303 (accessed June 23, 2012).

PubMed Health. "Celiac Disease - Sprue." U.S. National Library of Medicine. http://www.ncbi.nlm.nih.gov/pubmedhealth/PMH0001280 (accessed June 23, 2012).

ORGANIZATIONS

American College of Gastroenterology, 6400 Goldsboro Rd., Ste. 200, Bethesda, MD 20817, (301) 263-9000, info@acg.gi.org, http://www.gi.org.

Celiac Sprue Association, PO Box 31700, Omaha, NB 68131, (877) 272-4272, celiacs@csaceliacs.org, http://www.csaceliacs.org.

National Digestive Diseases Information Clearinghouse, 2 Information Way, Bethesda, MD 20892–3570, (800) 891–5389, TTY: (866) 569–1162, Fax: (703) 738–4929, nddic@info.niddk.nih.gov, http://www.digestive.niddk.nih.gov.

Tish Davidson, AM
David Newton

Central American and Mexican diet

Definition

The traditional diets in Mexico and Central America (Guatemala, Nicaragua, Honduras, El Salvador, Belize, and Costa Rica) have several commonalities, though great variances exist in methods of preparation and in local recipes. The basis of the traditional diet in this part of the world is corn (maize) and beans, with the addition of meat, animal products, local fruits, and vegetables. As in other parts of the world, the diets in this area have expanded to include more processed foods. In many parts of Mexico and Central America, access to a variety of foods remains limited, and undernutrition, particularly among children, is a major problem. Although access to an increased variety of foods can improve the adequacy of both macronutrient and micronutrient status, there is evidence that the use of processed foods is contributing to the rapidly increasing prevalence of **obesity** and diet-related chronic diseases such as diabetes.

Origins

The traditional diet of Mexico and Central America is based on corn and beans but offers a wide diversity of preparations. The central staple in the region is maize, which is generally ground and treated with lime and then pressed into flat cakes called *tortillas*. In Mexico and Guatemala, these are flat and thin, while tortillas in other Central American countries are thicker. In El Salvador, for example, small, thick cakes of maize, filled with meat, cheese, or beans, are called *pupusas*. Maize is also used in a variety of other preparations, including tacos, tamales, and a thin gruel called atole. The complementary staple in the region is beans (*frijoles*), most commonly black or pinto beans. Rice is also widely used, particularly in the southernmost countries, such as El Salvador, Honduras, Nicaragua, and Costa Rica. Historically, major changes in the traditional diet occurred during colonial times, when the Spaniards and others introduced the region to wheat bread, dairy products, and **sugar**. Wheat is commonly consumed in the form of white rolls or sweet rolls, or, in the northern part of Mexico, as a flour-based tortilla. Noodles (*fideos*), served in soups or mixed with vegetables, have also become popular.

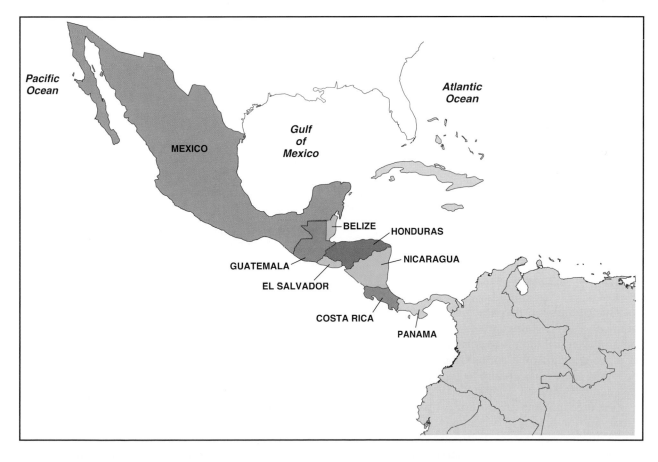

Map of Central America. *(Map by Electronic Illustrators Group. © 2013 Cengage Learning.)*

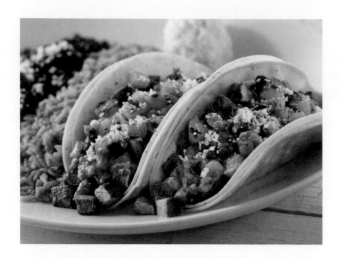

Traditional tacos. (© John Kelly/Alamy)

The consumption of meat and animal products, although popular, is often limited due to their cost. Beef, pork, chicken, fish, and eggs are all used. Traditional cheeses are prepared locally throughout the region as *queso del pais*, a mild, soft, white cheese, and milk is regularly used in *café con leche* and with cereal gruels.

The region is a rich source of a variety of fruits and vegetables. Best known among these are the chile peppers, tomatoes, and tomatillos that are used in the salsas of Mexico. Avocado is also very popular in Mexican and Central American cuisines. Other commonly used vegetables include *calabaza* (pumpkin), carrots, plantains, onions, locally grown greens, and cacti. Fruits are seasonal but abundant in the rural areas and include guavas, papayas, mangoes, melons, pineapples, bananas, oranges, and limes, as well as less known local fruits such as *nances*, *mamey*, and *tunas* (prickly pears from cacti). Traditional drinks (*frescos*, *chichas*, or *liquados*) are made with fruit, water, and sugar.

Description

Methods of cooking

The traditional preparation of maize involves boiling and soaking dried maize in a lime-water solution and then grinding it to form a soft dough called *masa*. Soaking in lime softens the maize and is an important source of **calcium** in the diet. The masa is shaped and cooked on a flat metal or clay surface over an open fire. In some areas, lard or margarine, milk, cheese, and/or baking powder may be added to the tortilla during preparation. Beans are generally boiled with seasonings such as onion, garlic, and sometimes tomato or chile peppers. They are served either in a

soupy liquid or are "refried" with lard or oil, which makes the beans drier but also higher in fat.

Meat, poultry, and fish are commonly prepared in local variations of thin soup (*caldo* or *sopa*) or thicker soups or stews (*cocido*) with vegetables. In Mexico and Guatemala, grilled meats are cut into pieces and eaten directly on corn tortillas as tacos. These are often served with a variety of salsas based on tomato or tomatillo with onion, chile, coriander leaves (cilantro), and other local seasonings. Tamales are made with corn (or corn and rice) dough that is stuffed with chicken and vegetables. The tamales are steamed after being wrapped in banana leaves. Salvadorian *pupusas* are toasted tortillas filled with cheese, beans, or pork rind eaten with coleslaw and a special hot sauce.

Central American and Mexican dishes

Beyond the basic staples, the cuisine of Mexico and Central America is rich with many regional variations. The tortilla-based Mexican preparations familiar in the United States are generally simpler in form in Mexico. *Tacos* are generally made with meat, chicken, or fish grilled or fried with seasoning and served on tortillas; *enchiladas* are filled tortillas dipped in a chile-based sauce and fried; and *tostadas* are fried tortillas topped with refried beans or meat, and sometimes with vegetables and cream. *Chiles rellenos* are made with the large and sweet chile *poblano* and filled with ground meat. Examples of specialty dishes include *mole*, a sauce made with chocolate, chile, and spices and served over chicken, beef, or enchiladas, and *ceviche*, raw marinated fish or seafood made along the coast throughout Central America and Mexico.

Influence of Central American and Mexican culture

When two cultures intermingle, the foods and preparations from each tend to infiltrate the other. This is clearly the case near the U.S.-Mexican border, where Mexican immigrants and return immigrants have incorporated foods from U.S. diets into their traditional diets. The result has been a modified form of Mexican cuisine popularly known as "Tex-Mex." Beyond the border, this Americanized version of popular Mexican foods has spread throughout the United States with the popularity of Mexican restaurants. In the United States, tacos and tostadas tend to have less Mexican seasoning but include lettuce and shredded processed cheese. Flour (rather than corn) tortillas are more widely used along the border. Many foods, such as soups and chiles, prepared along the border have become known for their spicy hotness, due to the Mexican-influenced use of chiles and chile powder.

Function

Coupled with locally available fruits, vegetables, meat, and dairy products, the diets of Mexico and Central America can be highly nutritious. However, poverty frequently limits access to an adequate variety of quality foods, resulting in **malnutrition**. At the same time, the increasing use of processed foods is contributing to obesity, diabetes, and other chronic conditions in this region. The balance between improving access to variety and maintaining dietary quality poses a challenge for public health.

Benefits

The staple diet of the region—corn and beans, supplemented with meat, dairy products, and local fruit and vegetables—is nutritionally complete and well suited to a healthful lifestyle. The combination of tortilla and beans provides an excellent complement of amino acids, thus supplying necessary amounts of complex **protein**. Maize is a source of calcium and **niacin**, and the process of liming the maize makes these nutrients even more bioavailable. In addition, the traditional preparation of tortillas with a hand mill and grinding stones appears to add **iron** and **zinc** to the tortilla. Beans are excellent sources of B **vitamins**, **magnesium**, **folate**, and **fiber**. The tomato and chile-based salsas, along with several of the tropical fruits such as limes and oranges, are important sources of **vitamin C**, and the variety of vegetables and yellow fruits such as papaya, melon, and mango provide excellent sources of **carotenoids**, which are precursors of **vitamin A**.

Risks

Unfortunately, limited financial access to a wide variety of foods for many people in Central America and Mexico means that their diets often do not include sufficient levels of vitamins and **minerals**. For low-income households, lack of access to animal products contributes to deficiencies in iron, zinc, vitamin A, and other nutrients. When animal products are included, there has been a tendency to choose high-fat products such as sausage and fried pork rinds (*chicharron*) over leaner meats. The use of lard and a preference for fried foods also contributes to high intakes of saturated fat and cholesterol among subsets of the population. The Central America Diabetes Initiative's 2010 *Survey of Diabetes, Hypertension, and Chronic Disease Risk Factors*, published by the U.S. Centers for Disease Control and Prevention and the World Health Organization, found that rates of diabetes and hypertension in Central America were 8.5% and 25.4%, respectively.

> **KEY TERMS**
>
> **Bioavailability**—The degree to which a compound (such as a vitamin or mineral) can be absorbed and used by the body.
>
> **Hypertension**—High blood pressure.
>
> **Macronutrient**—Nutrient needed by the body in large quantities.
>
> **Malnutrition**—Condition characterized by a chronic lack of sufficient nutrients to maintain health.
>
> **Micronutrient**—Nutrient needed by the body in very small quantities (such as vitamins and minerals)
>
> **Undernutrition**—Condition characterized by food intake too low to maintain adequate energy expenditure without weight loss.

Changes in dietary practices

Throughout the world, the diets of traditional cultures have experienced what has been called the "nutrition transition." In Mexico and Central America, as elsewhere, this transition has been fueled by globalization and urbanization. According to a study published in the July 2009 issue of *Globalization and Health*, food imports into Central America more than doubled between 1990–92 and 2000–05, due largely in part to reduced tariffs. The study found the increase in imports correlated with an increase in chronic disease. Major dietary changes include an increased use of animal products and processed foods that include large amounts of sugar, refined flour, and hydrogenated **fats**, with a decline in the intake of **whole grains**, fruit, and vegetables. While the increased variety of foods has improved micronutrient status for many low-income groups, the inclusion of more animal fat and refined foods has contributed to a rapid increase in obesity and cardiovascular disease throughout the region.

These changes are more evident among immigrants to the United States, where adoption of U.S. products has been shown to have both positive and negative impacts on nutritional status. Studies that compared diets of Mexican residents to newly arrived Mexican American immigrants and to second-generation Mexican Americans have documented both nutritionally positive and negative changes with acculturation. On the positive side, acculturated Mexican Americans consume less lard and somewhat more fruit, vegetables, and milk than either newly arrived immigrants or Mexican residents. On the negative side, they also consume less tortillas, beans, soups, stews, gruels, and fruit-based drinks, with greater use of meat, sweetened ready-to-eat breakfast cereals, soft drinks, candy, cakes, ice cream, snack chips, and salad dressings.

Resources

PERIODICALS

Mattei, J., F.B. Hu, and H. Campos. "A Higher Ratio of Beans to White Rice is Associated with Lower Cardiometabolic Risk Factors in Costa Rican Adults." *American Journal of Clinical Nutrition* 94, no. 3 (2011): 869–76.

Rhee, J.J., J. Mattei, and H. Campos. "Association between Commercial and Traditional Sugar-Sweetened Beverages and Measures of Adiposity in Costa Rica." *Public Health Nutrition* (April 12, 2012): e-pub ahead of print. http://dx.doi.org/10.1017/S1368980012001000 (accessed June 27, 2012).

Romero-Gwynn, Eunice, et al. "Dietary Acculturation among Latinos of Mexican Descent." *Nutrition Today* 28, no. 4 (1993): 6–12.

Thow, Anne Marie, and Corinna Hawkes. "The Implications of Trade Liberalization for Diet and Health: A Case Study from Central America." *Globalization and Health* 5, no. 5 (July 2009): online only. http://dx.doi.org/10.1186/1744-8603-5-5 (accessed June 27, 2012).

WEBSITES

National Heart, Lung, and Blood Institute. "Guatemala—Institute of Nutrition of Central America and Panama." U.S. National Institutes of Health. http://www.nhlbi.nih.gov/about/globalhealth/centers/guatemala-center-of-excellence.htm (accessed June 27, 2012).

ORGANIZATIONS

Pan American Health Organization (PAHO), Regional Office for the Americas of the World Health Organization, 525 23rd St. NW, Washington, DC 20037, (202) 974-3000, Fax: (202) 974-3663, http://new.paho.org.

Katherine L. Tucker

Central European and Russian diet

Definition

The Central European and Russian diet is comprised mainly of animal **protein**, vegetables, and fruits. Foods are prepared most often either baked or boiled. Garlic, cabbage, pumpkin, and onion are staples of diets in these regions. Dairy is often consumed as milk,

sour cream, cheese, and yogurt. Popular herbs and spices include basil and paprika.

Origins

The socioeconomic situation in the democratic part of Europe, the Soviet bloc, and in the United States after World War II played a part in the development of the central European and Russian diet. The United States and the European democratic states were prosperous countries with effective economies and a rich variety of all kinds of foods. The Communist states, however, had ineffective centralized economies and lower standards of living. The amount of various foods, especially foods of animal origin, was almost always insufficient in the USSR and the majority of its satellite countries. Data on food consumption compiled by the Food and Agricultural Organization (FAO) confirm that meat consumption between 1961 and 1990 was substantially lower in the USSR, Poland, Romania, and Bulgaria than in Western Europe or the United States. Similarly, the consumption of milk and butter in Bulgaria, Hungary, and Romania was significantly lower in comparison with Western and Northern Europe.

Description

Diets from this region have developed in response to numerous factors including climate, environmental agriculture, and influences of neighboring countries and cultures.

Borshch is a traditional soup of the region and is made primarily with beets, vegetables, and meat. Pastries called pirozhki may include fillings of potatoes, cabbage, meat, or cheese. Fish is also a staple, including caviar.

Function

Grain products serve as a foundation for hearty food substances, such as breads and cereals, providing **fiber** and **carbohydrates** in the diet. Meat and fish allow for high intake of protein and **minerals**. Dairy products, such as eggs and cheese, serve as important sources of **calcium**.

Benefits

With the collapse of Communism, higher consumption of healthful food has occurred, including a substantial increase in the consumption of fruit and vegetables, a decrease in butter and fatty milk consumption, and an increase in the consumption of vegetable oils and high-quality margarines.

Precautions

High prevalence of smoking and alcoholism has been an important factor in high cardiovascular disease mortality rates, especially in Russia. Alcoholism has evidently played a key role in the extremely high incidence of cardiovascular disease mortality, as well as in the numbers of accidents, injuries, suicides, and murders. There is no way to determine a reliable estimation of the actual consumption of alcohol in Russia, since alcohol is being smuggled into the country on a large scale.

Risks

Trends in lifestyle, smoking, food selection, **alcohol consumption**, and other areas will be determined by both economic and political factors. The successfulness of continued economic transformation will be a key factor in improving diet choices, nutritional options, and the health status in post-Communist countries.

Research and general acceptance

Traditional cuisine of the central European and Russian diet has long been adhered to by individuals of these regions, dating back to Medieval days, with continued intake of many of the same foods during modern times. Individuals from these regions maintain celebrations (such as Maslenitsa) and feasts that still include foods and favorite dishes from long-held traditions.

Resources

BOOKS

Bender, David A. *A Dictionary of Food and Nutrition*. New York: Oxford University Press, 2009.

Counihan, Carole, and Penny Van Esternik, eds. *Food and Culture*. 3rd ed. New York: Routledge, 2012.

WEBSITES

World Health Organization. "European Health for All Database." http://www.euro.who.int/hfadb (accessed August 14, 2012).

ORGANIZATIONS

World Health Organization, Avenue Appia 20, 1211 Geneva 27, Switzerland, + 41 22 791-2111, Fax: + 41 22 791-3111, info@who.int, http://www.who.int.

Emil Ginther
Laura Jean Cataldo, RN, EdD

ChangeOne diet

Definition

The aim of "ChangeOne: Lose Weight Simply, Safely, and Forever" is to provide a simple, straightforward plan for gradual, permanent weight loss. The book features a twelve-week eating plan that outlines portion sizes, recipes, and meal suggestions designed to achieve weight loss. A major distinguishing feature of the ChangeOne plan is its emphasis on making lifestyle changes gradually over a three-month interval, rather than advocating a complete, abrupt transformation of existing eating patterns. The diet is based on everyday foods, both home-prepared and available in restaurants, and does not require purchase of special foods or supplements.

Origins

ChangeOne is published by the Reader's Digest Association, a New York–based company that also owns and operates *Reader's Digest*, the best-selling consumer magazine in the United States. ChangeOne has been dubbed "The Official Reader's Digest Diet." The lead author is John Hastings, a senior staff editor for health at *Reader's Digest*. Co-authors are Peter Jaret, a health journalist, and Mindy Hermann, a registered dietitian.

The principles underlying this diet reflect the influence of the *Dietary Guidelines for Americans* set by the U.S. Department of Agriculture. These guidelines emphasize moderation, portion control, and the use of plant foods—grains, fruits, and vegetables—as the basis for meals.

Description

The cornerstone of this diet is the progressive, gradual nature in which it promotes behavior change. Readers are advised to approach weight loss one meal at a time, one day at a time, beginning with a week-long focus on breakfast. The reader starts out by completing a quiz assessing readiness for permanent lifestyle changes.

Meal plans are designed to meet the following daily intakes:

- calories: 1,300–1,600
- calories from fat: 30%–35% of total calories
- saturated and hydrogenated ("trans") fats: no more than 10% of calories
- fiber: at least 25 grams
- calcium: approximately 1,000 milligrams
- fruits and vegetables: at least five servings

The ChangeOne diet is flexible in letting readers set their own calorie target within the recommended range and adjust it throughout the program to suit their needs. Those who are physically inactive or weigh less than 190 pounds are advised to aim for the lower end of the calorie range. Readers who weigh more than 190 pounds or get more than thirty minutes of daily vigorous exercise are advised to aim for the higher calorie intake.

A key idea underlying the ChangeOne plan is that all foods can fit within a balanced plan for long-term weight management. The authors recognize that food restrictions tend to intensify **cravings**; for this reason, no foods are forbidden on this plan. The crux of the diet lies in portion control. Household items such as tennis balls, golf balls, and checkbooks are suggested for gauging portions. The reader is not required to count **calories**, but must adhere to the recommended food types and portion sizes. Presumably, if the portion sizes are followed correctly, the day's total calories will fall within the targeted range.

The ChangeOne program advocates eating at a slow pace, both to enhance enjoyment of meals and to help the body properly assess hunger and satisfaction levels while eating. The authors recommend a high consumption of water and other calorie-free beverages for their satisfying effect. For the same reason, an unlimited intake of non-starchy vegetables, such as those used in salads and stir-fries, is allowed. Alcohol intake is allowed but limited to one standard serving of beer or wine per day. Each chapter features recipes to complement the meal plan, as well as "Fast Track" suggestions for accelerating progress, such as increasing minutes spent on physical activity or using a journal to keep track of foods eaten. Readers learn to use rewards to reinforce positive behavior changes until the weight loss provides the necessary reinforcement.

The Program at a Glance

WEEK ONE: BREAKFAST. Eating a morning meal is cited as being crucial to weight management. The authors refer to data from the National Weight Control Registry that suggest that eating breakfast every day is associated with losing weight and keeping it off. The ChangeOne breakfast plan encourages a balance of starchy foods, fruit, and a calcium-rich food. High-fiber foods are promoted for their satisfying quality and nutrient density. Sample recipes include vegetable frittata and dried cranberry scones with orange glaze.

WEEK TWO: LUNCH. The second week of the program has dieters planning ahead for both home-prepared and purchased lunches that are satisfying and portion-controlled. The mid-day meal is comprised of a small portion of lean meat, fish, or a vegetarian alternative, along with a starchy food, one fruit, and unlimited vegetables. Restaurant meals can fit the plan as long as recommended portion sizes are honored. Readers are encouraged to anticipate the difficulty of making healthy restaurant choices by creating a list of ChangeOne meals that can be ordered in restaurants. This chapter provides an overview of best options in fast food restaurants. Sample recipes include grilled turkey Caesar salad and roasted vegetable wraps with chive sauce.

WEEK THREE: SNACKS. On the ChangeOne regime, dieters plan for two snacks each day. The authors point to scientific evidence that eating frequently throughout the day can assist with weight management by regulating blood sugar levels and warding off cravings and intense hunger. This chapter teaches readers to properly interpret hunger cues and encourages an awareness of emotional eating. It offers strategies to manage hunger and appetite. Sample recipes include chocolate snacking cake and multigrain soft pretzels.

WEEK FOUR: DINNER. The fourth week of the program places as much emphasis on how to eat as it does on what and how much to eat. The author provides an overview of the principles of effective goal setting, advising that goals have clear deadlines and be realistic, inspiring, and measurable. This chapter provides plenty of practical suggestions for meal preparation, including tips for low-fat cooking, such as the use of marinades to tenderize lean cuts of meat and the use of seasonings and herbs to add flavor without calories. The dinner meal plan features a small serving of lean meat or another protein-rich food, paired with a starchy side dish and unlimited vegetables. Sample recipes include Thai noodle salad and red snapper with Spanish rice. By the end of the fourth week, dieters should have all three meals and two snacks under good control.

WEEK FIVE: DINING OUT. The authors recommend eating in restaurants at least twice in the fifth week of the program in order to gain practice navigating menus and making healthy choices. This chapter opens with an eye-opening discussion of how restaurant meals distort our understanding of sensible portions. The keys to sticking with the ChangeOne plan when eating out, the authors contend, is being both prepared and discerning. When possible, reviewing the menu prior to arriving at the restaurant is recommended. Readers are advised to keep a list of restaurants on hand that are known to offer good tasting options that are lower in calories. Dieters are encouraged to be assertive when ordering by requesting ingredient substitutions and smaller portions. Discipline is required to stick to the portion sizes recommended in the meal plans, leaving excess food uneaten. The chapter outlines best menu options for such favorites as Italian, Mexican, and Chinese restaurants; surf and turf; diners; and coffee shops.

WEEK SIX: WEEKENDS AND HOLIDAYS. ChangeOne is realistic in acknowledging that routines tend to change over the weekend. The authors advise against viewing weekends as vacations from the healthy eating patterns implemented during the workweek; to do so implies that the diet is merely a temporary effort to improve eating habits. This chapter encourages enlisting friends and family for support but warns against saboteurs and others who will apply pressure to abandon new healthy eating habits. Strategies are offered for staying on track during the holidays (for example, having low-calorie snacks on hand and directing activities that do not involve food). The recipe section features calorie-wise alternatives to traditional holiday fare, including a revamped turkey dinner and Sunday brunch.

WEEK SEVEN: FIXING YOUR KITCHEN. The challenge this chapter proposes is taking stock of the food supplies in the kitchen so that they support the reader's new healthy eating habits. The first step advised to get the kitchen diet-ready is purging the shelves of anything that might sabotage healthy eating efforts. The authors offer strategies for smart grocery shopping such as not shopping on an empty stomach, sticking to planned purchases, and spending the most time shopping around the store's perimeter, avoiding aisles

laden with processed foods. The reader is advised to inspect foodstuffs and "read the small print," but specifics on how to read and interpret nutrition labels are not offered. The chapter closes with a few recipes that feature basic ingredients found in most pantries.

WEEK EIGHT: HOW AM I DOING? This week serves as a checkpoint for assessing progress and provides an opportunity to reshape goals and renew commitment. The authors guide in trouble-shooting common stumbling blocks like portion distortion and lack of meal planning. Practical suggestions are offered for dealing with emotional stress and the temptation to quit. The authors advise their readers to revisit their expectations for what constitutes weight loss success. Dieters are taught to pace their long-term goals by setting more tangible milestones and rewarding small successes along the way.

WEEK NINE: STRESS RELIEF. In week nine, dieters are encouraged to consider the relationship between weight management and stress management. The authors explain how high levels of stress affect the body's hormonal balance, triggering food cravings and promoting fat deposition. Readers are advised to analyze the stressors in their lives and begin brainstorming solutions. The authors emphasize participation in physical activity and the support of friends as effective stress management tools. Readers are encouraged to try a step-by-step 20-minute daily relaxation routine to relieve tension and enhance coping. This week's featured recipes are calorie-reduced versions of traditional comfort foods such as meatloaf, chicken pot pie, and beef stew.

WEEK TEN: STAYING ACTIVE FOR SUCCESS. In the program's tenth week, healthy eating and active living are shown to be synergistic. The author presents research showing that dieters who exercise regularly enjoy greater success in their weight-loss programs than those who are physically inactive. Rather than advocating intense gym workouts, the authors highlight the calories expended in activities of daily living and encourage being active in ways that are enjoyable. For optimal fat burning, however, readers are advised to check their pulse and aim for an intensity equivalent to 60% to 80% of maximum heart rate. The chapter is consistent with the book's message of making changes gradually; it encourages starting out with 10 to 15 minute walks each day and slowly working up to 30 minutes of daily physical activity.

WEEK ELEVEN: KEEPING ON TRACK. This week's goal is developing strategies for monitoring progress and trouble-shooting areas of difficulty in order to avoid set-backs. Readers are advised to anticipate small weight fluctuations but to take action before a few pounds of weight gain become a full relapse. The authors provide a diagnostic checklist for identifying areas of difficulty. They advise weekly weigh-ins to gauge long-term progress. Dieters are encouraged to monitor and make a written record of mood states in order to uncover their relationship to emotional eating.

WEEK TWELVE: AVOIDING BOREDOM AND MAINTAINING CHANGES. ChangeOne acknowledges that boredom with a set routine is a big obstacle in maintaining changes over the long term. The authors encourage their readers to break their routine slightly every week to foster continued enjoyment of eating. Suggestions include trying a new food every week, creating a salad bar at home for dinner and concocting signature flavor combinations for standbys like home-made pasta and pizza. Again, dieters are reminded to keep the process from becoming tedious by setting rewards for small steps taken towards the achievement of the ultimate goal.

Part Two of the ChangeOne book is a collection of resources, including meal plans, recipes, and an eight-week fitness program complete with color photographs of aerobic, strengthening, and stretching exercises.

Function

The ChangeOne diet promotes a gradual calorie deficit by remodeling eating habits one meal at a time. Ultimately, three low-calorie meals plus two small snacks provide a total of 1,300 to 1,600 calories per day, which represents a significant reduction in calorie consumption for the average North American adult.

Meal plans are presented in a style that allows the reader to mix and match set amounts of preferred foods. This flexibility allows the reader to create enjoyable meals that are calorie-controlled, thus promoting weight loss.

Part Two of the ChangeOne book includes recipes and daily menus to support readers who desire the structure of a set meal plan.

Benefits

The ChangeOne diet promises "no fads, no risks, no craziness." It is based on nutrition principles that are scientifically sound, and it echoes the nutrient balance endorsed by the U.S. Department of Agriculture. Meals consist of lean **protein**, high-fiber starchy foods, fruits, vegetables, and low-fat dairy. No foods are disallowed, and no special foods or supplements are necessary. Meals can be prepared at home or purchased in restaurants. Varied meal plans and tasty menus, combined with numerous recipes and cooking tips, make the book practical and informative.

ChangeOne is written in a straightforward, engaging manner. Changes are promoted in a step-wise fashion, in contrast to the "all-or-nothing" approach sometimes espoused by other diets. Rather than simply providing guidance on what to eat, ChangeOne encourages exploration of the reasons for eating.

Precautions

The ChangeOne program is a suitable weight loss plan for most adults. However, they should consult with their physician before beginning any weight-loss program. The upper limit of 1,600 calories per day may be insufficient for people who engage in regular physical activity. The use of **artificial sweeteners** is not appropriate for everyone. Readers should get clearance with their doctors regarding ideal exercise type, intensity, and duration before beginning any exercise program.

Risks

Because this diet emphasizes sound patterns of healthy eating, there are no significant risks in following its principles. Dieters should note that the program is not designed for rapid weight loss.

QUESTIONS TO ASK YOUR DOCTOR

- What is a healthy weight for me?
- Do I need to lose weight?
- Is it safe for me to start doing physical activity?
- Are there any artificial sweeteners that I should avoid?
- Can you refer me to a registered dietitian?

Research and general acceptance

The ChangeOne program echoes the principles of healthy eating promoted in the USDA Food Guidelines for Americans. In particular, the diet mirrors the National Academy of Sciences' Acceptable Macronutrient Distribution Ranges (AMDR) for fat, **carbohydrates**, and protein, which are 20%–35% of total calories, 45%–65% of total calories, and 10%–35% of total calories, respectively. The recommended intake of fat, as well as calories from saturated fat, *trans* fat, **fiber**, and **calcium**, also complies with the recommendations set by the National Academy of Sciences.

Much of the advice and strategies recommended in ChangeOne has a strong scientific basis. The authors substantiate their recommendations by quoting research from reputable sources such as Harvard University, Penn State University, the Journal of the American Medical Association, and the Center for Science in the Public Interest. The authors also draw data from the National Weight Control Registry, the largest study of its kind investigating factors associated with successful weight loss and maintenance.

Lead author John Hastings notes that physicians served as advisors in the development of the eating plan. The diet was pilot-tested by volunteers, mostly from the Reader's Digest workforce. Participants lost an average of 17 pounds over the 12 week program. There is no mention of the number of participants involved in testing the diet and whether these results bear any statistical significance.

Resources

BOOKS

Hastings, John. *ChangeOne: Lose Weight Simply, Safely and Forever*. Pleasantville, NY: Reader's Digest Association, 2003.

Katz, David, and Gonzalez, Maura. *The Way to Eat: A Six Step Path to Lifelong Weight Control*. Naperville, IL: Sourcebooks, 2004.

Larson Duyff, Roberta, and the American Dietetic Association. *American Dietetic Association Complete Food and Nutrition Guide*. Hoboken, NJ: John Wiley & Sons, 2006.

Napier, Kristine, and the American Dietetic Association. *American Dietetic Association Cooking Healthy Across America*. Hoboken, NJ: John Wiley & Sons, 2005.

Tribole, Evelyn, and Resch, Elyse. *Intuitive Eating: A Revolutionary Program That Works*. New York: St. Martin's Press, 2003.

PERIODICALS

Avenell, Alison, Naveed Sattar, and Mike Lean. "Management: Part I-Behavior Change, Diet, and Activity." *British Medical Journal* 333, no. 7571 (Oct 7, 2006): 740–43.

Kaplan, Lee. "Keeping the Weight Off." *Weigh Less, Live Longer (Harvard Special Health Report)* (Sept 2006): 40.

Melanson, Kathleen. "Food Intake Regulation in Body Weight Management: A Primer." *Nutrition Today* 39, no. 5 (Sep–Oct 2004): 203–15.

Solo, Sally. "Ditch Your Diet." *Real Simple* 8, no. 2 (Feb 2007): 162.

WEBSITES

Mayo Clinic staff. "Weight-Loss Help: Gain Control of Emotional Eating." http://www.mayoclinic.com/health/weight-loss/MH00025 (accessed September 27, 2012).

Reader's Digest. "Best You." http://mybestyou.com (accessed September 27, 2012).

U.S. Department of Agriculture and U.S. Department of Health and Human Services. *Dietary Guidelines for Americans, 2010*. 7th ed. Washington, DC: U.S. Government Printing Office, December 2010. http://health.gov/dietaryguidelines (accessed September 27, 2012).

ORGANIZATIONS

Academy of Nutrition and Dietetics, 120 South Riverside Plz., Ste. 2000, Chicago, IL 60606-6995, (312) 899-0040, (800) 877-1600, amacmunn@eatright.org, http://www.eatright.org.

British Nutrition Foundation, High Holborn House, 52-54 High Holborn, London, United Kingdom WC1V 6RQ, 44 20 7404 6504, Fax: 44 20 7404 6747, postbox@nutrition.org.uk, http://www.nutrition.org.uk.

Dietitians of Canada, 480 University Ave., Ste. 604, Toronto, Ontario, Canada M5G 1V2, (416) 596-0857, Fax: (416) 596-0603, centralinfo@dietitians.ca, http://www.dietitians.ca.

National Weight Control Registry, Brown Medical School/The Miriam Hospital Weight Control & Diabetes Research Center, 196 Richmond St., Providence, RI 02903, (800) 606-NWCR (6927), tmnwcr@lifespan.org, http://www.nwcr.ws.

Marie Fortin, MEd, RD

Chicken soup diet

Definition

The chicken soup diet is a seven-day diet that allows the dieter to eat one of five approved breakfasts each day and as much chicken soup as desired.

Origins

The origins of the chicken soup diet are not clear. It seems to circulate mostly from person to person and on the Internet. For many years, people have believed that chicken soup has various health properties. Many different cultures give versions of chicken soup to people who are sick. This belief in the health benefits of chicken soup may have something to do with its popularity as a diet food.

Description

The chicken soup diet is a diet that is designed to be followed for seven days, although many versions of the diet say that it can be followed for as long as

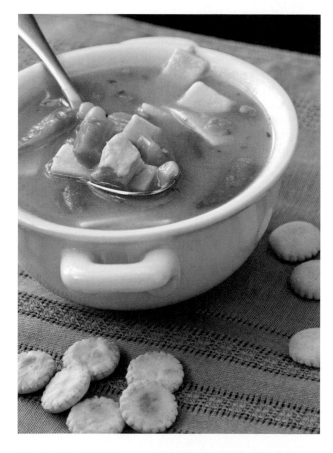

Homemade chicken soup. *(Jill Battaglia/Shutterstock.com)*

desired or repeated at any time. It consists of a soup recipe and five breakfast choices. After breakfast, the only thing that the dieter is allowed to eat until the next morning is the soup. This diet also tells dieters what they may or may not drink while on the diet.

The soup

The recipe for the soup is as follows:

- 2 tablespoons of oil (olive oil is recommended)
- 4 parsnips (about 1 lb.) cut into 1/2 inch pieces
- 4 ribs of celery
- 1 turnip (about 3/4 lb.) cut into 1/2 inch pieces
- 1 jalapeno pepper, seeded and chopped
- 1 tablespoon of chopped garlic
- 2 teaspoons of salt
- 1/2 teaspoon of cayenne pepper
- 16 cups of reduced fat, low sodium chicken broth
- 7 (5 oz.) cans of chicken or 1 1/2 pounds (5 cups) cooked fresh chicken
- 1 bag (16 oz.) frozen carrots
- 1 box (10 oz.) frozen broccoli florets
- 1 box (10 oz.) frozen chopped collard greens
- 1 1/2 cups frozen chopped onions
- 1/4 cup of lemon juice
- 1/4 cup chopped fresh dill or 1 tablespoon dried dill

Heat the oil over medium heat in a large soup pot. Add the garlic, salt, cayenne pepper, jalapeno, parsnips, celery, and turnip to the pot. Cook these until the vegetables are tender but still crisp, which will take approximately 15 minutes. Next, add the carrots, collard greens, broccoli, onions, chicken broth, and lemon juice to the pot. Bring to a boil, then reduce the heat and allow the soup to simmer for 5 minutes. This recipe is said to make approximately 26 one-cup servings. There may be slightly different versions of this recipe, but this one is the most common.

Breakfast

The chicken soup diet allows dieters to chose one breakfast each day from five possible breakfasts. Most versions of the diet encourage dieters to eat each breakfast once for the first five days, and then choose the breakfast they liked best and repeat them for days six and seven. The breakfasts are:

1. 1 cup of nonfat vanilla yogurt and 1/2 cup of fruit salad sprinkled with wheat germ
2. 1 cup of ricotta cheese combined with 1/2 teaspoon of sugar and a dash of cinnamon, along

with 2 pieces of toasted whole-grain bread and 3 dried figs

3. 1.5 cups of Total brand cereal, along with 1/2 cup of nonfat milk and 1/2 cup of calcium-enriched orange juice

4. 1 small whole-wheat bagel topped with 1 ounce of melted fat-free cheddar cheese, along with 1/2 cup of prune juice

5. 1.5 cups of cooked Wheatena brand cereal along with 1/2 cup of nonfat milk

After the dieter eats one of these breakfasts, only the chicken soup may be consumed for the rest of the day.

Function

The chicken soup diet does not make any claims about how much weight a dieter can lose during the seven days of the diet, although it is usually implied that the dieter will be able to lose a substantial amount of weight. It does include any exercise or healthy living recommendations. Some versions of the diet suggest that it would be a good diet to use if a dieter wanted to "jump start" a more comprehensive dieting plan, or if a dieter needed to lose a large amount of weight quickly for an upcoming special event.

Benefits

Although the soup recipe is healthy, the chicken soup diet is not a well-balanced diet and is not recommended. Weight is best lost at a safe, moderate pace through a combination of healthy eating and exercise. There are many conditions for which **obesity** is considered a risk factor, including type 2 diabetes and heart disease. The risk of these and other diseases may be reduced through weight loss. This is especially

true for people who are very obese, who are generally thought to be at the greatest risk. The chicken soup diet is not a form of long-term moderate weight loss.

Precautions

The chicken soup diet is very restrictive and should not be followed for an extended period of time. Anyone thinking of beginning a new diet should consult a doctor or other medical practitioner. Requirements of **calories**, fat, and nutrients can differ from person to person, depending on gender, age, weight, and other factors such as the presence of diseases or conditions. The chicken soup diet does not allow very many different foods, and although the soup may be healthy, it is unlikely to be able to provide all the **vitamins** and **minerals** needed for healthy adults each day. Pregnant or **breastfeeding** women especially should not follow this or any other restrictive diet, because deficiencies of vitamins and other nutrients can negatively impact a fetus.

Risks

There are some risks associated with any diet. The chicken soup diet does not allow the dieter to eat very many different foods each day. This means that it is unlikely to provide enough of the vitamins and minerals required each day for good health. Anyone thinking of beginning this diet should first consult with a health-care practitioner. The risk of developing nutrient deficiencies increase the longer the diet is followed.

Research and general acceptance

The chicken soup diet has not been the subject of any significant scientific studies. In 2000, researchers at the University of Nebraska Medical Center found that chicken soup may have anti-inflammatory properties. The research was very preliminary and was done in a laboratory, not using human subjects, so it is not clear what the effect on the immune system of a human would actually be. The soup used in the research was not made using the recipe given in this diet, although it did contain some of the same ingredients.

The U.S. Department of Agriculture makes recommendations for how many servings of each type of food most adults need to eat each day for good health. These recommendations are represented by **MyPlate**, which replaced the former food pyramid. The chicken soup diet is extremely limited in what foods it allows dieters to eat and does not include all of the recommended food groups, such as fruit, dairy, and **carbohydrates**. The diet is likely to be especially unhealthy if followed for a long time or repeated frequently.

Resources

BOOKS

Larsen, Laura, ed. *Diet and Nutrition Sourcebook*. Detroit, MI: Omnigraphics, 2006.

Willis, Alicia P. ed. *Diet Therapy Research Trends*. New York: Nova Science, 2007.

WEBSITES

"Chicken Soup Diet." http://www.faddiet.com/chicsoupdiet.html (accessed September 27, 2012).

"Chicken Soup Diet." http://www.thedietchannel.com/Chicken-soup-diet.htm (accessed September 27, 2012).

U.S. Department of Agriculture. "MyPlate." http://www.choosemyplate.gov (accessed September 27, 2012).

ORGANIZATIONS

U.S. Department of Agriculture, 1400 Independence Ave. SW, Washington, DC 20250, (202) 720-2791, http://www.usda.gov.

Helen M. Davidson

Childhood nutrition

Definition

Childhood nutrition concerns the dietary needs of healthy children ages 2 through 11. Children younger than 2 and older than 11 have different nutritional requirements and concerns. In addition, parents of children with special health needs or dietary restrictions require individualized diet advice. They should consult a pediatrician or a registered dietitian about their child's diet.

Purpose

Proper nutrition for a healthy child should provide sufficient essential nutrients, **fiber**, and energy (**calories**) to maintain normal growth, maximize

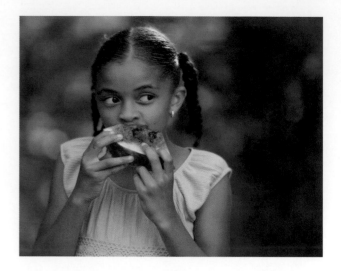

Fruits and vegetables are healthy snack options for kids.
(© iStockphoto.com/Glenda Powers)

cognitive development, and promote health. Diet should be balanced so that foods rich in some nutrients do not displace foods that are rich in other nutrients, and so low-nutrient foods ("empty calories") do not displace nutrient-dense foods. A child's diet should provide sufficient energy for proper physical and mental growth and development while preventing excess weight gain.

Description

Childhood is a time where many food likes and dislikes are determined, largely based on what food choices the family makes, socioeconomic status, budget, cultural and/or religious experiences, time constraints, and other various factors. For children, the food environment in which they are raised has a significant effect on food choices later in life. Parents, guardians, and others need to pay special attention to nutrition and food choices to support a wide variety of tastes and preferences.

Healthy eating habits in childhood have been shown to prevent chronic undernutrition and physical and cognitive growth problems as well as nutritional concerns such as iron-deficiency anemia and dental caries (cavities). A healthy diet in childhood can help prevent **obesity** and weight-related diseases, such as type 2 diabetes, which is increasingly diagnosed in children in the United States.

USDA guidelines and MyPlate

In 1980, the first edition of *Dietary Guidelines for Americans* was released by the U.S. Department of Agriculture (USDA). The most recent version, the

2010 *Dietary Guidelines for Americans*, was released on January 31, 2011. The 2010 version was developed specifically to help combat the increasing obesity problem in the United States. It focuses on providing recommendations that are easy for busy people to put into practice in their daily lives.

Some general guidelines from the 2010 directive include:

• Enjoy your food, but eat less.

• Avoid oversized portions.

• Make half your plate fruits and vegetables.

• Drink water instead of sugary drinks.

• Switch to fat-free or low-fat milk.

The 2010 guidelines also include a wide variety of other recommendations. The two overarching themes of the recommendations are: (1) maintain calorie balance over time to achieve and sustain a healthy weight, and (2) focus on consuming nutrient-dense foods and beverages. From the 2010 guidelines, the USDA developed and introduced **MyPlate**, which replaced the food pyramid. MyPlate offers a visual for families to create a nutritional plate for each meal based on dividing a plate into roughly 30% grains, 30% vegetables, 20% fruits, and 20% **protein**. A smaller circle separate from the plate represents dairy products.

Although MyPlate's general recommendations apply to almost all age groups, there are also suggestions for specific groups, including infants, preschoolers, and children. These suggestions include information about specific food groups, as well as suggested menus and tips for improving eating habits. Some general guidelines for kids ages 2–11 include:

• Make half of each plate fruits and vegetables. Kids 2–11 years old should have about 1–1.5 cups fruit and 1–2 cups vegetables per day.

• Switch to skim or 1% milk. Kids 2–11 years old should have 2–3 8-ounce glasses per day.

• Make at least half of all grains consumed whole. Kids 2–11 years old should have about 3–6 one-ounce equivalents of grains per day.

• Vary protein food choices. Kids 2–11 years old should have about 2–5 one-ounce equivalents of meat or meat substitutes per day.

• Choose foods and drinks with little or no added sugars.

• Look out for salt (sodium) in foods.

• Eat fewer foods that are high in solid fats.

KEY TERMS

Cholesterol—A waxy substance made by the liver and also acquired through diet. High levels in the blood may increase the risk of cardiovascular disease.

Fiber—Also known as roughage or bulk. Insoluble fiber moves through the digestive system almost undigested and gives bulk to stools. Soluble fiber dissolves in water and helps keep stools soft.

Hypertension—Persistently high blood pressure.

Osteoarthritis—The most common form of arthritis, characterized by erosion of the cartilage layer that lies between the bones in weight-bearing joints. It occurs mainly in older people.

Type 2 diabetes—In this form of diabetes, either the pancreas does not make enough insulin or cells become insulin resistant and do not use insulin efficiently. Formerly only seen in adults, it is becoming increasingly common in overweight children and young adults.

Precautions

The USDA guidelines are based on the most current research by nutrition scientists and have a very high level of acceptance by health professionals. For healthy children, there are no perceived precautions or risks associated with following these guidelines. Children younger than 2 or older than 11 should follow the recommendations for their particular age groups. Children of any age who have special health concerns or dietary restrictions may not be able to adhere to the USDA guidelines and should follow the advice of their pediatrician or a registered dietitian (RD).

Complications

In addition to addressing children's energy needs, the guidelines take into consideration the need for specific nutrients to avoid the development of undernutrition or **malnutrition**. For example, adequate intake of **calcium** and **vitamin D** in children helps build strong bones and is a preventative measure against osteopenia and rickets (and later in life, osteoporosis). Adequate calcium and vitamin D intake is crucial during adolescence and early adulthood to reach peak bone mass. Failure of children to meet the requirements, in combination with a sedentary lifestyle, makes achievement of maximal skeletal growth and bone mineralization challenging. Recommendations include several servings a day of low-fat or nonfat milk and dairy products (such as yogurt) in a child's diet.

GALE ENCYCLOPEDIA OF DIETS, 2ND EDITION   **217**

Iron deficiency has negative effects on children's cognitive development and can affect their capacity to do well in school. Adequate intake of foods high in iron, such as meats and fortified breakfast cereals, will help ensure that iron requirements are met.

While nutrient intake is important, overconsumption of nutrients can cause other problems. High saturated-fat intake is associated with increased low-density lipoprotein (LDL or "bad") cholesterol in childhood. This ultimately can increase the risk of cardiovascular disease and type 2 diabetes. A diet that includes lean meats (e.g., skinless chicken breasts) and low-fat or nonfat dairy products and limits foods high in saturated fat can help implement healthy habits and decrease a child's risk of developing type 2 diabetes or cardiovascular disease later in life.

Research has found that children who are obese experience psychological stress, decreased **body image** scores, lower self-esteem, and potentially more health problems than normal weight children of the same age. They are also more likely than normal-weight children to become obese adults. This increases their risk of cardiovascular disease, **hypertension**, type 2 diabetes, non-alcoholic fatty liver disease, gallbladder disease, osteoarthritis, and some cancers. Childhood nutritional guidelines emphasize nutrient-dense foods that provide enough calories for growth and activity while limiting foods of low nutritional value and high calorie content to avoid these health issues.

Parental concerns

Before children are two, parents' focus is on making sure their infant or toddler is consuming enough calories and nutrients to support growth and development. As the child ages, a shift occurs, and parents become more focused on the types of food their child is eating. There is a transition from the higher-fat foods needed in infancy to the lower or nonfat versions. During this time, children are highly influenced by flavor and will be guided to eat foods for taste instead of nutrition content, so parents need to be aware of what their children are eating and should limit foods high in fat and added **sugar**. Parents are also responsible for making sure that the foods offered are safe and appropriate for the child and their developmental skills.

For parents, childhood can be a time of "food quarrels" as their child is becoming more independent in their eating. When children are young, parents are responsible for what, when, and where the child eats. It is important that parents be attentive to the nutritional needs of their children and ensure that they are supplying appropriate foods in amounts that meet nutritional requirements. For younger children, having a set schedule of meal and snack times may help achieve nutritional balance. Parents should also be aware that kids may be unpredictable in the amounts of food, and they should allow their children to determine when and how much to eat and not to force them to eat.

As habits are being formed during these years, it is important for meals and snacks to be a social and a pleasant time. Televisions, video games, and other distractions should try to be avoided. Eating the same healthy foods as the child and encouraging them to try new foods will help provide a model of healthy eating. Parents should also not use food as a reward for good behavior, as a bribe, or for entertainment.

Children with **food allergies** or intolerances or other medical concerns may display poor growth, poor eating skills, inadequate food intake, developmental delays, elimination problems, or metabolic disorders. A parent who is concerned about their child's health should visit a pediatrician and express their concerns. If a problem is found to be related to the child's diet, a referral to a specialist is important for early intervention so that it will not affect long-term growth and health.

Resources

Nitzke, Susan. *Rethinking Nutrition: Connecting Science and Practice in Early Childhood Settings*. St. Paul, MN: Redleaf Press, 2010.

Satter, Ellyn. *Secrets of Feeding a Healthy Family: How to Eat, How to Raise Good Eaters, How to Cook*. Kelcy Press, 2008.

WEBSITES

American Academy of Family Physicians. "Kids: Eating & Nutrition." FamilyDoctor.org. http://familydoctor. org/familydoctor/en/kids/eating-nutrition.html (accessed September 21, 2012).

Centers for Disease Control and Prevention. "BMI Percentile Calculator for Child and Teen." http://apps.nccd.cdc.gov/dnpabmi/Calculator.aspx (accessed September 21, 2012).

Mayo Clinic staff. "Nutrition for Kids: Guidelines for a Healthy Diet." MayoClinic.com. http://www.mayoclinic.com/health/nutrition-for-kids/NU00606 (accessed September 21, 2012).

Paul, Maya W., and Lawrence Robinson. "Nutrition for Children and Teens: Helping Your Kids Eat Healthier." HelpGuide.org. http://helpguide.org/life/healthy_eating_children_teens.htm (accessed September 21, 2012).

U.S. Department of Agriculture. "Health and Nutrition Information for Preschoolers." ChooseMyPlate.gov. http://www.choosemyplate.gov/preschoolers.html (accessed September 21, 2012).

U.S. Department of Agriculture and U.S. Department of Health and Human Services. *Dietary Guidelines for Americans, 2010.* 7th ed. Washington, DC: U.S. Government Printing Office, December 2010. http://health.gov/dietaryguidelines (accessed February 22, 2012).

ORGANIZATIONS

Academy of Nutrition and Dietetics, 120 South Riverside Plz., Ste. 2000, Chicago, IL 60606-6995, (312) 899-0040, (800) 877-1600, amacmunn@eatright.org, http://www.eatright.org.

American Academy of Pediatrics (AAP), 141 Northwest Point Blvd., Elk Grove Village, IL 60007, (847) 434-4000, (800) 433-9016, Fax: (847) 434-8000, http://www.aap.org.

Center for Nutrition Policy and Promotion, U.S. Department of Agriculture, 3101 Park Center Drive, 10th Fl., Alexandria, VA, 22302, (703) 305-7600, Fax: (703) 305-3300, support@cnpp.usda.gov, http://www.cnpp.usda.gov.

U.S. Department of Agriculture, 1400 Independence Ave. SW, Washington, DC 20250, (202) 720-2791, http://www.usda.gov.

Weight-Control Information Network (WIN), 1 WIN Way, Bethesda, MD 20892-3665, (202) 828-1025, (877) 946-4627, Fax: (202) 828-1028, win@http://win.niddk.nih.gov, http://win.niddk.nih.gov.

Tish Davidson, AM
Megan C.M. Porter, RD, LD, CDE

Childhood obesity

Definition

Childhood **obesity** is the condition of being severely overweight between the ages of 2 and 19 years. The U.S. Centers for Disease Control and Prevention defines overweight as "having an excess body weight for a

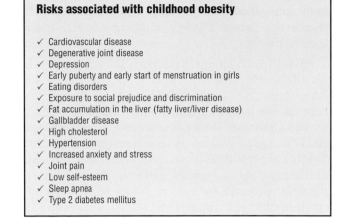

Risks associated with childhood obesity

✓ Cardiovascular disease
✓ Degenerative joint disease
✓ Depression
✓ Early puberty and early start of menstruation in girls
✓ Eating disorders
✓ Exposure to social prejudice and discrimination
✓ Fat accumulation in the liver (fatty liver/liver disease)
✓ Gallbladder disease
✓ High cholesterol
✓ Hypertension
✓ Increased anxiety and stress
✓ Joint pain
✓ Low self-esteem
✓ Sleep apnea
✓ Type 2 diabetes mellitus

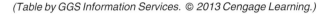

(Table by GGS Information Services. © 2013 Cengage Learning.)

particular height." The excess weight can come from bone, fat, muscle, water, or a combination of all four. Obesity is defined as "having excess body fat."

Demographics

There is no doubt that American children are getting heavier. In 2008, the CDC estimated that one-third of American children and adolescents were overweight or obese. Other surveys have found the total obesity rate among American children and adolescents to be between 21% and 24%. Although the problem of excessive weight is growing fastest in the United States, the trend toward heavier children is occurring in most developed countries.

In the United States, the National Center for Health Statistics has tracked children's weight for several decades and recorded the following changes in the percentage of children who are obese:

• Children ages 2–5: 1976 5.0%, 2008 10.4%
• Children ages 6–11: 1976 6.5%, 2008 19.6%
• Children ages 12–19: 1976 5.0%, 2008 18.1%

The number of children who are overweight or obese differs significantly among different races and ethnic groups. Significantly more Hispanic-American boys are obese than non-Hispanic black or white boys. Significantly more Hispanic American girls and non-Hispanic black girls are obese than white girls. Native American and Native Hawaiian children also have higher rates of obesity than whites.

Description

Childhood obesity is of increasing concern as a public health problem in the United States. Most healthcare professionals calculate obesity using the **body mass index** (BMI). BMI is a calculation that compares a person's weight and height to arrive at a specific number.

BMI for children is calculated the same way it is for adults, but, unlike for adults, age and gender are taken into consideration. The BMIs of children between the ages of 2 and 19 are compared against growth charts based on age and gender, referred to as BMI-for-age percentiles. A child's percentile indicates how his or her weight compares to other children who are the same age and gender. For example, if a boy is in the 65th percentile for his age group, 65 of every 100 children who are his age weigh less than he does and 35 of every 100 weigh more than he does.

The BMI weight categories for children are:

• below the 5th percentile: underweight
• 5th to less than the 85th percentile: healthy weight
• 85th to less than the 95th percentile: overweight
• 95th percentile and above: obese

In the early 2000s, many health organizations avoided applying the term "obese" to children. Children between the 85th and 95th percentile were classified as "at risk for overweight" and children above the 95th percentile were called "overweight." No child was labeled obese, in part because of the social stigma the word carries.

Children who are classified in the top 15th percentile are at risk of developing weight-related health problems. However, one criticism of BMI is that it does not take into consideration factors like muscle mass. Certain adolescent athletes, such as wrestlers or weightlifters, may be categorized as overweight or obese when using BMI calculations, even if they are fit and in good health.

Causes and symptoms

At its simplest, obesity is caused by taking in more **calories** than the body uses. This difference is called the "energy gap." A 2006 study done by the Harvard School of Public Health and published in the journal *Pediatrics* found that, on average, American children consumed between 110 and 165 more calories every day than they used. Over a 10-year period, these extra calories add 10 lb. to their weight. However, already overweight teens took in an average of 700–1,000 extra calories every day, resulting in an average of 58 extra pounds.

Causes

There are many reasons why the energy gap exists. These reasons are related to both increased food intake and decreased energy use. Food intake reasons include:

• increased consumption of sugary beverages and decreased consumption of milk
• tendency to supersize portions; in some fast food restaurants portions have almost tripled since the 1970s
• more meals eaten away from home
• more use of prepared foods in the home
• increased snacking between meals along with fewer meals eaten together as a family
• heavy advertising of high-sugar, high-fat foods to children
• decrease in children carrying their lunch to school from home
• poor eating habits such as skipping breakfast and later snacking on high-fat, sugary foods

Inadequate energy use reasons include:

• more time spent watching television, playing video games, or using the computer than playing outside
• fewer physical education requirements at school— many schools do not require or provide a regularly scheduled recess
• fewer children walking to school—in 1969, half of all schoolchildren walked or biked to school, but by 2003 (the date of the most recent CDC study), the rate had dropped to 15%
• fear of crime, which limits outdoor activities of children and walking to school
• more affluence—teen access to cars has increased over the past 30 years

According to a 2012 study published in the *Journal of Teaching in Physical Education*, only six states required at least 150 minutes of physical activity in elementary schools and only two states required 225 minutes in middle schools, the amounts recommended by the National Association of Sport and Physical Education. No states met the guidelines for high schools, which were also 225 minutes of activity per week. The U.S. Centers for Disease Control and Prevention recommends that children 6–17 participate in at least one hour of physical activity each day.

Other factors that affect childhood obesity include an inherited tendency toward weight gain; mental illness; **binge eating** disorder; eating in response to stress, boredom, or loneliness; poor sleeping habits; and having at least one obese parent.

In rare cases, medical or genetic disorders can cause obesity. For example, Prader-Willi syndrome is a genetic disorder that causes an uncontrollable urge to eat. The only way to prevent a person with Prader-Willi disorder from constant eating is to keep them in an environment where they have no free access to food. Other genetic and hormonal disorders (e.g., hypothyroidism) can cause obesity. Certain medications also can cause weight gain (e.g., cortisone, tricyclic antidepressants), but these situations are the exception. Researchers estimate that fewer than 10% of cases of childhood obesity are associated with hormonal or genetic causes. Most children are too heavy because they eat too much and/or exercise too little.

Symptoms

The most obvious symptom of obesity is an accumulation of body fat. Other symptoms involve changes in body chemistry. Some of these changes cause disease in children, while others put the child at risk for developing health problems later in life. Children who are obese are at increased risk of:

- type 2 diabetes; this disease is appearing in adolescents and young adults at an alarmingly high rate, whereas in the past, it was usually seen in older adults
- high blood pressure (hypertension)
- fat accumulation in the liver (fatty liver/liver disease)
- sleep apnea
- early puberty; early start of menstruation in girls
- eating disorders
- joint pain
- depression
- increased anxiety and stress
- low self-worth
- exposure to social prejudice and discrimination

Diagnosis

Diagnosis of obesity is usually made based on the child's BMI. To better assess the problem, the physician will take a family history and a medical history and do a complete physical examination, including standard blood and urine tests. A thyroid hormone test may be done to rule out hypothyroidism as the cause of obesity. Based on the physician's findings, other tests may be performed to rule out medical causes of obesity.

Treatment

Obese children and their parents may be referred to a registered dietitian or nutritionist who can help them develop a plan to replace high-fat/energy foods with nutrient-rich, low-calorie foods. Nutrition education usually involves the entire family. Children may be asked to keep a food diary to record everything that they eat in order to determine what changes in behavior and diet need to be made. Typically, children are encouraged to increase their level of physical activity rather than to drastically reduce calorie intake.

Drug therapy and weight-loss surgery are very rarely used in children, except in the most extreme cases of health-threatening obesity when other methods of weight control have failed. Some teenagers may benefit from joining a structured weight-loss program such as **Weight Watchers** or Jenny Craig. They should check with their physician before joining.

Nutrition and dietary concerns

Teaching children how to eat a healthy diet sets a framework for their lifetime eating habits. A nutritionist or dietitian can help families to understand how much and what kinds of food are appropriate for their child's age, weight, and activity level.

The American Heart Association has adapted the following dietary suggestions for children over two. Separate guidelines exist for infant nutrition.

- For children over three, limit fat intake to 25%–30% of total calories. Fat sources should be low in saturated and *trans* fats.
- Consume a variety of colorful fruits and vegetables daily, but limit fruit juice due to its sugar content.
- Select high-fiber, whole-grain cereals and breads.
- Limit sugary drinks and foods, such as carbonated soft drinks, candy, and baked goods.
- Drink fat-free or low-fat milk after age two. Children younger than two have higher energy requirements and need the benefits of dietary fat, including improved absorption of fat-soluble vitamins, for proper growth and development of the nervous system. Other good sources of calcium include low-fat or fat-free yogurt and cottage cheese.
- Eat a variety of foods, including fish and shellfish; oily fish such as salmon provide healthy fats.
- Do not add extra salt to foods and reduce overall sodium intake.
- Balance calories consumed with regular physical activity to help maintain a healthy weight.

It is often difficult for parents to understand how much food their child should eat at a particular age. Parents tend to overestimate the amount of food small children need. The daily amounts of some common foods that meet the American Heart Association guidelines for different ages are based on children who are sedentary or physically inactive. Active children will need more calories and slightly larger amounts of food. Calorie and serving recommendations are as follows:

- children ages 2–3—total daily calories, 1,000; milk, 2 cups; lean meat or beans, 2 ounces; fruits, 1 cup; vegetables, 1 cup; grains, 3 ounces
- girls ages 4–8—total daily calories, 1,200; milk, 2 cups; lean meat or beans, 3 ounces; fruits, 1.5 cups; vegetables, 1 cup; grains, 4 ounces
- boys ages 4–8—total daily calories, 1,400; milk, 2 cups; lean meat or beans, 4 ounces; fruits, 1.5 cup; vegetables, 1.5 cups; grains, 5 ounces
- girls ages 9–13—total daily calories, 1,600; milk, 3 cups; lean meat or beans, 5 ounces; fruits, 1.5 cups; vegetables, 2 cups; grains, 5 ounces
- boys ages 9–13—total daily calories, 1,800; milk, 3 cups; lean meat or beans, 5 ounces; fruits, 1.5 cups; vegetables, 2.5 cups; grains, 6 ounces
- girls ages 14–18—total daily calories, 1,800; milk, 3 cups; lean meat or beans, 5 ounces; fruits, 1.5 cups; vegetables, 2.5 cups; grains, 6 ounces
- boys ages 14–18 years—total daily calories, 2,200; milk, 3 cups; lean meat or beans, 6 ounces; fruits, 2 cups; vegetables, 3 cups; grains, 7 ounces

Therapy

Children who are overweight or obese may have accompanying psychological and social problems that may be helped with psychotherapy in addition to nutritional counseling. Cognitive-behavioral therapy (CBT) is designed to confront and change thoughts and feelings about one's body and behaviors toward food. CBT is relatively short-term and does not address the origins of those thoughts or feelings. CBT may include strategies to maintain self-control with regard to food. Family therapy may help children who overeat for emotional reasons related to conflicts within the family. Family therapy teaches strategies for reducing conflict, disorder, and stress that may be factors in triggering emotional eating.

Prognosis

The younger the child is when weight control strategies begin, the better the chance that the child will be able to maintain a normal weight. When it comes to weight control, one advantage children have over adults is that they grow. If a child can maintain his weight without gaining, he may grow into a normal weight as he becomes taller.

Parents need to be careful about how they approach weight loss in children. Critical comments

---

about weight from parents or excess zeal in putting their child on a rigorous diet can trigger **eating disorders** such as **anorexia nervosa** or **bulimia nervosa** in some children, especially adolescent girls. Instead of placing their child on a diet, parents should promote healthy eating and prepare meals that include lots of fruits and vegetables, **whole grains**, and low-fat dairy and **protein**. It is helpful for parents to lead by example, so that the child does not feel isolated. Criticism and focus on losing weight as opposed to getting healthy may lead to a negative **body image**.

Children who remain overweight or obese have a much greater likelihood of being overweight or obese adults with all the health problems that obesity brings. Studies have found that 26%–41% of preschoolers who are obese become obese adults. In school-aged children, 42%–63% of children with obesity become obese adults. The relationship between obesity in early life and adulthood is strongest for adolescents, so it is important to deal with childhood obesity as soon as possible.

Prevention

Parents must take the lead in preventing obesity in children. Starting good eating habits in children when they are young may help them carry such practices into adult life. Some of the ways parents can promote healthy habits are:

- serve a healthy variety of foods; keep healthy snacks on hand
- choose low-fat cooking methods such as broiling or baking
- eliminate high-fat and high-calorie snack food and sugary beverages from the house; this removes temptation and eliminates the need to nag

QUESTIONS TO ASK YOUR DOCTOR

- To what degree is my child overweight or obese?
- Should my child be on a formal diet?
- Can you recommend a nutritionist or dietitian to help our family eat better?
- Would behavioral therapy help my child handle his/her food issues better?
- In what ways is my child's weight affecting his/her health?

- eat meals together as a family rather than grabbing something quick on the run
- limit visits to fast-food restaurants
- limit television, computer, and video game time
- plan family activities that involve physical activity, such as hiking, biking, or swimming
- encourage children to become more active in small ways such as walking to school, biking to friends' houses, or doing chores such as walking the dog or mowing the lawn
- avoid using food as a reward
- pack healthy homemade lunches on school days
- encourage school officials to eliminate soda machines on campus, bake sales, and fundraising with candy and cookies
- set realistic goals for weight control and reward children's efforts (but not with food)
- model the eating behaviors and active lifestyle you would like your child to adopt

Resources

BOOKS

Fletcher, Anne M. *Weight Loss Confidential: How Teens Lose Weight and Keep It Off—And What They Wish Parents Knew.* Boston: Houghton Mifflin Harcourt, 2008.

Hassink, Sandra. ed. *A Parent's Guide to Childhood Obesity: A Road Map to Health.* Elk Grove Village, IL: American Academy of Pediatrics, 2006.

Okie, Susan. *Fed Up!: Winning the War Against Childhood Obesity.* Washington, DC: Joseph Henry Press, 2005.

Schumacher, Donald, and J. Allen Queen. *Overcoming Obesity in Childhood and Adolescence: A Guide for School Leaders.* Thousand Oaks, CA: Corwin Press, Sage, 2007.

Waters, Elizabeth. *Preventing Childhood Obesity: Evidence Policy and Practice (Evidence-Based Medicine).* Hoboken, NJ: Blackwell, 2010.

PERIODICALS

Kakinami, Lisa, et al. "Association Between Different Growth Curve Definitions of Overweight and Obesity and Cardiometabolic Risk in Children." *Canadian Medical Association* 184, no. 10 (2012): E539–E550. http://dx.doi.org/10.1503/cmaj.110797 (accessed July 11, 2012).

McCullick, Bryan A., et al. "An Analysis of State Physical Education Policies." *Journal of Teaching in Physical Education* 31, no. 2 (2012): 200–210.

Park, M.H., et al. "The Impact of Childhood Obesity on Morbidity and Mortality in Adulthood: A Systematic Review." *Obesity Reviews* (June 26, 2012): e-pub ahead of print. http://dx.doi.org/10.1111/j.1467-789X.2012.01015.x (accessed July 11, 2012).

Sanchez-Villegas, Almudena, et al. "Perceived and Actual Obesity in Childhood and Adolescence and Risk of Adult Depression." *Journal of Epidemiology & Community Health* (July 5, 2012): e-pub ahead of print. http://dx.doi.org/doi:10.1136/jech-2012-201435 (accessed July 11, 2012).

Verstraeten, Roosmarijn, et al. "Effectiveness of Preventive School-Based Obesity Interventions in Low- and Middle-Income Countries: A Systematic Review." *American Journal of Clinical Nutrition* (July 3, 2012): e-pub ahead of print. http://dx.doi.org/10.3945/ajcn.112.035378 (accessed July 11, 2012).

OTHER

American Heart Association. *Understanding Childhood Obesity: 2011 Statistical Sourcebook.* Dallas: AHA and American Stroke Association, 2011. http://www.heart.org/idc/groups/heart-public/@wcm/@fc/documents/downloadable/ucm_428180.pdf (accessed July 11, 2012).

U.S. Department of Agriculture and U.S. Department of Health and Human Services. *Dietary Guidelines for Americans, 2010.* 7th ed. Washington, DC: U.S. Government Printing Office, December 2010. http://health.gov/dietaryguidelines (accessed February 22, 2012).

WEBSITES

American Heart Association. "Dietary Recommendations for Healthy Children." http://www.heart.org/HEARTORG/GettingHealthy/NutritionCenter/Dietary-Recommendations-for-Healthy-Children_UCM_303886_Article.jsp (accessed July 11, 2012).

Mayo Clinic staff. "Childhood Obesity." MayoClinic.com. http://www.mayoclinic.com/health/childhood-obesity/DS00698 (accessed July 9, 2012).

MedlinePlus. "Obesity in Children." U.S. National Library of Medicine, National Institutes of Health. http://www.nlm.nih.gov/medlineplus/obesityinchildren.html (accessed July 9, 2012).

National Heart, Lung, and Blood Institute. "How Are Overweight and Obesity Diagnosed?" U.S. National Institutes of Health. http://www.nhlbi.nih.gov/health/health-topics/topics/obe/diagnosis.html (accessed July 10, 2012).

Schwartz, Steven M. "Obesity in Children." Medscape Reference. January 26, 2012. http://emedicine.medscape.com/article/985333-overview (accessed July 9, 2012).

U.S. Centers for Disease Control and Prevention. "BMI Percentile Calculator for Child and Teen." http://apps.nccd.cdc.gov/dnpabmi/Calculator.aspx (accessed July 9, 2012).

———. "Childhood Overweight and Obesity." http://www.cdc.gov/obesity/childhood (accessed July 9, 2012).

———. "How Much Physical Activity Do Children Need?" http://www.cdc.gov/physicalactivity/everyone/guidelines/children.html (accessed July 9, 2012).

ORGANIZATIONS

Academy of Nutrition and Dietetics, 120 South Riverside Plz., Ste. 2000, Chicago, IL 60606-6995, (312) 899-0040, (800) 877-1600, amacmunn@eatright.org, http://www.eatright.org.

American Academy of Pediatrics (AAP), 141 Northwest Point Blvd., Elk Grove Village, IL 60007, (847) 434-4000, (800) 433-9016, Fax: (847) 434-8000, http://www.aap.org.

Center for Nutrition Policy and Promotion, U.S. Department of Agriculture, 3101 Park Center Drive, 10th Fl., Alexandria, VA, 22302, (703) 305-7600, Fax: (703) 305-3300, support@cnpp.usda.gov, http://www.cnpp.usda.gov.

Centers for Disease Control and Prevention, 1600 Clifton Rd. NE, Atlanta, GA 30333, (800) CDC-INFO (232-4636), TTY: (888) 232-6348, cdcinfo@cdc.gov, http://www.cdc.gov.

The Obesity Society, 8757 Georgia Ave., Ste. 1320, Silver Spring, MD 20910, (301) 563-6526, Fax: (301) 563-6595, http://www.obesity.org., http://www.obesity.org/resources-for/consumer.htm.

Weight-Control Information Network (WIN), 1 WIN Way, Bethesda, MD 20892-3665, (202) 828-1025, (877) 946-4627, Fax: (202) 828-1028, win@http://win.niddk.nih.gov, http://win.niddk.nih.gov.

Tish Davidson, AM

Children's diets

Definition

Childhood diets are ways of treating overweight and **obesity** in children ages 2–19 years by changing eating and exercise habits.

Healthy snack foods for children

- Applesauce cups (unsweetened)
- Apples or pears and low-fat cheese
- Baby carrots and celery
- Baked potato chips or tortilla chips with salsa
- Cereal, dry or with low-fat milk
- Cucumber or zucchini slices
- Dried fruits such as raisins, apple rings, or apricots
- Fresh fruit
- Fruit canned in juice or light syrup
- Fruit juice
- Fruit salad
- Frozen fruit bars
- Frozen grapes
- Low-fat chocolate milk
- Low-fat frozen yogurt with fresh berries
- Low-fat yogurt with fruit
- Nonfat cottage cheese with fruit
- Popcorn, air popped or low fat
- Pretzels (lightly salted or unsalted) and a glass of low-fat milk
- Raw vegetable sticks with low-fat yogurt dip, cottage cheese, or hummus
- Rice cakes with peanut butter
- Smoothies with low-fat milk or yogurt and sliced bananas or strawberries
- String cheese and fruit (canned or fresh)
- Whole-grain crackers or English muffin with peanut butter
- Whole-wheat crackers with cheese or peanut butter

SOURCE: Center for Science in the Public Interest, "Healthy School Snacks," http://cspinet.org/nutritionpolicy/healthy_school_snacks.html.

(Table by PreMediaGlobal. © 2013 Cengage Learning.)

Background

There is no doubt that American children are getting heavier. In 2008, the United States Centers for Disease Control and Prevention (CDC) estimated that one-third of American children and adolescents were overweight or obese. Other surveys have found the total obesity rate among American children and adolescents to be between 21% and 24%. Although the problem of excessive weight is growing fastest in the United States, the trend toward heavier children is occurring in most developed countries.

In the United States, the National Center for Health Statistics has tracked children's weight for several decades and recorded the following changes in the percentage of children who are obese:

- Children ages 2–5: 1976 5.0%, 2008 10.4%
- Children ages 6–11: 1976 6.5%, 2008 19.6%
- Children ages 12–19: 1976 5.0%, 2008 18.1%

The number of children who are overweight or obese differs significantly among different races and ethnic groups. Significantly more Mexican American boys are obese than non-Hispanic black or white boys. Significantly more Mexican American girls and non-Hispanic black girls are obese than white girls. Native

American and Native Hawaiian children also have higher rates of obesity than whites.

Calculating obesity

Most healthcare professionals calculate overweight and obesity using the **body mass index** (BMI). BMI is a calculation that compares a person's weight and height to arrive at a specific number. See the body mass index entry for details on how to calculate BMI.

BMI for children is calculated the same way it is for adults. However, children between the ages of 2 and 19 are assigned a percentile ranking for their age group, while adults are simply assigned a BMI number and weight category. The percentile ranking indicates how a child's weight compares to that of other children who are their same age and gender. For example, if a boy is in the 65th percentile for his age group, 65 of every 100 children who are his age weigh less than he does and 35 of every 100 weigh more than he does. The percentiles are based on growth charts last modified in 2000, so it is possible that, with the increase in **childhood obesity**, the rankings are now inaccurate or skewed.

The BMI weight categories for children are:

- below the 5th percentile: underweight
- 5th percentile to less than the 85th percentile: healthy weight
- 85th percentile to less than the 95th percentile: overweight
- 95th percentile and above: obese

In the early 2000s, many health organizations avoided applying the term "obese" to children. Children between the 85th and 95th percentile were classified as "at risk for overweight" and children above the 95th percentile were called "overweight." No child was labeled obese, in part because of the social stigma the word carries.

By 2010, the CDC and some other influential health organizations had changed the way they defined overweight and obesity in children ages 2–19. As of 2012, the CDC defined overweight in children as "having an excess body weight for a particular height." The excess weight can come from bone, fat, muscle, water, or a combination of all four. Obesity was defined as "having excess body fat." These changes came about in part because certain adolescent athletes such as weightlifters were being categorized as overweight or obese when they scored above the 85th percentile using BMI calculations, despite the fact that they were fit and in good health. Whatever term is used to describe children in the top 15th percentile, these children are at higher risk of developing health problems because of their weight. A child whose BMI falls above the 85th percentile for age and gender should be evaluated for secondary complications of obesity, including **hypertension** (high blood pressure) and hyperlipidemias (high level of **fats** in the blood).

Problems of childhood obesity

Childhood obesity can cause both immediate and long-term health problems. Common obesity-related medical conditions include cardiovascular disease, type 2 diabetes, and joint disorders.

Orthopedic complications include slippage of the head of the thigh bone (capital femoral epiphysis) where it meets the pelvis at the hip. This can occur during the adolescent growth spurt. It is not common but occurs most frequently in obese children. The slippage causes a limp and/or hip, thigh, and knee pain and can result in considerable disability.

Blount's disease (tibia vara) is a growth disorder of the tibia (shin bone). The inner part of the tibia, just below the knee, fails to develop normally. This causes the growing bone to angle inward, so that the child appears bowlegged. The cause is unknown, although it is related to the effects of excess weight on the growth plate and is associated with obesity.

Research has shown that about 25% of obese, inactive children test positive for sleep-disordered breathing or sleep apnea. The long-term consequences of sleep-disordered breathing on children are unknown. In adults, obstructive sleep apnea is associated with many complications, including headaches, daytime sleepiness, high blood pressure, and other heart and lung problems.

Obesity is a risk factor for gallbladder disease in adults. Gallbladder disease causes abdominal pain and tenderness. Although the risk of gallbladder disease is much lower in children than in adults, obese children are at greater risk than those of normal weight. Obese children may develop **gallstones** because they have higher levels of cholesterol.

Noninsulin-dependent **diabetes mellitus** (NIDDM), commonly called type 2 diabetes, is a hormone disorder strongly related to obesity. Type 2 diabetes has become increasingly common in children, whereas a generation ago it was extremely rare. The link between obesity and **insulin** resistance, which causes type 2 diabetes, has been very clearly documented.

Obese children are at risk for hypertension (high blood pressure), and hyperlipidemias (high blood fats). These conditions increase the risk of cardiovascular disease in adulthood. Hypertension and **hyperlipide-mia** often go undiagnosed or untreated in children because they cause no obvious symptoms.

Childhood obesity also affects the social and emotional development of children. In a society that places a high premium on thinness, obese children often become targets of early and systematic bullying and discrimination that can seriously hinder healthy development of **body image** and self-esteem.

Causes

Less than 10% of childhood obesity is associated with a hormonal or genetic defect. The remaining 90% of cases are caused by lifestyle and dietary factors.

At its simplest, obesity is caused by taking in more **calories** than the body uses. This difference is called the "energy gap." There are many reasons why the energy gap exists. These reasons are related to both increased food intake and decreased energy use. Reasons related to food intake include:

- increased consumption of sugary beverages and decreased consumption of milk
- super-sized portions—some fast food restaurants' portions have almost tripled since the 1970s
- more meals eaten away from home
- more use of prepared foods in the home
- increased snacking between meals along with fewer meals eaten together as a family
- heavy advertising of high-sugar, high-fat foods to children
- decrease in children bringing their lunch to school
- poor eating habits such as skipping breakfast and later snacking on high-fat, sugary foods

Inadequate energy use reasons include:

- more time spent watching television, playing video games, or using the computer
- fewer physical education requirements at school
- fewer children walking to school
- decreased recess time in grades 1–5
- fear of crime, which limits outdoor activities of children and walking to school
- increase in the number of teenagers with their own cars

Other factors that affect childhood obesity include an inherited tendency toward weight gain, mental illness, **binge eating** disorder, eating in response to stress, boredom, loneliness, poor sleeping habits, and having at least one obese parent.

KEY TERMS

Body mass index (BMI)—Also known as BMI, the index determines whether a person is at a healthy weight, underweight, overweight, or obese.

Hypertension—High blood pressure.

Treatment

Before putting a child on a diet, parents should always seek the advice of a pediatrician and/or dietitian. Inappropriate dieting in children can negatively affect their physical growth and cognitive development. Current medical thinking is that overweight and obesity in children are often best treated by establishing healthy eating habits and increasing physical activity. Many experts suggest children should not diet to reach a specific target weight, but rather be encouraged to change their lifestyle habits and hold their weight steady. With growing children, keeping weight steady as the child grows is often enough bring to the child into a healthy weight range. Any complications of obesity such as hypertension should be treated under the direction of a physician.

Depending on their age and health, some children who are obese should diet under medical supervision. Some children may be resistant, and if their weight is adversely affecting their health, an intervention may be necessary. When weight loss goals are set by a medical professional, they should be moderate and allow for normal growth. Goals should initially be small; one-quarter of a pound to a maximum of two pounds per week. An appropriate weight goal for all obese children is a BMI below the 85th percentile, although such a goal should be secondary to the primary goal of weight maintenance via healthy eating and increased activity.

Many studies have demonstrated that obesity runs in families. For this reason, it is important to involve the entire family when treating obesity in children. The long-term effectiveness of a weight control program is significantly improved when the intervention is directed at the parents/caregivers as well as the child. Some positive guidelines for safe weight-loss programs include:

- Develop attainable and safe weight-loss goals; a rate of 1–4 lb. per month.
- Provide dietary management tools to both parent and child.
- Match recommended physical activity to the child's fitness and mobility level, with an ultimate goal of 60 minutes per day of structured movement.

- Incorporate behavior modification techniques such as self-monitoring tools, nutritional education, identification and modification of stimulus controls, family role modeling, positive reinforcements, and non-food rewards.
- Involve the entire family in creating healthier eating patterns and a more active lifestyle.

Therapy

Children who are overweight or obese often have psychological and social problems that can be helped with psychotherapy (talk therapy) in addition to nutritional counseling. Types of therapy include:

- Cognitive behavior therapy (CBT) is designed to confront and then change the individual's thoughts and feelings about his or her body and behaviors toward food, but it does not address why those thoughts or feelings exist. Strategies to maintain self-control may be explored. This therapy is relatively short-term.
- Family therapy may help children who eat for emotional reasons related to conflict within the family. Family therapy teaches strategies to reduce conflict, disorder, and stress that may be factors in triggering emotional eating.
- Although drugs are rarely prescribed for weight control in children, many overweight children have depression and anxiety. Drug therapy to treat these conditions may help the child to better deal with his or her weight and become more involved in physical activities and weight loss strategies.

Precautions

As the problem of childhood obesity has come into focus, commercial diet companies have begun touting diets for children. Parents should be very wary of these products. Some are appropriate for certain children who meet specific criteria. The best programs require a note from a physician stating that it is safe for the child to participate. However, many **fad diets** found on the Internet can be quite harmful when used by children. The best way to avoid negative health complications and achieve weight-loss success is to consult a health-care professional before starting any child on a diet.

There is a clear association between obesity and low self-esteem in adolescents. This relation brings other concerns that include the psychological or emotional harm a weight-loss program may cause in a child. **Eating disorders** may arise, although a supportive, nonjudgmental approach to therapy and attention to the child's emotional state minimizes this risk. A child or parent's preoccupation with the child's

---

QUESTIONS TO ASK YOUR DOCTOR

- Where is my child on the growth chart compared to other kids his/her age?
- Should my child be placed on a formal diet?
- Can you recommend a registered dietitian to help our family eat better?
- Would behavioral therapy help my child handle his/her food issues better?
- Is my child's weight affecting his/her health?

---

weight may damage the child's self-esteem. If weight, diet, and activity become areas of conflict, the relationship between the parent and child may deteriorate.

Prevention

Children who remain overweight or obese have a much greater likelihood of being overweight or obese adults with all the health problems that obesity brings. Studies have found that 26%–41% of preschoolers who are obese become obese adults. In school-aged children, 42%–63% of children with obesity become obese adults. The more overweight a child is, the higher the likelihood that the child will continue to be overweight into adulthood.

Eating habits are often established early in life. Building healthy eating and exercise habits early on can help prevent unhealthy weight gain. Strategies for building a healthy relationship to food and body image include:

- Respect a child's appetite. Children know when they are no longer hungry and do not need to finish every bottle or meal.
- Prepare and supply fresh, non-processed foods often. Avoid foods with added sugar as much as possible.
- Limit the amount of high-calorie foods kept in the home. Do not supply sodas, sugar flavored drinks, candy, cakes, or cookies in the home.
- Provide low-fat foods such as lean proteins, and low-fat or nonfat dairy products, and choose lower fat options for foods when available. Skim milk may safely replace whole milk at two years of age.
- Choose high-fiber foods by selecting whole grains, legumes, and fresh fruit and vegetables.
- Do not provide food for comfort or as a reward. Instead, use positive reinforcement.

- Do not insist that a child eat his or her meal in order to get dessert.
- Limit the amount of sedentary activities such as television viewing, computer time, and video games to two hours or less per day.
- Encourage active play by offering the support needed for the child to be active.
- Establish regular family activities such as daily walks, walk your child to school, or plan other regular outdoor activities.

Resources

BOOKS

Hassink, Sandra. ed. *A Parent's Guide to Childhood Obesity: A Road Map to Health.* Elk Grove Village, IL: American Academy of Pediatrics, 2006.

Weight Watchers International. *Weight Watchers Eat! Move! Play!: A Parent's Guide for Raising Healthy, Happy Kids.* Hoboken, NJ: John Wiley, 2010.

PERIODICALS

Wang, Y. Claire, et al. "Estimating the Energy Gap among U.S. Children: A Counterfactual Approach." *Pediatrics* 118, no. 6 (2006): e1721–1733. http://dx.doi.org/10.1542/peds.2006-0682 (accessed September 14, 2012).

WEBSITES

Centers for Disease Control and Prevention. "BMI Percentile Calculator for Child and Teen." http://apps.nccd.cdc.gov/dnpabmi/Calculator.aspx (accessed September 14, 2012).

———. "Clinical Growth Charts." http://www.cdc.gov/growthcharts/clinical_charts.htm (accessed September 14, 2012).

Mayo Clinic staff. "Nutrition for Kids: Guidelines for a Healthy Diet." http://www.mayoclinic.com/health/nutrition-for-kids/NU00606 (accessed September 14, 2012).

MedlinePlus. "Obesity in Children." http://www.nlm.nih.gov/medlineplus/obesityinchildren.html (accessed September 14, 2012).

Paul, Maya, and Lawrence Robinson. "Nutrition for Children and Teens: Helping Your Kids Develop Healthy Eating Habits." HelpGuide.org. http://helpguide.org/life/healthy_eating_children_teens.htm (accessed September 14, 2012).

U.S. Department of Agriculture and U.S. Department of Health and Human Services. *Dietary Guidelines for Americans, 2010.* 7th ed. Washington, DC: U.S. Government Printing Office, December 2010. http://health.gov/dietaryguidelines (accessed September 14, 2012).

ORGANIZATIONS

Academy of Nutrition and Dietetics, 120 South Riverside Plz., Ste. 2000, Chicago, IL 60606-6995, (312) 899-0040, (800) 877-1600, amacmunn@eatright.org, http://www.eatright.org.

American Academy of Pediatrics (AAP), 141 Northwest Point Blvd., Elk Grove Village, IL 60007, (847) 434-4000, (800) 433-9016, Fax: (847) 434-8000, http://www.aap.org.

U.S. Department of Agriculture, 1400 Independence Ave. SW, Washington, DC 20250, (202) 720-2791, http://www.usda.gov.

Weight-Control Information Network (WIN), 1 WIN Way, Bethesda, MD 20892-3665, (202) 828-1025, (877) 946-4627, Fax: (202) 828-1028, win@http://win.niddk.nih.gov, http://win.niddk.nih.gov.

Megan Porter, RD, LD
Tish Davidson, AM

Chinese diet *see* **Asian diet**

Chocolate diet

Definition

The chocolate diet is a weight-loss plan that includes the daily consumption of limited amounts of dark chocolate. The phrase "chocolate diet" may also refer to the consumption of chocolate for its health benefit claims, such as lowering cholesterol.

Origins

Chocolate originated during the Classic Period of the Maya civilization (250–900 AD) in Mesoamerica, an area that encompassed the Tropic of Cancer in Mexico, Guatemala, Belize, El Salvador, and parts of Honduras, Nicaragua, and Costa Rica. The Maya and their ancestors developed a method of converting the beans from the *Theobroma cacao* tree into a chocolate

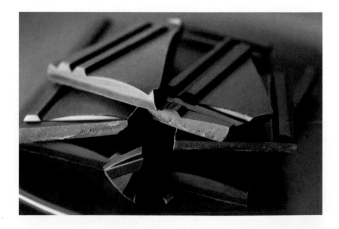

Dark chocolate contains flavonols, which are thought to have health benefits. *(© Istockphoto.com/ NightAndDayImages)*

beverage. This process started with the harvesting, fermenting, and roasting of the beans. The beans were then ground into a paste and mixed with ingredients including water, chile peppers, and corn meal.

The Maya and the Aztecs in the fifteenth century used the bitter-tasting beverage in religious and royal ceremonies. Christopher Columbus saw that some of the Amerindians used cacao beans as currency. He took some cacao beans back to Queen Isabella and King Ferdinand. Later explorers brought back the knowledge about how to convert the beans into a beverage. The Spanish added spices like cinnamon and **sugar** to the beverage to make it sweeter. The new beverage remained Spain's secret for a century.

Other Europeans eventually found out about the chocolate drink. It was an expensive indulgence, only affordable to the upper classes. That changed with the Industrial Revolution of the 1800s. Mass production brought down the cost of manufacturing treats, including solid chocolate. Another milestone occurred in 1875 when Daniel Peter and Henri Nestlé created milk chocolate by adding condensed milk to chocolate.

Chocolate diets

During the 1990s and in subsequent years, researchers began investigating the health benefits of chocolate. At around the same time, several books began promoting weight-loss plans that involved chocolate. In 1999, the book *The Pasta-Popcorn-Chocolate Diet* was published (now out of print). Sally Ann Voak's *The Chocolate Diet* was published in 2001. Voak, a British journalist, targeted her diet toward "chocoholics," people who have trouble resisting chocolate. Her book included six diets and the promise that people could eat chocolate and lose weight. The book is also now out of print.

Two other books titled "The Chocolate Diet" have been published as of 2012; one in 2011 by Drs. John Ashton and Lily Stojanovska, and another in 2012 by Rachel Henderson. Both books emphasize the health benefits of chocolate and how in moderation it can be included in a diet that results in weight loss.

Description

Cocoa beans contain approximately 50% fat; one ounce (oz.) (28 grams [g]) of chocolate contains approximately 150 **calories** and 8.5 g of fat. While the calorie and fat gram counts can contribute to weight gain if too much is eaten, the cocoa butter in chocolate contains oleic acid, which is a monounsaturated, or "healthy" fat. Chocolate also contains forms of saturated fat known as stearic and palmitic acids. Palmitic acid in particular has been linked to higher

levels of low-density lipoprotein (LDL). Also known as "bad" cholesterol, increased LDL cholesterol can clog arteries, raising the risk for heart disease. Palmitic acid forms one-third of the fat calories in chocolate; stearic acid appears to have no effect on cholesterol levels.

Cacao beans contain flavonoids, a broad category of plant products that act as **antioxidants**. Antioxidants are thought to be effective in helping to prevent cancer, heart disease, and strokes. Sources of flavonoids include citrus fruits, onions, **green tea**, red wine, and dark chocolate with a cocoa content of 70% or higher. Flavonoids also relax the blood vessels, allowing blood to circulate. Chocolate belongs to a subgroup of flavonoids called flavonols.

The presence of plant chemicals like flavonoids is related to the color of the chocolate. There are more flavonoids in dark chocolate than there are in milk or other types of chocolate. Dark chocolate is also known as semisweet or bittersweet chocolate because it contains little or no sugar. It is frequently categorized by its cocoa content, which ranges from 30% for sweet dark chocolate to 70% or sometimes above 80%. A higher percentage indicates a higher degree of bitterness.

Milk chocolate contains fewer flavonoids than dark chocolate but tastes sweeter. American chocolate contains milk, while European varieties often contain condensed milk. White chocolate lacks flavonoids because there are no cocoa solids in it. It is considered a chocolate because cocoa butter is usually an ingredient. Some white chocolate is made with vegetable **fats**.

Chocolate also contains **caffeine** and theobromine, a chemical similar to caffeine. Phenylethylamine is a stimulant found in chocolate, but there is an insignificant amount of this chemical in the processed form of chocolate.

Chocolate diets

The premise of most chocolate diets is that by allowing foods (in this case, chocolate) that are usually forbidden in other diets, dieters will be more likely to stick to their weight-loss plans. Though the chocolate diet is generally considered a fad diet, the notion of allowing "treats" may be beneficial to weight-loss goals. Believing that certain foods are "forbidden" may increase the desire to consume those foods, resulting in **binge eating** and **weight cycling** or weight gain. Instead, people should aim to eat a healthy and balanced diet, incorporating lots of fruits, vegetables, **whole grains**, and lean **protein**, with sweets or other treat foods allowed in moderation.

CocoaVia

CocoaVia is a line of cocoa extract supplements developed by Mars Botanicals, a division of Mars Incorporated. The CocoaVia brand came on the market in 2003 in chocolate bar form and claimed that the bars supported heart health. In 2006, the U.S. Food and Drug Administration (FDA) issued a warning to the company citing adulteration (for containing folic acid as a food additive) and misbranding—due to the significant amount of saturated fat in the recommended daily serving of two chocolate bars, the heart-healthy benefits were negated. By 2009, the CocoaVia chocolate bars were no longer manufactured.

After significantly changing the CocoaVia product, packaging, and labeling, it reentered the marketplace as a cocoa extract supplement in single-serve powder packets (to be added to food and drinks). Suggestions include adding it to oatmeal, yogurt, tea, or smoothies. According to the nutritional label, each serving of the cocoa extract supplement contains 250 mg of cocoa flavonols extracted from 100% pure cocoa. The dark chocolate flavors have 30 calories, 0.5 g fat, and 0 g sugar. Fruit flavors have 20 calories, 0 g fat, and 0 g sugar.

Function

Chocolate diets are used to satisfy dieters' **cravings** by allowing limited amounts of chocolate. Consuming dark chocolate may also provide health benefits. It is important to distinguish, however, between dark and milk chocolate, as the latter is generally more processed and higher in sugar.

QUESTIONS TO ASK YOUR DOCTOR

- What is your opinion of the chocolate diet for weight loss?
- Could eating dark chocolate help lower my cholesterol?
- What type of exercise program do you recommend in addition to the chocolate diet?
- Do I have any health conditions that would be affected by following this type of eating plan?
- What specific kinds of chocolate offer the best health benefits?
- Are cocoa extract supplements safe and beneficial for me?

Benefits

Research related to diets that include consumption of moderate amounts of dark chocolate has been increasing. Eating flavonol-rich chocolate may lower blood pressure and lessen the risk of heart disease. Including chocolate in a diet plan may also help keep dieters motivated to stay on track.

Precautions

People who are allergic to chocolate should not consider any form of diet involving chocolate. People with other conditions, such as elevated LDL or total cholesterol levels, should consult their physicians before beginning a diet or health regimen involving the daily consumption of chocolate. It may be necessary to have their cholesterol tested. Overweight or obese people should ask their health professionals whether it is wise to include chocolate in their diets.

Research and general acceptance

A meta-analysis of studies on chocolate, published in *BMJ* in 2011, found that participants who regularly consumed dark chocolate were 37% less likely to develop heart disease and 29% less likely to have a stroke. A study published in the *Archives of Internal Medicine* in 2012 evaluated the relationship between chocolate consumption and a lower **body mass index**. Although further research is required, the preliminary study found that participants who consumed moderate amounts of chocolate tended to lose more weight than those who did not consume any chocolate or ate it less frequently. This may have been because, by being permitted an indulgence, the dieters did not feel deprived. Though more research is needed, chocolate eaten in moderation can certainly fit into a healthy diet.

Resources

BOOKS

Ashton, John, and Lily Stojanovska. *The Chocolate Diet: How A Delicious Food Can Be Healthy Too.* Kindle Edition: HarperCollins, 2011.

Orey, Cal. *The Healing Powers of Chocolate.* New York: Kensington Books, 2010.

Voak, Sally Ann. *The Chocolate Diet.* London: Blake Publishing, Ltd., 2001.

PERIODICALS

Buitrago-Lopez, Adriana. "Chocolate Consumption and Cardiometabolic Disorders: Systematic Review and Meta-Analysis." *BMJ* 343 (August 29, 2011). http://dx.doi.org/10.1136/bmj.d4488 (accessed September 14, 2012).

Djoussé, L., et al. "Chocolate Consumption is Inversely Associated with Prevalent Coronary Heart Disease: The National Heart, Lung, and Blood Institute Family Heart Study." *Clinical Nutrition* 30, no. 2 (April 2011): 182–7.

Golomb, Beatrice, Sabrina Koperski, and Halbert White. "Association Between More Frequent Chocolate Consumption and Lower Body Mass Index." *Archives of Internal Medicine* 172, no. 6 (March 26, 2012): 519–21.

WEBSITES

"Cocoa Flavanols and Health." MARS, Inc. http://www.cocoavia.com/mars-and-cocoa-flavanols (accessed September 14, 2012).

Doheny, Kathleen. "Choose Dark Chocolate for Health Benefits." WebMD. http://www.webmd.com/diet/news/20120424/pick-dark-chocolate-health-benefits (accessed September 14, 2012).

O'Connor, Anahad. "The Chocolate Diet?" *Well* (blog), *New York Times*, March 26, 2012. http://well.blogs.nytimes.com/2012/03/26/the-chocolate-diet (accessed September 14, 2012).

ORGANIZATIONS

Academy of Nutrition and Dietetics, 120 South Riverside Plz., Ste. 2000, Chicago, IL 60606-6995, (312) 899-0040, (800) 877-1600, amacmunn@eatright.org, http://www.eatright.org.

American Heart Association, 7272 Greenville Ave., Dallas, TX 75231, (800) 242-8721, http://www.heart.org.

Center for Science in the Public Interest, 1220 L St., NW, Ste. 300, Washington, DC 20005, (202) 332-9110, http://www.cspinet.org.

Liz Swain

Cholesterol *see* **Dietary cholesterol**
Cholesterol-lowering diet *see* **TLC diet**

Choline

Definition

Choline is a nutrient required by the body. It does not meet the classic definition of a vitamin—a nutrient that the body needs in small amounts to remain healthy but cannot manufacture for itself—because the body makes some choline, but it does not make enough. The remainder must be acquired through diet. Choline is often grouped with the B-complex **vitamins** because it is a water-soluble compound that performs some similar functions to these vitamins.

Purpose

Choline has several actions in the body. It is incorporated into the fat-containing structures in cell membranes and is necessary for the formation of certain signaling chemicals made by cells to activate other molecules. Choline is also necessary for the formation of acetylcholine. Acetylcholine is a neurotransmitter that transfers information from nerves to muscles.

Choline

Age	Adequate intake (mg)	Tolerable upper intake level (mg)
Children 0–6 mos.	125	Not established
Children 7–12 mos.	150	Not established
Children 1–3 yrs.	200	1,000
Children 4–8 yrs.	250	1,000
Children 9–13 yrs.	375	2,000
Boys 14–18 yrs.	550	3,000
Girls 14–18 yrs.	400	3,000
Men 19≤ yrs.	550	3,500
Women 19≤ yrs.	425	3,500
Pregnant women 18≥ yrs.	450	3,000
Pregnant women 19≤ yrs.	450	3,500
Breastfeeding women 18≥ yrs.	550	3,000
Breastfeeding women 19≤ yrs.	550	3,500

Food	Choline (mg)
Beef liver, fried, 3 oz.	356
Egg, 1 large	147
Beef, chuck roast, 3 oz.	101
Brussels sprouts, cooked, 1 cup	63
Broccoli, cooked, 1 cup	62
Soymilk, 1 cup	58
Peanut butter, 2 tbsp.	20
Milk chocolate, 1.5 oz.	20

mg = milligram

SOURCE: U.S. Department of Agriculture, National Agricultural Library, Food and Nutrition Information Center and USDA Agricultural Research Service.

(Table by PreMediaGlobal. © 2013 Cengage Learning.)

Acetylcholine is thought to be important to memory and learning in the brain.

Like several of the B vitamins, choline is active in the metabolic pathway that breaks down homocysteine and removes it from the body. Homocysteine is an amino acid that circulates in the blood. Research has shown that people who have high levels of homocysteine in the blood are more likely to develop cardiovascular diseases such as coronary artery disease and stroke, and too much homocysteine may also adversely affect fetal health and development.

Description

Choline has not been studied as much as many of the other micronutrients, and it was not declared to be an essential nutrient until 1998. Research suggests that the body makes only between 10% and 20% of the choline it needs to maintain health, so the rest must come from diet.

Dietary requirements

The Food and Nutrition Board of the United States Institute of Medicine (IOM), a part of the National Academy of Sciences, develops values called **Dietary Reference Intakes (DRIs)** for many vitamins, **minerals**, and essential micronutrients. The **DRIs** consist of three sets of numbers: the recommended dietary allowance (RDA), which defines the average daily amount of the nutrient needed to meet the health needs of 97%–98% of the population; adequate intake (AI), an estimate set when there is not enough information to determine an RDA; and tolerable upper intake levels (UL), the average maximum amounts that can be taken daily without risking negative side effects. The DRIs are calculated for children, adults, and pregnant and **breastfeeding** women.

The IOM has not set RDAs for choline because of the scarcity of large, long-term dietary studies on this micronutrient. Instead, AI levels have been established for all age groups based on the best research information available. For choline, the AI level was established as the average daily amount needed to prevent the development of a condition called fatty liver, and it may not be the amount needed for other conditions. A 2008 study on Mexican American men found that higher levels were needed to accommodate rises in homocysteine. The IOM's recommended AI and UL levels of choline for each age group (in milligrams) are:

- children birth–6 months: AI 125 mg; UL not established
- children 7–12 months: AI 150 mg; UL not established

- children 1–3 years: AI 200 mg; UL 1,000 mg
- children 4–8 years: AI 250 mg; UL 1,000 mg
- children 9–13 years: AI 375 mg; UL 2,000 mg
- boys 14–18 years: AI 550 mg; UL 3,000 mg
- girls 14–18 years: AI 400 mg; UL 3,000 mg
- adult men age 19 and older: AI 550 mg; UL 3,500 mg
- adult women age 19 and older: AI 425 mg; UL 3,500 mg
- pregnant women: AI 450 mg; UL 3,500 mg (3,000 mg for women younger than 19)
- breastfeeding women: AI 550 mg; UL 3,500 mg (3,000 mg for women younger than 19)

Choline for children younger than 12 months should come from breast milk and infant formula or food and never from **dietary supplements**.

Sources of choline

Foods rich in choline include beef liver, egg yolks, peanuts, and soybeans. Most choline in foods is in the form of phosphatidylcholine, which is also known as lecithin. Most people can meet the AI levels of choline through their normal diet. Sources of choline include:

- beef liver, fried, 3 ounces: 355 mg
- egg, 1 large: 147 mg (choline is concentrated in the yolk)
- ground beef, cooked, 3 ounces: 70 mg
- cod, cooked, 3 ounces: 68 mg
- Brussels sprouts, cooked, 1 cup: 63 mg
- broccoli, cooked, 1 cup: 62 mg
- turkey, roasted, 1/2 cup: 58 mg
- baked potato, with skin: 30 mg
- peanut butter, 2 tablespoons: 20 mg

Choline chloride and choline bitartrate are also sold as a dietary supplements. Choline is also found in dietary supplements marketed as lecithin. Soybeans are the most common source for lethicin in dietary supplements. These supplements contain a much smaller and more variable amount of choline than choline chloride or choline bitartrate supplements. Consumers should read the lethicin labels carefully. Some children's multivitamins also contain choline.

Precautions

Moderate choline deficiency is associated with an increase in the blood levels of homocysteine. High levels of this molecule are known to increase the risk of cardiovascular disease. Extreme choline deficiency can result in a condition called fatty liver. Fat accumulates in liver cells where, in the absence of choline, it cannot be packaged and transported through the body. As a result, **fats** in the blood called **triglycerides** increase, creating an increased risk of heart disease and other health problems. Choline deficiency in pregnant women appears to have a negative effect on the development of the fetal brain and may cause learning, memory, and attention problems later in life.

Large excesses (10 g or more) of choline can cause nausea and extreme sweating. However, the most noticeable symptom of excess is the development of a highly unpleasant fishy body odor that results from the excretion of a choline breakdown product from the skin, urine, and breath. Large doses of choline dietary supplements do not appear to improve either physical or mental performance, nor do they appear to confer any specific health benefits.

Interactions

Methotrexate, a drug used to treat **cancer**, psoriasis, and rheumatoid arthritis, causes choline deficiency in laboratory animals. Individuals taking this drug should discuss possible side effects with their physician. Choline also is involved in many of the same metabolic pathways as other B-complex vitamins. Deficiencies or excesses of any of these B vitamins may potentially alter choline **metabolism**.

Complications

No complications are expected when choline is taken in amounts equal to or exceeding the AI level. Doses much higher than the UL level have been tolerated without any obvious serious negative side effects (but also without any observed benefits). Adequate levels of choline are obtained through a healthy diet, and supplementation is not needed unless recommended by a physician.

Parental concerns

Animal studies suggest that choline has a positive effect in stimulating the developing brain of the fetus and that choline supplements given after birth may offset some of the effects of fetal alcohol exposure. Some dietary supplement sellers have exaggerated these results, calling choline a "miracle brain supplement." Pregnant and breastfeeding women do need to eat a diet that provides adequate intake of choline, as choline deficiency may adversely affect brain development. However, there is no evidence that choline supplements will produce the opposite effect and increase an infant's intelligence.

Resources

BOOKS

Brown, Paul. "Choline, Inositol, and Related Nutrients." In *Encyclopedia of Food and Culture*, edited by Solomon H. Katz. New York: Charles Scribner's Sons, 2003.

Wildman, Robert E. C., ed. *Handbook of Nutraceuticals and Functional Foods*. 2nd ed. Boca Raton, FL: CRC/ Taylor & Francis, 2007.

PERIODICALS

Signore, Caroline, et al. "Choline Concentrations in Human Maternal and Cord Blood and Intelligence at 5 Years of Age." *American Journal of Clinical Nutrition* 87, no. 4 (2008): 896–902.

Thomas, Jennifer D., et al. "Choline Supplementation Following Third-Trimester Equivalent Alcohol Exposure Attenuates Behavioral Alterations in Rats." *Behavioral Neuroscience* 121, no. 1 (Feb 2007): 120–30.

Veenema, K., et al. "Adequate Intake Levels of Choline Are Sufficient for Preventing Elevations in Serum Markers of Liver Dysfunction in Mexican American Men but Are Not Optimal for Minimizing Plasma Total Homocysteine Increases after a Methionine Load." *American Journal of Clinical Nutrition* 88, no. 3 (2008): 685–92.

Zeisel, Steven H., and Kerry-Ann da Costa. "Choline: An Essential Nutrient for Public Health." *Nutrition Reviews* 67, no. 11 (2009): 615–23. http://

dx.crossref.org/10.1111%2Fj.1753-4887.2009.00246.x
(accessed August 15, 2012).

WEBSITES

Contie, Vicki. "Choline Deficiency May Hinder Fetal
Brain Development." National Institutes of Health.
http://www.nih.gov/researchmatters/july2010/
07262010choline.htm (accessed August 15, 2012).

Higdon, Jane, and Victoria J. Drake. "Choline." Linus
Pauling Institute, Oregon State University. http://
lpi.oregonstate.edu/infocenter/othernuts/choline
(accessed August 15, 2012).

U.S. Department of Agriculture, National Agricultural
Library. "DRI Tables." Food and Nutrition Information
Center. http://fnic.nal.usda.gov/dietary-guidance/
dietary-reference-intakes/dri-tables (accessed August 16,
2012).

ORGANIZATIONS

Food and Nutrition Information Center, National Agricultural Library, 10301 Baltimore Ave., Rm. 105, Beltsville, MD 20705, (301) 504-5414, Fax: (301) 504-6409, fnic@ars.usda.gov, http://fnic.nal.usda.gov.

Institute of Medicine, National Academy of Sciences, 500
Fifth St. NW, Washington, DC 20001, (202) 334-2352,
iomwww@nas.edu, http://www.iom.edu.

Helen M. Davidson

Chromium

Definition

Chromium is a mineral that is essential to humans. It is found naturally in a variety of foods and is available as a supplement in capsule or tablet form. Supplements are prepared using a number of formulas, including chromium (III), chromium aspartate, chromium chloride, chromium citrate, chromium nicotinate, chromium picolinate, GTF chromium, and trivalent chromium.

Purpose

Chromium supports the normal function of **insulin**, which is a hormone secreted by the pancreas. Insulin helps transport glucose from the bloodstream into liver, muscle, and fat cells. Once it is inside these cells, the **sugar** is metabolized into a source of energy. Insulin is also involved in regulating **protein**, fat, and catalytic enzyme processes. Diabetes is a condition in which the body either produces no or very little insulin or cannot properly use the insulin that is produced. As a result, sugar builds up in the bloodstream, causing serious health consequences. Numerous scientific studies have

Chromium

Age	Adequate intake (mcg/day)
Children 0–6 mos.	0.2
Children 7–12 mos.	5.5
Children 1–3 yrs.	11
Children 4–8 yrs.	15
Boys 9–13 yrs.	25
Girls 9–13 yrs.	21
Boys 14–18 yrs.	35
Girls 14–18 yrs.	24
Men 19–50 yrs.	35
Women 19–50 yrs.	25
Men 50< yrs.	30
Women 50< yrs.	20
Pregnant women 18≥ yrs.	29
Pregnant women 19≤ yrs.	30
Breastfeeding women 18≥ yrs.	44
Breastfeeding women 19≤ yrs.	45

Food	Chromium (mcg)
Broccoli, ½ cup	11
Grape juice, 1 cup	8
English muffin, whole wheat, 1	4
Garlic, dried, 1 tsp.	3
Potatoes, mashed, 1 cup	3
Basil, dried, 1 tbsp.	2
Beef cubes, 3 oz.	2
Orange juice, 1 cup	2
Turkey breast, 3 oz.	2
Whole wheat bread, 2 slices	2
Red wine, 5 oz.	1–13
Apple, unpeeled, 1 med.	1
Banana, 1 med.	1
Green beans, ½ cup	1

mcg = microgram

SOURCE: U.S. Office of Dietary Supplements, National Institutes of Health.

(Table by PreMediaGlobal. © 2013 Cengage Learning.)

shown that chromium may be useful in treating insulin resistance (**metabolic syndrome**) and type 2 diabetes. Diabetic peripheral neuropathy, a form of nerve damage that is a direct result of diabetes, is indirectly related to a lack of sufficient chromium.

Chromium has been studied as a potential treatment for polycystic ovarian syndrome (PCOS), but evidence has been insufficient.

Description

Chromium occurs naturally in meat, seafood, dairy products, eggs, **whole grains**, black pepper, and almonds. A complete lack of chromium is rare. According to the U.S. Office of Dietary Supplements, most adults consume enough chromium through diet, and supplementation is not needed unless recommended by a physician.

Several studies have shown that chromium supplements may improve insulin sensitivity and lower blood glucose and elevated body fat. Chromium has been studied as a potential therapy for insulin resistance, a condition that occurs when the body fails to respond properly to the insulin it already produces. People who are insulin resistant may have the ability to overcome this problem by producing more insulin. However, if the body cannot produce sufficient amounts of insulin, glucose levels in the bloodstream rise, ultimately resulting in type 2 diabetes.

Through its involvement with insulin function, chromium plays an indirect role in lowering blood lipids. This has led some researchers to believe that chromium supplementation may reduce the risk of cardiovascular (heart) disease in men, and may help decrease total cholesterol and triglyceride levels. However, results have been conflicting. Many factors contribute to heart disease, including **obesity** and high cholesterol, and a person is not likely to achieve reduced heart disease risk simply by taking chromium supplements. Studies in animals suggest chromium supplementation may reduce **hypertension** (high blood pressure) and insulin resistance caused by a high-fat diet, but these results have not been replicated in humans.

Chromium supplements in high doses—1,000 mcg or more a day—are sometimes used in weight loss and muscle development. However, a number of scientific studies have found that chromium supplements are not effective in these areas. In fact, precautions warn against chromium doses exceeding 1,000 mcg per day. Chromium's primary function is insulin regulation and control, so when insulin is well regulated and controlled, potential effects like weight loss, muscle development, or lowered blood pressure may not occur.

Recommended intake

The Food and Nutrition Board of the United States Institute of Medicine (IOM), a part of the National Academy of Sciences, develops values called **Dietary Reference Intakes (DRIs)** for many **vitamins**, **minerals**, and essential micronutrients. The **DRIs** consist of three sets of numbers: the recommended dietary allowance (RDA), which defines the average daily amount of the nutrient needed to meet the health needs of 97%–98% of the population; adequate intake (AI), an estimate set when there is not enough information to determine an RDA; and tolerable upper intake levels (UL), the average maximum amounts that can be taken daily without risking negative side effects. The DRIs are calculated for children, adults, and pregnant and **breastfeeding** women.

The IOM has set the following AI levels for chromium based on the best research available:

- children birth–6 months: 0.2 mcg
- children 7–12 months: 5.5 mcg
- children 1–3 years: 11 mcg
- children 4–8 years: 15 mcg
- boys 9–13 years: 25 mcg
- girls 9–13 years: 21 mcg
- boys 14–18 years: 35 mcg
- girls 14–18 years: 24 mcg
- adult men 19–50 years: 35 mcg
- adult women 19–50 years: 25 mcg
- adult men 51 and older: 30 mcg
- adult women 51 and older: 20 mcg
- pregnant women: 30 mcg (29 mcg for women younger than 19)
- breastfeeding women: 45 mcg (44 mcg for women younger than 19)

Precautions

People with type 2 diabetes may wish to consult with a physician regarding chromium supplementation. General doses of 200–1,000 mcg are suggested. However, people should only take doses at these levels at the recommendation of a doctor. Pregnant or breastfeeding women are advised to consult a physician before taking chromium supplements. Chromium should not be taken in doses exceeding 1,000 mcg a day. Increased dietary sugar may be associated with higher urinary excretion of chromium.

Interactions

People who are taking antacids are advised to talk with a physician before taking chromium supplements. Studies in animals suggest that antacids, especially those containing **calcium** carbonate, may reduce the body's ability to absorb chromium. Chromium may enhance the effectiveness of drugs taken by people who have type 2 diabetes or insulin resistance. These drugs include glimepiride, glipizide, glyburide, insulin, and metformin. Individuals taking these drugs should discuss chromium supplementation with a physician, as any improvements in insulin regulation may necessitate medication dosage changes.

KEY TERMS

Diabetes—A condition in which the body either does not make or cannot respond to the hormone insulin. As a result, the body cannot use glucose (sugar).

Glucose—A simple sugar that results from the breakdown of carbohydrates. Glucose circulates in the blood and is the main source of energy for the body.

Hypertension—High blood pressure, which, if untreated, can lead to heart disease and stroke.

Insomnia—The inability to sleep.

Insulin—A hormone made in the pancreas that is essential for the metabolism of carbohydrates, lipids, and proteins, and that regulates blood sugar levels.

Insulin resistance—A condition in which normal amounts of insulin in the blood are not adequate to produce an insulin response from fat, muscle, and liver cells. Insulin resistance is often a precursor of type 2 diabetes.

Complications

Several studies have noted occasional reports of irregular heartbeats with chromium use. Infrequently, chromium has been reported to cause such sleep pattern changes as insomnia and increased dream activity. Irritability has also been reported. In rare instances, people may be allergic to a chromium formula. The symptoms of an allergic reaction include difficulty breathing, chest pain, hives, rash, and itchy or swollen skin. If this happens, the affected person should seek medical care immediately. High doses may also cause liver and kidney damage or gastric irritation, although these side effects are rare.

Resources

BOOKS

"Chromium." In *Meyler's Side Effects of Drugs: The International Encyclopedia of Adverse Drug Reactions and Interactions*. 15th ed., vol. 2, edited by J.K. Aronson and M.N.G. Dukes. Amsterdam: Elsevier, 2006.

Evans, Gary. *All About Chromium Picolinate: Frequently Asked Questions*. Garden City Park, NY: Avery, 1999.

Icon Health Publications. *Chromium Picolinate: A Medical Dictionary, Bibliography, and Annotated Research Guide to Internet References*. San Diego, CA: Icon Health Publications, 2003.

Juturu, Vijaya. "Chromium Picolinate." In *Encyclopedia of Obesity*, vol. 1, edited by Kathleen Keller. Thousand Oaks, CA: Sage Publications, 2008.

PERIODICALS

Hua, Y., et al. "Molecular Mechanisms of Chromium in Alleviating Insulin Resistance." *Journal of Nutritional Biochemistry* 23, no. 4 (2012): 313–19.

Machender, Reddy Kandadi, et al. "Chromium (d-Phenylalanine)3 Alleviates High Fat-Induced Insulin Resistance and Lipid Abnormalities." *Journal of Inorganic Biochemistry* 105, no. 1 (2011): 58–62. http://dx.cross ref.org/10.1016%2Fj.jinorgbio.2010.09.008 (accessed August 15, 2012).

Sharma, S., et al. "Beneficial Effect of Chromium Supplementation on Glucose, HbA1C And Lipid Variables in Individuals with Newly Onset Type-2 Diabetes." *Journal of Trace Elements in Medicine and Biology* 25, no. 3 (2011): 149–53.

Ward, Elizabeth M. "Top 10 Supplements for Men." *Men's Health*. (December 2003): 106.

WEBSITES

MedlinePlus. "Chromium." U.S. National Library of Medicine, National Institutes of Health. http://www.nlm.nih.gov/medlineplus/druginfo/natural/932.html (accessed August 15, 2012).

National Institute of Diabetes and Digestive and Kidney Diseases (NIDDK). "Insulin Resistance and Prediabetes." National Diabetes Information Clearinghouse (NDIC). http://diabetes.niddk.nih.gov/dm/pubs/insulinresistance (accessed August 15, 2012).

Office of Dietary Supplements. "Dietary Supplement Fact Sheet: Chromium." U.S. National Institutes of Health. http://ods.od.nih.gov/factsheets/Chromium-Health Professional (accessed August 15, 2012).

University of Maryland Medical Center. "Chromium." http://www.umm.edu/altmed/articles/chromium-000294.htm (accessed August 15, 2012).

U.S. Food and Drug Administration. "Qualified Health Claims: Letter of Enforcement Discretion - Chromium Picolinate and Insulin Resistance (Docket No. 2004Q-0144)." August 25, 2005. http://www.fda.gov/Food/LabelingNutrition/LabelClaims/Qualified HealthClaims/ucm073017.htm (accessed August 15, 2012).

ORGANIZATIONS

Food and Nutrition Information Center, National Agricultural Library, 10301 Baltimore Ave., Rm. 105, Beltsville, MD 20705, (301) 504-5414, Fax: (301) 504-6409, fnic@ars.usda.gov, http://fnic.nal.usda.gov.

National Diabetes Information Clearinghouse, 1 Information Way, Bethesda, MD 20892-3560, (800) 860-8747, TTY: (866) 569-1162, Fax: (703) 738-4929, ndic@info.niddk.nih.gov, http://diabetes.niddk.nih.gov.

Office of Dietary Supplements, National Institutes of Health, 6100 Executive Blvd., Rm. 3B01, MSC 7517, Bethesda, MD 20892-7517, (301) 435-2920, Fax: (301) 480-1845, ods@nih.gov, http://ods.od.nih.gov.

Ken R. Wells

Clean eating *see* **Eat-Clean diet**
Cleveland Clinic 3-day diet *see* **3-day diet**
Cobalamin *see* **Vitamin B12**
Compulsive overeating *see* **Binge eating**

Constipation

Definition

Constipation is a symptom characterized by either having fewer than three bowel movements a week or having difficulty passing stools that are often hard, small, and dry.

Description

Food in the process of being digested moves through the intestines as a slurry or watery mush. In the small intestine, nutrients are absorbed from this material. After most of the nutrients have been absorbed, the material passes into the colon, or large intestine. Here, much of the water in the slurry is absorbed back into the bloodstream, and the remaining solid material is eliminated as waste or stool. Constipation occurs when too much water is removed from the slurry and it becomes difficult or painful to eliminate the stool. The most common reason why too much water is removed is that the material stays too long in the colon.

The frequency of bowel movements varies greatly from person to person and is influenced by age, health, diet, and lifestyle. It is a common misperception that a daily bowel movement is necessary for health. This is not true. For some healthy people, it is normal to have three bowel movements a day, while other healthy people have only three a week. Determining whether an individual is constipated must start with knowing what frequency of bowel movements is normal for that person.

Demographics

Constipation is a very common complaint. About 2% of Americans complain of frequent or constant constipation. In 2011, constipation accounted for about 2.5 million visits to the doctor. In the United States, more black Americans report being constipated than white Americans. In Africa, the reverse is true, suggesting that diet plays a more important role than race in determining who develops constipation. This presumption is also supported by the fact that very few Asians who eat an **Asian diet** report being constipated, while those who adopt a Western diet report constipation much more frequently. Complaints about constipation are more likely to come from women than from men, and from people over age 65. Pregnant women are at higher risk to become constipated, as are people who have had surgery and who are taking narcotic painkillers.

Causes and symptoms

Constipation is not a disorder, but a symptom of a health problem, like a fever or a cough. There are two general categories of constipation: idiopathic constipation, and functional constipation. Idiopathic means "of unknown origin." Idiopathic constipation is constipation that arises from an unknown cause. It may be related to hormonal abnormalities, nerve or muscle damage, or something physicians do not yet understand. Functional constipation occurs when the bowel is healthy, but constipation develops because of diet, lifestyle habits, psychological disorders, or abnormalities in the rectum or anus.

Symptoms of constipation may include:

- bowel movements that occur less frequently than normal
- straining to eliminate stools
- small, hard, dry, painful stools

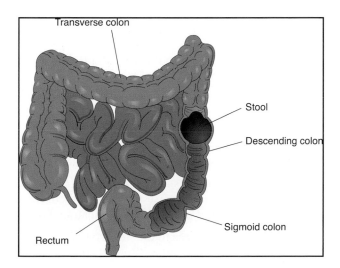

Constipation is an acute or chronic condition in which bowel movements occur less often than usual or consist of hard, dry stools that are painful or difficult to pass. *(Illustration by Electronic Illustrators Group. © 2013 Cengage Learning.)*

- a feeling of pressure in the rectum
- a feeling of abdominal fullness or bloating
- leakage of small amounts of liquid stool. This occurs when there is a blockage or impaction and the colon is abnormally stretched.

Constipation has many causes. The most common cause in the United States is poor diet. A diet that increases the chances of developing constipation is one that is high in meat, dairy products, and refined **sugar** and low in dietary **fiber**. Other causes include:

- little physical exercise—a particular problem in the elderly.
- medications, especially narcotic drugs used to treat pain, but also antidepressants, antacids containing aluminum, iron supplements, tranquilizers, antispasmodics, and anticonvulsants
- pregnancy
- change in routine; for example, traveling
- irritable bowel syndrome
- not drinking enough fluids (dehydration)
- laxative abuse (where people become dependent on laxatives and need higher and higher doses to avoid constipation)
- poor bowel habits, such as ignoring the urge to have a bowel movement or refusal to use public toilets
- tumor or other mechanical blockage
- eating disorders, such as anorexia nervosa or bulimia nervosa, where there is low calorie intake and (for bulimia) vomiting
- stroke, or other conditions causing nerve damage, such as multiple sclerosis, Parkinson's disease, and spinal cord injuries
- disorders that affect the muscles that cause material to move through the colon
- hormonal disorders, such as diabetes, hypercalcemia (too much calcium), and hypothyroidism (too little thyroid hormone)
- abnormalities of the rectum or anus
- iron supplements

Diagnosis

Diagnosis begins with a medical history so that the physician can determine the normal frequency of bowel movements and the length of time the individual has been constipated. The clinical definition of constipation requires that it be present for at least 12 weeks out of the past 12 months. The 12 weeks do not have to be consecutive.

Diagnosis also requires a physical examination, including a rectal exam and blood tests. Other tests, such as a thyroid hormone test, may be necessary to rule out other disorders. When symptoms are severe or do not improve with treatment, the physician may order specialized tests to determine how long material stays in the colon, evaluate the condition of the muscles of the rectum and anus, and look for evidence of **cancer** or other disease. These tests may include a sigmoidoscopy, barium enema x ray, colorectal transit study, and anorectal function tests.

Treatment

The first choice in treating constipation is a change of diet. People with constipation are advised to eat more foods high in dietary fiber; to decrease dairy, egg, and meat products to a healthy balance; and to increase the amount of water and non-caffeinated beverages they drink. They are also encouraged to increase their level of physical activity and to respond promptly to the urge to have a bowel movement.

When changes in diet and exercise do not work, laxatives can be used to stimulate movement of the bowels. Many types of laxatives can be purchased without a prescription. Americans spend about $725 million annually on laxatives. However, laxative dependency can become a problem. People who have been using laxatives regularly and wish to stop should reduce their use gradually. Each type of laxative has benefits and drawbacks. Individuals should discuss which one is best for them with their healthcare provider or pharmacist. Laxatives usually take 6–12 hours to stimulate a bowel movement.

Bulk-forming or fiber supplement laxatives are generally the safest type of laxative. Some common brand names of fiber-supplement laxatives are Metamucil, Citrucel, Fiberall, Konsyl, and Serutan. These must be taken with water. They provide extra fiber that absorbs water and helps keep the stool soft. The extra bulk also helps move materials through the colon.

Stool softeners help prevent the stool from drying out. They are recommended for people who should not strain to have a bowel movement, for example, people recovering from abdominal surgeries or childbirth. Brand names include Colace and Surfak.

Stimulant laxatives such as Dulcolax, Senokot, Correctol, and Purge increase the rhythmic contractions of the colon and move the material along faster.

Lubricants add grease to the stool so that it moves more easily through the colon. Mineral oil is the most common lubricant.

Saline laxatives, such as milk of magnesia, draw water from the body into the colon to help soften and move the stool.

In the case of serious constipation, prescription drugs such as tegaserod (Zelnorm) may be used under the supervision of a doctor. Other medical treatment involves treating the underlying cause of the constipation, such as changing a medication, removing tumors, or correcting a hormonal imbalance.

Some foods and supplements containing **probiotics** claim to alleviate irregularity and constipation. However, studies on probiotics as a treatment for constipation have had conflicting results, and further research is needed. Patients should consult with their physicians before taking any **dietary supplements**.

Nutrition and dietary concerns

The major cause of constipation is poor diet. Studies find that the average American eats only 5–14 grams of fiber daily. The United States Institute of Medicine (IOM) of the National Academy of Sciences has issued the following guidelines for daily consumption of fiber.

- men age 50 and younger: 38 grams (1.34 ounces)
- women age 50 and younger: 25 grams (0.88 ounces)
- men age 51 and older: 30 grams (1.058 ounces)
- women age 51 and older: 21 grams (0.74 ounces)

There are two types of dietary fiber, and both play a role in controlling constipation. Insoluble fiber passes through the intestines undigested, adds bulk to stool, and increases the speed with which it moves through the colon. Good sources of insoluble fiber include many **whole grains** such as wholemeal bread, brown rice, and high bran cereals. Soluble fiber dissolves in water and forms a gel that keeps the stool soft. It also has health benefits, such as lowering cholesterol (see entry for high fiber diet). Good sources of soluble fiber include oats, apples, beans, peas, citrus fruits, barley, and carrots.

The **Academy of Nutrition and Dietetics** and several other health organizations encourage people to increase the amount of fiber in their diet for many health reasons, not just to control or prevent constipation. The following list gives the fiber content of some common foods:

- split peas, cooked, 1 cup: 16.3 g (0.57 oz)
- lentils, cooked, 1 cup: 14.6 g (0.515 oz)
- kidney beans, cooked, 1 cup: 13.1 g (0.462 oz)
- brown rice, cooked, 1 cup: 3.5 g (0.123 oz)
- 100% bran cereal, 1/2 cup: 8.4 g (0.296 oz)
- oatmeal, 1 cup: 4.0 g (0.141 oz)
- peas, cooked, 1/2 cup: 3.6 g (0.127 oz)
- carrots, cooked, 1/2 cup: 2.3 g (0.081 oz)
- potato, baked with skin: 2.5 g (0.088 oz)

- potato, baked without skin: 1.4 g (0.049 oz)
- apple with skin: 3.5 g (0.123 oz)
- apple without skin: 2.7 g (0.095 oz)
- pear with skin, 1/2: 3.1 g (0.109 oz)
- pear without skin, 1/2: 2.5 g (0.088 oz)
- prunes, 3: 3.0 g (0.105 oz)
- wholemeal bread, 1 slice: 1.9 g (0.067 oz)
- popcorn, air popped, 2 cups: 2.4 g (0.084 oz)
- peanuts, 10: 1.4 g (0.049 oz)

Therapy

Biofeedback training may help individuals whose constipation is caused by dysfunctional control of the muscles that control the anus.

Prognosis

Many people have short bouts of constipation, especially when traveling, after childbirth or surgery, or with a change in lifestyle. These episodes usually can be resolved through attention to diet and exercise. People who have chronic idiopathic constipation, **irritable bowel syndrome**, and the elderly (especially those who are bed or wheelchair bound) often continue to have long-term problems with constipation, despite attention to diet, and become dependent on laxatives. Since many people self-treat constipation with over-the-counter laxatives, rates of improvement are difficult to determine.

Some people develop **hemorrhoids** and cracks in their skin at the anus (anal fissures) as the result of constipation. These are painful, but not usually medically serious. Some people also develop rectal prolapse from straining to produce a bowel movement. In this case, the lining of the rectum bulges out through the anus. The most serious complication from constipation is an impaction, which is a hard mass of stool that blocks the colon. Removing an impaction often requires professional medical intervention.

Prevention

A diet high in fiber, whole grains, fruits, and vegetables, and low in sugar, **fats**, and refined grains helps promote good bowel health in most people. Adequate amounts of fluid and regular exercise also help prevent constipation from becoming a problem.

Resources

BOOKS

Peikin, Steven R. *Gastrointestinal Health: The Proven Nutritional Program to Prevent, Cure, or Alleviate Irritable Bowel Syndrome (IBS), Ulcers, Gas, Constipation, Heartburn, and Many Other Digestive Disorders*. 3rd ed. New York: Collins, 2005.

Sauers, Joan and Joanna McMillan-Price. *Get to Know Your Gut: Everything You Wanted to Know About Burping, Bloating, Candida, Constipation, Food Allergies, Farting, and Poo but Were Afraid to Ask*. New York: Marlowe, 2005.

Sierpina, Victor S. *The Healthy Gut Workbook: Whole-Body Healing for Heartburn, Ulcers, Constipation, IBS, Diverticulosis & More*. Oakland, CA: New Harbinger Publications, 2010.

Wexner, Steven D. and Graeme S. Duthie, eds. *Constipation: Etiology, Evaluation and Management*. 2nd ed. New York: Springer, 2006.

PERIODICALS

Bassotti, G., V. Villanacci, and S. Bologna. "Evaluating Slow-Transit Constipation in Patients Using Laxatives: A Better Approach or Do We Need Improved Patient Selection?" *Expert Review of Gastroenterology & Hepatology* 6, no. 2 (April 2012): 145–47.

Chmielewska, Anna, and Hania Szajewska. "Systematic Review of Randomised Controlled Trials: Probiotics for Functional Constipation." *World Journal of Gastroenterology* 16, no. 1 (2010): 69–75.

Mota, D. M., et al. "Characteristics of Intestinal Habits in Children under Four Years of Age: Detecting Constipation." *Journal of Pediatric Gastroenterology and Nutrition* (February 29, 2012) [e-pub ahead of print]. http://dx.doi.org/10.1097/MPG.0b013e 318251482b (accessed June 20, 2012).

WEBSITES

Basson, Mark D. "Constipation." Medscape Reference. http://www.emedicine.com/article/184704-overview (accessed June 20, 2012).

Levitt, Marc A. "Management of Severe Pediatric Constipation." Medscape Reference. http://www.emedicine.com/article/937030-overview (accessed June 20, 2012).

Mayo Clinic staff. "Dietary Fiber: Essential for a Healthy Diet." MayoClinic.com. http://www.mayoclinic.com/health/fiber/NU00033 (accessed June 20, 2012).

MedlinePlus. "Constipation." U.S. National Library of Medicine. http://www.nlm.nih.gov/medlineplus/constipation.html (accessed June 20, 2012).

National Digestive Diseases Information Clearinghouse. "Constipation." National Institute of Diabetes and Digestive and Kidney Diseases (NIDDK). http://digestive.niddk.nih.gov/ddiseases/pubs/constipation (accessed June 20, 2012).

ORGANIZATIONS

American Gastroenterological Association, 4930 Del Ray Ave., Bethesda, MD 20814, (301) 654-2055, member@gastro.org, http://www.gastro.org.

International Foundation for Functional Gastrointestinal Disorders, PO Box 170864, Milwaukee, WI 53217, (414) 964-1799, (888) 964-2001, Fax: (414) 964-7176, iffgd@iffgd.org, http://www.iffgd.org.

National Digestive Diseases Information Clearinghouse, 2 Information Way, Bethesda, MD 20892–3570, (800) 891–5389, TTY: (866) 569–1162, Fax: (703) 738–4929, nddic@info.niddk.nih.gov, http://www.digestive.niddk.nih.gov.

Tish Davidson, AM
David Newton

Copper

Definition

Copper is an essential mineral that plays an important role in **iron** absorption and transport. It is considered a trace mineral because it is needed in very small amounts. Only 70–80 milligrams (mg) of copper are found in the body of a normal healthy person.

Copper

Age	Recommended dietary allowance (mcg/day)
Children 0–6 mos.	200 (AI)
Children 7–12 mos.	220 (AI)
Children 1–3 yrs.	340
Children 4–8 yrs.	440
Children 9–13 yrs.	700
Adolescents 14–18 yrs.	890
Adults 19≤ yrs.	900
Pregnant women	1,000
Breastfeeding women	1,300

Food	Copper (mcg)
Beef liver, 3 oz.	1,240
Oysters, raw, 6 med.	240
Mushrooms, shiitake, cooked, 1 cup	130
Chocolate, semisweet, 1 cup	118
Soybeans, boiled, 1 cup	70
Cashews, dry roasted, 1 oz.	63
Beans, white, canned, 1 cup	61
Sunflower seeds, ¼ cup	59
Chickpeas, cooked, 1 cup	58
Baked beans, with pork, 1 cup	54
Lentils, cooked, 1 cup	50
V-8 juice, canned, 1 cup	48
Potato skin, baked, 1	47
Raisins, seedless, 1 cup	46
White rice, enriched, 1 cup	41

AI = Adequate intake
mcg = microgram

SOURCE: U.S. Department of Agriculture, National Agricultural Library, Food and Nutrition Information Center and USDA Agricultural Research Service.

(Table by PreMediaGlobal. © 2013 Cengage Learning.)

Even though the body needs very little, it is necessary to many vital body functions.

Purpose

Copper is essential for normal development of the body. Copper:

- participates in a wide variety of important enzymatic reactions in the body and is a component of or a cofactor for approximately 50 different enzymes
- is essential for iron absorption and transport; copper deficiency is often linked to iron-deficiency anemia
- protect bones and joints by helping to build elastin and collagen, important components of bones and connective tissues
- is required for melanin production
- promotes wound healing and is a key mineral for the immune system
- attacks free radicals (acts as an antioxidant)

- participates in oxidative reactions that break down fats in fat tissue to produce energy for the body
- is necessary for normal functioning of insulin
- is needed for normal functioning of the cardiovascular system
- protects the structure and function of the nervous system, including the brain, by maintaining myelin, the insulating sheath that surrounds nerve cells
- aids in the transmission of nerve signals in the brain

Description

Certain diseases or conditions may reduce copper absorption or transport or increase its requirements, resulting in abnormally low copper blood levels. Increased copper intake through diet or supplementation may be necessary in the following conditions:

- premature infants fed only cow's milk
- pregnant women
- malnutrition
- celiac disease, sprue, cystic fibrosis, or short-bowel syndrome (these diseases cause poor absorption of dietary copper)
- kidney disease
- high consumption of zinc or iron (these minerals interfere with copper absorption)
- Menkes syndrome (copper deficiency is caused by genetic defects of copper transport; patients cannot use copper supplied by the diet efficiently)

Symptoms of copper deficiency include:

- anemia
- malnourished infants
- prominently dilated veins
- pale hair or skin
- poorly formed bones
- nervous system disorders
- high cholesterol levels
- heart disease
- loss of taste
- poor blood glucose control
- increased susceptibility to infections
- infertility
- birth defects

Copper supplements may be beneficial in treating or preventing copper deficiency. Copper deficiency used to be relatively rare because the body requires so little of it, only about 2 mg per day. In addition, it is available naturally in a variety of foods such as **whole grains**, shellfish, nuts, beans, and leafy vegetables. Additional sources of copper are copper water pipes that run through homes or copper cookware. These sources leach copper into the water and food, and levels of copper in drinking water can sometimes become so high that it becomes a public concern. However, scientists have realized that copper deficiency, especially borderline cases, is more common than once thought due to a decrease of whole foods in the diet and high consumption of fatty and processed foods. Most of the naturally occurring copper is stripped from these foods during processing.

Disease prevention

Copper is a good antioxidant. It works together with an antioxidant enzyme, superoxide dismutase (SOD), to protect cell membranes from being destroyed by free radicals. Free radicals are any molecules that are missing one electron. Because this is an unbalanced and unstable state, a radical is desperately looking for ways to complete its pair. It reacts to any nearby molecules to either steal an electron or give away the unpaired one. In the process, free radicals initiate chain reactions that destroy cell structures. Like other **antioxidants**, copper scavenges or cleans up these highly reactive radicals and changes them into inactive, less harmful compounds. Free radicals are implicated in the development of **cancer**. In 2001, a study reported that concentrations of copper sulfate and ascorbate may inhibit breast cancer growth. However, further research is needed.

Copper may also help prevent degenerative diseases or conditions such as premature aging, heart disease, autoimmune diseases, arthritis, cataracts, Alzheimer's disease, or diabetes.

OSTEOPOROSIS. Copper may play a role in preventing osteoporosis. **Calcium** and **vitamin D** have long been considered the mainstays of osteoporosis treatment and prevention. However, they may be even more effective in increasing bone density and preventing osteoporosis if they are used in combination with copper and two other trace **minerals**, **zinc** and **manganese**.

RHEUMATOID ARTHRITIS. Copper has been a folklore remedy for rheumatoid arthritis since 1500 BC in ancient Egypt. Some people believe that wearing jewelry made of copper may relieve arthritic symptoms. Researchers suggest that copper contained in the bracelets is dissolved in sweat and then absorbed through the skin. They suspect that this may be related to copper's role as an antioxidant and that it may also function as an anti-inflammatory agent.

Supplementation

Copper is contained in many multivitamin/mineral preparations. It is also available as a single ingredient in the form of tablets. These tablets should be swallowed whole with a cup of water, preferably with meals, to avoid stomach upset. A person may choose any of the following preparations: copper gluconate, copper sulfate, or copper citrate. However, copper gluconate may be the least irritating to the stomach.

Recommended intake

The U.S. Institute of Medicine (IOM) of the National Academy of Sciences has developed values called **Dietary Reference Intakes (DRIs)** for many **vitamins** and minerals. The **DRIs** consist of three sets of numbers: recommended dietary allowance (RDA), which defines the average daily amount of the nutrient needed to meet the health needs of 97%–98% of the population; adequate intake (AI), an estimate set when there is not enough information to determine an RDA; and tolerable upper intake level (UL), the average maximum amount that can be taken daily without risking negative side effects. The DRIs are calculated for children, adult men, adult women, pregnant women, and **breastfeeding** women.

The RDAs for copper are as follows:

- children birth–6 months: 200 micrograms (mcg) (AI); no UL established
- children 7–12 months: 220 mcg; UL not established
- children 1–3 years: 340 mcg; UL 1 mg
- children 4–8 years: 440 mcg; UL 3 mg
- children 9–13 years: 700 mcg; UL 5 mg
- teens 14–18 years: 890 mcg; UL 8 mg
- adults 19 and older: 900 mcg; UL 10 mg
- pregnant women 14–18 years: 1,000 mcg (1 mg); UL 8 mg
- pregnant women 19 and older: 1,000 mcg (1 mg); UL 10 mg
- breastfeeding women 14–18 years: 1,300 mcg; UL 8 mg
- breastfeeding women 19 and older: 1,300 mcg; UL 10 mg

Precautions

People should talk to their doctors before adding copper supplements to their diets. Copper toxicity due to excessive doses of copper supplements has been reported. Pregnant or breastfeeding women should not take copper or any other supplements or drugs without first consulting with their doctors.

Because individual antioxidants often work together as a team to defend the body against free radicals, the balance between copper, zinc, and iron must be maintained. Excessive intake of one nutrient might result in a deficiency of other minerals and

KEY TERMS

Antioxidants—Antioxidants are nutrients that deactivate reactive molecules (free radicals) and prevent harmful chain reactions.

Minerals—Inorganic chemical elements that are found in plants and animals and are essential for life. There are two types of minerals: major minerals, which the body requires in large amounts, and trace elements, which the body needs only in minute amounts.

decreased resistance to infections and increased risk of heart disease, diabetes, arthritis, and other diseases. For example, zinc and copper compete with each other for absorption in the gastrointestinal tract. Excessive copper intake may cause zinc deficiency and vice versa. A person taking zinc and copper supplements together should take them in ratios of 10:1 or 15:1.

Exceeding the daily requirement for copper can result in copper toxicity, a very serious medical problem. Acute toxicity due to ingestion of too much supplement, for example, may cause nausea, vomiting, abdominal pain, diarrhea, dizziness, headache, and a metallic taste in the mouth. Chronic toxicity is often caused by genetic defects of copper **metabolism**, such as **Wilson disease**. In this disease, copper is not eliminated properly and is allowed to accumulate to toxic levels. Copper is therefore present at a high concentration in a place it should not be, such as in the liver, lens of the eye, kidneys, or brain. Other diseases may cause copper deficiency. Premature infants or children with genetic copper defects are at high risk of infections.

Disorders and conditions known to increase copper levels include:

- recent heart attacks
- lupus erythematosus
- cirrhosis of the liver
- schizophrenia
- leukemia and some other forms of cancer
- viral infections
- ulcerative colitis
- Wilson disease

People with these conditions should not take copper supplements as they may cause copper toxicity.

In certain areas, drinking water may contain high levels of copper. Periodic checks of copper levels in drinking water may be necessary.

Complications

A person should stop taking copper supplements and seek medical help immediately if having the following signs or symptoms:

- anemia
- nausea
- vomiting
- abdominal pain

Resources

BOOKS

Lieberman, Shari, and Nancy Bruning. "Copper." In *The Real Vitamin & Mineral Book: Using Supplements for Optimum Health.* Garden City Park, NY: Avery Publishing Group, 1997.

Passwater, Richard A. *All About Antioxidants.* Garden City Park, NY: Avery Publishing Group, 1998.

PERIODICALS

de Romaña, D L., et al. "Risks and Benefits of Copper in Light of New Insights of Copper Homeostasis." *Journal of Trace Elements in Copper and Biology* 25, no. 1 (2011): 3–13.

Gonzalez, M.J, et al. "Inhibition of Human Breast Carcinoma Cell Proliferation by Ascorbate and Copper." *The Journal of Nutrition* 131, no. 11 (November 2001): 3142S.

Hunt, Janet R., and Richard A. Vanderpool. "Apparent Copper Absorption from a Vegetarian Diet." *American Journal of Clinical Nutrition* 74, no. 6 (December 2001): 803–5.

Reginster, Jean-Yves, Anne Noel Taquet, and Christiane Gosset. "Therapy for Osteoporosis: Miscellaneous and Experimental Agents." *Endocrinology and Metabolism Clinics* (June 1998): 453–463.

Uauy, Ricardo, Manuel Olivarez, and Mauricio Gonzales. "Essentiality of Copper in Humans." *American Journal of Clinical Nutrition* 67, suppl (1998): 952S–959S.

WEBSITES

American Cancer Society. "Copper." Food and Nutrition Information Center. http://www.cancer.org/Treatment/TreatmentsandSideEffects/ComplementaryandAlternativeMedicine/HerbsVitaminsandMinerals/copper (accessed September 27, 2012).

MedlinePlus. "Copper in Diet." U.S. National Library of Medicine, National Institutes of Health. http://www.nlm.nih.gov/medlineplus/ency/article/002419.htm (accessed September 27, 2012).

———. "Wilson Disease." U.S. National Library of Medicine, National Institutes of Health. http://www.nlm.nih.gov/medlineplus/wilsondisease.html (accessed September 27, 2012).

U.S. Department of Agriculture, National Agricultural Library. "DRI Tables." Food and Nutrition Information Center. http://fnic.nal.usda.gov/dietary-guidance/dietary-reference-intakes/dri-tables (accessed August 16, 2012).

ORGANIZATIONS

Academy of Nutrition and Dietetics, 120 South Riverside Plz., Ste. 2000, Chicago, IL 60606-6995, (312) 899-0040, (800) 877-1600, amacmunn@eatright.org, http://www.eatright.org.

Institute of Medicine, National Academy of Sciences, 500 Fifth St. NW, Washington, DC 20001, (202) 334-2352, iomwww@nas.edu, http://www.iom.edu.

U.S. Department of Agriculture, 1400 Independence Ave. SW, Washington, DC 20250, (202) 720-2791, http://www.usda.gov.

U.S. Food and Drug Administration, 10903 New Hampshire Ave., Silver Spring, MD 20993-0002, (888) INFO-FDA (463-6332), http://www.fda.gov.

Mai Tran
Teresa Odle

Coronary heart disease

Definition

Coronary heart disease is the narrowing or blockage of the arteries and vessels that provide oxygen and nutrients to the heart. It is caused by a condition called atherosclerosis, which is the gradual buildup of fatty materials on the arteries' inner linings. The blockage that results from the buildup restricts blood flow to the heart. When the blood flow is completely cut off, a heart attack can occur.

Description

Coronary heart disease also may be called coronary artery disease or simply heart disease. It is the leading cause of death in the United States among men and women.

When the heart works harder and needs more oxygen, the coronary arteries expand. But buildup of fatty materials, or plaque, from atherosclerosis causes the arteries to harden and narrow. If the arteries are unable to expand because of coronary artery disease, the heart is deprived of oxygen. The heart muscle cannot work properly without oxygen. The reduced blood flow and oxygen supply may cause angina, which is pain in the chest. It also may cause shortness of breath or other symptoms. Complete blockage or clotting at the site where the blood enters the heart can cause a heart attack.

Coronary heart disease can worsen over time. The heart muscles may weaken, even though no symptoms may be evident. Eventually, this leads to heart failure. In heart failure, the heart does not suddenly stop, but

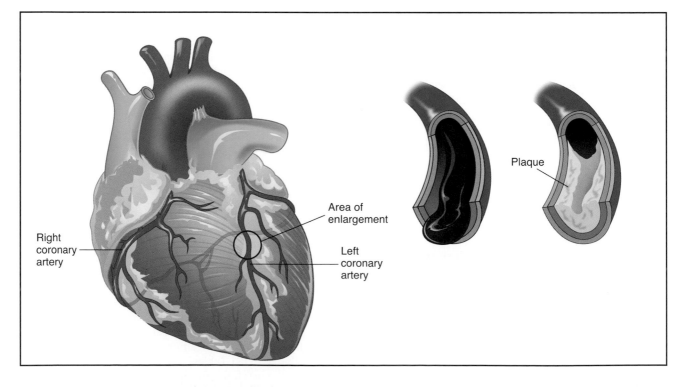

Coronary heart disease is caused by plaque build-up in the arteries. *(Illustration by Electronic Illustrators Group. © 2013 Cengage Learning.)*

it fails to pump blood to the body the way that it should. Coronary heart disease also can lead to heart arrhythmias, or changes in the normal rhythm of heartbeat. These can be serious.

Demographics

According to the American Heart Association, coronary heart disease caused more than 250,000 deaths in 2004. But the number of deaths from the disease declined 33% from 1994 to 2004. Although about 325,000 people a year die of coronary attacks in hospital emergency departments without even being hospitalized, more than 15 million people in America live with a history of heart attack, angina pectoris, or both. More of these are males, but not by a wide margin. Black males have a higher death rate per 100,000 than white males, and men generally have a higher chance of dying from coronary heart disease than women.

Causes and symptoms

Coronary heart disease is caused by atherosclerosis. Some risk factors for coronary heart disease cannot be changed, whereas others are tied to lifestyle choices.

Causes

Age is a major risk factor for death from coronary heart disease. Over 83% of people who die from coronary heart disease are over age 65. Gender plays a role too, since men have a higher risk of heart attacks. Men tend to get heart disease earlier than women. While men are at higher risk for coronary heart disease by about age 45, women are at risk for heart disease later in life, beginning at about age 55. People whose parents had heart disease also are at higher risk for coronary heart disease. Certain racial groups have higher risk as well, often because of a greater tendency toward **obesity**, high blood pressure, or diabetes.

Other risk factors can be affected by diet and lifestyle changes. Smoking is a big contributor to coronary heart disease. Not only do smokers have a risk two to four times that of nonsmokers of developing coronary heart disease, but they also have a higher risk of heart attack from the disease. In fact, a smoker with coronary heart disease is twice as likely as a nonsmoker with coronary heart disease to die suddenly from the disease.

Elevated blood cholesterol levels are a risk factor for developing coronary heart disease. Risk of developing coronary heart disease rises steadily as levels of low-density lipoprotein (LDL) cholesterol rise or if a person has high cholesterol levels combined with high blood pressure and smoking. The body produces cholesterol, and a person's age, sex, and heredity can affect their blood cholesterol levels. The most important dietary factor influencing blood cholesterol is intake of saturated fat found in fatty meats, full-fat dairy products, butter, ghee, and coconut and palm oils.

Other diseases and conditions contribute to risk of coronary heart disease. High blood pressure makes the heart work harder and weakens it over time. **Diabetes mellitus** can be a serious risk for coronary heart disease and cardiovascular disease, which includes other disease to other arteries throughout the body. About three-fourths of people with diabetes die from heart disease or blood vessel disease.

Weight and physical activity play a role in risk of coronary heart disease. Being overweight makes the heart work harder to do its everyday job of pumping blood to the body. Even when people have no other risk factors, obesity greatly increases risk of heart disease, particularly if weight is concentrated at the waist. Excess weight also raises blood pressure and affects cholesterol and triglyceride levels. Losing as little as 10 pounds can decrease risk for coronary heart disease, though maintaining a healthy weight is best. Being inactive contributes to weight gain and all of the associated conditions that then lead to coronary heart disease.

Stress also may play a role in coronary heart disease risk. However, the real problem is how people react to stress. For instance, overeating in response to stress leads to risk factors listed above. Drinking too much alcohol can cause some of the conditions listed above and lead to heart failure. However, studies have shown that moderate amounts of alcohol, described as about 1.5 fluid oz. of 80-proof spirits, 1 fluid oz. of 100-proof spirits, 4 fluid oz. of wine, or 12 fluid oz. of beer per day, may be good for the heart. The American Heart Association does not recommend that people who do not drink begin drinking or that anyone increase alcohol intake to meet these amounts, however.

Symptoms

The restricted blood flow to the heart caused by narrowing arteries may not produce any symptoms at first and many people are completely unaware that they have coronary heart disease. As the plaque builds up, symptoms begin to develop. One of the first signs may be chest pain that is triggered by physical or emotional stress. This pain often is referred to as angina. The pain feels much like pressure or tightening in the chest or it may be felt in the arm, neck, jaw, shoulder, or back. Sometimes the pain is confused with indigestion. Women may notice pain more often in the back or arm than in the chest and the pain may be brief and pass quickly.

Shortness of breath also is a symptom of coronary heart disease. This results from the heart's decreasing ability to pump enough blood to the body to meet its needs. The person with shortness of breath also may feel very tired.

The most serious symptom of coronary heart disease is heart attack. Although some heart attacks start suddenly and are clearly occurring, most start slowly with uncertain symptoms. Discomfort in the center of the chest that lasts for several minutes that feels like squeezing, fullness, or pain is a sign that a heart attack is occurring or about to occur. The pain also may go away and come back. The pain may occur in one or both upper arms, the back, neck, jaw, or stomach. A person may experience shortness of breath with or without chest pain. Some people break out in a sweat or experience nausea or lightheadedness.

Diagnosis

A physician will ask questions about medical history, symptoms, and relatives with heart disease, as well as diet and lifestyle. A physical examination and routine blood tests also may be ordered as part of the evaluation. In addition, several examinations can be done to diagnose and evaluate coronary heart disease. These include:

- Resting electrocardiogram (ECG or EKG). This records electrical signals as they travel through the heart and usually is performed in a physician's office. It is noninvasive and involves placing electrodes on the body.
- Holter monitoring. Also called ambulatory electrocardiography, this involves wearing a portable EKG unit for 24 hours to monitor inadequate blood flow to the heart as a person goes about everyday activities.
- Exercise stress test. This test takes an EKG reading while a person is walking on a treadmill or riding a stationary bicycle. It often is used to evaluate people who experience symptoms when exercising. A nuclear stress test may be used as well. In this examination, the patient exercises and the flow of blood to the heart while at rest and during exercise is measured by injecting minor amounts of a radioactive material into the bloodstream. A special camera can show which parts of the heart may receive less blood flow than normal.
- Angiogram. This is an x ray of the heart taken when a small tube, or catheter, is inserted into the arteries through a blood vessel in the groin or arm. The tip of the catheter can be guided to the coronary arteries and contrast is released. The contrast will be visible on x rays and will help show blood flow in the heart's chambers. Today, angiograms can be performed through the use of contrast and imaging with computed tomography or magnetic resonance imaging.
- Computed tomography (CT) scan. A CT scan, which is a cross-sectional x ray of the body or an organ of the body, can show images of the arteries to determine atherosclerosis. Ultra-fast CT imaging also can detect calcium within plaque.
- Magnetic resonance imaging (MRI). This noninvasive method may be used to examine the tissues of the heart. MRI uses no radiation. Magnetic resonance angiography provides an alternative to the more invasive method that involves introducing a catheter into the body.
- Other imaging methods may be used to detect coronary heart disease, such as single photon emission computed tomography (SPECT).

Treatment

There are many ways to treat coronary heart disease, and the choice of treatment depends on the cause of the disease and its severity. Treatment ranges from lifestyle changes and use of medication to surgical procedures. People with less severe disease and fewer risk factors may be able to manage their disease through lifestyle changes and drug therapy. Changes in diet and an increase in exercise, as well as quitting smoking, can gain control of coronary heart disease. Often all treatment procedures are used. Lifestyle factors such as diet and exercise are first line prevention and treatment methods. They are to be continued even after beginning medications and following surgery.

Medications used to treat coronary heart disease include:

- cholesterol-lowering medicines such as statins and fibrates
- blood thinners, or anticoagulants, to prevent blood clots from forming
- aspirin, also to help prevent clotting
- blood pressure medicines to lower blood pressure, such as angiotensin-converting enzyme (ACE) inhibitors
- calcium channel blockers, to relax blood vessels and lower blood pressure
- beta blockers, to slow heart rate and lower blood pressure

Surgery or other procedures also may be recommended to treat coronary heart disease. A physician may be able to use a catheter to guide a tiny balloon into the artery. Once in place, the balloon is inflated and used to widen the artery by pushing the plaque up against the artery wall, Next, a stent, or mesh tube, is placed in the widened area to help keep the artery opened and clear for adequate blood flow.

Coronary artery bypass surgery reroutes, or bypasses, blood flow around the arteries that have clogged to improve blood flow to the heart. To perform the procedure, the surgeon takes a healthy blood vessel from another part of the body and uses it to create a detour around the clogged artery. This procedure requires open heart surgery and is reserved for people with multiple areas of artery blockage.

Heart attacks from coronary heart disease require emergency medical treatment.

Nutrition and dietary concerns

Nutrition is key to preventing and controlling coronary heart disease. The American Heart Association recommends that adults get no more than 300 mg of cholesterol a day in their diet and that those with heart disease get no more than 200 mg a day. In terms of blood cholesterol, it is most important to limit intake of saturated **fats**. Eating fat-free or low-fat dairy and meat products and opting for oils rich in polyunsaturated or monounsaturated fatty acids (e.g., olive, sunflower, rapeseed oils) will help to keep cholesterol levels in check.

Controlling blood pressure helps prevent or manage coronary heart disease. A diet low in **sodium** (salt) and high in fruits, vegetables, and **whole grains** helps to control blood pressure. The **DASH diet** is a balanced approach to controlling **hypertension**.

Eating lots of sugars and simple **carbohydrates** can contribute to weight gain and raise blood triglyceride levels, increasing risk of coronary heart disease. It is important for people with diabetes to control their intake of white bread, bagels, cakes, soft drinks, and other carbohydrates. Whole-wheat breads, brown rice, and legumes provide more fiber and slowly absorbed carbohydrate than refined carbs and can aid in appetite control and help regulate blood glucose levels. People with high intakes of whole-grain foods seem to be at lower risk of suffering from coronary heart disease.

In the past, there have been recommendations to follow high-protein, high-fat diets to control coronary heart disease. While these diets are generally successful in the short term, not enough is known about their effects in the long term on controlling weight or reducing coronary heart disease. Research has shown that diets lower in carbohydrates and higher in vegetable sources of fat and protein moderately reduce the risk of coronary heart disease in women. Certain foods, such as fish (especially oily fish, which are rich in **omega-3 fatty acids**) and foods high in **fiber** (whole grains, fruits, and fresh vegetables) are healthy foods for the diets of people with coronary heart disease. Protein-rich foods help promote satiety (a feeling of fullness), which can aid in weight control.

The most important aspect of nutrition and diet for people with coronary heart disease is a balanced diet that helps them to lose and manage weight. The U.S. Department of Agriculture (USDA) and the U.S. Department of Health and Human Services (HHS) revised the *Dietary Guidelines for Americans* in 2010. The guidelines are science-based and outline advice for choosing a nutritious diet and maintaining a healthy weight. The 2010 guidelines also address physical activity and **food safety** and make recommendations for special population groups. Finally, calorie requirements and servings are based more on gender, age, and level of physical activity, while in 2000, the servings were more uniform for all adults. The USDA also revised the traditional food pyramid to make it customized for individuals. The new guidelines are known as MyPlate. These guidelines form the basis for healthy eating. The American Heart Association and the Academy of Nutrition and Dietetics also offer heart healthy diet recommendations, as do family physicians and cardiologists.

Therapy

Some patients with coronary heart disease will be referred for cardiac rehabilitation, particularly following bypass surgery or if they have experienced angina or a heart attack. The rehabilitation may consist of an exercise plan to help regain stamina safely based on individual ability and needs, education, counseling, and training. Training may include ways to better manage stress, as well as how to manage other lifestyle factors that contribute to coronary heart disease.

Prognosis

Coronary heart disease can be successfully managed and treated in many cases. Advances in diagnosis and techniques such as stenting have helped to improve the lives of people with the disease, bringing

KEY TERMS

Angina pectoris—Chest pain or discomfort. Angina pectoris is the more common and stable form of angina. Stable angina has a pattern and is more predictable in nature, usually occurring when the heart is working harder than normal.

Atherosclerosis—The hardening and narrowing of the arteries caused by the slow build-up of fatty deposits, or plaque, on the artery walls.

Triglyceride—A fat that comes from food or is made up of other energy sources in the body. Elevated triglyceride levels contribute to the development of atherosclerosis.

about a significant decline in death rates from coronary heart disease since the mid-1980s. However, as the leading cause of death in the United States, coronary heart disease is a serious condition that is best prevented and that requires careful management and attention once diagnosed. The more risk factors a person has, the worse the prognosis.

Prevention

Preventing coronary heart disease begins with identification of common risk factors and taking action to reduce the impact of these factors (e.g., cholesterol or blood pressure reduction). Management of the primary contributing factors that can be avoided goes a long way in preventing the advancement of atherosclerosis and eventual coronary heart disease. By quitting smoking, moderating alcohol use, controlling blood pressure, preventing diabetes, and maintaining healthy cholesterol levels, people can prevent many of the causes of coronary heart disease. Maintaining a healthy body weight by eating a balanced diet with healthy-sized portions and participating in regular physical activity helps to prevent the disease. Those with known hereditary or other risk factors for coronary heart disease should have regular physical examinations with their physicians and should pay careful attention to the signs and symptoms of coronary heart disease and heart attack.

Omega-3 fatty acids have been found to help prevent heart disease in people at high risk. The American Heart Association recommends eating two servings of fatty fish (e.g., salmon, herring, trout, mackerel, sardines, tuna) every week. People who do not eat fish may wish to talk to their doctors about taking fish oil supplements.

Resources

BOOKS

American Heart Association No-Fad Diet: A Personal Plan for Healthy Weight Loss. Clarkson Potter Publishers, 2005.

Bybee, Kevin A., et al. *Cardiovascular Disease in Women Essentials 2011.* Sudbury, MA: Jones & Bartlett Learning, 2011.

Fuster, Valentin, Eric J. Topol, and Elizabeth G. Nabel. *Atherothrombosis and Coronary Artery Disease.* 2nd ed. Philadelphia: Lippincott, Williams, and Wilkins, 2005.

PERIODICALS

Janssen, V., et al. "Lifestyle Modification Programmes for Patients With Coronary Heart Disease: A Systematic Review and Meta-Analysis of Randomized Controlled Trials." *European Journal of Preventive Cardiology* (September 28, 2012): e-pub ahead of print. http://dx.doi.org/10.1177/2047487312462824 (accessed October 2, 2012).

Roger, V.L., et al. "Heart Disease and Stroke Statistics—2012 Update: A Report from the American Heart Association." *Circulation* 125, no. 1 (February 2012): e2–220.

WEBSITES

American Heart Association. "Coronary Artery Disease—Coronary Heart Disease." http://www.heart.org/HEARTORG/Conditions/More/MyHeartandStrokeNews/Coronary-Artery-Disease—The-ABCs-of-CAD_UCM_436416_Article.jsp (accessed October 2, 2012).

———. "Fish and Omega-3 Fatty Acids." http://www.heart.org/HEARTORG/GettingHealthy/NutritionCenter/HealthyDietGoals/Fish-and-Omega-3-Fatty-Acids_UCM_303248_Article.jsp (accessed October 2, 2012).

National Heart, Lung, and Blood Institute. "What is Coronary Heart Disease?" National Institutes of Health. http://www.nhlbi.nih.gov/health/health-topics/topics/cad (accessed September 28, 2012).

PubMed Health. "Coronary Heart Disease." U.S. National Library of Medicine. http://www.ncbi.nlm.nih.gov/pubmedhealth/PMH0004449 (accessed October 2, 2012).

U.S. Department of Agriculture and U.S. Department of Health and Human Services. *Dietary Guidelines for Americans, 2010.* 7th ed. Washington, DC: U.S. Government Printing Office, December 2010. http://health.gov/dietaryguidelines (accessed September 27, 2012).

ORGANIZATIONS

American Heart Association, 7272 Greenville Ave., Dallas, TX 75231, (800) 242-8721, http://www.americanheart.org.

British Heart Foundation, Greater London House, 180 Hampstead Rd., London, United Kingom NW1 7AW, +44 20 7554 0000, http://www.bhf.org.uk.

Centers for Disease Control and Prevention, Division for Heart Disease and Stroke Prevention, 4770 Buford Hwy NE, Mail Stop F-72, Atlanta, GA 30341-3717, (800) CDC-INFO (232-4636), TTY: (800) 232-6348, Fax: (770) 488-8151, cdcinfo@cdc.gov, http://www.cdc.gov/dhdsp.

Heart Foundation (Australia), 80 William St., Level 3, Sydney NSW, Australia 2011, +61 2 92 19 2444, http://www.heartfoundation.org.au.

National Heart, Lung, and Blood Institute, PO Box 30105, Bethesda, MD 20824-0105, (301) 592-8573, TTY: (240) 629-3255, Fax: (240) 629-3246, nhlbiinfo@nhlbi.nih.gov, http://www.nhlbi.nih.gov.

Teresa G. Odle

Cravings

Definition

Craving is defined as a desire or overwhelming yearning to consume a food even when one is not hungry. **Pica** is a rare condition when an individual develops a craving that leads to the intentional consumption of things commonly considered as inedible, such as chalk, paper, soil, and other substances that can cause significant health risks.

Purpose

Food cravings have been the study of research for decades by anthropologists, dietitians, doctors, and others. Food cravings are still not well understood

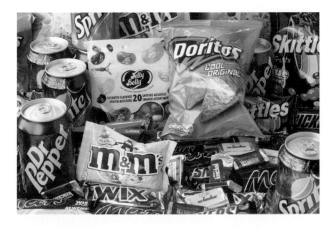

Many people tend to crave sweet or salty foods.
(© Istockphoto.com/nkbimages)

and they have distinct biological and cultural themes. Some research suggests that cravings for **carbohydrates** occur in an effort to elevate mood. This theory hypothesizes that food, usually carbohydrates or chocolate, is being used as a form of self-medication to decrease unpleasant moods. It is thought that these foods increase the brain neurotransmitter serotonin, which is known to have a positive impact on mood. However, evidence for specific macronutrient cravings as a form of self-medication appears to be inconsistent in research.

Description

Cravings for foods are extremely common, with up to 97% of women and 68% of men reporting episodes of food cravings. Chocolate, the most frequently craved food in North America, is the choice of 40% of women and 15% of men when having a craving. Women in particular report extreme cravings for foods that are both sweet and high in fat (e.g., chocolates, cakes or pastries, and ice cream), especially during their menstrual cycle. Dieters are another group who experience stronger cravings that are more difficult to resist than the general population, and for foods they were restricting themselves in eating.

There are a number of theories as to why people crave certain foods, including:

- self-imposed food restriction
- a psychological desire for a "comfort" food
- hormonal changes
- gender differences
- response to stress

FOOD RESTRICTION. The theory of food restriction holds that people desire those foods that they feel should be avoided. According to research, the ability to stop a food craving does not cause weight gain, but a low self-control for cravings does.

COMFORT FOODS. Certain foods are usually served during holidays or special occasions. These foods become associated with comfort and happy times, eliciting feelings of relaxation and reduced stress, and are thus called "comfort foods." Comfort foods vary among cultures and are those foods that are traditionally prepared during social times. One's cultural background plays a large part in comfort food choices. Mood also plays a role in cravings for comfort food. Women are more likely to eat when they are sad, mad, or anxious, while men look to food when bored or lonely.

Those who find themselves reaching for comfort foods frequently should ask themselves if they are truly hungry, or whether they are using food to soothe themselves. For those who are feeding emotions with food, it is helpful to begin to replace the food with healthier activities, such as taking a walk, participating in a favorite form of exercise, getting together with a friend, or reading a good book.

HORMONES. For women, these cravings can be more intense than for men. Hormonal changes tied to the menstrual cycle are often a cause of cravings. Immediately prior to the menstrual period, the body's estrogen level drops, as does the serotonin level in the brain.

SEROTONIN. Serotonin is a neurotransmitter, or brain chemical, that plays a role in maintaining a relaxed feeling. When the level decreases, irritability and mood swings increase, as does the craving for carbohydrate- and fat-rich foods, such as chocolate, cookies, cake, potato chips, and roasted nuts. There is nothing wrong with eating a piece of chocolate, of course, but when chocolate and other craved foods become the mainstay of the diet and healthier choices get overlooked, the cravings have gotten out of control and health may be compromised.

GENDER DIFFERENCES. Men tend to crave salty or savory foods, like potato chips or meat dishes, while women tend to crave sweet foods, like chocolate. Registered dietitian Debra Waterhouse attributes these differences to sex hormones and body composition. Men have larger amounts of the hormone testosterone and about 40 pounds (18 kg) more muscle mass than women. They eat increased amounts of **protein** to build, repair, and synthesize muscle.

STRESS RESPONSE. Many people today lead stressful lives, which can lead to stress eating. Increased stress results in a need for carbohydrates to provide energy for the stress response, also known as the *fight-or-flight* response (a defense reaction of the body that prepares it to fight or flee by triggering certain cardiovascular, hormonal, and other changes). When coping with stress, a person needs increased energy to deal with the demands placed on the body. Carbohydrates provide a fairly rapid source of fuel to the body by raising blood-glucose levels. However, when life becomes hectic and feels out of control, it is common to reach for any available food, regardless of **calories** or nutritional content.

Conquering cravings

Life will always have its stresses, but dealing with stress in a healthful, nutritional way can have a positive impact on self-esteem, energy level, emotional

---

KEY TERMS

Calorie—Unit of food energy.

Estrogen—Hormone that helps control female development and menstruation.

Neurotransmitter—Molecule released by one nerve cell to stimulate or inhibit another.

Serotonin—Chemical used by nerve cells to communicate with one another.

Testosterone—Male sex hormone.

---

outlook, and weight. Positive methods for dealing with cravings include:

- Start the day off with breakfast, which helps to prevent overwhelming hunger later in the day.
- Eliminate feelings of guilt related to labeling food as either "good" or "bad." Some choices are healthier than others, but snacks and treats can be consumed in reasonable amounts.
- Plan ahead for each new week; think about school, work, and activity schedules and how healthful snacks can be incorporated into each day.
- Keep healthful snacks close at hand, both at home and at work.
- Try not to go for long periods of time without eating.
- Combine lean protein foods with high-fiber carbohydrate sources to provide energy that lasts for several hours, such as a slice of vegetable pizza or a bean burrito.

Cravings can be the exception instead of the rule when it comes to one's diet. Developing a lifestyle that includes healthful food selections and regular meals and snacks can help control cravings. The extra time it takes in planning meals or snacks, whether eating at home or eating on the run, is easily made up for in increased energy and improved mood.

Precautions

Food cravings are particularly relevant to health because they may contribute to excessive overeating; unhealthy snacking behavior; poor adherence to diets where calories are being restricted; increased frequency of eating fast foods or prepared foods, such as cookies and candy; or **binge eating**. There is also a growing amount of literature suggesting that chronic dieters, or people eliminating foods for weight loss, are prone to food cravings that lead to increased food intake over time and thus weight gain or regain.

cravings may lead to weight gain, making the person less motivated to quit the substance.

Cravings have also been shown to be more predominant in those with reported **bulimia nervosa**, premenstrual syndrome, seasonal affective disorder, major depression, and substance abuse. It has also been reported that individuals who do not get enough sleep, skip breakfast, or go long periods of time without eating will crave foods more. For those who experience pica, it may be an important sign of **iron** deficiency or a more serious mental health issue that should not be ignored.

Aftercare

When having a craving, studies have shown that cognitive defusion (CD), the process of reducing distress from thoughts about cravings by training people to focus on their process of thinking rather than its content or meaning, is a simple and efficient approach to manage food cravings and, potentially, other behavioral contributors to **obesity**, such as overeating. Other studies have shown that smelling an odor may help alleviate the craving; for example, smelling jasmine while having a craving for chocolate can reduce or diminish the craving.

Complications

High-energy density and high-fat foods, as well as foods with low protein and **fiber** contents, have been identified as frequently craved foods. If a person has multiple cravings weekly, weight gain may occur over time if he or she gives into each craving. Portion size of craved foods and frequency of giving in to food cravings are important considerations in weight loss or management. Cravings may also be triggered for high-calorie, sweet foods when a person decides to quit using cigarettes, alcohol, or drugs, and the

Parental concerns

Children who have repeated incidents of eating indigestible substances, such as chalk, dirt, sand, wax crayons, soap, feces (either their own or animal feces), or other non-edible items may be experiencing unusual cravings (pica). This may be an indication of nutritional deficiencies or even mental illness and parents should discuss with their primary physician for further evaluation.

For women who are pregnant, their food cravings may have a future impact on their baby. Research has shown that pregnant women who gorge on junk food are more likely to give birth to a child with a sweet tooth, a love of **fats**, and a craving for salt. If they eat nutritious foods, such as fruits, vegetables, and **whole grains**, their child could have more of a taste for these foods as well.

If a child is having many food cravings, the parents should also look into the nutrient value of all foods served and eaten, but also if the child is going too long without eating, is skipping meals, or is watching too much television. Proper nutrition and timing of meals, as well as setting limits on how much television and what type of television the child watches to decrease food commercial viewing, may help with food cravings.

Resources

BOOKS

Waterhouse, Debra. *Why Women Need Chocolate*. New York: Hyperion, 1995.

PERIODICALS

Gilhooly, C.H., et al. "Food Cravings and Energy Regulation: The Characteristics of Craved Foods and Their Relationship with Eating Behaviors and Weight Change During 6 Months of Dietary Energy Restriction." *International Journal of Obesity* 31, no. 12: (2007): 1849–58.

Massey, A., and A. J. Hill. "Dieting and Food Craving. A Descriptive, Quasi-Prospective Study." *Appetite* 58, no. 3 (2012): 781–85.

Moffit, R., et al. "A Comparison of Cognitive Restructuring and Cognitive Defusion as Strategies for Resisting a Craved Food." *Psychology & Health* (June 12, 2012): e-pub ahead of print. http://dx.doi.org/10.1080/08870446.2012.694436 (accessed September 10, 2012).

Yanovski, S. "Sugar and Fat: Cravings and Aversions." *The American Society for Nutritional Sciences* 133, no. 3 (2003): 8355–75.

WEBSITES

Burrell, Diana. "Stop the Cravings!" Academy of Nutrition and Dietetics. http://www.eatright.org/Public/content. aspx?id = 6442469608&terms = cravings (accessed September 10, 2012).

Hellmich, Nanci. "Stress Can Put on Pounds." *USA Today*, January 2, 2002. http://www.usatoday.com/news/ health/diet/2002-01-02-usat-diet.htm (accessed September 10, 2012).

Rolnick, Alyssa. "Curb Your Kid's Food Cravings." Canadian Heart and Stroke Foundation. http:// www.heartandstroke.on.ca/site/apps/nlnet/content2. aspx?c = pvI3IeNWJwE&b = 5063573&ct = 6616317 (accessed September 7, 2012).

University of Georgia, Division of Student Affairs. "Nutrition: Healthy Eating When Busy or Stressed." http://www. uhs.uga.edu/stress/strategies.html (accessed September 10, 2012).

ORGANIZATIONS

Academy of Nutrition and Dietetics, 120 South Riverside Plz., Ste. 2000, Chicago, IL 60606-6995, (312) 899-0040, (800) 877-1600, amacmunn@eatright.org, http:// www.eatright.org.

Susan Mitchell
Megan Porter, RD

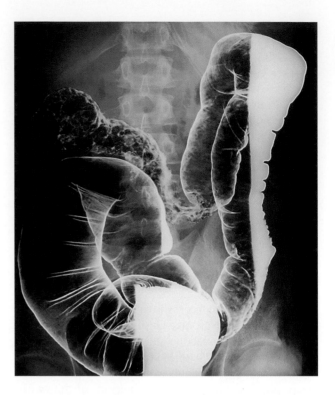

X ray of the colon of a patient with Crohn's disease. The x ray shows ulceration of the intestinal tract (upper left). *(Zephyr/ Photo Researchers, Inc.)*

Crohn's disease

Definition

Crohn's disease is a chronic inflammatory disorder that affects the digestive tract. It is characterized by cramping pains, diarrhea, and sometimes nausea or vomiting.

Demographics

It is estimated that there are about 500,000 people with Crohn's disease in the United States. Another statistic given by some doctors is 7 cases per 100,000 in the general population in Canada and the United States. Crohn's disease is primarily a disorder found in adults, most often beginning in late adolescence or the early adult years. The most common age at onset is between 15 and 30 years, although the disorder may begin at any age.

The rate of Crohn's disease in North America has been increasing since the 1960s, although the reasons for the increase are not well known. Southern Europe, South America, Africa, and Asia have considerably lower rates of the disease—as low as 0.08–0.5 cases per 100,000 people. Around the world, rates of Crohn's disease are higher in cities than in rural areas, and higher among people with higher incomes than among lower-income groups.

One argument for the presence of a genetic factor in Crohn's disease is that it runs in some families; people who have a sibling with the disease are 30 times more likely to develop it than the normal population. Crohn's disease is also relatively common among certain ethnic groups, particularly Jews of Eastern European origin. A two- to four-fold increase in the frequency of Crohn's disease has been found among the Jewish population in the United States, Europe, and South Africa compared to other ethnic groups.

Description

Crohn's disease is named for Dr. Burrill Bernard Crohn (1884–1983) who, with his colleagues, first described the disease in 1932. Crohn's disease can affect any part of the digestive system, but it develops most often in the section of the small intestine just before the large intestine begins. This region is called the ileum, and Crohn's disease that develops there is sometimes called ileitis. The other common site for Crohn's disease is in the colon or large intestine.

Crohn's disease is one of several inflammatory bowel diseases. It can be mistaken for ulcerative colitis, as both these diseases cause watery or bloody diarrhea and abdominal cramps or pain. However, ulcerative colitis affects only the layer of cells that line the intestine, forming sores or **ulcers** on this surface. Crohn's disease begins in these same surface cells, but eats its way inward, damaging all four layers of the intestine and sometimes creating a hole (fistula) through the intestine and into other tissue. Another major difference between Crohn's disease and ulcerative colitis is that Crohn's disease can develop simultaneously in several spots in the digestive tract, resulting in areas damaged with patches with healthy tissue in between. Ulcerative colitis, on the other hand, spreads uniformly across an area. Crohn's disease is somewhat treatable, but not curable, and can cause many complications beyond the digestive system. Eventually, the walls of the intestine thicken, and blockages may occur that can only be corrected by surgery.

In some cases of Crohn's disease, the underlying layers of intestinal tissue are damaged also, leading to complete perforation (puncturing) of the wall of the intestine. This form of the disease is sometimes called penetrating Crohn's disease. Penetrating disease may cause a serious infection in the abdomen or the formation of fistulas. In Crohn's disease, fistulas are most likely to form in the area around the anus, leading to the formation of abscesses (pus-filled sores). About 30 percent of patients with Crohn's disease develop fistulas.

Another subtype of Crohn's disease is called stricturing disease. Stricture is the medical term for an abnormal narrowing of a hollow organ such as the bowel. In stricturing disease, the inflammation and swelling of tissue inside the bowel leads to changes in the size of the patient's stools and eventual blockage of the intestinal passages. Severe abdominal cramping is often an indication of stricturing disease, as are nausea and vomiting.

Risk factors

Risk factors for Crohn's disease include a family history of the disorder, a history of heavy smoking, and Eastern European Jewish ethnicity.

Causes and symptoms

Causes

At one time, researchers thought that stress and diet caused Crohn's disease, particularly high-fat foods. Now researchers know that these are not factors, although both stress and diet can worsen symptoms in people who already have the disease. What researchers do know is that Crohn's disease is caused by an inappropriate immune system reaction that affects cells in the digestive tract. Beyond that, the reasons why some people develop the disease are not clear, although smoking does increase the risk.

There is almost certainly an inherited component that predisposes some people to the disease. Individuals who are blood relatives of a parent, sibling, or child with Crohn's disease are 30 times more likely to develop the disease than the general population. Scientists believe multiple genes are involved in development of the disease. However, more than genetics determines who gets Crohn's disease, because only about 44% of identical twins both develop the disease. Researchers have found mutated (altered) genes in many, but not all, people who have Crohn's disease but do not yet have a clear understanding of what these genes do.

The current thinking is that interactions among genes, the environment, the individual's health, and body chemistry affect a person's risk of developing Crohn's disease. When foreign materials (antigens) enter the body, the immune system produces antibodies, which are proteins that neutralize the foreign invader. One theory about Crohn's disease is that some foreign organism or material stimulates an immune system response in the digestive system, and then through an error in genetic control, the response cannot be "turned off." A second theory suggests that the cells of the immune system mistake good bacteria, food, or some other substance that is normally present in the digestive tract and make antibodies against this material as if it were a foreign substance. Either way, an inappropriate immune system response occurs that appears to be the root cause of the symptoms people with Crohn's disease experience.

Symptoms

Symptoms of Crohn's disease vary, depending on the location of the damaged cells and the length of time the individual has had the disease. Symptoms can be mild or severe. They can develop suddenly or gradually, and they may improve or even disappear, and then worsen many times throughout an individual's life. Some people may have only occasional episodes of diarrhea, for example, while others may have 20–30 bowel movements in a single day that interfere with sleep, work, school, or other activities. In general, symptoms can be divided into those that affect the digestive tract and those that affect the rest of the body.

psychotherapy (talk therapy), guided by a psychologist or psychiatrist experienced in the stresses of chronic illness, can help them make a better adjustment to life with Crohn's disease.

Prognosis

Crohn's disease is a lifelong disease. Symptoms may improve or disappear for periods, but overall, symptoms and complications tend to worsen. Most people with Crohn's disease eventually need surgery as the disease becomes less and less responsive to medication. Living with Crohn's disease can be a difficult challenge that requires major lifestyle adjustments. The chance of a shortened life span or serious complications increases with the duration of the illness; patients with Crohn's disease also have an increased risk of colorectal **cancer**. The disease itself, however, is rarely fatal.

Prevention

Crohn's disease cannot be prevented.

Resources

BOOKS

Sklar, Jill. *The First Year: Crohn's Disease and Ulcerative Colitis: An Essential Guide for the Newly Diagnosed*, 2nd ed. New York: Marlowe and Company, 2007.

Steinhart, Hillary *Crohn's and Colitis: Understanding the Facts About IBD*. West Toronto, ON: Robert Rose, 2006.

Tessmer, Kimberly A. *Tell Me What to Eat If I Have Inflammatory Bowel Disease: Nutritional Guidelines for Crohn's Disease and Colitis*. Pompton Plains, NJ: New Page Books, 2012.

Warner, Andrew S., and Amy Barto. *100 Questions & Answers About Crohn's Disease and Ulcerative Colitis: A Lahey Clinic Guide*. Sudbury, MA: Jones and Bartlett Publishers, 2007.

Zonderman, Jon, and Ronald Vender. *Understanding Crohn Disease and Ulcerative Colitis*. Jackson, MS: University Press of Mississippi, 2006.

PERIODICALS

American Academy of Family Practice (AAFP). "Patient Information: Crohn's Disease." *American Family Physician* (2003). Available online at http://www.aafp.org/afp/20030815/717ph.html.

Bakalar, Nicholas. "Crohn's Disease and Colitis Are Linked to Mutant Gene." *New York Times*, November 7, 2006.

Bernard, André. "A Systematic Review of Patient Inflammatory Bowel Disease Information Resources on the World Wide Web." *American Journal of Gastroenterology* (September 2007): 2070–77.

Clark, M., et al. "American Gastroenterological Association Consensus Development Conference on the Use of Biologics in the Treatment of Inflammatory Bowel Disease." *Gastroenterology* (July 2007): 312–39.

Feagan, Brian G., et al. "Health-Related Quality of Life During Natalizumab Maintenance Therapy for Crohn's Disease." *American Journal of Gastroenterology* (December 2007): 2737–46.

Lucendo, A.J., and L.C. De Rezende. "Importance of Nutrition in Inflammatory Bowel Disease." *World Journal of Gastroenterology* 15 (May 7, 2009): 2081–88.

Noomen, C.G., D.W. Hommes, and H.H. Fidder. "Update on Genetics in Inflammatory Disease." *Best Practice and Research. Clinical Gastroenterology* 23, no. 2 (2009): 233–43.

Van Limbergen, Johan, et al. "The Genetics of Inflammatory Bowel Disease." *American Journal of Gastroenterology* (December 2007): 2820–31.

WEBSITES

Crohn's & Colitis Foundation of America. "Living with Crohn's & Colitis." http://www.ccfa.org/living-with-crohns-colitis (accessed February 27, 2012).

———. "What is Crohn's Disease?" http://www.ccfa.org/info/about/crohns (accessed August 2, 2012).

Gardner, Amanda. "Omega-3 Fatty Acids Won't Prevent Crohn's Relapse." ABC News, April 9, 2008. http://abcnews.go.com/Health/Healthday/story?id=4613371 (accessed August 2, 2012).

Mayo Clinic staff. "Crohn's Disease." MayoClinic.com. http://www.mayoclinic.com/health/crohns-disease/DS00104 (accessed August 2, 2012).

MedlinePlus. "Crohn's Disease." U.S. National Library of Medicine, National Institutes of Health. http://www.nlm.nih.gov/medlineplus/crohnsdisease.html (accessed August 2, 2012).

National Digestive Diseases Information Clearinghouse (NDDIC). "Crohn's Disease." http://digestive.niddk.nih.gov/ddiseases/pubs/crohns/index.aspx (accessed August 2, 2012).

ORGANIZATIONS

American College of Gastroenterology, 6400 Goldsboro Rd., Ste. 200, Bethesda, MD 20817, (301) 263-9000, http://www.gi.org.

Crohn's & Colitis Foundation of America, 386 Park Ave. S., 17th Fl., New York, NY 10016, (800) 932-2423, info@ccfa.org, http://www.ccfa.org.

National Institute of Diabetes and Digestive and Kidney Diseases (NIDDK), Bldg. 31, Rm. 9A06, 31 Center Dr., MSC 2560, Bethesda, MD 20892, (301) 496-3583, http://www2.niddk.nih.gov/Footer/Contact-NIDDK.htm, http://www2.niddk.nih.gov.

Tish Davidson, AM
David Edward Newton, EdD
Rebecca J. Frey, PhD

CSIRO total wellbeing diet

Definition

The CSIRO total wellbeing diet (TWD) is a high-protein, low-fat, moderate-carbohydrate weight-loss and maintenance diet developed by Australia's national science agency, the Commonwealth Scientific and Industrial Research Organization (CSIRO). It is a very structured, calorie-controlled, and nutritionally balanced diet that includes exercise and large amounts of **protein** from meat, fish, and poultry.

Origins

The TWD was developed by CSIRO researchers at its Clinical Research Unit in Adelaide, South Australia. The CSIRO research was initiated in response to a large number of inquiries from dietitians concerning popular high-protein diets, whose use did not appear to be supported by scientific evidence. Previous CSIRO research had suggested that high-protein, low-fat diets were at least as effective for weight loss as high-carbohydrate, low fat diets.

In research partially funded by Meat and Livestock Australia and Dairy Australia, the CSIRO team, led by Dr. Manny Noakes, developed the TWD for overweight and obese women. Dr. Grant Brinkworth was the exercise/nutrition physiologist on the team. The TWD was the culmination of eight years of research on diet composition, weight loss, and risks for developing diabetes and heart disease, conducted at CSIRO's Human Nutrition Clinic. In initial clinical studies the researchers claimed to have found clear health benefits and significant weight loss associated with their high-protein, **low-fat diet**. They further claimed that clinical studies showed the diet to be superior to a high-carbohydrate, low-fat diet with identical caloric intake, at least in a subset of women.

Meat and Livestock Australia distributed a booklet about the CSIRO diet in a women's magazine. The publisher Penguin then commissioned Noakes and Dr. Peter Clifton, director of the CSIRO Nutrition Clinic, to write the book *The CSIRO Total Wellbeing Diet*. It was a runaway bestseller in Australia upon its publication in 2005. A sequel was published in 2006.

Description

The key components of the TWD are:

- high amounts of protein from lean meat, fish, and low-fat dairy products
- moderate amounts of carbohydrates
- low fat
- adequate fiber from whole grains, fruits, and vegetables
- caloric restriction
- exercise

With the exception of its emphasis on meat, the TWD recommendations follow standard nutritional guidelines. The diet offers a variety of healthy food choices, including large amounts of fruits and vegetables, along with moderate exercise.

The basic daily TWD consists of:

- lean dinner protein, 7 oz. (200 g) raw weight of lean red meat (beef, lamb, veal) four times per week, fish twice per week, chicken once per week
- lean lunch protein, up to 4 oz. (110 g)
- whole-grain bread, two 1 oz. (28-g) slices
- fruit, two medium pieces
- high-fiber cereal, 1.5 oz. (42 g) or about one cup
- low-fat dairy, three servings
- salad, one-half cup
- vegetables, four one-half-cup servings
- oil or margarine, three teaspoons
- indulgence foods, two servings per week
- exercise, 30 minutes daily

Levels

The TWD has four different diet levels, which are designed to cover the varying energy requirements of the majority of people. Level 1 is approximately 1,337 **calories** (5,600 kilojoules) per day. Levels 3 and 4 have higher allowances of lean protein, low-fat dairy, and high-fiber cereal. Before choosing a level, CSIRO recommends that people calculate their basal metabolic rate (BMR), which is based on height, weight, age, and gender. The Harris-Benedict Equation then uses the BMR and a factor based on a person's activity level to determine daily energy expenditure in calories or kilojoules.

In general, the level 1 and 2 plans are suitable for women and the level 3 and 4 plans are suitable for men, who tend to be taller and heavier than women. A basic daily TWD for men consists of:

- 7–9 oz. (200–250 g) raw weight of lean meat, chicken, or fish for dinner
- 4 oz. (110 g) cooked weight of meat, ham, chicken, or tuna for lunch
- whole-grain bread, two slices
- fruit, two pieces

- high-fiber cereal, 1.5 oz. (40–50 g)
- low-fat dairy, three servings
- vegetables, two cups
- margarine/oil, four teaspoons
- one optional glass of wine

Protein

The TWD calls for a high amount of lean protein to prevent hunger. For dinner, the TWD recommends 28 oz. (800 g) raw weight of red meat per week or an average of 4 oz. (110 g) per day, as well as at least 14 oz. (400 g) of fish per week, or 2 oz. (56 g) per day, and 7 oz. (200 g) per week of skinless chicken with the fat removed. The diet calls for another 3.5 oz. (100 g) of protein for lunch, based on the cooked weight of processed meat, chicken, or tuna.

An extra serving of dairy can be substituted for 1.7 oz. (50 g) of protein at lunch. One dairy serving is:

- a low-fat or diet yogurt
- a dairy dessert, 7 oz. (200 g)
- low-fat milk, 8.5 oz. (250 mL)
- cheddar or other full-fat cheese, 1 oz. (28 g)
- reduced-fat cheese (10% fat), 1.7 oz. (50 g)

Carbohydrates

The TWD contains moderate amounts of slow-releasing **carbohydrates** that are necessary for energy and maintaining blood glucose levels. These carbohydrates, primarily fruit and dairy, tend to have a low glycemic index (GI). They are digested slowly and help to keep blood glucose levels steady. Since total carbohydrate is limited to 40% of the total calories or kilojoules in the diet, the TWD has a low glycemic load (GL).

Fruits are limited to 11 oz. (300 g) per day, as two servings of unsweetened fresh or canned fruit (5.3 oz., 150 g) or unsweetened juice (5 oz., 150 mL). Equal amounts of dried or frozen fruit, vegetables, or unsweetened vegetable juice (5 oz., 150 mL) may be substituted for one serving of a fruit or vegetable.

Simple sugars and refined carbohydrates are not recommended. **Sugar** or honey as sweeteners can be used only in small amounts. Small amounts of sweeteners or thickeners can be used occasionally in cooking. One level teaspoon of sugar is equivalent to 10–14 calories (40–60 kilojoules).

Fats

The TWD contains very small amounts of fatty foods and oils. It calls for less than 30% of calories from fat or about 50 g of fat per day. The TWD assumes that low-fat foods contain no more than 3 g of fat per 3.5 oz. (100 g) of solid food or 1.5 g of fat per 3.5 oz. (100 g) of liquid. Fat-free foods contain no more than 0.15 g of fat per 3.5 oz. (100 g). Reduced/low-fat milk contains 1%–2% fat and skim/nonfat milk contains less than 0.16% fat.

The TWD recommends that the daily fat allowance be consumed as:

- canola oil
- olive oil
- sunflower oil
- soft/light margarine
- avocados
- nuts and seeds

Two teaspoons of light margarine is equal to one teaspoon of oil. Three teaspoons of oil is equivalent to 2 oz. (56 g) of avocado or 0.7 oz. (20 g) of nuts.

Snacks

Allowable snacks include:

- leftover portions from main meals
- low-calorie soup
- a cappuccino or café latte with skim milk from the milk allowance
- low-fat yogurt or custard
- fresh fruit from the fruit allowance

Alcohol

The level 1 TWD allows for two glasses (10 oz., 300 mL) of wine or about 205 calories (860 kilojoules) per week. Equivalent amounts of other alcohol or treats, such as 1.5 oz. (40 g) of chocolate, may be substituted. It is suggested that **alcohol consumption** be kept to a minimum during the first few weeks of the diet because alcohol can increase the appetite. Presuming that other medical conditions do not limit the acceptable alcohol intake, other TWD levels and the maintenance diet allow for increased amounts. However, alcohol intake should not exceed the recommended two standard drinks per day for women and four for men.

"Free" food

The TWD includes a "free" food list with minimal calories. Diet or low-calorie soups are an optional daily extra. Packet soups containing about 38 calories (160 kilojoules) per serving or vegetable soups made from the "free" list are appropriate daily. The TWD includes an average of 2 to 2.5 cups of vegetables, or about 14 oz. (400 g), per day. Since vegetables tend to be very low in calories, eating more vegetables is acceptable and many vegetables are included in the "free" list.

Foods that can be consumed as desired include:

• all green, orange, yellow, red, and most white vegetables, except potatoes and sweet potatoes
• diet soft drinks, unflavored bottled water, teas, coffee, cocoa
• stock cubes and clear soups
• diet jellies
• oil-free salad dressing
• sauces such as tomato, chili, and soy
• condiments
• garlic
• lemons
• herbs and spices

Substitutions and adjustments

Allowable diet adjustments include swapping the mid-day and evening meals or distributing the diet components differently over the course of the day. However, the quantities and total intake should be the same each day. Other lean protein food can be substituted for meat. For example, a dinner might include 3.5 oz. (100 g) of meat, chicken, or fish and a vegetable protein such as 4.5 oz. (130 g) of cooked beans or 3.5 oz. (100 g) of tofu. Eggs are protein foods and one egg can be substituted for 1.7 oz. (50 g) of lean meat, chicken, turkey, ham, pork, fish, or low-fat cheese. Soymilk products or low-lactose milk products may be used for the dairy requirement.

Allowable substitutions within food groups include:

• eggs for other protein
• non-dairy products for dairy
• rice or beans for bread
• toast for cereal
• frozen, canned, or dried fruit or vegetables for fresh fruit
• milk or yogurt for other dairy
• fruit juice for fruit
• vegetable juice for vegetables
• avocados or nuts for fats and oils
• other drinks or snacks for wine

Whole-grain bread should be high in **fiber**, containing at least 3 g per serving. Whole grain means that all of the components of the grain—the bran, germ,

and endosperm—are present. One of the two daily slices of bread may be replaced with:

• 1/3 or 1/2 cup of chickpeas, lentils, or beans
• two pieces of crispbread
• one medium potato (about 5.3 oz. or 150 g)
• one-third cup of cooked rice or noodles
• one-half cup of cooked pasta

A low-fat coffee drink may be substituted for a similar drink such as tea with low-fat milk. Cocoa and herbal tea are on the "free" list.

Vegetarians

Vegetarians can substitute cooked beans or lentils (9 oz., 260 g) or tofu (7 oz., 200 g) for meat, chicken, or fish (7 oz., 200 g). One egg can be substituted for 1.7 oz. (50 g) of meat, ham, pork, chicken, turkey, fish, or low-fat cheese. Legumes, including beans, split peas, lentils, and chickpeas, or tofu or other **soy** products can also be substituted for red meat. Vegetarians can substitute two eggs or 3.5 oz. (100 g) of low-fat cheese for 3.5 oz. (100 g) of the lunch protein requirement.

Eating out

When choosing from a restaurant menu, the TWD recommends foods that are:

• grilled
• steamed
• poached
• stir-fried

Foods to be avoided include:

• deep-fried
• pan-fried
• battered
• crumbed
• sauces with cheese, oil, butter, or cream
• fried potatoes

Maintenance diet

The weekly menu plans are repeated until the desired weight loss is achieved and then a maintenance plan is implemented. The maintenance plan is the same as the weekly diet plan with the addition of about 120 calories (500 kilojoules) to the diet, as long as weight is not regained. Each week the following foods can be added back in any order:

• week 1: two slices of whole-grain bread daily
• week 2: one-half cup cooked rice or pasta

- week 3: extra milk such as low-fat milk, yogurt, ice cream
- week 4: an extra potato
- week 5: an extra snack food
- week 6: one extra restaurant meal

Snack choices for the maintenance diet include:

- 0.7 oz. (20 g) of nuts
- two plain sweet biscuits
- one to two whole-grain biscuits or crackers and low-fat cheese
- 2 oz. (56 g) of chips in canola or olive oil
- part of an avocado
- one fruit bar

On the maintenance diet the following foods may be exchanged:

- 8 oz. (250 mL) of wine or 2 fl oz. (60 mL) of other alcohol for one snack
- one medium potato with skin, 2 oz. (56 g) of fries, or 0.7 oz. (20 g) of pretzels for one slice of bread or one piece of fruit
- three-quarter cup of boiled pasta or rice for two slices of bread
- 2 oz. (56 g) or ten small squares of chocolate for one snack
- one fruit bar for one piece of fruit

Books

The CSIRO Total Wellbeing Diet explains and details the diet and contains over 100 recipes. *Book 2* includes some revisions and additions:

- The caloric intake is slightly higher.
- Calcium intake is increased by an extra daily serving of dairy.
- The daily folic-acid intake is increased to 400 mcg for adults and 600 mcg for pregnant and breastfeeding women.
- Eighty new recipes and substitutions have been added.
- Twelve weeks of sample menu plans give examples of how to organize the diet.
- New tips on eating out and packing a lunch are included.
- A simple, structured, do-anywhere exercise plan has been added.
- There is a section on maintaining focus on the diet.

Function

The TWD is designed to result in a weight loss of 1–2 lbs (0.5–1 kg) per week. The subsequent maintenance diet is designed to maintain the desired weight. The higher protein in the TWD helps control appetite and prevent muscle loss. The TWD can be used to feed an entire family, although family members who do not need to lose weight may eat more carbohydrates with their meals, such as extra bread, pasta, rice, or potatoes.

Benefits

Because the TWD diet is high in protein, it tends to satisfy hunger and prevent overeating. Men, in particular, seem to appreciate the amount of meat in this diet. It provides nutrients such as **iron**, **zinc**, and **calcium** that may be minimal on a lower-protein diet. There are additional benefits from a high-protein meat diet:

- Lean red meat is the best source of well-absorbed iron and meat is rich in zinc.
- Iron and zinc, which help boost the immune system, are more easily absorbed from meat than from plant foods.
- Meat, poultry, fish, and eggs are excellent sources of vitamin B_{12}, which is not found in plants.
- Fish and seafood are the best sources of omega-3 fats, which help protect the heart. Beef and lamb are the next best sources.

The TWD can significantly reduce **triglycerides** and LDL ("bad") cholesterol. Sustained weight loss, exercise, and moderate alcohol intake can increase HDL ("good") cholesterol. Therefore CSIRO researchers believe that the high protein in the TWD may help prevent heart disease and type 2 diabetes. Some experts also consider the TWD superior to other diets because it calls for a fiber intake in excess of 28 g per day.

The TWD has other advantages:

- It includes a large variety of foods.
- It is a very flexible diet and allows many substitutions.
- Daily meals can be consumed in any order.
- Tested recipes and menus are available online.
- Shopping lists can be downloaded from the CSIRO Website.
- The TWD is designed for long-term maintenance.

Basal metabolic rate—BMR; the rate of energy consumption when at complete rest.

Calorie—The heat- or energy-producing value of food when it is oxidized in the body; the amount of food having an energy-producing value of one calorie. Also called a large calorie or kilocalorie; equivalent to 4.2 kilojoules.

Carbohydrates—Sugars, starches, and celluloses produced by plants and ingested by animals.

Cholesterol—A steroid alcohol in animal cells and body fluids that controls the fluidity of membranes and functions as a metabolic precursor.

Fiber—Roughage; a complex mixture found in plant foods that includes the carbohydrates cellulose, hemicellulose, gum, mucilages, and pectins, as well as lignin.

Glycemic index—GI; a measure of the rate at which an ingested carbohydrate raises the glucose level in the blood.

Glycemic load—GL; a measure of the GI of a given food.

HDL cholesterol—High-density lipoprotein containing cholesterol in a healthy form.

Kilojoule—1,000 joules; a unit equivalent to 0.239 calories.

LDL cholesterol—Low-density lipoprotein containing a high proportion of cholesterol that is associated with the development of arteriosclerosis.

Metabolic rate—The BMR adjusted by an activity factor with the Harris-Benedict Formula to determine total daily energy expenditure in calories or kilojoules.

Omega-3 fatty acids—A type of polyunsaturated fat that may be beneficial for the heart.

Syndrome X—Metabolic syndrome; a metabolic condition characterized by excess abdominal fat, high blood pressure, low HDL cholesterol, high fasting blood-glucose levels, and high blood triglycerides, that may affect at least one in four women and increase their risk of developing type 2 diabetes and heart disease.

Triglycerides—Neutral fats; lipids formed from glycerol and fatty acids that circulate in the blood as lipoproteins.

Precautions

Dr. Rosemary Stanton, a leading Australian nutritionist, has pointed out that the high amount of red meat in the TWD contradicts the Australian government's own recommendations. Whereas the *Australian Guide to Healthy Eating* recommends 2–4 oz. (56–112 g) of lean red meat three or four times per week, the TWD prescribes more than twice that amount. Consumers may be confused by these discrepancies. In addition, the trade organization Meat and Livestock Australia provided CSIRO with research funds and heavily promoted the book, suggesting possible conflicts of interest. Vegetarians in particular may have a difficult time following the TWD.

The TWD was based on clinical studies of overweight women, some of whom had metabolic dysfunction. Therefore the advantages of the TWD for men and healthy women are unclear.

CSIRO claims that the TWD is suitable for pregnant and **breastfeeding** women. However, breastfeeding women may need up to 700 extra calories (3,000 extra kilojoules) per day. CSIRO recommends that breastfeeding women should start with level 1 or 2 and include three servings of dairy for calcium. Additional bread and fruit can be added to satiate hunger

and increase energy. Furthermore, because of the large amount of fish and seafood in the diet, pregnant women should check for the types of fish that are safe to eat during pregnancy.

The TWD is suitable for overweight children, as long as it includes three units of dairy. However, a registered dietitian should adjust the number of calories for the age, size, and activity level of the child.

CSIRO claims that the TWD can be used effectively by people with diabetes, **celiac disease** (gluten intolerance), **fructose intolerance**, and **irritable bowel syndrome**. However, people with diabetes should consult their doctor or a registered dietitian before using the TWD. People with gluten intolerance should choose gluten- or wheat-free substitutes or substitute rice, beans, chickpeas, or lentils for bread. Those with irritable bowel syndrome may substitute a lower-fiber cereal and take psyllium supplements of 30 g per day to obtain adequate fiber. CSIRO recommends that a registered dietitian be consulted if significant adjustments to the diet are required.

The TWD was designed for foods readily available to Australians and assumes the intake of significant amounts of processed foods. It is not suitable for

D

Danish diet *see* **Scandinavian diet**
Dark chocolate *see* **Chocolate diet**

DASH diet

Definition

DASH stands for Dietary Approaches to Stop Hypertension. The DASH diet is based on DASH study results published in 1997. The study showed that a diet rich in fruits, vegetables, and low-fat dairy foods, with reduced saturated and total fat, could substantially lower blood pressure. It is the diet recommended by the National Heart, Lung and Blood Institute (part of the National Institutes of Health) for lowering blood pressure.

Origins

High blood pressure affects about one in three adults in the United States and is defined as blood pressure consistently above 140/90 mmHg. The top number, 140, is the systolic pressure exerted by the blood against the arteries while the heart is contracting. The bottom number, 90, is the diastolic pressure in the arteries while the heart is relaxing or between beats. The concern is the higher the blood pressure, the greater the risk for developing heart disease, kidney disease, and stroke. High blood pressure is known as the silent killer as it has no symptoms or warning signs.

The DASH study by the National Heart, Lung, and Blood Institute (NHLBI), published in the *New England Journal of Medicine* in 1977, was the first study to look at the effect a diet rich in potassium, **magnesium**, and **calcium**, not supplements, had on blood pressure.

The study involved 459 adults with and without high blood pressure. Systolic blood pressures had to be less than 160 mmHg and diastolic pressures 80 to 95 mmHg. Approximately half the participants were women and 60% were African American. Three eating plans were compared. The first was similar to a typical American diet—high in fat (37% of **calories**) and low in fruit and vegetables. The second was the American diet but with more fruits and vegetables. The third was a plan rich in fruits, vegetables, low-fat dairy foods, and low in overall fat (less than 30% of calories). It also provided 4,700 milligrams (mg) potassium, 500 mg magnesium, and 1,240 mg calcium per 2,000 calories. This has become known as the DASH diet. All three plans contained equal amounts of **sodium**, about 3,000 mg of sodium daily, equivalent to 7 grams (g) of salt. This was approximately 20% below the average intake for adults in the United States and close to the current salt recommendations of 4–5 g. Calorie intake was adjusted to maintain each person's weight. These two factors were included to eliminate salt reduction and weight loss as potential reasons for any changes in blood pressure. All meals were prepared for the participants in a central kitchen to increase compliance with the diets.

Results showed that the increased fruit and vegetable and DASH plans lowered blood pressure, but the DASH plan was the most effective. For participants without high blood pressure, it reduced systolic pressure by 6 mmHg and diastolic by 3 mmHg. The results were better for participants with high blood pressure—the drop in systolic and diastolic was almost double, at 11 mmHg and 6 mmHg, respectively. These results showed that the DASH diet appeared to lower blood pressure as well as a 3 g salt-restricted diet, but more importantly, had a similar reduction as seen with the use of a single blood pressure medication. The effect was seen within two weeks of starting the DASH plan, which is also comparable to treatment by medication, and continued throughout the trial. This trial provided the first experimental evidence that potassium, calcium, and magnesium are important dietary factors in affecting blood pressure, rather than just sodium alone.

DASH Eating Plan

Food group	Daily servings	Serving sizes
Grains*	6–8	1 slice bread 1 oz. dry cereal[†] ½ cup cooked rice, pasta, or cereal
Vegetables	4–5	1 cup raw leafy vegetable ½ cup cut-up raw or cooked vegetable ½ cup vegetable juice
Fruits	4–5	1 medium fruit ¼ cup dried fruit ½ cup fresh, frozen, or canned fruit ½ cup fruit juice
Fat-free or low-fat milk and milk products	2–3	1 cup milk or yogurt 1½ oz. cheese
Lean meats, poultry, and fish	6 or less	1 oz. cooked meats, poultry, or fish 1 egg[‡]
Nuts, seeds, and legumes	4–5 per week	⅓ cup or 1½ oz. nuts 2 Tbsp. peanut butter 2 Tbsp. or ½ oz. seeds ½ cup cooked legumes (dry beans and peas)
Fats and oils§	2–3	1 tsp. soft margarine 1 tsp. vegetable oil 1 Tbsp. mayonnaise 2 Tbsp. salad dressing
Sweets and added sugars	5 or less per week	1 Tbsp. sugar 1 Tbsp. jelly or jam ½ cup sorbet, gelatin 1 cup lemonade

*Whole grains are recommended for most grain servings as a good source of fiber and nutrients.
[†]Serving sizes vary between ½ cup and 1 ¼ cups, depending on cereal type. Check the product's Nutrition Facts label.
[‡]Since eggs are high in cholesterol, limit egg yolk intake to no more than four per week.

SOURCE: National Heart, Lung and Blood Institute, *Your Guide to Lowering Your Blood Pressure with DASH: DASH Eating Plan*, rev. ed., NIH publication no. 06-4082, Washington, DC: National Institutes of Health, Department of Health and Human Services, 2006.

(Table by PreMediaGlobal. © 2013 Cengage Learning.)

The original DASH plan did not restrict sodium. As a result, a second DASH-sodium trial from 1997–1999 (published in 2001) studied the effect the DASH diet had on blood pressure using different sodium levels (3,300, 2,300 or 1,500 mg). This is known as the DASH-sodium diet. The highest amount of salt recommended by the U.S. Department of Agriculture's (USDA) 2010 *Dietary Guidelines for Americans* is 2,300 mg. The amount recommended by the Institute of Medicine, as a minimum to replace the amount lost through urine and to achieve a diet that provides sufficient amounts of essential nutrients, is 1,500 mg. The results showed that the combined effect of a lower

sodium intake with the DASH diet was greater than just the DASH diet or a low salt diet. Like earlier studies, the greatest effect was with the lower sodium intake of 1,500 mg, particularly for those without hypertension. For this group, the systolic dropped about 7 mmHg and the diastolic about 4 mmHg. However, the reduction in blood pressure for people with hypertension was about 12 mmHg for systolic and 6 mmHg for diastolic, quite similar to the reductions seen with the DASH diet.

Description

The diet is based on 2,000 calories a day with the following nutritional profile:

- Total fat: 27% of calories
- Saturated fat: 6% of calories
- Protein: 18% of calories
- Carbohydrate: 55% of calories
- Cholesterol: 150 mg
- Sodium: 2,300 mg
- Potassium: 4,700 mg
- Calcium: 1,250 mg
- Magnesium: 500 mg
- Fiber: 30 g

These percentages translate into more practical guidelines using food group servings.

- Grains and grain products: Seven to eight servings per day. One serving is equivalent to one slice of bread, half a cup of dry cereal, or cooked rice or pasta. These foods provide energy, carbohydrates, and fiber.
- Vegetables: Four to five servings per day. One serving size is one cup leafy vegetables, half-cup cooked vegetables, or half-cup vegetable juice. Fruits and vegetables provide potassium, magnesium, and fiber. Consuming the full number of vegetable servings is a key component of the diet.
- Fruits: Four to five servings per day. One serving is one medium fruit, half-cup fruit juice, or one-quarter cup dried fruit.
- Low-fat dairy foods: Two to three servings per day. One serving is equivalent to one cup milk or yogurt or one ounce (30 g) cheese. Dairy provides rich sources of protein and calcium.
- Meat, fish, poultry: Two or fewer servings per day. One serving is 2.5 ounces (75 g). The emphasis is on lean meats and skinless poultry. These provide protein and magnesium.
- Nuts, seeds, and beans: Four to five servings per week. Portion sizes are half a cup of cooked beans

and two tablespoons of seeds. These are good vegetable sources of protein, as well as magnesium and potassium.

- Fats and oils: Two to three servings per day. One serving is one teaspoon (tsp.) of oil or soft margarine. Fat choices should be heart healthy unsaturated sources (canola, corn, olive, or sunflower). Saturated and *trans* fat consumption should be decreased.
- Sweets: Five servings per week. A serving is one tablespoon of pure fruit jam, syrup, honey, and sugar. The plan still allows for treats, but the healthier the better.

An example breakfast menu is: cornflakes (one cup) with 1 tsp. **sugar**, skim milk (one cup), orange juice (1/2 cup), a banana, and a slice of whole wheat bread with one tablespoon jam. Suggested snacks during the day include dried apricots (1/4 cup), low-fat yogurt (one cup), and mixed nuts (1.5 oz. or 40 g).

These guidelines are available in the National Institutes of Health (NIH) updated booklet, "Your Guide to Lowering Your Blood Pressure with DASH," which also provides background information, weekly menus, and recipes.

Although the DASH diet provides two to three times the amount of some nutrients currently consumed in the average American diet, the recommendations are not dissimilar to the 2010 U.S. **dietary guidelines**, published by the U.S. Department of Agriculture (USDA) and U.S. Department of Health and Human Services. The main difference is the emphasis on more fruit and vegetable servings. In addition, it separates nuts, seeds, and beans from the meat, fish, and poultry food groups and recommends four to five weekly servings of nuts, seeds, and dry beans.

The DASH diet was not designed for weight loss, but it can be adapted for lower calorie intakes. The NIH booklet provides guidelines for a 1,600-calorie diet. Vegetarians can also use the diet, as it is high in fruits, vegetables, beans, seeds, and low-fat dairy, which are the main sources of **protein** in a vegetarian diet.

Function

The DASH meal plan is a healthy diet recommended for those with and without high blood pressure.

Benefits

The DASH diet may lower blood pressure as much as taking medication, but without the risk of unwanted side effects. The dietary changes can also have immediate effects comparable with drug therapy. A blood pressure reduction of the degree seen in the

DASH study is estimated to reduce the incidence of coronary artery disease by 15% and stroke by 27%.

The DASH plan may also lower blood pressure just as well as restrictive low-salt diets of 3–4 g of salt per day. Many people find low-salt foods be bland, and with 7%–80% of salt intake coming from processed foods, including baked foods such as breads, people may have trouble adhering to low-salt diets. The DASH diet is an adaptation to healthy eating, so it has no restrictions but instead follows standard dietary guidelines for the general public.

Precautions

Adding high-fiber foods to the diet should be done gradually to avoid side effects such as gas, bloating, and diarrhea. It is important to increase fluid at the same time, as **fiber** draws water into the bowel. High fiber intake with inadequate fluid can cause hard stools and **constipation**.

Increasing fruits and vegetables increases the potassium content of the diet. For healthy people with normal kidney function, a higher potassium intake from foods does not pose a risk as excess potassium is excreted in the urine. However, individuals whose urinary potassium excretion is impaired, such as those with end-stage renal disease, severe heart failure, or adrenal insufficiency, may be at risk of hyperkalemia (high levels of potassium in the blood). Hyperkalemia may cause cardiac arrhythmias (irregular heartbeat), which could be serious. Some common drugs can also decrease potassium excretion. Individuals at risk should consult a doctor before staring the DASH diet, as higher potassium intakes in the form of fruit and vegetables may not be suitable. Care should also be taken with potassium containing salt substitutes.

Risks

Currently, there are no known risks associated with the DASH diet. However, the long-term effects of the diet on morbidity and mortality are still unknown.

Research and general acceptance

Studies over the years have suggested high intakes of salt play a role in the development of high blood pressure. Dietary advice for the prevention and lowering of high blood pressure has focused primarily on reducing sodium or salt intake. A 1989 study looked at the response an intake of 3–12 g of salt per day had on blood pressure. The study found that modest reductions in salt, 5–6 g salt per day, caused blood pressures to fall in people with hypertension. The best effect was seen with only 3 g of salt per day, with blood pressure decreasing by an average of 11 mmHg systolic and 6 mmHg diastolic. More recently, the use of low-salt diets for the prevention or treatment of high blood pressure has come into question. The Trials of Hypertension Prevention Phase II in 1997 indicated that energy intake and weight loss were more important than the restriction of dietary salt in the prevention of hypertension. A 2006 Cochrane review, which looked at the effect of longer-term modest salt reduction on blood pressure, found that modest reductions in salt intake could have a significant effect on blood pressure in those with high blood pressure, but a lesser effect on those without. It was agreed that the 2007 public health recommendations of reducing salt intake from levels of 9–12 g/day to a moderate 5–6 g/day would have a beneficial effect on blood pressure and cardiovascular disease.

The effectiveness of the DASH diet for lowering blood pressure is well recognized. The 2010 Dietary Guidelines for Americans recommends the DASH Eating Plan as an example of a balanced eating plan consistent with the existing guidelines and it forms the basis for the USDA **MyPlate**. DASH is also recommended in other guidelines such as those advocated by the British Nutrition Foundation, American Heart Association, and American Society for Hypertension.

Although reducing sodium and increasing potassium, calcium, and magnesium intake play a key role in lowering blood pressure, the reasons why the DASH eating plan has a beneficial effect remains uncertain. The researchers suggest it may be because whole foods improve the absorption of the potassium, calcium, and magnesium or it may be related to the cumulative effect of eating these nutrients together rather than the individual nutrients themselves. It is also speculated that it may be something else in the fruits, vegetables, and low-fat dairy products that accounts for the association between the diet and blood pressure.

The Salt Institute supports the DASH diet but without the salt restriction. They claim that the DASH diet alone, without reduced sodium intake from manufactured foods, would achieve the desired blood pressure reduction. Their recommendation is based on the fact that there are no evidence-based studies supporting the need for dietary salt restriction for the entire population. The Cochrane review in 2006 showed that modest reductions in salt intake lowers blood pressure significantly in people with hypertension but has less of an effect on individuals with normal blood pressure. Restriction of salt for those without hypertension is not recommended.

There is a continued call for the food industry to lower their use of salt in processed foods from governments and health associations. The New York City Health Department has spearheaded the National Salt Reduction Initiative in the United States, and a number of other health-related organizations have joined this effort. Their goal is to reduce the consumption of salt by 20% in the United States by 2014. The coalition works closely with food manufacturers and restaurants that voluntarily agree to reduce sodium levels in their products. In addition, the U.S. Department of Health and Human Services, along with several other federal and private sector organizations, are leading the Million Hearts initiative. Their goal is to prevent the occurrence of one million heart attacks and strokes in the United States between 2012 and 2017. Reduction of sodium levels in the diet to aid in lowering blood pressure is a major component of this initiative as well.

Researchers have evaluated other dietary modifications, such as the role of potassium, magnesium, and calcium on blood pressure. Substantial evidence shows that individuals with diets high in fruits and vegetables—and hence potassium, magnesium, and calcium—tend to have lower blood pressures. However, in studies where individuals have been supplemented with these nutrients, the results of their effects on blood pressure have been inconclusive.

There is some debate on whether patients can follow the diet long-term. The 2003 PREMIER Clinical Trial (a multi-center trial), studied the effects of

QUESTIONS TO ASK YOUR DOCTOR

- Could the DASH diet help lower my blood pressure?
- Can I follow the DASH diet even if I already have low blood pressure?
- Will following this diet allow me to stop taking medication for high blood pressure?

diet on blood pressure and found that the DASH diet results were less than the original study. This difference was thought to be because participants in the DASH study were supplied with prepared meals, while participants in the PREMIER study prepared their own foods. As a result, only half the fruit and vegetable intake was achieved in the PREMIER study, which affected the overall intakes of potassium and magnesium. The researchers concluded that compliance with the DASH diet in the long term is questionable, but agreed that patients should still be encouraged to adopt healthy interventions such as the DASH diet, as it does offer health benefits.

In terms of heart health, the DASH diet lowered total cholesterol and LDL cholesterol, but it was also associated with a decrease in high-density lipoprotein (HDL), the "good" cholesterol. Low HDL levels are considered to be a risk factor for **coronary heart disease**, while high levels are thought to reduce the likelihood of heart disease. The decrease was greatest in individuals who started with a higher level of the protective HDL. Researchers agree that the reasons for the decrease in HDL levels need further review, but concluded that the overall effects of the DASH diet are beneficial in terms of preventing heart disease.

While the long-term health effects of the DASH diet are yet to be established, the diet closely resembles the **Mediterranean diet**, which has been shown to have other health benefits including a reduced risk for heart disease and **cancer** rates. It is thought that the DASH diet is likely to offer similar health benefits.

Resources

BOOKS

Hella, Marla. *The DASH Diet Action Plan.* New York: Grand Central Life & Style, 2011.

Moore, Thomas. *The DASH Diet for Hypertension.* New York: Pocket Books, 2003.

PERIODICALS

Appel, Lawrence J., et al. "Dietary Approaches to Prevent and Treat Hypertension: A Scientific Statement From the American Heart Association." *Hypertension* 47 (2006): 296. http://hyper.ahajournals.org/cgi/content/full/47/2/296 (accessed September 13, 2012).

———. "Effects of Comprehensive Lifestyle Modification on Blood Pressure Control: Main Results of the PREMIER Clinical Trial." *The Journal of the American Medical Association (JAMA)* 289, no. 16 (2003): 2083–2093.

He, F. J., and G. A. MacGregor. "Effect of Longer-Term Modest Salt Reduction on Blood Pressure (Review)." *Cochrane Database of Systematic Reviews* no. 1 (2004).

Lasser, V. I., J. M. Raczynski, et al. "The Trials of Hypertension Prevention TOHP Collaborative Research Group." *Annals of Epidemiology* 5, no. 2 (1995): 156-164.

Obarzanek, E., Frank M. Sacks, et al. "Effects on Blood Lipid of a Blood Pressure Lowering Diet: The Dietary Approaches to Stop Hypertension (DASH) Trial." *American Journal of Clinical Nutrition* 74, no. 1 (2001): 80-89.

Sacks, Frank M., Bernard Rosner, and Edward H. Kass. "Blood Pressure in Vegetarians." *American Journal of Epidemiology* 100, no. 5 (1974): 390-398

Sacks, Frank M., Laura P. Svetkey, et al. "Effects on Blood Pressure of Reduced Dietary Sodium and the Dietary Approaches to Stop Hypertension (DASH) Diet." *The New England Journal of Medicine* 344, no. 1 (2001): 3-10.

WEBSITES

Heller, Maria. "The DASH Diet Eating Plan." http://dashdiet.org (accessed September 13, 2012).

National Institutes of Health (NIH). *Your Guide to Lowering Your High Blood Pressure with DASH.* 1998. NIH Publication No. 06-4082. 2006. http://www.nhlbi.nih.gov/health/public/heart/hbp/dash/new_dash.pdf (accessed September 13, 2012).

ORGANIZATIONS

American Heart Association, 7272 Greenville Ave., Dallas, TX 7523, (800) 242-8721, http://www.heart.org.

American Society for Hypertension, 45 Main St., Ste. 712, Brooklyn, NY 11201, (212) 696-9099, http://www.ash-us.org.

British Heart Foundation (BHF), Greater London House, 180 Hampstead Rd., London, UK NW1 7AW, http://www.bhf.org.uk.

British Nutrition Foundation, High Holborn House, 52-54 High Holborn, London, UK WC1V 6RQ, 44 020 7404 6504, http://www.nutrition.org.uk.

The Cochrane Collaboration, Summertown Pavilion, 18-24 Middle Way, Oxford, UKOxfordshire OX2 7LG, 441865 516300, Fax: 44 18 6551 6311, http://www.cochrane.co.uk.

Food Standards Agency UK (FSA), Aviation House, 125 Kingsway, London, UK WC2B 6NH, http://www.food.gov.uk.

National Lung, Blood and Heart Institute (NHLBI), PO Box 30105, Bethesda, MD 20824-0105, (301) 592-8573, http://www.nhlbi.nih.gov.

Salt Institute, 700 N. Fairfax St., Ste. 600, Alexandria, VA 22314-2040, http://www.saltinstitute.org.

Tracy J. Parker, RD
Stacey J. Chamberlin

Dean Ornish's Eat More, Weigh Less

Definition

Dean Ornish's Eat More, Weigh Less diet focuses primarily on eating a **low-fat diet** of plant products and simple **carbohydrates** to achieve weight loss and better health without feelings of deprivation and hunger. It also emphasizes stress reduction techniques and light exercise. Creator Dean Ornish claims that the diet could prevent and even reverse some forms of heart disease.

Origins

Ornish received his Bachelor of Arts degree in humanities from the University of Texas at Austin and received training in internal medicine at Baylor College of Medicine and Harvard Medical School. He received further medical training at Massachusetts General Hospital. While Ornish was a medical student, he became interested in heart disease. In 1978, he began doing research on patients with **coronary heart disease**.

Ornish created a diet that was very low in fat and completely vegetarian and studied its effects on the symptoms experienced by the patients. This was the beginning of Ornish's research on the effects of low fat, low or no-meat diets on weight loss, health, and heart disease. This original diet was the basis for his "Eat More, Weigh Less" diet, as well as his other diets.

Over the years, Ornish published numerous books and articles and expanded his diets. All of his diets revolve around the same basic principles, with additions or changes depending on a person's goals. For example, Ornish's heart disease prevention diet allows small amounts of lean meat or fish, while his heart disease reversal diet is completely vegetarian.

Eat More, Weigh Less: Dr. Dean Ornish's Advantage Ten Program for Losing Weight Safely while Eating Abundantly was published in 2001. Six years later, *The Spectrum: A Scientifically Proven Program to Feel Better, Live Longer, Lose Weight, and Gain Health* was published. The spectrum includes diet, exercise, stress reduction, and other factors.

As of July 2012, Ornish was a professor of clinical medicine at the University of California, San Francisco, and a practicing physician. He founded and served as president of the Preventive Medicine Research Institute (PMRI) located in Sausalito, California.

Description

Eat More, Weigh Less

The main focus of Ornish's diets is eating more vegetable products and fewer meat products. The diet for people trying to lose moderate amounts of weight may permit small amounts of lean chicken or fish as well as some skim milk or egg whites. For people with higher weight-loss goals, the diet may be almost completely vegan and contain no meat or animal products.

The diet is extremely low in fat, with fewer than 10% of **calories** coming from fat. The strictest forms of the diet do not allow any nuts, seeds, or avocados. The only oil allowed is a small amount of fish oil each day due to its cardioprotective benefits.

Foods that are encouraged include nearly all fruit and vegetable products, especially leafy green vegetables, **soy** products, and **whole grains**. Processed and animal products usually contain many more calories and fat than similarly sized portions of vegetables, whole grains, fruits, and soy. This is the key concept of Ornish's diet—a person may be able to actually eat more and still lose weight. Eating foods with low caloric densities (calories per quantity) helps promote satiety (feeling of fullness) and prevent feelings of hunger.

Ornish Spectrum

The Ornish Spectrum diet expands upon the concept of the spectrum from Ornish's original diet. The Spectrum includes nutrition, stress reduction, and physical activity, as well as factors like emotional support. The Ornish Spectrum Program focuses on preventing conditions like high cholesterol and high blood pressure, both of which increase the risk for heart disease. The Ornish Program for Reversing Heart Disease is aimed at slowing, halting, and reversing the progression of heart disease and other chronic diseases. Nutrition choices are more limited for people in this group because of their health conditions.

Individuals can also develop a personal spectrum plan. Objectives include losing weight, lowering blood pressure, decreasing cholesterol, or preventing or reversing the progression of conditions such as diabetes, heart disease, or **cancer**.

SUPPLEMENTS. Ornish recommends that people take a daily multivitamin along with fish oil (if not eating seafood). People should not start taking **dietary supplements** without first consulting with their physician.

FITNESS. People are encouraged to do an aerobic exercise such as walking, bicycling, or swimming for a minimum of 30 minutes each day or for an hour every other day. The goal is to do three to five hours of exercise each week. People may increase the amount of time exercising and the intensity of the physical activity if they are physically able. Ornish also recommends resistance training, also known as strength training, two to three times weekly.

Function

Ornish's Eat More, Weigh Less diet and the Spectrum diet are used for weight loss and disease prevention. People trying to reverse heart disease or other chronic diseases should only undergo the diet with the consent of their physician.

Benefits

Because the Eat More, Weigh Less diet includes almost only plant products, it is high in **antioxidants** and **fiber** and low in saturated fat and cholesterol. Ornish also claims that his diet can help prevent or reverse heart disease.

Precautions

Anyone thinking about beginning a new diet and exercise plan should first consult their primary physician. Patients with heart disease or other chronic conditions should be especially cautious. Although Ornish has published data about how his diet may be able to prevent or reverse heart disease, no major dietary changes should be made without consulting a physician. Ornish's diet is not a replacement for medications prescribed by a doctor. In addition, the diet does not replace any medically recommended procedures. It is important to discuss all possible options with a physician and to make decisions based on professional recommendations.

If a person is not used to eating large amounts of fiber, additional fiber should be added to the diet slowly to avoid intestinal problems. Drinking fluids with fiber will help move the fiber through the intestines.

KEY TERMS

Antioxidant—A molecule that prevents oxidation. In the body, antioxidants attach to other molecules called free radicals and prevent the free radicals from causing damage to cell walls, DNA, and other parts of the cell.

Coronary artery—The arteries that supply blood to the tissues of the heart from the aorta.

Coronary heart disease—A progressive reduction of blood supply to the heart muscle due to narrowing or blocking of a coronary artery.

Vegan—A diet containing no meat or animal products.

Risks

If people on the Ornish diet stop eating meat and animal products, they should make sure that they are still receiving enough dietary **protein** and other nutrients. Discussing the diet plan with a physician or registered dietitian will help ensure that nutritional needs are being met.

Because of the very low fat allowance of some versions of the Ornish diet, there is some concern that people on this diet may not get enough **vitamin E**.

Research and general acceptance

The benefits of any diet that is low in fat and includes many different fruits, vegetables, and whole grains are generally accepted. Ornish has led many controlled research studies to test his diet and has published the results in peer-reviewed journals such as the *Journal of the Society of Behavioral Medicine*, the *Lancet*, and the *Journal of the American Medical Association*.

In 1990, Ornish and several coauthors published an article titled "Can Lifestyle Changes Reverse Coronary Heart Disease? The Lifestyle Heart Trial" in the *Lancet*. This was the first study to investigate whether changes in lifestyle alone, without the use of prescription drugs, could stop the progression of, or even reverse, coronary heart disease. The patients selected to participate had severe coronary heart disease and were divided randomly into two groups: those who would follow Ornish's program, and those who would follow the usual recommendations for such patients, including moderate lifestyle changes and cholesterol-lowering medications, if necessary.

QUESTIONS TO ASK YOUR DOCTOR

- Is this diet the best diet to meet my goals?
- Is it safe for me to go on this diet?
- What other diets do you recommend?
- Will I need to take a multivitamin or other dietary supplement on this diet?
- What signs or symptoms might indicate a problem while on this diet?
- Is it safe for me to start an exercise program?

Ornish's regimen included a diet that was very low in fat and completely vegetarian. It also emphasized moderate exercise, stress-reduction techniques, and quitting smoking (if applicable). The diameter of the coronary artery was measured at the beginning of the study and again at the end of the study one year later. For people following the usual recommendations for coronary patients, the average percentage of narrowing was 42.7% at the beginning of the study and increased to 46.1% at the end of the study. For patients on Ornish's plan, the average percentage of constriction was reduced 2.2% during the period of the study, from 40.0% to 37.8%. For the patients with the most constriction, the difference was even greater.

Since the 1990 study, Ornish and various coauthors have continued to research how lifestyle changes alone can positively affect heart disease in both the long- and short-term. In 2007, he published a study in the *Journal of the Society of Behavioral Medicine* that found reductions in the risk factors of coronary heart disease in just three months.

Resources

BOOKS

Larsen, Laura, ed. *Diet and Nutrition Sourcebook*. Detroit, MI: Omnigraphics, 2011.

Ornish, Dean. *Dr. Dean Ornish's Program for Reversing Heart Disease: The Only System Scientifically Proven to Reverse Heart Disease Without Drugs or Surgery*. New York: Random House, 1990.

———. *Eat More, Weigh Less: Dr. Dean Ornish's Advantage Ten Program for Losing Weight Safely while Eating Abundantly*. New York: Quill, 2001.

———. *Love and Survival: The Scientific Basis for the Healing Power of Intimacy*. Thorndike, ME: Thorndike Press, 1998.

———. *Stress, Diet, and Your Heart*. New York: Holt, Rinehart, and Winston, 1983.

———. *The Spectrum: A Scientifically Proven Program to Feel Better, Live Longer, Lose Weight, and Gain Health*. New York: Ballantine, 2007.

Willis, Alicia P. ed. *Diet Therapy Research Trends*. New York: Nova Science, 2007.

PERIODICALS

Dansinger, Michael L., et al. "Comparison of the Atkins, Ornish, Weight Watchers, and Zone Diets for Weight Loss and Heart Disease Risk Reduction." *Journal of the American Medical Association* 293 (January 5, 2005): 43–53.

Feingold, Linda. "Dr. Dean Ornish Covers The Spectrum: A Scientifically Proven Program to Feel Better, Live Longer, Lose Weight and Gain Health." *American Fitness* 26, no. 4 (July/August 2008): 35.

Gardner, Christopher D., et al. "Comparison of the Atkins, Zone, Ornish, and LEARN diets for Change in Weight and Related Risk Factors Among Overweight Premenopausal Women: The A to Z Weight Loss Study: A Randomized Trial." *Journal of the American Medical Association* 297, no. 9 (March 7, 2007): 969–77.

Hellmich, Nanci. "Bill Clinton Declares Vegan Victory." *USA Today*, August 23, 2011. http://yourlife.usatoday. com/fitness-food/diet-nutrition/story/2011-08-23/Bill-Clinton-declares-vegan-victory/50111212/1 (accessed July 13, 2012).

Koertge, Jenny, et al. "Improvement in Medical Risk Factors and Quality of Life in Women and Men with Coronary Artery Disease in the Multicenter Lifestyle Demonstration Project." *American Journal of Cardiology* (June 1, 2003): 1316–22.

Ornish, Dean. "Low-Fat Diets." *The New England Journal of Medicine* 338 (January 8, 1998): 127–29.

WEBSITES

"Dr. Dean Ornish Program for Reserving Heart Disease." West Virginia University. http://www.hsc.wvu.edu/Wellness/Dr-Dean-Ornish-Program (accessed September 23, 2012).

Harvard School of Public Health. "The Best Diet Is the One You'll Follow." The Nutrition Source, Department of Nutrition, Harvard University. http://www.hsph.harvard.edu/nutritionsource/healthy-weight/best-weight-loss-diet (accessed September 27, 2012).

"Ornish Diet." *U.S. News & World Reports*. http://health.usnews.com/best-diet/ornish-diet (accessed July 13, 2012).

"The Ornish Spectrum." http://www.ornishspectrum.com (accessed September 27, 2012).

Preventive Medicine Research Institute. "Research Highlights." http://www.pmri.org/research.html (accessed September 27, 2012).

Zelman, Kathleen M. "Review: Dean Ornish's *The Spectrum*." WedMD. http://www.webmd.com/diet/features/review-dean-ornish-the-spectrum (accessed July 23, 2012).

———. "Review: Eat More, Weigh Less." WebMD. http://www.webmd.com/content/pages/9/3068_9408.htm (accessed July 23, 2012).

ORGANIZATIONS

American Heart Association, 7272 Greenville Ave., Dallas, TX 75231, (800) 242-8721, http://www.americanheart.org.

Centers for Disease Control and Prevention, Division for Heart Disease and Stroke Prevention, 4770 Buford Hwy NE, Mail Stop F-72, Atlanta, GA 30341-3717, (800) CDC-INFO (232-4636), TTY: (800) 232-6348, Fax: (770) 488-8151, cdcinfo@cdc.gov, http://www.cdc.gov/dhdsp.

National Heart, Lung, and Blood Institute, PO Box 30105, Bethesda, MD 20824-0105, (301) 592-8573, TTY: (240) 629-3255, Fax: (240) 629-3246, nhlbiinfo@nhlbi.nih.gov, http://www.nhlbi.nih.gov.

Helen Davidson
Liz Swain

Dehydration

Definition

Dehydration is a condition in which the body loses too much water, usually as a result of excess sweating, vomiting, and/or diarrhea.

Description

Dehydration occurs because more fluid is lost from the body than is taken in. Water is essential for life. Transporting nutrients throughout the body, removing wastes, regulating body temperature, lubrication of joints and membranes, and chemical reactions that occur during cellular **metabolism** all require water.

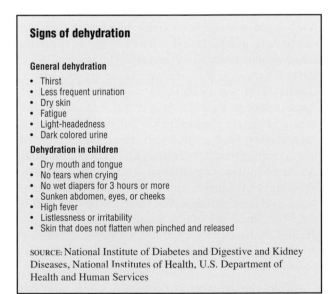

Signs of dehydration

General dehydration
- Thirst
- Less frequent urination
- Dry skin
- Fatigue
- Light-headedness
- Dark colored urine

Dehydration in children
- Dry mouth and tongue
- No tears when crying
- No wet diapers for 3 hours or more
- Sunken abdomen, eyes, or cheeks
- High fever
- Listlessness or irritability
- Skin that does not flatten when pinched and released

SOURCE: National Institute of Diabetes and Digestive and Kidney Diseases, National Institutes of Health, U.S. Department of Health and Human Services

(Table by GGS Information Services. © 2013 Cengage Learning.)

The amount of water a person needs to prevent dehydration varies widely depending on the individual's age, weight, level of physical activity, and the environmental temperature. The individual's health and the medications they take may also affect the amount of water a person needs. Most dehydration results from an acute, or sudden, loss of fluids. However, slow-developing chronic dehydration can occur, most often in the frail elderly and in infants and young children, who must rely on others to supply them with liquids.

Healthy people lose water from urination, elimination of solid wastes, sweating, and breathing out water vapor. This water must be replaced through diet. Water makes up about 75% of the body weight of infants, 65% of the weight of children, and 60% of the weight of an adult. In 2004, the United States Institute of Medicine (IOM) recommended that relatively inactive adult men take in about 3.7 liters (about 15 cups) of fluids daily and that women take in about of 2.7 liters (about 10 cups) to replace lost water. These recommendations are for total fluid intake from both beverages and food. Highly active adults and those living in very warm climates need more fluids.

About 80% of the water the average person needs is replaced by drinking liquids. The other 20% is found in food. Below are some foods and the percentage of water that they contain:

- iceberg lettuce, 96%
- squash, cooked, 90%
- cantaloupe, raw, 90%
- 2% milk, 89%
- apple, raw, 86%
- cottage cheese, 76%
- potato, baked, 75%
- macaroni, cooked, 66%
- turkey, roasted, 62%
- steak, cooked, 50%
- cheese, cheddar, 37%
- bread, white, 36%
- peanuts, dry roasted, 2%

Dehydration involves more than just water deficiency. **Electrolytes** are ions that form when salts dissolve in water or body fluids. In order for cells to function correctly, the various electrolytes, such as **sodium** (Na+) and potassium (K+), must remain within a very narrow range of concentrations. Often electrolytes are lost along with water. For example, sodium is lost in sweat. To prevent the effects of dehydration, both water and electrolytes must be replaced in the correct proportions.

Demographics

The very young and the very old are most likely to become dehydrated. Young children are at greater risk because they are more likely to get diseases that cause vomiting, diarrhea, and fever. Worldwide, dehydration is the leading cause of death in children. In the United States, 400–500 children under the age of 5 die every year of dehydration. The elderly are at risk because they are less likely to drink when they become dehydrated. The thirst mechanism often becomes less sensitive as people age. Also, their kidneys lose the ability to make highly concentrated urine. Older individuals who are confined to wheelchairs or bed and cannot get water for themselves (e.g., nursing home and hospital patients) are at risk of developing chronic dehydration.

Causes and symptoms

Diarrhea, often accompanied by vomiting, is the leading cause of dehydration. Both water and electrolytes are lost in large quantities. Diarrhea is often caused by bacteria, viruses, or parasites. Fever that often accompanies disease accelerates the amount of water that is lost through the skin. The smaller the child, the greater the risk of dehydration. Worldwide, acute diarrhea accounts for the death of about 4 million children each year. In the United States, about 220,000 children are hospitalized for dehydration caused by diarrhea annually.

Heavy sweating also causes dehydration and loss of electrolytes. Athletes, especially endurance athletes, and individuals with active outdoor professions such as roofers and road crew workers are at high risk of becoming dehydrated. Children who play sports can also be vulnerable to dehydration.

Certain chronic illnesses that disrupt fluid balance can cause dehydration. Kidney disease and hormonal disorders, such as diabetes, adrenal gland, or pituitary gland disorders, can cause fluid and electrolyte loss through excessive urination. Disorders such as cystic fibrosis or other genetic disorders resulting in inadequate absorption of nutrients from the intestines can cause chronic diarrhea that leads to dehydration. Individuals with **eating disorders** who abuse laxatives, diuretics, and enemas, or regularly cause themselves to vomit are vulnerable to severe electrolyte imbalances and dehydration. The same is true of people with alcoholism. People who have severe burns over a large part of their body also are likely to become dehydrated because they no longer have skin to act as a barrier to evaporation.

Dehydration can be mild, moderate, or severe. Mild dehydration occurs when fluid losses equal 3%–5%. At this point, the thirst sensation is felt and is often accompanied by dry mouth and thick saliva.

Moderate dehydration occurs when fluid losses equal 6%–9% of body weight. This can occur rapidly in young children who are vomiting and/or have diarrhea. In an infant, a loss of as little as 2–3 cups of liquids can result in moderate dehydration. Signs of moderate dehydration include intense thirst, severely reduced urine production, sunken eyes, headache, dizziness, irritability, and decreased activity.

Severe dehydration occurs when fluid losses are 10% or more of body weight. Severe dehydration is a medical emergency for individuals of any age. A loss of fluids equaling 20% of a person's body weight is fatal. Signs of severe dehydration include all those of moderate dehydration as well as lack of sweating, little or no urine production, dry skin that has little elasticity, low blood pressure, rapid heartbeat, fever, delirium, or coma.

Diagnosis

Dehydration is diagnosed by physical symptoms. A healthcare professional or observant adult can usually tell by looking at someone that they are moderately or severely dehydrated. Blood tests and a urinalysis may be done to check for electrolyte imbalances and to determine if the kidneys are damaged. However, visual signs are enough to begin treatment.

Treatment

The goal of treatment is to restore fluid and electrolyte balance. For individuals with mild dehydration, this can be done in infants and children by giving them oral rehydration solutions such as Pedialyte, Infalyte, Naturalyte, Oralyte, or Rehydralyte. These are available in supermarkets and pharmacies without a prescription. These solutions have the proper balance of salts and sugars to restore the electrolyte balance. Water, apple juice, chicken broth, sodas, and similar fluids are effective in treating mild dehydration. Oral rehydration fluids can be given to young children in small sips as soon as vomiting and diarrhea start. They may continue to vomit and have diarrhea, but some of the fluid will be absorbed. Breastfed infants should continue to nurse on demand. Babies who are formula fed should continue to get their regular formula unless directed otherwise by a pediatrician.

Older children who are dehydrated can be given oral rehydration solutions or sports drinks such as Gatorade for moderate and severe dehydration, otherwise general

KEY TERMS

Diabetes—A condition in which the body either does not make or cannot respond to the hormone insulin. As a result, the body cannot use glucose (sugar). There are two types, type 1 and type 2.

Diuretic—A substance that removes water from the body by increasing urine production.

Electrolyte—Ions in the body that participate in metabolic reactions. The major human electrolytes are sodium $(Na+)$, potassium $(K+)$, calcium $(Ca 2+)$, magnesium $(Mg2+)$, chloride $(Cl-)$, phosphate $(HPO4 2-)$, bicarbonate $(HCO3-)$, and sulfate $(SO4 2-)$.

Laxative—A substance that stimulates movement of food through the bowels. Laxatives are used to treat constipation.

fluids are fine. Athletes who are dehydrated should be given sports drinks. According to the American College of Sports Medicine, sports drinks are effective in supplying energy for muscles, maintaining blood sugar levels, preventing dehydration, and replacing electrolytes lost in sweat. Adults who are mildly or moderately dehydrated usually improve by drinking water and avoiding coffee, tea, and soft drinks that do not contain **caffeine**.

Individuals of all ages who are seriously dehydrated need to be treated by a medical professional. In the case of severe dehydration, the individual may be hospitalized and fluids given intravenously (IV; directly into the vein).

Nutrition and dietary concerns

Dehydration is usually an acute condition, and once fluid balance is restored, there are no additional nutritional concerns. In the mobility-impaired elderly, the main concern is making sure that they have adequate access to fluids.

Prognosis

Most people recover from dehydration with few complications so long as rehydration fluids are available and treatment begins before the condition becomes severe. However, severe dehydration can be fatal.

Prevention

The best way to prevent dehydration is to be alert to situations in which it could occur, such as exercising in hot weather or vomiting and diarrhea in infants and young children. Athletes and people who work in hot conditions should drink regularly, whether or not they feel thirsty. Rehydration of young children should begin at the first sign of fluid loss. A healthcare provider should be consulted before the situation becomes serious. Mobility-impaired elderly and infants and young children who cannot get water for themselves should be offered fluids on a regular basis.

Resources

BOOKS

Batmanghelidj, F. *Water: For Health, for Healing, for Life: You're Not Sick, You're Thirsty!* New York: Warner Books, 2003.

Panel on Dietary Reference Intakes for Electrolytes and Water, Standing Committee on the Scientific Evaluation of Dietary Reference Intakes, Food and Nutrition Board. *DRI, Dietary Reference Intakes for Water, Potassium, Sodium, Chloride, and Sulfate.* Washington, DC: National Academies Press, 2005.

PERIODICALS

Adan, A. "Cognitive Performance and Dehydration." *Journal of the American College of Nutrition* 31, no. 2 (2012): 71–78.

Kenney, Larry. "Dietary Water and Sodium Requirements for Active Adults." *Sports Science Exchange 92* 17, no. 1 (2004).

Wellbery, Caroline. "Diagnosing Dehydration in Children." *American Family Physician* 71, no. 5 (March 1, 2005): 1010.

WEBSITES

Mayo Clinic staff. "Dehydration." MayoClinic.com. http://www.mayoclinic.com/health/dehydration/DS00561 (accessed September 24, 2012).

Nemours Foundation. "Dehydration." TeensHealth.org. http://kidshealth.org/teen/safety/first_aid/dehydration.html (accessed September 24, 2012).

PubMed Health. "Dehydration." U.S. National Library of Medicine. http://www.ncbi.nlm.nih.gov/pubmedhealth/PMH0001977 (accessed September 24, 2012).

ORGANIZATIONS

American Academy of Pediatrics (AAP), 141 Northwest Point Blvd., Elk Grove Village, IL 60007, (847) 434-4000, (800) 433-9016, Fax: (847) 434-8000, http://www.aap.org.

American College of Sports Medicine, 401 West Michigan St., Indianapolis, IN 46202-3233, (317) 637-9200, Fax: (317) 634-7817, http://www.acsm.org.

Tish Davidson, AM

Dental health *see* **Oral health and nutrition**

Detoxification diets

Definition

Detoxification diets, or detox diets for short, are a group of short-term diets intended to release accumulated toxins and waste products from the body. They are based on a theory of digestion and elimination usually associated with naturopathy, an alternative medical system that emphasizes the role of nutrition in restoring or improving the body's own self-healing properties. In general, detox diets emphasize the following:

- Minimal intake of chemicals on or in food by choosing organic or non-processed foods
- Increased intake of fruits, vegetables, and other foods thought to aid the process of detoxification
- Increased intake of foods and fluids that speed up the processes of urination and defecation

Detoxification diets can be categorized into several subgroups: raw food diets, which are based on the premise that uncooked foods prevent the accumulation of toxins in the digestive system; mono diets, in which the dieter consumes only one or two foods (sometimes in liquid form only) for a period of 10–14 days; juice fasting, in which the dieter consumes large quantities of fruit and vegetable juices along with water and herbal teas for one to three days; and vegetarian or semi-vegetarian detox diets, which allow the dieter some variety of cooked **whole grains**, steamed vegetables, fresh fruit, and small amounts of **protein** foods as well as several glasses of water and herbal teas each day.

Origins

Detoxification diets as a general practice can be traced back over 5,500 years to an annual ritual of bodily and spiritual preparation known as *pancha karma*, which is part of the practice of Ayurvedic medicine in India. Ayurveda is a traditional system of health care that dates back to about 3500 BC; its name is Sanskrit for "science of long life." Pancha karma is undergone for disease prevention, which in Ayurvedic practice requires spiritual renewal and the breaking of negative emotional patterns as well as physical purification. It has three phases: a preparation phase, in which the person eliminates sweets, caffeinated drinks, and processed foods from the diet, as well as spending more time in meditation and taking walks in natural surroundings; the cleansing phase, which includes bloodletting, emesis (forced vomiting), nasal cleansing, and the use of enemas and laxatives as well as a very restricted diet of grains and vegetables; and a rejuvenation phase, in which solid foods are gradually reintroduced to the diet. Practitioners of Ayurveda in Canada and the United States generally omit vomiting and bloodletting in the second phase of pancha karma.

In Europe and North America the most important factor in the popularity of detoxification diets is naturopathy, an alternative approach to health care developed out of the natural healing movement in Germany and North America in the late nineteenth century. Naturopathy is closely connected with **vegetarianism**, particularly its raw-food offshoot. Naturopaths of the twenty-first century use a variety of techniques in treating patients, including hydrotherapy, spinal manipulation, and physical therapy as well as nutrition and dietary advice. There has been a revival of interest in naturopathy in the United States since the 1980s.

Naturopaths frequently recommend detoxification diets as a way of ridding the body of various toxins that they identify as coming from several sources:

- Heavy metals. These include such substances as cadmium, arsenic, nickel, aluminum, chromium, mercury, vanadium, strontium, antimony, cobalt, and lead, which are used in various manufacturing processes and some medical procedures as well as being present in batteries, electronic equipment, coins, cookware, food containers, and other common household items.
- Toxic chemicals taken directly into the digestive tract through alcoholic beverages, pesticide residues on supermarket produce, additives in processed foods, or drugs of abuse; or taken into the respiratory tract through breathing household solvents (nail polish remover, spot or stain removers containing benzene, etc.).
- Toxins in the digestive tract produced by yeast and other microorganisms. Ridding the body of this group of toxins is frequently cited as a reason for combining laxatives or enemas with detoxification diets. Mainstream physicians dispute the notion that normal digestion produces toxic substances in the colon that must be removed by a laxative or enema.
- Ammonia, urea, and other breakdown products of protein metabolism. Naturopaths often recommend a vegetarian lifestyle as well as periodic intensive detoxification practices in order to minimize the production of these byproducts of meat and dairy consumption.

A third factor that has contributed to interest in detox diets in the 1990s and early 2000s is the environmental movement. Some people who are concerned about the impact on the environment of raising animals for food use detox diets as a transition into a long-term vegetarian or vegan lifestyle. In addition, growing awareness of the effects of exposure to industrial chemicals, pesticides, secondhand tobacco smoke, and other contaminants in the home environment as well as the workplace has led many people to consider detoxification diets as a preventive health practice to lower their risk of arthritis and other degenerative diseases.

Description

Practitioners of alternative medicine generally recommend the warmer months as the best time of year for a detox diet, although some dieters prefer January in order to counteract the effects of overindulgence in food and drink during the holidays. Many people suggest beginning a detox diet on the weekend or scheduling time off from work in order to allow time for extra rest if needed. Detox diets are usually used only once or twice a year.

Many detoxification diet books include a questionnaire or symptom checklist to help readers evaluate whether they need detoxification. The following list is typical; more than four "yes" answers indicates the individual could benefit from a detox diet:

- Do you have only one bowel movement per day, or only one every other day?
- Do you take prescription, recreational, or over-the-counter drugs?
- Do you eat meat more than twice a week?
- Do you eat fast foods or processed foods?
- Do you smoke, or are you exposed to secondhand smoke?
- Do you have any skin problems or digestive gas and bloating?
- Do you drink alcohol?
- Do you live in a major city?
- Do you drink tap water, coffee, or soda?
- Do you feel tired, sleep poorly, or have low energy?

Individuals considering a detox diet should prepare by cutting down gradually on caffeinated beverages a week to 10 days before the diet, as sudden elimination of these drinks often causes headaches. Dieters should also reduce their intake of sugary foods, chocolate, alcohol, dairy products, foods high in fat, foods containing wheat or yeast, and grains containing gluten (an elastic protein found in barley and rye). Recommended foods for detox diets (except the mono diets) include fresh organic fruits and vegetables; rice (both brown and basmati rice), rice cakes, and rice pasta; other grains such as millet, quinoa, and buckwheat; beans, lentils, and dried green or yellow peas; unsalted nuts; seeds;

olive oil; and herbal teas. The dieter should plan to drink at least eight glasses of filtered or other non-tap water per day on a detox diet.

At the end of a detox diet, the dieter should return gradually to a full diet, perhaps vegetable soup or steamed vegetables the first day. They should not add fruits or vegetables until the second or third day.

Raw food diets

Raw food detox diets consist of foods that have not been heated above 92° to 118°F (33° to 48°C). These diets are based on the belief that raw foods have higher nutrient value and contain enzymes that assist digestion, allowing the other enzymes in the body to regulate other biological processes. Raw foodists also believe raw foods prevent **obesity** by lowering excessive food consumption, and their high **fiber** content helps detoxify the body by speeding up digestion and elimination.

Juice fasting

In a juice fast, the dieter is instructed to drink between 32 and 64 oz. of fruit or vegetable juice per day, in addition to six glasses of warm filtered water. Although some modified **juice fasts** allow a small quantity of steamed vegetables, most are short-term **liquid diets**. Some therapists recommend one or more cups of herbal tea each day in addition to the juice and water. The juice must be fresh, obtained from organic fruits and vegetables processed through a juicer or juice extractor. Prepackaged juices cannot be used for a juice fast because they have been pasteurized. In addition, fresh juice must be consumed within a half hour of extraction; it cannot be refrigerated.

Mono diets

Mono diets are detox diets in which the dieter consumes only one food, usually apples, grapes, or some other fruit or vegetable, or one liquid, for a period of 10 to 14 days. The oldest mono diet is the so-called Miracle Grape Cure, attributed to Johanna Brandt, a woman from South Africa who claimed that eating grapes cured her of stomach **cancer**. In a book she published in 1928, Brandt stated that she alternated 12 hours of drinking only natural (unchlorinated) water with 12 hours of eating only purple grapes or drinking grape juice made from purple grapes. Recent modifications of this diet recommend following Brandt's plan to the letter for five weeks, followed by one week of a raw-food vegetarian diet.

The best-known mono diet is variously known as the Master Cleanser, lemonade diet, or maple syrup diet. Stanley Burroughs is generally credited with inventing this diet in 1941, although he did not publish it in book form until 1976. His book, which is only about fifty pages long, is still in print even though Burroughs died in 1991. The Master Cleanser involves drinking a mixture of lemon juice, cayenne pepper, and grade B maple syrup for a period of 10 to 14 days. The lemon/maple syrup drink is then followed by drinking a "saltwater flush," which is supposed to purge toxins from the stomach and bowels. This diet was popularized in the early 2000s by a book by Peter Glickman titled *Lose Weight, Have More Energy and Be Happier in 10 Days*, which is a modernization of Burrough's regimen.

Vegetarian or semivegetarian diets

Less stringent detox diets that allow some protein foods have been published; a typical example is the following diet plan for a week-long detox regimen by Elson Haas. Haas begins with general guidelines for the dieter:

- Eat slowly and chew the food well.
- Relax for a few minutes before and after each meal.
- Eat in a comfortable sitting position.
- Drink only herbal teas (peppermint, chamomile, or pau d'arco) after dinner.

The daily diet plan:

- Morning: two glasses of filtered or spring water, one glass with half a lemon squeezed into it.
- Breakfast: One piece of fresh fruit at room temperature, followed 15 to 30 minutes later by a bowl of cooked whole grains (millet, buckwheat, quinoa, brown rice, or amaranth), flavored with 2 Tbsp. of fruit juice.
- Lunch: One or two medium bowls of steamed vegetables, using a variety of root vegetables, leafy vegetables, asparagus, cabbage, kale, or others. A maximum of 3 tsp. daily of a mixture of butter and canola or olive oil can be used for seasoning.
- Dinner: Same as lunch.
- Midmorning and midafternoon: One or two cups of vegetable water saved from the steamed vegetables, with a little sea salt or kelp added.
- A small portion (3 or 4 oz) of a protein food (fish, organic chicken, lentils, black beans, or garbanzo beans) may be eaten midafternoon if the dieter feels weak or extremely hungry.

Supplemental recommendations

An important part of many detoxification diets is the use of laxatives or enemas to cleanse the lower digestive tract. The removal of wastes is considered essential to prevent toxins in the intestines from being reabsorbed into the bloodstream. Some alternative therapists recommend mixtures of slippery elm or other herbs to cleanse the colon; others prefer salt-water laxatives, enemas, or colonics for cleansing the bowel. A colonic is a procedure in which a large amount of water, sometimes as much as 20 gal (76 L), is infused into the colon through the rectum a few pints at a time. It differs from an enema in that much more fluid is used; and a colonic is infused into the colon, whereas an enema infuses water or a cleansing solution into the rectum only. Mainstream physicians do not recommend colonics on the grounds that they are unnecessary, based on a nineteenth-century misunderstanding of the process of digestion, and very often uncomfortable for the patient. In some cases they pose serious risks to health.

Some therapists recommend the use of such **dietary supplements** as multivitamins, **vitamin C**, **choline** and methionine, milk thistle, or a laxative tea known as Smooth Move during a detox diet. These supplements are supposed to aid liver function and decrease such side effects of detox diets as headaches and nausea.

Many advocates of detox diets suggest the use of meditation, affirmations, yoga, and other spiritual practices in order to improve the mental and emotional well-being. Others recommend undertaking the detox diet at a health spa, where such services as massage therapy, sauna baths, and whirlpool therapy or other forms of hydrotherapy are available.

Function

The primary function of detoxification diets is physical purification—removal of toxic substances from the body including the skin and respiratory system as well as the digestive tract—in order to raise energy levels; relieve such minor health complaints as poor skin, bad breath, or headaches; and improve the body's ability to heal from various diseases. These diets are not primarily intended as weight reduction regimens.

Spiritual or religious practice

Some people undertake detoxification diets as part of a general religious or spiritual retreat. The first stage of Ayurvedic pancha karma includes extra time given to meditation and nature walks as well as gradual exclusion of stimulants and solid foods from the diet. Many people also report relief from insomnia or other symptoms of emotional stress as a side benefit of detoxification diets.

Treatment of specific illnesses

Detoxification diets are sometimes recommended for the treatment of specific diseases and disorders,

Amaranth—An herb cultivated as a food crop in Mexico and South America. Its grains can be toasted and mixed with honey or molasses as a vegetarian treat.

Ayurveda—The traditional system of natural medicine that originated in India around 3500 BC. Its name is Sanskrit for "science of long life." Some historians of medicine think that detoxification diets can be traced back to Ayurvedic practice.

Choline—A compound found in egg yolks and legumes that is essential to liver function.

Colonic—Sometimes called colonic hydrotherapy, a colonic is a procedure similar to an enema in which the patient's colon is irrigated (washed out) with large amounts of water. This procedure is discouraged by mainstream physicians because of its potential risks to health.

Fruitarian—A vegetarian who eats only plant-based products (fruits, seeds, and nuts) that can be obtained without killing the plant.

Methionine—A crystalline amino acid found in many protein foods. It is sometimes taken as a supplement during a detox diet.

Mono diet—A type of detoxification diet based on the use of only one food or beverage, such as apples, grapes, lemonade, or other raw fruits or vegetables.

Naturopathy—A system of disease treatment that emphasizes natural means of health care, such as water, natural foods, dietary adjustments, massage and manipulation, and electrotherapy, rather than conventional drugs and surgery. Naturopaths (practitioners of naturopathy) often recommend detox diets as a way of cleansing the body.

Pancha karma—An intensive one- to two-week ritual of detoxification practiced in Ayurvedic medicine that includes enemas, bloodletting, and nasal irrigation as well as fasting.

Pasteurization—A process for partial sterilization of milk or other beverages by raising the liquid to a temperature that destroys disease organisms without changing the basic taste or appearance. Raw foodists avoid pasteurized food products.

Pau d'arco—A medicinal bark derived from a tree native to the Amazon rainforest. Pau d'arco is often brewed as a tea and taken as a diuretic or anti-inflammatory preparation.

Quinoa—An herb native to the Andes that produces starchy seeds that can be ground into flour and used as food.

Raw foodism—A term that refers to a group of dietary regimens composed entirely of foods that have not been raised above a certain temperature. Many raw foodists are vegans, although some eat raw meat or fish and use unpasteurized dairy products.

Vegan—A vegetarian who excludes all animal products from the diet, including those that can be obtained without killing the animal. Vegans are also known as strict vegetarians.

---

most commonly arthritis, autoimmune disorders, and depression, but they have also been claimed to be an effective treatment for severe infections (including AIDS) and cancer. However, there is insufficient evidence to support such claims.

Benefits

Claimed benefits of detox diets include higher energy levels, increased mental clarity and ability to concentrate, clearer skin, improved digestion, and more restful sleep. Many of these improvements may simply be due to better **hydration** as such diets encourage high fluid intake. Some people also lose weight on detox diets, but emphasize that weight reduction should never be the primary purpose of following one of these regimens.

Precautions

In general, anyone considering a detoxification diet should consult a health professional beforehand. Some serious diseases, including cancer, may have minor symptoms at onset, including headaches, low back pain, and fatigue. These symptoms can easily be misattributed to stress or poor eating habits. Some therapists recommend requesting blood, urine, stool, and liver function tests from a physician before undergoing a detoxification diet.

Individuals who should not undertake a detoxification diet are:

• Pregnant or lactating women.

• Children.

• People with diabetes, hypothyroidism, heart disease, anorexia or bulimia nervosa, kidney or liver disease, stomach ulcers, impaired immune function, epilepsy, cancer, terminal illness, active infections, or ulcerative colitis.

- People who are underweight.
- People with alcohol or drug addictions.
- People who have recently undergone surgery or treatment for severe burns.

Prescription medications should be taken as usual during a detoxification diet. The dieter should not discontinue medications or reduce dosages without consulting a physician.

Anyone on a detoxification diet who feels faint or dizzy, develops an abnormal heart rhythm, feels nauseated or vomits, or has signs of low blood pressure should discontinue the fast and consult their doctor at once.

Detox diets may encourage yo-yo dieting, which is detrimental to health. They should not be undertaken more than three times a year without medical supervision.

Risks

The major risks to health from detoxification diets include metabolic crises in patients with undiagnosed diabetes; flare-ups or worsening of stomach **ulcers**; dizziness or fainting due to sudden lowering of blood pressure; diarrhea that may result in **dehydration** and an imbalance of **electrolytes** in the body; and protein or **calcium** deficiencies from unsupervised long-term juice fasts. Some people develop dental erosion from raw-food detoxification diets.

Other side effects reported include headaches (often caused by sudden withdrawal from **caffeine**), fatigue, **constipation** (from extra fiber combined with inadequate water intake), acne, irritability, dysmenorrhea (painful periods) in women, and intense hunger.

Raw-food detoxification diets increase the risk of contracting parasites or other foodborne illnesses caused by organisms normally destroyed in cooking or pasteurization. In addition, some raw vegetables, such as rhubarb leaves and stalks, buckwheat greens, kidney beans, kidney bean sprouts, and raw potatoes that have turned green are toxic, particularly if consumed in large quantities.

People on detoxification diets who undergo colonics are at risk of contracting an infection from improperly sterilized colonic equipment; of serious illness or death from electrolyte imbalances in the blood; or of serious illness or death resulting from perforation of the intestinal wall by improperly inserted equipment. Colonics can also worsen the symptoms of ulcerative colitis.

QUESTIONS TO ASK YOUR DOCTOR

- What type of detoxification diet would you recommend for me?
- What is your opinion of alternative practitioners' explanations of the need for detoxification?
- Have any of your other patients ever tried a mono diet? If so, did they develop any health problems?

Research and general acceptance

Detoxification diets are generally dismissed as fads by such professional organizations as the Academy of Nutrition and Dietetics and other mainstream medical groups. Most physicians point out that the human body is a remarkably efficient organism that can rid itself of toxins through normal digestion, respiration, and excretion without elaborate diets or the assistance of enemas and laxatives. In addition, some fruits and vegetables may contain more toxins than meat, fish, and other protein-rich foods usually condemned by proponents of detoxification diets. Lastly, many physicians object to the naturopathic view of the digestive tract as a source of illness or toxicity.

Resources

BOOKS

Brandt, Johanna. *The Grape Cure*. New York: The Order of Harmony, 1928.

Burroughs, Stanley. *The Master Cleanser with Special Needs and Problems*. N.p.: Burroughs Books, 1976.

Calbom, Cherie, and John Calbom. *Juicing, Fasting, and Detoxing for Life: Unleash the Healing Power of Fresh Juices and Cleansing Diets*. New York: Hachette Book Group, 2008.

Gittleman, Ann Louise. *The Fat Flush Cookbook*. New York: McGraw-Hill, 2003.

Jensen, Bernard. *Dr. Jensen's Guide to Diet and Detoxification*. Los Angeles: Keats Publishing, 2000.

Karas, Jim, and Carolyn Griesse. *The Raw Foods Diet: The Vital Gift of Enzymes*. Piscataway, NJ: New Century, 1981.

Kenton, Leslie. *Leslie Kenton's 10 Day Clean-up Plan: Detoxify Your Body for Natural Health and Vitality*. London: Century, 1986.

Meyerowitz, Steve. *Juice Fasting and Detoxification: Use the Healing Power of Fresh Juice to Feel Young and Look Great*, 6th ed. Great Barrington, MA: Sproutman Publications, 1999.

Pelletier, Kenneth R. *The Best Alternative Medicine*. New York: Fireside Books, 2002. See esp. Chapter 7, "Naturopathic Medicine," and Chapter 10, "Ayurvedic Medicine and Yoga."

Vasey, Christopher. *The Detox Mono Diet: The Miracle Grape Cure and Other Cleansing Diets*. Translated from the French by Jon E. Graham. Rochester, VT: Healing Arts Press, 2006.

Wigmore, Ann. *The Sprouting Book*. Wayne, NJ: Avery Publishing Group, 1986.

PERIODICALS

Griffin, J. "Health and Fitness Series—Popular Dietary Fads: How Should Health Professionals Respond?" *Journal of Family Health Care* 13, no. 3 (2003): 65–67.

"I've Heard Celebrities and Others Talk about Detox Diets. What Are They, and Do They Have Any Health Benefits?" *Mayo Clinic Women's Healthsource* 13, no. 7 (2009): 8.

WEBSITES

"Scientists Dismiss Detox Schemes." *BBC News*, January 3, 2006. http://news.bbc.co.uk/2/hi/health/4576574.stm (accessed September 28, 2012).

Zeratsky, Katherine. "Do Detox Diets Offer Any Health Benefits?" MayoClinic.com. http://www.mayoclinic.com/health/detox-diets/AN01334 (accessed September 28, 2012).

ORGANIZATIONS

American Association of Naturopathic Physicians (AANP), 818 18th St. NW, Ste. 250, Washington, DC 20006, (866) 538-2267, member.services@naturopathic.org, http://www.naturopathic.org.

American Holistic Medical Association, 27629 Chagrin Blvd., Ste. 213, Woodmere, OH 44122, (216) 292-6644, info@holisticmedicine.org, http://www.holisticmedicine.org.

American Vegan Society (AVS), 56 Dinshah Lane, PO Box 369, Malaga, NJ 08328, (856) 694-2887, http://www.americanvegan.org/index.htm.

National Center for Complementary and Alternative Medicine Clearinghouse, PO Box 7923, Gaithersburg, MD 20898, (888) 644-6226, Fax: (866) 464-3616, info@nccam.nih.gov, http://nccam.nih.gov.

National Institute of Ayurvedic Medicine (NIAM), 584 Milltown Rd., Brewster, NY 10509, (845) 278-8700, http://niam.com.

Rebecca J. Frey, PhD

DHEA

Definition

Dehydroepiandrosterone (DHEA) is a precursor (prohormone) of the sex hormones estrogen and testosterone. It is a steroid produced naturally by the adrenal glands and is also sold as a dietary supplement.

Purpose

Many claims have been made for DHEA including that it fights aging, burns fat, increases muscle mass, boosts the immune system, eliminates symptoms of menopause, prevents Alzheimer's disease, and can treat everything from inflammatory bowel syndrome to cocaine withdrawal. There is little or highly questionable evidence to support most of these claims. DHEA does have medical uses in treating adrenal insufficiency (Addison's disease) and systemic lupus erythematosus (SLE).

Description

DHEA is a supplement with a long history of controversy. In the 1980s it was promoted by supplement makers as a "miracle" product that would improve athletic performance, build muscle, burn fat, restore sexual potency, and prevent aging. Many of these claims are still made by supplement makers today. In 1985, the Food and Drug Administration (FDA) banned DHEA for sale in the United States because of its potential for abuse and the high risk of serious side effects. DHEA was also banned by several sports organizations including the International Olympic Committee and the National Football League. However, in 1994, the U.S. Congress passed the Dietary Supplement Health and Education Act (DSHEA). Under this law, DHEA met the definition of a dietary supplement and could once again be sold without a prescription in the United States.

DSHEA regulates supplements such as DHEA in the same way that food is regulated. Like food manufacturers, manufacturers of **dietary supplements** do not have to prove that their product is either safe or effective before it can be sold to the public. Manufacturers of conventional pharmaceutical drugs, however, must prove both safety and effectiveness in humans before a new drug is approved for use. With dietary supplements, the burden of proof falls on the FDA to show that the supplement is either unsafe or ineffective before it can be restricted or banned.

DHEA tablets. *(James Keyser/Time Life Pictures/Getty Images)*

WEBSITES

Boyles, Salynn. "Anti-Aging Hormone a Bust, Study Shows." WebMD.com, October 18, 2006. http://www.webmd.com/news/20061018/antiaging-hormone-bust-study-shows (accessed September 28, 2012).

MedlinePlus. "DHEA." U.S. National Library of Medicine, National Institutes of Health. http://www.nlm.nih.gov/medlineplus/druginfo/natural/331.html (accessed September 28, 2012).

National Center for Complementary and Alternative Medicine. "DHEA Information." http://nccam.nih.gov/taxonomy/term/123 (accessed September 28, 2012).

Natural Standard. "DHEA." MayoClinic.com. http://www.mayoclinic.com/health/dhea/NS_patient-dhea (accessed September 28, 2012).

University of Maryland Medical Center. "Dehydroepiandrosterone (DHEA)." http://www.umm.edu/altmed/articles/dehydroepiandrosterone-000299.htm (accessed September 28, 2012).

ORGANIZATIONS

National Center for Complementary and Alternative Medicine Clearinghouse, PO Box 7923, Gaithersburg, MD 20898, (888) 644-6226, Fax: (866) 464-3616, info@nccam.nih.gov, http://nccam.nih.gov.

National Institute on Aging, 31 Center Dr., Bldg. 31, Rm. 5C27, Bethesda, MD 20892, (800) 222-2225, TTY: (800) 222-4225, niaic@nia.nih.gov, http://www.nia.nih.gov.

Tish Davidson, AM

Diabetes mellitus

Definition

Diabetes mellitus is a condition in which the pancreas no longer produces enough **insulin** or cells stop responding to the insulin that is produced, so that glucose in the blood cannot be absorbed into the cells of the body. Symptoms include frequent urination, lethargy, excessive thirst, and hunger. Treatment can include changes in diet, oral medications, and daily injections of insulin, especially with type 1 diabetes.

Description

Diabetes mellitus is a chronic disease that causes serious health complications including renal (kidney) failure, heart disease, stroke, and blindness. Approximately 17 million Americans have diabetes. Unfortunately, as many as one-half are unaware they have it, and rates are expected to continue to increase due to the high prevalence of obesity in the United States.

Background

Every cell in the human body needs energy in order to function. The body's primary energy source is glucose, a simple **sugar** resulting from the digestion of foods containing **carbohydrates** (sugars and starches). Glucose from the digested food circulates in the blood as a ready energy source for any cells that need it. Insulin is a hormone or chemical produced by cells in the pancreas, an organ located behind the stomach. Insulin binds to a receptor site on the outside of a cell and acts like a key to open a doorway into the cell through which glucose can enter. Some of the glucose can be converted to concentrated energy sources like glycogen or fatty acids and saved for later use. When there is not enough insulin produced or when the doorway no longer recognizes the insulin key, glucose stays in the blood rather entering the cells.

The body will attempt to dilute the high level of glucose in the blood, a condition called hyperglycemia, by drawing water out of the cells and into the bloodstream in an effort to dilute the sugar and excrete it in the urine. It is not unusual for people with undiagnosed diabetes to be constantly thirsty, drink large quantities of water, and urinate frequently as their bodies try to get rid of the extra glucose. This creates high levels of glucose in the urine.

At the same time that the body is trying to get rid of glucose from the blood, the cells are starving for glucose and sending signals to the body to eat more food, thus making patients extremely hungry. To provide energy for the starving cells, the body also tries to convert **fats** and proteins to glucose. The breakdown of fats and proteins for energy causes acid compounds called ketones to form in the blood. Ketones also will be excreted in the urine. As ketones build up in the blood, a condition called ketoacidosis can occur. This condition can be life threatening if left untreated, leading to coma and death.

Types of diabetes mellitus

Type 1 diabetes, sometimes called juvenile diabetes, begins most commonly in childhood or adolescence. In this form of diabetes, the body produces little or no insulin. It is characterized by a sudden onset and occurs more frequently in populations descended from Northern European countries (Finland, Scotland, Scandinavia) than in those from Southern European countries, the Middle East, or Asia. In the United States, approximately three people in 1,000 develop type 1 diabetes. This form is also called insulin-dependent diabetes because people who develop this type need to have daily injections of insulin.

Brittle diabetes is a subgroup of type 1 where patients have frequent and rapid swings of blood sugar levels between hyperglycemia (a condition where there is too much glucose or sugar in the blood) and hypoglycemia (a condition where there are abnormally low levels of glucose or sugar in the blood). These patients may require several injections of different types of insulin during the day to keep the blood sugar level within a fairly normal range.

The more common form of diabetes, type 2, occurs in approximately 3%–5% of Americans under 50 years of age, and increases to 10%–15% in those over 50. More than 90% of people with diabetes in the United States have type 2. Sometimes called age-onset or adult-onset diabetes, this form of diabetes occurs most often in people who are overweight and who do not exercise. It is also more common in people of Native American, Hispanic, and African-American descent. People who have migrated to Western cultures from East India, Japan, and Australian Aboriginal cultures also are more likely to develop type 2 diabetes than those who remain in their original countries.

Type 2 is considered a milder form of diabetes because of its slow onset (sometimes developing over the course of several years) and because it usually can be controlled with diet and oral medication. The consequences of uncontrolled and untreated type 2 diabetes, however, are just as serious as those for type 1. This form is also called noninsulin-dependent diabetes, a term that is somewhat misleading. Many people with type 2 diabetes can control the condition with diet and oral medications, however, insulin injections are sometimes necessary if treatment with diet and oral medication is not working.

Another form of diabetes called **gestational diabetes** can develop during pregnancy and generally resolves after the baby is delivered. This diabetic condition develops during the second or third trimester of pregnancy in about 2% of pregnancies. In 2004, incidence of gestational diabetes was reported to have increased 35% in 10 years. Children of women with gestational diabetes are more likely to be born prematurely, have hypoglycemia, or have severe jaundice at birth. The condition usually is treated by diet, however, insulin injections may be required. These women who have diabetes during pregnancy are at higher risk for developing type 2 diabetes within 5–10 years.

Diabetes also can develop as a result of pancreatic disease, alcoholism, **malnutrition**, or other severe illnesses that stress the body.

Causes and symptoms

Causes

While the causes of diabetes mellitus are unclear, there seem to be both hereditary (genetic factors passed on in families) and environmental factors involved. Research has shown that some people who develop diabetes have common genetic markers. In type 1 diabetes, the immune system, the body's defense system against infection, is believed to be triggered by a virus or another microorganism that destroys cells in the pancreas that produce insulin. In type 2 diabetes, age, **obesity**, and family history of diabetes play a role.

In type 2 diabetes, the pancreas may produce enough insulin, however, cells have become resistant to the insulin produced and it may not work as effectively. Symptoms of type 2 diabetes can begin so gradually that a person may not know that he or she has it. Early signs are lethargy, extreme thirst, and frequent urination. Other symptoms may include sudden weight loss, slow wound healing, urinary tract infections, gum disease, or blurred vision. It is not unusual for type 2 diabetes to be detected while a patient is seeing a doctor about another health concern that is actually being caused by the yet undiagnosed diabetes.

Individuals who are at high risk of developing type 2 diabetes mellitus include people who:

- are obese (more than 20% above their ideal body weight)
- have a relative with diabetes mellitus
- belong to a high-risk ethnic population (African-American, Native American, Hispanic, or Native Hawaiian)
- have been diagnosed with gestational diabetes or have delivered a baby weighing more than 9 lbs (4 kg)
- have high blood pressure (140/90 mmHg or above)
- have a high density lipoprotein cholesterol level less than or equal to 35 mg/dL and/or a triglyceride level greater than or equal to 250 mg/dL
- have had impaired glucose tolerance or impaired fasting glucose on previous testing

Several common medications can impair the body's use of insulin, causing a condition known as secondary diabetes. These medications include treatments for high blood pressure (furosemide, clonidine, and thiazide diuretics), drugs with hormonal activity (oral contraceptives, thyroid hormone, progestins, and glucocorticoids), and the anti-inflammation drug indomethacin. Several drugs that are used to treat mood disorders (such as anxiety and depression) also can impair glucose absorption. These drugs include

Purified human insulin is most commonly used, however, insulin from beef and pork sources also are available. Insulin may be given as an injection of a single dose of one type of insulin once a day. Different types of insulin can be mixed and given in one dose or split into two or more doses during a day. Patients who require multiple injections over the course of a day may be able to use an insulin pump that administers small doses of insulin on demand. The small battery-operated pump is worn outside the body and is connected to a needle that is inserted into the abdomen. Pumps can be programmed to inject small doses of insulin at various times during the day, or the patient may be able to adjust the insulin doses to coincide with meals and exercise.

Regular insulin is fast-acting and starts to work within 15–30 minutes, with its peak glucose-lowering effect about two hours after it is injected. Its effects last for about four to six hours. NPH (neutral protamine Hagedorn) and Lente insulin are intermediate-acting, starting to work within one to three hours and lasting up to 18–26 hours. Ultra-lente is a long-acting form of insulin that starts to work within four to eight hours and lasts 28–36 hours.

Hypoglycemia, or low blood sugar, can be caused by too much insulin, too little food (or eating too late to coincide with the action of the insulin), **alcohol consumption**, or increased exercise. A patient with symptoms of hypoglycemia may be hungry, cranky, confused, and tired. The patient may become sweaty and shaky. Left untreated, the patient can lose consciousness or have a seizure. This condition is sometimes called an insulin reaction and should be treated by giving the patient something sweet to eat or drink like a candy, sugar cubes, juice, or another high sugar snack.

Surgery

Transplantation of a healthy pancreas into a diabetic patient is a successful treatment, however, this transplant is usually done only if a kidney transplant is performed at the same time. Although a pancreas transplant is possible, it is not clear if the potential benefits outweigh the risks of the surgery and drug therapy needed.

Alternative treatment

Since diabetes can be life-threatening if not properly managed, patients should not attempt to treat this condition without medical supervision. A variety of alternative therapies can be helpful in managing the symptoms of diabetes and supporting patients with the disease. Acupuncture can help relieve the pain associated with diabetic neuropathy by stimulation of certain points. A qualified practitioner should be consulted. Herbal remedies also may be helpful in managing diabetes. Although there is no herbal substitute for insulin, some herbs may help adjust blood sugar levels or manage other diabetic symptoms. Some options include:

- fenugreek (*Trigonella foenum-graecum*) has been shown in some studies to reduce blood insulin and glucose levels while also lowering cholesterol
- bilberry (*Vaccinium myrtillus*) may lower blood glucose levels, as well as help to maintain healthy blood vessels
- garlic (*Allium sativum*) may lower blood sugar and cholesterol levels
- onions (*Allium cepa*) may help lower blood glucose levels by freeing insulin to metabolize them
- cayenne pepper (*Capsicum frutescens*) can help relieve pain in the peripheral nerves (a type of diabetic neuropathy)
- ginkgo (*Ginkgo biloba*) may maintain blood flow to the retina, helping to prevent diabetic retinopathy

Any therapy that lowers stress levels also can be useful in treating diabetes by helping to reduce insulin requirements. Among the alternative treatments that aim to lower stress are hypnotherapy, biofeedback, and meditation.

Prognosis

Uncontrolled diabetes is a leading cause of blindness, end-stage renal disease, and limb amputations. It also doubles the risks of heart disease and increases the risk of stroke. Eye problems including cataracts, glaucoma, and diabetic retinopathy also are more common in people with diabetes.

Diabetic peripheral neuropathy is a condition where nerve endings, particularly in the legs and feet, become less sensitive. Diabetic foot ulcers are a particular problem since the patient does not feel the pain of a blister, callous, or other minor injury. Poor blood circulation in the legs and feet contribute to delayed wound healing. The inability to sense pain along with the complications of delayed wound healing can result in minor injuries, blisters, or callouses becoming infected and difficult to treat. In cases of severe infection, the infected tissue begins to break down and rot away. The most serious consequence of this condition is the need for amputation of toes, feet, or legs due to severe infection.

Heart disease and kidney disease are common complications of diabetes. Long-term complications may include the need for kidney dialysis or a kidney transplant due to kidney failure.

Babies born to diabetic mothers have an increased risk of birth defects and distress at birth.

Prevention

Research continues on diabetes prevention and improved detection of those at risk for developing diabetes. While the onset of type 1 diabetes is unpredictable, the risk of developing type 2 diabetes can be reduced by maintaining ideal weight and exercising regularly. The physical and emotional stress of surgery, illness, pregnancy, and alcoholism can increase the risks of diabetes, so maintaining a healthy lifestyle is critical to preventing the onset of type 2 diabetes and preventing further complications of the disease.

Resources

BOOKS

American Diabetes Association. *American Diabetes Association Complete Guide to Diabetes.* 5th ed. Alexandria, VA: American Diabetes Association, 2011.

PERIODICALS

Abbasi, A., et al. "Prediction Models for Risk of Developing Type 2 Diabetes: Systematic Literature Search and Independent External Validation Study." *BMJ* 18, no. 345 (September 18, 2012): e5900. http://dx.doi.org/10.1136/bmj.e5900 (accessed October 2, 2012).

American Diabetes Association. "Standards of Medical Care in Diabetes—2012." *Diabetes Care* 35, suppl. 1 (2012): S11–63.

Babbington, Gabrielle. "Metformin Tops Diabetes Trial." *Australian Doctor* (July 27, 2007): 3.

Buchanan, Thomas A., et al. "What is Gestational Diabetes?" *Diabetes Care* (July 2007): S105–S111.

Malik, Vasanti S., et al. "Sugar-Sweetened Beverages, Obesity, Type 2 Diabetes Mellitus, and Cardiovascular Disease Risk." *Circulation* 121 (2010): 1356–64. http://dx.doi.org/10.1161/CIRCULATIONAHA.109.876185 (accessed October 2, 2012).

"Research: Lower Chromium Levels Linked to Increased Risk of Disease." *Diabetes Week* (March 29, 2004): 21.

"Standards of Medical Care for Patients with Diabetes Mellitus: American Diabetes Association." *Clinical Diabetes* (Winter 2003): 27.

WEBSITES

American Diabetes Association. "Diabetes Basics." http://www.diabetes.org/diabetes-basics (accessed September 9, 2012).

———. "Low-Carb Diet for People with Diabetes." http://www.diabetes.org/news-research/research/access-diabetes-research/Ma-low-carb-diet.html (accessed October 3, 2012).

Centers for Disease Control and Prevention. "Diabetes Public Health Resource." http://www.cdc.gov/diabetes/ (accessed October 2, 2012).

Mayo Clinic staff. "Diabetes." MayoClinic.com. http://www.mayoclinic.com/health/diabetes/DS01121 (accessed October 2, 2012).

MedlinePlus. "Diabetes." U.S. National Library of Medicine, National Institutes of Health. http://www.nlm.nih.gov/medlineplus/diabetes.html (accessed October 2, 2012).

ORGANIZATIONS

Academy of Nutrition and Dietetics, 120 South Riverside Plz., Ste. 2000, Chicago, IL 60606-6995, (312) 899-0040, (800) 877-1600, amacmunn@eatright.org, http://www.eatright.org.

American Diabetes Association, 1701 North Beauregard St., Alexandria, VA 22311, (800) DIABETES (342-2383), askADA@diabetes.org, http://www.diabetes.org.

Canadian Diabetes Association, National Life Building, 1400–522 University Ave., Toronto, Ontario, Canada M5G 2R5, (800) 226-8464, info@diabetes.ca, http://www.diabetes.ca.

Centers for Disease Control and Prevention, 1600 Clifton Rd. NE, Atlanta, GA 30333, (800) CDC-INFO (232-4636), TTY: (888) 232-6348, cdcinfo@cdc.gov, http://www.cdc.gov.

Juvenile Diabetes Research Foundation International, 26 Broadway, 14th Fl., New York, NY 10004, (800) 533-CURE (2873), Fax: (212) 785-9595, info@jdrf.org, http://www.jdrf.org.

National Diabetes Education Program, One Diabetes Way, Bethesda, MD 20814-9692, (301) 496-3583, http://www.ndep.nih.gov.

National Diabetes Information Clearinghouse, 1 Information Way, Bethesda, MD 20892-3560, (800) 860-8747, TTY: (866) 569-1162, Fax: (703) 738-4929, ndic@info.niddk.nih.gov, http://diabetes.niddk.nih.gov.

Altha Roberts Edgren
Teresa G. Odle

Diabetic diet

Definition

The diabetic diet is a diet designed to control the level of glucose (sugar) in the blood of people who have diabetes or prediabetes.

Origins

Diabetes mellitus is a disease that is characterized by abnormally high levels of glucose in the blood. **Carbohydrates** (sugars and starches) are broken down during digestion into glucose, a monosaccharide time the amount and consumption of those foods in a way that helps them maintain a healthy blood glucose level. By keeping blood glucose within healthy limits, the individual decreases the risk of serious side effects and long-term complications of the disease, including heart and blood vessel (cardiovascular) disease, which can lead to heart attack and stroke; kidney failure; blindness (diabetic retinopathy); and nerve damage (neuropathy). In people with prediabetes, following a diabetic diet can stop or slow the progression to diabetes and can also help overweight and obese individuals lose weight. Regular physical activity is recommended in tandem with the diabetic diet. Even people without diabetes can benefit from this diet, as it falls in line with dietary recommendations from federal and medical organizations.

Precautions

There are no specific precautions related to this diet. The most important thing is for individuals to understand how the diet works and to follow it. Before beginning the diabetic diet, individuals must consult their doctor and set targets for their blood glucose levels both before meals and after eating. They must acquire and learn how to use equipment to take their own blood glucose readings up to several times daily. Consultation with a registered dietitian and attendance at diabetic education classes are strongly recommended, and regular checkups with a physician are mandatory. Family members also may benefit from a diabetic education classes in order to better understand the diet and medication regimen that their loved one should follow.

Risks

This diet is a healthy diet. There are no risks when following it correctly. Both long- and short-term health risks may occur, however, if a person with diabetes strays from the diet. People with diabetes should know the signs of overly high or overly low glucose levels and know how to correct these problems promptly.

Research and general acceptance

The diabetic diet is accepted by physicians, registered dietitians, and other healthcare professionals throughout the United States, as well as recommended by the American Diabetes Association. This healthy, non-controversial diet is acceptable for everyone over the age of three (unless they have special dietary considerations). Parents of children younger than age three should consult with their pediatrician about modifications in the diet needed to accommodate the rapid growth of young children.

Resources

BOOKS

Geil, Patti, and Tami A. Ross. *What Do I Eat Now?: A Step-by-Step Guide to Eating Right with Type 2 Diabetes.* Alexandria, VA: American Diabetes Association, 2009.

Mayo Clinic. *The Mayo Clinic Diabetes Diet.* Intercourse, PA: Good Books, 2011.

Powers, Margaret A. *American Dietetic Association Guide to Eating Right When You Have Diabetes.* New York: J. Wiley & Sons, 2003.

Prevention editors, with Ann Fittante. *Prevention's Diabetes Diet Cookbook.* Emmaus, PA: Rodale Books, 2008.

WEBSITES

American Diabetes Association. "Artificial Sweeteners." http://www.diabetes.org/food-and-fitness/food/what-can-i-eat/artificial-sweeteners (accessed September 16, 2012).

———. "Carbohydrate Counting." http://www.diabetes.org/food-and-fitness/food/ planning-meals/carb-counting (accessed September 16, 2012).

———. "Carbohydrates: Fiber." http://www.diabetes.org/food-and-fitness/food/what-can-i-eat/carbohydrates.html#Fiber (accessed September 16, 2012).

———. "Fat and Diabetes." http://www.diabetes.org/food-and-fitness/food/what-can-i-eat/fat-and-diabetes.html (accessed September 16, 2012).

———. "Glycemic Index and Diabetes." http://www.diabetes.org/food-and-fitness/food/planning-meals/glycemic-index-and-diabetes.html (accessed September 16, 2012).

Diabetes UK. "Ten Steps to Eating Well." http://www.diabetes.org.uk/Guide-to-diabetes/Food_and_recipes/Eating-well-with-Type-2-diabetes/Ten-steps-to-eating-well (accessed September 16, 2012).

Mayo Clinic staff. "Diabetes Diet: Create Your Healthy-Eating Plan." MayoClinic.com. http://www.mayoclinic.

com/health/diabetes-diet/DA00027 (accessed September 16, 2012).

———. "Your Diabetes Diet: Exchange lists." MayoClinic.com. http://www.mayoclinic.com/health/diabetes-diet/DA00077 (accessed September 16, 2012).

MedlinePlus. "Diabetes and Meal Planning [Interactive Tutorial]." U.S. National Library of Medicine, National Institutes of Health. http://www.nlm.nih.gov/medlineplus/tutorials/diabetesmealplanning/htm/index.htm (accessed September 16, 2012).

———. "Diabetic Diet." http://www.nlm.nih.gov/medlineplus/diabeticdiet.html (accessed September 16, 2012).

National Diabetes Information Clearinghouse (NDIC). "What I Need to Know About Eating and Diabetes." National Institute of Diabetes and Digestive and Kidney Diseases (NIDDK), U.S. National Institutes of Health. http://diabetes.niddk.nih.gov/dm/pubs/eating_ez/index.htm (accessed September 16, 2012).

ORGANIZATIONS

Academy of Nutrition and Dietetics, 120 S Riverside Plaza, Ste. 2000, Chicago, IL 60606, (312) 899-0040, (800) 877-1600, amacmunn@eatright.org, http://www.eatright.org.

American Diabetes Association, 1701 N Beauregard St., Alexandria, VA 22311, (800) 342-2383, askADA@diabetes.org, http://www.diabetes.org.

Diabetes UK, Macleod House, 10 Pkwy., London, United Kingdom NW1 7AA, +44 20 7424 1000, Fax: +44 20 7424 1001, info@diabetes.org.uk, http://www.diabetes.org.uk.

Juvenile Diabetes Research Foundation International, 26 Broadway, 14th Fl., New York, NY 10004, (800) 533-2873, Fax: (212) 785-9595, info@jdrf.org, http://www.jdrf.org.

National Diabetes Education Program, One Diabetes Way, Bethesda, MD 20814, (301) 496-3583, http://www.dep.nih.gov.

National Diabetes Information Clearinghouse, 1 Information Way, Bethesda, MD 20892, (800) 860-8747, TTY: (866) 569-1162, Fax: (703) 738-4929, ndic@info.niddk.nih.gov, http://diabetes.niddk.nih.gov.

Tish Davidson, AM

Diarrhea diet

Definition

A diarrhea diet is used to help alleviate diarrhea and replenish any fluids and **electrolytes** lost from this condition. Diarrhea is characterized by unusually frequent and loose (watery) bowel movements. More than four soft or watery bowel movements per day is considered abnormal. Diarrhea is classified into four subgroups: acute, intractable, osmotic, and secretory.

Causes of diarrhea	
Causes	**Examples**
Viral infections	Rotavirus, Norwalk virus
Bacterial infections	E. coli, Vibrio cholerae, Campylobacter, Shigella
Parasites	Giardia, Entamoeba
Helminths (intestinal worms)	Strongyloides
Allergic	Lactose intolerance, celiac sprue, medication side effects
Autoimmune	Ulcerative colitis, Crohn's disease
Malabsorptive	Pancreatic deficiency, biliary disease
Nutritional	Zinc deficiency, vitamin A deficiency, enteral feedings consisting of liquid nutritional formulas delivered straight to the bowels
Functional	Irritable bowel syndrome, short bowel syndrome, cancer

(Table by GGS Information Services. © 2013 Cengage Learning.)

Origins

Diarrhea is a symptom that is not only uncomfortable but also potentially dangerous to health. Recurrent diarrhea is usually indicative of an underlying infection or condition. Acute diarrhea is one of the most common types of diarrhea. It usually resolves within three weeks and is caused by bacteria. Intractable diarrhea is chronic (ongoing) and has a greater nutritional impact. Osmotic diarrhea is caused by the presence of osmotically active particles in the intestinal lumen, which occurs due to malabsorption or maldigestion. Fluid loss can be great and lead to **dehydration** quickly. Secretory diarrhea occurs when a disease causes the secretion of large amounts of fluid into the intestines. The diarrhea diet is comprised of techniques known to help alleviate symptoms of diarrhea. However, people experiencing diarrhea should visit a doctor to find out the underlying cause.

Description

Diarrhea is a symptom of many diseases and conditions. Some possible causes of diarrhea include:

- antibiotic use
- bacterial or viral infections (common causes include *Campylobacter jejuni*, *Salmonella*, *Shigella*, *Escherichia coli* O157:H7, rotavirus, Norwalk virus, and cytomegalovirus)
- certain diseases and conditions (e.g., celiac disease, Crohn's disease, diverticulitis, dysentery)
- excessive exercise
- food poisoning

- giardiasis (infection of the intestine by the parasite *Giardia intestinalis*)
- irritable bowel syndrome (IBS)
- lactose intolerance
- malabsorption
- traveler's diarrhea
- ulcerative colitis
- viral gastroenteritis (stomach flu)

The underlying condition and the type of diarrhea that a person is experiencing will determine the best diet to help resolve the diarrhea. If a person is experiencing diarrhea due to lactose intolerance, for example, avoiding lactose in the diet and replacing fluid losses will help reduce the symptoms.

A clear liquid diet may be used to help alleviate diarrhea. However, this diet is not nutritionally complete and is seldom followed for more than one or two days. Foods are slowly added back in as symptoms subside. The clear liquid diet allows water, fat-free broth or bouillon, diluted fruit juices, plain gelatin, popsicles, mineral water, and decaffeinated beverages. A full liquid diet consists of the clear liquid diet along with strained cream or broth soups, custard, and plain yogurts (especially important to add beneficial microorganisms back into the gut). A soft diet includes all of these foods plus rice, pastas, white bread, rolls, crackers, potatoes (not fried), eggs, milk, cheeses, tender meats, and low-fiber fruits and vegetables. Once the diarrhea has stopped, foods in the regular diet can be added back in, so long as symptoms do not recur. Sometimes milk products may aggravate the condition and will need to be avoided. Other foods and drinks that may worsen diarrhea include **caffeine**, foods high in **fiber** or fat, and spicy foods.

Some specific types of diarrhea may have their own dietary requirements, such as avoiding dairy products in lactose intolerance or gluten in **celiac disease**. Diarrhea caused by antibiotics can be reduced by consuming **probiotics** in foods or supplements. Foods that contain probiotics are usually labeled as having "live and active cultures." Supplements should not be taken without first consulting with a physician.

Function

The primary function of a diarrhea diet is to assist in preventing dehydration and replenishing lost electrolytes.

Benefits

Following a diarrhea diet will help reduce the risk of dehydration, electrolyte loss, and nutritional deficiencies. The diet may also provide the intestines some time to recover and heal and will help in rebuilding beneficial bacteria in the gut. It may be necessary to rebuild the intestinal flora, especially if antibiotics were taken. Eating probiotic yogurt (with acidophilus) helps restore the intestinal flora so that digestion can occur as normal.

Precautions

Diarrhea diets do not provide the full range of nutrients required by the body and should only be followed for a short period of time. An anti-diarrheal diet may not be appropriate in all cases of diarrhea. If a person is having diarrhea, they should seek medical attention to find the root cause and receive appropriate treatment. If diarrhea is severe, food may be withheld for 24 hours, or the person may be restricted to a clear liquid diet. Chronic diarrhea can lead to nutritional deficiencies, so adequate replacement of nutrients is highly important. A high-calorie, **high-protein diet** with supplements is usually the most beneficial in these cases.

Infants, small children, and the elderly are at great risk for dehydration and usually will need an oral rehydration solution. If electrolytes are not replaced and diarrhea is not treated, dehydration, hyponatremia (low serum **sodium**), hypokalemia (low serum potassium), and acidosis can occur. Very severe cases can lead to death. If the diarrhea is caused by fat-malabsorption, a deficiency in the fat-soluble **vitamins** can occur, as well as deficiencies in **calcium**, **magnesium**, **zinc**, **manganese**, **selenium**, and **chromium**.

Due to the amount of gastrointestinal infections in the world, the World Health Organization of the United Nations has developed an oral rehydration solution with common ingredients that is used for infants with less than 5% dehydration and no vomiting. If dehydration is greater than 5% in an infant, parents should seek medical attention.

For most people, any liquid should be adequate to bring fluid levels back to normal (rehydration). Too much water alone can be harmful, because water does not have any **sugar** or important electrolytes, such as sodium. A person's diet must include foods and beverages that restore electrolyte levels. Mineral water is recommended. For infants, a pediatrician may recommend solutions such as Pedialyte, which contains the necessary salts lost with diarrhea. Salt tablets should never be used as they may worsen diarrhea.

Diarrhea is often caused by foodborne or waterborne pathogens. The Mayo Clinic offers the following advice to prevent **food contamination** at home:

KEY TERMS

Acidophilus—Bacteria found in yogurt that, when ingested, helps restore the normal bacterial populations in the human digestive system.

Acute—Acute means sudden or severe. Acute symptoms appear, change, or worsen rapidly. It is the opposite of chronic.

Bacteria—Microorganisms found in the environment. Bacteria can multiply quickly in food, and can cause foodborne illnesses. Not all bacteria are harmful: some are used to make yogurt and cheese.

Celiac disease—Digestive disease that causes damage to the small intestine. It results from the inability to digest gluten found in wheat, rye, and barley.

Chronic—Chronic refers to a symptom or disease that continues or persists over an extended period of time.

Contamination—The undesired occurrence of harmful microorganisms or substances in food.

Crohn's disease—Inflammatory disease that usually occurs in the last section of the small intestine (ileum), causing swelling in the intestines. It can also occur in the large intestine.

Digestive tract—The tube connecting and including the organs and paths responsible for processing food in the body. These are the mouth, the esophagus, the stomach, the liver, the gallbladder, the pancreas, the small intestine, the large intestine, and the rectum.

Diverticulitis—Inflammation of small pouches (diverticula) that can form in the weakened muscular wall of the large intestine.

Dysentery—Inflammation of the intestine with severe diarrhea and intestinal bleeding, resulting from drinking water containing a parasite called *Entamoeba histolytica*.

Electrolytes—Chemicals such as salts and minerals required for various functions in the body.

Intestinal flora—The sum of all bacteria and fungi that live in the intestines. It is required to break down nutrients, fight off pathogens, and help the body build the vitamin E and K. An unbalanced intestinal flora can lead to many health problems.

Irritable bowel syndrome (IBS)—A chronic colon disorder that involves constipation and diarrhea, abdominal pain, and mucus in the stool.

Lactose intolerance—A condition in which the body does not produce enough lactase, an enzyme needed to digest lactose (milk sugar).

Malabsorption—Poor absorption of nutrients by the small intestine.

Microorganism—A general term for bacteria, molds, fungus, or viruses that can be seen only with a microscope.

Pathogen—A disease-causing microorganism.

Traveler's diarrhea—Diarrhea resulting from eating or drinking food or water contaminated by infected human bowel waste. Travelers to developing countries of the world are especially at risk.

Ulcerative colitis—Inflammation of the inner lining of the colon, characterized by open sores that appear in its mucous membrane.

• Wash hands, utensils, and food surfaces often to prevent cross-contamination, or the transfer of harmful bacteria from one surface to another.

• Keep raw foods separate from ready-to-eat foods.

• Cook foods to kill harmful organisms (to temperatures between 140° F [60° C] and 180° F [82° C]).

• Refrigerate or freeze perishable foods to avoid rapid growth of harmful bacteria.

• Drink water only from a trusted source.

• When in doubt, throw food out.

Risks

There are minimal risks associated with a diarrhea diet or with drinking liquids that replenish fluid levels as long as electrolytes are also provided. If diarrhea is not corrected and results in dehydration, vitamin and/or mineral deficiencies or loss of weight can occur. Signs of dehydration include:

• thirst

• dry mouth and tongue, parched throat

• reduced need to urinate

• dry skin and hair

• lack of energy, fatigue

• light-headedness

• dark, foul smelling urine

• fast heartbeat

• flushed or hot feeling in absence of a temperature

Research and general acceptance

The Division of Digestive Diseases and Nutrition at the National Institute of Diabetes and Digestive and Kidney Diseases (NIDDK) supports basic and clinical research into gastrointestinal conditions, including diarrhea. Among other areas, NIDDK researchers are studying how the processes of absorption and secretion in the digestive tract affect the content and consistency of stool, the relationship between diarrhea and pathogenic bacteria, motility in chronic diarrhea, and chemical compounds that may be useful in treating diarrhea. Research has shown that consuming probiotics may decrease the duration of diarrhea and help rebuild healthy gut bacteria. Probiotic strains include *Lactobacillus bulgaricus*, *Lactobacillus reuteri*, *Lactobacillus GG*, and *Lactobacillus acidophilus*. Yogurt with live and active cultures contains two or more of these strains and may help with diarrhea. *L. acidophilus* supplements are also commercially available in powder, liquid, capsule, or chewable tablet forms.

Resources

BOOKS

Banerjee, Bhaskar. *Nutritional Management of Digestive Disorders.* Boca Raton, FL: CRC Press, 2011.
Ericsson, C. D., H. L. Dupont, and R. Steffen. *Traveller's Diarrhea.* Hamilton, ON: B.C. Decker, 2003.
Guandalini, Stefano, and Haleh Vaziri. *Diarrhea: Diagnostic and Therapeutic Advances.* New York: Humana Press, 2011.
Wood, G. K. *The Complete Guide to Digestive Health: Plain Answers About IBS, Constipation, Diarrhea, Heartburn, Ulcers, and More.* Peachtree City, GA: FC&A Publishing, 2006.
Yarnell, Eric. *Natural Approach to Gastroenterology.* Seattle: Healing Mountain Publications, 2011.

PERIODICALS

Hempel, Susanne, et al. "Probiotics for the Prevention and Treatment of Antibiotic-Associated Diarrhea: A Systematic Review and Meta-analysis." *JAMA* 307, no. 18 (2012): 1959–69. http://dx.doi.org/10.1001/jama.2012.3507 (accessed September 24, 2012).

WEBSITES

Mayo Clinic staff. "Diarrhea." MayoClinic.com. http://www.mayoclinic.com/health/diarrhea/DS00292 (accessed September 24, 2012).
National Digestive Diseases Information Clearinghouse (NDDIC). "Diarrhea." National Institute of Diabetes and Digestive and Kidney Diseases. http://digestive.niddk.nih.gov/ddiseases/pubs/diarrhea (accessed September 24, 2012).

ORGANIZATIONS

American Gastroenterological Association, 4930 Del Ray Ave., Bethesda, MD 20814, (301) 654-2055, Fax: (301) 654-5920, member@gastro.org, http://www.gastro.org.
International Foundation for Functional Gastrointestinal Disorders, PO Box 170864, Milwaukee, WI 53217, (414) 964-1799, (888) 964-2001, Fax: (414) 964-7176, iffgd@iffgd.org, http://www.iffgd.org.
National Digestive Diseases Information Clearinghouse, 2 Information Way, Bethesda, MD 20892–3570, (800) 891–5389, TTY: (866) 569–1162, Fax: (703) 738–4929, nddic@info.niddk.nih.gov, http://www.digestive.niddk.nih.gov.

Monique Laberge, PhD
David Newton

Diet and disease prevention

Definition

Research has shown that diet has a tremendous impact on short- and long-term health. Poor diet can lead to nutritional deficiencies and chronic diseases such as **obesity**, **diabetes mellitus**, and **coronary heart disease**. A good diet combined with exercise promotes a healthy weight, reduces many health risks, and increases both physical and mental well-being.

Purpose

The concept of diet quality in relation to health has changed over time. In the early 1900s, lack of refrigeration, frozen food technology, and reliable transportation meant that people ate what grew locally and what was available seasonally. At that time, nutrition scientists focused on preventing specific nutrient and calorie deficiencies. Today, most people in developed countries have access to a large quantity and variety of foods. Nutrition researchers have shifted their focus to exploring the relationships among diet, chronic disease, longevity, and quality of life.

Well-nourished people have more energy, are more resistant to disease, and are better able to tolerate treatments and to recover from acute illnesses, surgery, and trauma. Consumption of a wide variety of foods, with appropriate amounts of **protein**, carbohydrate, fat, **vitamins**, and **minerals**, forms the basis of a healthy diet. However, many acute and chronic conditions are related to inadequate dietary intake. Obesity, a major public health concern, and many of the leading causes of death in the United States, including coronary heart disease, stroke, diabetes mellitus, and some cancers, are at least partially attributable to poor diet and **alcohol consumption**. Diet education has become a focus of public health outreach programs.

Description

The position of the **Academy of Nutrition and Dietetics** (formerly the American Dietetic Association) on the role of nutrition and diet in health promotion and disease prevention programs includes steps for primary, secondary, and tertiary prevention. These steps include the following guidelines:

• Primary prevention (health promotion): Health promotion is a population-based approach that encourages behaviors for better health. For example, taking nutrition classes at a local adult education center would be considered a primary prevention measure.

• Secondary prevention (risk appraisal and risk reduction): For people at risk of illness who are beginning to encounter health-related problems, secondary prevention encompasses risk appraisal and screening to detect preclinical disease and early intervention to promote health and well-being. Cholesterol screening for people with a family history of cardiovascular disease is an example of a secondary prevention measure.

• Tertiary prevention (treatment and rehabilitation): For people experiencing illness, injury, or disability, tertiary prevention includes treatment and rehabilitation to promote maximum health and prevent further disability and secondary conditions resulting from the initial health problem. Examples of tertiary prevention include medical nutrition therapy or diabetes education for people diagnosed with type 2 diabetes mellitus.

Dietary guidelines

The seventh edition of the *Dietary Guidelines for Americans*, published in 2010 by the U.S. Department of Agriculture (USDA) and Health and Human Services (HHS), provides an overall view of good nutrition along with specific recommendations for improved dietary habits. These dietary guidelines include:

• Make half your plate fruits and vegetables.

• Switch to fat-free or low-fat (1%) milk (for people over age 2).

• Drink water instead of sugary drinks.

• Compare sodium in foods like soup, bread, and frozen meals and choose the foods with lower numbers.

• Avoid oversized portions.

• Enjoy your food, but eat less.

MyPlate recommendations

More than one hundred years ago, in 1894, the USDA published its first set of national nutrition guidelines. **MyPlate**, replacing the former MyPyramid, is the most recent set of guidelines. The MyPlate design was simplified from the food pyramid to help consumers visualize the actual breakdown of each meal. Half of the plate is devoted to vegetables and fruits; slightly less than one-quarter is made up of protein (no longer meat and beans); and the remaining amount is dedicated to grains. A side of dairy is also featured, and the previous "fats and oils" category is obsolete. The MyPlate ethos emphasizes lifestyle factors such as exercise in addition to nutrition.

MyPlate is intended to help Americans become more aware of what they eat and what their nutrient requirements are. It is designed to help people learn how to eat a healthy diet, live an active lifestyle, and maintain or gradually move in the direction of a healthy weight, which will reduce the risk of weight-related diseases. MyPlate personalizes the specific amounts needed in each category based on the individual's age, gender, and activity level.

The MyPlate website, ChooseMyPlate.gov, provides detailed information on the five food categories along with additional guidelines on oils, calories, and physical activity. MyPlate assumes that people will eat from all food categories. The personalized recommendations about quantities to eat for each group do not take into consideration special diets for people with

members and especially the individual being treated must commit to achieving optimum health through medical nutritional therapy. Prioritized goals are critical when developing the nutrition treatment plan. Continuous assessment is made by the individual and healthcare team members to evaluate the importance of these and other goals. Physicians must understand the dietary approaches an individual is using and reinforce this diet therapy when interacting with the individual. The position of the Academy of Nutrition and Dietetics is that medical nutritional therapy is effective in treating disease and preventing disease complications.

Resources

BOOKS

Colson, Janet M. *Taking Sides: Clashing Views in Food and Nutrition.* New York: McGraw-Hill, 2012.

Dunn, Carolyn. *Nutrition Decisions: Eat Smart, Move More.* Burlington, MA: Jones & Bartlett Learning, 2013.

Hales, Dianne R. *An Invitation to Health: Build Your Future.* Belmont, CA: Wadsworth, 2013.

Haugen, David M., and Susan Musser. *Nutrition.* Detroit: Greenhaven Press, 2012.

WEBSITES

National Heart, Lung, and Blood Institute. "National Cholesterol Education Program." National Institutes of Health. http://www.nhlbi.nih.gov/about/ncep/index.htm (accessed September 20, 2012).

U.S. Department of Agriculture. "MyPlate." ChooseMyPlate.gov. http://www.choosemyplate.gov (accessed on September 16, 2012).

U.S. Department of Agriculture, National Agricultural Library. "DRI Tables." Food and Nutrition Information Center. http://fnic.nal.usda.gov/dietary-guidance/dietary-reference-intakes/dri-tables (accessed August 16, 2012).

U.S. Department of Agriculture and U.S. Department of Health and Human Services. *Dietary Guidelines for Americans, 2010.* 7th ed. Washington, DC: U.S. Government Printing Office, December 2010. http://health.gov/dietaryguidelines (accessed February 22, 2012).

U.S. Department of Health and Human Services. Healthy People.gov. http://www.healthypeople.gov/2020/default.aspx (accessed on September 16, 2012).

ORGANIZATIONS

Academy of Nutrition and Dietetics, 120 South Riverside Plz., Ste. 2000, Chicago, IL 60606-6995, (312) 899-0040, (800) 877-1600, amacmunn@eatright.org, http://www.eatright.org.

Food and Nutrition Information Center, National Agricultural Library, 10301 Baltimore Ave., Rm. 105, Beltsville, MD 20705, (301) 504-5414, Fax: (301) 504-6409, fnic@ars.usda.gov, http://fnic.nal.usda.gov.

Food Standards Agency, Aviation House, 125 Kingsway, London, United Kingdom WC2B 6NH, + 44 20 7276 8000, http://www.food.gov.uk.

International Food Information Council Foundation, 1100 Connecticut Ave., NW Ste. 430, Washington, DC 20036, (202) 296-6540, info@foodinsight.org, http://www.foodinsight.org.

U.S. Department of Agriculture, 1400 Independence Ave. SW, Washington, DC 20250, (202) 720-2791, http://www.usda.gov.

Tish Davidson, AM

Diet apps

Definition

Diet apps are software applications for tracking nutritional intake and managing diets for fitness, weight maintenance, weight loss, and weight gain. The apps can also be used for **food sensitivities**, allergies, and medical conditions, such as diabetes, high blood pressure, and heart disease. Most diet apps are tools for mobile devices, such as smart phones and tablets.

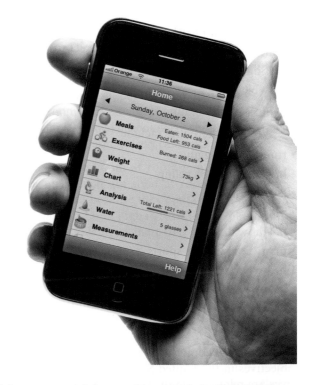

Diet apps on smartphones allow users to track their daily meals, calories, and physical activity. (© *incamerastock/ Alamy*)

Purpose

Millions of people worldwide follow weight loss diets or must track their nutritional intake or avoid certain types of food for medical reasons. With the proliferation of smart phones and other mobile devices, apps have made following these prescribed diets significantly easier and more convenient.

Approximately two-thirds of adults in the United States are overweight or obese and more than one-third are considered obese, compared with only 15% in 1980. About 17% of American children and adolescents are obese, three times the prevalence in 1980, and one-third are either overweight or obese, including almost 40% of African American and Hispanic children. Diet apps can be very powerful tools for helping people track **calories** and lose weight while maintaining balanced nutrition. Not only do diet apps make it easy to monitor calories and intake of **carbohydrates**, proteins, **fats**, and other nutrients, many of them perform calculations and provide information that was previously unavailable to the typical consumer.

Some diet apps function as companion tools for diet books or for online or in-person weight-management programs, such as **Weight Watchers**. In late 2010, Weight Watchers switched to the PointsPlus system, a different way of tracking food intake compared with their previous Points system. Based on the theory that the nutritional content of foods is at least as important as calorie counting, PointsPlus allocates points to individual foods based on their carbohydrate, **protein**, fat, and **fiber** content. Under PointsPlus, all fruits and most vegetables are "free," whereas processed and fast foods, as well as alcohol, rack up many more points than in the old system. The Weight Watchers diet app lets users track their daily points and also lets them calculate a food's point value by inputting the nutritional info.

In addition to weight loss, diet apps can be very useful for a variety of other purposes, including weight maintenance and weight gain. There are specific diet apps for patients with diabetes, **celiac disease** or gluten intolerance, **food allergies** and sensitivities, and various other medical conditions. Diet apps are particularly useful for consultations with dietitians and physicians, who can upload or receive e-mails of patients' logs and use the app to design individualized diets.

Description

There are thousands of diet and nutrition apps available for smart phones, tablets, and other devices, with new apps and new versions of older apps appearing almost daily. By mid-2012, the Apple "App Store" alone offered more than 1,300 diet apps, and there were even apps for choosing diet apps. While some diet apps are dual- or multipurpose, many are designed for specific purposes and goals, such as maintaining a low-carbohydrate diet, managing diabetes, or losing weight at a specific rate, such as 0.5–2 lb. (0.2–0.9 kg) per week. Some diet apps have different language selections or are designed specifically for travelers.

Databases

Many diet apps include nutritional databases that are either built-in to the app or accessed via the Internet. These databases vary in size and in the reliability of their information. Some diet apps utilize huge databases containing more than one million different foods and are updated daily, while others soon fall out of date. Although some databases include brand-name foods and even specific restaurant foods, diet apps tend to vary in their coverage of even the most common foods. Users can add new foods, recipes, and food data to some app databases, sometimes using a built-in barcode scanner. Depending on the app's specific purpose, the size, accessibility, and reliability of its database can, to a large extent, determine its usefulness.

Many diet apps, both in the United States and elsewhere, use national nutrient databases from the Beltsville Human Nutrition Research Center (BHNRC), part of the Agricultural Research Service (ARS) of the U.S. Department of Agriculture (USDA). These science-based nutritional databases can be downloaded free of charge by both commercial and nonprofit application developers. The National Nutrient Database for Standard Reference (SR), maintained by the Nutrient Data Laboratory (NDL) of the BHNRC, is considered the authoritative source on food composition and serves as the foundation for most food and nutrition databases used in the United States. The SR includes 7,900 profiles of the nutrients in single- and multiple-ingredient foods, including raw, cooked, processed, and prepared foods, from raw eggs to frozen lasagna. Many diet apps also utilize the USDA-ARS Food and Nutrient Database for Dietary Studies (FNDDS).

Procedures

Procedures for using diet apps vary as much as the apps themselves, starting with their registration and navigation functions. Some are designed to be used in conjunction with specific weight-loss programs. Others are better used under the guidance of a registered dietitian, especially if disease management requires a carefully controlled diet. Some diet apps readily integrate with social media, such as Facebook and Twitter.

Most diet apps involve keeping food logs, either by typing in the foods consumed over the course of the day or by scanning bar codes, although some apps allow voice logging. Calories, foods, nutrients, weight, and exercise may be tracked on a daily, weekly, or monthly basis, depending on the app, and graphs may show weight and progress over time. Tracking may include:

- food intake
- calories consumed
- calories burned during activities
- remaining calories available for consumption throughout the day, based on individual goals
- sources of the day's calories
- total consumed carbohydrates, proteins, and fats
- specific nutrients, such as fiber, saturated and trans fats, sugar, or cholesterol
- vitamins and minerals, such as iron, calcium, and potassium
- nutrition facts labels for brand-name and generic foods
- dietary supplements
- water intake
- alcohol intake
- exercise and fitness goals
- body weight
- measurements, including the neck, bust, arms, waist, hips, thighs, and calves

Some diet apps calculate an individual's **body mass index** (BMI), basal (resting) metabolic rate, and the thermal effects of exercise, based on gender, age, height, weight, and activity level. These apps may then calculate target caloric intakes or design customized daily meal plans for a given weight-loss rate or specific target date. Some apps include recipes, shopping lists, tips, reminders, and rewards for meeting goals. They may even assist users in choosing options, such as a healthier pizza or a different cocktail. Some apps send daily informational and inspirational articles and success stories. Some include databases of physical activities, fitness exercises, and the calories burned. Others include online communities and forums for support and enable users to add friends.

Specialized diet apps

Apps for managing diabetes, celiac disease, food allergies, or other conditions generally include functions in addition to those listed for weight loss. Managing diabetes requires careful and consistent logging.

In addition to total calories, diabetes management apps track intake of carbohydrates, fat, protein, fiber, specific foods, and water, as well as activities and exercise over the course of the day. They usually track blood sugar and set target ranges, quickly identify unsafe readings, show trends over time, and even schedule meals. They may track **insulin** injections and dosages, as well as other medications. The apps send hypoglycemia and hyperglycemia alerts and may note abnormalities in medication, exercise, fat or alcohol intake, or meal times. They may even track blood pressure and pulse. The apps may include diabetes management education, diabetes-appropriate foods and recipes, and connections to online diabetes management communities. Of particular benefit, diabetes apps export logs directly to healthcare providers for review and analysis.

Diet apps for people with food allergies or sensitivities can be customized with lists of specific restrictions. Some specialized apps—such as **gluten-free diet** apps—can be adapted for other sensitivities and even for vegan diets. Such apps often include special diets, menus, and shopping lists. They may include lists of allergens and specific allowable products and certifications. By scanning bar codes, they may be able to determine the safety of foods based on specific allergen restrictions. Some specialized diet apps include medication guides, information on **food additives**, links to tips and other resources, and sites for sharing experiences and recommendations. They may rate restaurants based on their ability to accommodate dietary restrictions and may even provide directions via GPS.

Brand names

There are thousands of weight-loss and weight-management apps available worldwide. Some of those that have won awards or been reviewed online include:

- Calorie Counter, by About, Inc.
- Calorie Counter, by MyNetDiary, 4Technologies Corp.
- Calorie Counter & Diet Tracker, by MyFitness Pal, LLC
- Calorie Counter: Diets & Activities, by Arawella Corp.
- Calorie Tracker, by Livestrong.com
- Daily Burn, by Daily Burn, Inc.
- GoodFoodNearYou, by Global Fitness Media
- iBody, winner of a Mobie Award for best healthcare and fitness app
- Lose It!, by FitNow, Inc.
- Nutrition Menu, by shroomies.com

- SparkPeople Food and Fitness Tracker, by Spark-People, Inc.
- Weight Watchers Mobile, by Weight Watchers International, Inc.

Apps for managing diabetes include:

- Bant, by University Health Network
- Blood Sugar Tracker, by Healthy Cloud LLC
- Carb Master Free, by Deltaworks Ltd.
- Diabetes Buddy Lite, by BHI Technologies, Inc.
- Diabetes Companion, by dLife
- Diabetes Log, by Distal Thoughts
- GluCoMo, by Artificial Life, Inc.
- Glucose Buddy, by OneAppOneCause
- Vree for Diabetes, by Merck & Co., Inc.
- WaveSense Diabetes Manager, by AgaMatrix, Inc.

Apps for gluten-free diets include:

- AllergyEatsMobile, by AllergyEats LLC
- CeliacFeed, by Daljit Ghag
- Eating Out G-Free, by Hachette Book Group, Inc.
- Find Me Gluten Free, by JATX Teck, LLC
- Food Additives 2: Free, by IGRASS PTY, Ltd.
- FoodWiz, by Food Angels UK, Ltd.
- Gluten Free Daily, by Visual Identify Group, Inc.
- Gluten Free Restaurant Cards from CeliacTravel.com, by Pepper Stuff
- Gluten Freed—Gluten Free Dining for Health and Celiac, by Magnolia Labs, Inc.
- iGlutenfree, by i3G Software, Inc.

Diet apps for kids

Diet apps for kids are a feature of First Lady Michelle Obama's "Let's Move" initiative, a comprehensive program aimed at solving **childhood obesity** within a generation. The "Apps for Healthy Kids" contest, a Let's Move program sponsored by the USDA's Center for Nutrition Policy and Promotion (CNPP), challenged software developers, game designers, students, and the general public to come up with fun and engaging applications for encouraging children, especially "tweens" aged 9–12, to improve their eating habits and increase their physical activity. The apps had to incorporate the SR, FNDDS, or a third CNPP database. Winning submissions had to be provided free to the public for one year. The winner in the tools category was Pick Chow! from the ZisBoomBah website, designed with the assistance of food, nutrition, and health experts. Pick Chow! enables children to design meals by clicking and dragging foods onto a virtual plate. Meters add up the nutritional values of

---

KEY TERMS

Basal metabolic rate (BMR)—Resting metabolic rate; the energy expended or calories used while at rest.

Body mass index (BMI)—A measure of body fat; the ratio of weight in kilograms to the square of height in meters.

Calorie—A unit of food energy.

Celiac disease—A digestive disease that causes damage to the small intestine. It results from the inability to digest gluten found in wheat, rye, and barley.

Diabetes—A condition in which the body either does not make or cannot respond to the hormone insulin. As a result, the body cannot use glucose (sugar). There are two types, type 1, also called juvenile onset, and type 2, also called adult onset.

Fiber—Indigestible material in food, also known as roughage or bulk. Insoluble fiber moves through the digestive system, giving bulk to stool; soluble fiber dissolves in water and helps keep stool soft.

Gluten—The protein in wheat, barley, and rye that makes dough sticky and triggers intolerance or celiac disease in some people.

Hyperglycemia—An abnormally high blood glucose level.

Hypoglycemia—An abnormally low blood glucose level.

Let's Move—First Lady Michelle Obama's initiative for combating childhood obesity.

Obesity—Excessive weight due to accumulation of fat, usually defined as a body mass index of 30 or above or body weight greater than 30% above normal on standard height-weight tables.

Overweight—A body mass index between 25 and 30.

Saturated fat—Hydrogenated fat; fat molecules that contain only single bonds, especially animal fats.

Trans fat—Fat that is produced by hydrogenation during food processing; trans fats increase bad cholesterol and decrease good cholesterol.

Wi-Fi—Wireless Internet.

---

the foods and rate the meal. Parents are sent e-mails with their children's choices, along with menus, recipes, a shopping list, and coupons. The runner-up tool was PapayaHead (http://www.papayahead.com), a family meal-planning app.

Precautions

Even diet apps that are designed for similar purposes vary greatly in their capabilities, information, databases, graphics quality, ease and convenience of use, and help and support functions. Some apps are much faster than others, and some are more reliable. Some require Internet access. Although many diet apps track intake of calories and at least some nutrients, such as carbohydrates, protein, and total fats, many do not track other important nutrients, such as saturated fats, fiber, or **sodium**.

Although many diet apps are inexpensive or free for download, their capabilities may be quite limited. Some are free for a limited trial, but user-entered information may be lost unless the app is purchased.

Complications

Diet apps can be awkward or confusing to use. The databases may be limited or may provide information that is confusing, overly technical, or misleading. Some apps list amounts in only one system, such as only ounces or only grams, which may be unfamiliar to some users. While some diet apps offer Wi-Fi backup and restore functions, others may lack a system for automatically backing up records. Some apps have problems scanning bar codes. Free versions of diet apps may contain advertisements.

Diet apps can have privacy and security issues, although some are password protected. In particular, diet apps that access Twitter or online forums or communities can raise serious privacy issues. They can also put the user at risk for false or misleading information.

Resources

PERIODICALS

O'Brien, Jeffrey M. "How to Count a Calorie." *Wired* (January 2012): 90–95, 110.

WEBSITES

Ahearn, Meghan. "10 Top Diet and Fitness Web Apps." *Woman's Day.* http://www.womansday.com/health-fitness/diet-weight-loss/10-top-diet-fitness-web-apps-70723 (accessed August 22, 2012).
Berrier, Christy. "16 Top Nutrition & Diet Apps." Franciscan Alliance News & Blog (Franciscan Alliance Hospitals of Northern Indiana), May 1, 2012. http://franciscanalliancenwi.wordpress.com/2012/05/01/16-top-nutrition-diet-apps (accessed August 22, 2012).
Moore, Marisa, Jessica Crandall, and Sarah Krieger. "Consumer and Lifestyle App Reviews." Academy of Nutrition and Dietetics. http://www.eatright.org/appreviews (accessed August 22, 2012).

U.S. Department of Agriculture (USDA) Agricultural Research Service. "Monitoring Food-Supply Nutrients." *The Second Step—Conservators of the National Nutrient Database.* http://www.ars.usda.gov/is/AR/archive/mar12/nutrients0312.htm (accessed August 22, 2012).
U.S. General Services Administration. "Apps for Healthy Kids." Challenge.gov. http://appsforhealthykids.com (accessed August 22, 2012).

ORGANIZATIONS

Academy of Nutrition and Dietetics, 120 South Riverside Plz., Ste. 2000, Chicago, IL 60606-6995, (312) 899-0040, (800) 877-1600, amacmunn@eatright.org, http://www.eatright.org.
Center for Nutrition Policy and Promotion, U.S. Department of Agriculture, 3101 Park Center Drive, 10th Fl., Alexandria, VA 22302, (703) 305-7600, Fax: (703) 305-3300, support@cnpp.usda.gov, http://www.cnpp.usda.gov.

Margaret Alic, PhD

Diet drugs

Definition

Diet drugs are medications that may help obese people lose weight when the drugs are used together with a program of diet and exercise. Historically, many drugs have been used as weight loss aids, and some ineffective products have been marketed with claims of helping in a program of weight loss.

Purpose

All diet drugs are intended to reduce caloric intake or increase calorie usage, however the methods vary.

Description

Appetite suppressants (anorexiants)

Most FDA-approved weight loss drugs suppress appetite by affecting one or more neurotransmitters in the brain. These are hormones that control appetite and mood. The model for these drugs is amphetamine, although there are many closely related drugs including the botanical product ephedrine. The mechanism of action of amphetamines on appetite suppression is not fully understood. It is known that amphetamines and amphetamine-like drugs cause the release of norepinephrine and dopamine. Although they are stimulants, amphetamines do not increase the basal metabolic rate, the rate at which the body uses energy

Diet pills approved by the U.S. Food and Drug Administration

Generic name	Trade name(s)	Drug type	FDA approval date
Approved for short-term use			
benzphetamine hydrochloride	Didrex	appetite suppressant	1960
diethylpropion	Tenuate, Tenuate Dospan	appetite suppressant	1959
phendimetrazine	Bontril, Plegine, Prelu-2, X-Trozine, Adipost, Melfiat	appetite suppressant	1982
phentermine	Adipex-P, Fastin, Ionamin, Oby-trim, Pro-Fast, Zantryl	appetite suppressant	1959
Approved for long-term use			
lorcaserin	Belviq	appetite suppressant	2012
orlistat	Xenical, Alli	lipase inhibitor	1999
phentermine and topiramate extended-release	Qsymia	appetite suppressant	2012

Note: The drug sibutramine (Meridia) was previously included in this list but was removed from U.S. markets in 2010 at the request of the FDA.

SOURCE: U.S. Food and Drug Administration.

(Table by PreMediaGlobal. © 2013 Cengage Learning.)

while in a resting state. Phenylpropanolamine had been approved by the U.S. Food & Drug Administration as an over-the-counter aid to diet in 1983, but this approval was withdrawn after several reports of hemorrhagic stroke associated with use of the drug.

Most weight loss drugs are approved for only a few weeks, and weight rapidly returns once the drug is discontinued. Long-term studies do indicate that continued use of weight loss drugs may be effective in maintaining weight loss, but in most cases long-term studies have not been conducted to adequately demonstrate safety. This was a particular problem with amphetamine and its derivatives, which are classified as controlled substances. Sibutramine, sold under the brand name Meridia, was approved by the FDA in 1997 but was removed from U.S. markets in 2010 due to increased risk of heart attack and stroke.

High-**fiber** foods have also been advocated as appetite suppressants. A typical example is glucomannan, a dietary fiber derived from the root of the elephant yam or konjac plant, which is native to Asia. The theory behind use of foods that contain indigestible fiber had been that these foods caused abdominal distention, or swelling of the stomach, which was believed to cause a feeling of fullness without increasing calorie intake. Studies and reviews of the effects of glucomannan and other non-nutritive fiber products such as bran have had varying results, but several of these studies have been encouraging. One Norwegian study compared three different kinds of fiber along with a highly calorie-restricted diet and reported "glucomannan induced body weight reduction in healthy overweight subjects, whereas the addition of guar gum and alginate did not seem to cause

additional loss of weight." A British study reviewed the effects of guar gum, a fiber which is often used as a thickening agent in food products, for its value in weight reduction. The researchers concluded that guar gum was not effective in aiding weight loss and the risks associated with taking guar gum outweighed its benefits. It appears that fiber, or the stomach expansion which fiber causes, is not adequate to reduce calorie intake. If there is a special benefit to glucomannan as indicated by the positive studies, its mechanism of action has not been explained.

Past evidence indicated that elevated blood glucose reduced appetite. This belief was the basis for the claim that sweets before meals would ruin an appetite. High glucose diet aids were marketed based on this concept. One example was the Ayds diet candy, which contained more **sugar** than regular candy, and was widely marketed in the 1970s. These products were found to be ineffective as an adjunct to diet and exercise in a weight loss regimen. While Ayds was reformulated to contain phenylpropanolamine, the similarity of the name to the disease AIDS eventually drove this product off the market.

Two new drugs were approved in 2012: lorcaserin (Belviq) and phentermine and topiramate extended release (Qsymia).

Topical anesthetics

In 1983, the Food and Drug Administration approved the use of benzocaine, a topical anesthetic widely used in first aid sprays, as an aid to weight-loss programs. The claim was that benzocaine, in the form of lozenges or gums, would anesthetize the tongue, making food less attractive. More recent studies have

GALE ENCYCLOPEDIA OF DIETS, 2ᴺᴰ EDITION

failed to show any significant benefit to benzocaine for weight loss.

Lipase inhibitors

In 1999, the FDA approved orlistat—the first of a new class of anti-obesity drugs called lipase inhibitors—for long-term use. **Orlistat**, marketed under the brand name Xenical, inhibits the pancreatic enzyme lipase that breaks down dietary fat. This decreases the body's absorption of dietary fat by as much as 30%. The undigested fat is excreted in the stool.

Orlistat is prescribed for overweight or obese patients who also have:

- high cholesterol
- diabetes
- high blood pressure
- heart disease

On February 7, 2007, the FDA approved orlistat for non-prescription sale.

Other agents

A large number of other agents have been offered for over-the-counter sale as weight loss agents, however they have not been either adequately studied or properly standardized, and so cannot be recommended. One typical example is chitosan, a fibrous material made of shellfish shells. This material may absorb **fats**, preventing their digestion, and thereby reducing caloric intake. Several studies have reported favorably on the effects of chitosan, but a careful analysis of these studies indicates that in the best conducted studies, the overall weight reduction benefits are trivial, and preparations containing chitosan cannot be recommended.

Many of the products marketed as herbal have been found to be adulterated with active drugs, including sibutramine and amphetamine. People taking these agents under the impression that they are safe because they are labeled as natural products may be taking inappropriate doses of active drugs. One Chinese remedy was found to contain Aristolochic acid which was found to be responsible for six deaths due to kidney failure among patients at a Belgian health spa.

Another reviewer examined studies relating to complimentary and alternative treatments for **obesity**. None of the drugs reviewed appeared to show convincing evidence of value based on published studies, although hypnotherapy did appear to be of potential value in weight reduction. While the overwhelming majority of complimentary and alternative medicines marketed for weight reduction are harmless, the lack

---

KEY TERMS

Anorexiant—A drug that causes loss of appetite.

Caloric—Relating to heat or calories; also, full of calories, and so likely to be fattening.

Dopamine—A neurotransmitter and precursor of norepinephrine; found in high concentrations in the brain.

Fiber—Nutrients in the diet which are not digested by enzymes. Insoluble fiber travels through the digestive tract and has a laxative effect.

Glucomannan—A plant substance composed of long chains of the sugars glucose and mannose. It is not digested, and may be used as a laxative. The material has been claimed to provide a feeling of abdominal and intestinal fullness.

Hemorrhagic—Relating to escape of blood from the vessels; bleeding.

Homeopathic—Relating to homeopathy, a system of treating diseases by giving people very small doses of natural substances which, in healthy people, cause the same symptoms as the disease being treated.

Norepinephrine—A hormone that constricts blood vessels.

Stroke—The sudden death of brain cells when the blood supply is disrupted either through blockage or bleeding.

Thermogenic—Producing heat. Relating to diet drugs, the term is used to indicate a drug which causes increased use of calories without exercise.

---

of evidence of efficacy makes their use inadvisable as there is no reason to accept any risk.

Some products claim to increase the body's thermogenesis. These claims purport that the body will burn more **calories** in the resting state, leading to increased weight loss. Some herbal remedies are based on seaweed, which has a high iodine content. As iodine is needed for the normal function of the thyroid gland, it is claimed that these drugs may help speed up metabolism. However, there is no research to show that providing more iodine will have this effect. At one time, thyroid hormone was prescribed for this purpose, but because of the very high risks associated with thyroid, this use has been discontinued. Comparable claims have been made for **green tea** extract, but the weight loss benefits of these products are not clear. In one study, patients taking green tea had greater weight loss than the subjects in the control group, but on careful review, it was found that patients in the active group were exercising more than patients taking placebo. No studies yet support these claims.

Homeopathic remedies have been offered as weight loss products. Homeopathy itself is controversial at best, and there have been no reputable studies indicating that homeopathic remedies have any value in weight reduction.

Starch blockers are products which inhibit the digestion of starch, and so reduce its caloric value. This, in theory, should lead to reduced effective calorie intake, however the value of these products has not been demonstrated. Because these products are made from bean husks, there has been an ongoing dispute in the courts. The manufacturers argue that their products are animal feed, and not subject to regulation as drugs, while the FDA has argued that the intended use of the starch blockers is as a drug, and should be subject to regulation. The courts have been divided on how these products should be defined.

Precautions

Because of the lack of standardization and high frequency of adulteration in some products marketed as herbal or natural weight loss remedies, people choosing to buy products of this type should deal only with a known and reputable supplier.

No weight loss product has demonstrated the ability to induce weight loss without diet, exercise, and behavioral modification. Although orlistat has been approved for long-term use, this is defined as up to two years, and in controlled studies, patients taking the drug showed increases in weight during the second year.

Aftercare

Weight-loss drugs are used as short-term adjuncts to programs of diet, exercise, and behavioral changes, such as portion control, that are intended to maintain lifetime weight goals. These behaviors must be continued after the drugs are discontinued.

Parental concerns

Weight-loss drugs are not normally indicated for children under the age of 16. Children should not use these drugs without proper medical supervision.

Resources

PERIODICALS

Birketvedt, G.S., et al. "Experiences with Three Different Fiber Supplements in Weight Reduction." *Medical Science Monitor* 11 (January 2005): PI5–8.

Greenway, F., et al. "Double-Blind, Randomized, Placebo-Controlled Clinical Trials with Non-Prescription Medications for the Treatment of Obesity." *Obesitye Research* (July 1999): 370–78.

Keithley, J., and B. Swanson. "Glucomannan and Obesity: A Critical Review." *Alternative Therapeutic Health Medicine* (Nov–Dec 2005): 30–34.

Ni Mhurchu, C., C.A. Dunshea-Mooij, D. Bennett, and A. Rodgers. "Chitosan for Overweight or Obesity." *Cochrane Database Syst Rev* (July 2005): CD003892.

Opala, T., et al. "Efficacy of 12 Weeks Supplementation of a Botanical Extract-Based Weight Loss Formula on Body Weight, Body Composition and Blood Chemistry in Healthy, Overweight Subjects—A Randomised Double-Blind Placebo-Controlled Clinical Trial." *European Journal of Medical Research* 11 (August 2006): 343.

Pittler, M.H., and E. Ernst. "Complementary Therapies for Reducing Body Weight: A Systematic Review." *International Journal on Obesity (London)* (September 2005): 1030–38.

————. "Guar Gum for Body Weight Reduction: Meta-Analysis of Randomized Trials." *American Journal of Medicine* 15 (June 2001): 724–30

WEBSITES

Aleccia, JoNel. "FDA OKs First New Weight-Loss Pill in 13 Years." NBC News, June 27, 2012. http://vitals.nbcnews.com/_news/2012/06/27/12440533-fda-oks-first-new-weight-loss-pill-in-13-years (accessed October 3, 2012).

MedlinePlus. "Sibutramine." U.S. National Library of Medicine, National Institutes of Health. http://www.nlm.nih.gov/medlineplus/druginfo/meds/a601110.html (accessed October 3, 2012).

U.S. Food and Drug Administration. "FDA Approves Belviq to Treat Some Overweight or Obese Adults." http://www.fda.gov/NewsEvents/Newsroom/PressAnnouncements/ucm309993.htm (accessed October 3, 2012).

————. "FDA Approves Weight-Management Drug Qsymia." http://www.fda.gov/NewsEvents/Newsroom/PressAnnouncements/ucm312468.htm (accessed October 3, 2012).

ORGANIZATIONS

The Obesity Society, 8757 Georgia Ave., Ste. 1320, Silver Spring, MD 20910, (301) 563-6526, Fax: (301) 563-6595, http://www.obesity.org, http://www.obesity.org/resources-for/consumer.htm.

U.S. Food and Drug Administration, 10903 New Hampshire Ave., Silver Spring, MD 20993-0002, (888) INFO-FDA (463-6332), http://www.fda.gov.

Samuel D. Uretsky, PharmD

Dietary cholesterol

Definition

Cholesterol is a soft, white, waxy substance found in the lipids of the bloodstream and in the cells of the body. There are two sources of cholesterol. The first is the body, mainly the liver, which produces typically about one gram per day. The second are cholesterol-containing foods from animal sources, especially egg yolks, meat, poultry, fish, seafood, and whole-milk dairy products. Cholesterol in foods is called dietary cholesterol.

Purpose

Cholesterol is found in every cell of the body. It has several important functions in maintaining health, such as:

- keeping cell membranes intact
- boosting mental performance
- helping digestion
- building strong bones
- building muscle
- maintaining energy, vitality, and fertility
- regulating blood sugar levels
- repairing damaged tissue
- protecting against infectious diseases

Dietary cholesterol

Food	Cholesterol (mg)
Beef liver, cooked, 3 oz	331
Beef sweetbreads, cooked, 3 oz.	250
Squid, cooked, 3 oz.	227
Egg, whole, large	212
Shrimp, cooked, 3 oz.	166
Ice cream, gourmet, 1 cup	90
Salmon, baked, 3.5 oz.	87
Lamb chop, cooked, 3 oz.	75
Chicken breast, cooked, 3 oz.	72
Beef, round, cooked, 3 oz.	71
Beef, sirloin, cooked, 3 oz.	71
Pork chop, cooked, 3 oz.	71
Chicken, dark meat, cooked, 3 oz.	70
Beef, rib eye, cooked, 3 oz.	65
Ham, regular, cooked, 3 oz.	50
Tuna, water packed, drained, 3.5 oz.	42
Milk, whole, 1 cup	33
Butter, 1 tbsp.	31
Ice cream, light, 1 cup	31
Cheese, cheddar, 1 oz.	30
Scallops, cooked, 3 oz.	27
Hot dog, beef, 1 frank	24
Cheese, reduced fat, 1 oz.	6
Yogurt, part skim, 1 cup	6

(Table by GGS Information Services. © 2013 Cengage Learning.)

However, excess cholesterol has been shown to accumulate in the bloodstream and on the walls of arteries, forming "plaques" that can clog the blood vessels (atherosclerosis) and lead to heart attack or stroke. Because high blood cholesterol is one of the major risk factors for heart disease, dietary cholesterol has been the focus of much debate over what constitutes healthy or unhealthy levels of cholesterol in the blood and how to lower cholesterol in the diet.

Description

Dietary cholesterol is found in animal food sources such as meat, poultry, seafood, and dairy products. Foods from plants, such as fruits, vegetables, vegetable oils, grains, cereals, and nuts and seeds do not contain cholesterol. Major sources of dietary cholesterol include meats and poultry (beef, chicken, pork, lamb), seafood (squid, salmon, tuna), and dairy products (eggs, ice cream, cheese, milk, butter).

Cholesterol does not dissolve in blood. It has to be transported to and from the cells by special carriers called lipoproteins, which are present in blood plasma. The most important forms of lipoproteins are:

- Very high-density lipoprotein (VHDL). VHDL consists of proteins and a high concentration of free fatty acids.
- High-density lipoprotein (HDL). HDL helps remove fat from the body by binding with it in the bloodstream and carrying it back to the liver for excretion in the bile and disposal. High levels of HDL may lower chances of developing heart disease or stroke.
- Intermediate-density lipoprotein (IDL). IDLs are formed during the degradation of very-low-density lipoproteins; some are cleared rapidly into the liver and some are broken down to low-density lipoproteins.
- Low-density lipoproteins (LDL). LDL transports cholesterol from the liver and small intestine to tissues outside the liver (extrahepatic) and other parts of the body. High LDL levels may increase chances of developing heart disease.
- Very low-density lipoprotein (VLDL). VLDLs carry triglycerides from the intestine and liver to fatty (adipose) and muscle tissues. A high VLDL level can cause a buildup of cholesterol in the arteries and increase the risk of heart disease and stroke.
- Chylomicrons. Chylomicrons are proteins that transport cholesterol and triglycerides from the small intestine to tissues after meals.

Generally speaking, LDL levels should be low because LDL deposits cholesterol in the arteries and causes them to become clogged. HDL levels should be high because HDL helps clean fat and cholesterol from arteries, carrying it to the liver for removal from the body. This is why HDL is often called the "good cholesterol" and LDL the "bad cholesterol," although studies conducted in 2012 began to challenge this belief.

American Heart Association recommendations

The American Heart Association (AHA) endorses the following dietary recommendations for people with high blood cholesterol:

- total fat: 25% of total calories
- saturated fat: less than 7% of total calories
- polyunsaturated fat: up to 10% of total calories
- monounsaturated fat: up to 20% of total calories
- carbohydrates: 50%–60% of total calories
- protein: about 15% of total calories
- cholesterol: less than 200 mg/dL
- plant sterols: 2 g
- soluble fiber such as psyllium: 10–25 g

Categories of appropriate foods include:

- lean meat or fish: less than 5 oz/day
- eggs: less than two yolks per week (whites unlimited)
- low-fat dairy products (1% fat): 2–3 servings/day
- grains, especially whole grains: 6–8 tsp/day
- vegetables: less than 6 servings per day
- fruits: 2–5 servings per day

Tips for preventing high cholesterol

Making smart dietary choices can prevent cholesterol levels from being too high. Some **fats**, such as mono- and polyunsaturated fats, may lower LDL cholesterol levels. Other fats, such as saturated and *trans* fats, raise cholesterol. Sources of fats include:

- monounsaturated fats (lower LDL, raise HDL): olives, olive oil, canola oil, nuts, avocados
- polyunsaturated fats (lower LDL, raise HDL): corn, soybeans, safflowers, cottonseed oils, fish
- saturated fats (raise both LDL and HDL): whole milk, butter, cheese, ice cream, red meat, chocolate, coconuts
- trans fats (raise LDL): most margarines, vegetable shortening, partially hydrogenated vegetable oil, deep-fried chips, many fast foods, most commercial baked goods

Other suggested guidelines include:

- Select lean meats and poultry. Choose chicken and turkey without skin or remove skin before eating. Dry peas, beans, and tofu are low in saturated fat

---

KEY TERMS

Artery—A blood vessel that carries blood from the heart to the body.

Atherosclerosis—Clogging, narrowing, and hardening of the large arteries and medium-sized blood vessels. Atherosclerosis can lead to stroke, heart attack, eye problems, and kidney problems.

Blood plasma—The pale, yellowish, protein-containing fluid portion of the blood in which cells are suspended. 92% water, 7% protein and 1% minerals.

Extrahepatic—Originating or occurring outside the liver.

Fatty acid—Any of a large group of monobasic acids, especially those found in animal and vegetable fats and oils, having the general formula CnH.

Heart attack—A heart attack occurs when blood flow to the heart muscle is interrupted. This deprives the heart muscle of oxygen, causing tissue damage or tissue death.

Lipids—Group of chemicals, usually fats, that do not dissolve in water, but dissolve in ether.

Omega-3 fatty acid—Any of several polyunsaturated fatty acids found in leafy green vegetables, vegetable oils, and fish such as salmon and mackerel, capable of reducing serum cholesterol levels and having anticoagulant properties.

Saturated fat—A type of fat that comes from animals and that is solid at room temperature.

Stroke—The sudden death of some brain cells due to a lack of oxygen when the blood flow to the brain is impaired by blockage or rupture of an artery to the brain.

Triglyceride—A fat that comes from food or is made up of other energy sources in the body. Elevated triglyceride levels contribute to the development of atherosclerosis.

Unsaturated fat—A type of fat derived from plant and some animal sources, especially fish, that is liquid at room temperature.

---

and cholesterol and can be eaten as alternatives to meat.

- Egg yolks are high in dietary cholesterol (213 mg per yolk). They should be limited to no more than two per week, including the egg yolks in baked goods and processed foods. Egg whites have no cholesterol and can be substituted for whole eggs when baking.

- Choose low- or reduced-fat dairy products (milk, cheese, yogurt, ice cream) over those made with whole milk.
- Limit butter, lard, and solid shortenings.
- Eat lots of fruits and vegetables, which are low in fat and high in fiber.

Cholesterol-lowering foods

Some foods may actually lower a person's cholesterol. Soluble **fiber** has been shown to help reduce LDL cholesterol levels when eaten as part of a healthy diet. Specific cholesterol-lowering foods include:

- oatmeal
- fish high in omega-3 fatty acids, such as salmon
- nuts
- olive oil

Plant sterols and stanols, found in trace amounts in plant-based foods, have been found to reduce LDL cholesterol levels by up to 15%. Because the amounts obtained through dietary sources are low, foods fortified with plant sterols are available.

Precautions

The National Heart, Lung, and Blood Institute (NHLBI), through its National Cholesterol Education Program (NCEP), recommends that adults begin cholesterol screening at age 20 and repeat the screening every five years. People who have one or more risk factors for developing heart disease (for example: diabetes, kidney disease, high blood pressure, vascular disease, or a history of elevated cholesterol levels) should have their cholesterol levels checked more often.

Simple blood tests are done to check blood cholesterol levels. A lipoprotein test, also called a fasting lipid test, is commonly performed as part of a routine medical examination. A cholesterol test measures lipid levels and usually reports on four groups:

- total cholesterol (normal: 100–199 mg/dL)
- LDL (normal: less than 100 mg/dL)
- HDL (normal: 40–59 mg/dL)
- triglycerides (normal: less than 150 mg/dL)

Complications

If dietary cholesterol intake is excessive, it can lead to an elevation of lipid levels in the bloodstream, a condition known as **hyperlipidemia**. These lipids include cholesterol, phospholipids, and **triglycerides** (fats). Hypercholesterolemia is the term for high cholesterol levels, and **hypertriglyceridemia** is the term

---

QUESTIONS TO ASK YOUR DOCTOR

- What is the connection between cholesterol and heart disease?
- Do I need to take medication to lower my cholesterol?
- Are there any precautions I should take with, or side effects to be expected from, cholesterol-lowering medications?

---

for high triglyceride levels. Because cholesterol-rich foods are also usually high in saturated fat, hypercholesterolemia is often combined with hypertriglyceridemia. Hyperlipidemias have been shown to represent a major risk factor for heart disease, a leading cause of death in the United States.

See also TLC diet.

Resources

BOOKS

American Heart Association. *American Heart Association Low-Fat, Low-Cholesterol Cookbook, 4th Edition: Delicious Recipes to Help Lower Your Cholesterol.* New York: Clarkson Potter, 2010.

Freeman, M.W., and C.E. Junge. *Harvard Medical School Guide to Lowering Your Cholesterol.* New York: McGraw-Hill, 2005.

Goldberg, Anne C., and Vera A. Bittner. *100 Questions & Answers About Managing Your Cholesterol.* London: Jones & Bartlett, 2011.

Larson Duyff, R. *ADA Complete Food and Nutrition Guide.* 3rd ed. Chicago, IL: American Dietetic Association, 2006.

Mihaly, Mary. *The Complete Guide to Lowering Your Cholesterol: Your All-in-One Resource for a Heart-Healthy Life.* New York: St. Martins Paperbacks, 2011.

Truswell, A. Stewart. *Cholesterol and Beyond: The Research on Diet and Coronary Heart Disease 1900–2000.* New York: Springer, 2010.

PERIODICALS

AbuMweis, S.S., and P.J. Jones. "Cholesterol-Lowering Effect of Plant Sterols." *Current Atherosclerosis Reports* 10, no. 6 (2008): 467–72.

Kolata, Gina. "Doubt Cast on the 'Good' in 'Good Cholesterol.'" *New York Times* (May 16, 2012): A1. http://www.nytimes.com/2012/05/17/health/research/hdl-good-cholesterol-found-not-to-cut-heart-risk.html (accessed June 20, 2012).

Sabatê, Joan, Keiji Oda, and Emilio Ros. "Nut Consumption and Blood Lipid Levels: A Pooled Analysis of 25

Intervention Trials." *Archives of Internal Medicine* 170, no. 9 (2010): 821–27. http://dx.doi.org/10.1001/archinternmed.2010.79 (accessed June 20, 2012).

WEBSITES

American Heart Association. "Whole Grains and Fiber." http://www.heart.org/HEARTORG/GettingHealthy/NutritionCenter/HealthyDietGoals/Whole-Grains-and-Fiber_UCM_303249_Article.jsp (accessed June 20, 2012).

Centers for Disease Control and Prevention. "Dietary Cholesterol." http://www.cdc.gov/nutrition/everyone/basics/fat/cholesterol.html (accessed June 20, 2012).

Cleveland Clinic. "Plant Sterols and Stanols." http://my.clevelandclinic.org/healthy_living/cholesterol/hic_plant_sterols_and_stanols.aspx (accessed June 20, 2012).

Harvard School of Public Health. "What Should I Eat? Fats and Cholesterol." *The Nutrition Source*, Department of Nutrition, Harvard University. http://www.hsph.harvard.edu/nutritionsource/what-should-you-eat/fats-and-cholesterol/index.html (accessed June 20, 2012).

Mayo Clinic staff. "Cholesterol: Top 5 Foods to Lower Your Numbers." MayoClinic.com. http://www.mayoclinic.com/health/cholesterol/CL00002 (accessed June 20, 2012).

National Heart, Lung, and Blood Institute. *Your Guide to Lowering Your Cholesterol with Therapeutic Lifestyle Changes (TLC)*. NIH Publication No. 06-5235. Washington, DC: U.S. Department of Health and Human Services, National Institutes of Health, December 2005. http://www.nhlbi.nih.gov/health/public/heart/chol/chol_tlc.htm (accessed June 20, 2012).

ORGANIZATIONS

American Heart Association, 7272 Greenville Ave., Dallas, TX 75231, (800) 242-8721, http://www.heart.org/HEARTORG.

Centers for Disease Control and Prevention, Division for Heart Disease and Stroke Prevention, 4770 Buford Hwy NE, Mail Stop F-72, Atlanta, GA 30341-3717, (800) CDC-INFO (232-4636), TTY: (800) 232-6348, Fax: (770) 488-8151, cdcinfo@cdc.gov, http://www.cdc.gov/dhdsp.

National Heart, Lung, and Blood Institute, Attn: Website, PO Box 30105, Bethesda, MD 20824-0105, (301) 592-8573, TTY: (240) 629-3255, Fax: (240) 629-3246, nhlbiinfo@nhlbi.nih.gov, http://www.nhlbi.nih.gov.

Monique Laberge, PhD

Dietary counseling

Definition

Dietary counseling is individualized nutritional care and advice for modifying eating habits. It includes patient education and meal planning and can help prevent or treat nutrition-related illnesses. Dietary counseling for chronic diseases is sometimes called medical nutrition therapy (MNT).

Purpose

Today's major health care problems are increasingly the result of acute and chronic conditions related to poor nutrition and/or overconsumption. A large proportion of cardiovascular disease and cancers are attributable, at least in part, to unhealthy eating habits and **obesity**. Dramatic increases in obesity rates in the United States and around the world are leading to increases in various chronic diseases. Primary prevention, including dietary counseling, is the most effective and affordable way to prevent and reduce the risk of chronic diseases such as cardiovascular disease, **cancer**, obesity, diabetes, and **hyperlipidemia**. Prevention at all levels—primary (disease prevention), secondary (early diagnosis), and tertiary (preventing or slowing deterioration)—requires active patient participation with the guidance and support of counseling by a registered dietitian or physician. Dietary counseling has important roles in weight management, in treating **eating disorders**, and in preventing nutrition-related conditions.

Dietary counseling that includes education, motivation, and meal planning geared to the individual is most effective for engaging active patient participation. Individualized dietary counseling can provide patients with important insights into food-related illnesses and education regarding how various **macronutrients** (proteins, **carbohydrates**, **fats**) and alcohol affect obesity and illness. Dietary counselors are also concerned with the intake of micronutrients, especially **vitamins** and **minerals**. Intakes of certain vitamins and minerals that are too low or too high can lead to a nutrient deficiency or nutrient toxicity, respectively. Dietary counseling may be tailored to the needs of patients diagnosed with specific conditions. It can also help reduce complications and/or side effects of treatments and improve general well-being.

Although dietary counseling is most often used to treat obesity and obesity-related conditions, as well as conditions such as diabetes and eating disorders, it can be useful for a wide range of circumstances. For example, hospice agencies routinely provide dietary counseling for their patients. The U.S. Preventive Services Task Force recommends intensive behavioral dietary counseling for adult patients with hyperlipidemia and other risk factors for cardiovascular and other diet-related chronic diseases. This intensive counseling may be provided by primary-care physicians or through referrals to other specialists such as registered dietitians.

Precautions

Dietary counseling—whether provided by a registered dietitian (RD), a nutritionist, a physician, or other healthcare provider—has consistently been shown to be much more effective when it is tailored to the individual. "One size fits all" approaches to dietary counseling, such as are sometimes offered by commercial weight-loss programs and meal plans, are rarely effective for permanently modifying dietary habits. Furthermore, dietary counseling that is effective with one group of people may be less effective with other groups, especially underserved or economically disadvantaged populations or clients with different cultural beliefs and practices. Age, gender, health status, and various psychological factors also affect how dietary counseling should be pursued with different individuals.

Description

There are numerous goals that must be considered when planning appropriate dietary counseling:

- determining a reasonable weight goal, based on weight history, physical activity levels, and other factors, that both the patient and counselor agree is attainable and can be maintained over the long term
- providing adequate calories for attaining and maintaining a desirable weight for adults, ensuring normal growth and development rates for children and adolescents, and meeting increased energy and nutritional requirements during pregnancy and lactation or recovery from catabolic illness
- ensuring that the diet contains appropriate amounts of protein, carbohydrates, fat, vitamins, and minerals
- attaining and maintaining recommended blood lipid levels through a low-fat diet
- preventing, delaying, or treating nutrition-related risk factors and complications
- improving overall health through optimal nutrition

Resources

Dietary counselors often use the **dietary reference intakes (DRIs)** developed by the U.S. Department of Agriculture as a guide for macronutrient and micronutrient recommendations. The **DRIs** also include safe upper intake limits for each nutrient. The guidelines provided by the National Cholesterol Education Program are often followed for achieving and maintaining optimal or satisfactory blood lipid levels (total cholesterol, low-density lipoproteins [LDL], high-density lipoproteins [HDL], and triglycerides).

Both dietary counselors and self-counseling individuals utilize various other U.S. Government sources, including the *Dietary Guidelines for Americans, 2010* and Healthy People 2020. The *Guidelines* include 23 key recommendations for choosing an overall healthy diet, as well as six additional key recommendations for specific populations such as pregnant women. The three major goals of the *Guidelines* are:

- balancing calories with physical activity to manage weight
- consuming more fruits, vegetables, whole grains, fat-free and low-fat dairy products, and seafood
- consuming fewer foods containing sodium, saturated fats, trans fats, cholesterol, added sugars, and refined grains

Other popular sources for dietary counseling include the U.S. Department of Agriculture's "Choose MyPlate" guide and tracker and the Dietary Approaches to Stop Hypertension (DASH) Plan. These are not weight-loss diets. Rather, they are designed to integrate dietary recommendations into overall healthy eating patterns. Both of these plans follow the 2010 *Dietary Guidelines*. These and other Internet-based informational and meal-planning sites can be effective support tools for patients in dietary counseling.

Approaches

Dietary counseling that is tailored to individual needs and tastes is more helpful and appropriate than general dietary advice. However, the best means of encouraging patients to follow dietary recommendations and elicit beneficial changes are often unclear. Positive feedback or implementation of a reward system helps some patients comply with dietary advice. It is often easier to introduce new behaviors than to eliminate established ones. For example, recommending that a patient start exercising regularly for weight loss may be more effective than trying to make dramatic changes in current dietary habits. Multiple simultaneous changes may be easier than a single behavior change, since multiple smaller changes can yield faster, more perceptible results. Dietary counseling should stress that lifestyle changes are not an all-or-none phenomenon and that clients should not give up because of setbacks. Counselors should stress the importance of persistence, since behavioral studies have shown that lifestyle changes are often characterized by abrupt forward and backward cycles, as well as periods of spiraling and stasis. Finally, prioritized goals are a critical part of dietary counseling, as is ongoing assessment of progress.

The transtheoretical (stages of change) model is one of the most popular models for changing health behaviors. This model classifies individuals into stages according to their degree of readiness to consider change and identifies the factors that can induce transitions from one stage to the next. It utilizes different types of skill training and advice at different stages and has shown promising results for dietary modifications.

Cognitive-behavioral strategies are also used in dietary counseling. In cognitive-behavioral therapy (CBT), the counselor interacts with patients as individuals; conveys interest, understanding, and acceptance; and provides ample opportunity for patients to express themselves. The counselor identifies the patient's readiness to change behavior, using empathy to identify less desirable dietary practices, and helps the patient recognize circumstances and scenarios that contribute to the undesirable behaviors. Next, the patient must come to understand and accept the need for changing behaviors that may be linked to stressful situations, work, family, economics, education, social, and various other factors. The counselor must then help patients develop independence and self-motivation to overcome inertia and make ordinary daily efforts. Finally, the counselor must help patients handle resistance to change and deal with recidivism.

Excess weight is a significant problem among American children and adolescents, and dietary counseling is one component of a multi-faceted intervention that includes promoting physical activity, parent training and modeling, behavioral counseling, and nutrition education. Family-based programs are geared toward children ages 5 to 12, and school-based programs are usually aimed at teens.

Availability

In the United States, the Affordable Care Act of 2010 and new regulations require that new health plans offer obesity screening and prevention and control of obesity-related diseases, as well as dietary counseling from physicians for promoting sustained weight loss, all without copayments. It is assumed that these provisions will significantly increase utilization of dietary counseling. However, relatively few physicians currently refer their patients for dietary counseling. For example, one study found that only about 15% of obese patients received recommendations for dietary counseling. Among overweight and obese patients enrolled in the Cholesterol Education and Research Trial, only about 15%–20% were referred for nutrition counseling. Thus, for these new provisions to have a significant impact, physicians will need to take the initiative and begin either performing dietary counseling themselves or referring their patients for counseling.

MNT is nutritional diagnostic, therapeutic, and counseling services for disease management provided by RDs. Medicare, the U.S. healthcare program for seniors, covers outpatient MNT for beneficiaries with diabetes, chronic renal insufficiency/end-stage renal disease, and kidney transplants. Many private insurance companies also cover MNT for various diseases and conditions. Patients generally receive three hours of MNT in the first year and two hours in subsequent years. Medicare covers additional hours when a diagnosis, condition, or treatment changes.

Preparation

Selecting an appropriate approach to dietary counseling first requires a comprehensive assessment of the individual's health, nutrition, lifestyle, and goals:

- medical history, including any nutrition-related illnesses, other diseases or conditions, lipid profiles, blood pressure, weight history and goals
- dietary analysis of calories, macronutrients, and micronutrients in the current diet
- risk assessment for chronic disease from a high-fat diet or a diet low in antioxidants or fruits and vegetables
- food-related attitudes and behaviors and personal food preferences and choices
- lifestyle factors including exercise and activity levels, work schedules, housing, cooking facilities, and time available for food preparation
- sociological evaluation including financial resources, cultural practices, support of family and friends, and social aspects of food consumption
- patient's knowledge of nutrition, readiness to learn, learning style, and openness to change

There are various dietary assessment tools. Among the most common are food records, dietary recall, food frequency questionnaires, diet histories, and biochemical indices. A scientific assessment of nutritional status combines information from clinical evaluations, biochemical tests, and dietary assessment. The clinical evaluation includes anthropometric measurements—height, weight, **body mass index** (BMI), and percent body fat as determined by the skin-fold test or hydrostatic weighing. A clinical evaluation may also include any signs of nutrient deficiencies in the mouth, skin, eyes, or nails. Biochemical tests provide a comprehensive picture of the patient's current nutritional status and relative risk factors.

KEY TERMS

Body mass index (BMI)—A measure of body fat; the ratio of weight in kilograms to the square of height in meters.

Cholesterol—A fat-soluble steroid alcohol found in animal fats and oils and produced in the body from saturated fats; high blood levels of low-density lipoprotein (LDL) or "bad" cholesterol increase the risk of heart disease, whereas high-density lipoprotein (HDL) or "good" cholesterol may protect against cardiovascular disease.

Cognitive-behavioral therapy (CBT)—A treatment that identifies negative thoughts and behaviors and helps develop more positive approaches.

Dietary Approaches to Stop Hypertension (DASH)—A flexible, balanced eating plan to help lower blood pressure.

Dietary assessment—An analysis of food and nutrients consumed over a particular time period, including food records, dietary recall, food frequency questionnaires, and diet histories.

Dietary reference intake (DRI)—A system of nutritional recommendations used by the Institute of Medicine of the U.S. National Academy of Sciences and the U.S. Department of Agriculture.

Hyperlipidemia—Excess fats or lipids in the blood.

Macronutrients—Carbohydrates, proteins, and fat that are required in relatively high amounts in the diet.

Medical nutrition therapy (MNT)—Dietary counseling for treating chronic disease.

Micronutrients—Nutrients, such as vitamins and minerals, that are required in minute amounts for growth and health.

Obesity—Excessive weight due to accumulation of fat; usually defined as a body mass index of 30 or above or body weight greater than 30% above normal on standard height-weight tables.

Overweight—A body mass index between 25 and 30.

Registered dietitian (RD)—A health professional with at least a bachelor's degree in nutrition who has undergone practical training and is legally registered.

Saturated fat—Hydrogenated fat; fat molecules that contain only single bonds, especially animal fats.

Trans fat—Fat that is produced by hydrogenation during food processing; trans fats increase bad cholesterol and decrease good cholesterol.

Triglycerides—Neutral fats; lipids formed from glycerol and fatty acids that circulate in the blood as lipoprotein. An elevated triglyceride level is a risk factor for diabetes.

Aftercare

Permanent modifications in dietary habits are the desired end-product of dietary counseling and are ultimately the responsibility of the patient. Minimal weight loss, or none at all, or minimal reduction in serum lipids is usually due to the patient's failure to comply with recommendations and instructions.

Complications

There are systematic problems with self-reported food intake. Patients must rely on their ability to honestly recall or record their food and resist impulses to "cheat" out of embarrassment or guilt for failing to follow recommendations. Careful selection of appropriate dietary assessments and counseling approaches can help alleviate these problems.

Over the long term, behavior changes, such as making healthier food choices and increasing physical activity, are much more successful—and more pleasurable—than dieting. Furthermore, most people cannot permanently follow a restrictive diet, so their food intake and weight eventually increase unless energy expenditure is increased through exercise or other means. Dieting can encourage "yo-yo" weight loss and gain, in which, typically, more weight is gained back than was initially lost. In addition, regained weight is often even less favorable because it may have a higher fat-to-muscle ratio. Because muscle is metabolically active tissue, it utilizes more **calories** even while at rest. This is only one of the reasons why exercise is so important for maintaining body weight.

Results

Results of dietary counseling vary greatly and depend on a number of factors, especially the patient's commitment to set goals. In general, the success of dietary counseling is limited, particularly with regard to weight loss and control. Nevertheless, studies have found that MNT improves patient outcomes and quality of life and lowers health care costs for those with or at risk for chronic diet-related conditions and illnesses.

QUESTIONS TO ASK YOUR DOCTOR

- Should I have dietary counseling?
- Do you provide dietary counseling or can you recommend someone?
- How many sessions will I need?
- Will my insurance cover dietary counseling?
- What results can I expect from dietary counseling?

Health care team roles

Dietary counseling is generally performed by RDs and registered dietary technicians, who have sufficient knowledge and training to accurately assess the nutritional adequacy of a patient's diet. Although some RDs call themselves nutritionists, the term "nutritionist" is not regulated by law in some states, so that anyone can call themselves nutritionists. Some physicians with adequate backgrounds specialize in nutritional counseling. However, medical school training in nutrition is limited, and physicians' visits are usually too brief to include nutritional counseling.

RDs and dietary technicians perform counseling in both clinics and community and public health settings. MNT is usually performed by an RD as part of a medical team in a hospital, clinic, health-maintenance organization, or other health care facility or in private practice. RDs also advocate for funding and the inclusion of dietary counseling in programs and policies at all levels and play an important role in researching improvements in dietary counseling.

Resources

BOOKS

King, Kathy. *The Entrepreneurial Nutritionist.* 4th ed. Philadelphia: Wolters Kluwer Health/Lippincott William & Wilkins, 2010.

Lee, Robert D., and David C. Nieman. *Nutritional Assessment.* 6th ed. New York: McGraw-Hill Science/Engineering/Math, 2013.

Samour, Patricia Queen, and Kathy King. *Pediatric Nutrition.* 4th ed. Sudbury, MA: Jones & Bartlett Learning, 2012.

PERIODICALS

Appelhans, Bradley M., et al. "Time to Abandon the Notion of Personal Choice in Dietary Counseling for Obesity?" *Journal of the American Dietetic Association* 111, no. 8 (August 2011): 1130.

Colleran, Heather L., and Cheryl A. Lovelady. "Use of MyPyramid Menu Planner for Moms in a Weight-Loss Intervention during Lactation." *Journal of the Academy of Nutrition and Dietetics* 112, no. 4 (April 2012): 553.

Louzada, Maria Laura da Costa, et al. "Long-term Effectiveness of Maternal Dietary Counseling in a Low-Income Population: A Randomized Field Trial." *Pediatrics* 129, no. 6 (June 2012): e1477–84.

Masheb, Robin M., Carlos M. Grilo, and Barbara J. Rolls. "A Randomized Controlled Trial for Obesity and Binge Eating Disorder: Low-Energy-Density Dietary Counseling and Cognitive-Behavioral Therapy." *Behaviour Research and Therapy* 49, no. 12 (December 2011): 821.

Niinikoski, Harri, et al. "Effect of Repeated Dietary Counseling on Serum Lipoproteins From Infancy to Adulthood." *Pediatrics* 129, no. 3 (March 2012): e704–13.

WEBSITES

Academy of Nutrition and Dietetics. "What Services Do RDs Provide?" http://www.eatright.org/HealthProfessionals/content.aspx?id = 6858 (accessed August 29, 2012)

Franklin, Barry A. "Counseling Patients to Favorably Modify Dietary and Physical Activity Practices." July 12, 2010. http://my.americanheart.org/professional/General/Counseling-Patients-to-Favorably-Modify-Dietary-and-Physical-Activity-Practices_UCM_432570_Article.jsp (accessed August 29, 2012).

National Heart, Lung, and Blood Institute. "National Cholesterol Education Program." National Institutes of Health. http://www.nhlbi.nih.gov/about/ncep (accessed October 2, 2012).

National Heart, Lung, and Blood Institute. "What Is the DASH Eating Plan?" National Institutes of Health. http://www.nhlbi.nih.gov/health/health-topics/topics/dash (accessed October 2, 2012).

U.S. Department of Agriculture. "ChooseMyPlate.gov." http://www.choosemyplate.gov (accessed August 31, 2012).

U.S. Department of Agriculture, Agricultural Research Service. "USDA National Nutrient Database for Standard Reference." http://www.ars.usda.gov/Services/docs.htm?docid = 8964 (accessed August 29, 2012).

U.S. Department of Agriculture, National Agricultural Library. "DRI Tables." Food and Nutrition Information Center. http://fnic.nal.usda.gov/dietary-guidance/dietary-reference-intakes/dri-tables (accessed August 16, 2012).

U.S. Department of Agriculture and U.S. Department of Health and Human Services. *Dietary Guidelines for Americans, 2010.* 7th ed. Washington, DC: U.S. Government Printing Office, December 2010. http://health.gov/dietaryguidelines (accessed September 27, 2012).

U.S. Department of Health and Human Services. Healthy People.gov. http://www.healthypeople.gov/2020/default.aspx (accessed August 29, 2012).

ORGANIZATIONS

Academy of Nutrition and Dietetics, 120 South Riverside Plz., Ste. 2000, Chicago, IL 60606-6995, (312) 899-0040, (800) 877-1600, amacmunn@eatright.org, http://www.eatright.org.

Food and Nutrition Information Center, National Agricultural Library, 10301 Baltimore Ave., Rm. 105, Beltsville, MD 20705, (301) 504-5414, Fax: (301) 504-6409, fnic@ars.usda.gov, http://fnic.nal.usda.gov.

International Food Information Council Foundation, 1100 Connecticut Ave., NW Ste. 430, Washington, DC 20036, (202) 296-6540, info@foodinsight.org, http://www.foodinsight.org.

U.S. Department of Health and Human Services, 200 Independence Avenue SW, Washington, DC 20201, (877) 696-6775, http://www.hhs.gov.

Crystal Heather Kaczkowski, MSc
Margaret Alic, PhD

Dietary guidelines

Definition

The *Dietary Guidelines for Americans* are the foundation of the national nutrition policy for the United States. They are designed to help Americans make food choices that promote health and reduce the risk of disease. The guidelines are published jointly by the U.S. Department of Agriculture (USDA) and the U.S. Department of Health and Human Services (HHS). The first set of guidelines was published as *Nutrition and Your Health: Dietary Guidelines for Americans* in 1980. Since then, an advisory committee has been appointed to review and revise the guidelines every five years based on the latest research in nutrition and health.

Description

Early dietary advice in the United States

The first half of the twentieth century was a period of enormous growth in nutrition knowledge. The primary goal of nutrition advice at this time was to help people select foods to meet their energy (calorie) needs and prevent diseases caused by nutritional deficiencies. During the Great Depression of the 1930s, many people had little money to buy food. They needed to know how to select an adequate diet with few resources. In response to this need, the USDA produced a set of meal plans that were affordable for families of various incomes. To this day, a food guide for low-income families—the Thrifty Food Plan—is issued regularly by the USDA and used to determine allotments in the

---

Supplemental Nutrition Assistance Program (SNAP), formerly called food stamps. In addition to meal plans, the USDA develops food guides as tools to help people select healthful diets. These food guides have changed over the years, based on the most recent research and information available.

Food guides versus dietary guidelines

Food guides are practical tools that people can use to select a healthful diet. Food guide recommendations, such as how much **protein** to eat daily, are based on dietary guidelines that are overall recommendations for well-rounded diets. For example, the *Dietary Guidelines for Americans* issued in 2010 emphasized consuming fewer **calories** and included the recommendation that Americans "make half [their] plate fruits and vegetables." The current USDA food guide, based on the 2010 dietary guidelines, is called **MyPlate**. MyPlate was issued in June 2011. It replaced various versions of the food pyramid that had been used for 19 years. MyPlate simplifies food choice recommendations and shows them in a clear graphic of a plate divided into 30% grains, 30% vegetables, 20% fruits, and 20% protein. A smaller circle separate from the plate represents dairy products. Supplemental MyPlate recommendations include eating smaller portions, choosing **whole grains** over refined grains (e.g., brown rice instead of white rice), choosing dairy products made with skim or low-fat milk, and reducing **sugar** and salt intake. Adjustments are made for special groups, such as children under two and pregnant or **breastfeeding** women.

Evolution of the dietary guidelines

During the 1970s, scientists began identifying links between people's eating habits and their risk for developing chronic diseases, such as heart disease, type 2 diabetes, and **cancer**. They realized that a healthful diet was important not only to prevent diseases caused by nutrient deficiencies but also because it could play a role in decreasing the risk of developing chronic diseases. Since heart disease, diabetes, and cancer were, and still are, major causes of death and disability in the United States, there was a need to help Americans select diets that promoted good health. It

---

later became evident that a healthful diet is one of the most affordable and effective modes of treatment and management of chronic diseases.

The first major step in federal dietary guidance was the 1977 publication of *Dietary Goals for the United States* by the Senate Select Committee on Nutrition and Human Needs. The publication recommended an increased intake of **carbohydrates** and a reduced intake of fat, saturated fat, cholesterol, **sodium** (salt), and sugar. At the time, there was heated debate among nutrition scientists about these recommendations. Some nutritionists believed that not enough was known about effects of diet on health to make suggestions as specific as those given.

In 1980, the first edition of *Dietary Guidelines for Americans* was released by the USDA and HHS. The seven guidelines were:

1. Eat a variety of foods.
2. Maintain ideal weight.
3. Avoid too much fat, saturated fat, and cholesterol.
4. Eat foods with adequate starch and fiber.
5. Avoid too much sugar.
6. Avoid too much sodium (salt).
7. Drink alcohol only in moderation.

The second edition, released in 1985, made a few changes, but kept most of the guidelines intact. Two exceptions were the weight guideline, which was changed to "maintain desirable weight" and the last guideline, in which "alcohol" was changed to "alcoholic beverages."

Following publication of the second edition of the *Dietary Guidelines*, two influential reports concerning diet and health were issued. The *Surgeon General's Report on Nutrition and Health* was published in 1988, and the National Research Council's report *Diet and Health—Implications for Reducing Chronic Disease Risk* was published in 1989. These two reports supported the goal of the guidelines to promote eating habits to help people stay healthy. In 1990, the third edition of the guidelines took a more positive tone than previous editions, using phrases such as "choose a diet," or "use . . . only in moderation," rather than "avoid too much. . ." This was seen as a positive step by many nutrition educators.

The fourth edition was the first to include the Food Guide Pyramid, which had been introduced in 1992. It also was the first edition to address vegetarian diets and the recently introduced "Nutrition Facts" panel for food labels. The fifth edition, issued in 2000, expanded the number of guidelines to ten and

---

QUESTIONS TO ASK YOUR DOCTOR

- Do I have any diseases or conditions that require different dietary practices?
- Do you have any literature that could help me implement the guidelines in my own life?
- Do you have a registered dietitian on staff? Would my insurance cover a consultation?
- How would these guidelines change for the other members of my family?

---

organized them into three messages: "Aim for Fitness, Build a Healthy Base, and Choose Sensibly" (ABC).

With the sixth edition in 2005, a redesigned food pyramid called MyPyramid was introduced. MyPyramid was intended to help Americans become more aware of what they eat and their nutrient needs. It was designed to help people learn how to eat a healthy diet, live an active lifestyle, and maintain or gradually move in the direction of a healthy weight that would reduce the risk of weight-related diseases. Unlike earlier diet and nutrition guides, MyPyramid personalized dietary recommendations based on the individual's height, weight, age, gender, activity level, and weight goals. MyPyramid was not well received by many nutrition educators who felt the graphic was confusing and the advice so overwhelmingly detailed and specific that it would discourage the average person. MyPyramid was replaced in June 2011 with the simpler MyPlate graphic and guidelines.

The 2010 Dietary Guidelines for Americans

On January 31, 2011, the USDA and HHS announced the 2010 *Dietary Guidelines for Americans*. The 2010 release was the seventh edition of the guidelines and was developed specifically to help combat the increasing **obesity** problem in the United States. It focused on providing recommendations that were simple to understand and easy for busy people to put into practice in their daily lives.

Some of the guidelines from the 2010 directive include:

- Enjoy your food, but eat less.
- Avoid oversized portions.
- Make half your plate fruits and vegetables.
- Drink water instead of sugary drinks.
- Switch to fat-free or low-fat milk.

(AMDRs) for energy-yielding nutrients. AMDRs are expressed not as absolute numbers but as a percentage of total energy (calorie) intake.

DRIs are intended as guidelines for population groups, not individuals. Although they assign values for daily intake of nutrients, these values are intended to apply over time. Except in cases of acute megadoses, the effects of too much or too little of a nutrient develop gradually over time. In any given day, an individual may eat more or less than the DRI of a particular nutrient and still remain healthy, so long as their average intake over time complies with recommendations.

Precautions

DRIs are intended to be applied to a healthy population. Individuals under the supervision of a healthcare professional may be advised to take more or less of particular nutrients than the DRIs indicate. In this situation, the advice of the healthcare professional should be followed.

Certain people, such as vegans, have dietary needs that may be satisfied only with very carefully controlled diets or additional dietary supplements.

Interactions

Nutrients interact with each other and with pharmaceuticals and herbal remedies. These interactions are not entirely understood and may affect the absorption, utilization, and excretion of various vitamins and minerals in ways that change the RDA.

Complications

The four components of the DRI are intended to provide more guidance than a single number alone would provide. However, they are not without critics. Some criticism stems from statistical assumptions made in the calculations; other critiques are based on the fact that different forms of certain nutrients have a different bioavailability. For example, **iron** in meat is more easily absorbed than iron in plant foods, and the **vitamin E** in dietary supplements is more biologically active than vitamin E in food. Although this should not be a source of confusion to healthcare professionals, it can be confusing to the average consumer.

The greatest controversies among experts are over the UL. These center around five areas:

1. Very little experimental data is available about the upper limit of certain nutrients in special populations, such as children, pregnant women, and elderly individuals.

KEY TERMS

Amino acid—Molecules that are the basic building blocks of proteins.

Bioavailability—The degree to which a compound can be absorbed and used by the body.

Dietary supplement—A product, such as a vitamin, mineral, herb, amino acid, or enzyme, that is intended to be consumed in addition to (supplement) an individual's diet with the expectation that it will improve health.

Fatty acids—Complex molecules found in fats and oils. Essential fatty acids are fatty acids that the body needs but cannot synthesize. They are made by plants and must be present in the diet to maintain health.

Macronutrient—A substance needed in large quantities to maintain growth and health, such as the energy-producing molecules that come from proteins, carbohydrates, and fats.

Micronutrient—Substances that are needed in very small, even trace, amounts to maintain normal growth and health.

Mineral—An inorganic substance found in the earth that is necessary in small quantities for the body to maintain health. Examples include zinc, copper, and iron.

Toxic—Harmful or poisonous to the body.

Vitamin—A nutrient that the body needs in small amounts to remain healthy.

2. Some experts are not comfortable with the way the Institute of Medicine derived UL values. Experts point out that in some cases, the UL for one subgroup overlaps the RDA for another subgroup, and in other cases the typical intake of certain groups already exceeds the UL with no apparent harmful effects (e.g., iron in young children). The vitamin C UL appears to be especially controversial.

3. No distinction is made between short-term (acute) and long-term (chronic) overdose of nutrients.

4. The ULs do not take into consideration the genetic diversity of the population and are much less sensitive to the life stage of an individual than RDAs. (This is in part due to the limited data available for certain age groups.)

5. Much of the data used to determine the UL is based on short-term (a few days) intake information and therefore has a high degree of unreliability. Human experiments with potentially toxic megadoses of nutrients is generally unethical, making an adequate amount of reliable data in the UL range difficult to obtain.

DRIs continue to be researched and revised as more data becomes available. Despite any surrounding controversy, DRIs offer both healthcare professionals and individual consumers some guidelines about the benefits and dangers of nutrient consumption.

Parental concerns

Parents should discuss DRIs with a healthcare professional who can translate them into practical healthy eating tips for use in providing a healthy diet for their children. A diet high in fruits and vegetables and low in fats will meet most DRIs for both children and adults.

Resources

BOOKS

Otten, Jennifer J., Jennifer Pitzi Hellwig, and Linda D. Meyers, eds. *DRI, Dietary Reference Intakes: The Essential Guide to Nutrient Requirements*. Washington, DC: National Academies Press, 2006.

Panel on Dietary Antioxidants and Related Compounds, Subcommittees on Upper Reference Levels of Nutrients and of Interpretation and Use of Dietary Reference Intakes, and the Standing Committee on the Scientific Evaluation of Dietary Reference Intakes, Food and Nutrition Board, Institute of Medicine. *Dietary Reference Intakes for Vitamin C, Vitamin E, Selenium, and Carotenoids*. Washington, DC: National Academy Press, 2000.

Panel on Dietary Reference Intakes for Electrolytes and Water, Standing Committee on the Scientific Evaluation of Dietary Reference Intakes, Food and Nutrition Board. *DRI, Dietary Reference Intakes for Water, Potassium, Sodium, Chloride, and Sulfate*. Washington, DC: National Academies Press, 2005.

Panel on Macronutrients, Panel on the Definition of Dietary Fiber, Subcommittee on Upper Reference Levels of Nutrients, Subcommittee on Interpretation and Uses of Dietary Reference Intakes, and the Standing Committee on the Scientific Evaluation of Dietary Reference Intakes, Food and Nutrition Board, Institute of Medicine of the National Academies. *Dietary Reference Intakes for Energy, Carbohydrate, Fiber, Fat, Fatty Acids, Cholesterol, Protein, and Amino Acids*. Washington, DC: National Academies Press, 2005.

Panel on Micronutrients and the Standing Committee on the Scientific Evaluation of Dietary Reference Intakes, Food and Nutrition Board, Institute of Medicine. *DRI: Dietary Reference Intakes For Vitamin A, Vitamin K, Arsenic, Boron, Chromium, Copper, Iodine, Iron, Manganese, Molybdenum, Nickel, Silicon, Vanadium, and Zinc*. Washington, DC: National Academy Press, 2001.

Ross, Catharine A., et al, eds. *Dietary Reference Intakes for Calcium and Vitamin D*. Washington, DC: National Academies Press, 2011.

Sizer, Frances, and Eleanor Whitney. *Nutrition Concepts and Controversies*. 12th ed. Belmont, CA: Cengage Learning, 2010.

Standing Committee on the Scientific Evaluation of Dietary Reference Intakes and its Panel on Folate, Other B Vitamins, and Choline and Subcommittee on Upper Reference Levels of Nutrients, Food and Nutrition Board, Institute of Medicine. *Dietary Reference Intakes for Thiamin, Riboflavin, Niacin, Vitamin B$_6$, Folate, Vitamin B$_{12}$, Pantothenic Acid, Biotin, and Choline*. Washington, DC: National Academy Press, 1998.

PERIODICALS

Butte, N. F., et al. "Nutrient Intakes of U.S. Infants, Toddlers, and Preschoolers Meet or Exceed Dietary Reference Intakes." *Journal of the American Dietetic Association* 110, suppl. 12 (2010): S27–37

Hambidge, K. M. "Micronutrient Bioavailability: Dietary Reference Intakes and a Future Perspective." *American Journal of Clinical Nutrition* 91, no. 5 (2010): 1430S–32S.

Kniskern, M. A., and C. S. Johnston. "Protein Dietary Reference Intakes May Be Inadequate for Vegetarians If Low Amounts of Animal Protein are Consumed." *Nutrition* 27, no. 6 (2011): 727–30.

Kris-Etherton, P. M., J. A. Grieger, and T. D. Etherton. "Dietary Reference Intakes for DHA and EPA." *Prostaglandins, Leukotrienes, and Essential Fatty Acids* 81, nos. 2–3 (2009): 99–104.

Murphy, S. P., and S. I. Barr. "Practice Paper of the American Dietetic Association: Using the Dietary Reference Intakes." *Journal of the American Dietetic Association* 111, no. 5 (May 2011): 762–70.

Ross, A. C., et al. "The 2011 Dietary Reference Intakes for Calcium and Vitamin D: What Dietetics Practitioners Need to Know." *Journal of the American Dietetic Association* 111, no. 4 (2011): 524–27.

OTHER

U.S. Department of Agriculture and U.S. Department of Health and Human Services. *Dietary Guidelines for Americans, 2010*. 7th ed. Washington, DC: U.S. Government Printing Office, December 2010. http://www.health.gov/dietaryguidelines/dga2010/DietaryGuidelines2010.pdf (accessed August 19, 2012).

WEBSITES

Council Responsible for Nutrition. "Vitamin and Mineral Recommendations." http://www.crnusa.org/about_recs.html (accessed August 19, 2012).

Food and Nutrition Information Center. "Dietary Reference Intakes." National Agricultural Library, U.S. Department of Agriculture. http://fnic.nal.usda.gov/dietary-guidance/dietary-reference-intakes (accessed August 19, 2012).

(DDS or DMD), registered nurses (RN), licensed practical nurses (LPN), pharmacists, and similar health care professionals. Some dietary supplements are routinely used as an accepted part of conventional medicine. The most common of these are vitamin and mineral supplements taken in accordance with established **dietary reference intakes (DRIs)**. **DRIs** are a set of values for different nutrients that indicate the daily amount of that nutrient necessary to meet the needs of most individuals, as well as the largest amount of the nutrient that can be consumed daily without harmful effects. Other supplements, such as folic acid, are prescribed for pregnant women in order to decrease the risk of neural tube defects in their offspring. Still other supplements, such as enzymes, may be given when the body fails to produce adequate amounts of the enzyme as the result of a genetic disorder, such as cystic fibrosis. When taken under supervision of a conventional health care professional, dietary supplements tend to be extremely safe.

Dietary supplements in complementary and alternative medicine

Most dietary supplements are used within a system of complementary and alternative medicine (CAM). Complementary medicine uses treatments that are not part of conventional medicine to supplement conventional medicine. Alternative medicine uses treatments that are not part of conventional medicine as a complete replacement for conventional medicine. Alternative medicine includes well-established treatment systems, such as homeopathy, Traditional Chinese medicine (TCM), and Ayurvedic medicine (traditional Indian medicine), as well as newer fad-driven treatments. Many CAM treatments have their roots in tradition and folklore.

Herbs are some of the most common dietary supplements used in CAM. Many have been used for hundreds of years and show evidence of effectiveness. Others are ineffective or may harm the individual either directly or when used as a replacement for conventional drugs and treatments whose effectiveness has been proven. Vitamin and mineral supplements used as part of conventional medicine become part of the CAM system when they are used in megadoses that far exceed DRI values or when they are used to prevent or treat a specific condition, such as **vitamin C** to prevent colds. Likewise, enzymes and amino acids that have specific uses within conventional medicine become part of the CAM system of dietary supplements when they are used in non-conventional ways or in non-standard doses. Some dietary supplements, such as bee pollen, are used exclusively in CAM.

KEY TERMS

Alternative medicine—A system of healing that rejects conventional, pharmaceutical-based medicine and replaces it with the use of dietary supplements and therapies, such as herbs, vitamins, minerals, massage, and cleansing diets. Alternative medicine includes well-established treatment systems such as homeopathy, Traditional Chinese medicine (TCM), and Ayurvedic medicine.

Amino acid—Molecules that are the basic building blocks of proteins.

Botanical—An herb; a dietary supplement derived from a plant.

Complementary medicine—Includes many of the same treatments used in alternative medicine, but uses them to supplement conventional drug and therapy treatments, rather than to replace conventional medicine.

Conventional medicine—Mainstream or Western pharmaceutical-based medicine practiced by medical doctors, doctors of osteopathy, and other licensed health care professionals.

Enzyme—Proteins that change the rate of a chemical reaction within the body without themselves being used up in the reaction.

Herb—A plant used in cooking or for medical purposes. Examples include Echinacea and ginseng.

Mineral—An inorganic substance found in the earth that is necessary in small quantities for the body to maintain health. Examples include zinc, copper, and iron.

Vitamin—A nutrient that the body needs in small amounts to remain healthy but that the body cannot adequately manufacture for itself and must acquire through diet.

Precautions

It is difficult to determine whether dietary supplements are safe or effective because of the loose way that they are regulated. Many of the studies done on supplements are poorly designed, have a small sample size, or are sponsored by the manufacturer of the supplement, making the results questionable. Natural Standard is an independent organization that evaluates studies, scientific evidence, and expert opinion on CAM treatments and therapies and makes impartial judgments concerning their safety and effectiveness. The National Center for Complementary and

Alternative Medicine is a government organization within the National Institutes of Health that investigates CAM treatments and runs rigorous clinical trials to determine safety and effectiveness.

Individuals interested in using dietary supplements should consult their health care provider and other reputable sources of information before taking any new supplements. Pregnant or **breastfeeding** women should be especially careful to discuss the supplements they may want to take with their health care provider. Many herbs and other dietary supplements cross the placenta or are secreted into breast milk and may affect the fetus or nursing baby. In addition, care should be taken in giving children dietary supplements. Few studies have been done specifically on children and the recommended dosage for adults may be harmful to children. As with any medication, more is not necessarily better. Overdose is a common cause of adverse side effects in dietary supplements. In the event of side effects, the supplement should be stopped immediately and the side effects reported to a health care professional.

Interactions

Dietary supplements may interact with both conventional drugs and other herbs or dietary supplements. Individuals should seek information about specific interactions from their health care provider. Many dietary supplements should be stopped several days before surgery to reduce the risk of excess bleeding.

Complications

There is strong evidence that some dietary supplements can cause serious harm or death. For example, the weight-loss supplement **ephedra** was found to have contributed to the death of the Baltimore Orioles pitching prospect Steve Belcher in 2003. The FDA later banned ephedra-containing supplements. According to the American Association of Poison Control Centers, in 2009 there were more than 64,000 reports of adult vitamin poisonings. There were also over 19,000 cases in children under age five of poisoning by dietary supplements, herbal medicines, or homeopathic remedies; two children died. It should be remembered that "natural" does not mean safe; for example, many wild mushrooms are completely natural and cause death when eaten.

Complications may arise from dietary supplements themselves, their misuse, or poor regulation of the manufacturing process. This is especially true of those supplements imported into the United States

from developing countries. Independent laboratory analyses of dietary supplements have found:

• contamination with pesticides
• contamination with heavy metals
• presence of ingredients not listed on the label
• amount of dietary ingredients not the same as the amount listed on the label

Some health professionals believe the number of complications related to dietary supplements is severely under-reported.

Parental concerns

Parents should be aware that the recommended dietary allowances (RDAs) and tolerable upper intake levels (ULs) for vitamins and minerals are much lower for children than for adults. Accidental overdose may occur if children are given adult vitamins or dietary supplements.

Resources

BOOKS

Bonakdar, Robert A. *The H.E.R.B.A.L. Guide: Dietary Supplement Resources for the Clinician*. Philadelphia: Wolters Kluwer Health/Lippincott Williams & Wilkins, 2010.

PDR Staff. *PDR for Nonprescription Drugs, Dietary Supplements, and Herbs 2010*. 31st ed. PDR Network, 2010.

WEBSITES

MedlinePlus. "Dietary Supplements." U.S. National Library of Medicine, National Institutes of Health. http://www.nlm.nih.gov/medlineplus/dietarysupplements.html (accessed August 2, 2012).

———. "Herbal Medicine." U.S. National Library of Medicine, National Institutes of Health. http://www.nlm.nih.gov/medlineplus/herbalmedicine.html (accessed August 2, 2012).

National Center for Complementary and Alternative Medicine (NCCAM). "Dietary and Herbal Supplements." National Institutes of Health. http://nccam.nih.gov/health/supplements (accessed August 2, 2012).

QUESTIONS TO ASK YOUR DOCTOR

- Do I need to take dietary supplements?
- What form of supplements are more effective?
- Can I overdose on dietary supplements?
- What is missing from my diet that I need supplements?

Office of Inspector General, U.S. Department of Health and Human Services. *Dietary Supplements: Structure/Function Claims Fail To Meet Federal Requirements*, OEI-01-11-00210. October 2, 2012. https://oig.hhs.gov/oei/reports/oei-01-11-00210.asp (accessed August 2, 2012).

U.S. Office of Dietary Supplements. "Dietary Supplements: Background Information." National Institutes of Health. http://dietary-supplements.info.nih.gov/factsheets/dietarysupplements.asp (accessed August 2, 2012).

ORGANIZATIONS

American Botanical Council, PO Box 144345, Austin, TX 78714, (512) 926-4900, (800) 373-7105, Fax: (512) 926-2345, abc@herbalgram.org, http://abc.herbalgram.org.

Council for Responsible Nutrition, 1828 L St. NW, Ste. 510, Washington, DC 20036, (202) 204-7700, Fax: (202) 204-7701, webmaster@crnusa.org, http://www.crnusa.org.

National Center for Complementary and Alternative Medicine Clearinghouse, PO Box 7923, Gaithersburg, MD 20898, (888) 644-6226, Fax: (888) 464-3616, info@nccam.nih.gov, http://nccam.nih.gov.

Natural Standard, One Davis Sq., Somerville, MA 02144, (617) 591-3300, Fax: (617) 591-3399, questions@naturalstandard.com, http://www.naturalstandard.com.

Office of Dietary Supplements, National Institutes of Health, 6100 Executive Blvd., Rm. 3B01, MSC 7517, Bethesda, MD 20892-7517, (301) 435-2920, Fax: (301) 480-1845, ods@nih.gov, http://ods.od.nih.gov.

Tish Davidson, A.M.

Dietwatch

Definition

Dietwatch is an online weight-loss program that focuses on helping dieters lose weight at a moderate, healthy pace through healthy eating, regular exercise, and motivational support.

Origins

Dietwatch was launched in 1999. It is an online-only program, and can be found at http://www.dietwatch.com. In December 2000, Dietwatch acquired cyberdiet.com, which greatly expanded its operations. Since its launch, more than a million people have visited the website. Dietwatch has won a number of awards for excellence in Internet content, including a "Best of the Web Award" from *Forbes* magazine. It is operated by DietWatch.com, Inc., which is headquartered in East Rockaway, New York.

The nutritional aspects of Dietwatch are headed by Jennifer May, the manager of nutritional services.

She is a registered dietitian who holds both a masters degree in nutrition science and a masters degree in exercise physiology, both from Indiana University. The Mastering Eating program was developed by Dr. Roger Gould. Dr. Gould has published a variety of scholarly articles and was the head of the University of California, Los Angeles outpatient and community psychiatry department.

Description

Dietwatch is an online program designed to support and guide dieters to healthy, maintainable weight loss. It provides advice from fitness and nutrition experts, meal plans, and tips and motivation, as well as an online community where dieters can help each other through dieting's rough patches.

There are four options for meal plans provided by Dietwatch. It offers a "no restrictions" plan that is simply a reduced-calorie, well-balanced diet. Dietwatch says that this is the plan for dieters who do not have any specific concerns or preferences, as it includes a variety of types and styles of food. Another available plan is the "reduced carbs plan," which limits **carbohydrates** to 40% of a dieter's total caloric intake each day. This is not a low carbohydrate plan but a limited carbohydrate plan. Unlike popular low carb diets such as Atkins, it does not restrict carbohydrates to just a few grams each day.

Another diet option is the "heart healthy Mediterranean plan," which limits saturated and **trans fats** while including a high level of unsaturated **fats**. The style of the food and diet is Mediterranean and combines many flavors and food groups. The last meal plan alternative is the "vegetarian plan," which is a plan specially designed to meet the **protein** and other needs of vegetarians who are on a diet. The plan does include eggs and milk products, but no chicken, fish, or meat.

Customers can personalize the meal plans offered by Dietwatch by switching meals or ingredients to meet individual preferences. The program also offers shopping lists that are customized to the dieter's meal plan. This makes the meal plan easier to fit into a busy schedule.

In addition to meal plans, Dietwatch offers exercise and fitness plans and advice that the dieter can use to help customize a fitness plan to meet individual needs. There are a variety or strength training, aerobic, relaxation, and other suggested workouts available.

Motivation and emotional health are important aspects of Dietwatch. There are motivational tips from nutritionists and other experts, as well as discussion boards where dieters share frustrations, achievements, and tips. Dieters can search based on age, sex, weight, or other characteristics to find dieters to partner with for more one-on-one motivation and help.

Behavior understanding and modification is an important aspect of the Dietwatch program. Dr. Roger Gould developed a program called Mastering Food that is available to Dietwatch members. It is a 12-week program designed to help dieters overcome negative eating habits. Its goal is to help dieters discover why they eat when they are not hungry and find ways to deal with the problems underlying their eating behaviors. Overcoming emotional eating problems can help dieters be more successful in sticking to their diets and allow for more productive, successful weight loss.

Dietwatch also offers a variety of tools that can be used at the dieter's discretion. A food journal lets dieters track everything that they eat each day. The tracker can tally **calories**, fat grams, and other information to help dieters ensure that they are getting all the nutrients they need. Also available is a tool for tracking a dieter's daily calorie balance. This tool combines information about activity level and exercise with information about food eaten during the day to come up with the total calorie balance. This way dieters can check to see that they are burning more calories than they are taking in and if they are on track for their desired weight loss.

There is a wealth of information available on Dietwatch for dieters who are interested in learning more about health and nutrition. There is information about different nutrients and how they work in the body and explanations about why certain nutrients are required for good health. Also available is nutritional information for many foods, including information about a number of different restaurants. There is also general information about eating well and maintaining a healthy approach to food.

Function

Dietwatch is intended to help dieters make long-term comprehensive lifestyle changes that will help them lose weight and keep it off. To do this, it helps dieters with healthy eating and moderate exercise, as well as stress reduction and other techniques aimed at better emotional health. The newest program, the Mastering Eating program, is intended to help dieters identify and change negative eating habits for better control over food in their lives. Dietwatch is also intended to help dieters become more fit and to attain overall better health.

KEY TERMS

Dietary supplement—A product, such as a vitamin, mineral, herb, amino acid, or enzyme, that is intended to be consumed in addition to an individual's diet with the expectation that it will improve health.

Mineral—An inorganic substance found in the earth that is necessary in small quantities for the body to maintain health. Examples: zinc, copper, iron.

Vitamin—A nutrient that the body needs in small amounts to remain healthy but that the body cannot manufacture for itself and must acquire through diet.

Benefits

There are many benefits to losing weight if it is done at a moderate pace through healthy eating and increased exercise. **Obesity** is a risk factor for many diseases and conditions including type 2 diabetes, cardiovascular disease, and **hypertension**. People who are the most obese are generally at the greatest risk and are likely to have more severe symptoms if these diseases develop. Losing weight can reduce the risk of these and other obesity-related diseases, and in some cases it can help reduce the severity of symptoms if the diseases have already occurred.

The Dietwatch program is designed to provide dieters with support for all the phases and processes of weight loss. Many dieters may find having all this support and information available in one place to be very helpful. The nutritional information may help dieters make more informed eating decisions, especially when eating out. The inclusion of a vegetarian meal planning option makes this diet available for vegetarian dieters who may be underserved by other diets offering meal plans.

One of the main aspects of the Dietwatch program is motivation. This comes in many forms including helpful and motivational tips from nutritionists and other dieters. Many dieters may find that the opportunity to find a dieting buddy that shares their same goals and challenges provides support that is more personal and effective than is usually available in commercial diet programs. Many dieters may also appreciate the opportunity to ask dietitians and other health professionals specific questions instead of relying on general information.

Precautions

Anyone thinking of beginning a new diet should consult a doctor or other medical professional.

Individuals have different requirements for calories, **vitamins**, **minerals**, and other nutrients. Talking to a doctor can help dieters ensure that a new diet is the right diet to meet all their personal needs and that weight loss can be achieved without sacrificing good health. Pregnant and **breastfeeding** women should be especially cautious when beginning a new diet because what a mother eats can have a significant impact on a baby.

Risks

There are some risks to any diet. Eating a limited diet can make it difficult for a dieter to get all of the vitamins and minerals required for good health. Generally, when following a good diet that contains many different fruits and vegetables this risk is not too significant, but dieters may want to consult a doctor about taking a multivitamin or dietary supplement to help reduce the risk of deficiency.

When beginning a new exercise routine, it is important that dieters begin with light or moderate exercise and slowly increase the intensity of the activity over weeks or months. Suddenly beginning a strenuous exercise routine can have many risks, especially if the dieter has been inactive for many years. Less serious risks include the risk of straining or spraining a muscle, but more serious risks can even include heart attack if the exercise is very strenuous and is begun suddenly. Risk of injury during exercise can be reduced if proper warm up and cool down procedures are followed, including stretching all appropriate muscle groups. Dieters should consult a doctor before beginning any new exercise routine, especially if it is possible that they have heart disease or other cardiovascular problems that might put them at high risk for serious injury.

Research and general acceptance

The diets and activities recommended by Dietwatch generally meet the standards for moderate weight loss of 1–2 pounds a week. This weight loss can be achieved through moderately reduced calorie meal plans and regular exercise. This is the approach that most experts recommend to successfully achieve permanent weight loss and better health.

The U.S. Department of Agriculture provides dietary recommendations in its *Dietary Guidelines for Americans*, updated every five years. These recommendations are illustrated by **MyPlate**, which replaced the former food pyramid. Any diet that follows these basic guidelines for good health is generally considered a safe and healthy diet for most people. Dietwatch's personalized daily food log can help dieters determine how many calories, grams of fat, carbohydrates, and amounts of other nutrients are eaten each day. This can help dieters ensure that they are following guidelines for a healthy diet.

The Centers for Disease Control recommends that healthy adults get 30 minutes or more of light to moderate exercise each day for good health. Although Dietwatch does not make specific exercise plans for each individual, most of their recommendations meet or exceed this minimum recommendation. Studies have shown that exercise and diet are more effective at producing weight loss when done together than either diet or exercise done alone. Dietwatch encourages dieters not only to combine diet and exercise, but also to alter problem eating behaviors, which many experts believe is important for long-term weight loss.

QUESTIONS TO ASK YOUR DOCTOR

- Is this diet the best diet to meet my goals?
- Will I need to take a multivitamin or other dietary supplement on this diet?
- Do I have any special nutritional needs that this diet might not meet?
- Is it safe for me to start exercising?
- Does diet or exercise pose any special risks for me that I should be aware of?
- Is this diet appropriate for my entire family?
- Is it safe for me to follow this diet over a long period of time?
- Are there any signs or symptoms that might indicate a problem while on this diet?

Resources

BOOKS

Larsen, Laura, ed. *Diet and Nutrition Sourcebook*. Detroit, MI: Omnigraphics, 2006.

Willis, Alicia P., ed. *Diet Therapy Research Trends*. New York: Nova Science, 2007.

WEBSITES

"DietWatch." http://www.dietwatch.com (accessed September 28, 2012).

U.S. Department of Agriculture. "MyPlate." http://www.choosemyplate.gov (accessed September 28, 2012).

ORGANIZATIONS

DietWatch.com, Inc., 336 Atlantic Ave., Ste. 301, East Rockaway, NY 11518, http://www.dietwatch.com.

Tish Davidson, A.M.

Digestive diseases

Definition

Digestive diseases, also called gastrointestinal diseases, are diseases that affect the digestive system, which consists of the organs, pathways, and processes responsible for processing food in the body.

Demographics

According to the National Center for Health Statistics, 60 to 70 million people were affected by digestive diseases in 2010. In 2004, digestive diseases accounted for 13.5 million hospitalizations and 236,164 deaths. In 2006 (the last year for which data are available), 20 million had ambulatory surgical procedures and 5.5 million people underwent diagnostic and therapeutic in-patient procedures for digestive diseases. The resulting cost was as an estimated $141.8 billion direct and indirect dollars in health care.

Description

The digestive system, or digestive tract, includes the oral cavity, esophagus, stomach, small intestine, biliary tract, pancreas, large intestine, gallbladder, colon, rectum, and anus, which are all linked as a long twisting tube that starts at the mouth and ends at the anus. It also includes the liver and pancreas, two organs that produce substances needed for digestion, such as enzymes. The function of the digestive system is to transform ingested food for use by the cells that make up the body. Food enters through the mouth and proceeds to the gut (digestive tract), where it is chemically modified (digested) for absorption by the body or for waste disposal. Digestive diseases are numerous and can affect any part of the digestive system.

Oral cavity, esophagus, and stomach

Diseases of the oral cavity, esophagus, and stomach include:

- Poor oral health, including ailing teeth, tongue, or salivary glands. For many people with malnutrition, poor oral health is a causative factor.
- Poor esophageal health. Problems in the esophagus can affect the ability to swallow, which can place a person at risk for nutritional deficiencies if they are not consuming enough food.
- Dysphagia, or difficulty swallowing.
- Achalasia, characterized by a feeling of fullness in the chest with frequent vomiting.
- Stricture, which is a narrowing of the esophagus that interferes with food intake.

- Gastroesophageal reflux disease (GERD), a burning sensation in the chest or throat caused by the reflux of stomach acid.
- Hiatal hernia, which is the presence of the stomach in the chest cavity.
- Scleroderma, a connective tissue disease that often involves the GI tract and can cause gastroparesis; also called delayed gastric emptying.
- Gastroparesis, which causes slow digestion and emptying, vomiting, nausea, and bloating.
- Peptic ulcer. Ulcers are sores that can be as deep as the muscle layer lining the esophagus (esophageal ulcer) or stomach (gastric ulcer).
- Dumping syndrome, a group of symptoms that occur after eating a high amount of carbohydrates and results in a feeling of fullness, flushing, sweating, and low blood pressure.

Liver, pancreas, and gallbladder

Diseases of the liver, pancreas, and gallbladder include:

- Budd-Chiari syndrome, a rare liver disease in which the veins that drain blood from the liver are blocked or narrowed.
- Cholecystitis, an infection of the gallbladder.
- Cirrhosis, a life-threatening disease that scars liver tissue and damages its cells. It severely affects liver function, preventing it from removing toxins such as alcohol and drugs from the blood.
- Hepatitis, an inflammation of the liver that can result in permanent liver damage.
- Non-alcoholic fatty liver disease (NAFLD), an inflammation of the liver related to insulin resistance, obesity, type 2 diabetes, and high blood pressure.
- Pancreatitis, an irritation of the pancreas that can alter its structure and its function.
- Primary biliary cirrhosis (PBC), a liver disease that slowly destroys the bile ducts in the liver, thus preventing the release of bile.
- Primary sclerosing cholangitis (PSC), characterized by an irritation, scarring, and narrowing of the liver bile ducts. The accumulation of bile in the liver damages liver cells.

Small and large intestines

Diseases of the small and large intestines include:

- Appendicitis, characterized by an inflammation of the appendix, the small, finger-like structure attached to the first part of the large intestine.

products, it suggests lactose intolerance. Celiac disease is also accompanied by recurring abdominal pain.

- Bloating. Abdominal bloating is a symptom of lactose intolerance, celiac disease, IBS, and diverticulosis.
- Changes in bowel movements. Yellow and greasy stools that float are indicative of impaired pancreas function or celiac disease. Excess gas and loose, foul-smelling stools are a symptom of giardiasis or various bowel infections. Alternating loose and hard bowel movements are indicative of IBS.
- Bloody stools. Blood in the stools is one of the symptoms of Crohn's disease, colitis, dysentery, and hemorrhoids.
- Dark urine. Dark urine, accompanied by a yellowing of the skin or the eyes is indicative of hepatitis.
- Diarrhea. Watery bowel movements that occur many times throughout the day is diarrhea. If not caused by a bacterial or viral infection, diarrhea can be indicative of celiac disease, Crohn's disease, giardiasis, or colitis.
- Fever. Fever accompanies several digestive diseases, in particular infectious diarrhea, dysentery, appendicitis, and colitis.

Diagnosis

Because many digestive diseases share similar symptoms, diagnosis can be difficult. For instance, **celiac disease** is commonly misdiagnosed as IBS, Crohn's disease, or diverticulitis. Physicians believe that the key to an accurate diagnosis is careful and detailed history-taking during patient medical interviews. Tests and procedures used in diagnosis include:

- Barium enema. This test, also called a lower gastrointestinal (GI) series, uses x rays to detect abnormal growths, ulcers, polyps, and small pouches (diverticula) in the large intestine and rectum. An enema tube is inserted into the patient's rectum and a barium solution is allowed to flow in to improve the contrast of the x rays.
- Computed tomography (CAT or CT scan). This technique uses a computerized x-ray scanner to take multiple views of the abdominal organs. The information is analyzed by a computer that produces cross-sectional images of the scanned area. CT is used for viewing the more solid digestive organs such as the liver and pancreas.
- Colonoscopy. This test allows the physician to look inside the colon using a colonoscope, a long, flexible tube that has a miniaturized color camera at one end. It is inserted through the rectum into the colon and provides a view of the lining of the lower digestive

tract on a television monitor. The test is used to evaluate intestinal inflammation, ulceration, bleeding, diverticulitis, and colitis.

- Endoscopic retrograde cholangiopancreatography (ERCP). ERCP is a technique used to diagnose problems in the liver, gallbladder, bile ducts, and pancreas. It uses both x rays and an endoscope, which is a long, flexible, lighted tube inserted through the patient's esophagus, stomach, and duodenum. Using the endoscope, the examining physician can see the inside of the digestive tract and inject contrast dyes into the bile ducts and pancreas so that they can be seen with x rays.
- Endoscopic ultrasound (EUS). EUS is a technique that uses sound waves to create a picture of the inside of the body. It uses a special endoscope that has an ultrasound device at the tip. It is placed in the gastrointestinal tract, close to the area of interest.
- Esophagogastroduodenoscopy (EGD). EGD is a technique used to look inside the esophagus, stomach, and duodenum. It uses an endoscope to investigate swallowing difficulties, nausea, vomiting, reflux, bleeding, indigestion, abdominal pain, or chest pain.
- Flexible sigmoidoscopy. This technique allows a physician to look at the inside of the large intestine from the rectum through the last part of the colon, called the sigmoid colon. It is used to investigate diarrhea, abdominal pain, or constipation.
- Stool tests. Collection of stool is used to identify microorganisms that may be infecting the intestine. Stools are examined under a microscope or analyzed for the substances they contain. For example, normal stool contains almost no fat. In certain types of digestive diseases, however, fat is not completely absorbed and remains in the stool.
- Swallowing test. In this procedure, the patient is asked to drink a solution of barium before the x-ray examination of the upper digestive tract (esophagus, stomach, and small intestine).

Treatment

The treatment of digestive diseases varies depending on the condition being treated. Almost all treatment seeks the relief of symptoms and combines changes in eating habits with medications specific to the disease. In serious cases, surgical procedures may be used, which can involve the complete removal of the affected organ, if necessary.

GASTROESOPHAGEAL REFLUX DISEASE (GERD). Treatment may involve lifestyle and nutritional changes, such as avoiding alcohol, coffee, or teas if not tolerated; decreasing the fat intake in the diet to 45 grams or less per day; avoiding spicy, citrus, or high-fat/high-carbohydrate foods; eating more frequent but smaller meals; and losing weight. Antacid medication, such as Alka-Seltzer, Maalox, Mylanta, Pepto-Bismol, Rolaids, and Riopan, can help relieve **heartburn**. Other drugs, such as foaming agents (Gaviscon), work by covering the stomach contents with foam to prevent reflux. H2 blockers, such as cimetidine (Tagamet HB), famotidine (Pepcid AC), nizatidine (Axid AR), and ranitidine (Zantac 75), can help reduce acid production. Proton pump inhibitors, such as omeprazole (Prilosec), lansoprazole (Prevacid), pantoprazole (Protonix), rabeprazole (Aciphex), and esomeprazole (Nexium), are the most commonly used prescription medications. Surgery is also an option when medications do not work. The standard surgical treatment is fundoplication, which wraps the upper part of the stomach around the lower esophageal sphincter to strengthen it and prevent acid reflux.

GASTROPARESIS. When related to diabetes, treatment seeks to control the blood sugar levels with **insulin** and oral medications, such as metoclopramide (Reglan), to stimulate stomach muscle contractions which helps empty food. In severe cases, intravenous feeding may be required to bypass the stomach entirely. This is achieved by inserting a jejunostomy tube through the skin of the abdomen into the small intestine. The procedure allows nutrients and medication to be delivered directly into the small intestine.

PEPTIC ULCER. Ulcers caused by *Helicobacter pylori* are treated with drugs to kill the bacteria, reduce stomach acid, and protect the stomach lining. Antibiotics are usually prescribed. The acid-suppressing drugs commonly used are H2 blockers and proton pump inhibitors. Medications such as bismuth subsalicylate are also used in the case of stomach ulcers. Surgery may be required. A procedure known as a vagotomy cuts parts of the vagus nerve that transmits messages from the brain to the stomach. This interrupts messages to produce acid, reducing acid secretion. Dietary changes to reduce the acidity of the stomach include avoiding alcoholic beverages without food intake, limiting coffee intake to a few cups per day, and stopping food intake one to two hours before bedtime.

BUDD-CHIARI SYNDROME. Treatment usually involves **sodium** restriction, diuretics to control the accumulation of fluid in the abdominal cavity (ascites), and prescription of anticoagulants such as heparin and warfarin. Surgical shunts that divert blood flow around the obstruction or the liver may be required. In very serious cases, liver transplantation is the only effective treatment.

CHOLECYSTITIS. If acute, treatment may require hospitalization to reduce stimulation to the gallbladder. Antibiotics are usually prescribed to fight the infection as well as acid-suppressing medications. In some cases, the gallbladder may be surgically removed (cholecystectomy).

CIRRHOSIS. Treatment depends on the cause of the cirrhosis and complications that may be present. Alcoholic cirrhosis is first treated by completely abstaining from alcohol. Hepatitis-related cirrhosis is treated with medications specific to the different types of hepatitis, such as interferon for viral hepatitis and corticosteroids for autoimmune hepatitis. Treatment also includes medications to help remove fluid from the body. When complications cannot be controlled or when the liver becomes so damaged that it can no longer function, a liver transplant is required.

HEPATITIS. Hepatitis A is treated by bed rest and medications to relieve symptoms such as fever, nausea, and diarrhea. Hepatitis B is treated with a course of interferon injections, usually for many months. Additionally, drugs such as lamivudine and dipivoxil are prescribed for a period of one year. Over time, hepatitis B may cause the liver to stop functioning and require a liver transplant. Hepatitis C is treated with peginterferon, usually in combination with ribavirin. Hepatitis C may also require a liver transplant.

NON-ALCOHOLIC FATTY LIVER DISEASE (NAFLD). No single truly effective treatment has yet been found. Obese or overweight patients are encouraged to lose weight and to follow a balanced diet. Increasing physical activity and avoiding alcohol is also recommended.

PANCREATITIS. If no complications occur, pancreatitis usually improves on its own. Treatment seeks to support body functions and to prevent any complications if hospitalization is needed.

PRIMARY BILIARY CIRRHOSIS. No treatment has yet been shown beneficial in slowing the progression of PBC. Patients are usually prescribed **vitamins** and **calcium** to help prevent loss of bone (osteoporosis), a common complication.

PRIMARY SCLEROSING CHOLANGITIS. There is no cure for PSC, but effective treatment is available for certain symptoms, such as the itching resulting from too much bile in the bloodstream, which can be controlled with drugs such as Questran or Actigall. Swelling of the abdomen and feet, due to fluid retention, can be treated with diuretics. In some cases, surgical procedures may be used to open major blockages in bile ducts. In the most severe cases, a liver transplant is performed.

INFECTIOUS DIARRHEA. In normally healthy people, the usual practice is to let the illness take its course, which can last from a few days to a week. Drinking plenty of liquids is required and medications such as Pedialyte, Ceralyte, and Infalyte can be provided to replace electrolyte losses. Treatment with antibiotics is increasingly complicated by the bacteria having developed drug resistance.

CELIAC DISEASE. The only treatment for celiac disease is a **gluten-free diet.**

CROHN'S DISEASE. There is no cure for Crohn's disease. The goal of treatment is to control inflammation in the intestine and reduce the symptoms of pain, diarrhea, and bleeding. Medications prescribed to reduce inflammation include Azulfidine (sulfasalazine), mesalamine, or 5-ASA agents such as Rowasa, Pentasa or Asacol. Serious cases usually require more powerful drugs such as prednisone, antibiotics, or drugs that weaken the body's immune system such as Imuran (azathioprine), Purinethol (6-mercaptopurine, 6-MP), methotrexate, or remicade (Infliximab). Nutritional management is very important but must be individualized. In general, diet should provide 1.5–2.0 grams of **protein** per kilogram of body weight, plus the needed **calories** for growth and maintenance. Supplements of vitamins or **minerals** may be given. Low-fiber foods are usually tolerated well, and a low fat intake is usually helpful.

LACTOSE INTOLERANCE. Removing dairy and other products that contain lactose from the diet is the standard treatment. Lactase enzymes can also be added to milk or taken in capsule or chewable tablet forms prior to eating foods with lactose.

APPENDICITIS. Surgery is performed to remove the appendix, with prescription of pain medication.

ULCERATIVE COLITIS. Treatment seeks to control acute attacks, prevent new attacks, and promote healing of the colon. Corticosteroids are usually prescribed to reduce inflammation. Medications prescribed to decrease the frequency of attacks include mesalamine, azathioprine, and 6-mercaptopurine. In severe cases, the colon may be removed surgically.

DIVERTICULOSIS. A fiber-rich diet is helpful in long-term management. During an attack, a clear liquid diet followed by a low-fiber diet will allow the colon to rest so healing can occur. Specific treatment depends on symptoms. In severe cases, patients may require intravenous antibiotics or surgery to remove the affected portion of the colon.

DYSENTERY. Rest and drinking plenty of fluids is the usual treatment. Hospitalization may be required for intravenous therapy.

GIARDIASIS. Anti-infective medications such as metronidazole (Flagyl, Protostat) or quinacrine may be used. In pregnant women, treatment is not started until after delivery, because the drugs can be harmful to the fetus.

IRRITABLE BOWEL SYNDROME (IBS). IBS has no cure. Treatment for symptoms may include diet changes, medication, and stress-relief therapy; however, new research has shown that 75% of people affected by IBS may find relief by following the FODMAP diet, which stands for fermentable oligosaccharides, disaccharides, monosaccharides, and polyols. The diet avoids food containing these sugars.

HEMORRHOIDS. Corticosteroid creams and lidocaine ointments are used to reduce itching, pain, and swelling. For severe cases, surgical removal of the **hemorrhoids** may be performed (hemorrhoidectomy).

ANAL FISSURES. Treatment may include the application of a hydrocortisone cream to the anal area to help relieve irritation, oral pain medications such as acetaminophen, or a stool softener such as Colace or Surfak to prevent **constipation** until the fissure heals. Soaking the anal area in a warm chamomile infusion for 20 minutes may help prevent infection and provide soothing relief. Avoidance of strenuous effort to pass stool will prevent further complications. If a fissure does not respond to conservative treatment, surgery may be required, involving an operation that removes the area of the fissure and any underlying scar tissue.

PERIANAL ABSCESSES. Treatment involves surgical drainage of the abscess, as antibiotics are ineffective. A small incision is made over the area and pus is expelled with manual pressure. The wound is packed with iodophor gauze, removed after 24 hours, and the patient is instructed to take Sitz baths 3–4 times a day for up to two weeks.

Nutrition and dietary concerns

Some digestive diseases require special diets, while others require only that patients follow the rules of basic good nutrition, avoiding foods that cause problems. Vitamin supplements may be recommended if the disorder is affecting nutrient absorption. However, the medical profession advises against taking megadoses of vitamins, special herbal extracts, and other unproven therapies.

GASTROESOPHAGEAL REFLUX DISEASE. Diets recommended for **GERD** are usually low fat and include **whole grains**, vegetables, fruits, dairy products, and protein-rich foods. A **vitamin C** supplement may be needed if the patient cannot consume foods such as

Abdominal cavity—The terminal opening of the digestive tract.

Anus—The hollow part of the body that extends from the chest to the groin.

Ascites—Abnormal accumulation of fluid in the abdominal cavity.

Bacteria—Microscopic, single-celled organisms found in air, water, soil, and food. Only a few actually cause disease in humans.

Bile—Fluid made by the liver and stored in the gallbladder. Bile helps break down fats and gets rid of wastes in the body.

Bile ducts—Tubes that carry bile from the liver to the gallbladder for storage and to the small intestine for use in digestion.

Colon—Part of the large intestine, located in the abdominal cavity.

Colon polyps—Extra tissue that grows in the colon.

Diverticula—Small pouches in the muscular wall of the large intestine.

Duodenum—The first section of the small intestine, extending from the stomach to the jejunum, the next section of the small intestine.

Esophagus—Muscular tube through which food passes from the pharynx to the stomach.

Ileum—The last section of the small intestine located between the jejunum and the large intestine.

Insulin—Hormone secreted by the pancreas that regulates carbohydrate metabolism in the body. It regulates the liver's ability to store or release glucose.

Insulin resistance—Condition in which normal amounts of insulin are inadequate.

Large intestine—The terminal part of the digestive system, site of water recycling, nutrient absorption, and waste processing located in the abdominal cavity. It consists of the caecum, the colon, and the rectum.

Lower esophageal sphincter (LES)—Ring of muscle at the bottom of the esophagus that acts like a valve between the esophagus and stomach.

Pancreas—The pancreas is a flat, glandular organ lying below the stomach. It secretes the hormones insulin and glucagon that control blood sugar levels and also secretes pancreatic enzymes in the small intestine for the breakdown of fats and proteins.

Rectum—Short, muscular tube that forms the lowest portion of the large intestine and connects it to the anus.

Small intestine—The part of the digestive tract located between the stomach and the large intestine. It consists of the duodenum, the jejunum, and the ileum.

---

lemons, oranges, tomatoes, and grapefruits, which are high in vitamin C.

GASTROPARESIS. Patients are asked to avoid foods that are high in fat, which normally delay the emptying of the stomach. High-fiber foods such as broccoli, cabbage, and other fruits and vegetables also tend to stay in the stomach and are restricted when symptoms are severe. Liquids always leave the stomach faster than solid food, so liquid foods are recommended.

PEPTIC ULCER. In the past, physicians advised people with ulcers to avoid spicy, fatty, or acidic foods. Research has shown, however, that such diets are ineffective for treating ulcers. In most patients, no particular diet has yet emerged as being particularly helpful.

BUDD-CHIARI SYNDROME. A **low-sodium diet** is required for the control of ascites.

CHOLECYSTITIS. A **low-fat diet** is usually recommended, with research showing that the pectin in apples

may be beneficial, as well as the cellulose contained in celery and other crisp fruits and vegetables.

CIRRHOSIS. Regardless of the type of cirrhosis, a healthy, low-sodium diet is usually prescribed with total avoidance of alcohol.

HEPATITIS. Stimulants such as colas, chocolate, coffee, and tea can place stress on the liver and are restricted. Consumption of fruit juices should also be reduced due to high levels of concentrated sugar, which stress the digestive process and the pancreas while feeding the virus.

NON-ALCOHOLIC FATTY LIVER DISEASE (NAFLD). A healthy diet controlling elevated cholesterol, **triglycerides**, and blood sugar is considered beneficial.

PANCREATITIS. Dietary guidelines recommend foods low in fat and high in **carbohydrates** and protein to decrease the work load of the pancreas. Stimulants such as coffee, alcohol, and spicy or and gas-forming foods are restricted.

PRIMARY SCLEROSING CHOLANGITIS. A low-sodium diet is usually recommended to reduce fluid retention.

CELIAC DISEASE. Patients work with a dietitian to design a diet plan that is totally gluten-free. This means not eating foods that contain wheat, rye, and barley. Restrictions include most pasta, cereal, and processed foods.

INFECTIOUS DIARRHEA. Diarrhea causes the body to lose too much fluid (**dehydration**) and **electrolytes**. Drinking plenty of water is extremely important. Broth and soups that contain sodium and fruit juices, soft fruits, or vegetables that contain potassium will help restore electrolyte levels.

LACTOSE INTOLERANCE. If milk is removed from the diet, other sources of calcium are added. Sometimes, fermented milk products like yogurt can be tolerated. Non-dairy foods that are good sources of calcium include dark leafy green vegetables such as kale, collard greens, and broccoli. Foods fortified with added calcium, such as soymilk, juices, cereals, and pasta are also good sources of calcium.

COLITIS. Patients are advised to eliminate any foods or beverages from their diet that seem to make symptoms worse. This usually includes limiting dairy products, initiating a low-fat diet high in fibers, eating small meals, and drinking plenty of water.

DIVERTICULOSIS. Since a lack of **fiber** and bulk in the diet may contribute to diverticular disease, adding fiber and bulk to the diet is considered very important. Foods rich in fiber, such as bran cereals, whole wheat breads, beans, and fresh fruits and vegetables will help keep the stools soft and bulky.

DYSENTERY. Patients are asked to fast for as long as acute symptoms are present, taking only orange juice and water or buttermilk. After the acute phase, rice, curd, fresh ripe fruits (especially banana and pomegranate), and skim milk are allowed. Solid foods are reintroduced very carefully in the diet depending on the pace of recovery.

GIARDIASIS. Drinking water to prevent dehydration is recommended, as is replenishing the electrolytes lost as a result of diarrhea.

IRRITABLE BOWEL SYNDROME. People with IBS are usually asked to avoid food that is high in fat, insoluble fiber, **caffeine**, coffee, carbonated sodas, and alcohol.

HEMORRHOIDS, ANAL FISSURES, AND PERIANAL ABSCESSES. A **high-fiber diet** consisting of fruits, vegetables, and whole grains is usually recommended, along with fiber supplements such as Metamucil, Citrucel, and Fibercon. Drinking plenty of water daily will help prevent stool hardening.

QUESTIONS TO ASK YOUR DOCTOR

- What type of digestive disorder I have?
- Will I need to change my diet?
- Will diet changes alone help, or will medications be necessary?
- What side effects can I expect from these medications?

Therapy

The management and treatment of digestive diseases is disease specific, and pharmacologic and other therapies are tailored to individual cases accordingly, depending on severity and patient history.

Prognosis

Prognosis for some digestive diseases is excellent, such as the infectious diseases that clear up once the infectious agent is destroyed. Outcomes for most of the other diseases depend on the severity of complications and the underlying causes.

Prevention

A healthy diet can help to prevent some digestive diseases altogether and lessen the chances of developing others. Balanced nutrition is based on eating foods that meet the recommended dietary allowances (RDA) of the National Institute of Medicine (IOM). These foods should come from the five major food groups: dairy, protein, grains, fruits, and vegetables. Experts also recommend that people drink plenty of water daily to help eliminate ingested toxins and maintain the pH balance of the stomach.

Another important prevention area is food contamination, which is directly responsible for all the digestive infectious diseases. These diseases can be avoided by simple precautions such as washing fruits and vegetables, cooking meat thoroughly, drinking water taken only from trusted sources, and basic hygiene.

Resources

BOOKS

Best-Boss, Angie, and David Edelberg. *The Everything Digestive Health Book: What You Need to Know to Eat Well, Be Healthy, and Feel Great.* Avon, MA: Adams Media, 2009.

Blum, H. E., Richard H. Hunt, and Jüurgen Schöolmerich, eds. *Environment and Lifestyle: Effects on Disorders of the Digestive Tract.* Basel: Karger, 2011.

Gaeddert, Andrew. *Healing Digestive Disorders: Natural Treatments for Gastrointestinal Conditions.* 3rd ed. Berkeley, CA: North Atlantic Books, 2008.

Lipski, Elizabeth. *Digestive Wellness.* 4th ed. Chicago: Contemporary, 2010.

———. *Digestive Wellness for Children.* Laguna Beach, CA: Basic Health Publications, 2006.

Minocha, Anil, and Christine A. Adamec. *The Encyclopedia of the Digestive System and Digestive Disorders.* New York: Facts On File, 2011.

Wexler, Barbara. *Digestive Health.* Salt Lake City, UT: Woodland Publishing, 2009.

PERIODICALS

Gibson, Peter R., and Susan J. Shepherd. "Evidence-Based Dietary Management of Functional Gastrointestinal Symptoms: The FODMAP Approach." *Journal of Gastroenterology and Hepatology* 25, no. 2 (2010): 252–58.

OTHER

National Digestive Diseases Information Clearinghouse. *The Digestive Diseases Dictionary.* NIH Publication No. 09-2750. Bethesda, MD: National Institute of Diabetes and Digestive and Kidney Diseases, U.S. Department of Health and Human Services, National Institutes of Health, 2009. http://digestive.niddk.nih.gov/ddiseases/pubs/dictionary (accessed March 12, 2012).

WEBSITES

MedlinePlus. "Digestive Diseases." U.S. National Library of Medicine, National Institutes of Health. http://www.nlm.nih.gov/medlineplus/digestivediseases.html (accessed March 12, 2012).

National Digestive Diseases Information Clearinghouse. "Digestive Diseases: A–Z List of Topics and Titles." National Institute of Diabetes and Digestive and Kidney Diseases (NIDDK). http://digestive.niddk.nih.gov/ddiseases/a-z.aspx (accessed March 12, 2012).

ORGANIZATIONS

American Gastroenterological Association, 4930 Del Ray Ave., Bethesda, MD 20814, (301) 654-2055, Fax: (301) 654-5920, member@gastro.org, http://www.gastro.org.

International Foundation for Functional Gastrointestinal Disorders, PO Box 170864, Milwaukee, WI 53217, (414) 964-1799, (888) 964-2001, Fax: (414) 964-7176, iffgd@iffgd.org, http://www.iffgd.org.

National Digestive Diseases Information Clearinghouse, 2 Information Way, Bethesda, MD 20892–3570, (800) 891–5389, TTY: (866) 569–1162, Fax: (703) 738–4929, nddic@info.niddk.nih.gov, http://www.digestive.niddk.nih.gov.

Monique Laberge, PhD
David Newton

Diuretics and diets

Definition

Diuretics are a group of drugs given to help the body eliminate excess fluid through the kidneys in order to treat **hypertension** (high blood pressure), kidney and liver disorders, glaucoma, congestive heart failure (CHF), and idiopathic intracranial hypertension (pseudotumor cerebri), a condition characterized by increased fluid pressure within the blood vessels supplying the brain.

In addition to prescription diuretics, there are several types of diuretics available in over-the-counter formulations or commonplace beverages.

Purpose

Diuretics have several purposes in mainstream clinical medicine:

- To lower blood pressure in people with hypertension.
- To lower fluid pressure inside the eyeball in patients with glaucoma.
- To reduce increased cerebrospinal fluid pressure in idiopathic intracranial hypertension.
- To reduce blood pressure and swelling during surgical procedures.
- To reduce bloating and discomfort associated with fluid retention in the premenstrual phase of a woman's monthly cycle.

The connection between diuretics and dieting is twofold. First, many of the conditions that are treated by administration of prescription diuretics—particularly hypertension, CHF, and idiopathic intracranial hypertension—are more common in obese patients, more difficult to treat in the obese population, or both. Thus weight loss and lifestyle change are commonly recommended to these patients along with prescription diuretics.

The second connection is that many dieters use or abuse diuretics as a means to quick weight loss. Abuse of diuretics frequently coexists with self-induced vomiting and abuse of laxatives in patients with **eating disorders**. This combination of behaviors is called purging. Purging may occur in some patients with eating disorders as a means to a slender appearance, but it is also common in high school and college athletes participating in such weight-related sports as rowing, wrestling, gymnastics, and long-distance running. Athletes may also abuse diuretics like furosemide (Lasix) in order to mask the fact that they are taking other drugs to enhance performance in competition. People who abuse diuretics may take herbal preparations reported to have diuretic effects or over-the-counter preparations containing **caffeine** or pamabrom as well as prescription diuretics.

Description

Prescription diuretics

There are five major types of prescription diuretics.

LOOP DIURETICS. Loop diuretics are the strongest of the prescription diuretics. They take their name from the fact that they work in the ascending limb of the loop of Henle, a structure in the kidney in which **magnesium** and **calcium** are ordinarily reabsorbed. By disrupting the reabsorption of these two ions, loop diuretics bring about increased urine production, which in turn lowers blood volume, leading to lowered blood pressure. Loop diuretics also cause the veins to dilate, which lowers blood pressure mechanically. This vasodilation is independent of the drug's diuretic effect.

Loop diuretics are usually given to treat edema (accumulation of fluid in body tissues) associated with heart failure; cirrhosis of the liver; impaired kidney function or nephrotic syndrome (a condition in which the kidneys leak **protein** from blood into the urine); hypertension; or severe hypercalcemia (abnormally high levels of calcium in the blood). They are also given together with other drugs to treat edema of the brain or lungs, conditions that require rapid diuresis. Drugs classified as loop diuretics include furosemide (Lasix), bumetanide (Bumex), ethacrynic acid (Edecrin), and torsemide (Demadex).

THIAZIDE DIURETICS. Thiazide diuretics are derived from a chemical called benzothiadiazene. Unlike the loop diuretics, which work in the loop of Henle, thiazide diuretics work in a different structure called the distal convoluted tubule, although they function in a similar way to increase urine production by decreasing the kidney's reabsorption of **sodium** and calcium. They are not as strong as loop diuretics and have fewer adverse effects.

Thiazide diuretics are commonly prescribed to manage high blood pressure because they help to dilate blood vessels as well as lower blood volume by increasing urine output. They are also sometimes given to patients with high levels of calcium in the urine to prevent the formation of kidney stones and lower the risk of osteoporosis. They include such drugs as hydrochlorothiazide (HydroDIURIL, Esidrix), chlorothiazide (Diachlor, Diuril), and chlorthalidone (Hygroton, Hylidone).

POTASSIUM-SPARING DIURETICS. Potassium-sparing diuretics include such drugs as amiloride (Midamor) and triamterene (Dyrenium). They are usually given together with loop diuretics in treating CHF or high blood pressure to prevent the patient's potassium level from falling too low. They work by decreasing sodium reabsorption in the collecting tubules of the kidneys.

There are two formulations that combine the potassium-sparing diuretic triamterene with the thiazide diuretic hydrochlorothiazide in one pill—Maxzide and Dyazide—thus simplifying the patient's dosage schedule.

OSMOTIC DIURETICS. Osmotic diuretics are substances that cannot be reabsorbed in the kidney and so increase urine volume by osmosis. The most commonly used osmotic diuretic is mannitol, a **sugar** alcohol or polyol that is also added to sugar-free candies, mouthwashes, and similar products as an artificial sweetener. Mannitol (Osmitrol) is given intravenously to patients with glaucoma to lower fluid pressure inside they eyeball, and to patients with acute kidney failure following cardiovascular surgery.

Until early 2007, high-dose mannitol was recommended as treatment to reduce fluid accumulation inside the skull in cases of head trauma, on the basis of randomized trials conducted by a neurosurgeon in Brazil who committed suicide in 2005. His papers on the use of mannitol in head surgery were called into question in late 2006; neither his former coauthors nor the journal editors who published his studies were able to verify his data, and the university he claimed as his affiliation had never employed him.

CARBONIC ANHYDRASE INHIBITORS. Carbonic anhydrase inhibitors are a class of diuretics that increase water loss through the kidneys by changing the acidity of urine. Their most common use, however, is to treat glaucoma by lowering the fluid pressure inside the eyeball. The most common diuretic in this group, acetazolamide (Diamox), is also used as an anticonvulsant (drug given to prevent seizures). Other carbonic anhydrase inhibitors include dichlorphenamide (Daranide) and methazolamide (Neptazane).

Nonprescription diuretics

Nonprescription diuretics are often used by dieters to flush water from the body in the belief that this practice will promote rapid weight loss. According to the Centers for Disease Control and Prevention (CDC), 1% of adult male dieters in the United States and 2% of adult women have used over-the-counter diuretics as part of weight loss attempts.

CAFFEINE. Caffeine is a xanthine alkaloid found naturally in coffee beans, tea leaves, kola nuts, cocoa beans, and a few other plants. It is well known as a central nervous system (CNS) stimulant, enjoyed in brewed coffee, tea, hot chocolate, cola beverages, and energy drinks. It is also available in tablet form as an over-the-counter stimulant in such compounds as NoDoz. Caffeine is broken down in the liver to three substances, one of which is theobromine, which acts as a diuretic and increases urine volume. Some dieters drink coffee as much for its diuretic effects as for its effectiveness is counteracting the fatigue that often accompanies low-calorie diets.

HERBAL PREPARATIONS. Naturopaths and other practitioners of alternative medicine often recommend certain herbal preparations, including herbal teas, as diuretics available without a prescription. Herbs commonly recommended for their diuretic qualities include uva ursi, dandelion, hydrangea, parsley, butcher's broom, buchu, juniper, horsetail, buckthorn, and asparagus.

ALCOHOL. Beverage alcohol (ethanol) is known to have a diuretic effect; in fact, many of the symptoms of an alcohol hangover, such as headache, nausea, and diarrhea, are related to the **dehydration** resulting from alcohol intoxication. Many weight-reduction diets (the **Mediterranean diet** being a notable exception) forbid alcohol because it contains more **calories** than most people realize—7 calories per gram, in comparison to 9 calories per gram for fat and 4 calories per gram for protein. Some women, however, drink an occasional glass of wine or beer for its diuretic effect, to relieve the discomfort of fluid retention before the onset of their menstrual period.

PAMABROM. Pamabrom is a mild diuretic related chemically to theophylline, one of the breakdown products of caffeine. It is compounded with acetaminophen in a number of over-the-counter (OTC) remedies for premenstrual bloating and backache associated with fluid retention, including New Tylenol for Women, Backaid, and Diurex.

Precautions

Both prescription and nonprescription diuretics should be used with care.

Prescription diuretics

Prescription diuretics should be used only under a doctor's supervision and monitored in long-term users, as dosage requirements may change or the doctor may recommend **dietary supplements** to compensate for **electrolytes** and nutrients lost through the use of some diuretics. In addition, patients should not stop taking prescription diuretics or change the dosage without consulting their doctor.

- Loop diuretics. Patients taking loop diuretics may require supplemental potassium, folic acid, and vitamin B_1. In addition, they should learn to recognize the symptoms of potassium depletion, as loss of potassium is a common adverse effect of this type of diuretic.

- Thiazide diuretics. Nursing mothers should not use thiazide diuretics during the first month of breast-feeding, as they can pass into the milk and in some cases decrease the flow of milk. Thiazide diuretics should also be taken with food or milk to lower the risk of upset stomach. They should be used very cautiously in patients with diabetes, as they tend to raise blood sugar levels.

- Potassium-sparing diuretics. Patients should avoid the use of salt substitutes containing potassium while taking this type of diuretic, as it may lead to overly high levels of potassium in the blood. In addition, patients should be advised to avoid driving or operating dangerous machinery until they know how these drugs affect them, because potassium-sparing diuretics may cause dizziness and blurred vision.

- Osmotic diuretics. Sodium levels in the patient's blood should be closely monitored, particularly if the patient develops muscle cramps.

- Carbonic anhydrase inhibitors. Acetazolamide should not be given to patients with a history of liver or kidney disorders, Addison's disease, known sensitivity to sulfonamide drugs, or angle-closure glaucoma; and used cautiously in patients with diabetes or gout. The patient should be advised to take this type of diuretic in the morning to prevent sleep interruption.

Nonprescription diuretics

Nonprescription diuretics can still cause adverse effects even though they are weaker than prescription diuretics:

- Caffeine. A dose of caffeine higher than 400 milligrams (more than 3 or 4 cups of brewed coffee) will produce a state of caffeine intoxication in most adults. Over-the-counter caffeine tablets, however, typically contain more caffeine than brewed coffee, usually 100–200 mg per tablet. In very high doses (around 5 g), caffeine will produce nausea, coma, convulsions, and eventually death.

- Herbal preparations. Herbal preparations should be purchased only from reliable sources, as their potency may vary from batch to batch. In addition, herbal products made outside the United States may be adulterated with filler products or contaminated by industrial byproducts.

- Alcohol. Alcohol should always be consumed in moderation and never combined with driving or operating heavy machinery.
- Pamabrom. Pamabrom is a mild diuretic that causes skin rashes in a few people who take it for backache or menstrual cramps.

Interactions

Prescription diuretics may interact with some other prescription drugs as well as with herbal products:

- Loop diuretics. Loop diuretics are known to interact with licorice, digitalis, and buckthorn or alder buckthorn.
- Thiazide diuretics. Thiazide diuretics interact with insulin to inhibit its effects in lowering blood sugar, intensify the toxic side effects of lithium therapy, and increase the effects of corticosteroids in causing loss of potassium.
- Potassium-sparing diuretics. May increase the toxicity of lithium.
- Osmotic diuretics.
- Carbonic anhydrase inhibitors. Enhance the effects of amphetamines and tricyclic antidepressants; increase the excretion of lithium and phenobarbital; increase the risk of aspirin toxicity for patients taking aspirin or other salicylates.

Nonprescription diuretics

Nonprescription diuretics, particularly alcohol, may interact with a variety of substances:

- Caffeine. Caffeine is known to intensify the effects of cimetidine (a drug that lowers the secretion of stomach acid) and theophylline.
- Herbal preparations. Herbal preparations with diuretic effects should be strictly avoided by people taking prescription diuretics, as the herbs may intensify the effects of the prescription drugs and lead to various cardiovascular side effects.
- Alcohol. Alcohol is known to interact with a wide number of prescription medications. It should never be taken together with other drugs that depress the central nervous system. These types of medications include antidepressants, benzodiazepines (tranquilizers), barbiturates, other sleeping medications, narcotic pain relievers (codeine and other derivatives of opium), and antihistamines. Alcohol may interact with antipsychotic medications to cause liver damage, with aspirin to cause stomach bleeding, and with

some cardiovascular medications to cause dizziness and fainting.

Aftercare

Aftercare following abuse of diuretics varies according to the substance and the consumption pattern. Caffeine intoxication can usually be treated by tapering intake of caffeinated beverages and/or discontinuing use of caffeine tablets. Alcohol hangovers may require rehydration as well as administration of **vitamin B₆**. Abuse of diuretics in patients with eating disorders requires long-term medical nutrition therapy supervised by a professional nutritionist. The position statement of the Academy of Nutrition and Dietetics (formerly the American Dietetic Association) is as follows: "Nutrition education and nutrition intervention by a registered dietitian is an essential component of the team treatment of patients with **anorexia nervosa**, **bulimia nervosa**, and eating disorders not otherwise specified (EDNOS) during assessment and treatment across the continuum of care." Similarly, adolescents who abuse diuretics as part of athletic training regimens require supervision by a registered dietitian as well as by a specialist in sports medicine.

Complications

Prescription diuretics have a number of side effects:

- Loop diuretics. Loop diuretics may produce several different types of adverse reactions. The first type are related to diuresis and electrolyte balance. Loop diuretics may cause loss of potassium and magnesium from the body; the loss of magnesium may lead to the loss of additional potassium. Patients taking loop diuretics should be taught to recognize the signs of potassium deficiency (hypokalemia), which include weakness, loss of appetite, irregular heartbeat, constipation, muscle cramps, a weak or heavy feeling in the legs, mental confusion, or unusual tiredness. The second type of adverse reaction to loop diuretics is ototoxicity, or damage to the nerves in the ears that control hearing and the sense of balance. Symptoms of ototoxicity include ringing in the ears (tinnitus) and dizziness. The third type of adverse effect of loop diuretics is uncommon but may occur in patients who are also taking ACE inhibitors (medications to control blood pressure) and nonsteroidal anti-inflammatory drugs (NSAIDs). This so-called "triple whammy" may lead to kidney failure.

KEY TERMS

Caffeine—A plant alkaloid found in coffee, tea, hot chocolate, and some soft drinks that functions as a diuretic as well as a central nervous system stimulant.

Edema—Abnormal and excessive accumulation of fluid in body tissues or certain cavities of the body. Edema is a symptom of a number of different kidney, liver, and circulatory disorders and is commonly treated with diuretics.

Electrolyte—Any of several chemicals dissolved in blood and other body fluids that are capable of conducting an electric current. The most important electrolytes in humans and other animals are sodium, potassium, calcium, magnesium, chloride, phosphate, and hydrogen carbonate.

Ethanol—The chemical name of beverage alcohol.

Glaucoma—An eye disorder marked by increased fluid pressure within the eyeball that can lead to gradual loss of vision. Glaucoma is sometimes treated with diuretics.

Hypercalcemia—Abnormally high levels of calcium in the blood.

Hypertension—The medical name for high blood pressure.

Idiopathic intracranial hypertension—Increased fluid pressure within the blood vessels supplying the brain. Obese women are at increased risk of developing this disorder.

Nephrotic syndrome—A disorder marked by a deficiency of albumin (a protein) in the blood and its excretion in the urine.

Ototoxicity—Damage caused to the nerves in the ear that are involved in hearing or balance. Ototoxicity is a rare but serious adverse effect of loop diuretics.

Pamabrom—A mild diuretic found in several over-the-counter compounds for the relief of premenstrual discomfort and water retention.

Purging—A behavior associated with eating disorders that includes self-induced vomiting and abuse of laxatives as well as diuretics.

Theobromine—A breakdown product of caffeine that is responsible for the diuretic effect of coffee and tea.

• Thiazide diuretics. Thiazide diuretics may cause low blood potassium levels, impotence in men, and increased levels of blood cholesterol. They also cause photosensitivity in some people, which means that the person will be more sensitive to sunlight and sunburn more readily. Last, thiazide diuretics can raise the levels of glucose and uric acid in the blood, which increases the patient's risk of developing gout.

• Potassium-sparing diuretics. Adverse effects may include loss of interest in sex (in both men and women), visual disturbances and dizziness, shortness of breath, nausea, and vomiting.

• Osmotic diuretics. Use of mannitol causes high blood pressure, blurred vision, chills, fever, nausea, and vomiting in some patients.

• Carbonic anhydrase inhibitors. May depress the activity of bone marrow, leading to anemia; may contribute to liver dysfunction; increases the patient's risk of developing gout; may lead to overly low blood levels of sodium, potassium, magnesium, and calcium.

Nonprescription diuretics

Adverse effects from nonprescription diuretics may include:

• Caffeine. Adverse effects from high doses of caffeine include nervousness, insomnia, restlessness, twitching, tingling or flushing of the face, nausea or vomiting, diarrhea, and dehydration.

• Herbal preparations. Herbal preparations used as diuretics have a wide range of potential adverse effects, ranging from intensifying the effects of prescription diuretics to indigestion, skin rashes, headache, and diarrhea.

• Alcohol. Complications associated with ethanol consumption include the risks of dehydration and electrolyte imbalance caused by intoxication; alcohol abuse; trauma from alcohol-related accidents; and interactions with other medications.

• Pamabrom. Pamabrom has been reported to cause skin rashes and dependence in a very small minority of patients.

Parental concerns

Parents do not ordinarily need to be concerned about children or adolescents abusing prescription diuretics, as these drugs do not produce mood alteration or relieve pain. Adolescents, however, are likely to abuse nonprescription diuretics in relation to eating disorders or athletic competition; one study found that 64% of adolescents diagnosed with eating disorders were using herbal diuretics. A few adolescents may develop caffeine-related disorders apart from eating disorders or sports.

Eating disorders

Abuse of over-the-counter diuretics is common among adolescents with eating disorders accompanied by purging, although it is slightly less common than self-induced vomiting or abuse of laxatives. Although eating disorders are classified as mental health problems, they can have serious lifelong digestive and nutritional consequences, including erosion of tooth enamel, loss of bone density leading to eventual osteoporosis, and ongoing problems with water retention.

Athletic competition

Numerous reports of diuretic abuse among athletes in high school and college sports programs have accumulated since the late 1980s. Abuse of OTC diuretics is higher among both males and females in such weight-related sports as wrestling and rowing than among participants in sports that do not classify athletes by weight (distance running, swimming, basketball, etc.). More males than females abuse diuretics at both the high school and college levels; the average age of initial misuse of diuretics in one sample was 15.6 years for males and 16.2 years for females. Abuse of diuretics puts young athletes, particularly males, at risk of dehydration, chest pains, fainting, and irregular heart rhythms, particularly when combined with ephedrine or other stimulants.

Caffeine dependence and intoxication

According to *DSM-IV*, caffeine use typically begins in the mid-teens in the United States and Canada, with levels of consumption increasing into the early adult years (20s and 30s). Among teenagers, caffeine use is usually higher among boys than girls, and higher among smokers than nonsmokers. Most fatal cases of caffeine overdose occur among adults in their early 20s, usually as a result of taking OTC caffeine tablets by mouth or inhaling crushed tablets.

Resources

BOOKS

American Psychiatric Association. *Diagnostic and Statistical Manual of Mental Disorders*. 4th ed, text rev. Washington, DC: American Psychiatric Association, 2000.

American Society of Health-System Pharmacists (ASHP). *AHFS Drug Handbook*. 2nd ed. Philadelphia: Lippincott Williams & Wilkins, 2003.

Brown, David L. *Drugs: Athlete Career Killer—Supplements, Diuretics and PEDs*. Niles, OH: Parkway Press, 2010.

PERIODICALS

American Dietetic Association (ADA). "Position of the American Dietetic Association: Nutrition Intervention in the Treatment of Anorexia Nervosa, Bulimia Nervosa, and Other Eating Disorders." *Journal of the American Dietetic Association* 106 (December 2006): 2073–82.

Hoyng, P.F., and L.M. van Beek. "Pharmacological Therapy for Glaucoma: A Review." *Drugs* 59 (March 2000): 411–34.

Karlson, K.A., C.B. Becker, and A. Merkur. "Prevalence of Eating Disordered Behavior in Collegiate Lightweight Women Rowers and Distance Runners." *Clinical Journal of Sport Medicine* 11 (January 2001): 32–37.

Kerrigan, Sarah, and Tania Lindsey. "Fatal Caffeine Overdose: Two Case Reports." *Forensic Science International* 153 (October 4, 2005): 67–69.

Kiningham, R.B., and D.W. Gorenflo. "Weight Loss Methods of High School Wrestlers." *Medicine and Science in Sports and Exercise* 33 (May 2001): 810–13.

Kruger, J., D.A. Galuska, M.K. Serdula, and D.A. Jones. "Attempting to Lose Weight: Specific Practices among U.S. Adults." *American Journal of Preventive Medicine* 26 (June 2004): 402–6.

Orbeta, R. L., M. D. Overpeck, D. Ramcharran, et al. "High Caffeine Intake in Adolescents." *Journal of Adolescent Health* 38 (April 2006): 451–53.

Roerig, James L., James E. Mitchell, M. de Zwaan, et al. "The Eating Disorders Medicine Cabinet Revisited: A Clinician's Guide to Appetite Suppressants and Diuretics." *International Journal of Eating Disorders* 33 (May 2003): 443–57.

Steffen, Kristine J., James L. Roerig, James E. Mitchell, and Ross D. Crosby. "A Survey of Herbal and Alternative Medication Use among Participants with Eating Disorder Symptoms." *International Journal of Eating Disorders* 39 (August 2006): 741–46.

Thomas, M.C. "Diuretics, ACE Inhibitors, and NSAIDs—the Triple Whammy." *Medical Journal of Australia* 172 (February 21, 2000): 184–85.

Vertalino, M., M.E. Eisenberg, M. Story, and D. Neumark-Sztainer. "Participation in Weight-Related Sports Is Associated with Higher Use of Unhealthful Weight-Control Behaviors and Steroid Use." *Journal of the American Dietetic Association* 107 (March 2007): 434–40.

WEBSITES

Alliance for Eating Disorders Awareness. "Diuretics." http://www.allianceforeatingdisorders.com/diuretics (accessed October 2, 2012).

Mayo Clinic staff. "Diuretics." MayoClinic.com. http://www.mayoclinic.com/health/diuretics/HI00030 (accessed October 2, 2012).

ORGANIZATIONS

Academy of Nutrition and Dietetics, 120 South Riverside Plz., Ste. 2000, Chicago, IL 60606-6995, (312) 899-0040, (800) 877-1600, amacmunn@eatright.org, http://www.eatright.org.

American College of Sports Medicine, 401 West Michigan St., Indianapolis, IN 46202-3233, (317) 637-9200, Fax: (317) 634-7817, http://www.acsm.org.

U.S. Food and Drug Administration, 10903 New Hampshire Ave., Silver Spring, MD 20993-0002, (888) INFO-FDA (463-6332), http://www.fda.gov.

Rebecca J. Frey, PhD

Diverticular disease diet

Definition

A diverticular disease diet is a diet that increases dietary **fiber** to recommended levels.

Origins

Diverticulosis is a condition characterized by small pouches (diverticula) that form and push outward through weak spots in the large intestine. Once diverticula have formed, there is no way to reverse the process. When diverticula become infected, the condition is called diverticulitis. Most people with diverticulosis do not experience symptoms. As for diverticulitis, the most common symptom is abdominal pain with tenderness around the left side of the lower abdomen. Fever, nausea, vomiting, chills, cramping, and **constipation** may occur as well. Diverticular disease is common in industrialized countries, especially in the United States, Canada, the United Kingdom, and Australia. It affects about 50% of Americans by age 60 and nearly all by age 80. A low-fiber diet is believed to be the main cause of the disease. It was first described in the United States in the early 1900s, at the time when processed foods were introduced into the American diet, many of which contained refined flour. Unlike whole-wheat flour, refined flour has no wheat bran and is accordingly a low-fiber food. The prevalence of the disease in industrialized countries seems to confirm the connection of diverticular disease with a low-fiber diet, since it occurs rarely in Asia or Africa, where people eat high-fiber, vegetable-based diets.

Description

Research has shown that increasing the amount of fiber in the diet may reduce symptoms of diverticular disease. The **Academy of Nutrition and Dietetics** recommends a daily intake of 20–35 grams of fiber. A diverticular disease diet will accordingly seek to increase dietary fiber to these levels to prevent constipation and the undue colon pressure that causes diverticula. Examples of foods that contain fiber and can be part of a diverticular disease diet include (amounts of fiber shown for a medium fruit or 1 cup of vegetable, fruit or grain):

- apple, raw, with skin (3.3 g)
- peach, raw (1.5 g)
- pear, raw (5.1 g)
- pineapple (1.9 g)
- tangerine, raw (1.9 g)
- blueberries (4.0 g)
- cranberries (4.0 g)
- raspberries (8.3 g)
- asparagus, 4 spears, fresh, cooked (1.2 g)
- broccoli, fresh, cooked (5.2 g)
- Brussels sprouts, fresh, cooked (4 g)
- cabbage, fresh, cooked (3 g)
- carrot, fresh, cooked (4.6 g)
- cauliflower, fresh, cooked (3.4 g)
- celery, raw (2.1 g)
- romaine lettuce, raw (1.2 g)
- spinach, fresh, cooked (4.4 g)
- summer squash, cooked (2.5 g)
- tomato, raw (1 g)
- winter squash, cooked (5.7 g)
- baked beans, canned, plain (12.6 g)
- kidney beans, fresh, cooked (11.4 g)
- lima beans, fresh, cooked (13.2 g)
- potato, fresh, cooked (2.3 g)
- bread, whole-wheat, 1 slice (1.9 g)
- brown rice, cooked (3.5 g)
- cereal, bran flake (7.1 g)
- oatmeal, plain, cooked (4 g)
- white rice, cooked (0.6 g)

There are several types of dietary fiber, which makes it easy to include it in the diet:

- Cellulose. Found in bran, legumes, peas, root vegetables, the cabbage family, the outer covering of seeds, and most fruits.
- Hemicellulose. A major constituent of cereal fiber, found in bran and whole grains.
- Polyfructose. Examples are inulins and oligofructans, found in onions, garlic, artichokes, and soybeans.

- Gums. These are substances secreted by a plant at injury sites. They are composed of various sugars and sugar derivatives. Found in oatmeal, barley, and legumes.
- Mucilages. Gelatinous substances found in most plants.
- Pectins. Water-soluble and gel-forming substances found in apples, strawberries, and citrus fruits.
- Lignin. This is the primary noncarbohydrate component of fiber. It is highest in mature root vegetables like carrots or fruits with edible seeds like strawberries.
- Resistant starches. These are starches that are classified as fibers because they are not digested by the body. They are found in whole legumes, potatoes, bananas, and plantains.

To help increase dietary fiber in the diet, breakfast could include a bowl of porridge made with millet, oats, or brown rice; toast made with whole-grain bread instead of white bread; whole-grain ready-to-eat cereals with milk; or a bowl of fruit instead of fruit juice. During the day, snacks can include fresh fruit; dried fruits like raisins, prunes, dates, apricots; or a few whole-grain crackers. In meals, brown rice should replace white rice. Pasta dishes should include more vegetables and fruit to increase the fiber content of the meal. Serve fruit after meals instead of a dessert. Vegetables should also be eaten at each meal. Sandwiches should be made with whole-grain bread and include vegetables.

Besides adding fiber foods to a diverticular disease diet, the health practitioner may also prescribe a fiber supplement such as Citrucel or Metamucil once a day. These products supply 2–3.5 grams of fiber per tablespoon, mixed with 8 ounces of water. Some physicians also recommend avoiding nuts, popcorn, and sunflower, pumpkin, caraway, and sesame seeds as they believe that particles of these foods could enter, block, or irritate the diverticula. However, no scientific evidence supports this opinion. The seeds in tomatoes, zucchini, cucumbers, strawberries, and raspberries, as well as poppy seeds, are generally considered harmless. An eating plan for diverticular disease is usually based on what works best for each person. To help the colon rest, the treating physician may also recommend bed rest and a liquid diet.

Function

Fiber is the edible part of fruits, vegetables, and grains that the body cannot digest. Since they are not absorbed into the body, dietary fibers are not considered a nutrient. Some fiber dissolves easily in water and becomes soft in the intestines, while insoluble fiber passes almost unchanged through the intestines. Both kinds of fiber are required to make stools soft and easy to pass. Fiber also prevents constipation, which makes the bowel muscles strain to move stool that is too hard. This is believed to be the main cause of increased pressure in the colon that may cause the weak colon spots to bulge out and become diverticula.

Many plant foods contain both soluble and insoluble fibers. For example, psyllium husks contain a mixture of 70% soluble and 30% insoluble fibers. Despite the general use of the terms "soluble" and "insoluble" to describe the health benefits of dietary fiber, many nutrition experts are now using the terms "viscous" and "fermentable" to describe the functions and health benefits of dietary fiber. These include:

- Reducing blood cholesterol levels: Viscous fibers lower cholesterol levels by reducing the absorption of dietary cholesterol. In addition, they combine with bile acids, which are compounds produced by the liver from cholesterol that are required for the breakdown of fats. After combining with bile acids, the compounds are removed from circulation and do not make it back to the liver. As a result, the liver must use additional cholesterol to manufacture new bile acids. Soluble fiber may also reduce the amount of cholesterol manufactured by the liver.
- Normalizing blood sugar levels: Viscous fibers are also involved in controlling blood glucose levels because they slow down the rate at which food leaves the stomach and delay the absorption of glucose after a meal. Viscous fibers also increase insulin sensitivity. As a result, viscous fibers are believed to play a role in the prevention and treatment of type 2 diabetes.
- Supporting bowel regularity: Fermentable fibers are fermented by the intestinal flora, the bacteria and fungi that live in the intestines. The fermentation of dietary fiber in the large intestine produces a short-chain fatty acid called butyric acid, which is used as fuel by the cells of the large intestine and helps maintain the health of the colon. Fermentable fibers also help maintain healthy populations of bacteria in the intestinal flora. Fibers that are not fermentable help maintain bowel regularity by increasing the bulk of the feces and decreasing the time required by fecal matter to move through the intestines.

Benefits

Fiber keeps stool soft and lowers pressure inside the colon so that bowel contents can move through easily. This is the reason it is considered beneficial for

Abdomen—Part of the body that extends from the chest to the groin.

Abdominal cavity—The hollow part of the body that extends from the chest to the groin. It is located between the diaphragm, which is the thin muscle below the lungs and heart, and the pelvis, the basin-shaped cavity that contains the reproductive organs, bladder, and rectum. The abdominal cavity contains the abdominal organs.

Bile—Digestive juice secreted by the liver and stored in the gallbladder; helps in the digestion of fats.

Colon—Part of the large intestine, located in the abdominal cavity. It consists of the ascending colon, the transverse colon, the descending colon, and the sigmoid colon.

Diverticulitis—Inflammation of the small pouches (diverticula) that can form in the weakened muscular wall of the large intestine.

Feces—Waste product of digestion formed in the large intestine. About 75% of its mass is water; the remainder is protein, fat, undigested roughage, dried digestive juices, dead cells, and bacteria.

Gastrointestinal tract (GI tract)—The tube connecting and including the organs and paths responsible for processing food in the body. These are the mouth, the esophagus, the stomach, the liver, the gallbladder, the pancreas, the small intestine, the large intestine, and the rectum.

Insoluble—Cannot be dissolved.

Insulin—A hormone secreted by the pancreas and required for the regulation of the metabolism of carbohydrates and fats.

Intestinal flora—The sum of all bacteria and fungi that live in the intestines. It is required to break down nutrients and fight off pathogens and helps the body build the vitamin E and K. An unbalanced intestinal flora can lead to many health problems.

Inulin—Naturally occurring oligosaccharides (several simple sugars linked together) produced by many types of plants. They belong to a class of carbohydrates known as fructans.

Large intestine—The terminal part of the digestive system, site of water recycling, nutrient absorption, and waste processing located in the abdominal cavity. It consists of the caecum, the colon, and the rectum.

Mucilage—A sticky, gummy substance used as an adhesive; obtained from certain plants.

Nutrient—A chemical compound (such as protein, fat, carbohydrate, vitamins, or minerals) that makes up foods. These compounds are used by the body to function and grow.

Soluble—Capable of being dissolved.

Syndrome X—A group of risk factors that together put someone at higher risk of coronary artery disease. These risk factors include: central obesity (excessive fat tissue in the abdominal region), glucose intolerance, high triglycerides and low HDL cholesterol, and high blood pressure.

---

diverticular disease. Eating a **high-fiber diet** will not only treat diverticular disease, it is also believed to play a role in the prevention and treatment of the following health conditions:

- breast cancer
- cardiovascular disease
- colon cancer
- diabetes
- gallstones
- high cholesterol
- irritable bowel syndrome
- obesity
- syndrome X

Precautions

When increasing the fiber content of the diet, dietitians recommend adding fiber progressively, adding just a few grams at a time to allow the intestinal tract to adjust. Otherwise, abdominal cramps, gas, bloating, and diarrhea or constipation may result. Intake of dietary fiber exceeding 50 g per day may also lead to intestinal obstruction. Excessive intake of fiber can also cause a fluid imbalance, leading to **dehydration**. This is the reason that people who start increasing their fiber intake are often advised to also increase their water intake. Excessive intake of dietary fiber has been linked with reduced absorption of **vitamins**, **minerals**, proteins, and **calories**. However, it is unlikely that healthy people who consume fiber in amounts within the recommended ranges will have problems with nutrient absorption.

Parents are urged to use caution when adding extra fiber to their child's diet. Excessive amounts of high-fiber foods may cause a child to fill up quickly, reducing appetite and possibly depriving the child of needed nutrients from a well-balanced diet. Elderly people and those who have had gastrointestinal surgery should also exercise caution when increasing their dietary fiber intake.

Risks

Most people recover fully after treatment for diverticular disease. If not treated however, diverticulitis can lead to the following serious conditions:

- Intestinal perforation: The diverticula burst because of increased pressure within the intestine.
- Peritonitis: This is a serious infection of the abdominal cavity outside the intestine. It often occurs after perforation, when the contents of the intestine are leaked into the abdominal cavity.
- Abscess formation: Sacs of infected intestinal material and pus can form that are very difficult to cure.
- Fistula formation: An abnormal connection between the colon and another organ can form. This occurs when the colon, damaged by infection, comes in contact with other tissue, such as the bladder, the small intestine, or the inside of the abdominal wall, and sticks to it. Fecal material from the colon can then get into the other tissue.
- Blockage of the intestine: This can result from hard fecal matter escaping from diverticula.
- Bleeding in the intestine: Stool that is trapped in a diverticulum may cause bleeding.

Research and general acceptance

Most health practitioners agree that the lack of fiber and bulk in the diet is the major cause of diverticular disease. As foods are becoming more highly refined, more people are suffering from diverticular disease symptoms. Eating a high-fiber diet is accordingly the only requirement highly emphasized by the medical profession. Eliminating specific foods is not considered necessary as no research supports that it may improve the condition. A gradual switch to a diet with increased intake of soluble fiber (green vegetables, oat bran) usually leads to an improvement in bowel function. There is general agreement on food sources being more efficient fiber sources than supplements since they also supply additional nutrients. Excessive use of fiber supplements can also lead to acute digestive problems and blockages.

QUESTIONS TO ASK YOUR DOCTOR

- What tests will you perform to determine whether or not I have diverticulitis?
- What medications do you recommend for treating my diverticulitis, or will you limit your treatment to dietary changes?
- Based on my medical examination, what is your prognosis for my diverticulitis?
- Assuming that my diverticulitis can be cured, what is the likelihood of it reoccurring at some time in the future?
- Does exercise play a role—and, if so, what role—in preventing the return of my diverticulitis?

The latest public health recommendations for dietary fiber, established by the National Academy of Sciences, is for an Adequate Intake (AI) level of 14 g of total daily fiber for every 1,000 calories of food intake, which amounts to about 25 g per day for women and 38 g per day for men. The latest evidence suggests that adults in the United States get only about half this much fiber each day. The recommendation for children older than 2 years is to increase dietary fiber intake to an amount equal to or greater than their age plus 5 g/day. There are currently no published studies that indicate optimal dietary fiber intakes for infants and children under 2. Until more information becomes available, a sensible guideline is to introduce a variety of fruits, vegetables, and easily digested cereals after weaning.

It is understood that, as the body ages, the outer layer of the intestinal wall thickens, which narrows the intestine. As a result, stool moves more slowly through the colon, increasing the pressure. Hard stools, such as those produced by a diet low in fiber, can further increase pressure. Repeated straining during bowel movements also increases pressure and contributes to formation of diverticula. As for the cause of diverticulitis, there is broad agreement that it occurs when diverticula become infected or inflamed, but medical experts do not know precisely what causes the infection. It is believed to start when stool or bacteria are caught in the diverticula.

The United States Food and Drug Administration (FDA) has approved the following claims about dietary fiber that can be listed on food labels:

- Good Source of Fiber, Contains Fiber or Provides Fiber: Any food product that contains 2.5 to less than 5 g of fiber per serving (less than 20% of the daily value of dietary fiber) and is low in total fat (3 g or less fat per serving).
- High Fiber, Rich in Fiber, Excellent Source of Fiber: Any food product that contains at least 5 g or more of dietary fiber per serving (20% or more of the fiber daily value) and is low in total fat per serving (3 g or less fat per serving).

Resources

BOOKS

Black, Patricia K., and Christine H. Hyde. *Diverticular Disease*. New York: John Wiley & Sons, 2005.

Brumback, Roger A., and Mary H. Brumback. *The Dietary Fiber Weight Control Handbook*. Charleston, SC: BookSurge Publishing, 2006.

Gomez, Joan. *How to Cope Successfully with the Diverticulitis Diet*. Farnham, UK: Wellhouse, 2008.

Gottschall, Elaine Gloria. *Breaking the Vicious Cycle: Intestinal Health through Diet*. Baltimore, ON: Kirkton Press, 2010.

Lipski, Elizabeth. *Digestive Wellness*. 4th ed. Chicago: Contemporary, 2010.

Miskovitz, Paul, and Marian Betancourt. *The Doctor's Guide to Gastrointestinal Health: Preventing and Treating Acid Reflux, Ulcers, Irritable Bowel Syndrome, Diverticulitis, Celiac Disease, Colon Cancer, Pancreatitis, Cirrhosis, Hernias and more*. New York: Wiley, 2005.

WEBSITES

National Digestive Diseases Information Clearinghouse. "What I Need to Know About Diverticular Disease." National Institute of Diabetes and Digestive and Kidney Diseases (NIDDK). http://digestive.niddk.nih.gov/ddiseases/pubs/diverticular (accessed July 11, 2012).

ORGANIZATIONS

Academy of Nutrition and Dietetics, 120 South Riverside Plz., Ste. 2000, Chicago, IL 60606-6995, (312) 899-0040, (800) 877-1600, amacmunn@eatright.org, http://www.eatright.org.

Food and Nutrition Information Center, National Agricultural Library, 10301 Baltimore Ave., Rm. 105, Beltsville, MD 20705, (301) 504-5414, Fax: (301) 504-6409, fnic@ars.usda.gov, http://fnic.nal.usda.gov.

International Foundation for Functional Gastrointestinal Disorders, PO Box 170864, Milwaukee, WI 53217-8076, (414) 964-1799, (888) 964-2001, Fax: (414) 964-7176, iffgd@iffgd.org, http://www.iffgd.org.

National Digestive Diseases Information Clearinghouse, 2 Information Way, Bethesda, MD 20892–3570, (800) 891–5389, TTY: (866) 569–1162, Fax: (703) 738–4929, nddic@info.niddk.nih.gov, http://www.digestive.niddk.nih.gov.

Monique Laberge, PhD
David Newton

Dr. Feingold diet

Definition

The Dr. Feingold diet is a diet that eliminates many **food additives** and other compounds from the diet. It is intended to reduce the symptoms of attention deficit disorder (ADD) and attention deficit **hyperactivity** disorder (ADHD). Many proponents of the diet suggest that it can be used to improve other common problems as well.

Origins

The Dr. Feingold diet was developed by Dr. Ben F. Feingold during the 1970s. Dr. Feingold was born on June 15th, 1899, in Pittsburgh, Pennsylvania. He received his Bachelor of Science degree from the University of Pittsburgh in 1921, and his Medical Degree from the same institution in 1924. Following this, he did an internship from 1924 to 1925 at Passavant Hospital, also in Pittsburgh, and then a fellowship in pathology at the University of Goettingen in Germany. He then spent 1928 and 1929 working with children in Austria before returning to the United States to be an instructor of pediatrics at the Northwestern University School of Medicine.

Dr. Feingold continued to work with children, specifically in the developing area of allergy studies. During World War II he was a commander in the U.S. Navy and then returned from the war to be chief of pediatrics at Cedars of Lebanon Hospital in Los Angeles, California. He worked at various other hospitals and established all of the Departments of Allergy for Northern California for Kaiser Foundation Hospitals and Permanent Medical Group in 1951. He died on March 23, 1982.

During his career, Dr. Feingold mainly studied allergies in children. He noticed that the increase of children exhibiting symptoms of hyperactivity seemed to correspond with the increased consumption by children of various food additives. He hypothesized that these food additives were what was causing the symptoms he observed. During the 1970s he set out to study this relationship and believed he had found a link. In 1975, he published the book *Why Your Child is Hyperactive*. The Dr. Feingold diet is derived from this book. Since then, the children he called "hyperactive" have been identified as having ADD or ADHD.

Although Dr. Feingold died in 1982, his followers and adherents continue to update his diet and ideas. Although he intended his diet only for the treatment of hyperactivity, the Feingold Association of the United

States has identified many other problems that my be alleviated by the diet. They have also continued to update the foods and additives believed to cause behavior and other problems in children.

Description

The Dr. Feingold diet involves eliminating from the diet all forms of food additives and chemicals believed (by the diet's proponents) to be the cause of a variety of diseases and disorders, most generally ADD and ADHD. The diet occurs in two stages: the first stage involves eliminating all of the offending foods, and the second stage involves reintroducing them one at a time to see which ones can be eaten without causing symptoms.

There are four main groups of chemicals and additives that are eliminated during the Dr. Feingold diet. The first of these are all forms of synthetic coloring. These are often made from by-products of petroleum, and some people believe that they cause hyperactivity. This means that any food products that have artificial colors (which include many popular children's foods and treats) are strictly forbidden.

The second group is artificial flavorings. The Feingold Association believes that many of these additives have not been studied carefully and can cause unwanted behaviors in children. Of special concern is the artificial vanilla flavoring vanillin, which is often made from by-products of paper production.

The Dr. Feingold diet requires the elimination of aspartame, an artificial sweetener sold mainly under the brand name NutraSweet. This restriction is not as limiting as it may have been in the past because of the number of non-aspartame sweeteners now available.

Artificial preservatives are also eliminated completely when on this diet. These include the preservatives BHA (butylated hydroxyanisole) and BHT (butylated hydroxytoluene), which are derived from petroleum. The purpose of these preservatives is mainly to delay the oxidization of **fats** in foods. Oxidization makes fats go rancid, so these preservatives give foods a longer shelf-life.

During stage one of the diet many salicylates are removed, but they may be reintroduced during stage two. Salicylates are a group of chemicals, some of which occur naturally, that are related to aspirin. Foods that contain salicylates include apples, berries, grapes, oranges, peaches, plums, tangerines, and tomatoes, along with many others.

The Dr. Feingold diet can be very time consuming to follow, especially at first, because many of the forbidden substances occur under a variety of names on labels, all of which must be learned. The Feingold Association of the United States produces a set of materials intended to help people beginning the diet, including an 150-page food guide. These can be ordered for a fee from their website, http://feingold.org.

Function

The Dr. Feingold diet is generally used for children, although it may be effective for adults as well. It is intended to remove substances that some people believe cause ADD and ADHD. According to the Feingold Association of the United States, it can also be effective in reducing or eliminating impulsiveness, compulsiveness, disruptive behaviors, poor self-control, abusive or unpredictable behavior, and destructive behaviors. They also believe it can change workaholic habits, chewing on clothing or other inappropriate objects, depression, frequent crying, irritability, panic, low self-esteem, mood swings, impatience, distraction, inability to follow directions, poor muscle coordination, speech difficulties, tics, seizures, and difficulty with comprehension. The association states that it may help physical problems such as ear infections, asthma, bedwetting, and **constipation**, and sleep problems such as resistance going to bed, difficulty falling asleep, and nightmares.

Benefits

There are many benefits for children who eat a balanced diet including many fresh fruits and vegetables. Because the Dr. Feingold diet excludes many forms of artificial additives, it may limit the amount of processed food available to consume, leading to a more balanced diet that contains whole foods. However, many fresh fruits must be eliminated during stage one because of naturally occurring salicylates. The diet may result in reduced symptoms of ADD and ADHD and is reported by the American Feingold Association to be able to resolve other physical, emotional, and sleep complaints.

Precautions

When starting any diet there are some risks, especially when beginning a diet that is very restrictive. The Dr. Feingold diet is inflexible on the point that all foods containing offending additives or compounds be completely eliminated from the diet. It is important for all adults to eat a balanced diet, but this is especially important for children. Not getting the right amounts of **vitamins** and **minerals** each day can have negative effects on a child's growth and development.

This may be a concern for children on the Dr. Feingold diet because stage one limits many healthy fruits such as apples, oranges, and grapes.

One problem some families may find when on the Dr. Feingold diet is that it is very time intensive. A significant amount of time is required to learn all the rules of the diet and to learn how to identify the various forbidden additives in all of the forms in which they may appear on labels. Children have to learn which foods can be eaten and how to read labels. They also need to learn coping skills to be able to explain to other children and any adults who might be offering them food (such as their friend's parents) which foods are not allowed. It may be advisable to go over some skills to help children explain to friends and classmates why they are on a special diet in a way that is not upsetting or embarrassing to them. Parents may wish to inform their children's teachers, babysitters, and any other caregivers about the diet.

One concern for some parents may be that being on such a strict diet may make children feel different than their peers. It can be very hard for children who feel or seem different than those around them, and other children might not understand why they cannot eat candy or have to eat special meals brought from home. Another issue brought up by some people who were on the diet as children is that it puts children who do give into temptation into a very difficult position. Because the Feingold Association maintains the diet must be followed exactly at all times to be effective, children who have eaten something forbidden on the diet must decide whether to admit it or lie to their parents. It can put children and parents into an antagonistic relationship because sometimes if the diet does not cure the disease or disorder, it is assumed that it is because forbidden foods have been consumed. This can lead to a accusations, guilt, and anger. These problems certainly will not occur with every child in every family, but it may be something that parents considering this diet for their child or children would want to consider.

Risks

There are some risks associated with starting any diet. Although there are no significant scientifically documented risks for starting this diet, there is some chance that it may cause feelings of isolation in the child if he or she feels different than other children. There is some risk that this diet may put significant stress on the family because it is very time intensive and must be strictly followed. The diet may also cause some tension in parent-child relationships because the

child may react negatively to being put on the diet or may be tempted to eat forbidden foods.

Research and general acceptance

The Dr. Feingold diet is extremely controversial. Since the 1970s many different experiments have been done in an attempt to determine if it is capable of the results it claims. Dr. Feingold himself did some preliminary studies in the 1970s, the results of which are still hotly debated by many people. There are many methods used to determine the effectiveness of the diet. These include putting children on the diet and monitoring any improvement in behaviors. To study its effects in an opposite way, scientists have tried reintroducing additives thought to be harmful into the diets of children who have been on the diet and watching to see if behavior deteriorates. The evidence has been mixed, and studies are interpreted differently by each side of the debate. The Feingold Association of the United States cites many different studies on its websites and gives short excerpts or summaries of some of the evidence. The Association cites these studies as proof that the diet is effective for most children. There has not been any significant research done on whether the diet is effective in achieving positive results for problems not related to ADD or ADHD.

Many health professionals are not convinced that the diet can help children with ADD or ADHD. One common argument against the effectiveness of the diet is that there may be other causes for the improvement shown in children on the diet. Because the diet is extremely complicated and involves closely monitoring everything that is eaten (as well as exposure to some things such as soaps and perfumes), parents have to be extremely involved in their child's life while their child is on this diet. Some experts have argued that any improved behavior is probably a result of this increased parental participation and not strategies, bringing healthy food choices into the environment, and even removing large-size clothes from the closet.

Mastery over food

Dr. Phil's fourth key advises people to control habits by gaining mastery over food and through impulse control. The fourth key focuses on wiping bad, weight-gaining habits from their lives and replacing them with healthier behaviors. He lists weight-gaining behaviors and various payoffs they offer to people. The chapter concludes with suggested behaviors to replace the weight-gaining behaviors, as well as the payoffs from the healthier behaviors.

High-response, high-yield foods

In this key, Dr. Phil discusses the nutritional value of various foods by describing a "high-response cost, high-yield food" plan. Instead of offering meal plans or calorie-cutting, Dr. Phil's diet talks about and lists foods that take longer to prepare and eat, and therefore are healthier. He contrasts these foods with those that take little time to prepare and eat, which normally offer higher **calories** and less nutritional value. He also mentions vitamin and mineral supplements in addition to high-yield foods.

Exercise

Dr. Phil calls his sixth key to weight loss intentional exercise. He says that instead of becoming obsessed about exercise, people need to take a balanced approach of regular strength-building and heart-conditioning activities to burn calories. Dr. Phil says that intentional exercise can open the door to body control, a state where the body can better metabolize energy for losing weight and keeping weight off. He breaks exercise into categories of moderate activities and vigorous activities. In addition, the book lists the physical and psychological benefits of exercise.

Support

The final key to weight loss provided by Dr. Phil involves social control. He says people can gain this by having a circle of support. People in a circle of support encourage a person trying to lose or maintain weight and also provide accountability to help achieve weight loss goals. He points out that the key to social support is not just having supportive friends and family in the circle, but also staying away from people who sabotage weight loss efforts.

The book concludes with several appendices, such as food lists, a workout diary, and a sample exercise for stress relief and relaxation. Dr. Phil reminds readers that weight is managed, not cured. He explains danger zones that allow people to drift off course in managing their weight, then discusses avoiding these danger zones.

Function

Dr. Phil's weight loss solution is for people who want to lose or manage weight. He presents the diet as an alternative to crash and **fad diets**. As a psychologist, Dr. Phil approaches the diet from behavioral aspects as well as from the nutritional aspects.

Benefits

Dr. Phil says that in typical diets, the emotion fades soon after starting the diet. In interviews about his weight loss solution, Dr. Phil said that people have better chances of succeeding on weight loss efforts if they reprogram their lives and follow the seven keys to success. He said that fear keeps people from addressing the emotions involved in overeating. The diet also focuses on being healthy and having realistic expectations for a person's age.

Precautions

Some registered dietitians and scientists have questioned the evidence quoted by Dr. Phil for the success rate of his plan and nutritional products. Following any particular diet plan should be done only after consultation with a physician and/or registered dietitian. The advice of involving a nutritionist comes late in Dr. Phil's book.

Risks

Among concerns was the nutritional balance of some of the Shape Up food products. Although Dr. Phil's diet does not lean toward one food group and gives generally traditional diet advice of balanced diet mixed with exercise, it is best to involve a health care

---

professional or registered dietary professional to ensure that the strategies are healthful and successful.

Research and general acceptance

In the book, Dr. Phil cites a bibliography, a consulting nutritionist, and an 80% success rate. However, there are no specific scientific studies published or referred to that prove the success of the program or its individual strategies. After developing the Shape Up products, which consisted of herbal supplements, shakes, and snack bars, a lawsuit was filed stating that Dr. Phil had made false claims about their benefits. Reports showed that although the nutrition shakes were in good ranges for **carbohydrates** and fat, the nutrition bars were in relatively high carbohydrate and fat ranges. The lawsuit was filed in 2004 on behalf of three disappointed consumers. They said that Dr. Phil had defrauded fans, making false statements about the supplement pills. CSA Nutraceuticals agreed to stop making the supplements in early 2004 when it faced an investigation from the Federal Trade Commission concerning false-advertising claims. The plaintiffs sought class action status for the lawsuit and reached a $10.5 million settlement in September 2006.

In an article in *Food Processing* magazine, a diet expert at the University of California at Berkeley was quoted as saying that Dr. Phil's diet advice was not innovative. She added that the advice was common sense. A review in the *Tufts University Health & Nutrition Letter* said there were several flaws in the book's advice and that some of the advice contradicted other points in the book or did not make sense. The review listed some good points, including the fact that a dieter does not have to be strong 24 hours a day, seven days a week.

An **Academy of Nutrition and Dietetics** (formerly the American Dietetic Association) fact sheet said that some of the book's advice is good, such as behavior modification strategies that have been used in weight control programs for many years. But the review said that the book also contained nutrition and dietary recommendations that were mistaken or outdated.

The review also stated that the advice for dealing with complicated emotional and other eating-related issues is made seemingly simple, but that managing these issues alone is not easy.

Resources

BOOKS

McGraw, Phillip C. *The Ultimate Weight Solution: The Seven Keys to Weight Loss Freedom.* The Free Press, 2003.
———. *The Ultimate Weight Solution Cook Book.* The Free Press, 2004.
———. *The Ultimate Weight Solution Food Guide.* Pocket Books, 2005.

PERIODICALS

Neff, Jack. "Dr. Phil Goes to the Grocery Store: The Shape Up! Line of Diet Products Endorsed By Phil McGraw Has Generated Controversy and Questions: Can Anybody Create Diet Foods?" *Food Processing* (April 1, 2004).

WEBSITES

Dorfman, Lisa. "Dr. Phil's Ultimate Weight Solution." Academy of Nutrition and Dietetics. http://www.eatright.org/Media/content.aspx?id=6442451343 (accessed September 28, 2012).
Dr. Phil's official website. http://www.drphil.com (accessed September 28, 2012).

Teresa G. Odle

DRIs *see* **Dietary reference intakes**

Drop 10 diet

Definition

The Drop 10 diet is a diet plan created by *Self* magazine that promises ten or more pounds of weight loss over five weeks.

Origins

The Drop 10 Diet was created by the editor of *Self* magazine, Lucy Danziger. Around 2007, Danziger decided that she wanted to lose a few pounds, but she did not like the idea of the traditional diet with all of its restrictions. Instead, Danziger decided to focus on eating fewer packaged foods that had long shelf lives, and instead eat more fresh foods. She even made a rule that if it was a food she could grow (not that she necessarily grew it, but that she could have done so), she could eat an unlimited quantity of it.

Danziger found that simply by making these food choices she lost ten pounds in five weeks and even more weight in the months that followed. Danziger recommends that adults participate in a total of 2 hours and 30 minutes of moderate-intensity aerobic activity or 1 hour and 15 minutes of vigorous-intensity aerobic activity each week, along with 2 or more days of muscle strengthening activities. The exercise regimen recommended by the Drop 10 diet fits these guidelines.

Resources

BOOKS

Danziger, Lucy. *The Drop 10 Diet: Add to Your Plate to Lose the Weight*. New York, Ballantine Books, 2012.

DeBruyne, Kelly, Kathryn Pinna, and Eleanor Noss Whitney. *Nutrition and Diet Therapy: Principles and Practice*. 8th ed. Belmont, CA: Wadsworth, Cengage Learning, 2012.

Gandy, Joan, Angela Madden, and Michelle Holdsworth, eds. *Oxford Handbook of Nutrition and Dietetics*. 2nd ed. New York: Oxford University Press, 2012.

OTHER

U.S. Department of Agriculture and U.S. Department of Health and Human Services. *Dietary Guidelines for Americans, 2010*. 7th ed. Washington, DC: U.S. Government Printing Office, December 2010. http://health.gov/dietaryguidelines (accessed August 22, 2012).

WEBSITES

Danziger, Lucy. "'The Drop 10 Diet': The Smart Way to Ditch Unwanted Inches [excerpt]." MSNBC.com, March 20, 2012. http://today.msnbc.msn.com/id/46798689/ns/today-books/t/drop-diet-smart-way-ditch-unwanted-inches (accessed August 22, 2012).

"Drop 10 Diet" Self.com. http://www.self.com/about/drop-10-diet (accessed August 22, 2012).

Mayo Clinic staff. "Weight Loss: Choosing a Diet That's Right for You." MayoClinic.com. http://www.mayoclinic.com/health/weight-loss/NU00616 (accessed August 22, 2012).

Wilson, Jacque. "Eat More 'Superfoods' to Lose Weight." CNN.com, April 10, 2012. http://www.cnn.com/2012/04/10/health/superfoods-weight-loss-diet/index.html (accessed August 22, 2012).

ORGANIZATIONS

Academy of Nutrition and Dietetics, 120 South Riverside Plz., Ste. 2000, Chicago, IL 60606-6995, (312) 899-0040, (800) 877-1600, amacmunn@eatright.org, http://www.eatright.org.

Center for Nutrition Policy and Promotion, U.S. Department of Agriculture, 3101 Park Center Drive, 10th Fl., Alexandria, VA 22302, (703) 305-7600, Fax: (703) 305-3300, support@cnpp.usda.gov, http://www.cnpp.usda.gov.

Tish Davidson, AM

Dukan diet

Definition

The Dukan diet is a high-protein, low-carbohydrate diet with four phases in which **carbohydrates** are completely eliminated at first and then slowly reintroduced in limited quantities.

Origins

The Dukan diet was created by Pierre Dukan (1941–), a French doctor. While he began his medical practice as a neurologist, he became interested in the problem of **obesity** and how best to help overweight patients lose weight and keep it off. According to the Dukan diet website, as of mid-2012 Dukan had spent 35 years working in clinical nutrition and had worked with over 40,000 patients.

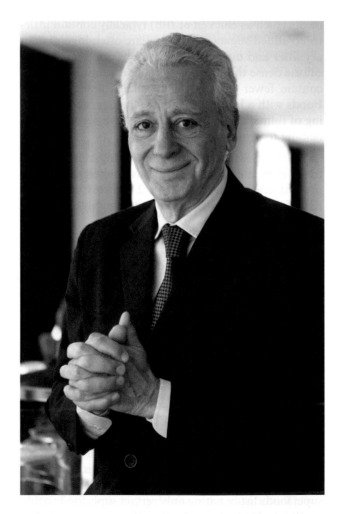

Dr. Pierre Dukan. (© *epa european pressphoto agency b.v./ Alamy*)

The Dukan diet was first introduced in France in 2000, when Dukan published his first diet book *Je ne sais pas maigrir*, which roughly translates to "I don't know how to lose weight." The book became widely successful in France, remaining a best seller for more than ten years, and was followed by many other books about the diet, including a variety of cookbooks.

In 2011, Dukan released *The Dukan Diet: 2 Steps to Lose the Weight, 2 Steps to Keep It Off Forever* in the United States, where it also became a best seller. As of 2012, Dukan's diet books had been published in more than 14 languages and sold over 7 million copies worldwide.

Description

The Dukan diet is a high-protein, low-carbohydrate (HPLC) diet that is divided into four phases. It completely restricts carbohydrates at first, and then slowly adds a small amount back into the diet. The final phase is intended to be a lifelong way of eating to help the dieter maintain the weight loss achieved during the previous phases.

The Dukan diet is different from another popular HPLC, the **Atkins diet**, in a few ways that Dukan emphasizes as being extremely important. The Dukan diet requires all dieters following his plan to drink at least 1.5 quarts (1.5 L) of water each day. Dukan suggests that this will help prevent the kidney problems often associated with HPLC diets. Also, the Dukan diet requires the dieter to eat a certain amount of oat bran each day. This, combined with the required water intake, may help prevent the **constipation** many dieters experience while on other HPLC diets. Additionally, the Dukan diet emphasizes lean sources of **protein** and does not allow high-fat meats such as bacon that other HPLC diets allow.

The Dukan diet also allows **artificial sweeteners** (but no **sugar**), diet soft drinks, teas, nonfat milk, and some other nonfat dairy products during each phase of the diet. It also recommends using spices, herbs, onions, shallots, vinegar, and other seasonings that do not contain any fat and no or very few **calories**. These are recommended to help dieters stick to the diet by providing them with ways to change the taste of the allowed high-protein foods so that they do not become bored with the available food options.

Phase 1: Attack

This is the first phase of the diet, and it is intended to "jump start" the dieter's weight loss. This phase lasts between 2 and 7 days. During this phase, no carbohydrates are allowed, except for a small amount of oat bran eaten each day. No fruits or vegetables are allowed during this phase. The dieter can, however, eat an unlimited amount of any of 68 high-protein foods. These foods include:

- beef (roasts or grilled items only, and not fatty cuts such as ribs)
- veal (cutlets, roast, or well-trimmed chops)
- buffalo
- venison
- chicken
- turkey
- other lean poultry
- eggs
- tofu

During this phase the dieter must consume 1.5 teaspoons of oat bran each day and should walk at a moderate pace for 20 minutes a day.

Phase 2: Cruise

The second phase of the Dukan diet lasts until the dieter has reached his or her goal weight. It generally lasts for about three days for each pound of weight loss desired. This phase allows all of the high-protein foods allowed in phase one. On alternate days, this phase also allows the inclusion of a small number of vegetables. The dieter is allowed to eat as much as he or she desires of all allowed foods. The allowed vegetables include:

- broccoli
- celery
- cucumber
- mushrooms
- spinach
- tomatoes

During this phase, no starchy vegetables, such as potatoes or corn, are allowed. The dieter must eat 2 tablespoons of oat bran each day and should increase his or her daily exercise to 30 minutes of brisk walking each day. This phase continues until the dieter has reached his or her goal weight.

Phase 3: Consolidation

Phase 3 begins after the dieter has reached his or her goal weight. The purpose of this phase is to ensure that the dieter does not regain the weight lost during the first two phases. This phase lasts for approximately five days for each pound the dieter lost in phase 2. During this phase, the dieter can introduce a small amount of foods that were previously not allowed, such as fruit and hard cheese. The dieter is print. http://dx.doi.org/10.1007/s00394-012-0338-0 (accessed August 25, 2012).

WEBSITES

"Dukan Diet." U.S. News & World Report: Health. http://health.usnews.com/best-diet/dukan-diet (accessed August 25, 2012).

"The Dukan Diet: Four Slimmers Give Their Verdict." BBC News Europe, July 5, 2011. http://www.bbc.co.uk/news/business-14020154 (accessed August 25, 2012).

Dukan diet official website. http://www.dukandiet.co.uk (accessed August 25, 2012).

Mayo Clinic staff. "Low-Carb Diet: Can It Help You Lose Weight?" MayoClinic.com http://www.mayoclinic.com/health/low-carb-diet/NU00279 (accessed August 25, 2012).

Zelman, Kathleen M. "'The Dukan Diet' Review." http://www.webmd.com/diet/features/dukan-diet-review (accessed August 25, 2012).

ORGANIZATIONS

Academy of Nutrition and Dietetics, 120 South Riverside Plz., Ste. 2000, Chicago, IL 60606-6995, (312) 899-0040, (800) 877-1600, amacmunn@eatright.org, http://www.eatright.org.

Center for Nutrition Policy and Promotion, U.S. Department of Agriculture, 3101 Park Center Drive, 10th Fl., Alexandria, VA 22302-1594, (703) 305-7600, Fax: (703) 305-3300, support@cnpp.usda.gov, http://www.cnpp.usda.gov.

Tish Davidson, AM

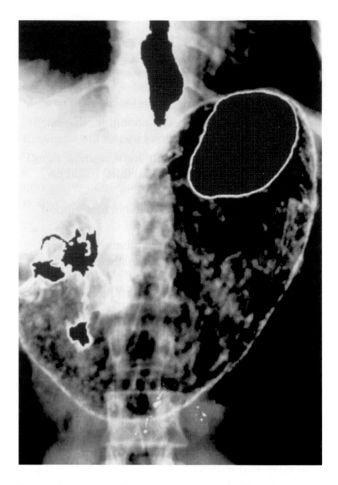

Stomach x-ray showing gastroesophageal reflux disease (GERD). The acid is shown traveling up the esophagus (in red), resulting in heartburn. *(Science Photo Library/CMSP)*

Dyspepsia

Definition

Dyspepsia is gastric upset due to the inability to properly digest food.

Origins

Dyspepsia is a word that has been used in English since the early eighteenth century not only for a variety of stomach ailments but also for bad moods or temper outbursts that were thought to be caused by indigestion. The English word comes from two Greek words meaning "hard or difficult" and "digestion." For many years dyspepsia was a catchall term for any kind of stomach upset characterized by burning, nauseous, or gassy sensations in the upper abdomen. Several phrases that are still used almost interchangeably for the condition are gastric indigestion, nervous dyspepsia, and impaired gastric function.

Dyspepsia was not defined more closely until the mid-1980s, when an international group of gastroenterologists (doctors who specialize in treating disorders of the digestive system) met in Rome to create a set of criteria for distinguishing dyspepsia from other disorders of the upper digestive tract (known as the Rome criteria); and to distinguish between organic dyspepsia—stomach upset that can be shown to have a physical cause (for example, stomach irritation caused by **alcohol consumption**), and functional dyspepsia (FD)—dyspepsia that cannot be traced to any specific physical cause. FD accounts for a majority of cases of dyspepsia, as many as 60% in some studies, and for 30%–50% of all referrals from primary care doctors to gastroenterologists.

Dyspepsia is considered a difficult condition to treat, even though it is widespread in the general population. An estimated 25%–40% of adolescents and adults in North America experience dyspepsia each year. Most people with the disorder do not seek medical treatment because it may be intermittent as well as persistent. FD is responsible for high health care costs in terms of prescription as well as over-the-counter medications, diagnostic tests, and time lost from work.

In the nineteenth and early twentieth centuries, FD was commonly treated with various forms of dietary therapies. Treatments commonly recommended by doctors in the 1920s included vegetarian diets as well as the use of laxatives and enemas to cure the patient of autointoxication—an imaginary disorder that originated in ancient Egypt and is based on the belief that the contents of the colon are toxic and capable of poisoning other body organs. Folk dietary remedies for dyspepsia included drinking peppermint tea or milk, eating spearmint leaves, or chewing mint-flavored chewing gum, which first became popular in the 1860s.

Although FD is not fully understood, there are several theories regarding its underlying mechanisms or possible causes:

- FD reflects greater than average sensitivity to uncomfortable sensations in the digestive tract. This theory holds that patients with FD perceive sensations in the stomach or intestines as painful that most people experience as ordinary or do not feel at all.
- FD is a motility disorder. FD may result from a decreased ability of the digestive system to contract and push food through the system. This, in turn, causes lower than normal stomach emptying.
- FD is caused by *Helicobacter pylori* infection. *H. pylori* is a spiral-shaped bacterium that is the only known microorganism that can live in the acidic environment of the stomach. It is now known to be a cause of peptic ulcers, but doctors do not yet agree on its role in functional dyspepsia.

Description

The Rome criteria for FD specify that the patient must have had 12 weeks (not necessarily consecutively) of the following symptoms in the previous 12 months:

- Persistent or recurrent pain or discomfort centered in the upper abdomen.
- No evidence of an organic disease (including findings from an endoscopy of the upper digestive tract) that is likely to explain the symptoms.
- No evidence that the dyspepsia is relieved exclusively by defecation or associated with the onset of a change in bowel habits.

The Rome criteria specify three subtypes of FD based on the most bothersome symptom: ulcer-like dyspepsia (pain in the upper abdomen); dysmotility-like dyspepsia (an unpleasant but nonpainful feeling of bloating, fullness, or nausea); and unspecified dyspepsia (patient's digestive discomfort does not fit either of the first two categories).

FD is widespread in the general population, however, the subtypes identified by the Rome working group appear to show slight gender differences. Ulcer-like dyspepsia appears to be more common in men and dysmotility-like dyspepsia more common in women. FD is equally widespread in all racial and ethnic groups.

Some medications other than aspirin and other over-the-counter pain relievers may cause dyspepsia: alendronate (Fosamax); codeine and aspirin fortified with codeine; **iron** supplements; metformin (Glucophage); oral antibiotics, particularly erythromycin; **orlistat** (Xenical); corticosteroids, especially prednisone; and theophylline. Patients should consult their doctors before discontinuing these drugs or changing the dosage.

Treatment

Dietary

Dietary treatment for dyspepsia generally consists of cutting down on alcohol intake; avoiding fatty or highly spiced foods; and avoiding any other food that appears to trigger episodes of dyspepsia. Therapeutic fasting, which is thought to give the digestive system a period of rest before making other changes in the patient's diet or beginning medication therapy, may be recommended.

Patients with FD may also benefit from discontinuing certain herbal remedies that produce symptoms of dyspepsia. These include garlic, ginkgo, saw palmetto, feverfew, chaste tree berry, and willow bark.

Medical

Medical management of FD in patients typically begins with either testing and treating the patient for infection with *H. pylori* or by prescribing medications to lower the level of stomach acid secretions for a trial period of 4–8 weeks. The two classes of medications most commonly prescribed to reduce acid secretion are H_2-receptor blockers and proton pump inhibitors (PPIs). The first group, which is the older of the two, was developed in the late 1970s and early 1980s and includes such drugs as cimetidine (Tagamet) and ranitidine (Zantac). The proton pump inhibitors are more

American Journal of Gastroenterology 100 (December 2005): 2743–2748.

Talley, Nicholas J., Nimish Vakil, and the Practice Parameters Committee of the American College of Gastroenterology (ACG). "Guidelines for the Management of Dyspepsia." *American Journal of Gastroenterology* 100 (October 2005): 2324–2337.

WEBSITES

American Academy of Family Physicians. "Dyspepsia." FamilyDoctor.org. http://familydoctor.org/familydoctor/en/diseases-conditions/dyspepsia.html (accessed September 29, 2012).

National Center for Complementary and Alternative Medicine (NCCAM). "Herbs at a Glance: Aloe Vera." National Institutes of Health. http://nccam.nih.gov/health/aloevera (accessed September 29, 2012).

———. "Herbs at a Glance: Peppermint Oil." National Institutes of Health. http://nccam.nih.gov/health/peppermintoil (accessed September 29, 2012).

———. "Herbs at a Glance: Turmeric." National Institutes of Health. http://nccam.nih.gov/health/turmeric/ataglance.htm (accessed September 29, 2012).

National Digestive Diseases Information Clearinghouse (NDDIC). "Indigestion." National Institute of Diabetes and Digestive and Kidney Diseases (NIDDK). http://digestive.niddk.nih.gov/ddiseases/pubs/indigestion (accessed September 29, 2012).

ORGANIZATIONS

American Gastroenterological Association, 4930 Del Ray Ave., Bethesda, MD 20814, (301) 654-2055, Fax: (301) 654-5920, member@gastro.org, http://www.gastro.org.

International Foundation for Functional Gastrointestinal Disorders, PO Box 170864, Milwaukee, WI 53217, (414) 964-1799, (888) 964-2001, Fax: (414) 964-7176, iffgd@iffgd.org, http://www.iffgd.org.

National Center for Complementary and Alternative Medicine Clearinghouse, PO Box 7923, Gaithersburg, MD 20898, (888) 644-6226, Fax: (866) 464-3616, info@nccam.nih.gov, http://nccam.nih.gov.

National Digestive Diseases Information Clearinghouse, 2 Information Way, Bethesda, MD 20892–3570, (800) 891–5389, TTY: (866) 569–1162, Fax: (703) 738–4929, nddic@info.niddk.nih.gov, http://www.digestive.niddk.nih.gov.

North American Society for Pediatric Gastroenterology, Hepatology, and Nutrition, PO Box 6, Flourtown, PA 19031, (215) 233-0808, Fax: (215) 233-3918, naspghan@naspghan.org, http://www.naspghan.org.

Rebecca J. Frey, PhD

E

East African diet *see* **African diet**

Eat More, Weigh Less *see* **Dean Ornish's Eat More, Weigh Less**

Eat Stop Eat *see* **Intermittent fasting**

Eat-Clean diet

Definition

The Eat-Clean diet is a weight loss and lifestyle plan that emphasizes eating unrefined (or "whole") foods in an attempt to eliminate all processed foods and refined ingredients, such as white flour or **sugar**, from the diet.

Origins

The Eat-Clean program is the brainchild of Tosca Reno. Reno, a Canadian, found herself overweight and with little energy at age 40. She lost weight and transformed herself into a fitness and lifestyle guru by exercising and following what became the Eat-Clean diet. She entered various fitness competitions and began publishing columns in fitness magazines, which eventually led to the publication of a dozen Eat-Clean books that she published with her husband, Robert Kennedy, as well as the *Clean Eating* magazine and a television program.

Description

The Eat-Clean organization emphasizes that clean eating is not a diet but a lifestyle. The program is structured so that participants eat five or six meals of 250–300 **calories** daily. Calorie counting is discouraged, however, and the program instead emphasizes portion control and limiting all processed and refined foods, alcohol, food colorings, preservatives, and saturated **fats**. Dieters are instructed to eat organic foods when possible,

choosing from lean meat (e.g., chicken, fish, turkey), vegetable proteins (e.g., soya, textured vegetable **protein**), **whole grains** (e.g., brown rice, quinoa, oats), and fresh fruits and vegetables. Other program guidelines include eating a small amount of protein with a complex carbohydrate at every meal, drinking at least eight glasses of water daily, never skipping a meal, and consuming small amounts of healthy fats. In addition, the program recommends certain **dietary supplements** and a weight-training program of at least 30 minutes three times a week, with additional exercise encouraged.

The Eat-Clean diet does not require the purchase of a membership, meeting attendance, or the purchase of pre-packaged foods. Dieters do have the option of purchasing any of the books and cookbooks written by Tosca Reno. Facebook and Twitter groups are available to offer support. Since the goal of this program is lifestyle change, there are no specific weight loss goals and no defined end to the program.

Function

The Eat-Clean diet is intended to promote weight loss, increase energy, and improve fitness. By eating many small meals, the diet strives to keep blood sugar levels constant and prevent hunger. The emphasis on chemical-free organic foods is intended to reduce the chemical burden on the body.

Benefits

The Eat-Clean program's emphasis on whole grains, lean proteins, and fresh fruits and vegetables is in line with conventional nutritional thinking on healthy eating. Vegetarians can go on this diet so long as they are careful about their protein consumption. This diet may be suitable for people with diabetes but should not be started without consulting a physician.

Limited portions and emphasis on exercise do lead to weight loss, as more calories are used than are taken in on the diet. The diet emphasizes a slow, steady weight loss of an average of 2 lb. (1 kg) per week, which is in line with most medical advice. Weight loss often increases energy and improves self-confidence and the general feeling of well-being.

The low cost of beginning the diet (Eat-Clean books cost about $17 per book) is another benefit, although participants may find they are spending more money at the grocery store to buy high-quality protein and organic foods.

Precautions

It is nearly impossible to eliminate all processed foods from the diet. People participating in the Eat-Clean program should understand that it is extremely difficult and should not feel as though they are unsuccessful if they do consume processed foods or ingredients.

Anyone beginning this diet should consult a healthcare professional, especially individuals with a chronic disease, such as diabetes or another ongoing health problem. If taking dietary supplements, participants should make sure that the supplements do not interact with any other medications (prescription, over-the-counter or herbal) that they are taking. Women who are, or who wish to become, pregnant should discuss the appropriateness of this diet and exercise program with their physician.

Risks

The greatest risk to participants is the difficulty in staying on the program. Dieters must give up many common foods and must eat frequently throughout the day. This can make work and socializing difficult. In addition, exercising is an essential part of the Eat-Clean program. Some suggested exercises may not be appropriate for everyone and could aggravate a pre-existing condition. Individuals should check with a healthcare professional about the type and level of exercise that is appropriate for their fitness levels.

Research and general acceptance

Many of the principles of the Eat-Clean diet are endorsed by the traditional medical establishment. This is not a fad diet. However, some healthcare professionals express reservations about the dietary supplements

recommended by the program, and other medical experts have also questioned the dietary fat restrictions imposed by the diet.

Resources

BOOKS

Reno, Tosca. *The Eat Clean Diet*. Robert Kennedy, 2006.
———. *The Eat-Clean Diet Recharged: Lasting Fat Loss That's Better than Ever!* Robert Kennedy, 2009.
———. *Tosca Reno's Eat Clean Cookbook: Delicious Recipes That Will Burn Fat and Re-Shape Your Body!* Robert Kennedy, 2009.

WEBSITES

Clean Eating magazine. http://www.cleaneatingmag.com (accessed August 24, 2012).
"Eat Clean Diet." Everydiet.org. http://www.everydiet.org/diet/clean-eat-diet (accessed August 24, 2012).
"Eat Clean Diet Recharged." Everydiet.org. http://www.everydiet.org/diet/eat-clean-diet-recharged (accessed August 24, 2012).
"The Eat-Clean Diet." http://www.eatcleandiet.com (accessed August 24, 2012).
Zelman, Katherine M. "The Eat-Clean Diet: Diet Review." WebMD.com. http://www.webmd.com/diet/features/eat-clean-diet-review (accessed August 24, 2012).

Tish Davidson, AM

Eating disorders

Definition

Eating disorders (EDs) are psychiatric disorders that have diagnostic criteria based on psychologic, behavior, and physiologic characteristics that usually

Symptoms of eating disorders		
Anorexia nervosa	**Bulimia nervosa**	**Binge eating disorder**
Resistance to maintaining body weight at or above a minimally normal weight for age and height	Recurrent episodes of binge eating, characterized by eating an excessive amount of food within a discrete period of time and by a sense of lack of control over eating during the episode	Recurrent episodes of binge eating, characterized by eating an excessive amount of food within a discrete period of time and by a sense of lack of control over eating during the episode
Intense fear of gaining weight or becoming fat, even though underweight	Recurrent inappropriate compensatory behavior in order to prevent weight gain, such as self-induced vomiting or misuse of laxatives, diuretics, enemas, or other medications (purging); fasting; or excessive exercise	The binge-eating episodes are associated with at least 3 of the following: eating much more rapidly than normal; eating until feeling uncomfortably full; eating large amounts of food when not feeling physically hungry; eating alone because of embarrassment by how much one is eating; feeling disgusted, depressed, or very guilty after overeating
Disturbance in the way in which one's body weight or shape is experienced, undue influence of body weight or shape on self-evaluation, or denial of the seriousness of the current low body weight	The binge eating and inappropriate compensatory behaviors both occur, on average, at least twice weekly for 3 months	Marked distress about the binge-eating behavior
Infrequent or absent menstrual periods (in females who have reached puberty)	Self-evaluation is unduly influenced by body shape and weight	The binge eating occurs, on average, at least 2 days a week for 6 months
		The binge eating is not associated with the regular use of inappropriate compensatory behaviors (e.g., purging, fasting, excessive exercise)

SOURCE: National Institute of Mental Health, National Institutes of Health, U.S. Department of Health and Human Services

(Table by PreMediaGlobal. © 2013 Cengage Learning.)

result in abnormal eating patterns that have a negative effect on health.

Demographics

According to the National Comorbidity Survey Replication study, reported lifetime prevalence rates for **anorexia nervosa** were 0.3% in men and 0.9% in women; for **bulimia nervosa**, 0.5% in men and 1.5% in women; and for **binge eating** disorder, 2% in men and 3.5% in women. In general, more women have eating disorders than men, and according to the National Eating Disorder Association, an estimated 10 million females in the United States have some form of eating disorder. The age at which a person develops an ED differs within conditions, with the greatest frequency of anorexia nervosa and bulimia nervosa occurring during adolescence, whereas binge eating disorder occurs well into adulthood. There are also clinical reports that show an increasing trend in EDs for middle-aged women. Longitudinal research has documented that 12% of adolescent girls aged 12 to 15 years, have experienced some form of ED. Anorexia athletica, muscle dysmorphic disorder, and orthorexia nervosa tend to be more common in men. Rumination, **pica**, and Prader-Willi syndrome affect men and women equally.

Anorexia nervosa begins primarily between the ages of 14 and 18 and affects mainly white girls. Bulimia usually develops slightly later, in the late teens and early twenties. Binge eating disorder is a problem of middle age and affects blacks and whites equally. Prader-Willi syndrome begins in the toddler years. Not enough is known about the more newly classified disorders—such as anorexia athletica, muscle dysmorphic disorder, and orthorexia nervosa—to determine when they are most likely to develop or which races or ethnic groups are most likely to be at risk.

Description

Eating disorders are largely psychological disorders. They develop when a person has an unrealistic attitude toward or abnormal perception of his or her body. This causes behaviors that lead to destructive eating patterns that have negative physical and emotional consequences. Individuals with eating disorders often hide their symptoms and resist seeking treatment. Depression, anxiety disorders, and other mental illnesses often are present in people who have eating disorders, although it is not clear whether these cause the eating disorder or are a result of it.

The two best-known eating disorders, anorexia nervosa and bulimia nervosa, have formal diagnostic criteria and are recognized as psychiatric disorders in the *Diagnostic and Statistical Manual for Mental Disorders*, fourth edition (*DSM-IV-TR*) published by the American Psychiatric Association (APA). Other eating disorders have recognized sets of symptoms, but have not been researched thoroughly enough to be considered separate psychiatric disorders as defined by the APA.

Well-known eating disorders

In North America and Europe, anorexia nervosa is the most publicized of all eating disorders. It gained widespread public attention with the rise of the ultra-thin fashion model. People who have anorexia nervosa are obsessed with body weight. They constantly monitor their food intake and starve themselves to become thin. No matter how much weight they lose, they continue to restrict their calorie intake in an effort to become ever thinner. Some people with anorexia overexercise or abuse drugs or herbal remedies that they believe will help them burn **calories** faster. A few purge their bodies of the few calories they do eat by abusing laxatives, enemas, and diuretics. In time, they reach a point where their health is seriously, and potentially fatally, impaired.

People with anorexia nervosa have an abnormal perception of their body. They genuinely believe that they are larger than they are, even if they are life-threateningly thin. People with anorexia may deny that they are too thin, or, if they admit they are thin, deny that their behavior is affecting their health. People with anorexia will lie to family, friends, and healthcare providers about how much they eat. Many vigorously resist treatment and accuse the people trying to cure them of wanting to make them fat. Anorexia nervosa is the most difficult eating disorder to recover from.

Bulimia nervosa is the only other eating disorder with specific diagnostic criteria defined by the (*DSM-IV-TR*). People with bulimia often consume unreasonably large amounts of food in a short time. Afterwards, they purge their body of calories. This is done most often by self-induced vomiting, often accompanied by laxative abuse. A subset of people with bulimia does not vomit after eating, but fast and exercise obsessively to burn calories. Both behaviors result in impaired health.

People with bulimia feel out of control when they are binge eating. Unlike people with anorexia, they recognize that their behavior is abnormal. Often they are ashamed and feel guilty about their behavior and will go to great lengths to hide their binge/purge cycles from their family and friends. People with bulimia are often of normal weight. Although their behavior results in negative health consequences, because they are less likely to be ultrathin, these consequences are less likely to be life-threatening.

The APA does not formally recognize binge eating as an eating disorder. Binge eating is quite common, but it only rises to the level of a disorder when bingeing occurs at least twice a week for three months or more. People with binge eating disorder may eat thousands of calories in an hour or two. While they are eating, they feel out of control and may continue to eat long after they feel full. Unlike bulimia, people with binge eating disorder do not purge or exercise to get rid of the calories they have eaten. As a result, many people with binge eating disorder are obese, although not all obese people are binge eaters.

People with binge eating disorder may feel ashamed of their behavior and may try to hide it by eating in secret or hoarding food for future binges. After a binge, they usually feel guilty about their eating behavior. They might promise themselves that they will never binge again but are usually unable to keep this promise. Binge eating disorder often follows this seemingly endless cycle—rigorous dieting followed by an eating binge followed by guilt and rigorous dieting, followed by another eating binge. The main health consequences of binge eating are the development of obesity-related diseases such as type 2 diabetes, sleep apnea, stroke, and heart attack.

Lesser-known eating disorders

Quite a few eating problems are called disorders even though they do not have formal diagnostic criteria. They fall under the APA definition of eating disorders not otherwise specified. Many have only recently come to the attention of researchers and have been the subject of only a few small studies. Some have been known to the medical community for years but are rare.

Purge disorder is thought by some experts to be a separate disorder from bulimia. It is distinguished from bulimia by the fact that the individual maintains a normal or near normal weight despite purging by vomiting or laxative, enema, or diuretic abuse.

Anorexia athletica is a disorder of compulsive exercising. The individual places exercise above work, school, or relationships and defines his or her self-worth in terms of athletic performance. People with anorexia athletica also tend to be obsessed less with body weight than with maintaining an abnormally low percentage of body fat. This disorder is common among elite athletes.

Muscle dysmorphic disorder is the opposite of anorexia nervosa. Where people with anorexia believe that they are always overweight, people with muscle dysmorphic disorder believe that they are too small. This belief is maintained even when a person is clearly well-muscled. Abnormal eating patterns are less of a problem in people with muscle dysmorphic disorder than damage from compulsive exercising (even when injured) and the abuse of muscle-building drugs such as anabolic steroids.

Orthorexia nervosa is a term coined by Steven Bratman, a Colorado physician, to describe "a pathological fixation on eating 'proper,' 'pure,' or 'superior' foods." People with orthorexia allow their fixation with eating the correct amount of properly prepared healthy foods at the correct time of day to take over their lives. This obsession interferes with relationships and daily activities. For example, they may be unwilling to eat at restaurants or friends' homes because the food is impure or improperly prepared. The limitations they put on what they will eat can cause serious vitamin and mineral imbalances. People with orthorexia may be judgmental about what other people eat to the point where it interferes with personal relationships. They justify their fixation by claiming that their way of eating is healthy. Some experts believe orthorexia may be a variation of obsessive-compulsive disorder.

Rumination syndrome occurs when an individual, either voluntarily or involuntarily, regurgitates food almost immediately after swallowing it, chews it, and then either swallows it or spits it out. Regurgitation syndrome is the human equivalent of a cow chewing its cud. The behavior often lasts up to two hours after eating. It must continue for at least one month to be considered a disorder. Occasionally the behavior simply stops on its own, but it can last for years.

Pica is the eating of non-food substances by people developmentally past the stage where this is normal (usually around age two). Earth and clay are the most common non-foods eaten, although people have been known to eat hair, feces, lead, laundry starch, chalk, burnt matches, cigarette butts, light bulbs, and other equally bizarre non-foods. This disorder has been known to the medical community for years, and in some cultures (mainly tribes living in equatorial Africa) is considered normal. Pica is most common among people with intellectual disability and developmental delays. It only rises to the level of a disorder when health complications require medical treatment.

Prader-Willi syndrome is a genetic defect that spontaneously arises in chromosome 15. It causes low muscle tone, short stature, incomplete sexual development, intellectual disability, and an uncontrollable urge to eat. People with Prader-Willi syndrome never feel full. The only way to stop them from eating themselves to death is to keep them in environments where food is locked up and not available. Prader-Willi syndrome is a rare disease, and although it is caused by a genetic defect, tends not to run in families, but rather is an accident of development. Fewer than 15,000 people in the United States have Prader-Willi syndrome.

"Drunkorexia," though not a medically recognized diagnosis, is the restriction of calories from food in order to consume greater amounts of alcohol without gaining weight. It is becoming increasingly common—a study conducted by professors at the University of Minnesota and published in the journal *Comprehensive Psychiatry* found that one in five students was substituting alcoholic beverages for meals. According to the U.S. Centers for Disease Control and Prevention, binge drinking is defined as having more than five drinks for men or four drinks for women in an short time frame. It is associated with a slew of adverse health effects, including higher risk of alcohol dependence, high blood pressure, stroke, heart disease, liver disease, neurological damage, sexual dysfunctions, injury (whether intentional or unintentional), and sexually transmitted diseases (due to lowered inhibitions while drunk). Replacing meals with alcohol can also place a person at risk of vitamin and nutrient deficiencies and **malnutrition**.

Causes and symptoms

Depression, low self-worth, and anxiety disorders are all common among people with eating disorders. Some disorders have obsessive-compulsive elements. The association between these psychiatric disorders and eating disorders is strong, but the cause and effect relationship is still unclear. Most specialists agree that eating disorders have multiple causes. There appears to be a genetic predisposition in some people toward developing an eating disorder. Biochemistry also seems to play a role. Neurotransmitters in the brain, such as serotonin, play a role in regulating appetite. Abnormalities in the amount of some neurotransmitters are thought to play a role in anorexia, bulimia, and binge eating disorder. Other disorders have not been studied enough to draw any conclusions.

Personality type can also put people at risk for developing an eating disorder. Low self-worth is common among people with eating disorders. Binge eaters and people with bulimia tend to have problems with impulse control and anger management. A tendency toward obsessive-compulsive behavior and black-or-white, all-or-nothing thinking also put people at higher risk.

Social and environmental factors also affect the development and maintenance of eating disorders and may trigger relapses during recovery. Relationship conflict, a disordered or unstructured home life, job or school stress, and transitional events such as moving or starting a new job are all potential triggers for some people to begin disordered eating behaviors. Dieting (nutritional and social stress) is the most common trigger of all. The United States in the early twenty-first century is a culture obsessed with thinness. The media constantly send the message through words and images that being not just thin, but ultrathin, is fashionable and desirable. Magazines aimed mostly at women devote thousands of words every month to diet and exercise advice that creates a sense of dissatisfaction, unrealistic goals, and through air-brushing models to make them look thinner, many women develop a distorted **body image**.

Research has documented that comorbid illnesses and EDs tend to be diagnosed as a cluster of diagnoses; that is, patients with EDs often experience other psychiatric disorders. Axis I psychiatric disorders (including depression, anxiety, body dysmorphic disorder, or chemical dependency) and Axis II personality disorders (particularly borderline personality disorder) are frequently seen in the ED population. The breadth of these conditions increases the complexity of treatment and the skill required of the counselors and medical providers involved in the treatment.

Diagnosis

Diagnosis involves four components: a health history, a physical examination which will rule out hormone abnormalities that may result in loss of weight, laboratory tests, and a mental status evaluation that also assesses suicidal risk. Health histories tend to be unreliable, because many people with eating disorders lie about their eating behavior, purging habits, and medication abuse. Based on the health history and a physical examination of the patient, the physician will order appropriate laboratory tests. Mental status can be evaluated using several different scales. The goal is to get an accurate assessment of the individual's physical condition and thinking in relationship to self-worth, body image, and food.

During the physical examination, other major medical complications may be diagnosed as well, such as cardiac arrhythmia, **dehydration** and electrolyte imbalances, delayed growth and development, endocrinological disturbances, gastrointestinal problems, oral health problems, osteopenia, osteoporosis, and protein/calorie malnutrition.

The mental health examination currently uses the *DSM-IV*, which provides diagnostic criteria for psychiatric disorders, including certain eating disorders. Expanded diagnostic criteria is under consideration for the fifth edition (*DSM-5*), expected to publish in 2013. The *DSM-IV* diagnostic criteria for anorexia nervosa includes an exaggerated drive for thinness, refusal to maintain a body weight above the standard minimum (e.g., 85% of expected weight), intense fear of becoming fat with self-worth based on weight or shape, and evidence of an endocrine disorder. The changes proposed for *DSM-5* include restricted energy

intake relative to requirements (leading to a markedly low body weight), intense fear of gaining weight or becoming fat or persistent behavior to avoid weight gain, and considerable distress regarding one's weight or body shape.

Criteria in the *DSM-IV* for bulimia nervosa include overwhelming urges to overeat and inappropriate compensatory behaviors or purging that follow the binge episodes (e.g., vomiting, excessive exercise, alternating periods of starvation, and abuse of laxatives or drugs). Similar to anorexia nervosa, individuals with bulimia nervosa also display psychopathology, including a fear of being overweight. New criteria proposed for *DSM-5* include recurrent episodes of binge eating with a sense of a lack of control with inappropriate compensatory behavior, self-evaluation that is unduly influenced by body shape and weight, and the specification that the behaviors do not occur exclusively during episodes of anorexia nervosa.

The *DSM-IV* is somewhat vague when discussing eating disorders that are not specifically classified, merely noting that they tend to be compensatory behaviors distinguished by binge eating and a lack of self-control. Proposals for *DSM-5* include better definitions and diagnostic criteria for unspecified eating disorders, including binge eating disorder, purging disorder, and night-eating syndrome.

Treatment

Treatment depends on a collaborative approach by an interdisciplinary team of mental health, nutrition, and medical specialists. The degree to which the individual's health and mental status is impaired can direct what type of treatment plan is appropriate for the individual. People with EDs may need to be hospitalized or attend structured day programs for an extended period. Some people are also prescribed medication, but the mainstay of treatment is psychotherapy. An appropriate therapy is selected based on the type of eating disorder and the individual's psychological profile. Some of the common therapies used in treating eating disorders include:

- Cognitive behavior therapy (CBT) is designed to confront and then change the individual's thoughts and feelings about his or her body and behaviors toward food, but it does not address why those thoughts or feelings exist. Research has shown that CBT is effective for those with binge eating behaviors by decreasing the frequency of binges through helping the person learn to normalize their thought patterns and find compensatory responses to binging. However, use of CBT with anorexia nervosa is compromised due to the addition of inborn disruptions in the person's neurotransmitter secretions, which places a limit on the extent to which CBT can assist in treatment.

- Psychodynamic therapy, also called psychoanalytic therapy, attempts to help the individual gain insight into the cause of the emotions that trigger their dysfunctional behavior. This therapy tends to be more long term than CBT.

- Interpersonal therapy is short-term therapy that helps the individual identify specific issues and problems in relationships. The individual may be asked to look back at his or her family history to try to recognize problem areas or stresses and work toward resolving them.

- Dialectical behavior therapy (DBT) consists of structured private and group sessions in which the therapist and patient(s) work at reducing behaviors that interfere with quality of life, finding alternate solutions to current problem situations, and learning to regulate emotions. In selected populations, some evidence suggests that DBT shows potential for decreasing binge eating and purging symptoms.

- Family and couples therapy can be helpful in dealing with conflict or disorders that may be a factor in perpetuating the eating disorder. Family therapy is especially useful in helping parents with anorexia to avoid passing on their attitudes and behaviors to their children. Self-esteem and assertiveness training may also be helpful in some patients with EDs.

Drugs

As of 2012, there were no medications approved by the U.S. Food and Drug Administration (FDA) for the specific treatment of anorexia nervosa. Medications prescribed for those with anorexia nervosa focus on either reducing anxiety or alleviating mood symptoms to assist the person in eating. For the treatment of bulimia nervosa, the Food and Drug Administration has approved fluoxetine after (or in conjunction with) behavior therapy.

Nutrition and dietary concerns

Eating disorders result in malnutrition that can have life-threatening consequences. Death may be due to cardiac arrhythmia, acute cardiovascular failure, gastric hemorrhaging, or suicide. Nutrition inadequacies commonly seen in the eating disorder group are low energy intake (which can be as severe as eating fewer than 500 calories per day), **protein** intake that results in clinical signs of protein deficiency, insufficient dietary **calcium** intake, fluid and electrolyte imbalances, and an array of vitamin and mineral insufficiencies.

KEY TERMS

Fast—A period of at least 24 hours in which a person eats nothing and drinks only water.

Type 2 diabetes—Sometimes called adult-onset diabetes, this disease prevents the body from properly using glucose (sugar).

Prognosis

Recovery from eating disorders can be a long, difficult process interrupted by relapses. About half of all people with anorexia relapse. Up to 20% die of complications of the disorder. The recovery rate for people with bulimia is slightly higher. Binge eaters experience many relapses and may have trouble controlling their weight even if they stop bingeing. Not enough is known about the other eating disorders to determine recovery rates. All eating disorders have serious social and emotional consequences. All except rumination disorder have serious health consequences. The sooner a person with an eating disorder gets professional help, the better the chance of recovery.

Prevention

Prevention involves both preventing and relieving stresses and enlisting professional help as soon as abnormal eating patterns develop. Some things that may help prevent an eating disorder from developing are listed below:

- Parents should not obsess about their weight, appearance, and diet in front of their children.
- Parents should not put their child on a diet unless instructed to by a pediatrician.
- Do not tease people about their body shapes or compare them to others.
- Make it clear that family members are loved and accepted as they are.
- Try to eat meals together as a family whenever possible; avoid eating alone.
- Avoid using food for comfort in times of stress.
- Monitor negative self-talk; practice positive self-talk.
- Spend time doing something enjoyable every day.
- Stay busy, but not overly busy; get enough sleep every night.
- Become aware of the situations that are personal triggers for abnormal eating behaviors and look for ways to avoid or defuse them.

QUESTIONS TO ASK YOUR DOCTOR

- My child keeps saying he/she is fat and is unhappy with the way he/she looks. Is there someone in your office who can talk with her?
- My child seems to be avoiding eating or is only eating a limited amount of food. Is there a way to evaluate him/her for an eating disorder?
- My child is a very picky eater. How can I assist him/her in trying new foods?
- Is my child's height and weight appropriate for his/her age?
- My daughter has not started her menstrual cycle, is this normal?
- Can you recommend a family therapist?

- Do not go on extreme diets.
- Be alert to signs of low self-worth, anxiety, depression, and drug or alcohol abuse. Seek help as soon as these signs appear.

Resources

BOOKS

Agras, W. Stewart. *Overcoming Eating Disorders: A Cognitive-Behavioral Therapy Approach for Bulimia Nervosa and Binge-Eating Disorder*. 2nd ed. New York: Oxford University Press, 2008.

Carleton, Pamela and Deborah Ashin. *Take Charge of Your Child's Eating Disorder: A Physician's Step-By-Step Guide to Defeating Anorexia and Bulimia*. New York: Marlowe & Co., 2007.

Heaton, Jeanne A. and Claudia J. Strauss. *Talking to Eating Disorders: Simple Ways to Support Someone Who Has Anorexia, Bulimia, Binge Eating or Body Image Issues*. New York: New American Library, 2005.

Kolodny, Nancy J. *The Beginner's Guide to Eating Disorders Recovery*. Carlsbad, CA: Gurze Books, 2004.

Liu, Aimee. *Gaining: The Truth About Life After Eating Disorders*. New York: Warner Books, 2007.

Messinger, Lisa, and Merle Goldberg. *My Thin Excuse: Understanding, Recognizing, and Overcoming Eating Disorders*. Garden City Park, NY: Square One Publishers, 2006.

Rubin, Jerome S., ed. *Eating Disorders and Weight Loss Research*. Hauppauge, NY: Nova Science Publishers, 2006.

Walsh, B. Timothy. *If Your Adolescent Has an Eating Disorder: An Essential Resource for Parents*. New York: Oxford University Press, 2005.

PERIODICALS

Osborne, V. A., K. J. Sher, and R. P. Winograd. "Disordered Eating Patterns and Alcohol Misuse in College Students: Evidence for 'Drunkorexia?'" *Comprehensive Psychiatry* 52, no. 6 (2011): e12. http://dx.doi.org/10.1016/j.comppsych.2011.04.038 (accessed September 7, 2012).

Wilson, Jenny, et al. "Surfing for Thinness: A Pilot Study of Pro-Eating Disorder Web Site Usage in Adolescents With Eating Disorders." *Pediatrics* 118, no. 6 (December 2006): e1635–43. http://dx.doi.org/10.1542/peds.2006-1133 (accessed September 7, 2012).

WEBSITES

Anorexia Nervosa and Related Eating Disorders (ANRED). "Table of Contents." http://www.anred.com/toc.html (accessed September 7, 2012).

Centers for Disease Control and Prevention. "Fact Sheets: Binge Drinking." http://www.cdc.gov/alcohol/fact-sheets/binge-drinking.htm (accessed September 7, 2012).

Jennings, Ashley. "Drunkorexia: Alcohol Mixes With Eating Disorders." ABC News, October 21, 2010. http://abcnews.go.com/Health/drunkorexia-alcohol-mixes-eating-disorders/story?id=11936398 (accessed September 7, 2012).

MedlinePlus. "Eating Disorders." U.S. National Library of Medicine, National Institutes of Health. http://www.nlm.nih/gov/medlineplus/eatingdisorders.html (accessed September 7, 2012).

National Association of Anorexia Nervosa and Associated Disorders. "About Eating Disorders." http://www.anad.org/get-information/about-eating-disorders (accessed September 7, 2012).

Pearce, Tralee. "'Drunkorexia' a Growing Problem as Female Students Favour Booze over Food." *Globe and Mail*, October 19, 2011.

ORGANIZATIONS

American Psychological Association, 750 First St. NE, Washington, DC 20002-4242, (202) 336-5500, (800) 374-2721, http://www.apa.org.

National Association of Anorexia Nervosa & Associated Disorders, 800 E. Diehl Rd. #160, Naperville, IL 60563, (630) 577-1333, (630) 577-1330 (helpline), anadhelp@anad.org, http://www.anad.org.

National Eating Disorders Association, 165 West 46th St., New York, NY 10036, (212) 575-6200, (800) 931-2237, info@NationalEatingDisorders.org, http://www.nationaleatingdisorders.org.

Tish Davidson, AM
Megan Porter, RD

Eating for Life

Definition

Eating for Life refers to a diet and nutrition plan that recommends eating six small, low-fat meals daily, popularized in the 2003 book *Eating for Life*, written by Bill Phillips.

A person who follows the Eating for Life program consumes about 40%–50% **protein**, 40%–50% **carbohydrates**, and small amounts of fat. Meals should be consumed about two to three hours apart. The program can be used as a way to lose or maintain weight or to supplement a fitness or resistance training regimen.

Origins

The Eating for Life plan was developed by Bill Phillips, a bodybuilder, former editor-in-chief of *Muscle Media* magazine, and former chief executive officer of EAS, a performance supplement company owned by Abbott Laboratories.

Prior to publishing Eating for Life in 2003, Phillips authored his first book, *Body for Life: 12 Weeks to Mental and Physical Strength*, a *New York Times* bestseller.

The Body-for-Life program began in the mid-1990s when Phillips first challenged dieters to make the best body transformation during a 12-week period, using the exercise and nutrition principles outlined in his now-defunct fitness magazine, *Muscle Media*. The first year of the challenge, Phillips offered his Lamborghini Diablo to the contestant who made the most radical transformation within 3 months. Every year since, individuals and couples compete for cash prizes and free exercise equipment in the annual Body-for-Life Challenge.

Description

Phillips, the author of *Eating for Life*, calls his program the "anti-diet," claiming that enjoying food and eating often are the keys to healthy weight loss and maintenance. Instead of focusing on the deprivation that typical accompanies weight-loss plan, Eating for Life claims to help its followers make wise eating choices that are sustainable over a long period of time. Phillips maintains that food is not the enemy, but rather, it's an essential part of an overall lifestyle choice.

The first ten chapters of *Eating for Life* that comprise Part I describe the extent of the overweight and **obesity** epidemic in the United States, identify common obstacles to health and fitness, such as easy access to fast food and restriction associated with traditional dieting, deconstruct popular dieting myths, and prepare the reader to begin using the Eating for Life nutrition plan and recipes.

The second part of the 405-page book includes photos and instructions for cooking the 150 recipes included in *Eating for Life*. The book includes recipes for dinner entrees, desserts, breakfasts, lunches, snacks, and nutrition shakes, as well as sample meal plans and a grocery guide. Sample recipes are also available on Phillips' Eating for Life website.

The final portion of the book includes motivational success stories of people who have lost weight with the Body-for-Life/Eating for Life diet and exercise plan, nutrition definitions, and tips for cooking healthy.

Six days a week, dieters are encouraged to eat six small meals consisting of one serving of protein and one serving of carbohydrate. Meals should be consumed about two to three hours apart. The benefit of this practice, according to Phillips, is that it keeps the **metabolism** elevated and energy levels stable.

Two of the daily meals should include vegetable servings, and 1 tablespoon of healthy fat is encouraged daily. Alternatively, three servings of fatty fish such as salmon could be consumed weekly to meet the healthy fat requirement.

On the seventh day, Eating for Life encourages a day of less restrained eating, in which dieters eat reasonable portions of unauthorized foods they've been craving throughout the week. Eating for Life does not prohibit particular foods, but encourages readers to save them for the "free day" and savor the pleasure they provide. This practice will help readers sustain healthy eating choices the rest of the time, Phillips maintains.

To aid in weight loss, Phillips says readers should choose from 82 "authorized foods," divided into five food categories, including proteins, vegetarian proteins, carbohydrates, vegetables, and **fats**. Recommended protein foods include lean red meat (including beef, buffalo, and venison), poultry (chicken and turkey), fish and shellfish, egg whites and egg substitutes, or low-fat cottage cheese; recommended carbohydrate sources include fruit, sweet potatoes, brown rice, oatmeal, barley, and whole-grain breads.

A sample daily menu might include:
- breakfast: zesty breakfast burrito
- midmorning: chocolate-mint nutrition shake
- lunch: grilled chicken soup
- midafternoon: strawberry-frost nutrition shake
- dinner: grilled salmon and potato
- late evening: cinnamon roll supreme nutrition shake

As part of the Eating for Life method, it is suggested that dieters plan their meals and grocery lists in advance and record their protein and carbohydrate servings daily. Phillips also suggests that dieters drink ten cups of water each day.

Eating for Life does not prohibit alcohol or **caffeine** consumption, but suggests limiting both.

Eating for Life also advocates portion control as an essential practice for weight loss. For example, a protein serving is about the size of a person's palm, whereas a carbohydrate serving should be about the size of the person's clenched fist. Counting **calories** or points or measuring food portions with a scale do not play a role in the Eating for Life plan.

Eating for Life also recommends readers participate in weight or resistance training three days a week and cardiovascular exercise three times a week. Doing so will help dieters build and maintain muscle mass, which is crucial for the body's ability to burn fat, Phillips says.

Function

Eating for Life is a program adopted by people who wish to lose weight or who are seeking a nutrition program to support their bodybuilding or resistance training efforts.

Benefits

Because of the six-day-a-week recommended exercise plan described in Body for Life, Eating for Life may work well for people who are serious about weight training for health and fitness. This plan may also benefit people who desire regimented eating and exercise programs as they attempt to lose weight.

The six small meals a day and regular exercise recommended in the Eating for Life plan are sound strategies for weight loss. However, the strict nature of the diet (readers are admonished to adhere to a list of authorized foods) may make it difficult for a person to maintain any weight loss long-term.

Precautions

Although *Eating for Life* does not formally require their use, supplements including meal replacement shakes and protein bars are frequently recommended by Phillips. Dieters are encouraged to consume up to three meal replacement products or shakes daily, such as the Myoplex brand marketed by EAS, the performance supplement company started by Phillips. These supplements can be difficult to find in conventional grocery outlets, as well as expensive. For example, 20 servings of the Myoplex protein powder often recommended in Eating for Life and Body for Life starts at $59.95 on the EAS website (www.eas.com). Myoplex and other supplements recommended by Phillips are also available at health food and supplement chain stores, such as GNC, or online.

KEY TERMS

Aerobic exercise—Moderate intensity exercise, done over a long duration, that uses oxygen. Aerobic exercise strengthens the cardiovascular system and lungs.

Bodybuilding—Developing muscle size and tone, usually for competitive exhibition.

Carbohydrate—A source of energy in the diet containing 4 calories per gram, often founds in foods such as breads, cereals, fruits, vegetables, and milk and dairy products. There are two kinds of carbohydrates: simple and complex.

Cardiovascular—Involving the heart and blood vessels.

Fat—A major source of energy in the diet. All food fats have 9 calories per gram. Fat is found in oils, nuts, seeds, avocados, meats, and high-fat dairy products, as well as in packaged, processed foods.

Protein—A nutrient that helps build many parts of the body, including muscle and bone. Protein provides 4 calories per gram. It is found in foods like meat, fish, poultry, eggs, dairy products, beans, nuts, and tofu.

Resistance training—Also called strength or weight training, this type of exercise increases muscle strength by working the muscles against a weight or force. Free weights, weight machines, resistance bands, or a person's body weight can be used in resistance training.

Eating for Life does not exclude vegetarian eaters, however, Phillips admits it may be difficult for vegans (people who do not eat any animal products, including eggs or dairy products) to find enough varied protein sources to eat according to the Eating for Life plan. Most of the recipes in the *Eating for Life* book include some type of meat, such as chicken, beef, turkey, or fish.

In addition, the weightlifting program advocated in *Body for Life* and *Eating for Life* may be daunting for the inexperienced beginner. With little regard for a person's cardiovascular fitness level, weightlifting experience, or propensity for injuries, Phillips advocates readers to begin exercising six days a week, even if they have been couch potatoes in the past. This "all-or-nothing" approach may be difficult for people to achieve or maintain over the suggested 12 weeks required for a Body for Life challenge, and someone who experiences an injury that prevents exercise may find it difficult to maintain their dieting motivation.

QUESTIONS TO ASK YOUR DOCTOR

- What are the potential benefits for me in adopting the Eating for Life plan?
- What are the potential health risks?
- Are there any health concerns associated with the protein intake recommended in Eating for Life?
- Is it advisable for me to take the meal replacements or supplements recommended in Eating for Life?
- Will I need to take a multivitamin or other dietary supplements if I eat according to the Eating for Life plan?
- Is it safe for me to start the strength and cardiovascular conditioning recommended by Eating for Life?

Risks

The protein intake suggested by Eating for Life, although not technically dangerous for most individuals, may be too much for the body to use on a daily basis. According to sports nutritionists, extra protein is broken down, the excess nitrogen is simply excreted in the urine, and the carbon skeleton is used/stored as energy. For some people, however, the amount of daily protein recommended by a plan such as Eating for Life may be a problem. People with preexisting kidney or liver disease, such as cirrhosis or fatty liver, should not attempt a popular diet plan such as Eating for Life without checking with their health care providers first.

In addition, dieters may need to be conscious of consuming enough fruits and vegetables while Eating for Life. Phillips encourages dieters to eat only two servings of vegetables daily; however, the U.S. Department of Agriculture (USDA) urges people eating about 2,000 calories a day to consume at least 4.5 cups of fruits and vegetables with their daily meals. Dieters may find it difficult to eat enough fruit and vegetable servings to satisfy the USDA recommendations while on the Eating for Life nutrition plan, especially since fruit servings count as carbohydrates on the plan, thereby limiting them to one per meal.

Research and general acceptance

Although there is no scientific data to point to Eating for Life's effectiveness, Phillips provides anecdotal stories and dramatic before-and-after photos of people who have successfully lost weight using Body for Life and the accompanying Eating for Life plan.

Some registered dietitians have also suggested that although the small meals and suggestions to exercise are important components of weight loss, in general the diet may be overly restrictive, making it difficult for dieters to maintain any losses long-term.

Resources

BOOKS

Phillips, Bill. *Body for Life: 12 Weeks to Mental and Physical Strength.* HarperCollins, 1999.
———. *Body for Life Success Journal.* HarperCollins, 2002.
———. *Eating for Life: Your Guide to Great Health, Fat Loss and Increased Energy!* High Point Media, 2003.
——— . *Transformation; How to Change Everything.* Carlsbad, CA: Hay House, Inc., 2007.

WEBSITES

"Bill Phillips Transformation." http://www.transformation.com/pages/public/welcome (accessed September 25, 2012).
Body-for-LIFE offical website. http://bodyforlife.com (accessed September 25, 2012).

Amy L. Sutton

Echinacea

Definition

Echinacea is a perennial plant native to North America that is farmed in both the United States and Europe for use in **dietary supplements**. Echinacea is a genus in the aster family containing nine plant species. Three species, *Echinacea angustifolia, E. purpurea,* and *E. pallida* are used in complementary and alternative medicine in the United States and Europe.

Echinacea species are commonly called coneflowers. The common name for *E. purpurea* is purple coneflower. *E. pallida* is known as pale purple coneflower and *E. angustifolia* as narrow-leaf coneflower. Echinacea is sold as an herbal dietary supplement under a variety of trade names. It is also a common ingredient in many supplements containing multiple ingredients.

Purpose

Echinacea has been used as a medicinal herb in North America for more than 400 years. Native Americans used echinacea to treat wounds, snakebites, infections, and as a general booster of health. In the 1930s, the herb was very popular in both the United States and Europe, as it was thought to fight infection by boosting the immune system. It was used to treat conditions as diverse as colds, influenza, eczema, many different types of infections, malaria, syphilis, **cancer**, and diphtheria. As antibiotics became more widely available after World War II, echinacea's popularity declined, only to rise again in the 1980s. It is one of the most frequently used herbal remedies in North America and Europe. Echinacea is especially popular in Germany, where many practitioners of conventional medicine accept it as a safe and effective treatment for cold symptoms. Echinacea is increasingly accepted for this use by conventional medical practitioners in the United States.

Description

Echinacea is a perennial herb with slender, rough leaves arranged opposite each other on a stem that grows to a height of about 18 in (45 cm) and produces a single large purplish flower. Both the above ground parts of the plant and the roots are used in dietary supplements. Fresh leaves are pressed and the resulting juice is used in extracts or tinctures, or it is combined with other ingredients to make a paste that can be applied to the skin. Dried leaves and roots are powered and made into tea or capsules. An injectable form of echinacea is available in Europe, but not in the United States. The active ingredients of echinacea have not been adequately identified. As a result, it is difficult to compare the strength and potency of different forms of the herb or the same formulation made by different manufacturers.

Safety and effectiveness of echinacea

Although echinacea has been used for hundreds of years, only recently have researchers started to examine its effectiveness in large, independent, rigorously controlled studies. Many early studies done in Germany suggested that the herb was effective in treating certain conditions. In the United States, the National Center for Complementary and Alternative Medicine (NCCAM), a government organization within the National Institutes of Health, continues to conduct studies on the safety and effectiveness of echinacea in treating a variety of conditions.

In the United States, the Food and Drug Administration (FDA) regulates dietary supplements such as echinacea using the same laws that regulate food, rather than the laws that regulate prescription and over-the-counter medications. Unlike conventional drugs, dietary supplements are not required to undergo rigorous testing to show that they are safe and effective before they are marketed to the public. One consequence of this is that there are many fewer studies of dietary

> **KEY TERMS**
>
> **Dietary supplement**—A product, such as a vitamin, mineral, herb, amino acid, or enzyme, that is intended to be consumed in addition to an individual's diet with the expectation that it will improve health.

supplements, and some of those studies are sponsored by the manufacturers who have an economic investment in positive outcomes. Too often, studies of dietary supplements are small, poorly designed, poorly controlled, or incompletely reported, making it is difficult to draw hard conclusions about the effectiveness and safety of the product.

The most common use of echinacea in the United States and Europe is to prevent, or shorten and reduce, the severity of symptoms of the common cold, including sneezing, runny, nose, cough, and fever. Natural Standard is an independent organization that evaluates studies, scientific evidence, and expert opinion on complementary and alternative treatments and makes impartial judgments concerning their safety and effectiveness. As of 2012, Natural Standard found that there was good scientific evidence to support the effectiveness of echinacea in preventing and treating cold symptoms.

For years, echinacea has been taken to improve general health and to treat a variety of infections because it is thought to boost the immune system. Laboratory analyses of the ingredients in echinacea and some animal studies have suggested that echinacea does stimulate immune system cells in humans. However, there is unclear evidence about whether this provides any health benefits.

Claims have also been made that genital herpes can be successfully treated with echinacea. Although there is some theoretical basis for this, both National Standard and the Natural Medicine Comprehensive Database consider echinacea ineffective when used for genital herpes.

There is not enough high-quality scientific evidence to rate echinacea's effectiveness in treating all other health problems including cancer, eye infection, migraine headaches, eczema, allergies, bee stings, attention-deficit-hyperactivity disorder and chronic fatigue syndrome.

Despite mixed evidence about the effectiveness of echinacea, the herb generally appears to be safe when taken by adults in moderate amounts for short periods. There is no standardization of the amount of active ingredient in products containing echinacea.

Guidelines of normal doses for a 150 lb. (70 kg) adult taken three times a day are:

- 1–2 g dried leaves or root brewed into tea
- 2–3 mL tincture
- 200 mg powdered extract

Lower doses of echinacea for children, based on the weight of the child, are generally thought to be safe. One study of pregnant women using echinacea found that moderate use of the herb during the first three months of pregnancy did not increase the likelihood of the baby being born with major birth defects, however, many physicians warn against taking herbal medicines during pregnancy because they are not as strictly regulated as pharmaceuticals and may contain undeclared ingredients. The safety of echinacea use in **breastfeeding** women has not been adequately studied.

Precautions

Individuals interested in taking echinacea should consult their health care provider and other reputable sources of information before starting the herb. Pregnant or breastfeeding women should be especially careful to discuss the use of echinacea and all other drugs and supplements with their health care provider.

As with any medication, more is not necessarily better, and the words "natural" or "organic" on the label do not mean the product is safe. Overdose can cause serious side effects. In the event of side effects, echinacea should be stopped immediately and the side effects reported to a health care professional. People with autoimmune diseases (e.g., AIDS, multiple sclerosis) are often counseled to avoid echinacea, because of theoretical, but unproven, negative effects on the immune system.

Interactions

Echinacea may interact with both conventional drugs and other herbs or dietary supplements, but few rigorous studies have been done on potential interactions. Individuals should tell their health care provider about all the conventional drugs and dietary supplements they are taking before beginning any new drug or supplement. There is some evidence that echinacea may slow the breakdown of many pharmaceutical drugs and **caffeine**.

Since echinacea may stimulate the immune system, individuals who are taking immune system suppressant drugs following cancer treatment or organ transplant should avoid echinacea.

QUESTIONS TO ASK YOUR DOCTOR

- Is echinacea better to take for a cold than over-the-counter drug remedies?
- Am I taking any drugs, herbs, or dietary supplements that might interact with echinacea?
- How long can I safely take echinacea?
- Is echinacea safe for my child to take?
- If I should avoid echinacea, what alternative remedies do you suggest?

Complications

People who are allergic to ragweed, chrysanthemums, marigolds, daisies, and related plants have a greater chance of being allergic to echinacea. Allergic reactions have been reported on rare occasions to be severe enough to cause breathing difficulties, especially in people with asthma. Much more common are allergic reactions consisting of a rash, sneezing, or runny nose.

Parental concerns

Parents should be aware that the safe dose of many herbal supplements has not been established for children. Accidental overdose may occur if children are give adult herbal supplements.

Resources

BOOKS

Mars, Brigitte. *The Desktop Guide to Herbal Medicine: The Ultimate Multidisciplinary Reference to the Amazing Realm of Healing Plants, in a Quick-Study, One-Stop Guide.* Laguna Beach, CA: Basic Health Pub., 2007.

PDR Staff. *PDR for Nonprescription Drugs, Dietary Supplements, and Herbs 2011.* PDR Network, 2011.

Wildman, Robert E.C., ed. *Handbook of Nutraceuticals and Functional Foods.* 2nd ed. Boca Raton, FL: CRC/Taylor &Francis, 2007.

WEBSITES

American Botanical Council. "Echinacea purpurea, E. Angustifolia/Compositae & E. pallida." http://www.herbmed.org/index.html#param.wapp?sw_page=viewHerb%3FherbID%3D6 (accessed September 29, 2012).

MedlinePlus. "Echinacea." U.S. National Library of Medicine, National Institutes of Health. http://www.nlm.nih.gov/medlineplus/druginfo/natural/981.html (accessed September 29, 2012).

National Center for Complementary and Alternative Medicine. "Echinacea." National Institutes of Health. http://nccam.nih.gov/health/echinacea/ataglance.htm (accessed September 29, 2012).

Natural Standard. "Echinacea." MayoClinic.com. http://www.mayoclinic.com/health/echinacea/NS_patient-echinacea (accessed September 29, 2012).

ORGANIZATIONS

American Botanical Council, 6200 Manor Rd., Austin, TX, (512) 926-4900, Fax: (512) 926-2345, http://abc.herbalgram.org.

National Center for Complementary and Alternative Medicine Clearinghouse, PO Box 7923, Gaithersburg, MD 20898, (888) 644-6226, Fax: (866) 464-3616, info@nccam.nih.gov, http://nccam.nih.gov.

Office of Dietary Supplements, National Institutes of Health, 6100 Executive Blvd., Rm. 3B01, MSC 7517, Bethesda, MD 20892-7517, (301) 435-2920, Fax: (301) 480-1845, ods@nih.gov, http://ods.od.nih.gov.

Tish Davidson, AM

eDiets

Definition

The eDiets.com website provides information on several diet programs, fitness regimens, as well as support from health professionals. The term ediets may be used to describe any diet program found on the Internet.

Origins

American Internet entrepreneur David R. Humble started eDiets.com in 1996. Unable to find investors for the site, Humble invested $500,000 of his own money to begin the company. Humble discovered a niche in the fee-based online dieting community. The eDiets website uses a unique software program to provide customized diet and fitness plans for individuals. From a small office in Deerfield Beach, FL, eDiets.com has grown into an international business with websites in Germany, Spain, and Portugal. Over two million members have joined eDiets.com since its inception. The company also operates eFitness.com and publishes *glee* Magazine*, a leading Internet magazine focusing on lifestyle issues. In spring 2004 and 2005, eDiets.com was named "Best of the Web" for diet and nutrition by *Forbes* and was selected as "Editors' Choice" by *PC Magazine*.

Description

The eDiets.com website asks prospective members to enter information about their physical description (height, weight, gender, body shape, etc.), activity level, and eating habits. This data is used to generate a customized weight-loss program based on the 24 specialized options available. Program options include the Mayo Clinic Plan, Atkins, the Glycemic Impact Diet, the New **Mediterranean Diet**, as well as eDiets own program. **Trim Kids** is available for children and teens. Members can indicate special dietary restrictions, such as lactose or wheat intolerance, low sodium, or vegetarian, which will be accounted for in the meal plans. The type of diet plan selected can be changed or modified at any time.

Pricing for the basic eDiets program is approximately $4 a day. This typically provides the member with customized weekly meal plans complete with grocery shopping lists, fitness program based on the member's profile, access to community forums, newsletters, and articles on a variety of mind and body issues. Features that require an additional monthly fee include the recipe club, online chat groups and meetings, and access to experts for advice or consultation.

New members are paired with an existing member as part of the eDiets mentor program. The mentor offers support and assistance with the program. In addition, members can choose to participate in online meetings, chat rooms, take advantage of 24-hour support, or find emotional support through interactive tools. These resources aim to provide community and accountability that can help individuals maintain their weight-loss program.

An online shopping section features fitness equipment, books, videos, nutritional supplements, and other health related products. To make the program even more convenient, a meal delivery plan is available allowing members to have their meals prepared and delivered to their door for approximately $15-25 per day.

Function

The premise of eDiets.com is to provide an informative and supportive environment available to members at their convenience. This type of weight-loss program appeals to individuals who are uncomfortable with face-to-face group programs or who cannot attend local support sessions. The flexibility and customization of meal and fitness plans is another highlight.

The eDiets.com proprietary software provides individuals with information on their **body mass index** (BMI) and offers diet plans based on the data entered. From the data provided in the member's profile, the program generates a meal guide that targets the member's optimal calorie intake to lose weight. A shopping list and recipe recommendations simplify food preparation. Additionally, members can switch from one weight-loss program to another at any time (such as from the New Mediterranean Diet to Atkins) while maintaining the other features and programs associated with their eDiets membership.

Benefits

An eDiets membership offers a wide array of support methods, meal preferences, fitness programs, and other features that help individuals stay motivated to reach their weight loss goals. The low monthly membership fee is attractive, typically half the cost of joining a local program such as **Weight Watchers**.

The option of adjusting the meal plan to accommodate eating habits is a great benefit. Menus can include convenience foods (including fast-food), self-prepared meals, or both. They can also be modified to account for special diets or dietary restrictions. A prepared shopping list that corresponds to the menu selections adds to the ease.

An important advantage is the fitness program component. A customized workout is created based on an individual's lifestyle, age, and other personal information provided. The option to work one-on-one with a trainer or have more personalized fitness plans developed are available for an additional monthly fee.

Member support is a significant part of eDiets. The website offers six different support areas:

- Support Groups—Over 120 specialized groups cover age groups, language spoken, women's issues, relationships, type of diet, etc.
- Mentor Program—New members are paired with existing members for 30 days of one-on-one support and guidance.
- Chat Rooms—24-hour communication with other members as well as online meetings are available, an additional monthly fee is usually required.
- Experts—A panel of experts moderate online support groups and meetings, provide feedback to individual members, and write articles for the eDiets newsletter.
- Circle of Winners—Small support groups created by members to find other members with similar needs or interests.
- Success Stories—Members share their success with eDiets.com to offer inspiration to other members.

Precautions

As with any weight-loss program, it is important to talk with a physician about the intended changes. A disclaimer on eDiets.com states that the advice and recommendations on the website are not intended to

be medical advice or take the place of a physician's advice. Recommendations for diet plans, optimal weight loss, and exercise programs on the website are calculated using a proprietary software program. They are based on data provided by the individual, and therefore are only as accurate as the information entered. It is imperative to be honest when entering the requested data.

If an individual already has an ideal weight, the program indicates additional weight loss is not necessary. However, the individual may choose to join in order to improve their eating habits and/or fitness level.

In general, members should use the eDiets website with the same caution as other websites. Articles and information presented should be reviewed for timeliness and reliability. Members must be careful when providing personal identification information, especially in e-mail or chat rooms with other members. Members who falsify their identities are a possibility.

Risks

Risks related to using eDiets.com are minimal. When registering for membership, individuals should carefully review the terms and conditions. Dissatisfied members complain about poor customer service and difficulty canceling membership. They also cite frustration with identifying plan pricing and fees for several features on the website.

Before beginning any of the diet plans or exercise programs, individuals should talk with a physician to identify risks specific to the type of diet or exercise selected.

Research and general acceptance

The University of Vermont Department of Nutrition and Food Sciences has performed several studies on the effectiveness of commercial online weight-loss programs versus more traditional weight-loss programs. Between February 2003 and March 2005 they studied the effectiveness of a structured Internet behavioral weight-loss program (VTrim) compared to a commercial Internet weight-loss program (eDiets.com). The results found the structured behavioral weight-loss program, led by a therapist, to be significantly more effective than the self-led commercial weight-loss program. VTrim participants lost twice as much weight throughout the study and were nearly twice as likely to have kept it off after 12 months. While the Internet is a practical medium for commercial weight-loss programs, their impact would be more noticeable if they integrated more structure such as that used in VTrim.

Another study at the University of Vermont involved participants using an Internet based behavioral weight-loss program for one year. All participants used the same program, but half supplemented with face-to-face meetings once a month. The study concluded that participants lost approximately the same amount of weight whether or not they attended meetings in person.

The University of Pennsylvania School of Medicine began a year-long controlled study in 2001 comparing eDiets.com to a weight loss manual to gage overall effectiveness for modifying an individual's lifestyle. Forty-seven female participants followed either eDiets.com or the LEARN Program for Weight Control. This small study concluded the manual had a greater impact on weight loss than eDiets since women following the manual lost approximately 4% of their body weight as compared to only 1% loss in women who used eDiets.com.

Research on the effectiveness of online diet programs remains limited. Studies at major universities demonstrate that websites such as eDiets.com can be effective tools for weight loss, but are usually most successful when coupled with personalized feedback.

Resources

PERIODICALS

Gold, Beth, et al. "Weight Loss on the Web: A Pilot Study Comparing a Structured Behavioral Intervention to a Commercial Program." *Obesity* 15, no. 1 (2007): 155–64.

Hansen, Matthew. "Print Works Better Than Web for Weight Loss, Research Suggests." *DOC News* 1, no. 2 (2004): 19.

Micco, N., et al. "Minimal In-Person Support as an Adjunct to Internet Obesity Treatment." *Annals of Behavioral Medicine* 33 (February 2007): 49–56.

Womble, Leslie G., et al. "A Randomized Controlled Trial of a Commercial Internet Weight Loss Program." *Obesity Research* 12, no. 6 (2004): 1011–18.

WEBSITES

"eDiets." http://www.ediets.com (accessed September 29, 2012).

Stacey L. Chamberlin

Electrolytes

Definition

Electrolytes are ions that form when salts dissolve in water or fluids. These ions have an electric charge. Positively charged ions are called cations. Negatively charged ions are called anions. Electrolytes are not evenly distributed within the body, and their uneven distribution allows many important metabolic reactions to occur. **Sodium** (Na^+), Potassium (K^+), **Calcium** ($Ca2+$), **Magnesium** ($Mg2+$), chloride (Cl^-), phosphate (HPO_42-), bicarbonate (HCO_3-), and Sulfate (SO_4-) are important electrolytes in humans.

Purpose

Electrolytes play a critical role in almost every metabolic reaction in the body. For example, they:

- Help control water balance and fluid distribution in the body
- Create an electrical gradient across cell membranes that is necessary for muscle contraction and nerve transmission
- Regulate the acidity (pH) of the blood
- Help regulate the level of oxygen in the blood
- Are involved in moving nutrients into cells and waste products out of cells

Description

Water is essential to life. **Dehydration** occurs when more water is lost from the body than is replaced. A loss of 20% of the body's water can be fatal. Water balance and electrolyte concentrations are closely

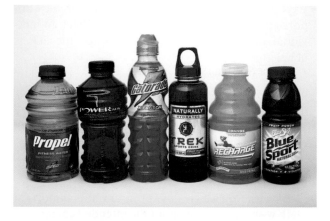

Sports drinks containing electrolytes. (© *Editorial Image, LLC/ Alamy*)

intertwined. Dehydration is a major cause of electrolyte imbalances.

Electrolytes, proteins, nutrients, waste products, and gasses are dissolved in fluid in the body. This fluid is not distributed evenly. About two-thirds of it is found inside cells (intracellular fluid). The rest is found in the spaces between cells (interstitial fluid), in the circulatory system, and in small amounts in other places such as the stomach. Changes in the concentration of electrolytes results in changes to the distribution of water throughout the body as water moves into or out of cells.

The components of body fluid—electrolytes, proteins, and so forth—are not evenly distributed either. Different types of cells have membranes that allow some electrolytes (and other components of the fluid) to pass across them while blocking others. This difference in the distribution of electrolytes (and thus electric charges) on either side of cell membranes makes it possible for many metabolic reactions to take place.

Water passes easily across cell membranes. When fluid with two different concentrations of electrolytes is separated by a cell membrane, there is pressure (called osmotic pressure) for water to flow across the membrane from fluid that contains fewer electrolytes (less concentrated) into fluid that contains more electrolytes (more concentrated). The cell uses energy to resist osmotic pressure and maintain different concentrations of electrolytes on either side of the membrane because even small changes in the concentrations and distribution of electrolytes can result in large movements of water in and out of cells. Maintaining this difference, or gradient, across cell membranes is a major part of the complex regulatory events called homeostasis that keep conditions within the body stable within very narrow limits. When there is an imbalance in electrolytes many systems in the body are affected and serious, even fatal, health problems can result.

Causes of electrolyte imbalances

An electrolyte imbalance occurs when the concentration of a specific electrolyte is either too high or too low. The concentration of electrolytes is strongly affected by the amount of fluid in the body. Fluid balance is largely controlled by hormones that act on the kidneys and regulate how much urine the kidneys produce. The average male adult loses about 1.5-2.5 L of water daily through urine production, sweating, breathing out water vapor, and bowel movements depending on exercise levels and environmental temperature. The United States Institute of Medicine recommends that adult men drink a minimum of 3 L of liquids a day,

and that women drink a minimum of 2.2 L to replace lost water.

Dehydration is a major cause of electrolyte imbalance. It occurs whenever water is lost from the body and not replaced fairly quickly. When fluids are lost, electrolytes in those fluids are lost too, increasing the risk of electrolyte imbalance. Dehydration can be caused in many ways. These include:

- Heavy exercise, especially in hot weather. Sodium and water are both lost through the skin with heavy sweating.
- Limited fluid intake. This is a particular problem with the elderly, especially those who are unable to walk or are bedridden.
- Severe vomiting and diarrhea. Large amounts of water and many electrolytes that would normally be absorbed in the intestines are lost with diarrhea and vomiting. Small children with diarrhea can become seriously dehydrated in less than one day. Infants can become dehydrated within hours.
- High fever. Increased water loss through the skin due to fever is especially serious in infants and young children.
- Severe burns. More water is lost from the surface of the body when the skin is not there to prevent evaporation, and damaged cells release their electrolytes into interstitial fluid, upsetting the electrolyte balance.

Electrolyte imbalances can have other causes unrelated to dehydration. These include:

- Kidney damage or kidney failure. This is a common cause of electrolyte imbalances in the elderly and can be fatal.
- Anorexia nervosa (self starvation) or bulimia nervosa (binge and purge eating).
- Excessive intake of water. Called water intoxication, this can result in swelling in the brain. In 2007, a Sacramento, California, woman died when she participated in a radio station contest that involved drinking large amounts of water in a short period of time.
- Some drugs, herbal supplements, and chemotherapy. Some medications/treatments selectively increase the excretion of certain electrolytes, cause the body to retain excess water, or stimulate the kidneys to produce excess urine.
- Hormonal imbalances in the production of hormones that regulate the kidneys. This causes too little or too much urine to be produced.
- Cancer. Some tumors produce chemicals that upset electrolyte balance.
- Abuse of electrolyte supplements.

Specific electrolyte imbalances

Each electrolyte has a special function in the body, although if one electrolyte is out of balance, the concentrations and actions of other electrolytes are often affected. The serum concentration of sodium, potassium, and chloride can be measured in a simple blood test. Sodium, chloride, potassium, and calcium concentrations can also be determined from a urine sample. A urine test helps show how well the kidneys are functioning. Electrolyte imbalances are most common among the seriously ill and the elderly. Kidney (renal) failure is the most common cause of electrolyte imbalances.

SODIUM. Sodium affects how much urine the kidney produces and is involved in the transmission of nerve impulses and muscle contraction. Too high a concentration of sodium in the blood causes a condition called hypernatremia. Causes of hypernatremia include excessive water loss (e.g., severe diarrhea), restricted water intake, untreated diabetes (causes water loss), kidney disease, hormonal imbalances, and excessive salt (NaCL) intake. Symptoms include signs of dehydration such as extreme thirst, dark urine, sunken eyes, fatigue, irregular heart beat, muscle twitching, seizures, and coma.

Too low a concentration of sodium in the blood causes hyponatremia. This is one of the most common electrolyte imbalances, and occurs in about 1% of hospitalized individuals. It can result from vomiting, diarrhea, severe burns, taking certain drugs that cause the kidneys to selectively excrete sodium, inadequate salt intake, water intoxication (a problem among the elderly with dementia), hormonal imbalances, kidney failure, and liver damage. Symptoms include nausea, vomiting, headache, tissue swelling (edema), confusion, mental disorientation, hallucinations, muscle trembling, seizures, and coma.

POTASSIUM. Potassium ions play a major role in regulating fluid balance in cells, the transmission of nerve impulses, and in muscle contractions. Too high a concentration of potassium causes a condition called hyperkalemia that is potentially life threatening. The most common cause is kidney failure. It can also result from severe burns or injury (excess potassium released from injured cells), inadequate adrenal hormones (Addison's disease), the use of certain medications, and excessive use of potassium supplements. Sometimes hyperkalemia occurs in conjunction with hypernatremia. Symptoms include nausea, diarrhea, weakness, muscle pain, irregular heart beat, coma, and death.

Abnormally low concentrations of potassium cause hypokalemia. Hypokalemia can result from excess adrenal hormones (Cushing's disease), kidney disease, long-term use of certain diuretic drugs, laxative abuse, bulimia, and kidney failure. Symptoms include increased production of urine, muscle pain, paralysis, irregular heart beat, and low blood pressure.

CALCIUM. Calcium is needed to build and maintain bones. It also plays a role in nerve impulse transmission and muscle contraction. Excess calcium results in a condition called hypercalcemia. Hypercalcemia can be caused by too much parathyroid hormone (PTH), certain cancers, some genetic disorders, and excessive use of antacids containing calcium in rare cases. Symptoms include bone and muscle pain, mental changes such as depression and confusion, increased urine production, fatigue, nausea, and vomiting.

Abnormally low concentrations of calcium cause hypocalcemia. Hypocalcemia can be caused by too little parathyroid hormone, kidney failure, and **vitamin D** deficiency. Vitamin D is necessary for the body to absorb calcium. Symptoms include muscle twitches and spasms, convulsions, mental changes such as depression and irritability, dry skin, and brittle nails.

MAGNESIUM. Magnesium is involved in **protein** synthesis and cellular **metabolism**. Abnormally high concentrations of magnesium, or hypermagnesemia, may occur with severe (end-stage) renal failure or by overdose of magnesium-containing intravenous fluids. Hypermagnesemia is rare. Symptoms include exhaustion, low blood pressure, depressed heart and breathing rate, and slow reflexes.

Abnormally low concentrations of magnesium, or hypomagnesemia, are most common among people with alcoholism and those who are severely malnourished. Other causes include digestive disorders that interfere with the absorption of magnesium from the intestines. Symptoms of hypomagnesemia include vomiting, weight lose, leg cramps, muscle spasms, seizures, and irregular heartbeat.

CHLORIDE. Chloride is involved in regulating blood pressure. High concentrations of chloride, called hyperchloremia, can be caused by kidney failure, kidney dialysis, and an overproduction of parathyroid hormone. Symptoms include weakness, headache, nausea, and vomiting. In people with diabetes, hyperchloremia makes it difficult to control blood glucose levels.

Hypochloremia often occurs along with hyponatremia or hypokalemia and is caused by excessive fluid loss (e.g., diarrhea). Serious deficiencies of chloride cause the blood to become less acidic, resulting in a condition called metabolic alkalosis. Symptoms of severe hypochloremia include confusion, paralysis, and difficulty breathing.

PHOSPHATE. Phosphate helps control the acidity level (pH) of the blood. Phosphate also causes calcium to be deposited in bones. High blood levels of phosphate, or hyperphosphatemia, often result in too low levels of calcium, or hypocalcemia. Hyperphosphatemia is usually caused by kidney failure. It can also result from kidney dialysis, parathyroid gland dysfunction, and several inherited diseases. Mild hyperphosphatemia usually produces no symptoms. Severe imbalance can cause tingling in the fingers, muscle cramps, and convulsions.

Hypophosphatemia, or abnormally low concentrations of phosphate in the blood, often occurs along with hypomagnesemia and hypokalemia. It can also be caused by kidney disease, kidney dialysis, vitamin D deficiency, and hormonal imbalances. Up to 30% of individuals admitted to hospital intensive care units have hypophosphatemia.

Electrolyte supplements

Most people get all the electrolytes and water they need from a normal diet. However, some individuals, such as athletes, people with severe diarrhea and vomiting, **cancer** patients, people with hormonal imbalances, and other very ill people, need fluid and electrolyte replacement therapy. Short-term therapy often quickly restores electrolyte balances.

Electrolyte replacement supplements can be sold either over-the-counter or by prescription. Prescription supplements are used for seriously ill or hospitalized patients and can be given by mouth or intravenously under supervision of a physician.

In North America, commonly used over-the-counter electrolyte replacements include:

- Sports drinks formulated to replace electrolytes lost through sweating. These drinks, such as Gatorade and Powerade, also contain sugars and sometimes caffeine. According to the American College of Sports Medicine, sports drinks are effective in supplying energy for muscles, maintaining blood sugar levels, preventing dehydration, and replacing electrolytes lost in sweat.
- Dietary supplements in the form of tablets and powders containing electrolytes. These are popular among athletes who participate in endurance sports. Some also contain herbs and flavorings. They are regulated by the United States Food and Drug Administration (FDA) as dietary supplements.
- Electrolyte replacements for children such as Pedialyte, Naturalyte, or Rehydralyte. These are sold in supermarkets and pharmacies and are used primarily in children who have lost fluids through vomiting

---

KEY TERMS

Diuretic—A substance that removes water from the body by increasing urine production.

Glucose—A simple sugar that results from the breakdown of carbohydrates. Glucose circulates in the blood and is the main source of energy for the body.

Homeostasis—The complex set of regulatory mechanisms that works to keep the body at optimal physiological and chemical stability in order for cellular reactions to occur.

Hormone—A chemical messenger produced by one type of cell that travels through the bloodstream to change the metabolism of a different type of cell.

Serum—The clear fluid part of the blood that remains after clotting. Serum contains no blood cells or clotting proteins, but does contain electrolytes.

---

and diarrhea. Children should not be given sports drinks for this purpose.

Precautions

As with any dietary supplement, electrolyte replacements can be abused. When used properly, they are of great benefit and have no undesirable side effects.

Sports drinks should not be given to children who need rehydration because of vomiting and diarrhea. Instead, oral rehydration liquids specially formulated for children should be used.

Interactions

The goal of electrolyte replacement therapy is to restore the body to its natural condition. When used this way, electrolyte replacement does not interfere with other drugs. Many drugs, however, have the potential to cause electrolyte imbalances. When starting a new drug, individuals should discuss possible side effects with their healthcare provider.

Complications

No complications are expected when electrolyte replacement therapy is used as directed. Seriously ill individuals and those using long-term electrolyte replacement therapy should have their electrolyte levels checked regularly.

Parental concerns

Dehydration is a real threat to children, especially infants and toddlers. Parents should be alert to dehydration caused by illness or athletic activity and begin oral fluid and electrolyte replacement therapy immediately. Parents of young children with vomiting, diarrhea, or high fever should consult their healthcare provider promptly about steps to take to prevent dehydration.

Resources

BOOKS

Hawkins, W. Rex. *Eat Right—Electrolyte: A Nutritional Guide to Minerals in Our Daily Diet.* Amherst, NY: Prometheus Books, 2006.

PERIODICALS

Allison, S.P., and D.N. Lobo. "Fluid and Electrolytes in the Elderly." *Current Opinion in Clinical Nutrition and Metabolic Care* 7, no. 1 (2004): 27–33.

Kenney, Larry. "Dietary Water and Sodium Requirements for Active Adults." *Sports Science Exchange 92* 17, no. 1 (2004). http://www.gssiweb.com/Article_Detail.aspx?articleID = 667 (accessed October 2, 2012).

WEBSITES

American Council on Exercise. "Electrolytes: Understanding Replacement Options." http://www.acefitness.org/certifiednewsarticle/715/electrolytes-understanding-replacement-options (accessed October 2, 2012).

"Electrolytes." Lab Tests Online. http://www.labtestsonline.org/understanding/analytes/electrolytes/glance.html (accessed October 2, 2012).

Mayo Clinic staff. "Dehydration: Treatments and Drugs." MayoClinic.com. http://www.mayoclinic.com/health/dehydration/ds00561/dsection = treatments-and-drugs (accessed October 2, 2012).

MedlinePlus. "Electrolytes." U.S. National Library of Medicine, National Institutes of Health. http://www.nlm.nih.gov/medlineplus/ency/article/002350.htm (accessed October 2, 2012).

———. "Fluid and Electrolyte Balance." U.S. National Library of Medicine, National Institutes of Health. http://www.nlm.nih.gov/medlineplus/fluidandelectrolytebalance.html (accessed October 2, 2012).

Micromedex. "Carbohydrate and Electrolyte Combination (Oral Route)." MayoClinic.com. http://www.mayoclinic.com/health/drug-information/DR602265 (accessed October 2, 2012).

ORGANIZATIONS

American Academy of Pediatrics (AAP), 141 Northwest Point Blvd., Elk Grove Village, IL 60007, (847) 434-4000, (800) 433-9016, Fax: (847) 434-8000, http://www.aap.org.

American College of Sports Medicine, 401 West Michigan St., Indianapolis, IN 46202-3233, (317) 637-9200, Fax: (317) 634-7817, http://www.acsm.org.

American Council on Exercise, 4851 Paramount Dr., San Diego, CA 92123, (888) 825-3636, support@acefitness.org, http://www.acefitness.org.

Gatorade Sports Science Institute, 617 West Main St., Barrington, IL 60010, (800) 616-4774, http://www.gssiweb.com.

Helen Davidson

Elimination diets

Definition

Elimination diets are diets in which people stop eating specific foods for a period and then challenge their body by adding the food back into their diet and evaluating how the body responds. Elimination diets are used to detect **food allergies** and food intolerances. They are not nutritionally balanced and are intended to be used only for diagnostic purposes.

Origins

For centuries it has been known that some people develop unpleasant symptoms (adverse reactions) to certain foods that other people can eat without any problems. However, it was not until the 1900s that food allergies began to be investigated in rigorous and scientific ways and studies on food allergies started appearing in reputable medical journals. Elimination diets developed out of this scientific interest in the effects of food on the body.

Description

Adverse reactions to food fall into two main categories: food allergies and food intolerances. Food allergies trigger a reaction from the immune system. When a person has a food allergy, his or her body responds to the allergen by treating it like a threatening foreign object. Immune system cells produce proteins called antibodies that work to disable the material. This process often causes inflammation and results in undesirable symptoms that range from mild and annoying to life threatening. It is not known for certain why some people respond negatively to certain foods and others do not, but genetics are likely a factor.

Food intolerances also cause adverse reactions, but these reactions do not involve the immune system and are not life threatening. Lactose (milk **sugar**) intolerance is an example of a food intolerance. It is caused by the body producing too little of the enzyme lactase, which is needed to digest lactose. Although surveys show that in the United States up to 30% of families believe they have at least one member with a food allergy, the actual documented rate of food allergies is about 6% in infants and children and 3.7% in adults. On the other hand, in Hispanic, Jewish, and Southern European populations, the rate of lactose intolerance is about 70%, and it reaches 90% or more in Asian and African populations. Food intolerances are much more common, but true food allergies tend to be much more severe. In this article, **food sensitivities** are used to include both food allergies and food intolerances.

The most common symptoms of food sensitivities are nausea, diarrhea, bloating, excessive gas, hives, rashes, eczema, headaches, migraine, asthma, wheezing, and hay fever-like symptoms. These symptoms may occur immediately after eating the trigger food or may not develop for hours. Most immediate reactions are severe allergic responses that can result in anaphylactic shock, a condition in which the airways swell shut and the person cannot breathe. Foods most likely to cause immediate reactions are peanuts, tree nuts, and shellfish.

Delayed symptoms are difficult to detect and are sometimes called "masked" food sensitivities. The most common foods that cause delayed sensitivities are dairy products, egg, wheat, and **soy**; however, sensitivities vary widely and can be caused by many foods. The amount of a trigger food that it takes to cause a response also varies considerably from person to person.

A true elimination diet is very rigorous and needs to be implemented under the direction of a physician often in consultation with a registered dietitian. For the elimination diet to be useful, the patient must follow the diet strictly. Cheating invalidates the results.

For 2–3 weeks, a person on the elimination diet cannot eat any of the following foods, according to the Institute of Functional Medicine (this list may be modified by the physician):

- grains: wheat, corn, oats, barley, spelt, kamut, rye; grains allowed include brown rice, quinoa, buckwheat, millet, amaranth
- proteins: pork, beef, veal, lunch meat, hot dogs, shellfish
- fruit: grapes and citrus fruits (oranges, grapefruit, lemons, limes)
- dairy: milk, cheese, eggs, cream, yogurt, ice cream
- legumes, nuts, and seeds: peanuts, pistachios, soy

- vegetables: mushrooms, corn, white potatoes, eggplant, tomatoes, peppers, some spices
- sweeteners and seasonings: white and brown sugar, maple syrup, corn syrup, honey, cane juice, succanat
- fats: butter, margarine, shortening, mayonnaise, salad dressing, processed oils (such as vegetable oil)
- beverages: alcohol, caffeinated beverages, soda

The individual must avoid all medicines containing aspirin (salicylates) and food colorings. After several weeks on these restricted foods, one new food is introduced in larger than normal amounts. This is the challenge food, and it is eaten for three days in a row. If no symptoms appear, the dieter continues to eat that food in normal amounts and adds another challenge food. If symptoms appear, the challenge food is stopped immediately and no new challenge food is introduced until symptoms disappear. During this time the dieter keeps a food journal, writing down everything that is eaten and any symptoms, either physical or emotional, that appear. It can take two to three months to work through all challenge foods.

Function

Elimination diets are the first part of a diagnostic technique for determining what foods are causing undesirable symptoms. Their purpose is to prepare the patient for the second part of the diagnostic process, the food challenge, by cleansing the body of all possible foods that could be causing the symptoms.

During the challenge phase, the patient eats the suspect food and waits to see if symptoms reappear. Elimination and challenge give healthcare professionals a way to reproducibly pinpoint exactly which foods are causing adverse reactions so that the patient can exclude these foods from their diet.

Benefits

People with symptoms that interfere with their daily life benefit greatly from pinpointing which foods are causing the symptoms so that these foods can be eliminated from the diet. People with less severe symptoms may find the process of elimination and challenge too costly and disruptive to make it worthwhile.

Precautions

Many people who suspect that certain foods are causing their symptoms try modified elimination diets found on the Internet or elimination diets they devise themselves. These diets have varying degrees of success. For example, many people try eliminating all dairy products to see if their symptoms of lactose intolerance—bloating, cramping, diarrhea, and gas—improve. This do-it-yourself approach may be adequate for people with mild sensitivities to only one food or food group, but it is risky for people with severe intolerances. People with moderate to severe sensitivities need professional guidance to eliminate non-obvious sources of the potential problem food.

Risks

One risk of all elimination diets is that they are not nutritionally balanced. They increase the risk that vitamin and mineral deficiencies will develop. Anyone going on a full elimination regimen needs to consult a registered dietitian about how to use **dietary supplements** to ensure adequate, balanced nutrition.

A second risk is that people who self-diagnose symptoms as food intolerances using a non-medically supervised elimination diet may be ignoring symptoms of more serious and progressive diseases such as **celiac disease**, **Crohn's disease**, **gastroesophageal reflux disease**, **irritable bowel syndrome**, and other health problems that need medical treatment.

Finally, anyone suspected of having a moderate to severe food allergy should be under the care of a physician. Food challenging is best done in a healthcare setting in case severe reactions occur.

QUESTIONS TO ASK YOUR DOCTOR

- Do my symptoms suggest a food allergy or a food intolerance?
- Do you think an elimination diet is the best way to determine which foods are causing my (or my child's) symptoms?
- I have to travel for my work, which means eating out. Can you give me some suggestions how to stay on this diet when eating in restaurants?
- What vitamins and minerals should I be taking while I am on this diet?

Research and general acceptance

The medical community accepts elimination diets as a standard way to diagnose food sensitivities. A true elimination diet is quite restrictive, is time intensive to implement, and should be supervised by a healthcare professional. Many shortcut, "do-it-yourself" elimination-style diets are available on the Internet. Although people who believe they have a food intolerance often try these diets, they are not accepted by healthcare professionals as diagnostically accurate, and they may cause short-term vitamin and mineral deficiencies.

Resources

BOOKS

Carter, Jill and Alison Edwards. *The Allergy Exclusion Diet: The 28-Day Plan to Solve Your Food Intolerances.* Carlsbad, CA: Hay House, 2003.
———. *The Elimination Diet Cookbook.* Rockport, MA: Element, 1997.
Scott-Moncrieff, Christina. *Overcoming Allergies: Home Remedies-Elimination and Rotation Diets-Complementary Therapies.* London: Collins & Brown, 2002.

PERIODICALS

Scarpellini, E., and J. Tack. "Food Allergy: From Diagnosis to Treatment." *Digestive Diseases* 30, no. 2 (2012): 224–31.

OTHER

Institute of Functional Medicine. "Comprehensive Elimination Diet." Applying Functional Medicine in Clinical Practice. http://www.functionalmedicine.org/content_management/files/ifm_Comp_Elim_Diet_091503.pdf (accessed September 5, 2012).

WEBSITES

Cleveland Clinic. "Elimination Diet and Food Challenge Test." http://my.clevelandclinic.org/services/allergy_

testing/hic_elimination_diet_and_food_challenge_test. aspx (accessed September 5, 2012).

Foodintol. "How To Do An Elimination Diet." http://www. foodintol.com/elimination-diet (accessed September 5, 2012).

Meyers, Suzzanne. "The Elimination Diet." http://www. eliminationdiet.com (accessed September 5, 2012).

Sicherer, Scott H. "Food Allergies." http://emedicine. medscape.com/article/135959-overview (accessed September 5, 2012).

WebMD. "Allergies: Elimination Diet and Food Challenge Test." http://www.webmd.com/allergies/allergies-elimination-diet (accessed September 5, 2012).

ORGANIZATIONS

Academy of Nutrition and Dietetics, 120 South Riverside Plz., Ste. 2000, Chicago, IL 60606-6995, (312) 899-0040, (800) 877-1600, amacmunn@eatright.org, http://www. eatright.org.

Chronic Fatigue and Immune Dysfunction Syndrome Association of America (CFIDS), PO Box 220398, Charlotte, NC 28222-0398, (704) 365-2343, http://www.cfids.org.

Institute for Functional Medicine, 505 S. 336th St., Ste. 500, Federal Way, WA 98003, (253) 661-3010, (800) 228-0622, Fax: (253) 661-8310, http://www.functionalmedicine.org.

Tish Davidson, AM

Encopresis

Definition

Encopresis is defined as the repeated passage or leaking of feces in inappropriate places in a child over four years of age that is not caused by a physical illness or disability.

Description

Over 80% of cases of encopresis begin with the child's experience of a painful bowel movement or passing a very large bowel movement. Over time, the child comes to associate using the toilet with pain and begins to hold in, or retain, his or her bowel movements to avoid the pain. The child may occasionally try to pass some of the hardened stool and develop a crack in the skin surrounding the anus known as an anal fissure. Anal fissures cause additional pain and usually reinforce the child's habit of retaining feces. As the mass of stool grows, the colon stretches to many times its normal diameter—a condition known as megacolon. The child also loses the natural urge to have a bowel movement because the muscles in the wall of the colon cannot contract and push the stool out.

Encopresis is thought to affect between 1%–2% of children in the United States below the age of ten. Boys are six times as likely to develop encopresis. It is not known to be related to race or social class, the size of the family, the child's birth order, or the age of the parents.

Treatment

There is no universal agreement among doctors as to the best method of treatment for encopresis, including dietary recommendations. It is a disorder resulting from the interaction of bodily, psychological, and social factors in the child's life. As a result, there have been no large-scale controlled studies of different treatment methods.

Dietary treatment

Dietary treatment of encopresis is intended to help the child develop regular bowel habits after disimpaction and to minimize the risk of recurrent **constipation**. Dietary modifications usually include:

• Reducing the child's intake of milk and other dairy products that tend to cause constipation. Some pediatricians recommend soymilk as a substitute for cow's milk during maintenance treatment.

• Adding dietary fiber to the child's diet in the form of high-fiber breads and cereals, vegetables and fruits that are high in fiber, or over-the-counter fiber supplements.

• Increasing the child's water intake, particularly during warm weather.

• Encouraging the child to participate in vigorous physical activity. Exercise helps to move food through the digestive system.

• Increasing the child's intake of fruit and fruit juices. Fruit juices, particularly prune juice, have a laxative effect. Fruit and fruit juices cannot be used by themselves as maintenance treatment for encopresis because few children are able to drink or eat the amounts required for laxative treatment. Fruit is recommended over fruit juice since it has more nutrients.

Medical approaches

Medical treatment of encopresis begins with disimpaction, or softening and removal of the mass of fecal material in the lower colon. Disimpaction may be accomplished by administering enemas or a series of enemas; one or a series of suppositories; laxatives taken by mouth; or a combination of these treatments. Commonly used enemas include homemade soap-and-water solutions and commercial saline preparations. Dulcolax (bisacodyl) and BabyLax are popular brands of suppositories. Laxatives, which work by increasing the amount of water in the large intestine to soften the impacted stool, include citrate of magnesia, Fleet Phospho-soda, Colyte, or GoLYTELY. Other laxatives sometimes used are mineral oil and senna, a plant native to the tropics that has been used to treat constipation for over three thousand years.

Following disimpaction, the child is given maintenance medications intended to produce soft stools once or twice daily to prevent constipation from recurring. They also help the child break the mental and emotional connection between defecation and pain. The child may be given glycerine or bisacodyl suppositories once or twice a day, or mineral oil, senna syrup (Senokot), milk of magnesia, lactulose, or sorbitol twice a day by mouth. Maintenance treatment typically takes several months.

Glucomannan, a complex **sugar** derived from the roots of the Japanese konjac plant, is an effective **fiber** supplement for children that appears to be well tolerated and has fewer side effects than many laxatives. Glucomannan is a water-soluble fiber that forms a gel-like mass in the digestive tract and helps to push fecal matter through the lower bowel more rapidly.

Psychological treatment

Psychological treatment is part of maintenance therapy for encopresis because of the emotional stress the condition causes the child and other family members. In many cases the child has become depressed or developed other behavioral problems as a result of punishment, teasing, or social rejection related to episodes of soiling. Psychological treatment begins with education; the doctor explains to the parents as well as the child how encopresis develops, what causes it, and why medications are used to treat it.

If the child's encopresis is involuntary, behavioral therapy is often used. This approach employs such techniques as star charts and daily diaries to teach the child to recognize the body's internal cues. Some doctors also recommend biofeedback for maintenance therapy in encopresis.

If the child's episodes of soiling are intentional rather than involuntary, he or she will usually be referred to a child psychiatrist for specialized evaluation and treatment.

Function

The function of dietary treatment for encopresis is as a form of maintenance therapy. The goal is to prevent stool from building up in the child's colon, allow the colon to return to its normal shape and muscular function, and to help the child have bowel movements in the toilet at appropriate times.

Benefits

The benefit of dietary treatment for encopresis is prevention of future episodes of constipation while providing adequate nutrition for the child. Medications are used to clear impacted fecal material from the colon and relieve discomfort associated with defecation.

Precautions

Parents should follow the doctor's advice about laxatives and enemas during maintenance treatment for encopresis, as some of these products have side effects or interact with other medications that the child may be taking.

Risks

There are no reported adverse effects of dietary treatment for encopresis.

Enemas and laxatives often produce side effects including abdominal cramping, intestinal gas, nausea, and vomiting. The child's doctor may be able to change the dosage or type of product for a child on maintenance treatment. Lactulose should not be given to patients with diabetes because it contains a form of sugar, while sorbitol may reduce the effectiveness of other medications. Mineral oil sometimes causes seepage into underwear and itching in the anal area. Senna and citrate of magnesia may lead to electrolyte imbalance if used in high doses over a long period of time.

Research and general acceptance

Disagreements regarding treatment for encopresis focus on three subjects: whether enemas are preferable to laxatives taken by mouth or whether enemas are emotionally traumatic to the child; whether or not adding fiber to the child's diet is useful; and whether placing the child on the toilet at set times helps in establishing bowel control or whether it creates emotional conflict between parent and child. Opinion is divided about the effectiveness of placing the child on the toilet at fixed times during the day; some doctors think that taking the child to the toilet after a meal helps to teach good bowel habits, while others think it is not a good idea if the child does not feel an urge to defecate.

There is no evidence that long-term use of laxatives creates dependency on them or causes colon **cancer**.

KEY TERMS

Anal fissure—A crack or slit that develops in the mucous membrane of the anus, often as a result of a constipated person pushing to expel hardened stool. Anal fissures are quite painful and difficult to heal.

Biofeedback—A technique for improving awareness of internal bodily sensations in order to gain conscious control over digestion and other processes generally considered to be automatic.

Constipation—Abnormally delayed or infrequent passage of feces. It may be either functional (related to failure to move the bowels) or organic (caused by another disease or disorder).

Enema—The injection of liquid through the anus into the rectum in order to soften hardened stools.

Impaction—The medical term for a mass of fecal matter that has become lodged in the lower digestive tract. Removal of this material is called disimpaction.

Laxative—A drug usually administered by mouth to produce a bowel movement. Laxatives are also known as cathartics.

Megacolon—A condition in which the colon becomes stretched far beyond its usual size. Children with long-term constipation may develop megacolon.

Suppository—A tablet or capsule, usually made of glycerin, inserted into the rectum to stimulate the muscles to contract and expel feces.

Resources

BOOKS

American Psychiatric Association. *Diagnostic and Statistical Manual of Mental Disorders.* 4th ed. Washington, DC: American Psychiatric Association, 2000.

Schaefer, Charles E. *Childhood Encopresis and Enuresis: Causes and Therapy.* Northvale, NJ: Jason Aronson, 1993.

"Toileting Problems." Chapter 298, Section 19. *Merck Manual of Diagnosis and Treatment,* 18th ed. Edited by Mark H. Beers and Robert Berkow. Whitehouse Station, NJ: Merck, 2007.

PERIODICALS

Biggs, Wendy S., and William H. Dery. "Evaluation and Treatment of Constipation in Infants and Children." *American Family Physician* 73 (February 1, 2006): 469–82.

Fishman, Laurie, Leonard Rappaport, Alison Schonwald, and Samuel Nurko. "Trends in Referral to a Single Encopresis Clinic over 20 Years." *Pediatrics* 111 (May 2003): 604–7.

Fleisher, David R. "Understanding Toilet Training Difficulties." *Pediatrics* 113 (June 2004): 1809–10.

Loening-Baucke, V., E. Miele, and A. Staiano. "Fiber (Glucomannan) Is Beneficial in the Treatment of Childhood Constipation." *Pediatrics* 113 (March 2004): 259–64.

McGrath, M.L., M.W. Mellon, and L. Murphy. "Empirically Supported Treatments in Pediatric Psychology: Constipation and Encopresis." *Journal of Pediatric Psychology* 25 (June 2000): 225–54.

Pashankar, Dinesh S., and Vera Loenig-Baucke. "Increased Prevalence of Obesity in Children with Functional Constipation Evaluated in an Academic Medical Center." *Pediatrics* 116 (September 2005): 377–80.

WEBSITES

Mayo Clinic staff. "Encopresis" MayoClinic.com. http://www.mayoclinic.com/health/encopresis/DS00885 (accessed September 28, 2012).

Nemours Foundation. "Soiling (encopresis)." KidsHealth.org. http://kidshealth.org/parent/general/sick/encopresis.html (accessed September 28, 2012).

North American Society for Pediatric Gastroenterology, Hepatology, and Nutrition (NASPGHAN). "Encopresis." http://www.naspghan.org/wmspage.cfm?parm1 = 104 (accessed September 29, 2012).

PubMed Health. "Encopresis." U.S. National Library of Medicine. http://www.ncbi.nlm.nih.gov/pubmedhealth/PMH0002537 (accessed September 28, 2012).

ORGANIZATIONS

American Academy of Child and Adolescent Psychiatry (AACAP), 3615 Wisconsin Ave. NW, Washington, DC 20016, (202) 966-7300, http://www.aacap.org.

American Academy of Pediatrics (AAP), 141 Northwest Point Blvd., Elk Grove Village, IL 60007, (847) 434-4000, (800) 433-9016, Fax: (847) 434-8000, http://www.aap.org.

American Gastroenterological Association, 4930 Del Ray Ave., Bethesda, MD 20814, (301) 654-2055, Fax: (301) 654-5920, member@gastro.org, http://www.gastro.org.

International Foundation for Functional Gastrointestinal Disorders, PO Box 170864, Milwaukee, WI 53217, (414) 964-1799, (888) 964-2001, Fax: (414) 964-7176, iffgd@iffgd.org, http://www.iffgd.org.

National Digestive Diseases Information Clearinghouse, 2 Information Way, Bethesda, MD 20892–3570, (800) 891–5389, TTY: (866) 569–1162, Fax: (703) 738–4929, nddic@info.niddk.nih.gov, http://www.digestive.niddk.nih.gov.

North American Society for Pediatric Gastroenterology, Hepatology, and Nutrition, PO Box 6, Flourtown, PA 19031, (215) 233-0808, Fax: (215) 233-3918, naspghan@naspghan.org, http://www.naspghan.org.

Rebecca J. Frey, PhD

English diet *see* **Northern European diet**

Ephedra

Definition

Ephedra is a genus of plants found worldwide. One species, *Ephedra sinica* or Chinese ephedra, has a long history of use in complementary and alternative medicine (CAM). In the late twentieth century, ephedra gained popularity as a weight-loss supplement. The herb can cause life-threatening side effects, and since April 2004, sale of products containing ephedra have been banned in the United States. In Traditional Chinese Medicine (TCM), ephedra is called *ma huang*.

Purpose

Ephedra (ma huang) has been used in TCM for about 5,000 years primarily to treat sneezing, runny nose, coughing and other symptoms of a cold, influenza, bronchitis, and allergy. In the 1990s, ephedra was marketed in the United States as a dietary supplement that stimulated weight loss. It was also marketed to adolescents as a mood-altering "herbal Ecstasy" and to athletes to improve performance. In 2005, use of ephedra-containing supplements in the United States was banned.

Description

Ephedra is an evergreen plant with tiny leaves that grows to a height of about 12 in. (30 cm). Many species of ephedra are found worldwide, but *E. sinica* used in herbal medicine grows mainly in dry, rocky areas of

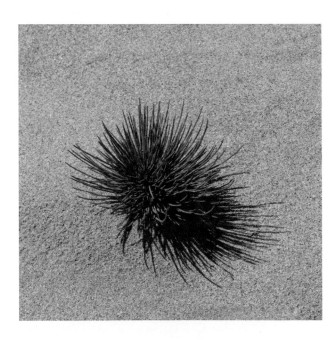

Ephedra plant. *(Nikita Tiunov/Shutterstock.com)*

Mongolia and northern China. The stems and roots of the plant are used medicinally. Many other species of ephedra, for example, *E. nevadensis* or Mormon tea that grows in the western United States, do not have the same active ingredients as *E. sinica*.

The active ingredients in ephedra are the alkaloids ephedrine and pseudoephedrine. These chemicals have effects similar to amphetamines. They stimulate the central nervous system and affect the heart and circulatory system. Ephedra causes blood vessels to narrow, increases heart rate, and raises blood pressure. These effects are enhanced when ephedra is taken with **caffeine**. Ephedra also expands the airways, making breathing easier. Researchers generally agree that ephedra is effective in treating cold and allergy symptoms.

Standardized amounts of manufactured ephedrine and pseudoephedrine, the active ingredients found in ephedra, are used in many cold and allergy products made by traditional pharmaceutical companies and approved for sale by the FDA. For years, these drugs were sold in the United States over the counter without restrictions. Beginning in the early 2000s, a movement developed to limit access to these drugs by placing them behind the counter at the pharmacy, limiting the amount an individual could buy, and requiring identification to purchase the drugs. This came about more because ephedrine and pseudoephedrine are used in the manufacture of illicit methamphetamines (e.g., crystal meth) than because of safety concerns about the drugs.

Ephedrine and pseudoephedrine are also effective appetite suppressants, especially when combined with caffeine. Many people who took diet pills containing ephedra or a combination of ephedra and caffeine did lose weight. However, they also experienced an increased risk of dangerous, sometimes fatal, side effects. Ephedra was brought to the attention of the FDA in the mid-1990s by a large increase in the number of reports from poison control centers and health care providers about serious adverse effects related to ephedra-containing weight-loss supplements. These side effects included dangerously high blood pressure, fast heart rate, stroke, and heart attack. By 2003, at least 155 deaths were linked to ephedra use, including that of Baltimore Oriole's pitching prospect Steve Belcher. That same year, an analysis of side effects related to herbal therapy published in the *Annals of Internal Medicine* found that ephedra accounted for less than 1% of all herbal supplement sales, but was responsible for 64% of all reported negative events caused by herbs.

Ephedra and the Law

The FDA regulates ephedra and other **dietary supplements** under the 1994 Dietary Supplement

Health and Education Act (DSHEA). At the time the act was passed, legislators felt that because many dietary supplements come from natural sources such as plants and because they have been used for hundreds of years by practitioners of CAM, these products did not need to be regulated as rigorously as prescription and over-the-counter drugs used in conventional medicine. The legislators decided that dietary supplements should be regulated the same way food is regulated. As a result, manufacturers of ephedra supplements, just like the manufacturers of cheese or cereal, did not have to prove that ephedra was either safe or effective before it could be sold to the public. They also were not required to tell the public about possible side effects of the herb. (Conventional pharmaceuticals must include potential side effects in their packaging.)

With ephedra and all other dietary supplements, the burden of proof falls on the FDA to show that the supplement is either unsafe or ineffective before the supplement can be restricted or banned. Information about a supplement's safety and effectiveness is normally gathered only after people using the product develop health problems or complain that the product does not work.

The FDA involvement with ephedra in weight-loss supplements began in 1996 after receiving more than 800 reports of adverse events in people taking products containing ephedra. In 1997 the FDA proposed regulating ephedra by requiring that the product carry a warning on the label stating that adults should take no more than 8 mg of ephedra at one time and no more than 24 mg in one day. The proposed regulation was fought by the diet supplement industry. During the course of public comment about the regulation, it became clear that there was little or no standardization of ephedra content among products or even within different batches of product from the same manufacturer. This lack of standardization made it difficult for consumers to know and control how much ephedra they were taking from day to day.

In 2002, the FDA commissioned an independent organization to study ephedra-related complications and deaths. As a result of this study, the FDA banned the uncontrolled sale of dietary supplements containing ephedra based on the what the FDA called an "unreasonable risk of illness or injury." The ban took effect on April 14, 2005.

Several supplement makers have challenged the ban on ephedra-containing supplements in federal and state courts. They argue that the FDA did not test supplements containing low doses of ephedra for safety and effectiveness and that a total ban on

ephedra supplements based only on high-dose products was illegal. The FDA took the position that it was unethical to do more human testing of ephedra given the findings that ephedra-containing supplements increase the risk of stroke, heart attack, irregular heart beat, and similar serious cardiovascular events. On October 18, 2006, after several legal challenges, the United States Court of Appeals Tenth Circuit upheld the FDA ban on all ephedra-containing supplements regardless of dose. Nutraceutical Corporation, the plaintiff in the case, vowed to file another a petition for review with the United States Supreme Court.

The ban on ephedra-containing supplements continues to be controversial. There is general agreement that ephedra does treat cold symptoms and does help people with short-term weight loss. However, these benefits do not, in the opinion of FDA scientists, outweigh the health risks associated with the ephedra-containing products. Ephedra continues to be legal in countries such as Germany, Japan, India, and China where it is widely used. Ephedra-containing supplements are easily available over the Internet, and it is estimated that several million Americans continue to use them.

Precautions

The FDA warns that no one should take dietary supplements that contain ephedra because they can cause serious, sometimes fatal, side effects. Some individuals choose to ignore this warning. In that case, people with high blood pressure, heart problems, thyroid problems, enlarged prostate, and glaucoma should avoid ephedra because there is a high risk the supplement will worsen their condition and could cause serious complications. Ephedra-containing supplements should not be given to children, pregnant women, or **breastfeeding** women.

Interactions

Studies have shown that ephedra interacts with many drugs used in conventional medicine, especially those used to treat heart problems and monoamine oxidase inhibitors (MAOI) used to treat mental depression, anxiety, and phobias.

Complications

At low doses, adverse side effects include headache, restlessness, anxiety, sleeplessness, nausea, difficulty urinating, and racing heart. At high doses, adverse reactions include sweating, enlarged pupils, fever, spasms, and death, usually through heart failure or stroke.

KEY TERMS

Alternative medicine—A system of healing that rejects conventional, pharmaceutical-based medicine and replaces it with the use of dietary supplements and therapies such as herbs, vitamins, minerals, massage, and cleansing diets. Alternative medicine includes well-established treatment systems such as homeopathy, traditional Chinese medicine, and Ayurvedic medicine, as well as more-recent, fad-driven treatments.

Amphetamine—A drug that stimulates the central nervous system and can be physically and psychologically addictive.

Complementary medicine—Includes many of the same treatments used in alternative medicine, but uses them to supplement conventional drug and therapy treatments, rather than to replace conventional medicine.

Conventional medicine—Mainstream or Western pharmaceutical-based medicine practiced by medical doctors, doctors of osteopathy, and other licensed health care professionals.

Dietary supplement—A product such as a vitamin, mineral, herb, amino acid, or enzyme, that is intended to be consumed in addition to an individual's diet with the expectation that it will improve health.

Traditional Chinese Medicine (TCM)—An ancient system of medicine based on maintaining a balance in the vital energy or qi that controls emotional, spiritual, and physical well being. In TCM, diseases and disorders result from imbalances in qi, and treatments such as massage, exercise, acupuncture, and nutritional and herbal therapy are designed to restore balance and harmony to the body.

Parental concerns

Ephedra is a dangerous herbal supplement and should not be given to children. Accidental use of ephedra by children can result in serious side effects. In the case of accidental poisoning in the United States, call the national poisoning hotline at 1-800-222-1222, the local hospital emergency room, or emergency services.

Resources

BOOKS

Fillon, Mike. *Ephedra Fact and Fiction: How Politics, the Press and Special Interests are Targeting Your Rights to Vitamins, Minerals, and Herbs.* Orem, UT: Woodland Pub., 2004.

PDR for Herbal Medicines. 3rd ed. Montvale, NJ: Thompson Healthcare, 2004.

Pierce, Andrea. *The American Pharmaceutical Association Practical Guide to Natural Medicines.* New York: William Morrow, 1999.

PERIODICALS

Bent, S., et al. "The Relative Safety of Ephedra Compared With Other Herbal Products." *Annals of Internal Medicine* 138, no. 6 (2003): 468–71.

Harrison, Todd. "Ephedra: The Real Story.(INDUSTRY NEWS)." *Nutraceuticals World* 9, no. 9 (2006): 24–25.

Shekell, P., et al. "Ephedra and Ephedrine for Weight Loss and Athletic Performance Enhancement: Clinical Efficacy and Side Effects." *Evidence Report/Technology Assessment No. 76* AHRQ Publication no. 03-E022, (February 2003).

WEBSITE

"Ma Huang." Drugs.com. http://www.drugs.com/mtm/ma_huang.html (accessed September 29, 2012).

Mayo Clinic staff. "Ephedra (*Ephedra sinica*)/Ma Huang." MayoClinic.com. http://www.mayoclinic.com/health/ephedra/NS_patient-ephedra (accessed September 29, 2012).

National Center for Complementary and Alternative Medicine. "Ephedra." http://nccam.nih.gov/health/ephedra (accessed September 29, 2012).

ORGANIZATIONS

National Center for Complementary and Alternative Medicine Clearinghouse, PO Box 7923, Gaithersburg, MD 20898, (888) 644-6226, Fax: (866) 464-3616, info@nccam.nih.gov, http://nccam.nih.gov.

Office of Dietary Supplements, National Institutes of Health, 6100 Executive Blvd., Rm. 3B01, MSC 7517, Bethesda, MD 20892-7517, (301) 435-2920, Fax: (301) 480-1845, ods@nih.gov, http://ods.od.nih.gov.

U.S. Food and Drug Administration, 10903 New Hampshire Ave., Silver Spring, MD 20993-0002, (888) INFO-FDA (463-6332), http://www.fda.gov.

Tish Davidson, A.M.

Ergogenic aids

Definition

Ergogenic aids are substances, foods, or training methods that enhance energy production, use, or recovery and provide athletes with a competitive advantage.

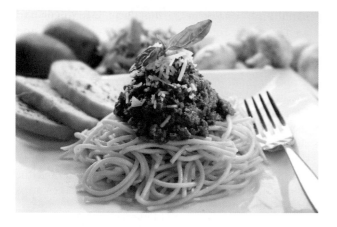

"Carbo-loading," or eating a meal heavy in carbohydrates the night before an athletic event, is a type of ergogenic aid. *(Hywit Dimyadi/Shutterstock.com)*

Purpose

New ergogenic products claiming to enhance performance appear on the market almost every week. Most ergogenic aids are sold as **dietary supplements**. The U.S. Food and Drug Administration (FDA) regulates dietary supplements under the 1994 Dietary Supplement Health and Education Act (DSHEA). Manufacturers of ergogenic aids sold as dietary supplements do not have to prove that their product is either safe or effective before it can be sold to the public. The contents of a product, its manufacturing process, and the claims on its label have not been evaluated by the FDA, and the burden of proof falls on the FDA to show that a supplement is either unsafe or ineffective before that supplement can be restricted or banned. Information about an ergogenic aid's safety and effectiveness normally is gathered only after people using the product develop health problems or complain that the product does not work.

Despite the fact that many ergogenic aids may have little or no scientific basis for their claims, surveys have shown that about three-quarters of college athletes and nearly 100% of professional bodybuilders take supplements. Athletes use ergogenic aids to improve their energy and performance and to gain a competitive edge. There are generally two types of aids: those that are legal and considered generally safe, and those that are considered dangerous. Aids in the latter group are usually prohibited in competitive sports. The best, and safest, ergogenic aids are proper training and rest, good nutrition, correct technique, and good coaching.

Description

Ergogenic aids generally viewed as safe include the following:

- Carbohydrate loading: Research shows that adequate intake of dietary carbohydrates in the days and hours before strenuous training and competition is critical to maintaining adequate glycogen levels in muscles. Increasing consumption of carbohydrates three days before an endurance-type event is therefore a safe way to enhance performance. Endurance athletes, such as marathon runners, rely on their stores of glycogen as a source of energy during competition and carbohydrate loading is a method for boosting the amount of glycogen in the body before a competition.

- Proper nutrition: Proper nutrition means making good food choices and following diets that lead to better health, good immunity, and reduce major risk factors for diseases. The estimated average daily calorie requirement is 1,940 calories per day for women and 2,550 for men. Caloric intake should be adjusted to compensate for an increased level of activity in athletes. A registered dietitian can develop a healthy and effective diet for competitive athletes that takes into consideration the amount, timing, and type of activities they perform.

- Sports drinks: According to the American College of Sports Medicine, as well as American and Canadian dietitians' associations, sports drinks are effective in supplying energy for the muscles, maintaining proper levels of blood sugar, and lowering the risk of dehydration or hyponatremia (low sodium levels). Some sports drinks have been formulated to ensure rapid provision of water, while others are formulated to optimize energy provision. Other researchers have noted that the flavoring added to sports drinks encourages athletes to drink more during periods of exercise, thus maintaining proper levels of hydration. A fluid loss equivalent to 2% of body weight can impair performance. A fluid loss of 5% of body weight can lead to heat exhaustion. Sports drinks, also called electrolyte replacement solutions, not only provide fluid but also contain a proper balance of the salts and minerals required for various functions by the body, which are lost in sweat. Examples of well-known brands include Gatorade, Lucozade, and Powerade.

- Increased protein consumption: Many weightlifters, bodybuilders, or others looking to increase muscle mass consume extra amounts of protein, often in the form of protein supplements. The protein may come from different sources, including whey, casein, soy, or certain plants. A number of studies have found that consuming protein after a workout can help promote both muscle growth and recovery. The Academy of Nutrition and Dietetics recommends that endurance athletes and weightlifters consume 1.2–1.7 g of protein per kg of body weight, in comparison to the 0.8 g/kg recommended for the average adult. The Academy recommends that these intakes be met through consumption of whole foods, as opposed to protein powders or bars.

- Stress management: The increased stress of competitive sports can affect athletes both physically and mentally such that their performance abilities are lowered. Stress may lead to excessive tension, increased heart rates, cold sweats, and anxiety about the outcome of the competition. Stress management techniques are recognized ergogenic aids that help maintain concentration, confidence, control, and commitment.

- Relaxation techniques: Relaxation is especially important for high performance athletic activities. It promotes rest, recovery, and recuperation while removing stress-related reactions, such as increased muscular tension. In addition, relaxation contributes to the maintenance of positive physical and mental states.

Precautions

Some ergogenic aids are known to have harmful side effects and this is the reason why they are banned by sports governing authorities because they are unsafe and unethical. The most abused aids include the following:

- Anabolic steroids: Anabolic steroids are a class of man-made drugs that are chemically related to the male hormone testosterone. They increase skeletal muscle mass and strength. Not a single anabolic steroid has been manufactured that is free of negative side effects. In many developing countries, anabolic steroids can be purchased without a prescription. However, in the United States, they have been controlled substances since 1991.

- Blood doping: This is another dangerous ergogenic aid. It involves taking blood or blood products, such as erythropoietin (EPO), a hormone that stimulates the bones to make red blood cells, to improve athletic endurance and speed. It can also have harmful side effects.

- Human growth hormone (HGH): HGH is a widely abused ergogenic aid by bodybuilders. Some body builders take large doses to decrease fat and increase muscle mass. Many adverse effects have been documented.

- Caffeine: Caffeine affects the central nervous system by increasing mental alertness and lowering fatigue. It has many positive benefits, the most recent identified as a possible preventative against Alzheimer's disease. It also helps increase endurance capacity and lower perceived pain. Excessive use can cause irritability, restlessness, diarrhea, insomnia, and anxiety. It is found in coffee, tea, chocolate, and some soft drinks.

- Ephedrine: Some athletes use ephedrine-containing supplements to improve their performance, have more energy, or decrease their body fat. Unfortunately, athletes who use ephedrine may find that while it helps them run farther and faster, research findings have shown that it also puts them at risk of potentially life-threatening side effects. The National Football League, the National Collegiate Athletic Association, and the International Olympic Committee have all taken steps to keep it off the playing fields.

- Gene doping: Gene doping is the non-therapeutic use of cells, genes, and genetic elements to improve athletic performance. Besides being a complex ethical and philosophical issue, the long-term effects on health have not been investigated.

- Megadoses of vitamins, minerals, and herbs: Vitamins, minerals, and some well-researched herbs all have a role in maintaining health. Nevertheless, intake of very large quantities of these materials can cause serious health problems; for example, high doses of vitamin C (more than 2,000 mg/day) can result in gastrointestinal upset. In the case of vitamins, minerals, and herbs, more is not necessarily better and can lead to reduced, rather than enhanced, performance.

Interactions

Athletes who train hard frequently complain about energy drain and fatigue. Because they are regularly reminded to consume adequate fluids and **calories** to minimize early fatigue and to maximize performance and recovery, many have turned to energy drinks. These are drinks, such as Red Bull or 5-Hour Energy, that contain fluids, large amounts of **caffeine**, and **sugar**. They are different from balanced sports drinks, such as Gatorade, that replenish fluids and **electrolytes** and provide energy in the form of sugar. Recent research sponsored by the Food and Nutrition Information Center of the United States Department of Agriculture (USDA) a has shown that some energy drinks contain herbs, amino acids, **protein**, and other substances in such small amounts that they are unlikely to have any noticeable effect on performance. Other energy drinks were found to have ingredients that can cause inefficient absorption of fluid and nutrients from the intestine, along with possible gastrointestinal distress.

Aftercare

Treatment for excessive use of ergogenic supplements starts with complete avoidance. Depending on the supplement used and the medical complications, aftercare is tailored to individual cases and depends on the nature of the resulting medical condition.

Complications

Many ergogenic aids are either illegal or have been banned by the organizations that oversee various sports. Urine and blood testing is now standard in many professional sports and in high-profile sporting events, such as the Olympics. Athletes caught using forbidden ergogenic aids can be stripped of their wins and banned from their sport.

Harmful effects have been reported for several ergogenic products. Anabolic steroids have very serious side effects. Anabolic steroids fool the body into thinking that testosterone is being produced in large quantities. Excessive use causes a harmful disturbance of the body's normal hormone levels and body chemistry. Cardiovascular side effects are the most common. They include increased heart rate (tachycardia); heart attack (myocardial infarction), even in young athletes; high blood pressure (**hypertension**), an increase in low-density lipoprotein (LDL or "bad" cholesterol); and a decrease in high-density lipoprotein (HDL or "good" cholesterol) that increases the risk of stroke. Other negative side effects may include liver damage, liver tumors (usually not cancerous), and a decrease in blood clotting factors. Young people may develop severe acne. Males may experience shrinking testes, falling sperm count, increased risk of infertility, enlarged breasts, and an enlarged prostate gland and baldness. In addition, the ends of long bones fuse together and stop growing, resulting in permanently stunted growth and short stature. Women frequently show signs of masculinity including the development of facial hair, lower voice, and male-type musculature. They may stop menstruating, may be at higher risk for certain types of **cancer**, and have an increased risk of birth defects in their children.

Anabolic steroids also affect mental health. Their use can cause drastic mood swings, inability to sleep, depression, and feelings of hostility. There is some evidence that young men may become more volatile and violent when taking these drugs, a condition known as "roid rage." Steroids also may be psychologically and physically addictive to some users. Withdrawal symptoms may include insomnia, fatigue, restlessness, reduced sex drive, depression, and suicidal thoughts.

Blood doping has been linked to strokes, allergic reactions, and infections. HGH adverse effects include heart and nerve diseases, glucose intolerance, and higher levels of blood **fats** (lipids). Other effects also come from the extra HGH levels in the body along with what is already produced by the pituitary glands. Ergogenic doses of caffeine may cause restlessness, nervousness, insomnia, tremors, and an increased heart rate. At least 17 deaths have been linked to products that combine caffeine and ephedrine.

Adverse effects have also been reported with carbohydrate supplementation. Increased **insulin** levels after carbohydrate consumption were shown to significantly decrease blood glucose levels in some athletes, and fructose-containing solutions have been associated with adverse gastrointestinal effects in some studies.

Parental concerns

Parents should educate their teenagers concerning the use of ergogenic aids, and strive to increase their awareness of illegal ones. Steroid abuse has spread downward from elite and professional athletes to college and high school athletes and younger. According to a survey by the U.S. Centers for Disease Control and Prevention (CDC) in 2005, 850,000 high school students in the United States had used anabolic steroid pills or shots without a prescription. A 2007 study found that 1.5% of eighth graders and 2.2% of twelfth graders (2.3% of boys and 0.6% of girls) had at some time used illicit steroids.

Resources

BOOKS

Greenwood, Mike, Douglas Kalman, and Jose Antonio, eds. *Nutritional Supplements in Sports and Exercise.* New York: Humana Press, 2010.

PERIODICALS

Academy of Nutrition and Dietetics. "Position of the American Dietetic Association, Dietitians of Canada, and the American College of Sports Medicine: Nutrition and Athletic Performance." *Journal of the American Dietetic Association* 109, no. 3 (2009): 509–27. http://dx.doi.org/10.1016/j.jada.2009.01.005 (accessed August 24, 2012).

Beelen, M., et al. "Nutritional Strategies to Promote Postexercise Recovery." *International Journal of Sport Nutrition and Exercise Metabolism* 20, no. 6 (2010): 515–32.

WEBSITES

National Institute on Drug Abuse. "Steroids (Anabolic)." U.S. National Institutes of Health. http://www.drugabuse.gov/drugs-abuse/steroids-anabolic (accessed August 24, 2012).

U.S. Department of Agriculture, National Agricultural Library. "Ergogenic Aids." Food and Nutrition Information Center. http://fnic.nal.usda.gov/dietary-supplements/ergogenic-aids (accessed August 24, 2012).

ORGANIZATIONS

American College of Sports Medicine, 401 West Michigan St., Indianapolis, IN 46202-3233, (317) 637-9200, Fax: (317) 634-7817, http://www.acsm.org.

Center for Food Safety and Applied Nutrition (CFSAN), U.S. Food and Drug Administration, 5100 Paint Branch Pkwy., College Park, MD 20740, (888) SAFE-FOOD (723-3366), consumer@fda.gov, http://www.fda.gov/Food/default.htm.

National Center for Drug Free Sport, 2735 Madison Ave., Kansas City, MO 64108, (816) 474-8655, Fax: (816) 502-9287, info@drugfreesport.com, http://www.drugfreesport.com.

National Institute on Drug Abuse, 6001 Executive Blvd., Rm. 5213, MSC 9561, Bethesda, MD 20892, (301) 443-1124, information@nida.nih.gov, http://www.drugabuse.gov.

Monique Laberge, PhD
Tish Davidson, AM

Essential fatty acids *see* **Omega-3 and omega-6 fatty acids**

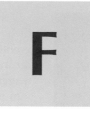

F

Fad diets

Definition

Fad diets are diets that promise quick weight loss results. These diets are generally not sustainable due to unrealistic expectations, and may even be harmful.

Purpose

Despite the popularity of dieting, the prevalence of overweight and obese individuals has increased steadily since the 1970s. In 2011, U.S. government health surveys showed that about 31% of adult men and 35% of adult women (a total of about 100 million people) in the United States were overweight or obese. Between 20%–25% of children under the age of 18 were overweight.

Fad diets are popular because they promise quick results, but the most effective and safe way to lose weight is by increasing physical activity over time and reducing caloric intake by choosing foods that are nutrient dense, such as fruits, vegetables, **whole grains**, lean proteins, and low- or nonfat dairy foods. Fad diets counter this combination and the information provided by science-based governmental and nongovernmental organizations.

Description

Fad diets seem relatively easy to implement and claim remarkable improvements in how their followers will look or feel. Unfortunately, the one thing most fad diets have in common is that they seldom promote safe and/or long-term weight loss efforts. More importantly, fad diets that do not incorporate healthful eating and exercise fall short in incorporating the needed behavior changes for long-term weight maintenance. It is realistic to state that most diets work in the short term, but most reports show that after five years, less than 10% of people maintain a 5% loss from their initial body weight. With so many conflicting diets available, it is not surprising that many are confused when it comes to information about how to lose weight safely and for the long term.

Types of fad diets

Fad diets take many forms. Over the years, fad diets have circulated around either the promotion of food in specific combinations or the elimination or increased consumption of certain macro- and/or micronutrients for the purpose of weight loss. Some of the most popular types of fad diets include:

- Fad diets that eliminate main food groups (e.g., the Cabbage Soup diet, the Grapefruit diet, the Lemonade diet). These diets offer quick weight loss based on a low-calorie diet with minimal nutrients. When followed for a short period of time, weight loss will occur, but if followed for longer periods of time, these diets may be harmful due to the severe caloric restrictions and macro- and micronutrient deficiencies.

- Fad diets that offer specific combinations of foods for weight loss (e.g., the Zone diet, the Food Combining diet). These diets are based on the theory that certain foods and/or nutrients are or are not digested beneficially when combined or eaten separately.

- Fad diets that rely on specific times that foods must be eaten (e.g., the Food Timing diet, the Rotation diet). These diets usually claim that when certain foods are eaten at specific times during the day that it will boost metabolism, thus helping in shedding pounds.

- Fad diets that recommend elimination of certain foods (e.g., the Atkins diet, the Dukan diet, Protein Power, the Carbohydrate Addict's diet, Life without Bread, and Sugar Busters!). This idea is the premise of most fad diets in one way or another, when a food is eliminated from the diet, especially if it is a food that consists of a large percentage of the calories eaten,

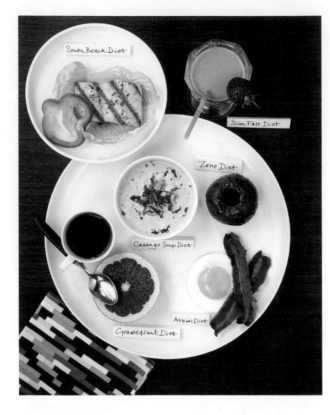

Representations of popular fad diets. (© Bon Appetit/Alamy)

weight loss will occur due to the decrease in total daily caloric intake.

• Fad diets that rely on eating certain foods and/or nutrients that are specific to a person's body chemistry to promote weight loss (e.g., hCG diet, Eat Right for Your Type, Paleo Diet, Neanderthin, Apple Cider diet. Açaí berry diet, Raw Food diet). These diets usually tie in health claims that lack scientific evidence that state that your body will function better if this food is either eaten or not consumed.

• Fad diets promoted by celebrities or that claim celebrities have followed the diet (e.g., Suzanne Somers' the Hollywood Cookie diet, Oprah diet). These diets consist of a plethora of different types of diets and usually are endorsed by a celebrity that has recently lost weight.

If fad diets resulted in long-term maintenance of weight loss efforts, the problem of **obesity** would likely have been solved long ago.

Some fad diets have been popular for many years (e.g., **Atkins Diet** Revolution). Books appear as "new, revised" editions and continue to sell millions of copies. Rarely is there anything new or revised about the diets; they simply appeal to a new generation of overweight, frustrated dieters.

The underlying reason why diets, including fad diets, work is that they result in decreased caloric intake. When energy intake is less than energy expenditure, people lose weight. Fad diets that lead to decreased caloric intake, whether by eliminating certain **macronutrients**, eating only a restricted amount of foods, or other various ways to decrease overall energy intake, will result in weight loss. If a person followed such a diet long term, he or she would keep the weight off, although general health would likely be impaired because these diets are not nutritionally balanced. Of course, few people want to live on cabbage soup or eliminate **carbohydrates** forever, so most people break the "diet" and gain back the weight they lost—and sometimes even more.

Recognizing fad diets

The American Heart Association provides some tips that can be used to recognize a fad diet. First, does the diet contain "magic" or "miracle" foods or proprietary ingredients? There are no "super foods" or "magic ingredients" that can undo the long-term effects of overeating and lack of activity. Next, beware of fad diets that claim rapid weight loss (e.g., "lose ten pounds this weekend!"). Though appealing, weight loss occurring this quickly is due to loss of fluid, not fat. Studies show that gradual weight loss increases a person's success at keeping weight off permanently. Sound weight loss plans aim for losing no more than one to two pounds per week.

Another sign of a fad diet is losing weight without exercise. Studies consistently show that an important variable that predicts long-term success at weight loss and maintenance (not gaining back the weight that was lost) is physical activity. Simple activities, such as walking or riding a bike, should be incorporated into daily life. Also, beware of the promotion of bizarre quantities of foods or the elimination of other types of foods (e.g., cabbage soup for breakfast, lunch, and dinner; avoiding dairy foods; or eliminating carbohydrates). Forbidding certain foods or entire food groups, in addition to being unhealthy, may increase the likelihood that one will cheat, binge, or just give up on the diet. Finally, a rigid menu or rigid schedule of eating is a good sign that one should avoid the diet. Limiting food choices and adhering to specific eating times is a daunting task. Rather, one should look for a plan that can be followed not for a week or a month, but for an entire lifetime.

Not all commercially advertised diets are fad diets. The **Weight Watchers** program, for example, is a diet and lifestyle program that follows sound medical and scientific advice.

Precautions

Knowledgeable practitioners do not recommend fad diets, because such diets do not work in the long term. Even though they might work initially, there is little value in losing weight if the weight is going to be regained after the diet ends (sometimes called the yo-yo effect). With repeated dieting, weight loss becomes more difficult and results in frustration, feelings of failure, loss of self-esteem and may be harmful to health.

From a nutritional standpoint, many fad diets lack important nutrients. For example, high-fat, low-carbohydrate diets (such as the Atkins Diet) are low in **vitamin A**, **vitamin B$_6$**, **vitamin E**, **thiamin**, **folate**, **calcium**, **magnesium**, **iron**, **zinc**, potassium, and dietary **fiber**. They also require the dieter to take **dietary supplements**. On the other hand, when individuals are allowed to choose foods from all food groups and control their portion size, and are encouraged to increase their physical activity, the diet is likely to be nutritionally adequate and sustainable.

Complications

Major concerns have been raised over the **weight cycling** of people who follow fad diets on and off over a period of years. Rapid weight loss and fluctuations of weight gain/loss have been shown in research studies to increase risk factors and the risk of mortality, especially cardiovascular deaths as well as **gallstones** and gallbladder problems. Further, some experts suspect that weight cycling may lower the metabolic rate, increase fat-to-lean ratio and waist-hip ratio, increase the appetite, and decrease a person's ability to lose weight in future attempts. There is also concern over the mental effects it may have on self-esteem and the relationship a person has with his or her own body. Over time, people who have not had long-term success in their weight-loss efforts may show more signs of depression.

Parental concerns

For some kids, their doctor may recommend weight loss or weight maintenance. A child or adolescent should not attempt a weight loss diet, especially a fad diet to lose weight. Children who need to lose weight should do so under the supervision of their doctor, which may also consist of a visit with a dietitian who can explain how to reduce **calories** safely, while still getting all the necessary nutrients for growth, puberty, and weight loss or weight maintenance.

QUESTIONS TO ASK YOUR DOCTOR

- Is this diet safe?
- Will I need to take any supplements while on this diet?
- Are there other diets that might be better suited for me?
- Are there any symptoms that might serve as a sign to stop the diet?
- How much weight is safe for me to lose?

Resources

BOOKS

American Heart Association. *American Heart Association No-Fad Diet: A Personal Plan for Healthy Weight Loss.* 2nd ed. New York: Clarkson Potter, 2011.

OTHER

U.S. Department of Agriculture. "Your Personal Health: Steps to a Healthier You!" MyPyramid.gov. http://www.choosemyplate.gov/food-groups/downloads/resource/MyPyramidBrochurebyIFIC.pdf (accessed July 9, 2012).

U.S. Department of Agriculture and U.S. Department of Health and Human Services. *Dietary Guidelines for Americans, 2010.* 7th ed. Washington, DC: U.S. Government Printing Office, December 2010. http://health.gov/dietaryguidelines (accessed February 22, 2012).

WEBSITES

American Heart Association. "No-Fad Diet Tips." http://www.heart.org/HEARTORG/GettingHealthy/WeightManagement/No-Fad-Diet-Tips_UCM_305838_Article.jsp (accessed August 14, 2012).

———. "Quick-Weight-Loss or Fad Diets." http://www.heart.org/HEARTORG/GettingHealthy/NutritionCenter/Quick-Weight-Loss-or-Fad-Diets_UCM_305970_Article.jsp (accessed August 14, 2012).

"Fad Diets." Everydiet.org. http://www.everydiet.org/fad_diets.htm (accessed July 9, 2012).

MedlinePlus. "Diets." U.S. National Library of Medicine, National Institutes of Health. http://www.nlm.nih.gov/medlineplus/diets.html (accessed July 9, 2012).

ORGANIZATIONS

Academy of Nutrition and Dietetics, 120 South Riverside Plaza, Ste. 2000, Chicago, IL 60606, (800) 877-1600, http://www.eatright.org.

American Heart Association, 7272 Greenville Ave., Dallas, TX 75231, (800) 242-8721, http://www.americanheart.org.

American Society for Nutrition, 9650 Rockville Pike, Bethesda, MD 20814, (301) 634-7050, Fax: (301) 634-7894, http://www.nutrition.org.

Obesity Prevention Center, University of Minnesota, 1300 South Second St., Ste. 300, Minneapolis, MN 55454, (612) 625-6200, umopc@epi.umn.edu, http://www.ahc.umn.edu/opc/home.html.

Overeaters Anonymous, PO Box 44020, Rio Rancho, NM 87174, (505) 891-2664, Fax: (505) 891-4320, http://www.oa.org.

The Obesity Society, 8758 Georgia Ave., Ste. 1320, Silver Spring, MD 20910, (301) 563-6526, Fax: (301) 563-6595, http://www.obesity.org.

Weight-Control Information Network (WIN), 1 WIN Way, Bethesda, MD 20892, (888) 232-6348, Fax: (202) 828-1028, win@info.niddk.nih.gov, http://win.niddk.nih.gov.

Marjorie R. Freedman
Tish Davidson, AM
Megan Porter, RD

Fat flush diet

Definition

The fat flush diet is a combination weight-loss and detoxification ("detox") or cleansing diet, formulated by the well-known nutritionist Ann Louise Gittleman. It is a low-carbohydrate, restricted-calorie diet, which is designed to boost **metabolism**, decrease water retention, and promote loss of fat.

Origins

Ann Louise Gittleman, a certified nutrition specialist with a PhD in holistic nutrition, first introduced the idea of "fat flush" in her 1988 book *Beyond Pritikin*. Gittleman created her diet after working as a nutritionist at the Pritikin Longevity Center in Florida, where she observed that many of her clients did very poorly on Nathan Pritikin's extremely **low-fat diet**. The author of approximately 25 books on nutrition, dieting, and health, Gittleman is America's self-described "First Lady of Nutrition." *The Fat Flush Plan* became a best-selling diet book in 2002. It received additional publicity in the 2006 film *Last Holiday* starring Queen Latifah.

Description

Theory

The theory behind the fat flush diet is that eating the correct combinations of foods and eating more often will increase the body's metabolism and lead to the efficient burning of fat. Therefore, rather than totally restricting fat, the fat flush diet calls for eating the correct **fats**, as well as the correct **carbohydrates** and proteins. However, in order to maximize the body's burning of stored body fat 24 hours per day, the liver and lymphatic system must first be detoxified.

According to Gittleman there are five "hidden factors" that sabotage weight loss, lower energy levels, and interfere with good health:

- A liver that is overloaded with toxins and functioning poorly cannot burn fat properly.
- Food sensitivities and intolerances lead to water retention and "waterlogged tissues." The fat flush diet eliminates foods that cause water retention and prescribes protein-rich foods, filtered water, and diuretics to remove excess water.
- People are afraid of eating fat. The fats in Gittleman's diet accelerate fat burning, satisfy hunger, and maintain lean muscle mass.
- Insulin is a fat-storing hormone, and excess insulin is caused by foods that are high in rapidly released carbohydrates.
- The stress hormone cortisol causes the body to store fat, particularly around the abdomen. Cortisol levels can be controlled by timing meals.

Diet components

The fat flush diet includes:

- 8 oz. (225 g) daily of lean protein as lean meat, eggs, and fish
- fruits and vegetables
- omega-3-rich fats such as flaxseed oil and evening primrose oil
- spices such as ginger, cayenne, mustard, and cinnamon, to speed up metabolism
- "long-life cocktail" consisting of one teaspoon of powdered psyllium husks or one tablespoon of ground or milled flaxseed in 8 oz. (237 mL) cranwater (one part unsweetened cranberry juice, four parts filtered water), a diuretic to speed the detoxification process and balance hormones
- a supplement called GLA

Gamma linolenic acid or GLA is an essential fat from black currant seed oil that Gittleman sells as 90 mg capsules. Gittleman claims that GLA-90 boosts weight loss by activating brown adipose tissue (BAT) and "balancing the body's sodium/potassium pump."

Specific fat flushing diet rules include:

- only one protein item per meal, with the exception of eggs
- no fruits and vegetables together

- no milk and meat together
- no water with meals, fluids only between meals
- eating about every three hours

There are three phases to the fat flush diet:

- Phase 1 is a two-week very restrictive cleansing diet.
- Phase 2 is a less restrictive diet that is continued until the desired weight or body size is achieved.
- Phase 3 is a typical low-carbohydrate diet that can be maintained for life.

PHASE 1. The two-week phase 1 of the fat flush diet is designed to detoxify the liver so that it can efficiently burn fat. It calls for eight glasses per day of cran-water to reduce water retention or "bloating," lose fat, cleanse the lymphatic system, and reduce cellulite. Caloric intake is restricted to 1,100–1,200 **calories** per day. So-called "metabolism blockers," such as wheat and dairy, are prohibited.

The phase 1 diet consists of:

- cran-water
- long-life cocktail
- one tablespoon twice daily of organic high-lignan flaxseed oil in non-heated food
- GLA supplements twice daily for a total of 360–400 mg
- hot water with the juice of half of a lemon before breakfast as a detox drink for the liver and kidneys
- 8 oz. (225 g) of lean protein daily
- one egg per day
- at least two portions of fruit daily
- unlimited raw or steamed vegetables
- one chicken, beef, or vegetable stock without salt for cooking
- herbs and spices

The lean **protein** may be:

- any fish or seafood
- lean beef, veal, or lamb
- skinless chicken or turkey
- tofu
- high-protein whey powder for thickening

Allowable vegetables include:

- asparagus
- aubergine
- bamboo shoots
- black olives without oil
- broccoli
- Brussels sprouts
- cabbage
- cauliflower
- celery
- cucumbers
- green beans
- mushrooms
- onions
- peppers
- radicchio
- spinach
- tomatoes
- water chestnuts

Acceptable fruits are:

- blackberries
- blueberries
- cherries
- cranberries
- grapefruit
- oranges
- nectarines
- peaches
- plums
- raspberries
- strawberries

Allowable herbs and spices are:

- anise
- apple cider vinegar
- bay leaf
- cayenne
- cinnamon
- cloves
- coriander, cilantro
- cumin
- dill
- dried mustard
- fennel
- garlic
- ginger
- parsley
- tumeric

Forbidden foods during phase 1 include:

- oils and fats, except flaxseed oil
- margarine
- grains
- bread
- cereal
- sugar

- starchy vegetables such as beans, potatoes, carrots, corn, and peas
- dairy products
- most herbs and spices
- alcohol

A sample phase 1 daily meal plan calls for:

- upon waking: a long-life cocktail
- before breakfast: 8 oz. (237 mL) of hot water with lemon juice
- breakfast: "vegetable scramble"—two scrambled eggs with spinach, green onions, scallions, and parsley; 8 oz. (237 mL) of cran-water
- snack: one-half of a large grapefruit
- 20 minutes before lunch: 8 oz. (237 mL) of cran-water
- lunch: 4 oz. (110 g) of salmon with lemon and garlic, warm asparagus, mixed-green salad with broccoli florets and cucumber, one tablespoon of flaxseed oil, 8 oz. (237 mL) of cran-water
- mid-afternoon snack: 16 oz. (474 mL) of cran-water
- 4 p.m. snack: one apple
- 20 minutes before dinner: 8 oz. (237 mL) of cran-water
- dinner: 4 oz. (110 g) of grilled lamb chop with a pinch of cinnamon and dried mustard, sautéed kale in broth, baked summer squash with a bit of clove, one tablespoon of flaxseed oil
- mid-evening: long-life cocktail

PHASE 2. This ongoing phase of the fat flush diet is designed for continued weight loss with a more moderate cleansing program and a slightly increased variety of foods. The caloric allowance is raised to 1200–1500 calories. Phase 2 is continued until the desired weight loss, or size, is achieved.

Carbohydrates that may be added back into the diet, at the rate of one per week, include:

- sweet potato
- brown rice
- fresh or frozen peas
- carrots
- butternut squash

PHASE 3. Phase 3 is a lifelong weight-maintenance plan with a daily caloric allowance of 1500 calories or more. The diet is made up of 40% carbohydrates, 30% protein, and 30% fat, and may include two dairy products and four carbohydrates per day. Some starchy vegetables, fruits, gluten-free grains, dairy products, and more oils are introduced into the diet one at a time, to check for any adverse reactions.

Other fat flush components

There are very few options for eating out on the fat flush diet, although choices such as fish tacos or grilled chicken sandwiches are possible. Since **caffeine** stresses the liver and, according to Gittleman, impedes fat burning, coffee should be tapered off and eventually replaced with one cup of herbal coffee per day. Alcohol is strictly forbidden during phases 1 and 2 because of its damaging effects on the liver.

Exercise is an important component of the fat flush plan. The first two phases call for brisk walking for 20–30 minutes five times per week and five minutes daily of 100 jumping jacks on a mini-trampoline. Exercise is increased in phase 3 and includes lifting weights for strength training twice per week.

The fat flush plan calls for exactly eight hours of sleep per night and for the dieter to keep a journal.

Kits

Gittleman runs residential fat flush and "Fast Track" cleansing programs and an online forum. She sells a line of organic processed foods and a 30-day fat flush detoxification kit that includes **vitamins** and **minerals**, GLA-90, and a weight-loss formula. The latter contains high amounts of **chromium** and L-carnitine. Chromium is a nutrient that can assist the body in utilizing protein, **sugar**, and fat. According to Gittleman, L-carnitine maximizes fat burning by helping the body transform food into energy. Her formula is also advertised to contain blood-sugar-stabilizing agents, appetite controllers, fat burners, and lipotropic nutrients and herbs.

Function

The fat flush diet first uses a detoxification regimen to improve fat burning and then implements a plan for losing weight rapidly, followed by a maintenance plan. It is considered to be a healthy weight-loss program. It is a balanced diet with a significant exercise component and is designed to be followed for life.

Benefits

Benefits of the fat flush diet may include:

- detoxification or cleansing of the liver and lymphatic system
- rapid weight loss of up to 10 lb. (4.5 kg) in the first two weeks
- elimination of bloating
- weight loss accompanied by body toning
- maintenance of weight loss
- decreased hips, waist, and thigh measurements

KEY TERMS

Brown adipose tissue—BAT; brown fat; a heat-producing tissue found primarily in human fetuses and infants and hibernating animals.

Cellulite—Fat deposited in pockets just below the surface of the skin around the hips, thighs, and buttocks.

Chromium—An essential mineral that must be obtained from the diet. It is important for the metabolism of fats and carbohydrates and for insulin metabolism, as well as for many enzymatic reactions in the body.

Cortisol—Hydrocortisone; a glucocorticoid that is produced by the adrenal cortex and regulates various metabolic processes and has anti-inflammatory and immunosuppressive properties. Blood levels may become elevated in response to stress.

Cran-water—A diuretic drink consisting of one part unsweetened cranberry juice in four parts filtered water.

Detoxification—Detox; cleansing; to remove toxins or poisons from the body.

Diuretic—An agent that increases urine excretion.

Evening primrose oil—Oil extracted from the seeds of the evening primrose, *Oenothera biennis*; contains GLA.

Flaxseed—Linseed; the seed of flax, *Linum usitatissimum*, used as a source of oil for treating inflammation of the respiratory, intestinal, and urinary tracts, and as a dietary supplement.

GLA—Gamma-linolenic acid; an essential fatty acid found in evening primrose oil.

Insulin—A hormone made in the pancreas that is essential for the metabolism of carbohydrates, lipids, and proteins, and that regulates blood sugar levels.

L-carnitine—A molecule in muscle that is responsible for transporting fatty acids across mitochondrial membranes; obtained from meat and milk.

Lignan—Compounds in plants that have antioxidant and estrogenic activities.

Lipotropic—Factors that promote the utilization of fat by the body.

Long-life cocktail—A drink consisting of one teaspoon of powdered psyllium husks or one tablespoon of ground or milled flaxseed in 8 oz. (237 mL) cran-water.

Omega-3 fats—A type of polyunsaturated fatty acids that appear to be beneficial for the heart.

Psyllium—Fleawort; plants of the genus *Plantago* whose seed husks have laxative activity.

According to Gittleman, this plan will also:

- increase metabolism
- permanently eliminate cellulite
- increase energy
- improve sleep
- improve health and appearance
- manage hormones and stabilize mood swings
- improve attitude
- create a healthy lifestyle

Precautions

The fat flush diet is only appropriate for people who can maintain a very strict diet for the first few weeks in order to lose weight rapidly. It may not be appropriate for vegetarians because it specifies animal protein. Vegans should add an amino-acid supplement and possibly protein powder. It is not known how often the fat flush diet leads to permanent weight loss. As with most diets, if healthy eating habits are not maintained long term, any weight lost will be regained and the other benefits will be lost.

Some experts advise against following diets that eliminate entire food groups and/or require the taking of supplements whose effects are unknown. The fat flush diet prohibits wheat and dairy during phases 1 and 2 and requires supplements. Whole-wheat grains are considered to be one of the best foods for reducing the risk of heart disease. Low-fat dairy products provide **calcium** and nutrients such as **magnesium** and **riboflavin** that may be hard to obtain from other foods. The fat flush diet requires expensive supplements including **flaxseed** oil, evening primrose oil, GLA, and protein powders.

Those following the fat flush diet should be aware of additional precautions:

- The caloric allowance in phase 1 may be too low for some people, particularly men.
- The calorie levels in phases 1 and 2 are too low to support a strenuous exercise regimen.
- The low calories may slow down, rather than speed up, metabolism.

- Although eight hours of sleep is sufficient for many people, other people require more sleep, particularly with 40 minutes of brisk walking per day and two strength-training sessions per week.
- Medications should be taken an hour before or after the long-life cocktail because the fiber in the cocktail may interfere with absorption of medicine.

Risks

The fat flush plan can disrupt menstrual cycles. Gittleman suggests using black currant seed oil rather than evening primrose oil as a GLA source to avoid this. According to Gittleman, black currant seed oil has a better omega-6 to omega-3 ratio for balancing hormones.

Gittleman's fast flush kit contains chromium, which has been linked to **ulcers** and liver and kidney damage. Large doses of chromium can be lethal.

Research and general acceptance

Research

There is little scientific evidence to support claims made for the benefits of detox diets. Gittleman claims that her plan speeds up metabolism, detoxifies the liver by flushing out waste and fat, and helps digest fatty globules in the lymphatic system. Registered dietitian Jane Kirby, in her book *Dieting for Dummies*, says that there is no scientific evidence that the liver is a "fat-burning furnace." She says: "It's just a low-calorie diet. Most people lose weight when calories are cut this low." Dr. Donald Hensrud of the Mayo Clinic was quoted in *O: the Oprah Magazine* in August of 2006: "There's no such thing as a metabolism-blocking food; the liver and lymphatic system have no link to weight loss that we know of; there's no medical purpose for cleansing the body with a diuretic; and while the fat-burning supplement recommended [GLA] has been tested in animals, there's very little data on its effect in humans."

General acceptance

The fat flush diet is very popular. Gittleman is a highly respected nutritionist who has written many articles and books on women's health, nutrition, and **detoxification diets**, and the fat flush diet has received much publicity in the popular press. Testimonials as to the success of the diet are abundant on the Internet. According to Gittleman's Website, some individuals have lost up to 12 in. (30 cm) from their buttocks, hips, and thighs in the two-week phase 1 of the diet. One individual claims that it eliminated 95% of her intractable chronic pain. The fat flush diet has proved so

popular that other entrepreneurs are selling their own fat flush kits.

QUESTIONS TO ASK YOUR DOCTOR

- Have you had other patients who have tried the fat flush diet?
- Is the calorie allowance in this diet adequate for my activity level?
- Is it healthy for me to completely eliminate grains and dairy from my diet?
- Is eight hours of sleep adequate for my needs?
- Should I be taking a diuretic?
- Should I take GLA and other supplements?
- Could the medications that I take interact with the herbs, supplements, and nutrients in the fat flush kit?
- Are there vitamin and mineral supplements that I should take while following this diet?

Resources

BOOKS

Gittleman, Ann Louise. *Beyond Pritikin*. New York: Bantam, 1988.

———. *The Fat Flush Cookbook*. New York: McGraw-Hill, 2003.

———. *The Fat Flush Fitness Plan*. New York: McGraw-Hill, 2004.

———. *The Fat Flush Foods*. New York: McGraw-Hill, 2004.

———. *The Fat Flush Journal and Shopping Guide*. New York: McGraw-Hill, 2002.

———. *Fat Flush for Life: The Year-Round Super Detox Plan to Boost Your Metabolism and Keep the Weight Off Permanently*. Cambridge, MA: Da Capo Press, 2010.

———. *The Fat Flush Plan*. New York: McGraw-Hill, 2002.

Kirby, Jane. *Dieting for Dummies*. New York: Wiley, 2004.

PERIODICALS

Callahan, Maureen. "Fat Flush Diet Review." *Health Magazine* (April 2004).

Lewis, Kristyn Kusek. "America's Next Diet Craze." *O: the Oprah Magazine* 7 (August 2006): 127–30.

Michelle, Lynne. "Health: The Fat Flush Diet; Do You Dream of Dropping a Dress Size in as Little as Two Weeks? Do You Want to Burn Fat Faster, Detox Your System and Send Your Energy Levels Sky-High—All in a Fortnight? Well, Here's the Healthy Eating Plan

You've Been Waiting For." *Sunday Mirror* (London) (January 12, 2003): 34.

WEBSITES

"Dr. Ann Louise (official website)."http://annlouise.com (accessed October 2, 2012).

"Fat Flush® (official website)."http://www.fatflush.com (accessed October 2, 2012).

"Fat Flush Diet." EveryDiet.org. http://www.everydiet.org/diet/fat-flush-diet (accessed October 2, 2012).

Margaret Alic, PhD

Fat Loss 4 Idiots diet *see* **Weight Loss 4 Idiots**

Fat replacers

Definition

Fat replacers, also called fat substitutes, are substances that take the place of all or some of the fat in a food and yet give the food a taste, texture, and mouth feel similar to the original full-fat food.

Purpose

Fat replacers serve two purposes. They reduce the amount of fat in food, and they usually reduce the calorie content of the food.

Description

Fat is not a single substance, but a collection of different compounds that are all made of a glycerol molecule and three varying fatty acids. Fat is a necessary part of a healthy diet. It provides essential fatty acids, helps regulate cholesterol **metabolism**, carries fat-soluble **vitamins** and **carotenoids** throughout the body, contains the building blocks for prostaglandins, and provides nine **calories** of energy per gram.

Although there is no official recommended daily allowance (RDA) for fat, the American Heart Association strongly recommends that **fats** provide no more than 30% of one's total daily calories. The average American gets about 34% of his or her calories from fat (down from about 41% in the 1950s).

As of 2000, there were more than 5,000 reduced-fat foods on the market. New reduced- and low-fat foods were being introduced at the rate of about 1,000 per year. Concern about heart disease, **obesity**, diabetes, and their relationship to diet has turned processed foods containing fat replacers into a multi-billion dollar industry.

To be labeled "low fat" a product must contain 3 g of fat or less per serving. To be labeled "reduced fat" or "reduced calorie," a product must contain 25% less fat or 25% fewer calories than the regular version of the product. "Light" foods contain half the fat or one-third the calories of the regular product. "Fat-free" means the food has less than 0.5 g of fat per serving. Fat enhances food flavor, adds volume, and gives food a particular texture and mouth feel. Removing fat from food usually results in unappealing, unmarketable products. To achieve fat and calorie reduction, processors have turned to fat replacers.

Types of fat replacers

Fat replacers are either carbohydrate-based, protein-based, or fat-based. Most foods use several different fat replacers that come from different sources. Many are substances that have been found in foods for years, but are now being used in different ways.

Carbohydrate-based fat substitutes include guar gum, polydextrose (Litesse), gum Arabic, xanthan gum, carrageenan (an extract from seaweed), dried plum paste, modified food starches, oat **fiber**, and wheat fiber. Carbohydrate-based fat replacers have the creaminess of fat. They absorb water, add volume, thicken, and stabilize foods. They are used in baked goods, frozen desserts, yogurts, cheeses, sour cream, low-fat puddings, processed meats, salad dressings, sauces, and spreads. Because fat contains nine calories per gram and **carbohydrates** contain only four calories per gram, every gram of fat replaced with a gram of a carbohydrate-based fat substitute reduces the calorie content of the food by five calories as well as reducing the fat content. Carbohydrate-based fat replacers cannot be used in frying.

Protein-based fat replacers (e.g., Simplesse) are made from milk **protein** and/or egg white protein. These proteins are heated and then whirled violently in blenders to produce very tiny particles in a process called microparticulation. These microparticles give protein-based fat replacers the same mouth feel as fats. Like carbohydrate-based substitutes, protein provides four calories per gram so they reduce the calorie content of food by five calories per gram of fat replaced. Protein-based fat replacers are used in butter, cheese, frozen dairy desserts, mayonnaise, soups, salad dressings, and sour cream. They do not work well in baked goods and cannot be used for frying.

Fat-based fat replacers (e.g., Caprenin, Benefat, Olean) are made of fat molecules that are modified so that they cannot be absorbed (Olean), or can be only partially absorbed (Caprenin, Benefat), in the intestine. Olestra, now marketed under the name Olean, is the best known of these products. Olestra is made of six to eight fatty acids bound to a sucrose (**sugar**) molecule. Normal fats have only three fatty acids. Adding the extra fatty acids makes the olestra molecule too large to be absorbed, so it simply passes through the intestine and is eliminated as waste. In this way, it adds no calories to food. Proctor & Gamble spent 25 years and more than $200 million developing this fat replacement.

Olestra has all the properties of regular fat and can be used in frying. It is used mainly in crunchy snack foods such as potato chips. Other fat-based fat replacers, such as Caprenin and Benefat, are partially absorbed by the body and contain about five calories per gram. Emulsifiers can also be used as fat replacers. They contain the same number of calories per gram as fat, but fewer grams of emulsifier are needed to achieve the same taste, texture, and mouth feel as fat.

Health considerations

All fat replacers on the market are on the generally recognized as safe (GRAS) list approved by the United States Food and Drug Administration (FDA). When olestra was first introduced for use in snack foods in 1996, it was required by the FDA to carry the following warning: "This Product Contains Olestra. Olestra may cause abdominal cramping and loose stools. Olestra inhibits the absorption of some vitamins and other nutrients. Vitamins A, D, E, and K have been added." In 2003, after additional controlled studies and consumer education, the FDA allowed the warning to be removed from olestra-containing foods. The FDA requires small amounts (far less than the RDA) of vitamins A, D, E, and K be added to foods containing olestra. This helps compensate for the small amount of these fat-soluble vitamins that dissolve in olestra and is carried out of the body rather than being absorbed. Other vitamins are not affected.

A diet too high in fat can increase levels of blood lipids and increase risk of plaque build up on the walls of arteries and result in the development of cardiovascular disease. Reducing the amount of fat intake along with other lifestyle changes can help reduce this risk. In addition, obesity increases the risk of developing diabetes and other health problems. Studies have shown reduced-fat foods can be part of an effective weight-loss program that combines a healthy diet, reduced calorie intake, and exercise. The American Heart Association states, "Within the context of a healthy dietary pattern, fat substitutes, when used judiciously, may provide some flexibility in dietary planning, although additional research is needed to fully determine the longer-term health effects."

Precautions

People who have disorders that interfere with the absorption of nutrients from the intestine, such as **celiac disease**, **Crohn's disease**, or **inflammatory bowel disease**, should consider avoiding foods containing olestra.

Fat replacers are often found in high-calorie foods. These foods may contain extra sugar to compensate for the absence of fat. Many reduced-fat products contain as many or almost as many calories as the full-fat equivalent. Consumers concerned about calorie intake should read the label and not assume that reduced-fat implies a reduced-calorie product.

Interactions

Olestra reduces the absorption of the fat-soluble vitamins A, D, E, and K, and carotenoids. Olestra-containing products have extra fat-soluble vitamins, but not carotenoids, added to compensate for this.

Complications

Large amounts of Olestra and the carbohydrate-based fat replacer polydextrose can cause loose stools and diarrhea in some people. Individuals should start with a small amount of foods containing these substances and see how they are affected.

Parental concerns

Reduced-fat foods may appear healthy, but they may contain as many calories and more sugar than the equivalent full-fat product. Parents should encourage their children to eat a healthy diet high in fruits and vegetables and low in fats and not rely on fat substitutes to control fat and calorie intake.

Resources

PERIODICALS

Academy of Nutrition and Dietetics. "Position of the American Dietetic Association: Fat Replacers." *Journal of the American Dietetic Association* 105, no. 2 (2005): 266–75.

Wylie-Rosett, Judith. "Fat Substitutes and Health." *Circulation* 105, no. 23 (June 11, 2002): 2800–2804.

WEBSITES

International Food Information Council Foundation. "Background on Dietary Fats and Fat Replacers." FoodInsight.org. http://www.foodinsight.org/Resources/Detail.aspx?topic=Background_on_Dietary_Fats_and_Fat_Replacers_ (accessed October 2, 2012).

———. "Questions and Answers About Fat Replacers." FoodInsight.org. http://www.foodinsight.org/Resources/Detail.aspx?topic=Questions_and_Answers_About_Fat_Replacers (accessed October 2, 2012).

U.S. Department of Agriculture. "Dietary Fat and Fat Replacers." Snap-ED Connection. http://snap.nal.usda.gov/professional-development-tools/hot-topics-z/dietary-fat-and-fat-replacers (accessed October 2, 2012).

ORGANIZATIONS

Academy of Nutrition and Dietetics, 120 South Riverside Plz., Ste. 2000, Chicago, IL 60606-6995, (312) 899-0040, (800) 877-1600, amacmunn@eatright.org, http://www.eatright.org.

International Food Information Council Foundation, 1100 Connecticut Ave., NW Ste. 430, Washington, DC 20036, (202) 296-6540, info@foodinsight.org, http://www.foodinsight.org.

U.S. Food and Drug Administration, 10903 New Hampshire Ave., Silver Spring, MD 20993-0002, (888) INFO-FDA (463-6332), http://www.fda.gov.

Tish Davidson, A.M.

Fat smash diet

Definition

The fat smash diet is a 90-day, four-phase weight-loss program that is designed to "smash" bad habits and make permanent lifestyle changes in eating and physical activity.

Origins

Dr. Ian Smith, M.D., developed the fat smash diet plan after he became weight-loss consultant and judge for the VH1 hit television program *Celebrity Fit Club.*

The plan was originally designed for celebrities trying to lose weight on the show. Smith's bestselling book, *The Fat Smash Diet: The Last Diet You'll Ever Need,* was published in 2006. In April of 2007 Smith published the *Extreme Fat Smash Diet,* an alternative program for people wanting to lose weight in a short period of time.

Description

Principles

According to Smith, the fat smash diet plan is designed to "rewire" the body and its relationship to food and physical activity. It is based on lifestyle changes that will enable people to maintain their weight once they have achieved their weight-loss goals. The aim of the plan is to eliminate bad habits, while enjoying food without overindulging. The fat smash diet is very flexible and utilizes a wide variety of healthy everyday foods, with the emphasis on **whole grains**, fresh produce, lean meat, fish, poultry, and healthy **fats**. Smith's book includes more than 50 quick and simple recipes. Although the diet does not involve calorie counting, quantities are suggested as a guide for keeping portions small.

The major principles behind the fat smash diet plan are:

- eating 4–5 small meals or large snacks daily, no more than 3–4 hours apart, with the last meal at least one and one-half hours before bedtime
- establishing a regular eating schedule to avoid hunger pangs
- eating small portions—just enough to feel full
- including fresh fruits and vegetables with meals
- eating "good" carbohydrates and avoiding "bad" carbohydrates
- eating foods raw, baked, steamed, or grilled
- a large exercise component, preferably with a partner
- avoidance of stress.

The rules for success on the fat smash diet are:

- not overeating
- always eating fruits and vegetables, regardless of the diet stage
- not eating fried foods
- not skipping meals
- continuing the exercise regimen
- maintaining emotional and mental focus.

Before beginning the fat smash plan dieters are instructed to:

- record their pre-diet weight
- determine their body mass index (BMI)
- take photographs of themselves.

The pyramid

The fat smash diet is constructed as a pyramid, with each of the four phases building on the previous phases:

- Phase 1 is the nine-day detoxification, "detox," stage to rid the body of impurities.
- Phase 2 is the three-week foundation stage.
- Phase 3 is the four-week construction stage.
- Phase 4 is the lifelong temple stage.

The fat smash diet is designed to allow for mistakes. Dieters who overindulge or eat a prohibited food can return to phase 1 for about a week and then pick up the diet at the phase where they left off.

PHASE 1—DETOXIFICATION. The nine-day natural detoxification stage is not a fasting diet. Rather it is a vegetarian diet consisting primarily of fruits and vegetables, with some dairy and egg whites allowed. There are no absolute restrictions on how much to eat. The diet is designed to rid the body of toxins from processed foods and the environment, including the elimination of **caffeine** and alcohol, to make it easier to lose weight. Phase 1 includes 30 minutes of aerobic exercise five times per week, with a suggested 20–25 minute walk after dinner to increase the **metabolism**.

Foods allowed during phase 1 include:

- all fresh fruits in any quantity
- all vegetables in any quantity, except white or red potatoes and avocados; vegetables should be raw or lightly cooked (steamed or grilled)
- one cup daily of fresh-squeezed—not canned—fruit or vegetable juice
- one cup daily of cooked unsweetened oatmeal, grits, farina, or cream of wheat
- up to four egg whites daily
- any dried beans such as lentils or chickpeas
- two cups daily of cooked brown rice
- tofu
- a maximum of two tablespoons per day of tahini (sesame paste)
- two cups daily of low-fat or nonfat milk or soymilk
- 6 oz. (170 g) of low-fat yogurt, maximum of 12 oz. (340 g) daily
- a maximum of two pickles per day
- 1–2 teaspoons of low-fat virgin olive oil for grilling vegetables
- low-fat dressing, no more than three tablespoons per salad
- herbs and spices
- hot-air popcorn without butter or margarine

- a maximum of two tablespoons per day of artificial sweetener
- two cups daily of unsweetened decaffeinated herbal or green tea
- unlimited water.

Foods prohibited during phase 1 include:

- meat
- bread
- cheese, including soy cheese
- fried food
- nuts
- fast food
- desserts
- soda
- coffee
- alcohol.

Canned foods should be rinsed thoroughly to remove excess salt.

Although phase 1 lasts only nine days, dieters can choose to stay with phase 1 for one to two extra weeks or longer.

PHASE 2—THE FOUNDATION. In phase 2 the quantity of food is increased slightly and exercise is increased by 10%–15% over phase 1, to 35 minutes five times per week. Weight lifting and other types of anaerobic exercise are not recommended during phase 2.

Foods added during phase 2 include:

- 3–4 oz. (85–110 g) daily of lean meat, turkey, chicken, or fish (no pork)
- an additional one-half cup of unsweetened hot cereal
- one and one-half cups of unsweetened cold cereal, such as shredded wheat
- one whole egg daily
- 1 oz. (28 g) of cheese
- two teaspoons of peanut butter
- one-half avocado
- up to four teaspoons of sugar or artificial sweetener or one tablespoon of honey per day
- up to two teaspoons of salt per day and unlimited herbs and spices.

PHASE 3—THE CONSTRUCTION. The four-week construction phase requires at least four meals per day. It adds **protein** and whole grains to the diet, allows for larger portions, and continues ample amounts of fruits and vegetables. Exercise levels are increased by another 25% to 45 minutes daily. Smith recommends exercising twice per day several days per week to boost metabolism.

Phase 3 allows:

- up to 5 oz. (140 g) of meat daily, although seafood remains at 3 oz. (85 g)
- two whole eggs daily
- four thin slices of whole-grain bread daily
- additional brown rice
- one cup of whole-wheat pasta
- up to 16 oz. (475 mL) of fresh-squeezed fruit juice
- up to three cups of skim or soymilk daily
- 1.3 oz. (37 g) of low-fat or fat-free cheese daily
- fat-free mayonnaise
- one daily dessert—one scoop of low-fat ice cream or two to three small chocolate-chip or oatmeal-raisin cookies or graham crackers
- two cans of diet soda daily
- 10 oz. (300 mL) of coffee.

Smith recommends that the phase 1 regimen be followed at least one day a week during phase 3 to expedite weight loss. If weight-loss goals have not been reached by the end of phase 3, phases 1–3 can be repeated as many times as necessary.

PHASE 4—THE TEMPLE. Any and all foods are allowed during the maintenance phase 4 including:

- white starches such as potatoes and white rice in limited amounts
- three glasses of wine or beer per week.

Phase 4 includes one hour of moderate to intense exercise, including weight training, five times per week. If weight is regained, the dieter can return to phase 1 for about a week.

Extreme fat smash

Smith's extreme fat smash diet is an alternative to the fat smash diet for people who want to lose weight rapidly by raising their metabolism, with a goal of losing up to 12 lb. (5.4 kg) in the first three weeks. He writes: "Extreme fat smash is for people who are determined to reach what they might've considered unthinkable success in a weight-loss journey. The idea is simple: if you want big results, then you'll have to push yourself beyond the normal limits to attain them."

Like the original fat smash, extreme fat smash utilizes healthy foods and relies on portion control—eating only to satisfy hunger, with the knowledge that another meal or snack will be coming soon. It differs from the fat smash in that it requires organizing the day around meals and exercise:

- The diet is very specific and must be followed exactly.
- Meals and snacks are on a schedule that must be followed exactly.

- Meals are simple but repetitive.
- The diet includes increased fiber and foods with a lower glycemic index (GI) to stabilize blood sugar levels.
- It includes a 40-minute workout with a specific exercise program for conditioning the heart, muscles, and lungs.

The book *Extreme Fat Smash Diet* includes:

- 75 simple recipes for easily prepared meals
- tips and strategies for sticking to the diet
- a newly designed maintenance plan
- meal plans and corresponding journal pages.

The extreme fat smash diet consists of three one-week cycles:

- The first cycle is a very strict diet with a set menu. Some fruits, such as bananas and pineapples, are prohibited.
- The second cycle adds back some fruit, bread, and peanut butter that were not allowed in the first week.
- The third cycle, although still a strict diet, is more flexible.

At the end of the three weeks, the dieter has the option of repeating the three cycles to lose more weight or of entering the maintenance phase. The same cycle cannot be followed for two weeks in a row.

There is an extensive snack food list that includes:

- fruit
- popcorn
- chocolate.

Unlike the original fat smash, the cycles are adjusted for individual body types, dieting profiles, and weight-loss goals of 5 lb. (2.3 kg), 10 lb. (4.5 kg), or 15 lb. (7 kg) and up. For example, an active person who has healthy eating habits but still cannot lose weight should:

- increase the cardiovascular exercise by 10 minutes on some days
- reduce the carbohydrate option by one-half cup on some days
- consume fewer calories.

Function

The fat smash diet is designed to make small but significant adjustments in food consumption and in attitudes toward food and physical activity. It can be followed easily by vegetarians and vegans as well as meat lovers. It is a diet for people who eat too much junk food and are not used to exercising very much;

KEY TERMS

Anaerobic exercise—Brief, strength-based activity, such as sprinting or weight training, in which anaerobic (without oxygen) metabolism occurs in the muscles.

Body mass index—BMI, a measure of body fat determined from the ratio of one's weight in kg to the square of one's height in meters; the BMI from weight in pounds and height in inches is determined from tables; an adult BMI of 25–29.9 is considered overweight and 30 or above indicates obesity.

Detoxification—Detox; cleansing; to remove toxins or poisons from the body.

Fiber—Roughage; a complex mixture found in plant foods that includes the carbohydrates cellulose, hemicellulose, gum, mucilages, and pectins, as well as lignin.

Glycemic index—GI; a measure of the rate at which an ingested carbohydrate raises the glucose level in the blood.

for people who need to lose anywhere from 50–100 lb. (23–46 kg) or more. It is probably too strict a diet for active people with only a few pounds to lose.

The extreme fat smash diet is for people who want to lose 10–25 lb. (4.5–11 kg) in a healthy manner in a short period of time and to maintain the weight loss.

Benefits

The fat smash diet is a healthy, well-balanced, and flexible plan. It is a sustainable diet that allows unlimited fruits and vegetables and relies on regular inexpensive foods. Its calorie control, via portion control, and emphasis on exercise should lead to weight loss. Smith claims that people can lose from 6–10 lb. (3–5 kg) during phase 1. He further claims that the fat smash diet:

• detoxifies the body
• promotes rapid weight loss
• teaches sustainable weight-maintenance skills
• reduces the risk of diet-related disease
• leads to a healthier lifestyle.

Portion control is a key to the fat smash diet and Smith claims that even people who eat unhealthy foods can lose 10–15 lb. (5–7 kg) in a year by practicing portion control—eating smaller meals that still satisfy hunger—without making any other changes.

Precautions

The fat smash diet may be difficult for some people to adhere to, particularly during the nine-day detoxification phase. The weight loss in phase 1 is due to its severe **calorie restriction**. There is little allowance for occasional indulgences. Eating out is almost impossible during phases 1 and 2. The recipes in the book are sometimes inconsistent, with some phase 1 recipes containing prohibited ingredients.

The extreme fat smash may be too extreme and inflexible for many people.

Risks

The fat smash plan is a healthy, well-balanced diet that should have few health risks. The extreme fat smash diet may produce too rapid of a weight loss for some people.

Research and general acceptance

Research

With its emphasis on fruits and vegetables, whole-grain foods, lean meats, portion control, and physical activity, the fat smash diet is considered to be scientifically sound. Tara Gidus of the Academy of Nutrition and Dietetics told *AOL Diet & Fitness*: "It helps people eat more low-calorie, nutrient dense foods, exercise more and get rid of unhealthy habits. I love that it encourages so much aerobic exercise." Although the fat smash detox is relatively moderate, there is no scientific evidence to show a person can detoxify their body through diet.

Most research suggests that slow, gradual, and consistent weight loss is the healthiest way to lose weight and increases the likelihood of maintaining the weight loss.

General acceptance

Although *The Fat Smash Diet* earned mixed reviews among diet critics, Ian Smith enjoys a high degree of credibility among his audience. He is a Harvard-trained medical doctor and on the board of directors of the American Council on Exercise. Before joining the *Celebrity Fit Club*, Smith was medical correspondent for the *Today* show and NBC News. Millions of viewers have watched celebrities lose as much as 41 lb. (19 kg) in a season of *Celebrity Fit Club*. Thus Smith's legions of fans have been accepting of his diet plan.

On April 7, 2007, Dr. Ian, as he is commonly called, launched an ongoing "50 Million Pound Challenge." Aimed primarily at the black community, he called on 5 million people to lose 10 lb. (4.5 kg) each. As of 2012, the program had 1.5 million members and

QUESTIONS TO ASK YOUR DOCTOR

- Is the fat smash diet plan a reasonable approach for me to lose weight?
- How much weight do I need to lose?
- Should I make any adjustments in following the plan?
- Should I take any vitamins or other supplements while on this plan?
- Is the exercise required by the plan suitable for me?
- Is the extreme fat smash diet a healthy option for me?

had achieved a collective weight loss of more than 5 million pounds.

Resources

BOOKS

Smith, Ian. *EAT: The Effortless Weight Loss Solution.* New York: St. Martin's Press, 2011.

————. *Extreme Fat Smash Diet.* New York: St. Martin's Griffin, 2007.

————. *The Fat Smash Diet: The Last Diet You'll Ever Need.* New York: St. Martin's Griffin, 2006.

————. *The Take-Control Diet: A Life Plan for Thinking People.* New York: Ballantine, 2001, 2005.

WEBSITES

"The Diet Channel Interviews VH1's Celebrity Fit Club Diet Expert Dr. Ian Smith, Author of *The Fat Smash Diet.*" The Diet Channel. http://www.thedietchannel.com/VH1-Celebrity-Fit-Club-Diet-Expert-Dr-Ian-Smith-Fat-Smash-Diet-Interview.htm (accessed October 2, 2012).

Ian Smith's official website. http://www.doctoriansmith.com (accessed October 2, 2012).

Jones, H.K. "Fat Smash Diet Review." HealthCastle.com. http://www.healthcastle.com/review_fat_smash_diet.shtml (accessed October 2, 2012).

Margaret Alic, PhD

Fats

Definition

Fats are also known as lipids but are truly a subset of the class of nutrients known as lipids. A lipid is a substance that is poorly soluble or insoluble in water. The term "dietary fat" encompasses many different types of fat. Over 90% of dietary fats are called triacylglycerols or **triglycerides**. Other dietary fats include cholesterol.

Triglycerides contain three fatty acids attached to a glycerol molecule. Fatty acids vary according to their length, which is composed of carbon and hydrogen atoms joined together to form a hydrocarbon chain. The number of double bonds that occur between the carbon molecules also varies. The chemical structure of each type of fatty acid determines its physical characteristics and its nutritional and physiological function. Regardless of the type of fatty acid present, all triacylglycerols provide 9 kcal (37 KJ) per gram (g); this makes fat the most concentrated source of energy in the diet. Fats come in a variety of different forms, from liquid (unsaturated) to solid (saturated) at room temperature.

Purpose

Some types of fatty acids are essential nutrients. They must be consumed in the diet for the body to function properly. Fats form the structure of cell membranes; they are involved in the transport, breakdown, and excretion of cholesterol; and they are the building blocks for many important compounds such as hormones, blood-clotting agents, and compounds involved in immune and inflammatory responses. Fats also transport fat soluble **vitamins** and **antioxidants**; provide the body with insulation and form a protective layer around organs; are a structural component of the brain and nervous system; and provide a reserve supply of energy in the form of adipose tissue (body fat). Excess amounts of adipose tissue defines **obesity** and may lead to health problems such as diabetes, **cancer**, and heart disease. Fats in our diet give food tenderness, aroma, flavor, and palatability. They also help us feel satisfied and full after a meal.

Description

Saturated fatty acids

Saturated fatty acids have a hydrocarbon chain where each carbon atom carries its maximum number of hydrogen atoms except for the end carboxyl group, and they do not have any double bonds, meaning that the fatty acid is carrying the maximum number of hydrogen atoms possible. The molecules are straight, allowing them to pack closely together. For this reason, they are solid at room temperature with a high melting point. Saturated fatty acids are chemically stable both within the body and in food.

Saturated fatty acids are named according to the number of carbon atoms they contain. Each one has a common name (e.g., stearic acid), a systematic name (e.g., octadecanoic acid because stearic acid has 18

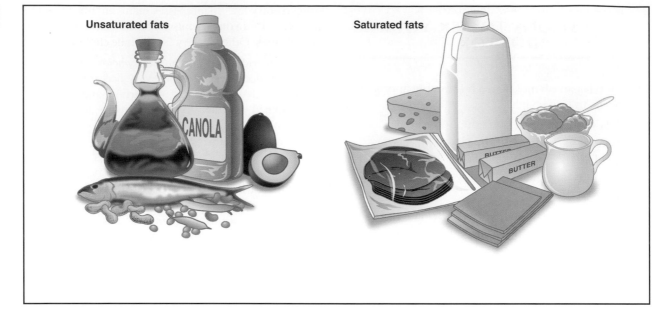

Unsaturated fats

Saturated fats

Unsaturated fats can be divided into polyunsaturated fats, which include cold-water fish, poultry, nuts, seeds, and vegetable and nut oils, and monounsaturated fats, which include olives, avocados, nuts, and beans. Saturated fats mainly come from animal sources of food such as dairy products and meat, as well as grain-based desserts and coconut, palm, and partially hydrogenated oils. *(Illustration by Electronic Illustrators Group. © 2013 Cengage Learning.)*

carbon atoms), and a notational name (e.g., 18:0 as stearic acid has 18 carbon atoms but no double bonds).

Animal products such as meat fat, meat drippings, beef tallow, lard, milk, butter, cheese, and cream are the primary sources of saturated fatty acids. Most plant products have a lower amount of saturated fat, with the exception of coconut, palm kernel, and palm oil.

SATURATED FATTY ACIDS AND HEALTH. Saturated fatty acids increase the body's levels of cholesterol, including low density lipoprotein (LDL) cholesterol. LDL cholesterol is commonly known as "bad" cholesterol. High levels of LDL cholesterol in the blood increase the risk of cardiovascular disease. LDL cholesterol transports excess cholesterol through the bloodstream where it can become deposited in the walls of the arteries and form a hardened plaque. This is called atherosclerosis. This thickening of the artery walls reduces the flow of blood supplying the heart, brain, and other organs. A heart attack or stroke is caused by a blood clot blocking these narrowed arteries. Saturated fatty acids also contribute to production of these blood clots as they are converted into substances that can increase the stickiness of the blood and increase its tendency to clot. For this reason **dietary guidelines** recommend that no more than 10% of dietary energy should come from saturated fatty acids. This means that on a daily basis approximately no more than 22 g of

saturated fat should be consumed by a woman consuming 2,000 **calories** a day, and no more than 28 g of saturated fat should be consumed by a man consuming 2,500 calories a day. A product is considered low in saturated fat if it contains less than 1.5 g per 100 g and high in saturated fat if it contains more than 5 g of fat per 100 g.

Monounsaturated fatty acids

Monounsaturated fatty acids have a hydrocarbon chain that contains one unsaturated carbon bond that is not fully saturated with hydrogen atoms. Instead, it has a double bond to the adjoining carbon atom. Double bonds are either in a *cis* or *trans* formation. In the *cis* formation the hydrogen atoms bonded to the carbon atoms in the double bond are positioned on the same side of the double bond. This creates a kink in the hydrocarbon chain. There is also a free electron or slightly negative charge surrounding the double bond, causing them to repel each other. The molecules are not packed closely together and become liquid (oil) at room temperature. In the *trans* formation the hydrogen atoms are on opposite sides of the carbon-carbon double bond resembling the characteristics of a saturated fatty acid. It should be noted that there is less kinking of the hydrocarbon chain and the fat is more solid at room temperature, and that *trans* bonds are rarely seen in nature.

Monounsaturated fatty acids are named according to the number of carbons they contain and the position of their double bond. Like saturated fatty acids, they each have a common name, a systematic name, and a notational name. Fatty acids with double bonds in the ninth position are sometimes called n-9s or omega-9s.

The most concentrated sources of monounsaturated fatty acids in the diet are olive oil and canola (rapeseed) oil. They are present in many other foods including nuts and seeds, avocados, eggs, fish, and meat fats, especially chicken.

MONOUNSATURATED FATTY ACIDS AND HEALTH. Monounsaturated fatty acids reduce the level of total cholesterol and LDL cholesterol when used in place of saturated fats. They also have a significant effect on increasing and maintaining the body's level of high density lipoprotein (HDL) cholesterol. HDL cholesterol is commonly known as "good" cholesterol because it removes cholesterol from the blood, transferring it to body tissues where it is used to make hormones and other substances the body needs. Therefore, higher levels of HDL cholesterol are associated with a reduction in the risk of cardiovascular disease. Monounsaturated fats are also typically high in **vitamin E**. Between 10%–20% of dietary energy should come from monounsaturated fats.

Polyunsaturated fatty acids

Polyunsaturated fatty acids have a hydrocarbon chain containing two or more double bonds not fully saturated with hydrogen atoms. The double bonds may either be in the *cis* or *trans* formation. The majority of naturally occurring polyunsaturated fats are in the *cis* form. In this form the hydrogen atoms bonded to the carbon atoms in the double bond are positioned on the same side of the double bond. This creates a kink in the hydrocarbon chain. There is also a free electron or slightly negative charge surrounding the double bond causing them to repel each other. The molecules are not packed closely together and become liquid (oil) at room temperature. The presence of one or more double bonds with free electrons and a negative charge makes them unstable molecules ready to react with other chemicals. Polyunsaturated fatty acids are susceptible to chemical changes or oxidation within food leading to cell damage in the body.

Polyunsaturated fatty acids are named just like other fatty acids. They have a common name, a systematic name, and a notational name. Fatty acids with double bonds starting in the sixth position are commonly known as n-6s or omega-6s.

POLYUNSATURATED FATTY ACIDS AND HEALTH. Polyunsaturated fatty acids are divided into two groups, omega-6s and omega-3s. There is one essential fatty acid in each of these groups from which all other fatty acids can be made in the human body. These essential fatty acids cannot be made by the body and must be obtained from the diet. They are a necessary component of the diet; without them deficiency symptoms and poor health would result. Linoleic acid (omega-6) and alpha-linolenic acid (omega-3) are the essential fatty acids. Linoleic acid should provide at least 1% of dietary energy and alpha-linolenic acid should provide 0.2% of dietary energy. These essential fatty acids are converted into longer chain fatty acids that form important substances in the body such as hormones, blood-clotting agents, and compounds involved in immune and inflammatory responses.

These long chain fatty acids are not technically essential, but they have an important role in the body. Examples of long chain fatty acids include arachidonic acid (AA), eicosapentaenoic acid (EPA), and docosahexaenoic acid (DHA). Long chain **omega-3 fatty acids** become essential if there is insufficient linoleic and alpha-linolenic acid available in the diet. These fats play a significant role in development of the brain, nervous system, and retina in fetal development and early life.

OMEGA-6. The most concentrated sources of omega-6 in the diet are vegetable oils, such as sunflower, safflower, corn, cottonseed, canola, and soybean oils. They are also present in plant seeds, nuts, vegetables, fruits, and cereals. In addition to being a source of linoleic acid, omega-6s have been shown to have a lowering effect on both LDL and HDL cholesterol. However, there are health concerns with excessive omega-6 intakes. Omega-6 fats are susceptible to oxidation within the body and may contribute to tissue damage that leads to atherosclerosis and cancer. Omega-6 fats should contribute no more than 10% of dietary energy. Antioxidant nutrients such as vitamin E are required to reduce this oxidation with higher intakes of omega-6 fats. Omega-6s compete with the more beneficial omega-3 fatty acids, so it is recommended that the omega-6:omega-3 ratio is reduced to 4:1.

OMEGA-3. Short chain omega-3 fats are found in **flaxseed** or linseed oil, walnut oil, and canola oil. They are also present in nuts, seeds, and wheat germ, but the best sources of long chain omega-3s are fish and fish oil.

Evidence suggests that consuming long chain omega-3 fats has cardiovascular health benefits. This is believed to be the result of their anti-clotting effect. Growing evidence also suggests that consuming long chain omega-3s has benefits beyond those achieved when consuming shorter chain fatty acids. The United Kingdom's Food Standards Agency recommends that oily fish be consumed at least once a week.

Antioxidant—A chemical that has the ability to neutralize free radicals and prevent damage that would otherwise occur through oxidation.

Atherosclerosis—A thickening of the artery walls that impedes the flow of blood supplying the heart, brain, and other organs.

Bile acids—Produced by the liver, from cholesterol, for the digestion and absorption of fat.

Carboxyl group—The carbon atom at the end of a fatty acid hydrocarbon chain is attached by a double bond to oxygen and by a single bond to hydrogen forming the chemical structure carboxyl.

Cis formation—The arrangement of atoms where hydrogen atoms sit on the same side of the carbon-to-carbon double bond.

Electron—A component of an atom or molecule. It has a negative charge when a free or unpaired electron exists, making it chemically unstable and likely to initiate chemical reactions.

Essential fatty acid—A molecule that cannot be made by the body and must be supplied by food in order to prevent deficiency.

Fatty acid—A molecule consisting of mainly carbon atoms joined together to form a carbon chain to which hydrogen atoms are attached. Fatty acids vary according to their degree of saturation (i.e., the number of hydrogen atoms attached and the length of the hydrocarbon chain).

High density lipoprotein (HDL)—One of several proteins in the blood that transports cholesterol to the liver and away from the arteries.

Hydrogenated—Usually refers to partial hydrogenation of oil, a process where hydrogen is added to oils to reduce the degree of unsaturation. This converts fatty acids from *cis* to *trans* fatty acids.

Omega-3—Polyunsaturated fatty acid where the first double bond occurs on the third carbon-to-carbon double bond from the methyl end of the hydrocarbon chain.

Omega-6—Polyunsaturated fatty acid where the first double bond occurs on the sixth carbon-to-carbon double bond from the methyl end of the hydrocarbon chain.

Omega-9—Polyunsaturated fatty acid where the first double bond occurs on the ninth carbon-to-carbon double bond from the methyl end of the hydrocarbon chain.

Oxidation—A chemical reaction in which electrons are lost from a molecule or atom. In the body these reactions can damage cells, tissues, and deoxyribonucleic acid (DNA), leading to cardiovascular disease or cancer.

Trans fatty acids—Monounsaturated or polyunsaturated fats where the double bonds create a linear formation. They are formed largely by the manufacture of partial hydrogenation of oils, which converts much of the oil into *trans* fat. Hydrogenated fats and *trans* fats are often used interchangeably.

There has been much interest in the effect of EPA and DHA deficiency and supplementation on behavior in children, particularly those with learning difficulties. Although there is some evidence of benefit with EPA, in 2006 the UK Food Standards Agency concluded that there was insufficient evidence to reach a firm conclusion and additional clinical trials were needed.

There is also interest in the anti-inflammatory properties of long chain omega-3s in inflammatory conditions such as **Crohn's disease** and rheumatoid arthritis. The role of omega-3s has been evaluated in treatment of depression and prevention of cognitive decline, but more research is needed to confirm these benefits.

Omega-3 fats have been shown to reduce blood pressure and triglyceride levels (another fat in the blood that contributes to raising the risk of cardiovascular disease). To achieve these benefits, omega-3s must be taken in pharmacological doses and there are small risks associated with these high doses such as

raised LDL cholesterol, poor control of diabetes, and increased risk of bleeding. Large doses of omega-3s should only be taken under the supervision of a qualified medical doctor.

Trans fatty acids

Trans fatty acids are monounsaturated or polyunsaturated fatty acids where the double bond is in the *trans* rather than *cis* formation. They occur naturally in small amounts in lamb, beef, milk, and cheese as they are created in the rumen of cows and sheep. The majority of *trans* fat in the diet comes from the partial hydrogenation of vegetable oils. This is a process in food manufacture that adds hydrogen atoms to unsaturated fatty acids so that oils become more hardened at room temperature. The process results in some of the double bonds of the fatty acid molecules becoming saturated and some of the remaining double bonds changing from a *cis* to a *trans* formation; for example, when partially hydrogenated oleic acid becomes elaidic acid or 9 *trans*-octadecenoic acid. ***Trans* fats** are semi-solid at room temperature and more stable within food. Partial hydrogenation of oils has traditionally been used to develop spreading fats and margarines, for fast food, and in cakes and biscuits. Manufacturers are using it less because of the health problems associated with it. In 2006, New York City adopted the United States' first major ban on all but trace amounts of artificial *trans* fats in restaurant cooking. As of July 2008, a serving of food must not contain more than half a gram of *trans* fat. Food legislation in the United States and the European Union states that hydrogenated or partially hydrogenated fats must be labeled in the ingredients of food and in some cases the amounts of *trans* fat must also be labeled.

TRANS FATTY ACIDS AND HEALTH. *Trans* fat raises LDL cholesterol in a similar way to saturated fat and it reduces HDL cholesterol. It may also raise blood triglyceride levels. The combination of both of these effects means that it is likely to increase cardiovascular risk. The World Health Organization recommends phasing out *trans* fat in food manufacturing and reducing *trans* fat consumption to no more than 1% of dietary energy or 2.5 g per day.

Cholesterol

Cholesterol is essential to the structure of cell membranes and production of bile acids for digestion, steroid hormones, and **vitamin D**. **Dietary cholesterol** has little effect on blood cholesterol levels because an increased dietary intake reduces the amount the body produces. Only extreme dietary levels of cholesterol need to be restricted. For most individuals, dietary measures that reduce saturated fat also avoid excessive cholesterol consumption. However, individuals with familial hypercholesterolemia may need to consume less than 300 milligrams (mg) per day, which requires avoidance of most animal products.

The most concentrated dietary sources of cholesterol include liver (foie gras), egg yolks and products made from egg yolk, caviar (fish roes), butter, and shrimp.

Recommended intake

U.S. and international (World Health Organization/Food and Agriculture Organization [WHO/FAO]) recommendations for fat intake are similar. Fatty acids should provide no more than 30%–35% of total calories, which equates to approximately no more than 70 g/day for adult women and no more than 90 g/day for adult men. Amounts for children are slightly higher, starting at 40%–60% for infants up to six months and then

gradually tapering off to 25%–35% by age two. Saturated fats should comprise no more than 10% of total energy intake in adults and 8% in children. Cholesterol intake should be less than 300 mg per day. A person should not drop his or her fat intake to less than 15% of calories unless prescribed by a medical professional and with guidance from a registered dietitian. People should also not increase fat intake to more than 35% unless being monitored by a doctor.

Typical high sources of fat in the diet include cooking fats and oils, fried food, fatty and processed meats, cheeses and whole-fat dairy products. These should form a small part of the diet. Care should be taken to reduce fried foods; avoid adding fats and oils during cooking; to grill food, which allows fat to drip out; and to choose lean meats and low fat dairy products. A product is considered to be low in fat if it contains less than 3 g fat per 100 g and high in fat if it contains more than 20 g fat per 100 g or 21 g fat per serving.

Precautions

The guidelines for the recommended levels of dietary fat are not appropriate for people under two years of age, who are ill or malnourished, or who have been diagnosed with a medical condition that requires higher or lower intake of dietary fat.

Parental concerns

A study conducted by the International Study of Asthma and Allergies in Childhood (ISAAC) found a strong correlation between *trans* fatty acids and increased occurrence of allergies in adolescents. Parents should provide healthy alternatives to foods containing fatty acids and monitor the amount and type of fats consumed in the diets of their children. These preventative measures may help avoid serious health problems, including heart disease and stroke, which can result from high levels of fatty acids in the diet.

Resources

BOOKS

Betteridge, John. *Hyperlipidaemia*. Oxford: Cardiology Library, 2012.

Lawrence, Glen D. *The Fats of Life*. Rutgers University Press, 2010.

PERIODICALS

Alcock, Joe, Melissa L. Franklin, and Christopher W. Kuzawa. "Nutrient Signaling: Evolutionary Origins of the Immune-Modulating Effects of Dietary Fat." *The Quarterly Review of Biology* 87, no. 3 (September 2012).

Chavarro, Jorge E., Janet W. Rich-Edwards, Bernard A. Rosner, and Walter C. Willett. "Recommended Dietary Reference Intakes, Nutritional Goals and Dietary Guidelines For Fat and Fatty Acids: A Systematic Review." *The British Journal of Nutrition* 107, suppl. 2 (June 2012): S8–S22.

de Oliveira Otto, Marcia C., D. Mozaffarian, D. Kromhout, et al. "Dietary Intake of Saturated Fat by Food Source and Incident Cardiovascular Disease: The Multi-Ethnic Study of Atherosclerosis." *American Journal of Clinical Nutrition* 96, no. 2 (2012): 397–404.

Mead, A., G. Atkinson, D. Albin, et al. "Dietetic Guidelines on Food and Nutrition in the Secondary Prevention of Cardiovascular Disease—Evidence from Systematic Reviews of Randomized Controlled Trials." *Journal of Human Nutrition and Dietetics* 19 (January 2007): 401–9.

Mozaffarian, D., et al. "Trans Fatty Acids and Cardiovascular Disease." *The New England Journal of Medicine* 354, no. 15 (2006): 1601–13.

OTHER

Food and Agriculture Organization of the United Nations. *Fats and Fatty Acids in Human Nutrition: Report of an Expert Consultation* 91 (2010). http://foris.fao.org/preview/25553-0ece4cb94ac52f9a25af77ca5cfba7a8c.pdf (accessed September 7, 2012).

WEBSITES

American Heart Association. "Fish and Omega-3 Fatty Acids." http://www.heart.org/HEARTORG/Getting Healthy/NutritionCenter/HealthyDietGoals/Fish-and-Omega-3-Fatty-Acids_UCM_303248_Article.jsp (accessed September 7, 2012).

Food and Drug Administration. "Guidance for Industry: *Trans* Fatty Acids in Nutrition Labeling, Nutrient Content Claims, Health Claims; Small Entity Compliance Guide." United States Department of Health and Human Services. http://www.fda.gov/Food/Guidance ComplianceRegulatoryInformation/Guidance Documents/FoodLabelingNutrition/ucm053479.htm (accessed September 7, 2012).

Higdon, Jane. "Essential Fatty Acids." *Micronutrient Information Center*. Linus Pauling Institute, Oregon State University. http://lpi.oregonstate.edu/infocenter/othernuts/omega3fa/ (accessed September 7, 2012).

Larsen, Joanne. "Fatty Acids." *Ask the Dietitian*. http://www.dietitian.com/fattyaci.html (accessed September 7, 2012).

ORGANIZATIONS

Academy of Nutrition and Dietetics, 120 South Riverside Plz., Ste. 2000, Chicago, IL 60606-6995, (312) 899-0040, (800) 877-1600, amacmunn@eatright.org, http://www. eatright.org.

American Heart Association, 7272 Greenville Ave., Dallas, TX 75231, (800) 242-8721, http://www.americanheart.org.

British Heart Foundation, Greater London House, 180 Hampstead Road, London, United Kingdom NW1 7AW, +44 020 7554 0000, http://www.bhf.org.uk.

British Nutrition Foundation, High Holborn House, 52-54 High Holborn, London, United Kingdom WC1V 6RQ, 44 20 7404 6504, Fax: 44 20 7404 6747, postbox@nutrition.org.uk, http://www.nutrition.org.uk.

Deborah Lycett, BSc(Hons) RD MBDA
Megan Porter, RD

Feingold diet *see* **Dr. Feingold diet**

Fen-Phen

Definition

Fen-Phen was an anti-obesity regimen composed of fenfluramine or the closely related drug dexfenfluramine (marketed under the brand name Redux) and phentermine (sold under several brand names including Adipex-P, Anoxine-AM, Fastin, Ionamin, Obephen, Obermine, Obestin-30 and Phentrol). The combination was found to cause damage to heart valves, and fenfluramine and dexfenfluramine were removed from the United States market in 1997.

Purpose

The combination of these two drugs had been reported to be significantly more effective than placebo in promoting weight loss when used in combination with diet, exercise and behavior modification.

Description

Phentermine was first approved for use by the United States Food & Drug Administration (FDA) in 1959. Its claimed advantage over other appetite suppressants available at the time was a reduced risk of abuse. While the drug was chemically related to the amphetamines, with the same side effects, the incidence of these side effects was reportedly lower than with the amphetamines.

Fenfluramine was approved by the FDA in 1973 and dexfenfluramine (Redux) was approved for use in 1996. Fenfluramine is the racemic form of dexfenfluramine. The drugs were approved for short term use as part of a program of diet and exercise. Although fenfluramine is chemically related to the amphetamines, its action appears to be based on increasing levels of *serotonin* in the brain and bloodstream. Dexfenfluramine had been marketed in Europe for over a decade without detection of an association between dexfenfluramine and heart valve problems; however, the FDA noted that the number of patients having heart valve problems was very low compared to the total number of patients using the drug, and heart valve screening is not a routine part of drug monitoring.

Neither fenfluramine nor phentermine had been approved for use in long term treatment or combination therapy. The drugs were indicated only as short term adjuncts in patients with **obesity**.

In 1992, a research group from the University of Rochester published reports indicating that the combination of fenfluramine and phentermine might be a valuable adjunct to diet and exercise in a controlled program of weight loss. A total of 121 patients were initially enrolled in the study, and 9 dropped out during the active study period. After the first 34 weeks of the study, patients on the fen-phen regimen had lost an average of 31 lb. (14.2 kg), compared with an 11 lb. (4.9 kg) weight loss in the placebo control group. The researchers noted that upon discontinuation of the drugs, patients regained most of the weight lost during the study, and after 210 weeks, the average weight loss was only 3 lb. (1.4 kg) below the baseline. Patients who had received active drug tended to regain weight more rapidly than those who received placebo. The authors concluded that despite long periods of time at weights much lower than baseline, permanent resetting of weight control mechanisms could not be shown for most participants.

In spite of the disappointing long-term results, these reports led to the wide use of the fen-phen regimen for people attempting to lose weight. In 1996, fenfluramine was the 46th most frequently prescribed drug in the United States, with sales of $176 million per year (roughly $209 million in 2006 dollars). No long-term studies were performed for these drugs, and they were never approved for use in combination therapy.

On July 8, 1997, *The New England Journal of Medicine* published a report from the Mayo Clinic describing 24 cases of *regurgitational valvular heart disease* in women who had been treated with fenfluramine and phentermine. By September 30, the FDA had received a total of 144 reports of heart value problems associated with fenfluramine, with or without phentermine.

On November 19, 1997, the Centers for Communicable Disease Control published a review of the cases of heart valve damage associated with fenfluramine:

… Of these 113 cases, 111 (98%) occurred among women; the median age of case-patients was 44 years (range: 22 68 years). Of these 113 cases, two (2%) used fenfluramine alone; 16 (14%), dexfenfluramine alone; 89 (79%), a combination of fenfluramine and phentermine; and six (5%), a combination of all three drugs. None of the cases used phentermine alone. The median duration of drug use was 9 months (range: 1 39 months). Overall, 87 (77%) of the 113 cases were symptomatic. A total of 27 (24%) case-patients required cardiac valve-replacement surgery; of these, three patients died after surgery….

The Food & Drug Administration removed fenfluramine from the market. Approximately 18,000 people sued American Home Products, which had marketed the drug, to recover damages, either from the costs of actual injuries, or the cost of tests to determine whether any damage had been done. In a class action lawsuit, American Home Products agreed to establish a trust fund with a reported value of $3.75 billion, with the money to be distributed among victims of the drug, depending on extent of injury. People exposed to fenfluramine must be monitored for heart valve problems for a period of 20 years.

Although fen-phen has been associated with another very important adverse effect, *primary pulmonary hypertension*, the focus of all regulatory and legal problems has been on the heart valve problems associated with the drug.

Precautions

Phentermine hydrochloride tablets and capsules are indicated only as short-term monotherapy for the management of exogenous obesity. The safety and efficacy of combination therapy with phentermine and any other drug products for weight loss, including selective serotonin reuptake inhibitors (e.g., fluoxetine, sertraline, fluvoxamine, paroxetine), have not been established. Therefore, coadministration of these drug products for weight loss is not recommended.

KEY TERMS

Anorectic—A drug that suppresses the appetite.

Dexfenfluramine—An anorectic drug formerly marketed under the brand name Redux.

Etiology—The cause of a disease or medical condition.

Fenfluramine—An anorectic drug formerly marketed under the brand name Pondimin.

Fluoxetine—An antidepressant drug, sold under the brand name Prozac.

Fluvoxamine—An antidepressant drug sold under the brand name Luvox.

Indicated—In medical terminology, reviewed and approved by the United States Food & Drug Administration, or the comparable agency in other nations, for a specific use.

Monoamine oxidase inhibitor—A class of antidepressant drugs that act by blocking an enzyme that destroys some of the hormones in the brain. These drugs have a large number of food and drug interactions.

Mitral valve—A heart valve, also called the bicuspid valve, that allows blood to flow from the left auricle to the ventricle, but does not allow the blood to flow backwards.

Paroxetine—An antidepressant drug sold under the brand name Paxil.

Phentermine—An anorectic drug sold under a large number of brand names.

Primary pulmonary hypertension—Abnormally high blood pressure in the arteries of the lungs, with no other heart disease causing this problem.

Racemic—A chemical term, relating to the way a compound turns a beam of light. Racemic compounds are composed of equal amounts of left-turning and right-turning molecules. Molecules that turn a beam of light to the right are *dextrorotatory*, while those that turn a beam to the left are *levorotatory*.

Regurgitational valvular heart disease—A type of damage to the heart valves which allows blood to leak back through the valve.

Serotonin—A hormone that stimulates brain cells and also causes blood vessels to constrict.

Sertraline—An antidepressant drug sold under the brand name Zoloft.

Serious regurgitant cardiac valvular disease, primarily affecting the mitral, aortic and tricuspid valves, has been reported in otherwise healthy people who had taken a combination of phentermine with fenfluramine or dexfenfluramine for weight loss. The etiology of these valvulopathies has not been established and their course in individuals after the drugs are stopped is not known. The possibility of an association between valvular heart disease and the use of phentermine alone cannot be ruled out; there have been rare cases of valvular heart disease in patients who reportedly have taken phentermine alone.

Tolerance to the anorectic effect usually develops within a few weeks. When this occurs, the recommended dose should not be exceeded in an attempt to increase the effect; rather, the drug should be discontinued.

Interactions

Phentermine hydrochloride may decrease the hypotensive effect of guanethidine.

Monoamine oxidase inhibitors (MAOIs) may increase the pressor response to the anorexiants. Possible hypertensive crisis and intracranial hemorrhage may occur. This interaction may also occur with furazolidone, an antimicrobial with MAOI activity. Avoid combining with phentermine hydrochloride. There should be a 14-day interval between use of any MAOI and phentermine.

Aftercare

For those patients who had been exposed to fenfluramine, aftercare depends on the extent of damage. For those patients with significant heart valve damage, surgical valve replacement may be in order. Those who received the drug but show no damage should be monitored by a cardiologist for the possibility of late onset damage.

Although phentermine alone has been associated with rare instances of valvular heart disease, there are no recommendations for routine aftercare or monitoring.

Resources

PERIODICALS

Connolly, H.M., et al. "Valvular Heart Disease Associated with Fenfluraminephentermine." *New England Journal of Medicine* 337 (December 1997): 581–87.

Weintraub, M., et al. "Long-Term Weight Control Study. II (Weeks 34 to 104). An Open-Label Study of Continuous Fenfluramine Plus Phentermine Versus Targeted Intermittent Medication As Adjuncts to Behavior Modification, Caloric Restriction, and Exercise." *Clinical Pharmacology and Therapeutics* 51, no. 5 (1992): 595–601.

————. "Long-Term Weight Control Study V (Weeks 190 to 210). Follow-Up of Participants after Cessation of Medication." *Clinical Pharmacology and Therapeutics* 51, no. 5 (1992): 615–18.

WEBSITES

Cohen, Katie. "Fen-Phen Nation." PBS *Frontline*, November 13, 2003. http://www.pbs.org/wgbh/pages/frontline/shows/prescription/hazard/fenphen.html (accessed October 2, 2012).

U.S. Food and Drug Administration. "Fen-Phen Safety Update Information."http://www.fda.gov/Drugs/Drug Safety/PostmarketDrugSafetyInformationforPatients andProviders/ucm072820.htm (accessed October 2, 2012).

ORGANIZATIONS

U.S. Food and Drug Administration, 10903 New Hampshire Ave., Silver Spring, MD 20993-0002, (888) INFO-FDA (463-6332), http://www.fda.gov.

Sam Uretsky, PharmD

Fiber

Definition

Dietary fiber is the collective name for a group of indigestible carbohydrate-based compounds found in plants. They are the materials that give the plant rigidity and structure. Two types of fiber are important to human health: insoluble fiber and soluble fiber.

Purpose

Fiber helps move food waste through the digestive system, preventing **constipation** and supporting bowel health. Fiber and high-fiber diets are also associated with a myriad of other health benefits:

- High-fiber diets may assist with weight management because they tend to be satisfying without being calorie dense.
- Soluble fiber has been shown to help lower blood cholesterol by binding to cholesterol molecules in the digestive tract, thus encouraging their elimination from the body.
- High consumption of fiber-rich whole grains is associated with a lower risk of developing type 2 diabetes.

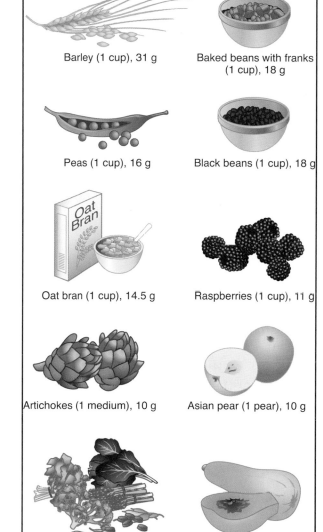

Barley (1 cup), 31 g

Baked beans with franks (1 cup), 18 g

Peas (1 cup), 16 g

Black beans (1 cup), 18 g

Oat bran (1 cup), 14.5 g

Raspberries (1 cup), 11 g

Artichokes (1 medium), 10 g

Asian pear (1 pear), 10 g

Mixed vegetables (1 cup), 8 g

Squash (1 cup), 6 g

Sources of fiber. *(Illustration by Electronic Illustrators Group. © 2013 Cengage Learning.)*

- Soluble fiber slows the emptying of food from the stomach to the small intestine, thus causing a gradual release of glucose into the bloodstream after a meal; this may promote better blood sugar management in people with diabetes.
- A low-fat, high-fiber diet combined with daily exercise appears to be associated with a reduced risk of developing breast cancer.
- Studies investigating whether a high-fiber diet is protective against colon cancer are inconclusive, but those that support the protective effect of fiber

Fiber

Age	Recommended intakes (g/day)
Children 1< yr.	Not established
Children 1–3 yrs.	19
Children 4–8 yrs.	25
Boys 9–13 yrs.	31
Girls 9–13 yrs.	26
Boys 14–18 yrs.	38
Girls 14–18 yrs.	26
Men 19–50 yrs.	38
Women 19–50 yrs.	25
Men 50< yrs.	30
Women 50< yrs.	21
Pregnant women	28
Breastfeeding women	29

SOURCE: U.S. Department of Agriculture (USDA) Food and Nutrition Information Center.

(Table by PreMediaGlobal. © 2013 Cengage Learning.)

suggest that fiber encourages the movement of food waste through the bowel, possibly reducing the body's exposure to carcinogens in the waste products.

• High-fiber foods tend to be rich in phytochemicals, which have been linked to cancer protection.

• High-fiber diets that are comprised of large amounts of fruits, vegetables, and whole grains are associated with better blood pressure control.

Many large, well-designed, long-term studies have been done on the health effects of a diet high in fiber. The almost universally accepted result is that health benefits result when individuals meet or exceed the **dietary reference intakes (DRIs)** for fiber for their age group. This concept is so well accepted that it has become the official position of the National Institutes of Health and other U.S. government agencies charged with improving the health of the nation. Increased fiber intake was included in the government-promoted goals for Healthy People 2010.

Description

Fiber is found only in foods of plant origin. It occurs in the skins, seeds, leaves, and roots of fruits and vegetables, and in the germ and bran layers of grains. Pectins, lignans, cellulose, gums, and mucilages are all different forms of fiber found in plant foods. Humans lack the digestive enzymes to break down fiber, and so it passes through the digestive tract largely unchanged.

Because insoluble dietary fiber is not digested, it does not provide energy (**calories**). Instead, fiber adds bulk to the waste (stool or feces) in the large intestine

(colon). Increased bulk causes the walls of the intestine to contract rhythmically (peristalsis) so that waste moves through the large intestine more rapidly. In the colon, most of the water in digested food is reabsorbed into the body, and then the solid waste is eliminated. By passing through the colon more rapidly, less water is reabsorbed from the waste. The stool remains soft and moist, and is easy to expel without straining.

Good sources of insoluble fiber include:

• whole grains and foods made of whole grains, such as whole wheat bread and whole wheat pasta, couscous, or bulgur

• bran and bran breakfast cereals

• brown rice

• carrots, cucumbers, and other raw vegetables

Soluble fiber is found dissolved in water inside plant cells. Like insoluble fiber, it is not digested and does not provide energy, although it may be consumed by bacteria that live in the digestive tract. In water, soluble fiber forms a gel-like substance. This gel absorbs water and helps to keep the stool soft. Good sources of insoluble fiber include:

• oatmeal and foods made with oats

• foods such as chili or split pea soup that contain dried beans and peas

• lentils

• apples

• pears

• citrus fruits

Foods rich in soluble fiber often are recommended to help improve blood glucose and cholesterol levels, while diets containing high amounts of insoluble fiber contribute to bowel regularity and may help prevent diverticular disease. Since high-fiber diets tend to be satisfying but relatively low in calories, they are often promoted for weight management.

Because fiber is so important in the diet, the amount of fiber in canned goods, frozen foods, and other processed foods sold commercially in the United States must be shown on the label. A food that is labeled "high in fiber" contains 5 or more grams of fiber per serving. As of 2012, manufacturers were required to show only the total amount fiber in each serving of food.

Recommended dosage

The average American consumes only 14 grams of fiber each day, despite extensive research that shows that higher levels of fiber provide increased health benefits.

The U.S. Institute of Medicine (IOM) of the National Academy of Sciences has set **DRIs** for fiber based on research data that applies to American and Canadian populations. DRIs provide nutrition guidance to both health professionals and consumers. The current daily DRIs for fiber are as follows:

• children ages 1–3: 19 grams
• children ages 4–8: 25 grams
• men ages 14–50: 38 grams
• men age 51 and older: 30 grams
• girls ages 9–18: 26 grams
• adult women ages 19–50: 25 grams
• women age 51 and older: 21 grams
• pregnant women: 28 grams
• breastfeeding women: 29 grams

Precautions

Fiber should be increased in the diet gradually. If fiber intake increases suddenly, abdominal pain, gas, and diarrhea may result. Also, when eating a **high-fiber diet**, it is important to drink at least eight glasses (64 ounces or 2 liters) of water or other fluids daily. People whose fluid intake must be restricted for medical reasons should avoid a high-fiber diet.

Interactions

Fiber supplements such as psyllium may reduce the absorption of certain medications when taken at the same time. In general, medications should be taken at least one hour before or two hours after fiber supplements.

QUESTIONS TO ASK YOUR DOCTOR

• How much fiber do I need?
• Is it safe to increase the amount of fiber I eat when I am pregnant?
• Am I taking any medications or do I have any medical conditions that conflict with eating a high-fiber diet?

Complications

Fiber and high-fiber diets have traditionally been thought to help prevent diverticulosis, a disease of the large intestine, but a study published in the February 2012 issue of *Gastroenterology* challenged this notion. Doctors previously believed that diverticula formed as a result of chronic constipation, but participants in the study were found to be less likely to develop diverticulosis when eating diets lower in fiber. While researchers will need to revisit the question of how and why diverticula are formed, the study does not undermine the overall importance of fiber in the diet.

Resources

BOOKS

Logue, Dick. *500 High Fiber Recipes: Fight Diabetes, High Cholesterol, High Blood Pressure, and Irritable Bowel Syndrome with Delicious Meals That Fill You Up and Help You Shed Pounds!* Beverly, MA: Fair Winds Press, 2009.

Shirk, Lynette Rhorer. *The Everything Whole Grain, High Fiber Cookbook: Delicious, Heart-Healthy Snacks and Meals the Whole Family Will Love.* Avon, MA: Adams Media, 2008.

PERIODICALS

Anderson, James W., et al. "Health Benefits of Dietary Fiber." *Nutrition Reviews* 67, no. 4 (2009): 188–205. http://dx.doi.org/10.1111/j.1753-4887.2009.00189.x (accessed September 5, 2012).

Strate, Lisa L. "Diverticulosis and Dietary Fiber: Rethinking the Relationship." *Gastroenterology* 142, no. 2 (2012): 205–7.

Tjønneland, Anne, and Anja Olsen. "Fibre and Prevention of Chronic Diseases." *British Medical Journal* 343 (November 2011). http://dx.doi.org/10.1136/bmj.d6938 (accessed September 5, 2012).

OTHER

American Institute for Cancer Research. *The Facts about Fiber.* Washington, DC: AICR. http://www.aicr.org/assets/docs/pdf/brochures/facts-about-fiber.pdf (accessed September 5, 2012).

WEBSITES

American Heart Association. "Whole Grains and Fiber." http://www.heart.org/HEARTORG/GettingHealthy/NutritionCenter/HealthyDietGoals/Whole-Grains-and-Fiber_UCM_303249_Article.jsp (accessed September 5, 2012).

Harvard School of Public Health. "Fiber: Start Roughing It!" *The Nutrition Source*, Department of Nutrition, Harvard University. http://www.hsph.harvard.edu/nutritionsource/what-should-you-eat/fiber/index.html (accessed September 5, 2012).

Mayo Clinic staff. "Dietary Fiber: Essential for a Healthy Diet." MayoClinic.com. November 19, 2009. http://www.mayoclinic.com/health/fiber/NU00033 (accessed September 5, 2012).

MedlinePlus. "Dietary Fiber." U.S. National Library of Medicine, National Institutes of Health. http://www.nlm.nih.gov/medlineplus/dietaryfiber.html (accessed September 5, 2012).

ORGANIZATIONS

Academy of Nutrition and Dietetics, 120 South Riverside Plz., Ste. 2000, Chicago, IL 60606-6995, (312) 899-0040, (800) 877-1600, amacmunn@eatright.org, http://www.eatright.org.

American College of Gastroenterology (ACG), 6400 Goldsboro Rd., Ste. 450, Bethesda, MD 20817, (301) 263-9000, info@acg.gi.org, http://www.acg.gi.org.

American Gastroenterological Association (AGA), 4930 Del Ray Ave., Bethesda, MD 20814, (301) 654-2055, Fax: (301) 654-5920, http://www.gastro.org.

National Digestive Diseases Information Clearinghouse (NDDIC), 2 Information Way, Bethesda, MD 20892-3570, (800) 891-5389, TTY: (866) 569-1162, Fax: (703) 738-4929, info@niddk.nih.gov, http://digestive.niddk.nih.gov.

Marie Fortin, MEd, RD
Tish Davidson, AM

Fit for Life diet

Definition

Fit for Life is a combination diet that emphasizes eating foods in the correct combination and avoiding the wrong combinations of foods rather than counting **calories** or controlling portion size. Several aspects of this diet have been disputed by dietitians.

Origins

Fit for Life is the creation of Harvey and Marilyn Diamond. The diet first came to the attention of the public in the mid-1980s with the publication of the book *Fit for Life*, which has sold millions of copies. On the official Fit for Life website, Diamond claims that the diet "spawned juice and salad bars, fruit sellers on the streets of New York, and the juice industry." He also claims the book "launched a nutritional awakening in the United States and other Western countries." These are impressive claims for a book written by a man whose "doctoral degree" came from the American College of Life Science, a non-accredited correspondence school founded in 1982 by a high school dropout.

Diamond has appeared on dozens of television talk shows explaining his theories on how eating foods in the correct combination and avoiding the "wrong" combinations of food can bring about weight loss without calorie counting or exercise. In the 2000s, the Fit for Life system added the Personalized FFL Weight Management Program. This program uses what they call Biochemical Analyzation, Metabolic Typing and Genetic Predispositions to individualize and personalize the dietary protocols. The resulting diet is said to be effective only for one specific individual and can be used for that person's entire life. Diamond has also begun selling nutritional supplements, many of which are strongly recommended in his newest version of the Fit for Life system.

Description

Fit for Life is a food combining diet based on the theory that to lose weight, one must not eat certain foods together. The philosophy behind the diet comes from Diamond's interest in natural hygiene, an offshoot of naturopathic medicine. In his original book, Diamond claimed that if a person ate foods in the wrong combination, they would "rot" in the stomach. He also categorized foods as "dead foods" that "clog" the body and "living foods" that cleanse the body. The newest version of Fit for Life talks less about rotting, dead, and living foods and more about "enzyme deficient foods." However, the general message about food combining is the same.

According to Diamond, dead foods are meats and starches. Living foods are raw fruits and vegetables. His diet plan requires that these foods not be eaten together. Some of the Fitness for Life rules include:

- Only fruit and fruit juice should be eaten from the time one awakes until noon. Fruits cleanse the body.
- Fruits are good for health only if they are eaten alone. They should never be eaten with any other food.
- Lunch and dinner can consist of either carbohydrates and vegetables or proteins and vegetables.
- Carbohydrates and proteins should never be put in the stomach at the same time.
- No dairy foods should ever be eaten.

KEY TERMS

Alternative medicine—A system of healing that rejects conventional, pharmaceutical-based medicine and replaces it with the use of dietary supplements and therapies such as herbs, vitamins, minerals, massage, and cleansing diets. Alternative medicine includes well-established treatment systems such as homeopathy, Traditional Chinese Medicine, and Ayurvedic medicine, as well as more recent, fad-driven treatments.

Cholesterol—A waxy substance made by the liver and also acquired through diet. High levels in the blood may increase the risk of cardiovascular disease.

Conventional medicine—Mainstream or Western pharmaceutical-based medicine practiced by medical doctors, doctors of osteopathy, and other licensed health care professionals.

Dietary fiber—Also known as roughage or bulk. Insoluble fiber moves through the digestive system almost undigested and gives bulk to stools. Soluble fiber dissolves in water and helps keep stools soft.

Dietary supplement—A product, such as a vitamin, mineral, herb, amino acid, or enzyme, that is intended to be consumed in addition to an individual's diet with the expectation that it will improve health.

Enzyme—A protein that changes the rate of a chemical reaction within the body without being depleted in the reaction.

Mineral—An inorganic substance found in the earth that is necessary in small quantities for the body to maintain health. Examples: zinc, copper, iron.

Naturopathic medicine—An alternative system of healing that primarily uses homeopathy, herbal medicine, and hydrotherapy and rejects most conventional drugs as toxic.

Vitamin—A nutrient that the body needs in small amounts to remain healthy but that the body cannot manufacture for itself and must acquire through diet.

- Water should never be drunk at meals.
- One day each week (the same day every week) is a free day, when the individual can eat whatever he or she wants.

Function

The goal of the Fit for Life diet is to help people lose weight and keep their body healthy through diet. Diamond states that people do not gain weight because they eat too many calories and exercise too little. Instead, he considers the cause of weight gain to be eating protein-rich foods at the same time as carbohydrate-rich foods. He argues that enzymes that digest proteins interfere with enzymes that digest **carbohydrates**, and therefore, these two foods should not be eaten together. His program makes little mention of the role of different types of fats—saturated, unsaturated, and *trans* fat—in diet, dietary **fiber**, the role of water in health, or of the need to exercise.

The Fit for Life program says it is a lifestyle program that will teach people to be healthier. Along with the personalized diet program, dieters get a "Clinical Manual" that claims to teach them how their body works, what is healthy for them, and what is not. The program is heavily infused with an alternative medicine approach to health and diet, and many of the explanations it gives for the way the body works are scientifically questionable and not accepted by practitioners of conventional medicine.

Benefits

The benefits claimed by Fit for Life are not supported by any scholarly research and are, in fact, refuted by some research (see below). The main claim, supported by testimonials and before and after pictures, is that people who follow Fit for Life will lose weight and keep it off. Along with weight loss will come a general improvement in health. The official Fit for Life Website claims an "86% success rate" and mentions "clinical trials" without providing any details.

Some benefits of the plan are that it encourages people to increase their consumption of fresh fruits and vegetables. Unlike some diets, Fit for Life does not require dieters to buy special foods, keeping food costs moderate. It does, however, encourage dieters to purchase enzyme supplements from Fit for Life Industries.

Precautions

The Fit for Life website is heavy on the theory behind the Fit for Life diet, but gives few specifics on how the diet cam be put into effect in daily life. Sample meal plans and approved food lists are not available until the dieter signs up for the program at a

QUESTIONS TO ASK YOUR DOCTOR

- Do I have health conditions that might be affected by this diet?
- Is there another diet that would meet my weight and health goals better?
- If I go on this diet, will I need to take dietary supplements? If so, which ones?
- Will this diet meet my long-term dietary needs?
- Does this diet pose any special risks for me that I should be aware of?
- Is this diet safe and effective for all members of my family?
- Would you recommend someone in your family going on this diet?

substantial fee. This is very different from programs such as Body for Life or **Weight Watchers**, which give potential program participants very specific information about diet, menus, and exercise before they pay for the plan.

Fit for Life claims that their rules for eating benefit everyone from young children to pregnant women to older adults. The diet is intended to be a diet for a lifetime, but it does not take into account changes in lifecycle nutrition.

Risks

Some registered dietitians feel that the Fit for Life diet can lead to serious vitamin and mineral deficiencies. Banning dairy products makes it extremely difficult for dieters to get the recommended daily allowance of **calcium**. Calcium is needed to keep bones strong and for many metabolic reactions in the body. Other potential vitamin deficiencies spotted by dietitians who have analyzed this diet include deficiencies in vitamin B and B_{12}.

Research and general acceptance

Many professionals in the nutrition community consider Fit for Life an unhealthy fad diet. The concept behind food combining was tested in a study published in the April 2007 issue of the *International Journal of Obesity*. In this study, participants were fed a 1,100 calorie a day diet to promote weight loss. One group ate balanced meals containing all the major food groups. The other group ate a similar diet, but tested the food-combining theory by avoiding eating certain food groups at the same time. At the end of six weeks, the blood sugar, cholesterol, **insulin**, and blood **fats** were the same for each group. The balanced-meal group had lost an average of 16.5 lb. and the food-combining group had lost 13.6 lb. This strongly suggests that eating a low-calorie diet is much more important than eating foods in certain combinations.

Resources

BOOKS

Bijlefeld, Marjolijn, and Sharon K. Zoumbaris. *Encyclopedia of Diet Fads*. Westport, CT: Greenwood Press, 2003.

Diamond, Harvey. *Fit for Life: A New Beginning: Your Complete Diet and Health Plan for the Millennium*. New York: Kensington Books, 2000.

Diamond, Harvey, and Marilyn Diamond. *Fit for Life*. New York: Fine Communications, 2002.

Icon Health Publications. *Fad Diets: A Bibliography, Medical Dictionary, and Annotated Research Guide to Internet References*. San Diego, CA: Icon Health Publications, 2004.

Scales, Mary Josephine. *Diets in a Nutshell: A Definitive Guide on Diets from A to Z*. Clifton, VA: Apex Publishers, 2005.

WEBSITES

Callahan, Maureen. "Fit for Life Diet Review." Health.com. http://www.health.com/health/article/0,,20410201,00.html (accessed October 5, 2012).

"Fit for Life Online Wellness Center." http://fitforlife.com (accessed October 5, 2012).

Mann, Denise. "It's the Calories That Count, Not the Food Combinations." WebMD.com. http://www.webmd.com/news/20000407/diets-combination-balanced (accessed October 5, 2012).

Tish Davidson, A.M.

5-Factor diet

Definition

The 5-Factor diet is part of an overall healthy lifestyle and fitness program devised by Harley Pasternak (1974–), a Canadian-born personal trainer for celebrities, as well as a nutrition and fitness expert. The diet regimen includes recommendations about exercise and cooking shortcuts, as well as meal plans and recipes. The diet itself is essentially a moderate-carbohydrate, high-fiber, and high-protein regimen that incorporates the glycemic index (GI) as a guide to choosing appropriate foods.

Origins

The 5-Factor diet originated with Harvey Pasternak, a Canadian-born and –educated sports and fitness expert who began his career as an exercise and nutrition scientist for Canada's Defence and Civil Institute for Environmental Medicine (DCIEM), where he worked between 2005 and 2007. Pasternak is somewhat unusual for writers of popular diet books in that he holds several academic credentials in physiology and nutrition. He completed high school at York Mills Collegiate Institute in Toronto and earned a master's degree in exercise physiology and nutritional science from the University of Toronto. Pasternak also holds a degree in kinesiology from the University of Western Ontario in London, Ontario. He has been certified as a personal trainer and health/fitness instructor by the American College of Sports Medicine (ACSM) and the Canadian Society for Exercise Physiology (CSEP).

Following his work with DCIEM, Pasternak became a personal trainer. His first book, published in 2004, was primarily concerned with fitness and exercise, along with some advice about diet and nutrition. The first two parts of the book are about fitness workouts, with an early version of the 5-Factor diet added as Part 3, titled "5-Factor Fuel." Pasternak's 2006 book is essentially an expansion of the third section of the earlier book with the exercise component reduced to a single chapter, "The New 5-Factor Hollywood Workout," and additional chapters on food selection and recipes. According to the introduction of *The 5-Factor Diet*, Pasternak struggled with weight issues himself as a youth, and became motivated to learn more about nutrition, human **metabolism**, and exercise at the graduate level not only because of his own weight problem but also because his two younger brothers had been diagnosed with type 1 diabetes.

According to Pasternak, the fitness program that he devised as a personal trainer brought him to the attention of a number of Hollywood and media celebrities who "wanted to tone up for upcoming roles." In addition to mentioning the names of some of these actors and musicians, Pasternak states that he wrote his 2006 book in response to "more than 5,000 e-mails from people who had purchased *5-Factor Fitness...* and wanted to know more about the 5-Factor Diet." Pasternak has since become a minor media celebrity in his own right, as a frequent guest on daytime talk shows and co-host of a short-lived health and lifestyle daytime television show on the ABC network called *The Revolution*, which aired from January to July 2012.

Description

As its name suggests, the 5-Factor diet is based on the number five, which is featured in the accompanying exercise program as well as the diet itself. The basic outline of the 5-Factor diet is to eat five meals per day every three to four hours (breakfast, a snack, lunch, a second snack, and dinner). Each meal is to contain only five main ingredients, take only five minutes to prepare, and to contain five components: a complex carbohydrate, a lean **protein**, a sugar-free beverage, **fiber**, and a "good" fat.

Pasternak's food choices are based on the glycemic index (GI), a measure of the effect of various types of **carbohydrates** on blood sugar levels that was developed at the University of Toronto in the early 1980s. The theory underlying the GI is that foods with a low GI help to control appetite because they break down slowly and raise blood glucose levels only gradually, in contrast to high-GI foods, which raise blood glucose levels rapidly and tend to leave a person feeling hungry again relatively quickly. Pasternak's book includes some advice about avoiding high-GI foods and choosing low-fat proteins—for example, avoiding dark poultry meat in favor of white meat.

The 5 Factor Diet provides five weeks of meal plans and recipes. A typical recipe, "Greek Pizza Roll Ups," uses the following ingredients:

- 4 ounces of reduced-fat feta cheese
- 1/2 cup tomato sauce
- 1/2 cup frozen spinach
- seasonings: garlic powder, pepper, red flakes
- 2 medium whole-wheat tortillas

The instructions are equally simple:

- Preheat oven to 350 degrees
- Cover a cookie sheet with aluminum foil and place the tortillas on it.
- Spread the tomato sauce on the tortillas to within 1 inch of the edges.
- Sprinkle the cheese and spinach over the tomato sauce and top with the seasonings as desired.
- Bake for 10 to 12 minutes or until completely heated. The tortillas can be eaten as is or rolled up to eat on the go.

Pasternak maintains that regular exercise is 50% of his weight-loss plan. The number five reappears in the form of five exercises to be performed for 5 minutes each for five days of the week, for a total of 25 minutes of physical exercise per day. The book includes photographs, as well as step-by-step instructions for the fitness exercises, which are a combination of cardiovascular and strength training: a cardiovascular warm-up, upper-body strength exercises, lower-body strength exercises, exercises for the core muscles, and a cardiovascular workout.

One distinctive feature of the 5-Factor diet is what Pasternak calls the "cheat" day: one day a week in which the dieter is free to eat favorite dishes that do not fit the 5-factor template, such as fried chicken legs or a glass of beer. Some dieters who feel deprived on less flexible diet plans may find that the "cheat" day will help them stick with the 5-Factor diet.

Function

The 5-Factor diet is essentially a moderate-carbohydrate, high-fiber, and **high-protein diet** combined with an exercise program intended to promote a moderate rate of weight loss and the adoption of more healthful eating habits in otherwise healthy people. It is not intended to treat any chronic medical conditions or disorders.

Benefits

The American Academy of Nutrition and Dietetics' (formerly the American Dietetic Association) review of the 5-Factor Diet recommends the plan as "a good, simple idea that sends a healthy message: Eat a variety of foods in appropriate amounts and you'll lose weight, be healthy and probably get most of the **vitamins** and other nutrients you need from your food." Other reviewers have noted that the 5-Factor diet is not a fad diet, as it does not exclude any basic food groups, allows users to adapt meal plans to their own tastes and preferences, and includes a regular workout program. Users of the diet will lose weight slowly rather than rapidly— an average of one or two pounds per week, which is not only healthful but better for long-term weight management than rapid weight loss.

Precautions

Although the 5-Factor diet is not a very low-calorie diet (VLCD), it is always a good idea for people who need to lose 30 pounds or more, are pregnant or nursing, are below the age of 18, or have a chronic disorder to check with their physician before starting any weight-reduction diet. The 5-Factor diet is not a good choice for people with diabetes, **hypertension**, or kidney disease.

Although Pasternak's book suggests five weeks as the duration of the diet, most reviewers have observed that anyone with more than 10 pounds to lose will need to remain on the diet longer than five weeks to

reach their desired weight. The 5-Factor diet is considered safe for long-term use.

One drawback of the 5-Factor diet is its one-size-fits-all approach to calorie content and portion size; the same meals and snacks are recommended for all dieters, without regard to age, sex, height, weight, or level of activity. The recipes also do not contain any other nutritional information.

Other criticisms of the diet include its lack of guidance for eating out; users are left on their own to estimate what restaurant foods might fit the 5-Factor pattern. In addition, the diet may not work well for people who are emotion-driven eaters or for those whose work and travel schedules make it difficult to eat or prepare five meals a day at Pasternak's recommended time intervals.

Risks

Some registered dietitians maintain that the 5-Factor diet is not appropriate for people with the following chronic health conditions:

• Diabetes—the 5-Factor diet does not allow enough carbohydrates for most adults with diabetes.

• Hypertension—Pasternak's menus contain more sodium than is healthful for those who must stick with a low-sodium diet.

• Kidney disease—the levels of potassium, phosphorus, and protein levels in the 5-Factor diet are too high for adults with kidney problems.

Research and general acceptance

One common criticism of the 5-Factor diet is its lack of clinical testing or other scientific evidence. No studies of the diet have been published in the mainstream medical literature as of 2012, which is ironic given Pasternak's academic background in nutrition and sports medicine. He is listed in the National Library of Medicine database as a coauthor on one scholarly article, a study of the effects of ephedrine and **caffeine** on muscular endurance that was published in 2003.

In addition to the absence of clinical studies of the 5-Factor diet, other dietitians have pointed out that the glycemic index, which is a prominent feature of Pasternak's diet, is controversial as a guide to weight loss for people without diabetes. Some researchers maintain that the total amount of carbohydrate in a person's diet is a more accurate indicator of nutritional status than the GI values of specific foods.

In addition to the lack of scholarly studies of the 5-Factor diet, Pasternak's role as a media star and his liberal use of celebrity endorsements has been criticized as diverting attention from the diet's genuine good points. A reviewer for the **Academy of Nutrition and Dietetics** remarked, "I wish every other page didn't quote celebrities in big letters about how wonderful the author and diet are. This makes the book seem gimmicky and less credible, which is unfortunate since the diet plan is quite good."

Resources

BOOKS

Pasternak, Harley. *The 5 Factor Diet*. Des Moines, IA: Meredith Books, 2006.

Pasternak, Harley, and Ethan Boldt. *5-Factor Fitness: The Diet and Fitness Secret of Hollywood's A-List*. New York: G.P. Putnam's Sons, 2004.

Pasternak, Harley, with Laura Moser. *The 5-Factor World Diet*. New York: Ballantine Books, 2009.

PERIODICALS

Jacobs, I., H. Pasternak, and D G. Bell. "Effects of Ephedrine, Caffeine, and Their Combination on Muscular Endurance." *Medicine and Science in Sports and Exercise* 35 (June 2003): 98–94.

WEBSITES

Bledsoe, Andrea. "The 5 Factor Diet." EverydayHealth.com. http://www.everydayhealth.com/diet-nutrition/5-Factor-diet.aspx (accessed September 7, 2012).

Bouchez, Colette. "The 5 Factor Diet: Can It Work for You?" WebMD.com. http://www.webmd.com/diet/features/the-5-Factor-diet-can-it-work-for-you (accessed August 24, 2012).

Harley Pasternak's 5 Factor. "What is 5-Factor?" http://www.5factor.com/Pages/The-Diet (accessed August 24, 2012).

Nonas, Cathy. "The 5-Factor Diet (Book Review)." Academy of Nutrition and Dietetics. http://www.eatright.org/Media/content.aspx?id=10439 (accessed August 24, 2012).

Scott, Jennifer R. "Information about the Five Factor Diet." About.com. http://weightloss.about.com/od/morediet1/a/5factordiet.htm (accessed August 24, 2012).

Sher, Lauren. "Get Fit in 2012 with Harley Pasternak's Full Body Toning Tips." ABCNews.com. http://abcnews.go.com/blogs/health/2011/12/22/get-fit-in-2012-with-harley-pasternaks-full-body-toning-tips (accessed August 24, 2012).

ORGANIZATIONS

Academy of Nutrition and Dietetics, 120 South Riverside Plz., Ste. 2000, Chicago, IL 60606-6995, (312) 899-0040, (800) 877-1600, amacmunn@eatright.org, http://www.eatright.org.

Canadian Society for Exercise Physiology (CSEP), 18 Louisa St., Ste. 370, Ottawa, Canada Ontario K1R 6Y6, (613) 234-3755, (877) 651-3755, Fax: (613) 234-3565, info@csep.ca, http://www.csep.ca/english/view.asp?x=1.

Rebecca J. Frey, PhD

Flaxseed

Definition

Flaxseed is the seed of the plant *Linum usitatissimum*. It is a rich source of alpha-linolenic acid (ALA), an omega-3 fatty acid that is an essential nutrient in the human diet. Flaxseed also contains linoleic acid (LA), an essential omega-6 fatty acid, and is rich in dietary **fiber** and lignans, a class of **phytonutrients**. Flaxseed oil is a vegetable oil derived from pressed flaxseed. Flaxseed and flaxseed oil have different properties and nutritional values.

Purpose

Flaxseed is most commonly used as a laxative, according to the National Center for Complementary and Alternative Medicine (NCCAM). This use is related to the fiber content of the seed. Due to the estrogen-like properties of lignans, it is also used as a treatment for hot flashes related to menopause and relief of breast

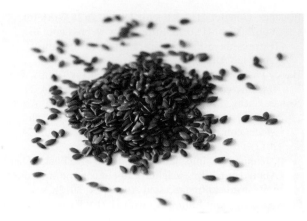

Golden flaxseeds. *(Goran Bogicevic/Shutterstock.com)*

pain. Flaxseed oil does not contain fiber or lignans, and it is used for conditions including the treatment of rheumatoid arthritis. Due to its omega-3 fatty acid content, flaxseed is sometimes taken as a supplement to help lower cholesterol and reduce the risk of heart disease. Evidence supports the use of flaxseed in lowering total cholesterol in people with high cholesterol and reducing menopause symptoms, but additional research is needed regarding the effectiveness of all other uses.

Description

L. usitatissimum is a slender plant with narrow leaves and blue flowers that grows anywhere from 8–45 in. (20–130 cm) tall. The plant originated in India but has been farmed across the world for thousands of years. Archaeologists discovered evidence that flax was cultivated in ancient Babylon as early as 3000 BC.

Flax is grown for both consumption and industrial use. The seed is about 42% oil. Solvent-extracted oil from flax seeds is used for industrial purposes and is often called linseed oil. It is used in manufacturing oil paints, varnishes, and linoleum. The material that remains after oil has been extracted from the seeds is called linseed cake or linseed meal. It is often added to animal feed as a **protein** and omega-3 fatty acid supplement. Omega-3 enriched eggs, for example, come from chickens fed flax. Omega-3 enriched pork is available in countries including the United States, Canada, and Japan.

Human consumption of flaxseed and flaxseed oil has increased substantially since the mid-1990s. Flaxseed oil for human consumption is produced through solvent-free cold pressing at low temperatures. Bottled flaxseed oil can be used to make salad dressing or added to already cooked foods. Flaxseed oil should not be used to fry food, however, because the oil

cannot withstand high temperatures. Flaxseed oil is also sold in capsule form as a dietary supplement. Flaxseeds come in brown, golden, and yellow varieties and have a slightly nutty flavor. Seeds are sold whole or are ground (milled) for consumption. Flaxseed flour, also called flaxseed meal or flaxmeal, is used in baking.

Nutritional information

Flaxseed is rich in fiber, **omega-3 fatty acids**, and lignans. According to the Flax Council of Canada, 1 Tbsp. (14.3 g) of ground flaxseed provides about 36 **calories**, 1.8 g of ALA, 1.6 g of protein, and 2.2 g of dietary fiber. One tsp. (4.5 mL) of flax oil provides 44 calories and 2.8 g of ALA, but contains no protein or fiber. The oil in flaxseed is high in polyunsaturated fat (a healthy fat) and contains no trans fat or cholesterol. Flaxseed also provides **vitamins** C, E, K, B_1 (**thiamin**), B_2 (**riboflavin**), and B_6, along with the **mineralscalcium, iron, magnesium,** phosphorous, **zinc, copper, manganese,** and **selenium.** Flaxseed is low in **sodium** and **carbohydrates.**

FIBER. Flaxseed, both whole and ground, contains dietary fiber. Fiber helps promote satiety and prevent **constipation**. Ground flax is preferred over whole seeds because it is easier to digest. If the seed is not broken down during digestion, the person will not obtain the health benefits of the seed. Flaxseed oil does not contain fiber.

POLYUNSATURATED FATTY ACIDS. According to the Flax Council of Canada, about 42% of the flaxseed is oil and more than 70% of that oil is polyunsaturated fat (PUFA). Of that fat content, 57% is ALA. PUFAs and monounsaturated **fats** are unsaturated fats, healthy fats that may help reduce blood cholesterol levels. Omega-6 is also a polyunsaturated fat, and flaxseed contains about 17% of this fat in the form of linolenic acid.

LIGNANS. Flaxseed is the richest dietary source of plant lignans, compounds found in plants that mimic the effect of estrogen. There are 85.5 mg of lignans in 1 oz. (28.35 g) of flaxseeds, according to the Linus Pauling Institute at Oregon State University. Lignans compete with estrogen for binding sites on cells. They may help alleviate symptoms of menopause by simulating estrogen response in the body.

Flaxseed supplements

Flaxseed is available in several forms: as whole seeds, ground flaxseed, flax meal, and flax oil. Whole seeds can be stored at room temperature for up to one year, and ground seeds can be kept in an airtight container in the refrigerator for up to three months. When ground flax is needed, it is preferable to grind whole seeds in a coffee grinder, blender, or food processor immediately before use.

According to the Mayo Clinic, ground seeds are preferred, because the body cannot break down the whole seeds to access the omega-3 oil. Ground flaxseed can be added to several foods, such as oatmeal, condiments, and baked goods. Flaxseed oil can be used to make salad dressing or added as an ingredient to food that is already cooked. Bottled flaxseed oil should be stored in the refrigerator to avoid the breakdown of the chemicals. Flaxseed oil supplements, which come in capsule form, usually range in strength from 1,000 to 1,300 mg.

Health claims and research

According to the National Center for Complementary and Alternative Medicine (NCCAM), flaxseed may produce a laxative effect and may reduce cholesterol in postmenopausal women and people with high cholesterol. As of August 2012, the NCCAM was funding additional studies on the potential role of flaxseed in preventing or treating atherosclerosis (hardening of the arteries), breast **cancer**, and ovarian cysts. While some studies showed that the omega-3 in fish and fish oil helped to reduce inflammation, more research was needed about the use of flaxseed for this treatment.

Flaxseed has also been studied as a potential treatment or deterrent for heart disease, rheumatoid arthritis, and cancer. However, there is not enough evidence that flaxseed helps treat or prevent any of these conditions.

MENOPAUSE. Ground flaxseed may help with symptoms of menopause such as hot flashes and night sweats. Menopause is defined as the time when a woman's menstrual periods stop, and menopause is the most common hormonal condition that causes hot flashes. Characterized by a sudden feeling of warmth, hot flashes are usually most intense around the face, neck, and chest, according to the Mayo Clinic. The skin may redden, and the woman may sweat profusely and then feel chilled. A woman may experience these symptoms several times a week or several times a day. When the symptoms occur at night, sleep is disrupted. In order to provide relief, 40 g of flaxseed must be consumed per day.

Precautions

People should discuss supplement intake with their physician before adding any supplements to their diet. This is especially important for women who are pregnant

---

KEY TERMS

Dietary supplement—A product, such as a vitamin, mineral, herb, amino acid, or enzyme, that is intended to be consumed in addition to an individual's diet with the expectation that it will improve health.

Fatty acids—Complex molecules found in fats and oils. Essential fatty acids are fatty acids that the body needs but cannot synthesize. Sources of essential fatty acids include plants.

Lignans—A group of compounds found in plants that have characteristics similar to the female hormone estrogen. They appear to have some anti-cancer and antioxidant effects.

Phytonutrients—A class of nutrients derived from plants that are believed to have positive effects on health.

Triglycerides—A type of fat found in the blood. High levels of triglycerides can increase the risk of coronary artery disease.

Vegan—A vegetarian who does not eat meat or dairy products.

---

or **breastfeeding** and for people with chronic conditions such as cancer. Parents should also discuss the use of supplements for their children. **Dietary supplements** do not undergo the same scrutiny as prescription medications. The U.S. Food and Drug Administration (FDA) does not require supplement manufacturers to prove that their products are safe and effective as long as the manufacturer does not make claims that the product can prevent, treat, or cure a specific disease.

Due to its fiber content, flaxseed should be taken with water, according to NCCAM. Too much fiber without water can lead to constipation or, in rare cases, intestinal blockage. Flaxseed can cause diarrhea.

Although flaxseed contains omega-3 fatty acids, fish is a richer source of the nutrient, according to the American Heart Association (AHA). The AHA recommends that people consume fish at least twice a week, especially fatty fish such as salmon, tuna, albacore tuna, and mackerel. Omega-3 fatty acids are thought to decrease triglyceride levels, prevent heart disease, and lower blood pressure.

Interactions

The fiber in flaxseed may lower the body's ability to absorb medications that are taken by mouth. Flaxseed should not be taken at the same time as other

QUESTIONS TO ASK YOUR DOCTOR

- Should I add flaxseed to my diet?
- Is there a limit to the amount of flaxseed that I can add to my food each day?
- Is it safe for me to take flaxseed oil supplements?
- What daily dosage of flaxseed oil supplements do you recommend?
- Will flaxseed interfere with the medications that I take?
- Is it safe for me to take flaxseed oil supplements if I am pregnant or breastfeeding?

medications or other dietary supplements without first consulting with a physician. Drugs that might interact with flaxseed include acetaminophen, antibiotic drugs, oral contraceptives, and diabetes medications, ibuprofen, aspirin, blood-thinning drugs such as warfarin (Coumadin), blood pressure medications, and herbal remedies.

Complications

Complications are unlikely to occur when flax products are used to meet daily dietary needs. Some studies have found a link between ALA and increased risk of prostate cancer, but other studies have found that flaxseed may reduce the risk of prostate cancer. Men who are at risk for prostate cancer may wish to consult with a physician before consuming flaxseed.

Parental concerns

Parents should be aware that a safe dosage of flaxseed supplements has not been established. They should consult with their child's pediatrician about recommended intake of flaxseed.

Resources

BOOKS

Muir, Alister D., and Neil D. Westcott, eds. *Flax: The Genus Linum.* New York: Routledge 2003.

PDR for Herbal Medicines. 3rd ed. Montvale, NJ: Thompson Healthcare, 2004.

Reinhardt-Martin, Jane. *The Amazing Flax Cookbook.* Moline: IL, TSA Press, 2004.

Wildman, Robert E. C., ed. *Handbook of Nutraceuticals and Functional Foods.* 2nd ed. Boca Raton, FL: CRC/Taylor &Francis, 2007.

PERIODICALS

Bloedon, L.T., et al. "Flaxseed and Cardiovascular Risk Factors: Results From a Double Blind, Randomized, Controlled Clinical Trial." *Journal of the American College of Nutrition* 27, no. 1 (2008): 65–74.

Covington, M.B. "Omega-3 Fatty Acids." *American Family Physician* 70, no. 1 (2004): 133–40.

OTHER

Edwards, Jane U. "Flaxseed: Agriculture to Health." North Dakota State University. http://www.ag.ndsu.edu/pubs/yf/foods/fn596.pdf (accessed August 21, 2012).

Morris, Diane H. "New Flax Facts: Food Sources of Alpha-Linolenic Acid." Flax Council of Canada. http://www.flaxcouncil.ca/english/pdf/Flax_FSht_FoodSourc08_R2.pdf (accessed August 21, 2012).

WEBSITES

American Cancer Society. "Flaxseed." http://www.cancer.org/Treatment/TreatmentsandSideEffects/ComplementaryandAlternativeMedicine/HerbsVitaminsandMinerals/flaxseed (accessed August 21, 2012).

Castle, Erik P. "Flaxseed: Does it Affect Risk of Prostate Cancer?" MayoClinic.com. http://www.mayoclinic.com/health/flaxseed/AN01712 (accessed August 21, 2012).

Higdon, Jane, and Victoria Drake. "Essential Fatty Acids." Linus Pauling Institute, Oregon State University. http://lpi.oregonstate.edu/infocenter/othernuts/omega3fa (accessed August 3, 2012).

———. "Lignans." Linus Pauling Institute, Oregon State University. http://lpi.oregonstate.edu/infocenter/phytochemicals/lignans (accessed August 21, 2012).

MedlinePlus. "Flaxseed." U.S. National Library of Medicine, National Institutes of Health. http://www.nlm.nih.gov/medlineplus/druginfo/natural/991.html (accessed August 21, 2012).

———. "Flaxseed Oil." U.S. National Library of Medicine, National Institutes of Health. http://www.nlm.nih.gov/medlineplus/druginfo/natural/990.html (accessed August 21, 2012).

National Center for Complementary and Alternative Medicine. "Flaxseed and Flaxseed Oil." U.S. National Institutes of Health. http://nccam.nih.gov/health/flaxseed/ataglance.htm (accessed August 21, 2012).

University of Maryland Medical Center. "Alpha-Linolenic Acid." http://www.umm.edu/altmed/articles/alpha-linolenic-000284.htm (accessed August 21, 2012).

———. "Flaxseed." http://www.umm.edu/altmed/articles/flaxseed-000244.htm (accessed August 21, 2012).

Zeratsky, Katherine. "Ground Flaxseed: Better than Whole?" MayoClinic.com. http://www.mayoclinic.com/health/flaxseed/AN01258 (accessed August 3, 2012).

ORGANIZATIONS

Flax Council of Canada, 465-167 Lombard Ave., Winnipeg, Canada Manitoba MB R3B 0T6, (204) 982-2115,

Fax: (204) 942-2128, flax@flaxcouncil.ca, http://
www.flaxcouncil.ca.
National Center for Complementary and Alternative
Medicine Clearinghouse, PO Box 7923, Gaithersburg,
MD 20898, (888) 644-6226, Fax: (866) 464-3616, info@
nccam.nih.gov, http://nccam.nih.gov.

Tish Davidson, A.M.
Liz Swain

Fluoride

Definition

Fluoride is a naturally occurring element found in
food and water. It occurs in the body as **calcium**
fluoride, primarily in the teeth and bones. Fluoride is
necessary for the development and maintenance of
strong teeth and bones and helps prevent tooth decay
(dental caries).

Purpose

The importance of fluoride for dental health has
been recognized since the 1930s, when an association
between the fluoride content of drinking water and the
prevalence of dental caries was first noted. Acids
found in food and released by bacteria that feed on
sugar in the mouth eat away at the enamel on the
surfaces of the teeth. Systemic fluoride enters the
bloodstream from food, water, and supplements and
is incorporated into the enamel as the teeth develop.
The enamel that covers the crown, the part of the tooth

Suggested amounts of dietary fluoride supplements

Age	Fluoride ion level in drinking water (ppm)*		
	<0.3 ppm	0.3–0.6 ppm	>0.6 ppm
Birth–6 months	None	None	None
6 months–3 years	0.25 mg/day**	None	None
3 years–6 years	0.50 mg/day	0.25 mg/day	None
6 years–16 years	1.0 mg/day	0.50 mg/day	None

* 1.0 part per million (ppm) 1 milligram/liter (mg/L)
** 2.2 mg sodium fluoride contains 1 mg fluoride ion

SOURCE: American Dental Association

**Children between the ages of 6 months to 16 years living in
non-fluoridated areas may require dietary fluoride
supplements. A dentist can prescribe the correct dosage
based on fluoride levels.** *(Table by GGS Information Services.
© 2013 Cengage Learning.)*

that is above the gum, is made of a substance called
hydroxyapatite. If enough fluoride reaches the teeth
while the enamel is forming, fluoride can replace a
component of the hydroxyapatite molecule to form
fluorapatite, becoming part of the tooth enamel. This
makes the tooth more acid-resistant. Fluoride in saliva
can also help repair enamel, making the new surface
stronger than the original enamel and better able to
resist decay, as well as reversing early decay. This
process is called tooth remineralization or recalcification. Fluoride also interferes with the **metabolism** of
bacteria in the mouth so that they produce less decay-
causing acids.

It is unlikely that sufficient fluoride from water
alone will be incorporated into the enamel during the
years of crown formation. Thus, topical fluoride is the
most effective means of remineralizing the surface
layers of tooth enamel and dentin as they wear out
and are eaten away by acids from food and bacteria.
Topical fluorides are applied directly to the surfaces of
fully formed teeth and help prevent tooth decay in
both children and adults. Topical fluorides include
fluoride toothpastes and mouthwashes and gels that
are applied to children's teeth during dental examinations. Systemic fluorides, such as fluoridated water,
can also provide topical protection, because they are
incorporated into the saliva that bathes the teeth.

It is estimated that fluoridated water is 20%–60%
effective in preventing cavities in children and adults.
Early studies suggested that water fluoridation was eliminating tooth decay in children; however, other factors
are now recognized as having contributed to the decline
in dental caries. The widespread use of fluoridated
toothpastes and mouthwashes has increased children's
fluoride intake significantly. Furthermore, awareness of
dental care and hygiene among both children and adults
has increased in recent decades.

Description

The element fluorine is the 17th most abundant
element in the earth's crust. It occurs as fluoride ion in
combination with other elements such as **sodium** and
calcium. Fluoride is present in small amounts in
almost all soils, plants, and animals. It is found naturally in seawater and at low levels in most drinking
water sources. Seawater contains about 1.5 parts per
million (ppm) fluoride. Fluoride dissolves in water to
form negatively charged fluoride ions (F^-). In the
body, this ion is absorbed into the bloodstream from
the small intestine. It then binds with calcium in teeth
and bones. The adult body contains less than 0.1 oz.
(about 2.8 g) of fluoride, and 95% of this is in teeth
and bones.

Fluoride requirements

The Institute of Medicine (IOM) of the U.S. National Academy of Sciences has developed dietary reference intake (DRI) values for many **vitamins** and **minerals**. The **DRIs** consist of three sets of numbers. The recommended dietary allowance (RDA) defines the average daily amount of a nutrient needed to meet the health requirements of 97%–98% of the population. The adequate intake (AI) is an estimate set when there is insufficient information available for determining the RDA. The tolerable upper intake level (UL) is the average maximum amount that can be taken daily without risking negative side effects. Similar recommendations have been established in other countries. The daily AIs and ULs for fluoride for healthy individuals are:

- children birth–6 months: AI 0.01 mg, UL 0.7 mg
- children 7–12 months: AI 0.5 mg, UL 0.9 mg
- children 1–3 years: AI 0.7 mg, UL 1.3 mg
- children 4–8 years: AI 1.0 mg, UL 2.2 mg
- children 9–13 years: AI 2.0 mg, UL 10 mg
- adolescents 14–18 years: AI 3.0 mg, UL 10 mg
- men over 18: AI 4.0 mg, UL 10 mg
- women over 18 and pregnant and breastfeeding women of all ages: AI 3.0 mg, UL 10 mg

Fluoridated water

Water is the major source of fluoride for most people. In the early twentieth century, Frederick McKay, a young dentist in Colorado Springs, Colorado, noticed that many local residents had brown stains on their permanent teeth and that their teeth were surprisingly resistant to decay. McKay eventually discovered that this tooth "mottling" resulted from high levels of naturally occurring fluoride in the drinking water.

The first fluoridation of a public water system was in Grand Rapids, Michigan, in 1945. Over the following decades, more and more communities fluoridated their water using by-products from the phosphate fertilizer industry. About two-thirds of Americans now drink fluoridated water. However, fluoridation quickly became mired in controversy, and it remains so in the second decade of the twenty-first century. Since the decision to fluoridate is usually made at the local level, by public officials or popular vote, fluoridation is a political as well as a scientific controversy. While some opponents reject existing scientific evidence and claim that fluoridation is ineffective and/ or harmful, for others, public water fluoridation is an issue of personal choice versus government control.

The levels of naturally occurring fluoride in fresh water range from less than 0.1 ppm to more than 13 ppm. The recommended level for preventing tooth decay is 0.7–1.2 ppm. Water fluoridation levels are usually at the low end of this range in warmer regions, where people tend to drink more water, and at the higher end of the range in colder regions. Filtered water and well water vary greatly in their fluoride content. Most bottled water contains only trace amounts of fluoride.

Dietary sources of fluoride

Dietary fluoride is obtained from food prepared with fluoridated water and from seafood, which usually contains significant amounts of fluoride. Fruits and vegetables may contain more than 0.2 mg of fluoride per serving, depending on where the food was grown and whether fluoridated water was used for irrigation and processing. The amount of fluoride in beverages and processed foods also depends on the fluoride content of the water used to produce them. A few other foods, such as tea leaves and gelatin, naturally contain significant amounts of fluoride. Approximate fluoride contents of some common foods include:

- tea, 3.5 oz. (104 mL), 0.1–0.6 mg
- canned sardines with bones, 3.5 oz. (100 g), 0.2–0.4 mg
- fish without bones, 3.5 oz. (100 g), 0.01–0.17 mg
- chicken, 3.5 oz. (100 g), 0.06–0.10 mg

Other fluoride sources

Many toothpastes and mouthwashes contain high amounts of fluoride. A tube of fluoride toothpaste may contain as much as 1–2 g of fluoride. Nonprescription mouthwashes can contain up to 120 mg of fluoride. Children between the ages of two and six swallow about 33% of the toothpaste they use; children between seven and 15 swallow about 20%. Thus, an average child using a typical amount of fluoride toothpaste will swallow or absorb 0.5–1.0 mg of fluoride per brushing, although much of this fluoride is excreted. In addition, many vitamin supplements and medications contain fluoride.

Precautions

The amount of fluoride occurring naturally in drinking water varies widely depending on the locale. People should be aware of whether their public water supply is fluoridated, and those with wells should have their water tested for fluoride. Bottled water suppliers can provide information about their water's fluoride content. Some built-in home water-softening systems may remove fluoride.

Although water fluoridation at levels that prevent tooth decay does not pose a health risk, high doses of fluoride can be toxic. Doses of 20–80 mg per day can cause bones to become chalky and brittle and can affect kidney function and possibly nerve and muscle function. Doses of 5–10 g per day can be fatal. In 2009, the American Association of Poison Control Centers reported 24,547 exposures involving fluoride toothpaste. Of these, 378 cases were treated in emergency departments, moderate effects were observed in 42 cases, and major effects in two cases. Most of these incidents involved children under age six who ate toothpaste. Too much fluoride in the diet is very rare.

At safe doses, fluoride does not appear to strengthen bones or prevent or delay osteoporosis (age-related thinning of the bones). Consequently, fluoride supplements are not an appropriate way to prevent or treat osteoporosis.

Interactions

Antacids containing aluminum hydroxide and calcium supplements can decrease the absorption of fluoride from the small intestine.

Complications

There are no expected complications from daily doses of fluoride falling between the AI and the UL. Too little fluoride leads to increased tooth decay. Too much fluoride can cause illness or death. Too much fluoride, especially in children, also results in a condition called dental fluorosis. The surfaces of the teeth become discolored by chalky white splotches. This is a cosmetic problem and does not affect the health of the teeth. Fluoride poisoning is much more serious. A 40 lb. (18 kg) child would probably start to show symptoms of fluoride poisoning after consuming about 55 mg of fluoride (3 mg/kg of body weight), and a dose of 290 mg (16 mg/kg of body weight) would likely be fatal. Symptoms of fluoride poisoning include nausea, vomiting, diarrhea, headaches, muscle spasms, irregular heartbeat, coma, and death. Besides toothpaste and mouthwash, fluoride is also found in pesticides, rodent poisons, and chrome polish for automobiles.

Parental concerns

Infants obtain fluoride through breast milk or infant formulas. However, most baby food is made with non-fluoridated water. For children who do not drink fluoridated water, the American Dental Association and the American Academy of Pediatrics recommend prescription fluoride supplements from the age of six months on. The supplements are supplied as

KEY TERMS

Adequate intake (AI)—The daily average intake level of a nutrient that is likely to be adequate for a healthy, moderately active individual, as determined by the Institute of Medicine.

Dietary reference intake (DRI)—A system of nutritional recommendations used by the Institute of Medicine of the U.S. National Academy of Sciences and the U.S. Department of Agriculture.

Enamel—The hard mineralized tissue covering the dentin of the crown of a tooth.

Fluorapatite—Fluoride-substituted hydroxyapatite.

Fluorosis—Mottling; spotting on the teeth due to excess fluoride during the forming of the tooth enamel.

Hydroxyapatite—$Ca_5(PO_4)_3OH$; the material of tooth enamel consisting of calcium, phosphorous, oxygen, and hydrogen.

Mottling—Fluorosis; spotting on the teeth due to excess fluoride as the tooth enamel is forming.

Recommended dietary allowance; RDA—The approximate amount of a nutrient that should be ingested daily.

Remineralization—Recalcification; the process by which minerals from saliva and food are added to the surface of the tooth enamel or to the dentin.

Systemic—A substance, such as fluoride, that is ingested, absorbed into the bloodstream, and distributed throughout the body.

Tolerable upper intake level (UL)—The highest daily intake level of a nutrient that is unlikely to cause adverse health effects in almost all individuals in the general population, as determined by the Institute of Medicine.

Topical—A substance, such as fluoride, that is applied directly to the teeth.

liquids and chewable tablets of varying strengths and are prescribed by a pediatrician, family physician, or dentist. In addition, dentists may apply fluoride pastes or varnishes directly to children's teeth for additional protection. This is usually done at six-month intervals during regular dental check-ups.

Rarely, infants who get too much fluoride before their teeth have broken through the gums have changes in the enamel that covers the teeth. Faint white lines or streaks may appear, but they are usually hard to see.

It is important to teach children to never eat toothpaste. This can be a problem, because toothpastes are formulated to taste good to kids. Adults should supervise tooth brushing by children under age six. Mouthwashes containing fluoride and prescription fluoride supplements should be kept out of the reach of children. A child who eats fluoridated toothpaste or drinks mouthwash should receive an immediate medical evaluation.

Resources

BOOKS

Buzalaf, Marília Afonso Rabelo. *Fluoride and the Oral Environment*. New York: Karger, 2011.

Connett, P. H., James S. Beck, and H. S. Micklem. *The Case Against Fluoride: How Hazardous Waste Ended Up in Our Drinking Water and the Bad Science and Powerful Politics That Keep It There*. White River Junction, VT: Chelsea Green, 2010.

Segrave, Kerry. *America Brushes Up: The Use and Marketing of Toothpaste and Toothbrushes in the Twentieth Century*. Jefferson, NC: McFarland & Co., 2010.

PERIODICALS

Brody, Jane E. "Personal Health: Dental Exam Went Well? Thank Fluoride." *New York Times*, January 24, 2012: D7.

Jagtap, Sneha, et al. "Fluoride in Drinking Water and Defluoridation of Water." *Chemical Reviews* 112, no. 4 (April 2012): 2454–66.

Woolston, Chris. "The Healthy Skeptic: A Brush with Fluoride-Free Toothpastes." *Los Angeles Times*, February 6, 2012: E3.

Zimmerman, Jonathan. "Science Fights Fluoride." *Los Angeles Times*, November 16, 2011: A19.

WEBSITES

American Dental Association. "Fluoride & Fluoridation." http://www.ada.org/fluoride.aspx (accessed September 2, 2012).

MedlinePlus. "Fluoride in Diet." U.S. National Library of Medicine, National Institutes of Health. http://www.nlm.nih.gov/medlineplus/ency/article/002420.htm (accessed September 2, 2012).

Nochimson, Geofrey. "Fluoride Toxicity." Medscape Reference. May 11, 2011. http://emedicine.medscape.com/article/814774-overview#showall (accessed September 2, 2012).

ORGANIZATIONS

Academy of Nutrition and Dietetics, 120 South Riverside Plaza, Ste. 2000, Chicago, IL 60606-6995, (312) 899-0040, (800) 877-1600, http://www.eatright.org.

American Academy of Pediatric Dentistry, 211 East Chicago Avenue, Ste. 1700, Chicago, IL 60611-2637, (312) 337-2169, Fax: (312) 337-6329, http://www.aapd.org.

American Dental Association, 211 East Chicago Ave., Chicago, IL 60611-2678, (312) 440-2500, http://www.ada.org.

Tish Davidson, AM
Margaret Alic, PhD

Folate

Definition

Folate is a naturally occurring water-soluble vitamin that the body needs to remain healthy. Folic acid is a stable synthetic form of folate that is found in **dietary supplements** and is added to fortified foods, such as flour and cereal. Humans cannot make folate or folic acid, so they must get it from foods in their diet or as a dietary supplement. Folic acid and folate are both converted into an active form that the body can use, although folic acid is more easily used (more bioavailable) in the body. Folic acid is also called vitamin B_9.

Purpose

Folate is necessary to create new DNA (genetic material) and RNA when cells divide. It plays a critical role in developing healthy red blood cells. Folate also helps protect DNA from damage that may lead to diseases such as **cancer**. Along with **vitamins** B_6 and B_{12}, folate helps regulate the level of the amino acid homocysteine in the blood. Homocysteine regulation is related to cardiovascular health. In the fetus, folate is necessary for the proper development of the brain and spinal cord.

Description

Folate is one of eight B-complex vitamins. Its function is closely intertwined with that of vitamins B_6 and B_{12}. Folate, from the Latin word *folium*, meaning leaf, was discovered in the late 1930s in yeast, and later found in spinach and other green leafy vegetables

Folate (Folic Acid)

Age	Recommended dietary allowance (mcg)	Tolerable upper intake level (mcg)
Children 0–6 mos.	65 (AI)	Not established
Children 7–12 mos.	80 (AI)	Not established
Children 1–3 yrs.	150	300
Children 4–8 yrs.	200	400
Children 9–13 yrs.	300	600
Children 14–18 yrs.	400	800
Adults 19+ yrs.	400	1,000
Pregnant women 14–18 yrs.	600	800
Pregnant women 19+ yrs.	600	1,000
Breastfeeding women 14–18 yrs.	500	800
Breastfeeding women 19+ yrs.	500	1,000

AI = Adequate Intake
mcg = microgram

SOURCE: Office of Dietary Supplements, "Dietary Supplement Fact Sheet: Folate," U.S. National Institutes of Health.

(Table by PreMediaGlobal. © 2013 Cengage Learning.)

and in liver. Starting in 1998, the U.S. Food and Drug Administration (FDA) required certain foods, such as flour, corn meal, bread, cereal, rice, and pasta, to be fortified with a folic acid. In Canada and Chile, fortification of flour is mandatory.

Folate's role in health

Folate is essential for the normal development of the neural tube in the fetus. The neural tube develops into the brain and spinal cord. It closes between the third and fourth week after conception. Too little folate at this time can lead to serious malformations of the spine (spina bifida) and the brain (anencephaly). Because many women do not realize that they are pregnant so soon after conception, the United States has included folic acid in its fortified foods program. Adding folic acid to common foods made with grains has substantially reduced the number of babies born with neural tube defects in the United States.

The body also needs folate to produce healthy red blood cells. When not enough folate is present, the red blood cells do not divide and instead grow to be abnormally large. These malformed cells have a reduced ability to carry oxygen to other cells in the body, a condition known as megaloblastic anemia. Folate also aids in the production of other new cells. Adequate supplies of folate are especially important in fetuses and infants because they are growing rapidly, but, since the lifespan of a red blood cell is only about four months, both children and adults need a continuous supply of folate throughout life to create healthy new replacement blood cells.

Folate acts together with **vitamin B$_6$** and **vitamin B$_{12}$** to lower the level of homocysteine in the blood. Homocysteine is an amino acid that is naturally produced when the body breaks down **protein**. Moderate to high levels of homocysteine in the blood are potentially linked to an increased risk of cardiovascular disease (e.g., atherosclerosis, heart attack, stroke). The trio of folate, vitamin B$_6$, and vitamin B$_{12}$ lower homocysteine levels. However, it is not clear whether taking large doses of these vitamins, either alone or in combination, will prevent heart disease from developing in healthy individuals. The official position of the American Heart Association in 2012 stated, "We don't recommend widespread use of folic acid and B vitamin supplements to reduce the risk of heart disease and stroke. We advise a healthy, balanced diet that's rich in fruits and vegetables, **whole grains**, and fat-free or low fat dairy products."

Damage to DNA appears to contribute to the development of many different cancers. Because folate helps protect against DNA damage, researchers have looked at whether it can reduce the risk of developing cancer. Results are mixed, with benefits seen for some cancers but not for others. The American Cancer Society position in 2012 was as follows: "Low levels of folic acid in the blood have been linked with higher rates of colorectal cancer and some other types of cancer, as well as with certain birth defects. It is not clear whether consuming recommended (or higher) amounts of folic acid—from foods or in supplements—can lower cancer risk in some people. These issues are being studied. High doses of folic acid can interfere with the action of some chemotherapy drugs, such as methotrexate."

Many clinical trials are underway to determine the safety and effectiveness of folate, both alone and in combination with other vitamins, in preventing cancer, cardiovascular disease, and dementias, such as Alzheimer's disease. Research is also underway on the effect of folate on schizophrenia and the feasibility of including folate in birth control pills. Individuals interested in participating in a clinical trial at no charge can find a list of open trials at http://www.clinicaltrials.gov.

Sources of folate

People need a continuous supply of folate from their diet because of the role it plays in creating new blood cells. Because folate is water-soluble, little is stored in the body, any excess is excreted in urine.

Selected food sources of folate and folic acid

Food	Micrograms (µg)	% daily value
*Breakfast cereals fortified with 100% of the DV, ¾ cup	400	100
Beef liver, cooked, braised, 3 ounces	215	54
Lentils, mature seeds, cooked, boiled, ½ cup	179	45
Spinach, frozen, cooked, boiled, ½ cup	115	29
*Egg noodles, cooked, enriched, ½ cup	110	28
*Breakfast cereals, fortified with 25% of the DV, ¾ cup	100	23
Great Northern beans, boiled, ½ cup	90	23
Asparagus, boiled, 4 spears	89	22
*Macaroni, cooked, enriched, ½ cup	84	21
*Rice, white, long-grain, enriched, cooked, ½ cup	77	19
Avocado, raw, all varieties, sliced, ½ cup	59	15
Spinach, raw, 1 cup	58	15
Papaya, raw, 1 cup cubes	52	13
Corn, sweet, yellow, canned ½ cup	52	13
Broccoli, chopped, frozen, cooked, ½ cup	51	13
Tomato juice, canned, 1 cup	49	12
Green peas, frozen, boiled, ½ cup	47	12
Orange juice, chilled, includes concentrate, 1 cup	47	12
*Bread, white, 1 slice	43	11
Peanuts, all types, dry roasted, 1 ounce	41	10
Broccoli, raw, 2 spears (each 5 inches long)	40	10
Wheat germ, crude, 2 tablespoons	40	10
Strawberries, raw, 1 cup	40	10
Cantaloupe melon, raw, 1 cup cubes	34	9
Lettuce, romaine, shredded, ½ cup	32	8
Vegetarian baked beans, canned, 1 cup	30	8
Orange, all commercial varieties, fresh, 1 small	29	7
Egg, whole, raw, fresh, 1 large	24	6
Banana, raw, 1 medium	24	6
*Bread, whole wheat, 1 slice	14	4

*Items are fortified with folic acid as part of the Folate Fortification Program.

SOURCE: U.S. Department of Agriculture (USDA) Agricultural Research Service, National Nutrient Database for Standard Reference, Release 24.

Available online at http://www.ars.usda.gov/ba/bhnrc/ndl.
(Table by PreMediaGlobal. © 2013 Cengage Learning.)

Since the folic acid fortification program began in 1998, most healthy Americans get enough folate from their diet. The exception is pregnant women who should, under medical supervision, take a folic acid supplement (400 mcg for most women and higher doses for those who have already had a baby with a neural tube defect). Good natural sources of folate include beef liver, green leafy vegetables, and dried beans. Cooking animal products does not reduce the folate content much, but cooking vegetables can reduce the amount of folate by up to 40%, depending on the vegetable and the cooking method.

The following list gives the approximate folate content of some common foods:

- asparagus, cooked, 1/2 cup: 132 mcg
- spinach, cooked, 1/2 cup: 131 mcg
- turnip greens, cooked, 1/2 cup: 135 mcg
- broccoli, steamed, 1/2 cup: 85 mcg
- beets, boiled, 1/2 cup: 68 mcg
- great northern beans, cooked, 1/2 cup: 90 mcg
- pinto beans, cooked, 1/2 cup: 147 mcg
- navy beans, cooked, 1/2 cup: 127 mcg
- tomato juice, canned, 6 oz: 35 mcg
- raspberries, 1/2 cup: 16 mcg
- corn, yellow, cooked, 1/2 cup: 37 mcg
- breakfast cereal, fortified 100%, 3/4 cup: 400 mcg
- bread, white or whole wheat, 1 slice: 25 mcg
- rice, white, enriched long-grain, cooked, 1/2 cup: 65 mcg
- bread, whole wheat, 1 slice: .07 mg
- bread, white, enriched, 1 slice: .09 mg

Recommended dosage

The U.S. Institute of Medicine (IOM) of the National Academy of Sciences has developed values called **Dietary Reference Intakes (DRIs)** for vitamins and **minerals**. The **DRIs** consist of three sets of numbers. The Recommended Dietary Allowance (RDA) defines the average daily amount of the nutrient needed to meet the health needs of 97%–98% of the population. The Adequate Intake (AI) is an estimate set when there is not enough information to determine an RDA. The Tolerable Upper Intake Level (UL) is the average maximum amount that can be taken daily without risking negative side effects. The DRIs are calculated for children, adult men, adult women, pregnant women, and breast-feeding women.

The IOM has not set RDAs for folate in children under one year old because of incomplete scientific information. Instead, it has set AI levels for this age group. RDAs and ULs for folate are measured in micrograms (mcg). Unlike the UL for many vitamins, the UL for folate refers only to folic acid that comes from fortified food or that is in folic acid dietary supplements, multivitamins, or B-complex vitamins. There is no UL for folate found in natural plant and animal foods. Dietary supplements containing more than 1,000 mcg (1 mg) of folic acid require a prescription. One mcg of folate from natural food sources is equal in biological activity in humans to 0.6 mcg of folic acid from supplements or fortified food.

The following are the daily RDAs and AIs and ULs for folic acid for healthy individuals:

- children birth–6 months: AI 65 mcg; UL not established
- children 7–12 months: AI 89 mcg; UL not established

- children 1–3 years: RDA 150 mcg; UL 300 mcg
- children 4–8 years: RDA 200 mcg; UL 400 mcg
- children 9–13 years: RDA 300 mcg; UL 600 mcg
- children 14–18 years: 400 RDA mcg; UL 800 mcg
- adults age 19 and older: RDA 400 mcg; UL 1,000 2mcg
- pregnant women: RDA 600 mcg; UL 1,000 mcg
- breastfeeding women: RDA 500 mcg; 1,000 mcg

Precautions

Since many pregnancies are unplanned and unrecognized until after the critical period for brain and spinal cord formation, any woman who may become pregnant should be careful to include enough folate in her diet, and folic acid supplements should be taken before and in the first trimester of pregnancy.

Folic acid may mask vitamin B_{12} deficiency. Folic acid supplements will reverse anemia symptoms, but they do not stop nerve damage caused by B_{12} deficiency. Permanent nerve damage may result. People with suspected folate deficiency who begin taking folic acid supplements should also be evaluated for vitamin B_{12} deficiency.

Interactions

The following is a partial list of medications that may interfere with the ability of the body to absorb and use folate. Individuals taking these medications should check with their physician about the effects they may have on folate levels in the body:

- seizure medications, such as dilantin, phenytoin, and primidone
- metformin (Fortamet, Glucophage, Glucophage XR, Riomet), used to treat type 2 diabetes
- sulfasalazine (Azulfidine, in the United States), used to treat Crohn's disease and inflammatory bowel disease
- triamterene (Dyrenium), a diuretic or "water pill"
- barbiturate sedatives
- methotrexate (Rheumatrex, Trexall), used to treat cancer, rheumatoid arthritis, and psoriasis
- drugs used to treat gastroesophageal reflux disease (GERD), such as omeprazole (Prilosec), lansoprazole (Prevacid), cimetidine (Tagamet), famotidine (Pepcid), nizatidine (Axid), or ranitidine (Zantac)

Complications

No complications are expected when folate or folic acid is taken within recommended levels.

KEY TERMS

Alzheimer's disease—An incurable disease of older individuals that results in the destruction of nerve cells in the brain and causes gradual loss of mental and physical functions.

Amino acid—Molecules that are the basic building blocks of proteins.

B-complex vitamins—A group of water-soluble vitamins that often work together in the body. These include thiamin (B_1), riboflavin (B_2), niacin (B_3), pantothenic acid (B_5), pyridoxine (B_6), biotin (B_7 or vitamin H), folate (B_9), and cobalamin (B_{12}).

Celiac disease—A chronic digestive disorder in which eating foods that contain the protein gluten (found in wheat flour, rye, and barley) causes an immune reaction that damages the small intestine and interferes with the absorption of food.

Deoxyribonucleic acid (DNA)—The genetic material in cells that holds the inherited instructions for growth, development, and cellular functioning.

Dietary supplement—A product—such as a vitamin, mineral, herb, amino acid, or enzyme—that is intended to be consumed in addition to an individual's diet with the expectation that it will improve health.

Diuretic—A substance that removes water from the body by increasing urine production.

Enzyme—A protein that changes the rate of a chemical reaction within the body without being depleted in the reaction.

Megaloblastic anemia—A type of anemia characterized by abnormally large red blood cells; usually caused by folate or vitamin B_{12} deficiencies.

Ribonucleic acid (RNA)—A molecule that helps decode genetic information (DNA) and is necessary for protein synthesis.

Water-soluble vitamin—A vitamin that dissolves in water and can be removed from the body in urine.

Folate deficiency

Most healthy people in the United States get enough folate in their diet because folate is added to many common foods, such as bread; however, this is not the case elsewhere. In Europe, low intakes are commonly reported, particularly in teenage girls and older people. Causes of folate deficiency include inadequate intake, impaired absorption (**celiac disease, Crohn's disease**, certain medications), inability of the body to use folate (enzyme deficiencies), increased

QUESTIONS TO ASK YOUR DOCTOR

- I would like to get pregnant. When should I begin taking folic acid supplements?
- I have celiac disease. Do I need a folic acid supplement?
- If I breast-feed my baby will he/she get enough folate?
- I am moving to a country that does not fortify its foods with folic acid. How can I make sure I am getting enough in my diet?

folate needs (pregnancy, cancer), or increased loss or excretion (kidney dialysis, alcoholism). The elderly are the largest group at risk to develop folate deficiency.

The major symptom of folate deficiency in pregnant women is having a baby born with a brain or spinal cord abnormality. Other symptoms of folate deficiency include slow growth in infants and children; megaloblastic anemia; digestive problems, such as diarrhea; sore tongue; irritability; forgetfulness; and changes in mental state. These changes also have other causes and should be evaluated by a healthcare professional.

Folate overdose

Complications of excess folic acid intake at levels above 1,000 mcg daily over an extended period can include seizures in individuals taking anticonvulsant medications and general irritability and restlessness in otherwise healthy individuals.

Parental concerns

Parents need to be aware that infants and rapidly growing children are at higher risk for folate deficiency. Parents of children with digestive disorders or allergies to wheat products (e.g., celiac disease) should discuss the need for a folic acid supplement with their pediatrician.

Resources

BOOKS

Bailey, Lynn B. *Folate in Health and Disease*. 2nd ed. Boca Raton, FL: CRC Press, Taylor & Francis Group, 2010.

Mason, Pamela. *Dietary Supplements*. 5th ed. Chicago: Pharmaceutical Press, 2011.

Webb, Geoffrey P. *Dietary Supplements and Functional Foods*. Chichester, West Sussex; Ames, IA: Wiley-Blackwell, 2011.

PERIODICALS

de Lourdes Samaniego-Vaesken, Maria, Elena Alonso-Aperte, and Gregorio Varela-Moreiras. "Vitamin Food Fortification Today." *Food & Nutrition Research* 6 (April 2, 2012): e-pub ahead of print. http://dx.doi.org/10.3402/fnr.v56i0.5459 (accessed August 14, 2012).

Kennedy, Deborah, and Gideon Koren. "Identifying Women Who Might Benefit from Higher Doses of Folic Acid in Pregnancy." *Canadian Family Physician* 58, no. 4 (2012): 394–97.

Xun, Pengcheng, et al. "Folate Intake and Incidence of Hypertension among American Young Adults: A 20-Year Follow-Up Study." *American Journal of Clinical Nutrition* 95, no. 5 (2012): 1023–1030. http://dx.doi.org/10.3945/ajcn.111.027250 (accessed August 14, 2012).

WEBSITES

American Cancer Society. "Folic Acid." http://www.cancer.org/Treatment/TreatmentsandSideEffects/ComplementaryandAlternativeMedicine/HerbsVitaminsandMinerals/folic-acid (accessed August 14, 2012).

American Heart Association. "Homocysteine, Folic Acid and Cardiovascular Disease." http://www.heart.org/HEARTORG/GettingHealthy/NutritionCenter/Homocysteine-Folic-Acid-and-Cardiovascular-Disease_UCM_305997_Article.jsp (accessed August 14, 2012).

Gentilli, Angela. "Folic Acid Deficiency." Medscape Reference. December 1, 2011. http://emedicine.medscape.com/article/200184-overview (accessed August 14, 2012).

Higdon, Jane. "Folic Acid." Linus Pauling Institute, Oregon State University. May 9, 2011. http://lpi.oregonstate.edu/infocenter/vitamins/fa (accessed August 14, 2012).

MedlinePlus. "Folic Acid." U.S. National Library of Medicine, National Institutes of Health. http://www.nlm.nih.gov/medlineplus/folicacid.html (accessed August 14, 2012).

University of Maryland Medical Center. "Vitamin B9 (Folic Acid)." http://www.umm.edu/altmed/articles/vitamin-b9-000338.htm (accessed August 14, 2012).

U.S. Office of Dietary Supplements. "Dietary Supplement Fact Sheet: Folic Acid." National Institutes of Health. http://ods.od.nih.gov/factsheets/Folate-Health Professional (accessed August 14, 2012).

ORGANIZATIONS

Academy of Nutrition and Dietetics, 120 South Riverside Plz., Ste. 2000, Chicago, IL 60606-6995, (312) 899-0040, (800) 877-1600, amacmunn@eatright.org, http://www.eatright.org.

Linus Pauling Institute, Oregon State University, 307 Linus Pauling Center, Corvallis, OR 97331, (541) 737-5075, Fax: (541) 737-5077, http://lpi.oregonstate.edu.

Office of Dietary Supplements, National Institutes of Health, 6100 Executive Blvd., Rm. 3B01, MSC 7517, Bethesda, MD 20892-7517, (301) 435-2920, Fax: (301) 480-1845, ods@nih.gov, http://ods.od.nih.gov.

Tish Davidson, AM

Folic acid *see* **Folate**

Food additives

Definition

The U.S. Food and Drug Administration (FDA) defines food additives as "any substance, the intended use of which results or may reasonably be expected to result, directly or indirectly, in its becoming a component or otherwise affecting the characteristics of any food." In other words, an additive is any substance that is added to food.

Purpose

Direct additives are those that are intentionally added to foods for a specific purpose, such as coloring. Indirect additives are those to which the food is exposed during processing, packaging, or storing. Preservatives are additives that inhibit the growth of bacteria, yeasts, and molds in foods.

Description

Additives and preservatives have been used in foods for centuries. When meats are smoked to preserve them, compounds such as butylated hydroxyanisole (BHA) and butyl gallate are formed and provide both antioxidant and bacteriostatic effects. Salt has also been used as a preservative for centuries. Salt lowers the water activity of meats and other foods and inhibits bacterial growth. Excess water in foods can enhance the growth of bacteria, yeast, and fungi. Pickling, which involves the addition of acids, such as vinegar, increases the acidity (lowers the pH) of foods to levels that slow bacterial growth. Some herbs and spices, such as curry, cinnamon, and chili pepper, also contain **antioxidants** and may provide bactericidal effects.

Uses of additives and preservatives in foods

Additives and preservatives are used to maintain product consistency and quality, improve or maintain nutritional value, maintain palatability and wholesomeness, provide leavening, control pH, enhance flavor, or provide color. Classes of food additives include:

- Antimicrobial agents prevent spoilage of food by mold or microorganisms. These include not only vinegar and salt but also compounds such as calcium propionate and sorbic acid, which are used in products such as baked goods, salad dressings, cheeses, margarines, and pickled foods.
- Antioxidants prevent rancidity in foods containing fats and damage to foods caused by oxygen. Examples of antioxidants include vitamin C, vitamin E, BHA, BHT (butylated hydroxytoluene), and propyl gallate.

- Artificial colors are intended to make food more appealing and to provide certain foods with coloring more indicative of their flavor (e.g., red for cherry, green for lime).
- Artificial flavors and flavor enhancers are the largest class of additives, and their function is to make foods taste better or to give them a specific taste. Examples are salt, sugar, and vanilla, which are used to complement the flavor of certain foods. Synthetic flavoring agents, such as benzaldehyde for cherry or almond flavor, may be used to simulate natural flavors. Flavor enhancers, such as monosodium glutamate (MSG), intensify the flavor of other compounds in a food.
- Bleaching agents such as peroxides are used to whiten foods, such as wheat flour and cheese.
- Chelating agents are used to prevent discoloration, flavor changes, and rancidity that might occur during the processing of foods. Examples are citric acid, malic acid, and tartaric acid.
- Nutrient additives include vitamins and minerals and are added to foods during enrichment or fortification. For example, milk is fortified with vitamin D, and rice is enriched with thiamin, riboflavin, and niacin.
- Thickening and stabilizing agents function to alter the texture of a food. Examples include the emulsifier lecithin, which keeps oil and vinegar blended in salad dressings, and carrageen, which is used as a thickener in ice creams and low-calorie jellies.

Regulating safety of food additives and preservatives

Based on the 1958 Food Additives Amendment to the Federal Food, Drug, and Cosmetic (FD&C) Act of 1938, the FDA must approve the use of all additives. Manufacturers bear the responsibility of proving that additives are safe for their intended uses. The Food Additives Amendment excluded additives and preservatives deemed safe for consumption before 1958, such as salt, **sugar**, spices, **vitamins**, vinegar, and monosodium glutamate. These substances are considered "generally recognized as safe" (GRAS) and may be used in any food, although the FDA may remove additives from the GRAS list if safety concerns arise. The 1960 Color Additives Amendment to the FD&C Act required the FDA to approve synthetic coloring agents used in foods, drugs, cosmetics, and certain medical devices. The Delaney Clause, which was included in both the Food Additives Amendment and Color Additives Amendment, prohibited approval of any additive that had been found to cause **cancer** in humans or animals. However, in 1996, the Delaney Clause was modified, and the commissioner of the FDA was charged with assessing the risk from

Food additives

Types of ingredients	What they do	Examples of uses	Names found on product labels
Preservatives	Prevent food spoilage from bacteria, molds, fungi, or yeast (antimicrobials); slow or prevent changes in color, flavor, or texture and delay rancidity (antioxidants); maintain freshness	Fruit sauces and jellies, beverages, baked goods, cured meats, oils and margarines, cereals, dressings, snack foods, fruits and vegetables	Ascorbic acid, citric acid, sodium benzoate, calcium propionate, sodium erythorbate, sodium nitrite, calcium sorbate, potassium sorbate, BHA, BHT, EDTA, tocopherols (Vitamin E)
Sweeteners	Add sweetness with or without the extra calories	Beverages, baked goods, confections, table-top sugar, substitutes, many processed foods	Sucrose (sugar), glucose, fructose, sorbitol, mannitol, corn syrup, high fructose corn syrup, saccharin, aspartame, sucralose, acesulfame potassium (acesulfame-K), neotame
Color additives	Offset color loss due to exposure to light, air, temperature extremes, moisture, and storage conditions; correct natural variations in color; enhance colors that occur naturally; provide color to colorless and "fun" foods	Many processed foods (candies, snack foods, margarine, cheese, soft drinks, jams/jellies, gelatins, pudding and pie fillings)	FD&C Blue Nos. 1 and 2, FD&C Green No. 3, FD&C Red Nos. 3 and 40, FD&C Yellow Nos. 5 and 6, Orange B, Citrus Red No. 2, annatto extract, beta-carotene, grape skin extract, cochineal extract or carmine, paprika oleoresin, caramel color, fruit and vegetable juices, saffron (Note: Exempt color additives are not required to be declared by name on labels but may be declared simply as colorings or color added)
Flavors and spices	Add specific flavors (natural and synthetic)	Pudding and pie fillings, gelatin dessert mixes, cake mixes, salad dressings, candies, soft drinks, ice cream, BBQ sauce	Natural flavoring, artificial flavor, and spices
Flavor enhancers	Enhance flavors already present in foods (without providing their own separate flavor)	Many processed foods	Monosodium glutamate (MSG), hydrolyzed soy protein, autolyzed yeast extract, disodium guanylate or inosinate
Fat replacers (and components of formulations used to replace fats)	Provide expected texture in reduced-fat foods	Baked goods, dressings, frozen desserts, confections, cake and dessert mixes, dairy products	Olestra, cellulose gel, carrageenan, polydextrose, modified food starch, microparticulated egg white protein, guar gum, xanthan gum, whey protein concentrate

[continued]

(Table by PreMediaGlobal. © 2013 Cengage Learning.)

consumption of additives that may cause cancer and making a determination as to the use of those additives.

In the United States, food additives and preservatives play an important role in ensuring that the food supply remains the safest and most abundant in the world. Despite consumer concerns about use of food additives and preservatives, there is very little scientific evidence that they are harmful at the levels at which they are used.

In Europe, food additives and preservatives are evaluated by the European Commission's Scientific Committee on Food. Regulations in the European Union countries are similar to those in the United States. The Food and Agricultural Organization (FAO) of the United Nations and the World Health Organization (WHO) Expert Committee on Food Additives work together to evaluate the safety of food additives, as well as contaminants, naturally occurring toxicants, and residues of veterinary drugs in foods. Acceptable Daily Intakes (ADIs) are established on the basis of toxicology and other information.

Precautions

Food additives can induce a wide range of adverse reactions in sensitive individuals. A prevalence of 0.03% to 0.23% is estimated. Before any substance can be added to food, the Food Safety and Inspection Service (FSIS) of the U.S. Department of Agriculture (USDA) share responsibility with the FDA to ensure the safety of food additives used in meat, poultry, and egg products. Initially, all additives are evaluated for safety by FDA.

Types of ingredients	What they do	Examples of uses	Names found on product labels
Nutrients	Replace vitamins and minerals lost in processing (enrichment), add nutrients that may be lacking in the diet (fortification)	Flour, breads, cereals, rice, macaroni, margarine, salt, milk, fruit beverages, energy bars, instant breakfast drinks	Thiamine hydrochloride, riboflavin (Vitamin B2), niacin, niacinamide, folate or folic acid, beta carotene, potassium iodide, iron or ferrous sulfate, alpha tocopherols, ascorbic acid, Vitamin D, amino acids (L-tryptophan, L-lysine, L-leucine, L-methionine)
Emulsifiers	Allow smooth mixing of ingredients, prevent separation, keep emulsified products stable, reduce stickiness, control crystallization, keep ingredients dispersed, help products dissolve more easily	Salad dressings, peanut butter, chocolate, margarine, frozen desserts	Soy lecithin, mono- and diglycerides, egg yolks, polysorbates, sorbitan monostearate
Stabilizers and thickeners, binders, texturizers	Produce uniform texture, improve texture	Frozen desserts, dairy products, cakes, pudding and gelatin mixes, dressings, jams and jellies, sauces	Gelatin, pectin, guar gum, carrageenan, xanthan gum, whey
pH Control agents and acidulants	Control acidity and alkalinity, prevent spoilage	Beverages, frozen desserts, chocolate, low-acid canned foods, baking powder	Lactic acid, citric acid, ammonium hydroxide, sodium carbonate
Leavening agents	Promote rising of baked goods	Breads and other baked goods	Baking soda, monocalcium phosphate, calcium carbonate
Anti-caking agents	Keep powdered foods from clumping, prevent moisture absorption	Salt, baking powder, confectioner's sugar	Calcium silicate, iron ammonium citrate, silicon dioxide
Humectants	Retain moisture	Shredded coconut, marshmallows, soft candies, confections	Glycerin, sorbitol
Yeast nutrients	Promote growth of yeast	Breads and other baked goods	Calcium sulfate, ammonium phosphate
Dough strengtheners and conditioners	Produce more stable dough	Breads and other baked goods	Ammonium sulfate, azodicarbonamide, L-cysteine
Firming agents	Maintain crispness and firmness	Processed fruits and vegetables	Calcium chloride, calcium lactate
Enzyme preparations	Modify proteins, polysaccharides, and fats	Cheese, dairy products, meat	Enzymes, lactase, papain, rennet, chymosin
Gases	Serve as propellant, aerate, or create carbonation	Oil cooking spray, whipped cream, carbonated beverages	Carbon dioxide, nitrous oxide

SOURCE: Center for Food Safety and Applied Nutrition, Food and Drug Administration, U.S. Department of Health and Human Services.

(Table by PreMediaGlobal. © 2013 Cengage Learning.)

Safe is defined by Congress as "reasonable certainty that no harm will result from use" of an additive in the food supply. Substances that are found to be harmful to either people or animals may be allowed as an additive, but only at the level of 1/100th of the amount that is considered harmful. This margin of safety is intended as a protection for the consumer by limiting the intake of dangerous substances. For example, some people are allergic to certain food additives, and their reaction can be mild or very severe when consumed.

Interactions

Nitrites are a controversial additive. When used in combination with salt, nitrites serve as antimicrobials and add flavor and color to meats. However, nitrite salts can react with certain amines in food to produce nitrosamines, many of which are known carcinogens. Food manufacturers must show that nitrosamines will not form in harmful amounts, or will be prevented from forming, in their products.

The flavoring enhancer MSG is another controversial food additive. MSG is made commercially from a natural fermentation process using starch and sugar. Despite anecdotal reports of MSG triggering headaches or exacerbating asthma, the Joint Expert Committee on Food Additives of the FAO, WHO, the European Commission's Scientific Committee for Food, the American Medical Association, and the National Academy of Sciences have all affirmed the safety of MSG at normal consumption levels.

Another controversial additive is ammonia, which is present in very small amounts in a number of foods, including ground beef and cheese. Ammonium hydroxide has been considered GRAS by the FDA since 1974, but many consumers are unaware of its presence in foods. If a substance is used during processing and is not considered to be part of the product, it is not required to be listed as an ingredient on the label.

KEY TERMS

Bacteria—Single-celled organisms without nuclei, some of which are infectious.

Bactericidal—A state that prevents growth of bacteria.

Bacteriostatic—A substance that kills bacteria.

Carcinogen—A cancer-causing substance.

Enrichment—The addition of vitamins and minerals to improve the nutritional content of a food.

Fermentation—A reaction performed by yeast or bacteria to make alcohol.

Fortification—The addition of vitamins and minerals to improve the nutritional content of a food.

Leavening—Yeast or other agents used for rising bread.

Microorganism—Bacteria and protists; single-celled organisms.

Complications

There are numerous difficulties that may be encountered by the FDA in assessing potential harm that may come from food additives. These are due to the inadequacies and complications of animal models and the variability of human exposure and reporting of adverse reactions. Typically, testing for food additive toxicity is designed so that the additive is administered to an animal model for the life of that animal in a range of doses, of which the highest dose is much greater than that expected to occur during the course of human exposure. It is also too complicated to predict all of the possible interactions or reactions that can occur with any given food additive, such as from the packaging, the heating or cooling process, other additions to the food, or consumption of the food.

The FDA continually monitors the safety of all food additives as new scientific evidence becomes available. For example, use of erythrosine (FD&C Red No. 3) in cosmetics and externally applied drugs was banned in 1990 after it was implicated in the development of thyroid tumors in male rats. However, the cancer risk associated with FD&C Red No. 3 is about 1 in 100,000 over a 70-year lifetime, and its use in some foods, such as candies and maraschino cherries, is still allowed. Tartrazine (FD&C Yellow No. 5) has been found to cause dermatological reactions ranging from itching to hives in a small population subgroup. Given the mild nature of the reaction, however, it still may be used in foods. In 2012, consumer groups, such as the

Center for Science in the Public Interest (CSPI), were seeking a ban on caramel coloring used in soft drinks (4-methylimidazole) due to its potential risk as a carcinogen. However, this claim was based on study of mice, and re-evaluations of the additive by the European Food Safety Authority did not find any risk to humans.

Resources

BOOKS

Minich, Deanna. *An A–Z Guide to Food Additives: Never Eat What You Can't Pronounce*. San Francisco: Conari Press, 2012.

Smith, Jim, Lily Hong-Shum. *A Consumer's Food Additive Data Book*. 2nd ed. Wiley-Blackwell, 2011.

Taub-Dix, Bonnie. *Read it Before You Eat it: How to Decode Food Labels and Make the Healthiest Choice Every Time*. New York: Penguin Group, 2010.

WEBSITES

European Commission, Directorate General for Health and Consumers. "Food Additives." http://ec.europa.eu/food/food/fAEF/additives/index_en.htm (accessed July 9, 2012).

Food Safety and Inspection Service. "Additives in Meat and Poultry Products." U.S. Department of Agriculture. http://www.fsis.usda.gov/Fact%5FSheets/Additives_in_Meat_&_Poultry_Products/index.asp (accessed July 9, 2012).

Geller, Martinne. "Ammonia Used in Many Foods, not Just 'Pink Slime.'" MSNBC.com. http://www.msnbc.msn.com/id/46958231/ns/health-diet_and_nutrition (accessed July 9, 2012).

International Food Information Council Foundation. "Questions and Answers about Caramel Coloring and 4-methylimidazole (4-MEI or 4-MI)." FoodInsight.org. http://www.foodinsight.org/Resources/Detail.aspx?topic=Questions_and_Answers_about_4_MEI (accessed July 9, 2012).

———. "The Rigorous Road to Food Ingredient Approval." FoodInsight.org. http://www.foodinsight.org/Newsletter/Detail.aspx?topic=The_Rigorous_Road_to_Food_Ingredient_Approval (accessed July 9, 2012).

Lembert, Phil. "The 5 Things you Need to Know About Deli Meats." TODAY Food, MSNBC.com. http://today.msnbc.msn.com/id/16361276/ns/today-food/t/things-you-need-know-about-deli-meats (accessed July 9, 2012).

U.S. Food and Drug Administration. "Color Additives." http://www.fda.gov/ForIndustry/ColorAdditives/default.htm (accessed July 9, 2012).

———. "Food Additives." http://www.fda.gov/food/foodingredientspackaging/foodadditives/default.htm (accessed July 9, 2011).

———. "Generally Recognized as Safe (GRAS)." http://www.fda.gov/Food/FoodIngredientsPackaging/GenerallyRecognizedas SafeGRAS/default.htm (accessed July 9, 2012).

ORGANIZATIONS

Center for Food Safety and Applied Nutrition (CFSAN), U.S. Food and Drug Administration, 5100 Paint Branch Pkwy., College Park, MD 20740, (888) SAFE-FOOD (723-3366), consumer@fda.gov, http://www.fda.gov/Food/default.htm.

European Commission, Directorate General for Health and Consumers, B-1049, Brussels, Belgium, 011 32 (2) 299-11-11, http://ec.europa.eu/dgs/health_consumer/index_en.htm.

Food Allergy and Anaphylaxis Network (FAAN), 11781 Lee Jackson Hwy., Ste. 160, Fairfax, VA 22033, (800) 929-4040, Fax: (703) 691-2713, faan@foodallergy.org, http://www.foodallergy.org.

Food and Nutrition Information Center, National Agricultural Library, 10301 Baltimore Ave., Rm. 105, Beltsville, MD 20705, (301) 504-5414, Fax: (301) 504-6409, fnic@ars.usda.gov, http://fnic.nal.usda.gov.

Food Safety and Inspection Service (FSIS), U.S. Department of Agriculture (USDA), 1400 Independence Ave. SW, Washington, DC 20250-3700, (888) 674-6854 (USDA Meat and Poultry Consumer Hotline), MPHotline.fsis@usda.gov, http://www.fsis.usda.gov.

Institute of Food Technologies, 525 W. Van Buren, Ste. 1000, Chicago, IL 60607, (312) 782-8424, Fax: (312) 792-8348, info@ift.org, http://www.ift.org.

International Food Information Council Foundation, 1100 Connecticut Ave., NW Ste. 430, Washington, DC 20036, (202) 296-6540, info@foodinsight.org, http://www.foodinsight.org.

U.S. Food and Drug Administration (FDA), 10903 New Hampshire Ave., Silver Spring, MD 20993, (888) 463-6332, http://www.fda.gov.

M. Elizabeth Kunkel
Tish Davidson, AM
Megan Porter, RD

Food allergies

Definition

Food allergies are the body's abnormal response to specific proteins found in food. These proteins normally are harmless but cause a reaction in some people. They can occur when food is either eaten or touched.

Demographics

About one-quarter of American households have a member with a food allergy. However, this statistic is derived from self-reported information rather than rigorous studies. Many people use the term "food allergy" to describe what is actually a food intolerance. A food intolerance is a reaction to food that does not involve

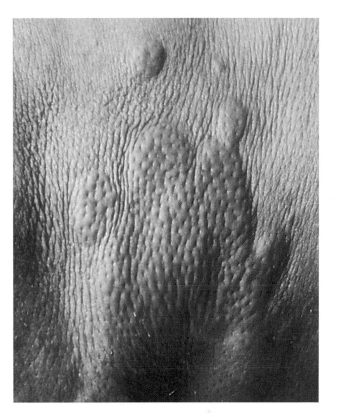

Hives on the back of a young woman's legs. The accompanying inflammation develops as an allergic reaction. The hives range in size from small spots to patches measuring several inches across. *(Caliendo/Custom Medical Stock Photography)*

the immune system. Lactose intolerance is a common food intolerance, while **celiac disease** is a food allergy.

Eight foods cause 90% of all food allergies. These are:

- milk
- eggs
- peanuts
- tree nuts (walnuts, cashews, pecans, almonds, etc.)
- fish
- shellfish
- soy
- wheat

Description

All food contains proteins that enter the body when the food is eaten, or in some cases if it is touched. Allergic reaction occurs when the body responds to these normally benign proteins as if they were harmful. The first time the food is consumed, the body reacts with an abnormal biological alarm. As the food is

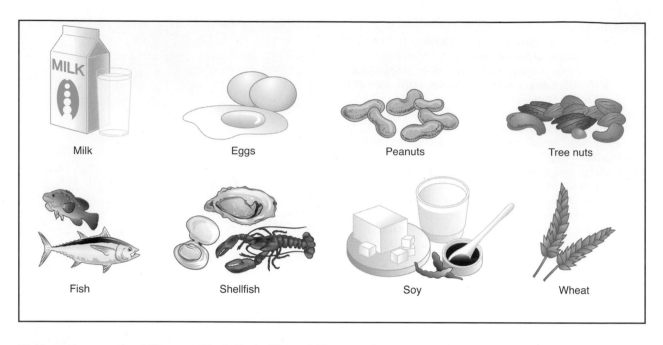

Eight most common food allergens. *(Illustration by Electronic Illustrators Group. © 2013 Cengage Learning.)*

digested and broken down into proteins that enter the bloodstream, protective cells, called antibodies, are formed. Usually, antibodies are used to attack germs, such as bacteria or viruses, that invade the body. In this case, antibodies protect from disease by destroying the germs. Antibodies prompt other reactions in the body, such as a fever to kill disease cells or the dilating of blood cells so that blood can reach infected areas of the body more rapidly.

The second time the food is ingested, the antibodies alert the body that an invader is present, and the body mounts an attack. The body's response causes the symptoms of an allergic reaction.

Causes and symptoms

When the body encounters an allergen, it releases large amounts of a chemical called histamine. This release of histamine is responsible for allergic symptoms. Symptoms of food allergy can range from mildly annoying to dangerous and life threatening. These symptoms include:

- tingling of the mouth
- tingling or numbness in arms or legs
- skin rash or hives
- itching
- abdominal cramps
- vomiting
- diarrhea

- breathing difficulties
- sudden drop in blood pressure (hypotension)
- swelling of the tongue
- swelling of the face and throat
- loss of consciousness
- death

The most serious symptom of food allergy is anaphylaxis. Anaphylaxis, also called anaphylactic shock, is a sudden and potentially life threatening allergic reaction in which the whole body reacts to an allergen. During anaphylaxis, the airway constricts, making breathing difficult. Swelling of the throat may block airways as well. Vomiting and diarrhea may occur. The face may swell and the skin may become itchy with a rash or hives. The heart may race and the heartbeat may become irregular.

Diagnosis

The offending food must be identified if food allergy reactions are to be avoided. To identify food allergies, a doctor will first record the patient's detailed medical history. It is a good idea for patients to keep a food diary documenting all foods eaten and when, as well as any physical symptoms and when they occurred. In most cases, patterns of reactions to specific foods can be seen in the food diary.

Other means of diagnosing food allergies include:

- Blood tests (RAST, CAP–RAST). In a blood test, a sample of blood is drawn and antibodies in the blood

Foods that may contain common allergens

Allergen	Food product
Milk	Butter (including butter flavor, butter fat, and butter oil)
	Buttermilk
	Casein
	Casemates
	Cheese
	Cream
	Cottage cheese
	Custard
	Ghee
	Goat milk
	Milk proteins (lactalbumin, lactalbumin phosphate, lactoglobulin, lactulose)
	Milk solids
	Pudding
	Sour cream
	Yogurt
Eggs	Albumin or albumen
	Eggnog
	Lecithin
	Lysozyme
	Marshmallows
	Marzipan
	Mayonnaise
	Meringue
	Nougat
	Pasta
	Surimi (fish product)
Peanuts	Any nut product (including nut butters and oils)
	Ethnic foods (especially African, Chinese, Indonesian, Mexican, Thai, and Vietnamese dishes)
	Many candies and baked goods
	Nougat
	Sunflower seeds

(Table by PreMediaGlobal. © 2013 Cengage Learning.)

are measured. These antibodies form in response to specific foods and occur only after the body has had an allergic reaction. An IgE test measures the level of Immunoglobulin E (IgE), which is specific for each food. Individual food allergies may be identified by this test.

- Skin tests. In a skin allergy test, a small amount of extract of a food that is suspected of causing an allergic reaction is placed on the skin. The skin is then scratched in that area and observed for reaction. If an allergy exists, a small bump (similar to a mosquito bite) will appear, usually within 15 minutes. The skin test is a rapid way to see if a food allergy exists.

- Food challenge. This is a food test in which neither the testing doctor nor the patient knows what food is given. Opaque capsules are filled (by an assistant or another doctor) with foods that are suspected of causing allergies and foods that are not. The capsules prevent the patient from tasting or smelling the food.

The patient swallows a capsule, and the doctor observes to see if a reaction occurs. This method of diagnosis is not appropriate for a person who has had a severe allergic reaction. It is time consuming and is usually performed when a doctor suspects the allergic reaction is not being caused by food. The test can rule out food as a cause for allergic reactions.

- Elimination diet. Similar to the food challenge, elimination diets help to determine which foods are responsible for allergy symptoms. All suspected foods are removed from the diet and then gradually added back in one at a time, to see which food item (if any) produces a response. Elimination diets may also discover food intolerances or sensitivities. They should not be used if the person has had a severe allergic reaction.

Treatment

Treatment for an allergic reaction is administration of an antihistamine drug. The most common antihistamine is diphenhydramine hydrochloride, which is found in over-the-counter drugs, such as Benadryl, and in some prescription drugs. If taken immediately, antihistamines can stop or moderate an allergic reaction.

In cases of a severe allergy or anaphylaxis, an injection of a strong antihistamine called epinephrine (also known as adrenaline) may be used. An auto-injectable form of epinephrine (Epi-Pen) that looks similar to a large ballpoint pen can be carried at all times if a person has a history of severe allergy. If a severe allergic reaction occurs, the auto-injector is held against the skin and the medication is self-administered as a shot. Epinephrine is a strong antihistamine; it often can stop anaphylaxis symptoms.

Nutrition and dietary concerns

A doctor and nutritionist should be consulted if a food allergy is suspected. Removing foods from the diet can cause an unbalanced diet that may be deficient in necessary nutrients. Since some of the most common foods that cause allergies include milk, eggs, and wheat, significant sources of **protein**, **calcium**, and **fiber** may be removed. With the assistance of healthcare professionals, diets can be modified and healthy substitutions identified to avoid nutrient deficiencies.

Individuals following a special diet to treat other medical conditions should always consult a doctor before altering that diet. Eliminating foods from a medically prescribed diet may aggravate an existing health condition and could be harmful.

Prognosis

There is no cure for food allergies, but allergic reactions can be prevented by avoiding food(s) that cause an allergic response.

Prevention

It is essential that individuals with serious food allergies read the labels of every food they eat. A federal law called the Food Allergen Labeling and Consumer Protection Act (FALPCA) took effect on January 1, 2006. This law mandates that all food containing milk, eggs, fish, crustacean shell fish, peanuts, tree nuts, wheat, or **soy** must note this on the label.

Ingredients that may cause allergies are listed on the label after the word "Contains." If these ingredients have names that are not readily known as versions of foods that may cause allergic reactions, the manufacturer will list the allergen in parentheses—for example, albumin (egg) or casein (milk). Additives for coloring or texture that may cause allergic reactions must also be listed.

Most individuals with food allergies are allergic to only one food; however, a peanut allergy may indicate reaction to tree nuts as well. Many manufacturers who process peanut products, process other nut products as well. Machines that handle and package these products may spread small pieces of peanut to other products. The FALPCA mandates that labels note this fact.

Resources

BOOKS

Hand, Carol. *Living with Food Allergies*. Minneapolis, MN: ABDO, 2012.

Nelson, Carmel and Amra Ibrisimovic. *The Food Allergy Cookbook: A Guide to Living with Allergies and Entertaining with Healthy, Delicious Meals*. New York: Skyhorse, 2011.

Welch, Michael J., ed. *Allergies and Asthma: What Every Parent Needs to Know*. 2nd ed. Elk Grove Village, IL: American Academy of Pediatrics, 2011.

WEBSITES

Li, James T.C. "What's the Difference between a Food Intolerance and Food Allergy?" MayoClinic.com. http://www.mayoclinic.com/health/food-allergy/AN01109 (accessed August 13, 2012).

MedlinePlus. "Food Allergy." U.S. National Library of Medicine, National Institutes of Health. http://www.nlm.nih.gov/medlineplus/foodallergy.html (accessed August 13, 2012).

Sicherer, Scott H. "Food Allergies." Medscape Reference. http://emedicine.medscape.com/article/135959-overview (accessed August 13, 2012).

ORGANIZATIONS

Allergy and Asthma Network: Mothers of Asthmatics (AANMA), 8201 Greensboro Dr., Ste. 300, McLean, VA 22102, (800) 878-4403, Fax: (703) 288-5217, http://www.aanma.org.

American Academy of Allergy, Asthma, and Immunology (AAAAI), 555 E Wells St., Ste. 1100, Milwaukee, WI 53202, (414) 272-6071, http://www.aaaai.org.

Asthma and Allergy Foundation of America, 8201 Corporate Dr., Ste. 1000, Landover, MD 20785, (800) 727-8462, info@aafa.org, http://www.aafa.org.

Food Allergy & Anaphylaxis Network, 11781 Lee Jackson Hwy., Ste. 160, Fairfax, VA 22033, (800) 929-4040, Fax: (703) 691-2713, http://www.foodallergy.org.

National Institute of Allergy and Infectious Diseases, Office of Communications and Government Relations, 6610 Rockledge Dr., MSC 6612, Bethesda, MD 20892, (301) 496-5717, TTY: (800) 877-8339, (866) 284-4107, Fax: (301) 402-3573, http://www3.niaid.nih.gov.

Deborah Nurmi, MS
Tish Davidson, AM

Food combining *see* **Hay diet**

Food contamination

Definition

Food contamination occurs when potentially harmful substances render food unsafe for consumption. Microorganisms—viruses, bacteria, and parasites—are the most common food contaminants. Naturally occurring or man-made chemicals can also contaminate food.

Demographics

Although widespread contamination is relatively rare in the United States, food contamination remains a serious public health concern throughout the world. In 2011, the U.S. Centers for Disease Control and Prevention (CDC) reported that about 48 million Americans—one in six—suffer the effects of food contamination every year, accounting for 128,000 hospitalizations and 3,000 deaths annually.

While disease-causing microorganisms are by far the most common contaminants in food, naturally occurring toxins sometimes contaminate shellfish and other organisms. Food can also be contaminated with heavy metals, man-made chemicals such as pesticides and herbicides, and radioactive **iodine** and cesium from nuclear accidents, such as the 2011 Fukushima Daiichi nuclear power plant disaster in Japan.

Although most food contamination is unintentional, sometimes contaminants are introduced as a means of "stretching" or extending the life of a product. Bioterrorism experts worry that disease-causing organisms or toxic chemicals could be intentionally introduced into food or water supplies to cause mass contamination. Scientists also worry that climate change may increase the risk of contamination of crops and seafood from biotoxins, pathogenic microbes, pesticides, and other chemicals.

Description

Of the more than 250 identified foodborne diseases, most are caused by pathogenic microorganisms. For example, the U.S. Food and Drug Administration (FDA) estimates that 90% of purchased raw poultry carries some disease-causing bacteria. Most pathogenic food contaminants originate from animal or human feces, and food contamination is directly responsible for many infectious **digestive diseases**.

In the United States, most food contamination is caused by one of eight pathogens:

- Noroviruses are responsible for 58% of illnesses and 11% of deaths from identified food contaminants. Unlike other foodborne pathogens, noroviruses are spread primarily by infected people, especially food-service workers. Noroviruses have been responsible for major outbreaks of foodborne illness on cruise ships and in nursing homes.

- *Salmonella* spp. are widespread intestinal bacteria that cause salmonellosis, a major cause of illness and death from food contamination.

- *Clostridium perfringens* is found throughout the environment, including human and animal intestines, and is common on raw meat and poultry.

- *Campylobacter* spp. are the most commonly identified cause of diarrheal illness worldwide. The bacteria live in the intestines of healthy birds and are found in most raw poultry. Undercooked chicken, foods contaminated with juices from raw chicken, and cross-contamination between raw and cooked foods are the most common sources of infection.

- *Staphylococcus aureus* is a bacterium in dust, air, and sewage. It is spread primarily through unsanitary food handling and can contaminate almost any food.

- *Toxoplasma gondii* is a single-celled parasite that causes toxoplasmosis, a potentially fatal condition that can result from consuming contaminated water or undercooked meat.

- *Escherichia coli* is a common, normally harmless bacterium in the human gut. However, some Shiga toxin-producing *E. coli* (STEC) strains, especially strain O157:H7, can cause severe food poisoning. O157:H7 is most often found in undercooked hamburger but has also contaminated produce and unpasteurized juice.

- *Listeria monocytogenes*, a ubiquitous bacterium in soil, groundwater, plants, and animals, can contaminate

---

Cutting boards and food safety

- **Type of boards**

  Choose either wood or a nonporous surface cutting board such as plastic, marble, glass, or pyroceramic. Nonporous surfaces are easier to clean than wood.

- **Avoid cross-contamination**

  Use one cutting board for fresh produce and bread and a separate one for raw meat, poultry, and seafood. This will prevent bacteria on a cutting board that is used for raw meat, poultry, or seafood from contaminating a food that requires no further cooking.

- **Cleaning cutting boards**

  To keep all cutting boards clean, wash them with hot, soapy water after each use; then rinse with clear water and air dry or pat dry with clean paper towels. Nonporous acrylic, plastic, or glass boards and solid wood boards can be washed in a dishwasher (laminated boards may crack and split).

  Both wooden and plastic cutting boards can be sanitized with a solution of 1 tablespoon of unscented, liquid chlorine bleach per gallon of water. Flood the surface with the bleach solution and allow it to stand for several minutes. Rinse with clear water and air dry or pat dry with clean paper towels.

- **Replace worn cutting boards**

  All plastic and wooden cutting boards wear out over time. Once cutting boards become excessively worn or develop hard-to-clean grooves, they should be discarded.

SOURCE: Food Safety and Inspections Service, U.S. Department of Agriculture

(Table by GGS Information Services. © 2013 Cengage Learning.)

food and cause listeriosis. Listeriosis appears to be on the increase in the United States—in 2011, at least 29 people died and at least 139 people across 28 states were sickened from eating contaminated cantaloupe that was traced to unsanitary conditions and poor handling at a single Colorado farm.

Other pathogenic food contaminants are serious problems worldwide:

- *Clostridium botulinum* is a rare bacterium that can contaminate food with a deadly paralytic nerve toxin called botulinum. Botulism is associated with improperly canned food, especially home-canned products, smoked fish, and honey.

- *Shigella* is a bacterial family that is a common cause of diarrhea in developing countries.

- *Vibrio cholera* is a fecal bacterial contaminant of food and water that is endemic in many parts of the world and causes deadly cholera outbreaks.

- *Vibrio vulnificus* and *Vibrio parahaemolyticus* are ocean bacteria that can contaminate filter-feeding shellfish such as oysters.

- *Yersinia enterocolitica* is a bacterium that can contaminate water, raw milk, and meat.

- Rotavirus is a major cause of diarrhea and death in infants and children.
- Hepatitis A virus can contaminate food.
- *Giardia lamblia* and *Cryptosporidium parvum* are intestinal parasites that contaminate water.
- *Entamoeba histolytica* is a parasite transmitted by contaminated water that causes amoebic dysentery and is prevalent in developing nations.
- *Cyclospora cayetanensis* is an emerging foodborne parasite.
- *Trichinella spiralis*, contracted from undercooked pork and wild game, is an intestinal roundworm that invades human muscle.
- *Taenia* spp. are parasitic tapeworms contracted from beef and pork.

Seafood contamination

Seafood can be contaminated in various ways, including via agricultural and other runoff, sewage, natural toxins, mercury, and chemical pollutants in water and the food chain. Filter-feeding shellfish, such as oysters, clams, scallops, and mussels, can accumulate toxins. Scombroid is caused by chemicals produced by bacteria in fish that are not refrigerated or frozen immediately.

Toxins associated with algal blooms called red and brown tides can accumulate in fish and shellfish:

- Ciguatera fish poisoning is caused by ciguatoxin or maitotoxin produced by various algal species.
- Paralytic shellfish poisoning (PSP) is caused by saxitoxins from several different red tide dinoflagellates.
- Neurotoxic shellfish poisoning is caused by brevetoxins from *Karenia brevis*, a dinoflagellate that accumulates in oysters, mussels, and clams.
- Amnesic shellfish poisoning is caused by domoic acid from *Pseudonitzschia* spp. of diatoms.

Causes and symptoms

Causes

Food can be contaminated at any point in the production chain—in the field, through animal feed, in the slaughterhouse or processing plant, during transport, in markets and restaurants, or in the home kitchen. Sources include:

- application of illegal or higher-than-approved pesticides or herbicides to crops
- waste disposal on agricultural land
- bacteria on growing fruits and vegetables

- molds and their toxic products that develop in grains during growth, harvesting, or storage

- during processing, improper handling of raw materials, contaminated water, inadequate or improper disinfection, equipment malfunctions, inadequate temperatures, rodent or insect infestations, or contamination with poisons used to control pests

- during transportation and storage, improper temperatures, inappropriate use of fumigants, inadequate sanitization of food-carrying tanker trucks, or contamination with insects or rodent droppings

- in stores and restaurants, improper temperatures, cross-contamination between raw and cooked foods, improper disinfection of food-preparation surfaces, transmission by infected food handlers, or improper hand washing by food handlers

- in the home, unhygienic food handling, food left at room temperature, inadequate cooking, cross-contamination between raw and cooked foods, or failure to properly reheat leftovers

Although any food can be contaminated, raw or undercooked meat, poultry, eggs, fish, and raw (unpasteurized) milk are the most common. Processed foods that pool ingredients from multiple sources are particularly prone to contamination. Washing raw fruits and vegetables reduces but does not eliminate contaminants. Improperly canned foods, luncheon and deli meats, soft cheeses, and any products containing raw eggs are subject to contamination. A few bacteria in alfalfa or bean seeds can multiply to contaminate an entire batch of sprouts. Refrigeration or freezing generally prevents bacteria from multiplying. However, *L. monocytogenes* and *Y. enterocolitica* can grow and multiply at refrigerator temperatures. High levels of salt, **sugar**, or acid prevent bacteria from growing in preserved foods and thorough cooking kills pathogenic microorganisms.

Symptoms

Although symptoms of food contamination depend on the type, abdominal pain and cramps, diarrhea, nausea, and vomiting are most common. After ingesting contaminated food, there is usually a delay before symptoms develop. However, symptoms of chemical **food poisoning** often appear very quickly, usually beginning with a tingling in the mouth, then in the arms and legs, followed by dizziness and possibly difficulty breathing. Symptoms of poisoning from man-made toxic chemicals that have accidentally contaminated food may develop rapidly or slowly and vary with the type of chemical and degree of exposure.

Treatment

Most illnesses caused by contaminated foods are mild and resolve on their own within one or a few days. Diarrhea and vomiting can cause **dehydration** if more fluids and salts (**electrolytes**) are lost than are taken in; oral medications, such as Ceralyte, Pedialyte, or Oralyte, can be used to replace fluid losses. An electrolyte replacement fluid can be made at home with one teaspoon of salt and four teaspoons of sugar per quart of water. Severe dehydration may require hospitalization and intravenous fluids. Drugs are sometimes prescribed to stop persistent vomiting. Over-the-counter medications to stop or slow diarrhea, such as Kaopectate, Pepto-Bismol, or Imodium, may provide some relief. Antibiotics are not usually required.

Botulism, shellfish poisoning, and chemical poisoning are medical emergencies. Botulism requires hospitalization, often in an intensive care unit. Adults are given botulism antitoxin if it can be administered within 72 hours of the appearance of symptoms. Patients may require mechanical ventilation to assist breathing, as well as intravenous feeding until the paralysis passes.

Prognosis

Most illnesses resulting from food contamination resolve quickly without complications. However, contaminated food can cause serious and potentially life-threatening complications, especially for the very young, the elderly, pregnant women and their unborn babies, and anyone with a weakened immune system. It is estimated that 2%–3% of acute illnesses from food contamination lead to secondary long-term illnesses and complications that may affect any part of the body, such as the joints, nervous system, kidneys, or heart. Listeriosis can be serious or even fatal in newborns, the elderly, and the immunocompromised and can cause miscarriage, stillbirth, or premature birth if contracted during pregnancy. *Campylobacter* infection can cause Guillain-Barré syndrome. STEC can cause hemolytic uremic syndrome (HUS), the most common cause of acute kidney failure in children. In the elderly, food contamination can even cause gastroenteritis-induced death.

Chemical food contamination is more likely to cause serious long-term health problems than the various forms of microbial contamination. Toxins in fish can cause permanent liver damage. Pesticides and other chemical contaminants can cause liver damage, kidney failure, and nervous system complications.

KEY TERMS

Botulism—A life-threatening paralytic illness from food contaminated with botulinum toxin from the bacterium *Clostridium botulinum*.

Campylobacter—A genus of bacteria that is found in almost all raw poultry.

Clostridium perfringens—A bacterium that is a common food contaminant.

Dehydration—The abnormal depletion of body fluids, as from vomiting and diarrhea.

Electrolytes—Ions—such as sodium, potassium, calcium, magnesium, chloride, phosphate, bicarbonate, and sulfate—that are dissolved in bodily fluids such as blood and regulate or affect most metabolic processes.

Gastroenteritis—Inflammation of the lining of the stomach and intestines.

Hemolytic uremic syndrome (HUS)—Kidney failure, usually in infants and young children, that can be caused by food contaminated with bacteria such as STEC or *Shigella*.

Listeriosis—Illness caused by food contaminated with the bacterium *Listeria monocytogenes*.

Norovirus—Norwalk virus; a large family of RNA viruses that are the most common cause of illness from contaminated food.

Parasite—An organism that survives by living with, on, or in another organism, usually to the detriment of the host.

Pathogen—A causative agent of disease, such as a bacteria, virus, or parasite.

Salmonellosis—Severe diarrhea caused by food contaminated with bacteria of the genus *Salmonella*.

Shiga toxin-producing E. coli (STEC)—Strains of the common, normally harmless, intestinal bacterium *Escherichia coli* that can contaminate food with Shiga toxin; *E. coli* O157:H7 is the most commonly identified STEC in North America.

spp.—Species.

Staphylococcus aureus—Staph; a bacteria that can contaminate food.

Toxoplasma gondii—A very common parasite that is a leading cause of death from food contamination; although it infects large numbers of people, *T. gondii* is usually dangerous only in immunocompromised patients and newly infected pregnant women.

Prevention

Avoiding food contamination requires vigilance at every level of the food-production process. Growers must use only approved pesticides and herbicides at no higher than recommended levels. Processors must use clean sources of water, regularly disinfect machinery, and use only safe pesticides around food. Canning requires high temperatures and pressure. Irradiation of meat and other foods destroys contaminating microbes. Bacterial toxins vary in their heat sensitivity. For example, although botulinum is completely inactivated by boiling, staphylococcal toxin is not.

Most food contamination is preventable, since the CDC estimates that about 97% of all poisonings from contaminated food result from improper food handling, such as undercooking or poor refrigeration. Simple precautions in restaurants, cafeterias, and home kitchens include:

- washing hands thoroughly with soap and water before, during, and after preparing food, and after using the bathroom or changing diapers
- preventing cross-contamination of foods by keeping hands, utensils, and food-preparation surfaces clean

- keeping raw foods, especially meat, poultry, fish, and shellfish, separated from ready-to-eat foods, such as fruits and vegetables
- washing all fruits and vegetables thoroughly before and after peeling
- discarding the outer leaves of lettuce and cabbage
- keeping foods above 140°F (60°C) or below 40°F (4°C)
- cooking food thoroughly to an internal temperature of 160°F (78°C), which kills most bacteria, viruses, and parasites
- cooking egg yolks until firm
- never placing cooked food on plates or surfaces that held raw food
- refrigerating or freezing perishable foods within two hours of purchasing or preparing them
- avoiding thawing and refreezing food
- defrosting food in the refrigerator, in cold water, or in a microwave and cooking immediately
- discarding any food or leftovers that have been at room temperature for more than two hours (or more than one hour in hot weather)

QUESTIONS TO ASK YOUR DOCTOR

- What are the best ways to avoid food contamination?
- Are there specific foods that I should avoid because of possible contamination?
- Should I avoid luncheon meats and fish during pregnancy?
- What type of oral rehydration fluid do you recommend for diarrhea and vomiting?
- Does illness from food contamination require medical attention?

- dividing large quantities of food into shallow containers to cool faster
- avoiding any suspect foods, such as raw meat, fish, and milk or unpasteurized juice and cider

As a general safety rule, "when in doubt, throw it out."

Parental concerns

Breastfeeding is the best way to protect infants from food contamination. Baby formula should never be left at room temperature and baby bottles must be kept clean and disinfected.

Infants and young children are particularly susceptible to dehydration from food contamination–induced diarrhea and vomiting, since they can lose water and electrolytes very quickly. Small sips of oral rehydration solution should be given to children as soon as vomiting or diarrhea begins. A physician should be consulted before giving antidiarrheal medicines to children.

Resources

BOOKS

Hewitt, Ben. *Making Supper Safe: One Man's Quest to Learn the Truth about Food Safety*. New York: Rodale, 2011.

Hwang, Andy, and Lihan Huang, eds. *Ready-to-Eat Foods: Microbial Concerns and Control Measures*. Boca Raton, FL: CRC, 2010.

Perrett, Heli. *The Safe Food Handbook: How to Make Smart Choices About Risky Food*. New York: Experiment, 2011.

PERIODICALS

"Don't Let Food Poisoning Spoil Your Picnic." *U.S. News & World Report* (May 2011). http://health.usnews.com/health-news/diet-fitness/diet/articles/2011/05/28/dont-let-food-poisoning-spoil-your-picnic (accessed July 9, 2012)

Dwoskin, Elizabeth. "Your Food Has Been Touched by Multitudes." *Bloomberg Businessweek*, August 29, 2011. http://www.businessweek.com/magazine/your-food-has-been-touched-by-multitudes-08252011.html (accessed July 9, 2012).

Kowalski, Kathiann. "How Safe is Your Food?" *Current Health Kids* 34, no. 7 (March 2011): 16–19.

Landro, Laura. "The Informed Patient: Food Illness and the Kitchen—Salmonella Infections Rose Last Year; Home Cooks Fail to Act Safely, Studies Say." *Wall Street Journal*, June 14, 2011, D3. http://online.wsj.com/article/SB10001424052702304665904576383582242952932.html (accessed July 9, 2012).

Lowenstein, Kate. "Not Safe to Eat." *Health* 25, no. 8 (October 2011): 86.

Park, Alice. "How to Stop the Superbugs." *Time*, June 20, 2011. http://www.time.com/time/magazine/article/0,9171,2076723,00.html (accessed July 9, 2012).

Rosenthal, Elisabeth. "My Salad, My Health." *New York Times*, June 12, 2011, WK3.

Tarshis, Lauren. "Delicious or DEADLY?" *Scholastic Scope* 60, no. 7 (January 9, 2012): 4–9.

"Tips for Safer Food." *Consumer Reports on Health* 23, no. 8 (August 2011): 8.

WEBSITES

American Academy of Family Physicians. "Food Poisoning." FamilyDoctor.org. http://familydoctor.org/familydoctor/en/diseases-conditions/food-poisoning.html (accessed July 9, 2012).

Centers for Disease Control and Prevention. "Questions and Answers About Foodborne Illness." National Center for Emerging and Zoonotic Infectious Diseases. http://www.cdc.gov/foodsafety/facts.html (accessed July 9, 2012).

Gammara, Roberto M. "Food Poisoning." Medscape Reference. http://emedicine.medscape.com/article/175569-overview (accessed July 9, 2012).

Mahon, Barbara. "Preventing Foodborne Illnesses." Centers for Disease Control and Prevention, Podcasts at CDC. April 15, 2010. http://www2c.cdc.gov/podcasts/player.asp?f=1266133 (accessed July 9, 2012).

MedlinePlus. "Foodborne Illness." http://www.nlm.nih.gov/medlineplus/foodborneillness.html (accessed July 9, 2012).

ORGANIZATIONS

National Agriculture Compliance Assistance Center, U.S. Environmental Protection Agency, 901 North 5th St., Kansas City, KS 66101, (888) 663-2155, Fax: (913) 551-7270, agcenter@epa.gov, http://www.epa.gov/agriculture.

Partnership for Food Safety Education, 2345 Crystal Dr., Ste. 800, Arlington, VA 22202, (202) 220-0651, Fax: (202) 220-0873, info@fightbac.org, http://www.fightbac.org.

U.S. Centers for Disease Control and Prevention, 1600 Clifton Rd., Atlanta, GA 30333, (800) CDC-INFO (232-4636), cdcinfo@cdc.gov, http://www.cdc.gov.

U.S. Department of Agriculture, 1400 Independence Ave. SW, Washington, DC 20250, (202) 720-2791, http://www.usda.gov/wps/portal/usdahome.

U.S. Food and Drug Administration, 10903 New Hampshire Ave., Silver Spring, MD 20993-0002, (888) INFO-FDA (463-6332), http://www.fda.gov.

Monique Laberge, PhD
Margaret Alic, PhD

Food intolerance *see* **Food sensitivities**

Food labeling

Definition

Responsibility for assuring that foods sold in the United States are safe relies on the U.S. Food and Drug Administration (FDA) who oversees that foods are wholesome and properly labeled. Foods produced both domestically, as well as foods from foreign countries, fall under the food labeling laws. The Federal Food, Drug, and Cosmetic Act (FD&C Act) and the Fair Packaging and Labeling Act are the federal laws governing food products under FDA's jurisdiction.

Purpose

Food labeling is designed to protect the health and well-being of consumers. It allows them to:

- know what ingredients are in a food or food product
- determine the relative amounts of each ingredient
- determine how much of selected vitamins, minerals, and other nutrients a food contains; this information may be given either by weight or as a percentage of a daily requirement value
- examine foods for potential allergens, additives, or ingredients that they wish to avoid
- learn about the conditions under which certain ingredients were produced (e.g., organic, free range)
- learn the country where the item was grown or raised
- compare the price per unit volume or weight of similar products
- determine if nutrients have been added or removed from the base food (e.g., enriched, reduced fat)

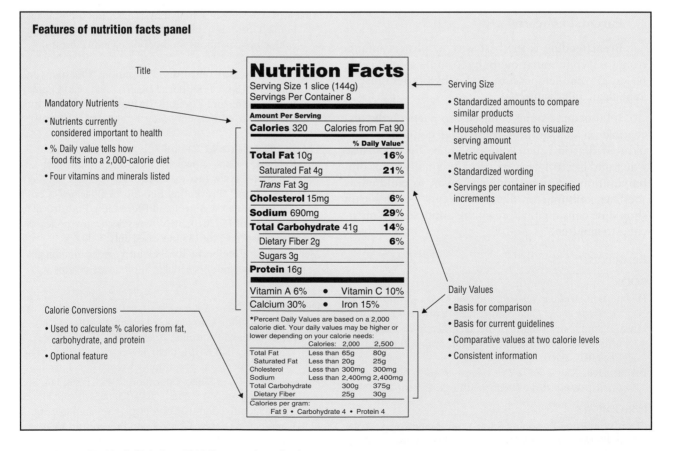

(Illustration by PreMediaGlobal. © 2013 Cengage Learning.)

Description

In the United States, food labeling is regulated by very specific, complex, and ever-evolving legislation. The U.S. Department of Agriculture (USDA) and the FDA are the federal agencies most involved with food-labeling issues and enforcement of food-labeling laws. The USDA is responsible for the labeling of meat, poultry, and egg products. The FDA regulates the labeling of most other foods, including seafood and **bioengineered foods**. The FDA also regulates **dietary supplements** and nutraceuticals. States also may regulate food labeling. For example, some states require sell-by or use-by information of food labels. When state and federal laws conflict, federal laws must be followed.

Different types of foods have different labeling requirements. For example, canned or frozen foods are required to have different information on their labels than fresh meat, poultry, and fish. Fresh vegetables must indicate their country of origin and additional labeling requirements if they are being sold as "organic" produce, other label information usually is voluntary. Legislation covers things as specific as the definitions of certain words used on the label (e.g., low fat), the size of the print used on the label, and where certain information must be placed on the package. Milk and milk products are often subject to additional regulation by state dairy boards. The federal Bureau of Alcohol, Tobacco, Firearms, and Explosives regulates labeling of alcoholic beverages. The U.S. Customs Service requires certain information on processed foods that are imported into the United States.

Basic mandatory information

Both the FDA and the USDA require certain information to be listed in English on the label of packaged food available for sale. This information includes:

- Name of the product. Laws regulating what some products may be called based on their content and processing. This explains why some substances that look like cheese are called "cheese food" or "processed cheese product," and some juice-like products are called "fruit drinks" or "fruit beverages" and not juice.

- Net quantity. This is the amount of food by weight in the package. It does not include the weight of the packaging. Meat and poultry labels are required to give the weight in imperial (avoirdupois) measures such as pounds or ounces. Other foods are required to give the weight in both English and metric (grams, kilograms) units.

- Serving size and number of servings the package contains.

- Nutrition facts. Calories, calories from fat, total fat, saturated fat, *trans* fat, cholesterol, sodium, total carbohydrates, dietary fiber, sugars, protein, vitamin A, vitamin C, calcium, and iron must be listed for a single serving of the food. This information is not required on fresh meat, fresh poultry, fresh seafood, or fresh fruit and vegetables.

- Ingredient list. Every ingredient must be listed in order from the greatest to least by weight. There are exceptions for certain artificial colors and flavorings, which may be listed generically by terms like "artificial coloring."

- Name of manufacturer or distributor. In some cases, a full street address is required.

- Country of origin. Imported foods must list the country of origin. Beginning in March 2009, fresh meats, poultry, fish, shellfish, and many fruits and vegetables were required to indicate their country of origin. Exceptions include vegetable mixtures, such as in bagged salads.

Supplemental required information

Certain foods are required to have additional information on the label:

- Foods containing the fat replacer olestra must state this on the label.

- Foods containing sorbitol or mannitol, both artificial sweeteners, must list the amount.

- Foods packaged under pressure must indicate that the contents are under pressure.

- Juices that have not been completely pasteurized must state that they have not been completely processed.

- Foods containing raw or not ready-to-eat meat or poultry products must be labeled as such.

- Juices must show the percentage of real juice that the product contains (e.g., 100% grapefruit juice).

- Foods enriched with vitamins and minerals must be labeled as such and specify the added nutrient(s).

Optional label information

Certain information on food labels is optional. However, any optional information on the label must follow set guidelines and not be misleading. Foods that are labeled as "low fat," "reduced calorie," "sugar free," or that make similar claims must meet the official FDA definition of these words. Foods may list a specific amount of a particular nutrient, such as "3 grams of carbohydrates," so long as it is not done in a misleading way. The FDA must approve any health claims that relate a specific ingredient to a specific disease, such as **calcium** helping to prevent osteoporosis.

Plant foods labeled "organic" are made from crops raised without synthetic fertilizers or sewage sludge fertilizer, and they have not been treated with most conventional pesticides or are not genetically engineered (bioengineered foods). Animal products that are labeled "organic" come from livestock that has been fed 100% organic feed and raised without growth hormones or antibiotics in an environment where they have access to the outdoors. There continues to be debate about the exact requirements to label animal products as "cage free," "free range," or "grass fed."

European regulations

Other countries have different requirements for what needs to be included on food labels. In Europe, the European Union (EU) mandates the information that needs to be present. Standard information includes the ingredients, ingredient amounts (in some cases), expiration dates, storage and cooking instructions, and allergen information. Countries in the EU are required to label foods containing genetically modified organisms (GMOs) and in 2014 will need to start listing the country of origin for meat and poultry products. Foods containing dyes (e.g., yellow, red) must display the warning "may have an adverse effect on activity and attention in children," though many countries have banned the use of these dyes altogether.

Reading a food label

The many descriptive words on a food label cannot be used unless they meet very specific legal requirements. Some of the common descriptions found on FDA-regulated foods include:

- fat free: less than 0.5 grams of fat per serving
- low fat: no more than 3 grams or less of fat per serving
- less fat: a minimum of 25% less fat than the comparison food
- light (fat): a minimum of 50% less fat than the comparison food
- cholesterol free: less than 2 mg of cholesterol and 2 g of saturated fat per serving
- low cholesterol: no more than 20 mg of cholesterol and 2 grams of saturated fat per serving
- reduced calorie: a minimum of 25% fewer calories than the comparison food
- low calorie: no more than 40 calories per serving
- light (calories): a minimum of one-third fewer calories than the comparison food
- sugar free: less than 0.5 grams of sugar per serving

- low sodium: no more than 140 mg of sodium per serving
- very low sodium: no more than 35 mg of sodium per serving
- high fiber: 5 or more grams of fiber per serving
- high, rich in, excellent source of: 20% or more of the daily value of the nutrient
- good source of: 10% or more of the daily value of the nutrient than the comparison food
- less, fewer, reduced: 25% or less of the named nutrient than the comparison food

The USDA also has specific requirements for words used in labeling meat and poultry. Some of these include:

- certified: inspected, evaluated, graded, and approved the USDA Food Safety and Inspection Service
- free range or free roaming: indicates that the animals have access to the outdoors
- fresh (poultry): the raw meat has never been held at a temperature below 26°F, although there are some adjustments to this that allow a temperature fluctuation of up to 2 degrees while poultry is in stores
- frozen (poultry): the temperature of the raw meat is 0°F or lower
- halal: prepared at a federally inspected meat-packing plant that also is overseen by an Islamic authority and meets the requirements of Islamic dietary law
- kosher: prepared at a federally inspected meat-packing plant that also is overseen by a rabbi and meets the requirements of Jewish dietary law
- natural: containing no artificial ingredients or added color and processed in a way that does not alter the raw product
- oven prepared: cooked and ready to eat without additional cooking
- oven ready: uncooked, but is ready to cook without additional preparation

Consumers may see a USDA grade on the label of cuts of beef and lamb. Pork, veal, and mutton are also graded, but the grades are not usually shown on store packaging. All USDA graded meat is inspected and wholesome, but some grades are more tender and better suited to certain cooking methods than others:

- Prime cuts are the highest quality and most tender and juicy cuts, but also the most expensive. Prime cuts contain the most fat and make excellent steaks and roasts.
- Choice cuts are very tender, juicy, and flavorful. Choice is the most popular grade of meat sold in the United States.

• Select cuts are very lean with less fat. They are best suited to long, moist cooking methods, such as soups and stews.

Two other lower grades of beef, standard and commercial, are sometimes sold as ungraded "store brand" meats. These cuts are wholesome and nutritious, but tend to be tougher and dryer than the higher grades. Utility, cutter, and canner beef, the lowest of the eight grades, are almost never seen in stores. These cuts of meat are used to make ground beef, hot dogs, and other processed meat products.

Understanding the nutrition facts panel

The Nutrition Labeling and Education Act of 1990 and subsequent revisions require certain nutritional information be clearly displayed on many foods. The Act does not apply to meat and poultry, raw fruits and vegetables, ready-to-eat foods (such as cookies or cakes sold at a bakery), foods sold by sidewalk vendors, and a few other exceptions. Counter cards can be used instead of packaging labels to provide voluntary nutrition information for many common fruits, vegetables, raw seafood, and wild game or exotic meats (e.g., ostrich). The nutrition facts panel is designed to encourage health eating. It gives consumers a way to compare the nutritional value of products and to see how specific products can help meet dietary needs.

The nutrition facts panel consists of several sections. The serving size is given in both familiar units, such as cups or ounces, and metric units. Serving sizes are standardized for similar foods so that consumers can make easy comparisons. If the package contains a single serving, the serving size is not required. Under the serving size, the servings per container lists the total number of servings contained in the package.

All information listed below the servings per container is given per single serving. People who eat more than one serving will take in more **calories** and nutrients than the amount listed on the label. Calories and calories from fat, the first nutrient listed, give the consumer a quick idea of how much energy the food provides and how healthful it is or isn't.

The next section of the nutrient facts panel deals with specific nutrients. The information is given by weight in metric units (grams or mg) and as a percent daily value. The percent daily value shows how much of each nutrient the food contributes toward meeting the daily recommended amount of each specific nutrient. Percent daily values are based on the recommended dietary allowances (RDAs) of the nutrient for a person who is eating a 2,000-calorie diet. Percent

daily values of 5% or less are considered low, and values of 20% or greater are considered high.

The nutrients listed next on the panel are ones that Americans generally eat enough or too much of and that they should try to limit. The first of these are total fat, saturated fat and *trans* fat. High consumption of saturated fat and *trans* fat are linked to the development of cardiovascular disease. People should try to consume as little of these **fats** as possible. *Trans* was not part of the original nutrient facts panel, but was added beginning January 1, 2006. Not enough information is available to calculate a percent daily value for *trans* fat. Cholesterol and **sodium** complete the list of nutrients that should be consumed in limited amounts.

The nutrient panel also lists total **carbohydrates**, dietary **fiber**, **protein**, and **sugar**. Americans should try to increase the amount of dietary fiber they consume. A percent daily value for protein is not required unless the food makes the claim that it is "high in protein." In that case, the daily value must be 20% or greater. There is no percent daily value for sugar.

At the bottom of the label, percent daily values, but no weights, are listed for four nutrients: **vitamin A**, **Vitamin C**, calcium, and **iron**. These percentages give consumers an idea how low or high the food is in these particular nutrients.

Larger labels have a footnote at the very bottom. The information in this footnote is always the same regardless of the type of food in the package. The footnote explains that the percent daily values are calculated based on a 2,000-calorie diet, and that an individual's needs may be greater or less than the listed percent daily value depending on the individual's energy (calorie) needs. The footnote provides the maximum recommended grams of fat, saturated fat, cholesterol, and sodium and the minimum grams of carbohydrates and dietary fibers for people on a 2,000- or 2,500-calorie diet. Whether this footnote is included in the label depends on the space is available.

Precautions

Not all foods require a Nutrition Facts label and due to the self-governing process, food labels may be out-of-date, improperly labeled, or misleading. The Nutrition Labeling and Education Act (NLEA), which amended the FD&C Act requires most foods to bear nutrition labeling and requires food labels that bear nutrient content claims and certain health messages to comply with specific requirements. Although final regulations have been established and are reflected in this guidance, there is a two-year phase-in period whenever labeling requirements are changed, lessening the financial impact on companies whose products require new labels. The responsibility to remain current with the legal requirements for food labeling relies upon the food industry. All new regulations are published in the Federal Register (FR) prior to their effective date and compiled annually in Title 21 of the Code of Federal Regulations (CFR).

Parental concerns

Special labeling requirements are in effect for foods designed to be consumed mainly by children age four and younger, and pregnant and lactating women. One of the most recent changes to the food label is the listing of food allergens. The Food Allergen Labeling and Consumer Protection Act of 2004 (Public Law 108–202), also known as FALCPA, addresses the labeling of foods that contain certain food allergens, among other issues. All foods labeled on or after January 1, 2006 have to comply and extends to foods packaged by a retail or foodservice establishment that are offered for human consumption. The FALCPA ensures that a food label lists any "major food allergen" ingredient that is one of the following five foods, or from one of the following three food groups, or is an ingredient that contains protein derived from one of the following:

- milk
- egg
- fish
- Crustacean shellfish
- tree nuts
- wheat
- peanuts
- soybeans

The FALCPA makes it easier for people who have restricted diets due to **food allergies** to properly and accurately identify whether a food contains an allergen, thus reducing the risks for complications due to food allergies.

Resources

BOOKS

Stewart, Kimberly Lord. *Eating Between The Lines: The Supermarket Shopper's Guide to the Truth Behind Food Labels.* New York: St. Martin's Griffin, 2007.

Taub-Dix, Bonnie. *Read It Before You Eat It: How to Decode Food Labels and Make the Healthiest Choice Every Time.* New York: Penguin Group, 2010.

WEBSITES

Associated Press. "Long-Sought Food Labeling Law Takes Effect Today." MSNBC.com, March 16, 2009. http://
www.msnbc.msn.com/id/29724685/ns/health-food_safety (accessed July 25, 2011).

Business Link. "Food Labelling and Packaging in International Trade: Understanding Food Labelling in the UK and the European Union." http://www.businesslink.gov.uk/bdotg/action/detail?itemId = 1080034063&type = RESOURCES (accessed July 25, 2012).

Center for Science in the Public Interest. "In Europe, Dyed Foods Get Warning Label." http://www.cspinet.org/new/201007201.html (accessed July 25, 2012).

European Commission. "GM Food & Feed—Labelling." http://ec.europa.eu/food/food/biotechnology/gmfood/labelling_en.htm (accessed July 25, 2012).

———. "New EU Law on Food Information to Consumers." http://ec.europa.eu/food/food/labellingnutrition/foodlabelling/proposed_legislation_en.htm (accessed July 25, 2012).

U.S. Department of Agriculture. "National Organic Program: Consumer Information." http://www.ams.usda.gov/AMSv1.0/ams.fetchTemplateData.do?template = TemplateC&navID = ConsumerlinkNOPConsumers&rightNav1 = ConsumerlinkNOPConsumers&topNav = &leftNav = NationalOrganicProgram&page = NOPConsumers&resultType = &acct = nopgeninfo (accessed July 25, 2012).

U.S. Food and Drug Administration. "Labeling & Nutrition: Food Labeling and Nutrition Overview." http://www.fda.gov/food/labelingnutrition/default.htm (accessed July 25, 2012).

ORGANIZATIONS

European Commission, Directorate General for Health and Consumers, B–1049, Brussels, Belgium, 01132(2) 299-11-11, http://ec.europa.eu/dgs/health_consumer/index_en.htm.

U.S. Food and Drug Administration, 10903 New Hampshire Ave., Silver Spring, MD 20993-0002, (888) INFO-FDA (463-6332), http://www.fda.gov.

Tish Davidson, AM

Food poisoning

Definition

Food poisoning—often called foodborne illness, disease, or infection—is illness caused by eating food or drinking water contaminated with disease-causing bacteria, viruses, parasites, or environmental toxins. Toxins may also be present within the food itself, such as the poisons in some mushrooms. Food poisoning is sometimes referred to as gastroenteritis or infectious diarrhea.

Microorganisms responsible for common foodborne illnesses

Microorganism	Foodborne illness	Symptoms	Common food sources	Incubation
Bacillus cereus	Bacterium	Watery diarrhea and cramps or nausea and vomiting	Cooked product that is left uncovered (milk, meats, vegetables, fish, rice, and starchy foods)	0.5–15 hours
Campylobacter jejuni	Bacterium	Diarrhea, sometimes accompanied by fever, abdominal pain, nausea, headache, and muscle pain	Raw chicken, foods contaminated by raw chicken, unpasteurized milk, untreated water	2–5 days
Clostridium botulinum	Bacterium	Lethargy; weakness; dizziness; double vision; difficulty speaking, swallowing, and/or breathing; paralysis; possible death	Inadequately processed or home-canned foods, sausages, seafood products, chopped bottled garlic, honey	18–36 hours
Clostridium perfringens	Bacterium	Intense abdominal cramps, diarrhea	Meats, meat products, gravy, Tex-Mex foods, other protein-rich foods	8–24 hours
Escherichia coli group	Bacterium	Watery diarrhea, abdominal cramps, low-grade fever, nausea, malaise	Contaminated water, undercooked ground beef, unpasteurized apple juice and cider, raw milk, alfalfa sprouts, cut melons	12–72 hours
Giardia lamblia	Parasite	Diarrhea, abdominal cramps, nausea	Water and foods that have come into contact with contaminated water	1–2 weeks
Hepatitis A	Virus	Jaundice, fatigue, abdominal pain, anorexia, intermittent nausea, diarrhea	Raw or undercooked molluscan shellfish or foods prepared by infected handlers	15–50 days
Listeria monocytogenes	Bacterium	Nausea, vomiting, diarrhea; may progress to headache, confusion, loss of balance and convulsions; may cause spontaneous abortion	Ready-to-eat foods contaminated with bacteria, including raw milk, cheeses, ice cream, raw vegetables, fermented raw sausages, raw and cooked poultry, raw meats, and raw and smoked fish	Unknown; may range from a few days to 3 weeks
Norwalk-type viruses	Virus	Nausea, vomiting, diarrhea, abdominal cramps	Shellfish grown in fecally contaminated water; water and foods that have come into contact with contaminated water	12–48 hours
Salmonella species	Bacterium	Abdominal cramps, diarrhea, fever, headache	Foods of animal origin or other foods contaminated through contact with feces, raw animal products, or infected food handlers; poultry, eggs, raw milk, meats are frequently contaminated	12–72 hours
Shigella	Bacterium	Fever, abdominal pain and cramps, diarrhea	Fecally contaminated foods	12–48 hours
Staphylococcus aureus	Bacterium	Nausea, vomiting, abdominal cramping	Foods contaminated by improper handling and holding temperatures—meats and meat products, poultry and egg products, protein-based salads, sandwich fillings, cream-based bakery products	1–12 hours
Trichinella spiralis	Parasite	Nausea, diarrhea, vomiting, fatigue, fever, abdominal cramps	Raw and undercooked pork and wild game products	1–2 days

SOURCE: U.S. Food and Drug Administration.

(Table by PreMediaGlobal. © 2013 Cengage Learning.)

Description

Foodborne illness is a serious public health concern in the United States and around the world. More than 250 different foodborne diseases have been identified, primarily infections caused by pathogenic microorganisms. In 2011, the U.S. Centers for Disease Control and Prevention (CDC) reported that about 48 million Americans—one in six—suffer from food poisoning every year. Although unpleasant, most cases are not severe enough to require medical treatment. Nevertheless, food poisoning results in 128,000 hospitalizations and 3,000 deaths annually in the United States and is estimated to cost $3–6 billion annually in direct medical care and lost productivity. The very young, the elderly, pregnant women, and people with weakened immune systems—such as HIV/AIDS, leukemia, and transplant patients—are more likely to suffer severe food poisoning that results in hospitalization and life-threatening complications.

Disease-causing organisms and chemicals can contaminate food at any point in the food-production chain. The majority of food poisonings result from contamination with animal or human feces during slaughter, processing, transport, storage, or preparation. The U.S. Food and Drug Administration (FDA) estimates that 90% of raw poultry sold at retail stores carries some disease-causing bacteria. Other raw meat products and eggs are contaminated to a lesser degree. Fruits and vegetables can also be contaminated in the field with feces or pesticides, as well as during harvesting, processing, distribution, and storage. Oysters and other filter-feeding shellfish can concentrate harmful bacteria that are normally present in seawater.

Although thorough cooking kills most bacteria, the CDC estimates that about 97% of food poisonings are due to improper food handling, such as undercooking or poor refrigeration, with 80% of such cases occurring in restaurants, cafeterias, or institutions such as nursing homes, schools, and prisons. The remaining 20% of cases come from improper food handling in the home.

Nevertheless, the U.S. food supply is probably the safest in the world, and serious outbreaks of food poisoning are relatively rare. Travel outside the United States, to countries with poorer sanitation, water purification, and food-handling practices, increases the risk of food poisoning. Bioterrorism experts are also concerned that disease-causing organisms could intentionally be introduced into the food or water supply to cause mass outbreaks of food poisoning.

Causes and symptoms

Food poisoning is primarily caused by a variety of different bacteria. According to the 2010 estimates, *Salmonella* infections accounted for the greatest number of hospitalizations (35%) and deaths (28%). In addition to *Salmonella*, other bacteria that commonly cause food poisoning include *Campylobacter*, *Toxoplasma*, *Escherichia coli* O157, , *Listeria*, *Clostridium perfringens*, *Staphylococcus aureus*, Shigella, and *Clostridium botulinum*. Each has a slightly different incubation period and duration, but all except *C. botulinum* cause inflammation of the intestines and diarrhea. Food and water also can be contaminated by viruses (e.g., norovirus, cholera, rotavirus), environmental toxins (e.g., heavy metals), and poisons produced within the food itself (e.g., mushroom poisoning, shellfish poisoning).

BACTERIA. Bacterial contamination is the leading cause of food poisoning. At room temperature, bacteria reproduce at astounding rates. A single bacterium that divides every half hour can produce 17 million offspring in 12 hours. Bacteria fall into two general categories. One group causes symptoms of food poisoning by directly infecting the intestines causing irritation and diarrhea. The other group

releases toxins (poisons) as they grow and reproduce. These toxins affect the digestive system and often cause vomiting first followed by diarrhea. Common bacteria include:

- Bacteria of the genus *Salmonella* are common in reptiles, birds, and mammals. They are found most often in eggs, poultry, dairy products, and beef. Infection with *Salmonella* causes nausea, vomiting, stomach cramps, headache, and low-grade fever. Symptoms begin anywhere from 6–48 hours after exposure and may last for seven days. In people with weakened immune systems, *Salmonella* infection can be life-threatening.

- Bacteria of the genus *Campylobacter* cause more diarrheal illnesses worldwide than any other group of bacteria. They produce fairly mild diarrhea, fever, and stomach cramps. *Campylobacter* bacteria are found in almost all raw chicken and turkey. Cross-contamination, that is putting cooked food down where raw food had been, is a leading cause of food poisoning from *Campylobacter*. These bacteria are also transmitted by water contaminated with animal feces.

- *Escherichia coli* are a large group of bacteria, only some of which cause food poisoning. *E. coli* food poisoning usually begins with watery diarrhea that later turns bloody. One strain of *E. coli* known as 0157:H7 is most often found in undercooked hamburger, but has also been found in ready-to-eat raw spinach. This particular strain can cause kidney failure and death, especially in children and the elderly.

- *Clostridium botulinum* is a bacteria that causes the disease botulism. *C. botulinum* produces a toxin that affects the nervous system and can cause difficulty breathing and paralysis. Symptoms do not appear until 1–4 days after exposure. Botulism is associated with improperly canned food (often home canned products), smoked fish, and honey. Infection with *C. botulinum* is uncommon but serious and often fatal. Proper cooking kills this bacterium.

- *Shigella* is a common cause of diarrhea in travelers to developing countries. It is associated with contaminated food and water, crowded living conditions, and poor sanitation. The bacterial toxins affect the small intestine. The disease runs its course in two to three days. Dehydration is a common complication. Most people recover on their own, although they may feel exhausted. Children who are malnourished or have weakened immune systems may die.

- *Staphylococcus aureus* is found in dust, air, and sewage. The bacteria are spread primarily by food handlers using poor sanitary practices. Almost any food can be contaminated, but salad dressings, milk products, cream pastries, and any food kept at room temperature, rather than hot or cold, are likely candidates.

It is difficult to estimate the number of cases of food poisoning from *Staphylococcus aureus* that occur each year, because its symptoms are so similar to those caused by other foodborne bacteria. Many cases are mild and the victim never sees a doctor.

- *Listeria monocytogenes* is a ubiquitous bacterium in soil, groundwater, plants, and animals that causes listeriosis.

VIRUSES. A large group of viruses called noroviruses are an extremely common cause of foodborne illness. In recent years, these viruses have caused major outbreaks of gastrointestinal disease on cruise ships and in nursing homes. They cause more vomiting than diarrhea than any other viruses. Unlike many of the other causes of food poisoning, these viruses are not usually naturally present in food. They are usually transferred from the hands of infected food handlers to the food that they are preparing, especially to foods such as salads and sandwiches.

Rotavirus infection is the leading cause of severe diarrhea in infants and children. Two vaccines that prevent most rotavirus infections are available for infants in the United States. One vaccine requires two doses, the other three. The first dose must be given after age 6 weeks and before age 15 weeks. In countries where a rotavirus vaccine is available, the number of cases of serious diarrhea and death from **dehydration** in infants has decreased substantially. This virus still remains a major killer of infants in underdeveloped countries.

PARASITES. Parasites that cause food poisoning usually come from contaminated water. They often cause mild symptoms that are slow to develop but last for several weeks. *Giardia* causes watery diarrhea and is often acquired by drinking untreated water from lakes or streams. *Cryptosporidium* is a parasite that causes large amounts of watery diarrhea for 3–4 days. Healthy people usually recover quickly, but in people with weakened immune systems, symptoms can persist for a long time. *Toxoplasma gondii* is a parasite that is responsible for 24% of food-poisoning deaths from identified agents.

NATURAL TOXINS. Natural poisons found in some wild mushrooms can cause anything from nausea and vomiting to hallucinations, coma, and death, depending on the amount and species of mushroom eaten. Mushroom poisoning is a medical emergency. People who believe they have eaten a poisonous mushroom should, if possible, take a sample of the mushroom or their vomit to the emergency room with them. Identifying the type of mushroom causing the illness can help determine the most effective treatment.

Oysters, clams, mollusks, and scallops can contain toxins that affect the nervous system. Symptoms usually begin with a tingling in the mouth, then the arms and legs. Individuals may become dizzy and may have difficulty breathing. Shellfish poisoning is a medical emergency because the muscles needed for breathing may become paralyzed. Similar symptoms result from eating the Japanese puffer fish which contains a natural poison that in its skin and digestive system that affects the nervous system.

MAN-MADE TOXINS. Man-made toxins include all pesticides, fertilizers, disinfectants, and any other chemicals remaining in food when it is eaten that can cause illness. Contamination is accidental, and often the result of ignorance or a misunderstanding of how to apply the chemical. Symptoms may develop rapidly or slowly depending on the type of chemical and the amount of exposure. Chemical poisoning requires prompt medical evaluation.

Other food-poisoning agents include toxins in poisonous mushrooms and reef fish, food contaminated with pesticides or herbicides, and certain communicable pathogens that are occasionally foodborne. The latter include the *Shigella* family of bacteria, hepatitis A virus, rotavirus, and the parasites *Giardia lamblia* and *Cryptosporidium*.

Ingested pathogens adhere to the intestinal lining and begin to multiply. Some types remain in the intestine and produce toxins that enter the bloodstream. Other pathogens invade deeper body tissues.

Emerging agents

The agents responsible for food poisoning evolve over time and require constant surveillance. Whereas typhoid fever, tuberculosis, and cholera were once common foodborne illnesses, improved food safety—including milk pasteurization, safer canning methods, and water treatment—have overcome these diseases in the developed world. However other sources of food poisoning have emerged. For example, in 1991, the parasite *Cyclospora* contaminated Guatemalan raspberries. In 1998, a new strain of the bacterium *Vibrio parahaemolyticus* contaminated oyster beds in Galveston Bay.

Some foodborne bacterial infections appear to be on the increase. In 2011, at least 29 people died and at least 139 people across 28 states were sickened from eating cantaloupe contaminated with *L. monocytogenes* and traced to unsanitary conditions and poor handling at a single Colorado farm. Both listeriosis and salmonellosis can be transmitted to a fetus, causing miscarriage, fetal or newborn death, premature delivery, or severe illness in mother and infant. Since most listeriosis outbreaks are caused by contaminated animal products, pregnant women are often advised to avoid deli meats.

Complications of some foodborne infections are now being recognized as the cause of certain serious medical conditions. For example, *Campylobacter* can cause Guillain-Barré syndrome and *E. coli* O157:H7 and related bacteria can cause hemolytic uremic syndrome (HUS), the most common cause of acute kidney failure in children.

Sources of contamination

Contamination can occur at any point in the food-production chain:

- in the field, by application of illegal or higher-than-approved pesticides or herbicides
- during processing, by improper handling of raw materials, contaminated water, inadequate disinfection, inadequate timing or temperature, or contamination with pest-control poisons
- during storage and transportation, by improper temperatures, inappropriate use of fumigants, inadequate sanitization of food-carrying tanker trucks, or contamination with insects or rodent droppings
- in stores and restaurants, with improper temperatures, cross-contamination between raw and cooked foods, improper disinfection of food-preparation surfaces, improper hand washing, or transmission by infected food handlers
- at home, by leaving food at room temperature, inadequate cooking, cross-contamination between raw and cooked foods, or failure to properly reheat leftovers

Raw or undercooked meat, poultry, eggs, fish—especially filter-feeding shellfish such as oysters, clams, scallops, and mussels—and raw (unpasteurized) milk are common sources of food poisoning. Raw fruits and vegetables may have been exposed to fresh manure or contaminated water, and washing will reduce but not eliminate pathogens. Misidentified wild mushrooms, improperly canned foods, luncheon and deli meats, and soft cheeses, such as brie and feta, are also associated with food poisoning.

Processed foods that pool ingredients from multiple sources are particularly dangerous, since a pathogen from one animal can contaminate an entire batch. For example, a single hamburger can include meat from hundreds of animals, a glass of raw milk may be the pooled milk of hundreds of cows, unpasteurized fruit juice can be made from many individual fruits, and a restaurant omelet can contain eggs from hundreds of chickens. An estimated one in every 20,000 eggs is contaminated with *Salmonella*. Egg-containing products, such as mayonnaise or raw cookie dough, also carry a risk.

Small numbers of bacteria in foods can multiply quickly under warm, moist conditions. A few bacteria in alfalfa or bean seeds can multiply to contaminate an entire batch of sprouts. Refrigeration or freezing generally prevents bacteria from multiplying. However *L. monocytogenes* and the foodborne bacterium *Yersinia enterocolitica* can grow and multiply at refrigerator temperatures. High levels of salt, **sugar**, or acid prevent bacteria from growing in preserved foods.

Symptoms

Food poisoning symptoms usually develop suddenly, within one to 48 hours after eating contaminated food, and resolve within one to a few days. Symptoms and their severity depend on the causative agent, the amount ingested, and the health of the individual; however food-poisoning symptoms tend to be similar, regardless of their cause:

- watery and sometimes bloody diarrhea
- nausea followed by forceful vomiting
- painful abdominal cramps
- fever
- headache
- dizziness
- blurred vision
- difficulty breathing

Children commonly vomit everything in their stomachs for three or four hours, followed by mild or moderate vomiting. Severe vomiting, especially in combination with diarrhea, can cause dehydration—the excessive loss of body fluids. Young children can become dehydrated very quickly.

Chemical food poisoning is a medical emergency. Natural poisons found in some wild mushrooms can cause, in addition to nausea and vomiting, hallucinations, coma, and death. Shellfish toxins and Japanese puffer fish poison affect the nervous system, beginning with tingling in the mouth, arms, and legs, followed by dizziness and possibly difficulty breathing. Poisoning with man-made toxic chemicals varies with the type of chemical and degree of exposure.

Diagnosis

In healthy people, food poisoning by a pathogen is usually a mild, short-lived illness that does not require specific diagnosis or medical treatment. Most mild food poisoning is diagnosed by the symptoms of vomiting, diarrhea, and stomach cramps coupled with information about what the individual has recently eaten. The length of time between eating the suspect food and the start of symptoms gives physicians a clue about what particular organism may be causing the food poisoning. Blood and urine tests may be ordered to determine the individual's degree of dehydration and electrolyte (chemical) imbalances. In most cases, determining the exact pathogen that is causing the food poisoning is relatively unimportant, as treatment tends to be the similar for most causes. However, if diarrhea is persistent, a stool culture may be done to provide more specific information.

Food poisoning can have serious complications in the very young, the elderly, and immunocompromised patients, and so it is sometimes necessary to identify the causative agent to begin appropriate treatment. The symptoms and length of time between consuming a suspected food and the onset of illness may suggest the culprit. However, unless the illness is part a known outbreak, laboratory tests may be required.

- Viral infections are usually identified by testing stool samples for genetic markers of a specific virus. However tests for noroviruses are not widely available, so this most common form of food poisoning is rarely diagnosed.
- Bacteria such as *Salmonella*, *Campylobacter*, and *E. coli* O157:H7 are usually identified from cultured stool samples. However, it is estimated that only one in 30 cases of salmonellosis is confirmed by a laboratory test. The CDC recommends that clinical laboratories test for both Shiga toxin and *E. coli* O157:H7 in the stools of all patients with community-acquired diarrhea or suspected HUS.
- Parasites are identified by examining stool samples under a microscope.
- Blood and urine tests can determine the extent of dehydration and electrolyte imbalances stemming from diarrhea and vomiting.

Treatment for poisoning from a natural or man-made toxin may require precise identification of the chemical. With suspected mushroom poisoning, a sample of the mushroom or the patient's vomit should be brought to the emergency department, if possible. In other cases, extensive blood tests are required or the stomach may be pumped and its contents tested. Sometimes activated charcoal is used to help absorb the poison in the stomach.

Treatment

Treatment for food poisoning usually involves preventing dehydration by replacing fluids and **electrolytes** lost through vomiting and diarrhea. Food poisoning can cause huge amounts of water and electrolytes to be lost very quickly, especially in infants and young children. The loss of 10%–15% of body fluid is very serious and the loss of 20% is fatal. Severe dehydration may require hospitalization and intravenous fluids. Drugs are sometimes prescribed to stop persistent vomiting. Vomiting and diarrhea in infants and young children require especially prompt professional treatment because small children can become dehydrated within hours.

Mild cases of food poisoning can usually be treated at home, especially if there is no fever. Dehydration can be prevented or treated with over-the-counter (OTC) oral-rehydration solutions such as Ceralyte, Pedialyte, or Oralyte. These are available in supermarkets and pharmacies without a prescription. An electrolyte-replacement fluid can be made at home with one teaspoon of salt and four teaspoons of sugar per quart of water. Small sips should be given to young children as soon as vomiting and diarrhea begin. Children may continue to vomit and have diarrhea, but some of the fluid will be absorbed. In the past, parents were told to withhold solid food from children who had diarrhea. New research indicates that it is better for children to be allowed to eat solid food should they want it, even though diarrhea continues.

Adults and older children with food poisoning should avoid drinking coffee, tea, and soft drinks, especially soft drinks that contain **caffeine**, as these liquids promote dehydration. Sports drinks, such as Gatorade, do not replace losses properly and should not be used to treat diarrheal illnesses. Over-the-counter medications to stop or slow diarrhea such as Kaopectate, Pepto-Bismol, or Imodium will not shorten the duration of the disease, but may give the individual some control over his or her bowels. Consult a physician before giving these over-the-counter medicines to children. They should not be used in the presence of high fever or blood in the stool.

Individuals of all ages who are seriously dehydrated need to be treated promptly by a medical professional. In the case of severe dehydration, the individual may be hospitalized and fluids given intravenously (IV; directly into the vein). Drugs may also be prescribed to stop persistent vomiting. Although bacteria cause many cases of food poisoning, antibiotics are not routinely used in treatment. Some studies have shown that antibiotics are necessary only in about 10% of cases.

Botulism is treated in a different way from other food poisonings. Botulism antitoxin is given to adults, but not infants, if it can be administered within 72 hours after symptoms are first observed. If given later, it provides no benefit. Both infants and adults require hospitalization, often in the intensive care unit. If the ability to breathe is impaired, patients are put on a mechanical ventilator to assist their breathing and are fed intravenously until the paralysis passes.

Individuals who think their food poisoning symptoms may be caused by chemicals or natural toxins should always seek emergency medical care immediately. These types of food poisoning are too serious to try to treat at home.

Although the food in the United States is very safe, occasionally major outbreaks of food poisoning occur that can be traced to a breakdown in the food handling system. Larger outbreaks can be identified and traced to their source because each state has a list of diseases that health professionals are required to report to the county public health service once positive diagnosis is made. Most states require that doctors and hospitals report confirmed cases of disease caused by *Salmonella* and *E. coli* 0157:H7 and several other food poisoning pathogens. This information is then passed on to the CDC.

Alternative treatment

Alternative practitioners offer the same advice as traditional practitioners concerning diet modification. In addition, they recommend taking charcoal tablets, *Lactobacillus acidophilus*, *Lactobacillus bulgaricus*, and citrus seed extract. An electrolyte replacement fluid can be made at home by adding one teaspoon of salt and four teaspoons of sugar to one quart of water. For food poisoning other than botulism, two homeopathic remedies, either *Arsenicum album* or *Nux vomica*, are strongly recommended.

In a recent review by the Cochrane Collaboration of 63 studies involving a total of 8,000 people, **probiotics** seems to be able to shorten the duration of diarrhea by 25 hours as compared with no treatment at all.

Prognosis

Most people have unpleasant gastrointestinal symptoms—vomiting and diarrhea—for a few days and then recover fully from food poisoning. In young children, dehydration is always a cause for concern. Worldwide, dehydration from diarrhea is the biggest killer of children under age 5. If dehydration can be controlled in young children with food poisoning, most recover with few complications. However, *E, coli* 0157:H7 can cause fatal renal failure in 3%–5% of children. This bacteria is most often acquired by eating

unpasteurized apple cider or apple juice, alfalfa or bean sprouts.

Botulism is the deadliest of the bacterial foodborne illnesses. With prompt medical care, the death rate is less than 10%.

More serious long-term health problems often result from chemical poisonings. Toxins found in some wild mushrooms and some fish can cause permanent liver damage requiring a liver transplant or death. Pesticides and other chemical contamination can cause liver damage, kidney failure, and nervous system complications. In 2007, chemical contamination of pet food caused the death of hundreds of dogs and cats in the United States.

Prevention

Healthcare professionals and individuals should report foodborne illnesses to their local health departments so that outbreaks can be detected, traced, and halted. However, most food poisonings are preventable by appropriate handling and processing at each level of the food-production chain. **Breastfeeding** is the best way to protect infants from food poisoning.

Growers should apply only approved pesticides and herbicides at no higher than recommended levels. Processors must use clean sources of water to wash produce, regularly disinfect processing machinery, and use only safe pesticides.

Proper refrigeration is required in stores, restaurants, and homes. Food should not be held under warming lights or at room temperature for long periods; they should be kept at above 140°F (60°C) or below 40°F (4°C). Fresh foods and leftovers should be promptly refrigerated or frozen. Frozen food should be defrosted in the refrigerator or microwave, rather than at room temperature, and cooked immediately. Food that has been at room temperature for 2–4 hours should be discarded. Large quantities of food should be divided into shallow containers to cool more rapidly.

Hands should be washed thoroughly with soap and water before, during, and after preparing food and after using the bathroom or changing diapers. Anyone with a diarrheal illness should not prepare food for others. Food preparation surfaces and utensils should be washed frequently during food handling. Produce should be washed thoroughly before and again after peeling to prevent salmonellosis. The outer leaves of lettuce and cabbage should be discarded. Cross-contamination of foods can be avoided by never placing cooked food on plates or surfaces that previously held raw food.

KEY TERMS

Botulism—Life-threatening paralytic food poisoning caused by botulinum toxin from the bacterium *Clostridium botulinum.*

Campylobacter—A genus of bacteria that can cause food poisoning and are found in almost all raw poultry.

Clostridium perfringens—A bacterium that is a common cause of food poisoning.

Dehydration—The abnormal depletion of body fluids, as from vomiting and diarrhea.

Diuretic—Medication that increases the urine output of the body.

Electrolytes—Ions—such as sodium, potassium, calcium, magnesium, chloride, phosphate, bicarbonate, and sulfate—that are dissolved in bodily fluids and regulate or affect most metabolic processes.

Gastroenteritis—Inflammation of the lining of the stomach and intestines.

Hemolytic uremic syndrome (HUS)—Kidney failure, usually in infants and young children, that can be caused by food poisoning with bacteria such as *Escherichia coli* or *Shigella.*

Lactobacillus acidophilus—This bacterium is found in yogurt and changes the balance of the bacteria in the intestine in a beneficial way.

Listeriosis—A usually mild illness caused by food poisoning with *Listeria monocytogenes*, but which can be serious or fatal in newborns, the elderly, and the immunocompromised and which can cause miscarriage, stillbirth, or premature birth if contracted during pregnancy.

Norovirus—Norwalk virus; a large family of RNA viruses that is the most common cause of food poisoning.

Salmonellosis—Food poisoning by bacteria of the genus *Salmonella*, which usually causes severe diarrhea and may be transmitted to the fetus.

Shiga toxin-producing E. coli (STEC)—Strains of the common, normally harmless, intestinal bacteria *Escherichia coli* that produce Shiga toxin, causing serious food poisoning; *E. coli* O157:H7 is the most commonly identified STEC in North America.

Staphylococcus aureus—A bacterium that causes food poisoning.

Toxoplasma gondii—A very common parasite that can cause toxoplasmosis and is a leading cause of death from food poisoning; although it infects large numbers of people, *T. gondii* is usually dangerous only in immunocompromised patients and in newly infected pregnant women.

Heating food to an internal temperature of 160°F (78°C), for even a few seconds, kills most bacteria, viruses, and parasites. *Clostridium* produces heat-resistant spores that must be destroyed with temperatures above boiling. Food thermometers should be used to check the internal temperature of cooked meat. Egg yolks should be cooked until firm. Bacterial toxins vary in their heat sensitivity. Although botulism toxin is completely inactivated by boiling, staphylococcal toxin is not. Milk, juice, and cider should be pasteurized. Irradiation of meat and other foods also destroys contaminating microbes.

Resources

BOOKS

Gillard, Arthur. *Food-Borne Diseases.* Detroit, MI: Greenhaven, 2011.

Hoorfar, J. *Rapid Detection, Characterization, and Enumeration of Foodborne Pathogens.* Washington, DC: ASM, 2011.

Juneja, Vijay K., and John Nikolaos Sofos. *Pathogens and Toxins in Foods: Challenges and Interventions.* Washington, DC: ASM, 2010.

Landau, Elaine. *Food Poisoning and Foodborne Diseases.* Minneapolis, MN: Twenty First Century Books, 2010.

Lew, Kristi. *Food Poisoning: E. coli and the Food Supply.* New York: Rosen, 2011.

Stille, Darlene R. *Recipe for Disaster: The Science of Foodborne Illness.* Mankato, MN: Compass Point, 2010.

Wiwanitkit, Viroj. *Focus on Emerging Food-Borne Infections.* Boca Raton, FL: Nova Science Pub., 2008.

PERIODICALS

"Don't Let Food Poisoning Spoil Your Picnic." *U.S. News & World Report* (May 2011): 1.

WEBSITES

American Academy of Family Physicians. "Food Poisoning." FamilyDoctor.org. http://familydoctor.org/familydoctor/en/diseases-conditions/food-poisoning.html (accessed January 12, 2012).

Centers for Disease Control and Prevention, National Center for Emerging and Zoonotic Infectious Diseases. "Questions and Answers About Foodborne Illness (Sometimes Called 'Food Poisoning')." http://www.cdc.gov/foodsafety/facts.html (accessed January 12, 2012).

Gammara, Roberto M. "Food Poisoning." Medscape Reference. December 20, 2011. http://emedicine.

medscape.com/article/175569-overview (accessed January 12, 2012).

Mahon, Barbara. "Foodborne Illness: A Handy Overview." CDC Expert Commentary, Medscape Today News. http://www.medscape.com/viewarticle/735505 (accessed January 12, 2012).

MedlinePlus. "Foodborne Illness." U.S. National Library of Medicine, National Institutes of Health. http://www.nlm.nih.gov/medlineplus/foodborneillness.html (accessed January 12, 2012).

ORGANIZATIONS

Center for Food Safety and Applied Nutrition (CFSAN), U.S. Food and Drug Administration, 5100 Paint Branch Pkwy., College Park, MD 20740, (888) SAFE-FOOD (723-3366), consumer@fda.gov, http://www.fda.gov/Food/default.htm.

Centers for Disease Control and Prevention, 1600 Clifton Rd. NE, Atlanta, GA 30333, (800) CDC-INFO (232-4636), TTY: (888) 232-6348, cdcinfo@cdc.gov, http://www.cdc.gov.

Food Safety and Inspection Service (FSIS), U.S. Department of Agriculture (USDA), 1400 Independence Ave. SW, Washington, DC 20250-3700, (888) 674-6854 (USDA Meat and Poultry Consumer Hotline), MPHotline.fsis@usda.gov, http://www.fsis.usda.gov.

National Digestive Diseases Information Clearinghouse, 2 Information Way, Bethesda, MD 20892–3570, (800) 891–5389, TTY: (866) 569–1162, Fax: (703) 738–4929, nddic@info.niddk.nih.gov, http://www.digestive.niddk.nih.gov.

Partnership for Food Safety Education, 2345 Crystal Drive, Ste. 800, Arlington, VA 22202, (202) 220-0651, Fax: (202) 220-0873, info@fightbac.org, http://www.fightbac.org.

U.S. Food and Drug Administration, 10903 New Hampshire Ave., Silver Spring, MD 20993-0002, (888) INFO-FDA (463-6332), http://www.fda.gov.

Crystal Kaczkowski, MSc.
Tish Davidson, AM
Margaret Alic

Food pyramid *see* **MyPlate**

Food safety

Definition

Food safety involves protecting food from all contamination—including pathogenic organisms, chemicals, toxins, and physical contaminants—at all stages of the food-production chain. This includes farming through harvesting or slaughtering, processing, packaging, distribution, retail sales, and meal preparation.

Safe cooking temperatures

Food	Internal temperature	
	Fahrenheit	Celsius
Ground meats		
Beef, veal, pork, lamb	160°	71°
Turkey, chicken	165°	74°
Fresh beef, veal, lamb		
Medium rare	145°	63°
Medium	160°	71°
Well done	170°	77°
Poultry		
Chicken, turkey, whole	165°	74°
Poultry breasts	165°	74°
Poultry thighs, wings	165°	74°
Duck, goose	165°	74°
Stuffing (cooked alone or in bird)	165°	74°
Fresh pork		
Medium	160°	71°
Well done	170°	77°
Ham		
Fresh (raw)	160°	71°
Pre-cooked (reheated)	140°	60°
Seafood		
Fish	145°	63°
Shellfish	Shells red and flesh opaque	
Clams, oysters, mussels	Shells open	
Scallops	Milky white or opaque and firm	
Eggs and egg dishes		
Eggs	Yolk and white firm	
Egg dishes	160°	71°
Leftovers and casseroles	165°	74°

(Table by GGS Information Services. © 2013 Cengage Learning.)

Purpose

The food supply in the United States is probably the safest in the world, and serious breaches of food safety are relatively rare. Nevertheless, the U.S. Centers for Disease Control and Prevention (CDC) reported in 2011 that about 48 million Americans—one in six—suffer from foodborne illness (**food poisoning**) every year. Internationally, **food contamination** and large-scale food recalls appear to be on the rise. The 2011 Fukushima Daiichi nuclear power plant disaster in Japan raised fears of radiation-contaminated food. Bioterrorism experts worry that disease-causing organisms or toxic chemicals could be intentionally introduced into food or water supplies causing mass contamination. Scientists worry that climate change may increase the risk of contamination from pesticides and other chemicals, biotoxins, and pathogenic microbes. Various groups question the safety of food derived from genetically modified organisms (GMOs).

Safe food storage limits

Category	Food	Refrigerator (40 °F or below)	Freezer (0 °F or below)
Salads	Egg, chicken, ham, tuna, and macaroni salads	3–5 days	Does not freeze well
Hot dogs	Opened package	1 week	1–2 months
	Unopened package	2 weeks	1–2 months
Luncheon meat	Opened package or deli sliced	3–5 days	1–2 months
	Unopened package	2 weeks	1–2 months
Bacon and sausage	Bacon	7 days	1 month
	Sausage, raw, from chicken, turkey, pork, beef	1–2 days	1–2 months
Ground meats	Hamburger, ground beef, turkey, veal, pork, lamb, and mixtures of them	1–2 days	3–4 months
Fresh beef, veal, lamb and pork	Steaks	3–5 days	6–12 months
	Chops	3–5 days	4–6 months
	Roasts	3–5 days	4–12 months
Fresh poultry	Chicken or turkey, whole	1–2 days	1 year
	Chicken or turkey, pieces	1–2 days	9 months
Soups and stews	Vegetable or meat added	3–4 days	2–3 months
Leftovers	Cooked meat or poultry	3–4 days	2–6 months
	Chicken nuggets or patties	3–4 days	1–3 months
	Pizza	3–4 days	1–2 months

SOURCE: U.S. Department of Health and Human Services, FoodSafety.gov.

(Table by PreMediaGlobal. © 2013 Cengage Learning.)

Although food safety includes preventing the contamination of crops with unsafe levels of pesticides and herbicides and avoiding poisonous mushrooms, mercury-contaminated fish, and shellfish contaminated with algal toxins, most illnesses resulting from food contamination are caused by pathogenic organisms—bacteria, viruses, and parasites. Although foodborne illnesses can be very unpleasant, they are usually mild and short-lived. However, they can cause serious complications and even death, particularly among the very young, the very old, pregnant women and their unborn children, and people with weakened or compromised immune systems. Foods that are tainted with natural toxins, synthetic chemicals, or physical contaminants can also cause serious or fatal illnesses.

Description

In the United States, the vast majority of food poisonings of known origin are caused by one of eight pathogens:

- noroviruses, a large group of viruses that are responsible for the majority of food poisonings of known origin, including major outbreaks on cruise ships and in nursing homes, and that, unlike most other food pathogens, appear to be spread primarily by infected food-service workers

- *Salmonella* spp., widespread intestinal bacteria that cause salmonellosis

- *Clostridium perfringens*, common bacteria found throughout the environment, including in human and animal intestines

- *Campylobacter* spp., bacteria present in most raw poultry and the most commonly identified cause of diarrheal illness worldwide

- *Staphylococcus aureus*, a bacterium in dust, air, and sewage that can contaminate almost any food

- *Toxoplasma gondii*, a parasite that can cause life-threatening illness

- certain strains of the normally harmless, human-gut bacterium *Escherichia coli*, called Shiga toxin-producing *E. coli* (STEC)

- *Listeria monocytogenes*, a bacterium that is ubiquitous in soil, groundwater, plants, and animals and that causes listeriosis

Contaminants that jeopardize food safety change over time, requiring constant surveillance. Improved food safety techniques—including milk pasteurization, safer canning methods, and water treatment—have helped overcome diseases, such as typhoid fever, tuberculosis, and cholera in the developed world. However, other foodborne diseases, such as listeriosis, appear to be on the rise. In 2011, at least 29 people died and at least 139 people across 28 states were sickened from eating cantaloupe contaminated with *L. monocytogenes*, which was traced to unsanitary conditions and poor handling at a single farm. There have been major recalls of ground beef, lettuce, and spinach contaminated with STEC. Strain O157:H7 is the most commonly identified STEC in the United States. There have also been nationwide recalls of peanut butter contaminated with salmonella.

Media reports of contaminated foods, frequent product recalls, and U.S. government initiatives have raised public awareness of food-safety issues. However, globalization of the food supply, industrial farming, concentrated animal feeding operations (CAFOs), and centralized slaughterhouses and processing facilities that pool ingredients from hundreds or thousands of plants and animals have made monitoring food safety very difficult.

The U.S. Food and Drug Administration's (FDA) Food Safety Modernization Act (FSMA) of 2011 was the most sweeping overhaul of food-safety laws in more than 70 years. It aimed to establish a comprehensive, prevention-based system of farm-to-table food safety. As of 2012, however, there were still more than a dozen federal agencies in charge of various aspects of food safety. For example, in the 2011 State of the Union address, President Barack Obama pointed out that the Interior Department is responsible for salmon while they are in fresh water, but once they hit saltwater, the Commerce Department takes over. The Food Safety and Inspection Service (FSIS) of the Department of Agriculture (USDA) is responsible for meat, poultry, and processed egg products that are produced in federally inspected facilities, while the FDA is responsible for the safety of most other foods. The Environmental Protection Agency (EPA) is in charge of pesticides and other toxic chemicals used in food production.

The FDA can request the recall of about 80% of foods consumed domestically, as well as contaminated animal feed. Additives and substances that contact food, such as packaging, must be approved by the FDA as safe. However, other food ingredients, including some that have been used for many years, do not require FDA approval. The FDA also regulates food irradiation that helps protect against disease-causing bacteria and delays spoilage. Irradiated foods include spices, red meat, poultry, some shellfish, and fresh iceberg lettuce and spinach.

Despite government regulation, almost all food safety testing is performed by the food companies themselves. This means that the responsibility of ensuring food is safe to eat falls upon food manufacturers and producers, as well as consumers. Cleanliness, food separation, and proper cooling and cooking are key to food safety.

Cleanliness

Frequent hand washing before, during, and after preparing and eating food is a central tenet of food safety. Hand washing is especially important after handling raw meat, poultry, eggs, and seafood. Hands should be rubbed together with soap under warm, running water for at least 20 seconds (two choruses of "Happy Birthday"). Soap should be rubbed between fingers, down to the wrists, and into fingernails. Paper towels should be used for drying, since cloths spread microbes.

Fresh fruits and vegetables should be washed under running water and scrubbed with a clean brush or with both hands just before cooking or eating. They should be washed both before and after peeling to prevent salmonellosis. Outside leaves of lettuce and cabbage should be discarded. Produce that is not eaten immediately should be dried with a clean cloth or disposable towel, since surface moisture can promote microbial growth. Raw meat and poultry should not be washed, because washing increases the danger of cross-contaminating surfaces.

Cutting boards, utensils, dishes, appliances, kitchen bins, and countertops should be carefully cleaned regularly with hot, soapy water. Dishtowels should be washed in hot water. Sponges should be disinfected in a chlorine bleach solution and replaced frequently. Two minutes in the microwave will kill harmful bacteria in wet sponges. Smelly sponges, cloths, utensils, or surfaces suggest microbial growth and require proper cleaning or disposal.

Food separation

Juices from raw meat, poultry, seafood, and eggs should never come in contact with uncooked, ready-to-eat foods, such as fruits and vegetables. Such foods should remain separated in the grocery cart, in bags, and in the refrigerator with their juices contained.

Cutting boards are a common source of cross-contamination. One cutting board should be set aside for raw meat, poultry, and seafood, and another for cutting vegetables, breads, and other ready-to-eat foods. Boards can be appropriately labeled or colored (e.g., green for vegetables). The meat board should be washed thoroughly with hot, soapy water or in a dishwasher immediately after use. Old cutting boards, especially wooden boards with cracks, crevices, and knife scars, should be discarded. Cross-contamination of cooked foods can occur when plates or surfaces that held raw meat, poultry, or seafood are reused for cooked food.

Cooling

Cold temperatures slow or halt bacterial growth. Although refrigerating leftovers might seem obvious, among the most common calls fielded by the USDA Meat and Poultry Hotline are college students asking whether it is safe to eat pizza that sat out overnight (it's not!). Refrigerators should be kept at 40°F (4°C) or below and freezers at 0°F (-18°C). A refrigerator thermometer can ensure the correct temperature. Raw meat, poultry, eggs, seafood, cut fruits and vegetables, and leftovers should not be left at room temperature for more than two hours or one hour at temperatures above 90°F (32°C). Refrigerators should be cleaned out often, since too much food can prevent cold air from circulating properly.

Foods are generally labeled with refrigeration/freezing instructions and expiration dates. Most foods are safe in the refrigerator for at least three to four days. Exceptions include stuffing, some cooked patties, gravies, and broths, which should only be kept for one to two days. Raw meats should be marinated in the refrigerator rather than at room temperature. Frozen foods should be defrosted in the refrigerator. Food defrosted in warm water or a microwave should be cooked immediately.

Cooking

Uncooked or undercooked meat, poultry, eggs, and egg products are potentially unsafe. Only a good meat thermometer—not the color of the meat or its juices—can determine whether meat is adequately cooked. The thermometer should be placed in the thickest portion of meat or poultry pieces, away from bone, fat, and gristle, and at the center of casseroles and egg dishes. Appropriate minimum temperatures include:

- hamburger patties and meatballs, 160°F (71°C)
- roasts and steaks, 165°F (74°C)
- chicken and turkey, 180°F (82°C)
- fish, 140°F (60°C)
- egg dishes and casseroles, 160°F (71°C)

Cold and hot spots must be avoided when cooking in a microwave. Stirring halfway through cooking evenly distributes the heat and ensures consistent temperature. Leftovers should be heated to at least 165°F (74°C). Leftover sauces, soups, and gravy should be brought to a boil.

Precautions

The most important food safety rule may be "when in doubt, throw it out." Although spoiled foods often have an unpleasant taste or smell, some people, especially

the elderly, may have difficulty telling whether food has gone bad by smell alone. Further, bacterial growth does not necessarily result in a bad taste or smell or discoloration. Dating foods when first refrigerated can help prevent the consumption of outdated items.

Consumers should be aware of updated food safety information and food recalls. Reports of suspect food should be made to the store where the food was purchased, to the manufacturer, or to the FDA or FSIS, depending on the type of food. Any identifying information on the packaging should be noted.

Complications

Ignorance of or disregard for food safety can lead to foodborne illness. Outbreaks of foodborne illness are common in restaurants, cafeterias, nursing homes, prisons, and family and community gatherings where large numbers of people are fed "from the same pot." Contaminated food usually causes diarrhea and often causes nausea, vomiting, abdominal cramps, and fever, which can pose significant health risks for infants, the elderly, and those with special medical conditions. Even moderate diarrhea and vomiting poses a risk for **dehydration**, especially in infants and young children. Although symptoms of food poisoning often occur soon after eating contaminated food, symptoms may not be apparent for up to a week.

Parental concerns

Pregnant women and their unborn babies, infants, and young children are particularly vulnerable to the effects of contaminated food. Thus, awareness of food safety, good food-hygiene practices, and possibly the avoidance of "high-risk" foods are especially important for pregnant women, parents, and caregivers. Vigilant food safety is particularly important when young children attend summer picnics, cookouts, and outdoor buffets.

Breast-feeding is the best food-safety practice for babies. Breast milk and infant formula must be carefully stored. Mixed formula should be kept in the refrigerator for no more than 24 hours. Expired formula and any formula or breast milk left in the bottle after feeding should be discarded. Bottles can become contaminated with salmonella within two hours at

room temperature. Infants under one year should never be given food containing honey, even if it is cooked, since honey can contain spores of *Clostridium botulinum*, the bacterium that produces the deadly paralytic toxin that causes botulism. Although the toxin is destroyed by boiling, the spores are not.

Baby food containers should always be checked to ensure that they have been well sealed and that the food has not reached its expiration date. Leftover food that has been contaminated with the spoon used to feed a baby should be discarded or moved to a dish that the same child will eat from again.

Resources

BOOKS

Bartos, Judeen, ed. *Food Safety*. Detroit: Greenhaven, 2011.
Benedict, Jeff. *Poisoned: The True Story of the Deadly E. coli Outbreak that Changed the Way Americans Eat*. Buena Vista, VA: Inspire, Mariner Media, 2011.
Hewitt, Ben. *Making Supper Safe: One Man's Quest to Learn the Truth about Food Safety*. New York: Rodale, 2011.
Juneja, Vijay K., and John Nikolaos Sofos. *Pathogens and Toxins in Foods: Challenges and Interventions*. Washington, DC: American Society for Microbiology, 2010.
Moby, and Miyun Park, eds. *Gristle: From Factory Farms to Food Safety (Thinking Twice About the Meat We Eat)*. New York: New Press, 2010.
Nestle, Marion. *Safe Food: The Politics of Food Safety*. Berkeley: University of California, 2010.
O'Reilly, James T. *A Consumer's Guide to Food Regulation & Safety*. New York: Oceana, 2010.
Paarlberg, Robert L. *Food Politics: What Everyone Needs to Know*. New York: Oxford University, 2010.
Wallace, Robert B., and Maria Oria. *Enhancing Food Safety: The Role of the Food and Drug Administration*. Washington, DC: National Academies, 2010.

PERIODICALS

Kowalski, Kathiann. "How Safe is Your Food?" *Current Health Kids* 34, no. 7 (March 2011): 16–19.
Palmer, Sharon. "8 Food Safety Myths Busted." *Environmental Nutrition* 34, no. 8 (August 2011): 2.
Roan, Shari, and Eryn Brown. "Q&A; Radiation and Food Safety." *Los Angeles Times*, March 22, 2011, A5.
Stacey, Michelle. "A Good Egg." *Prevention*, May 2011, 124–33.
Voelker, Rebecca. "FDA Tries to Catch Up on Food Safety." *Journal of the American Medical Association* 303, no. 18 (May 12, 2010): 1797.

WEBSITES

Food Safety and Inspection Service. "Food Safety Education." U.S. Department of Agriculture. http://www.fsis.usda.gov/Food_Safety_Education/index.asp (accessed August 19, 2012).
FoodSafety.gov. U.S. Department of Health & Human Services. http://www.foodsafety.gov (accessed August 19, 2012).

Partnership for Food Safety Education. "Safe Food Handling." http://www.fightbac.org/safe-food-handling (accessed August 19, 2012).

U.S. Centers for Disease Control and Prevention. "Food Safety at CDC." http://www.cdc.gov/foodsafety (accessed August 19, 2012).

U.S. Food and Drug Administration. "Food Safety." http://www.fda.gov/Food/FoodSafety/default.htm (accessed August 19, 2012).

———. "The New FDA Food Safety Modernization Act (FSMA)." http://www.fda.gov/food/foodsafety/fsma/default.htm (accessed August 19, 2012).

U.S. Food Safety and Inspection Service. "USDA Meat and Poultry Hotline." Food Safety Education. http://www.fsis.usda.gov/education/usda_meat_&_poultry_hotline/index.asp (accessed August 19, 2012).

ORGANIZATIONS

Academy of Nutrition and Dietetics, 120 South Riverside Plz., Ste. 2000, Chicago, IL 60606-6995, (312) 899-0040, (800) 877-1600, amacmunn@eatright.org, http://www.eatright.org.

Center for Food Safety, 660 Pennsylvania Ave. SE, Ste. 302, Washington, DC 20003, (202) 547-9359, Fax: (202) 547-9429, office@centerforfoodsafety.org, http://www.centerforfoodsafety.org.

Food Safety and Inspection Service (FSIS), U.S. Department of Agriculture (USDA), 1400 Independence Ave. SW, Washington, DC 20250-3700, (888) 674-6854 (USDA Meat and Poultry Consumer Hotline), MPHotline.fsis@usda.gov, http://www.fsis.usda.gov.

National Agriculture Center, U.S. Environmental Protection Agency, 901 N 5th St., Kansas City, KS 66101, (888) 663-2155, Fax: (913) 551-7270, agcenter@epa.gov, http://www.epa.gov/agriculture/agctr.html.

Partnership for Food Safety Education, 2345 Crystal Dr., Ste. 800, Arlington, VA 22202, (202) 220-0651, Fax: (202) 220-0873, info@fightbac.org, http://www.fightbac.org.

U.S. Centers for Disease Control and Prevention, 1600 Clifton Rd., Atlanta, GA 30333, (800) 232-4636, cdcinfor@cdc.gov, http://www.cdc.gov.

U.S. Food and Drug Administration, 10903 New Hampshire Ave., Silver Spring, MD 20993, (888) 463-6332, http://www.fda.gov/Safety/Recalls/default.htm.

Teresa G. Odle
Margaret Alic, PhD

Food sensitivities

Definition

Food sensitivities, also known as food intolerance or food hypersensitivity, are reproducible, adverse reactions to a food or food ingredient at a dose that is well

Common food sensitivities
• Eggs
• Milk and dairy
• Peanuts and other nuts
• Shellfish
• Soy
• Strawberries
• Wheat

Possible symptoms
• Abdominal pain and bloating
• Constipation
• Diarrhea
• Excess coughing
• Hyperactivity
• Infantile colic
• Irritable bowel syndrome
• Itchy skin
• Migraine
• Skin rash
• Sneezing
• Unexplained joint and muscle pain
• Vomiting
• Wheezing

(Table by GGS Information Services. © 2013 Cengage Learning.)

tolerated by most people. Food sensitivity is technically described as non-allergenic food hypersensitivity because it does not involve the immune system, unlike in cases of food allergy, where an immune response is involved. Typically the features of food sensitivity are less severe and take a longer time to manifest than food allergy, where symptoms can be potentially life threatening and occur soon after ingestion.

Demographics

Statistics on food sensitivities are difficult to obtain. Many factors—including that many healthcare professionals debate its prevalence, the lack of well-designed clinical trials, self-diagnosis, and that a person could be exempt of any symptoms—have made it difficult to establish the true incidence and prevalence of food sensitivities. As of 2012, the most common food sensitivity or intolerance in the United States was lactose intolerance, with up to 10% of individuals reporting (mostly self-diagnosed) intolerance to dairy products. Studies show that food intolerances most likely account for the majority of adverse food reactions and may be due to the pharmacologic properties of the food (e.g., headaches from tyramine in aged cheeses).

Description

Food intolerance can occur when the body is unable to digest a certain component of a food—such as lactose, the **sugar** in milk; monosodium glutamate (MSG); or sulfites, a preservative. An individual may be allergic to cow's milk due to an immunologic response to milk **protein**, casein, or alternatively, that individual may be intolerant to milk due to an inability to digest the sugar lactose. In the former situation, milk protein is considered an allergen because it triggers an adverse immunologic reaction. Inability to digest lactose leads to excess fluid production in the GI tract, resulting in abdominal pain, bloating, and diarrhea. This condition is termed lactose intolerance. Lactose is not an allergen because the response is not immune based.

A person's risk for developing food sensitivities or intolerances is increased if one or both of their parents have the condition.

The foods that tend to cause intolerance reactions in sensitive people include:

• dairy products, including milk, cheese, and yogurt
• chocolate
• eggs, particularly egg whites
• flavor enhancers, such as MSG
• food additives
• strawberries, citrus fruits, and tomatoes
• wine, particularly red wine
• histamine and other amines in some foods

Causes and symptoms

Food sensitivity or intolerance can occur for a variety of reasons as outlined in detail below:

• Enzyme deficiency: The most common example of a food sensitivity is lactose intolerance, resulting in intolerance of foods containing milk. This results from the genetic loss of the lactase enzyme needed to breakdown lactose found in milk and dairy foods. The undigested lactose is fermented by gut bacteria that produce large amounts of organic acids and gases, resulting in abdominal pain, distension, and diarrhea.
• Pharmacological: Some foods contain pharmacologically active substances that can cause adverse effects in some people. Good examples include caffeine, found in coffee and cola drinks, and monosodium glutamate, often used in manufactured foods and some Chinese meals.
• Histamine-release: Foods, such as shellfish and strawberries, contain histamine-releasing agents that can cause adverse reactions in sensitive individuals. Since histamine is also released during an allergic reaction, this can complicate distinguishing a food sensitivity from a food allergy.
• Irritant: Excessive consumption of foods such as onions, nuts, and prunes can act as an irritant to

the gastrointestinal tract (gut) and result in unpleasant symptoms such as cramping or gas.
• Toxic: A small number of foods contain naturally occurring toxic compounds, such as lectins, found in under-cooked kidney beans, which can be lethal.

Depending on the actual cause, food sensitivity can cause adverse effects throughout the body. If the gut is involved, symptoms can include vomiting, diarrhea, **constipation**, **irritable bowel syndrome**, infantile colic, **heartburn**, abdominal pain, and bloating. Other symptoms of food sensitivity can include skin rash, itchy skin, excessive coughing, sneezing, wheezing, migraine, and possibly **hyperactivity**, and unexplained joint and muscle pain. Symptoms and severity are usually related to the amount of the food consumed. When the food is consumed infrequently or in small quantities, symptoms may not occur until a certain amount (threshold level) of the food is eaten, but this amount varies for each person.

Diagnosis

In suspected cases of food sensitivity, the diet needs to be fully assessed to see what foods are included in the diet that could be triggering symptoms.

If a particular food, or food ingredient, is suspected, the tried and tested method for diagnosis is an exclusion diet. This diet consists of removing the suspect food from the diet for a time, followed by re-introduction of the food without the individual being tested knowing that it has been added back into the diet. The object is to see if the suspect food has any effect. This is usually followed by a second exclusion period. If the presence and absence of the food correlates with the presence and absence of symptoms, then a positive diagnosis can be made. This should only be the case if the testing is blinded, that is, if the person does not know whether the suspect substance is or is not in the diet at any given time. If a severe reaction is anticipated, re-introduction should be carried out under direct medical supervision.

In cases where multiple foods are suspected, a "few foods" diet, which consists of foods highly unlikely to cause a reaction (e.g., rice, lamb, pears), is followed until symptoms disappear. This is then followed by a systematic blinded re-introduction of single foods, one at a time, allowing the identification of any problem foods to be easily identified whilst avoiding unnecessary restrictions.

There are blood tests that may help in determining if a person has a food sensitivity, but some of these tests are not considered diagnostic and usually lead to confusion and unnecessary elimination of foods from a person's diet. Unstandardized food sensitivity tests, which can cost a person hundreds of dollars, are widely available and can be purchased by patients from a variety of health care providers, as well as some pharmacies. One common type of blood testing uses a measure of immunoglobulin G (IgG) antibody binding to specific foods. However, the presence of these antibodies may be part of the normal human response and indicate tolerance to these foods, rather than an intolerance or sensitivity resulting in an adverse reaction. People should be aware that there is no proven role for IgG testing in diagnosing intolerances or sensitivities to foods.

Treatment

The diet suitable for people with a food sensitivity will depend on which food or ingredient is causing the associated symptoms. Individuals with suspected or proven food intolerance who are excluding major food groups should seek the advice of a qualified dietitian to avoid compromising their nutrient intakes and consequently their physical and/or mental health.

Nutrition and dietary concerns

The diet suitable for food sensitivity benefits the individual by removing the offending food or food ingredient, leading to an improvement in symptoms. It is also worth noting that some types of food sensitivity can be transitory, and so re-introduction of the offending food is recommended every 3–6 months to test whether the sensitivity still persists.

Many people who have been motivated to change their diet in an attempt to relieve the effects of food sensitivity will remain interested in maintaining good nutritional health and continue to eat well. A well-balanced food sensitivity diet can still be rich in **fiber**, **vitamins**, and **minerals**, all of which are vital for good brain and body functioning, as well as reducing the risk of developing certain cancers and cardiovascular disease.

Very young children and babies should not have any dietary restrictions imposed upon them unless they are clinically indicated and are supervised by a doctor and dietitian. The restricted nutrient intake that might result can significantly compromise children's growth and development.

The same risk applies to older children and rapidly growing adolescents because of the high requirements needed to sustain good physical growth and mental development.

Women planning a pregnancy, or who are already pregnant or are **breastfeeding**, should also avoid any dietary restrictions, unless recommended by a doctor or dietitian. Nutrient restriction in these women can compromise the health of both the mother and the baby.

Individuals experiencing any chronic medical conditions, or recovering from surgery, should not follow a restricted diet without medical supervision as this can exacerbate symptoms and slow down recovery and wound healing.

The most nutritionally balanced diet is one that includes a wide range of different foods, and so the main risk attached to the food sensitivity diet depends on the particular restrictions involved. In some cases, avoidance of the offending foods is nutritionally insignificant and can be easily excluded (e.g., **caffeine** drinks or strawberries).

The greatest nutritional risk is associated with the exclusion of entire food groups, such as dairy foods and gluten-containing grains. Gluten-free diets can be low in fiber, which is needed for good bowel function and helps to protect against cardiovascular disease, and cow's milk-free diets can be low in **calcium** and **iodine**, which are important for bone strength and brain function.

Advice from a dietitian should be sought to ensure nutritional adequacy and allow discussion of suitable substitute foods and **dietary supplements**, where appropriate.

A final point worth mentioning is that substitute foods are not always available and are usually more expensive. Following a food sensitivity diet also can make eating out and social occasions more difficult.

Prognosis

In some cases, infants, children, and adults may, over time, develop the ability to consume the food without adverse symptoms occurring.

Prevention

There is no known cure for food sensitivities. The only prevention of the symptoms is by avoiding the food or foods that cause the symptoms. However, there may be remedies or medications that may be used to treat the condition. For example, in the condition of lactose intolerance, a person may take lactase, the enzyme that breaks down lactose, prior to eating/drinking foods containing lactose.

QUESTIONS TO ASK YOUR DOCTOR

- Do you think it is a food sensitivity or a food allergy?

- How do you plan to diagnose my suspected food intolerance/sensitivity?

- Are my other health conditions affected by this condition and/or treatment?

- How can I make sure my other doctors or members of my health care team know about my food intolerance/sensitivity?

- Can you recommend a specialist or dietitian to help me design a diet to eliminate the food I am sensitive to without any nutrient deficiencies?

- How long should I follow the exclusion diet for diagnostic purposes?

- Am I more likely to be intolerant or sensitive to other foods?

Resources

BOOKS

Skypala, Isabel and Carina Venter. *Food Hypersensitivity: Diagnosing and Managing Food Allergies and Intolerance.* Ames, IA: Blackwell Pub., 2009.

PERIODICALS

Lavine, Elana. "Blood Testing for Sensitivity, Allergy or Intolerance To Food." *Canadian Medical Association Journal* 184, no. 6 (2012): 666–68.

Lied, G.A., et al. "Perceived Food Hypersensitivity: A Review of 10 Years of Interdisciplinary Research at a Reference Center." *Scandinavian Journal of Gastroenterology* 46, no. 10 (2011): 1169–78.

Zopf, Y., et al. "The Differential Diagnosis of Food Intolerance." *Deutches Ärzteblatt International* 106, no. 21 (2009): 359–69 (article in English). http://dx.doi.org/10.3238/arztebl.2009.0359 (accessed August 23, 2012).

WEBSITES

Allergies Health Center. "Is It Food Allergy or Intolerance?" WebMD. http://www.webmd.com/allergies/foods-allergy-intolerance (accessed July 22, 2012).

Allergy UK. "Food Intolerance." http://www.allergyuk.org/food-intolerance/food-intolerance (accessed August 23, 2012).

Manners, Deborah. "Food Intolerance—Definition." http://www.foodintol.com/food-sensitivities (accessed August 23, 2012).

Mayo Clinic staff. "What's the Difference Between a Food Intolerance and Food Allergy?" MayoClinic.com.

http://www.mayoclinic.com/health/food-allergy/AN01109 (accessed July 22, 2012).

MedlinePlus. "Lactose Intolerance." U.S. National Library of Medicine, National Institutes of Health. http://www.nlm.nih.gov/medlineplus/lactoseintolerance.html (accessed July 22, 2012).

ORGANIZATIONS

Academy of Nutrition and Dietetics, 120 South Riverside Plz., Ste. 2000, Chicago, IL 60606-6995, (312) 899-0040, (800) 877-1600, amacmunn@eatright.org, http://www.eatright.org.

American College of Gastroenterology (ACG), 6400 Goldsboro Rd., Ste 450, Bethesda, MD 20817, (301) 263-9000, info@acg.gi.org, http://www.acg.gi.org.

British Nutrition Foundation, High Holborn House, 52-54 High Holborn, London, United Kingdom WC1V 6RQ, 44 20 7404 6504, Fax: 44 20 7404 6747, postbox@nutrition.org.uk, http://www.nutrition.org.uk.

International Foundation for Functional Gastrointestinal Disorders, PO Box 170864, Milwaukee, WI 53217-8076, (414) 964-1799, (888) 964-2001, Fax: (414) 964-7176, iffgd@iffgd.org, http://www.iffgd.org.

National Digestive Diseases Information Clearinghouse, 2 Information Way, Bethesda, MD 20892–3570, (800) 891–5389, TTY: (866) 569–1162, Fax: (703) 738–4929, nddic@info.niddk.nih.gov, http://www.digestive.niddk.nih.gov.

Emma Mills, RD
Tish Davidson, AM

Free-range, grass-fed, and cage-free animals

Definition

Free range, *cage free*, and *grass fed* are terms that describe how livestock and poultry are raised before their meat and eggs are used for food. Free-range animals and cage-free poultry are allowed to roam freely on a farm or ranch. Grass-fed animals receive the majority of their nutrients from grass during their lives. Products labeled "free range" and "grass fed" are regulated by the U.S. Department of Agriculture (USDA). The term "cage free" is a voluntary designation.

Purpose

The terms "free range," "grass fed," and "cage free" are used in two main contexts: federal standards for the identification and labeling of agricultural products and consumer advertising. The terms may be applied to eggs or dairy products as well as meat or poultry.

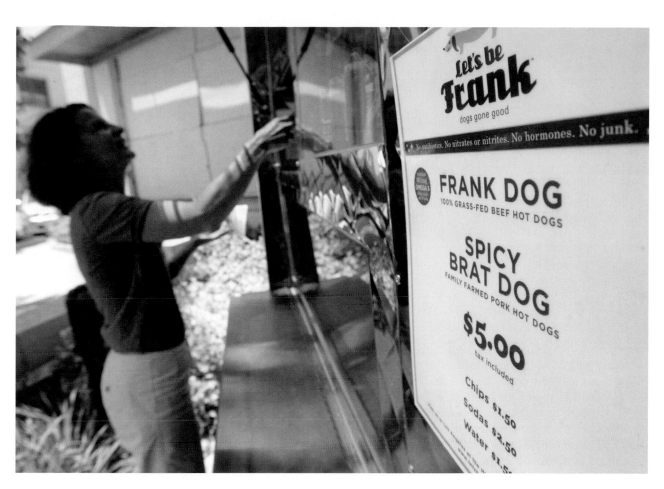

A woman purchases a hot dog made from grass-fed animals. *(AP Photo/Ric Francis)*

The terms are often associated with sustainable agriculture or the so-called alternative agriculture movement. Farmers or ranchers who practice free-range animal husbandry typically do so for one or more of five major reasons:

- humane considerations

- feed cost reduction

- happier and livelier animals

- higher-quality food products

- sustainable agriculture, which involves raising crops and livestock on the same parcel of land without exhausting the land or damaging the local environment

Terms like free range, grass fed, and cage free are used by advertisers to make food products more appealing to consumers. Several reasons motivate people to buy these products. They want animals that are raised in a natural manner, preferring animals raised on grass rather than corn. They want food from animals that were not given antibiotics or hormones; and these people do not want to eat food that was treated with pesticides.

Concern about the humane treatment of animals and poultry is another motivation for these consumers. Cage-free eggs come from hens that do not live in battery cages, stacked cages where each bird is in an area approximately the size of a small laptop computer. The quarters are so cramped that the hens cannot spread their wings.

Cage-free birds and free-range livestock are able to roam freely and perform natural activities. In addition, grass-fed livestock has health benefits that appeal to customers. Beef from grass-fed cattle has about half of the saturated fat found in corn-fed beef, according to *Consumer Reports*. Furthermore, some consumers want to support local farmers who raise free-range or grass-fed animals rather than buy products from large impersonal agribusinesses that may be hundreds of miles away.

Other terms used to label food include "pastured" and "organic."

Description

Free-range animal husbandry and pastured poultry raising are not new; they are the way that animals were raised for food products for millennia until the 1950s, when so-called factory farming was introduced as a way to maximize livestock and poultry production within a limited amount of space. Pastured poultry raising and free-range animal husbandry gained a new popularity in the United States beginning in the 1980s with Joel Salatin, a farmer in the Shenandoah Valley of Virginia. Salatin's system was based on feeding his livestock healthy grass and moving the cattle from one field to another for fresh forage rather than feeding them corn in a central location. After the cattle were moved from a specific pasture, chickens in portable coops were brought in behind them to live on grubs and other insects in the cow droppings. The chicken droppings were then used to fertilize the fields so that no chemical fertilizers were necessary to maintain the condition of the land.

Free range is sometimes misleading when applied to cattle, as it does not specify what the animals are fed. Many ranchers prefer the term grass fed, which indicates that their animals' primary lifelong diet is pasture grass rather than the concentrated mixture of grain, **soy**, and other supplements used in the feedlot method of raising cattle for the last three to four months of their lives. Some poultry farmers prefer the term pastured poultry to cage free on the grounds that it is a more accurate description of the fact that the birds are given pasture forage as their source of food.

Product labels

The U.S. Department of Agriculture (USDA) Agricultural Marketing Service National Organic Program website has labeling definitions that will help consumers understand the information on labels. These definitions include:

• Organic. Products labeled with the USDA organic seal are certified organic, meaning that the food or other agricultural product has been produced through approved methods. These methods integrate cultural, biological, and mechanical practices that foster cycling of resources, promote ecological balance, and conserve biodiversity. Synthetic fertilizers, sewage sludge, irradiation, and genetic engineering may not be used.

• Grass fed. Grass-fed animals receive a majority of their nutrients from grass throughout their lives, while organic animals' pasture diets may be supplemented with grain. Also USDA regulated, the grass-fed label does not limit the use of antibiotics, hormones, or pesticides. Meat products may be labeled as grass-fed organic.

• Free range. This labeling is regulated by the USDA. This label indicates that the flock was provided shelter in a building, room, or an area with unlimited access to food, fresh water, and continuous access to the outdoors during their production cycle. The outdoor area may or may not be fenced and/or covered with netting-like material.

• Cage free. The label indicates that the flock was able to freely roam a building, room, or enclosed area with unlimited access to food and fresh water during their production cycle.

• Natural. As required by the USDA, meat, poultry, and egg products labeled as natural must be minimally processed and contain no artificial ingredients. However, the natural label does not include any standards regarding farm practices and only applies to the processing of meat and egg products. There are no standards or regulations for the labeling of natural food products if they do not contain meat or eggs.

• Pasture raised. Due to the number of variables involved in pasture-raised agricultural systems, the USDA has not developed a labeling policy for pasture-raised products.

• Humane. Multiple labeling programs make claims that animals were treated humanely during the production cycle, but the verification of these claims varies widely. These labeling programs are not regulated.

Livestock and poultry in the United States

The cattle inventory in 2011 consisted of 92,582,400 animals, according to the USDA. The total included 30.9 million beef cows and 26.7 million feeder calves. There were 742,000 herds, with 90% of herds consisting of less than 100 cows. Herd size averaged 44 head of cattle.

At the start of the twenty-first century, there were only 50 grass-fed cattle operations in the United States, according to a 2010 National Public Radio (NPR) report. By the end of the decade, there were thousands of grass-fed operations, and the number was growing, according to reports by media including NPR. Market watchers say that consumer demand for grass-fed organic products is sparking the increase.

In 2012, 61 egg-producing companies with over 1 million hens (layers) represented approximately 87% of the total production in the United States, and cage-free production accounted for only 5.7% of U.S. flock size. Of those cage-free operations, 2.9% were organic. The amount of free-range layers tracked by United

Egg Producers (UEP), an organization representing approximately 95% of the egg-laying ownership in the country, has increased gradually. An August 12, 2007 *New York Times* article cited UEP statistics indicating that the amount of free-range hens was close to 5% in 2007, up from 2% a few years before that. At that time, businesses including Ben & Jerry's, Burger King, Whole Foods, Google, and chef Wolfgang Puck were implementing cage-free egg policies.

Some businesses were motivated by public attitudes about the humane treatment of poultry, as well as pressure from organizations opposed to battery cages, such as the Humane Society of the United States.

Benefits of free-range meat and poultry

Research has indicated that meat, dairy products, poultry and eggs from animals fed grass diets are lower in fat and cholesterol than animals fed grain-based diets. Grass-fed food also has more health benefits, according to studies that included findings from California State University in Chico. That study, described in a 2010 *Nutrition Journal* article, evaluated three decades of research into the comparisons of grass-fed and grain-fed beef.

The research showed that in addition to healthier levels of **fats** and cholesterol, beef from animals fed grass throughout their lives provided more of **vitamins** E and A and higher levels of conjugated linoleic acid (CLA), an acid that may help to fight **cancer** and reduce the risk of cancer and other health-related conditions. In addition, grass-fed beef is a better source of **omega-3 fatty acids** than grain-fed beef. However, the omega-3 levels in beef are lower than sources such as salmon and other fatty fish.

Some of those findings echoed research in a 2006 study by the Union of Concerned Scientists (UCS). The study stated the meat from grass-fed cattle was typically leaner (lower fat content) and lower in **calories** than meat from feedlot-fed cattle and also had a higher content of omega-3 fatty acids.

Meat from free-range chickens is reported to be chewier and less tender than meat from factory-farmed chickens, but it is lower in saturated fatty acids and higher in polyunsaturated fatty acids.

Precautions

In some cases, consumers may need to verify that food products labeled as free range, grass fed, or cage free are what they claim to be. Other precautions include standard procedures for the selection, safe

---

KEY TERMS

Agribusiness—A term that has two different meanings, depending on context. It is often used by farmers in a neutral way to refer simply to any business aspects of farm production, such as equipment purchasing, marketing, retail sales, and the like. It is also used, however, by opponents of large-scale factory farms to contrast these farms with smaller family-owned farms.

Animal husbandry—The practice of breeding and raising livestock (including poultry) for meat and other food products. It is also called animal science.

Factory farming—The practice of raising large numbers of animals indoors in close quarters with little or no mobility. It is also called intensive farming or corporate farming.

Feedlot—An enclosure in which beef cattle are finished prior to slaughter by being fed a specialized diet consisting of hay, sorghum, barley, soybean meal, and a variety of other products. Feedlots are also called feedyards or animal feeding operations (AFOs).

Forage—Plant material (usually leaves and stems) eaten by grazing livestock and poultry.

Sustainable agriculture—A term that refers to farming practices aimed at producing healthful crops and animal products while maintaining the soil in good condition and without doing long-term harm to the local environment.

Zoonosis—Any disease that can be transmitted to humans by animals.

---

storage, and safe preparation of perishable foods. These precautions are particularly necessary in the case of eggs, whose shells may be contaminated by *Salmonella* bacteria, a common source of **food poisoning**. However, cage-free or free-range poultry pose no higher risk than poultry raised using other methods.

Interactions

When people observe safe food-handling practices, there are usually no negative interactions when consuming free-range or grass-fed food, or when eating eggs from cage-free birds. While some people may be allergic to eggs, this allergy is to eggs in general and is not related to how the animals were raised.

QUESTIONS TO ASK YOUR DOCTOR

- What is your opinion of free-range meat, poultry, and dairy products? Are they safe?
- What is your opinion of cage-free eggs? Are they safe?
- What is your opinion of organic food? Is it healthier for me?
- Are these foods worth the extra expense?
- What are the risks of consuming these foods?

Complications

There may be a lower level of standardization in the taste and overall quality of free-range food products; that is, poultry or meat produced by a small farmer may not taste exactly the same each time it is purchased, or it may take slightly more or less time to cook. There is also the risk of food poisoning or other zoonosis if these foods are not stored or prepared properly; however, the risk is no higher with free-range foods than with food products produced using other methods.

Parental concerns

Parents may learn that their child has an allergy to eggs and will need to monitor the child's diet. However, the allergy is not related to whether the eggs are from cage-free hens or those raised in battery cages.

Research & general acceptance

Relatively little research has been done on free-range or pasture-fed animals or food products compared to their factory farm counterparts, most likely because direct comparisons are complicated by the number of variables (size of operation; geographic location, including altitude and the type of grass used for forage; specific breeds of animals involved, etc.). Another factor that makes direct comparisons difficult is that consumers appear to take ethical and other values into consideration when choosing food products from free-range or grass-fed animals, and these intangible concerns are harder to measure in a clinical study than nutrient values.

The Academy of Nutrition and Dietetics takes the position that research indicates that nutrient values appear to be similar for organic and conventional grains and vegetable crops, but that "more research is required to address systematically whether significant differences exist in nutrient content of organic and conventional produce, grain, meat and dairy products." The report produced by the UCS in 2006 also called for further research into the nutrient values of grass-fed meat and dairy products compared to those from factory-farmed animals.

Resources

BOOKS

American Pastured Poultry Producers Association (APPPA). *Raising Poultry on Pasture: Ten Years of Success.* Boyd, WI: APPPA, 2008.

Salatin, Joel. *Family Friendly Farming: A Multi-generational Home-based Business Testament.* Swoope, VA: Polyface, 2001.

———. *You Can Farm: The Entrepreneur's Guide to Start and Succeed in a Farm Enterprise.* Swoope, VA: Polyface, 1998.

Spilsbury, Richard, and Louise Spilsbury. *Feeding the World.* New York: PowerKids Press, 2010.

Williams, Jane, ed. *Complete Textbook of Animal Health and Welfare.* New York: Saunders/Elsevier, 2009.

PERIODICALS

Consumer Reports.org "Is 'Grass-fed' Beef a Healthier Choice?" *Consumer Reports* (May 1, 2008). http://news.consumerreports.org/health/2008/05/is-grass-fed-be.html (accessed August 10, 2012).

Daley, Cynthia A., et al. "A Review of Fatty Acid Profiles and Antioxidant Content in Grass-Fed and Grain-Fed Beef." *Nutrition Journal* (September 1, 2010). http://www.nutritionj.com/content/pdf/1475-2891-9-10.pdf (accessed August 10, 2012).

Dubey, J. P. "*Toxoplasma gondii* Infections in Chickens (*Gallus domesticus*): Prevalence, Clinical Disease, Diagnosis and Public Health Significance." *Zoonoses and Public Health* 57, no. 1 (February 2010): 60–73.

Husak, R. L., et al. "A Survey of Commercially Available Broilers Marketed as Organic, Free-range, and Conventional Broilers for Cooked Meat Yields, Meat Composition, and Relative Value." *Poultry Science* 87 (November 2008): 2367–2376.

Näther, G., et al. "Analysis of Risk Factors for *Campylobacter* Species Infection in Broiler Flocks." *Poultry Science* 88 (June 2009): 1299–1305.

Purdum, Todd S. "The High Priest of the Pasture." *New York Times Sunday Magazine* (May 1, 2005). http://query.nytimes.com/gst/fullpage.html?res=9D0CE7DF173EF932A35756C0A9639C8B63 (accessed August 10, 2012).

Severson, Kim. "Suddenly, the Hunt Is On for Cage-Free Eggs." *New York Times*, August 12, 2007. http://www.nytimes.com/2007/08/12/us/12eggs.html?pagewanted=all (accessed August 10, 2012).

OTHER

Clancy, Kate. *Greener Eggs and Ham: The Benefits of Pasture-Raised Swine, Poultry, and Egg Production.* Cambridge, MA: Union of Concerned Scientists (UCS), 2006. http://www.ucsusa.org/assets/documents/food_and_agriculture/greener-pastures.pdf (accessed August 10, 2012).

————. *Greener Pastures: How Grass-Fed Beef and Milk Contribute to Healthy Eating.* Cambridge, MA: Union of Concerned Scientists (UCS), 2006. http://www.ucsusa.org/assets/documents/food_and_agriculture/greener-eggs-and-ham.pdf (accessed August 30, 2012).

Food & Water Watch. *Factory Farm Nation: How America Turned Its Livestock Farms into Factories.* Washington, DC: Food & Water Watch, 2010. http://www.factoryfarmmap.org/wp-content/uploads/2010/11/FactoryFarmNation-web.pdf (accessed August 30, 2012).

U.S. Department of Agriculture, Food Safety and Inspection Service. "Animal Raising Claims in the Labeling of Meat and Poultry Products." http://origin-www.fsis.usda.gov/PDF/Claims_Poretta_101408.pdf (accessed August 30, 2012).

WEBSITES

Aubrey, Allison. "The Truth About Grass-Fed Beef." National Public Radio, April 8, 2010. http://www.npr.org/2010/04/08/125722082/the-truth-about-grass-fed-beef (accessed August 30, 2012).

Compassion in World Farming. "Your Food." http://www.ciwf.org.uk/your_food/default.aspx (accessed August 30, 2012).

United Egg Producers. "U.S. Egg Industry Stats." http://www.unitedegg.org/GeneralStats/default.cfm (accessed August 30, 2012).

U.S. Department of Agriculture, Agricultural Marketing Service. "National Organic Program." http://www.ams.usda.gov/AMSv1.0/ams.fetchTemplateData.do?template=TemplateA&navID=NationalOrganicProgram&page=NOPNationalOrganicProgramHome&resultType=&topNav=&leftNav=NationalOrganicProgram&acct=nop (accessed August 30, 2012).

U.S. Department of Agriculture, Food Safety and Inspection Service (FSIS). "Food Labeling: Meat and Poultry Labeling Terms." http://origin-www.fsis.usda.gov/Fact_Sheets/Meat_&_Poultry_Labeling_Terms/index.asp (accessed August 30, 2012).

U.S. Department of Agriculture and U.S. Department of Health and Human Services. *Dietary Guidelines for Americans, 2010.* 7th ed. Washington, DC: U.S. Government Printing Office, December 2010. http://health.gov/dietaryguidelines (accessed August 30, 2012).

ORGANIZATIONS

Academy of Nutrition and Dietetics, 120 South Riverside Plz., Ste. 2000, Chicago, IL 60606-6995, (312) 899-0040, (800) 877-1600, amacmunn@eatright.org, http://www.eatright.org.

American Grassfed Association Office, 4340 E Kentucky Ave., Ste. 311, Denver, CO 80246, (877) 774-7277, aga@americangrassfed.org, http://www.americangrassfed.org.

Compassion in World Farming, River Court, Mill Lane, GodalmingSurrey, United Kingdom GU7 1EZ, 440-1483-521-953, http://www.ciwf.org.uk.

Union of Concerned Scientists (UCS), Two Brattle Square, Cambridge, MA 02238, (617) 547-5552, http://www.ucsusa.org.

Rebecca J. Frey, PhD
Liz Swain

French diet *see* **Northern European diet**

French paradox

Definition

The French Paradox refers to the low rate of **coronary heart disease** (CHD) in France despite the diet being rich in saturated fat.

Origins

2002 data from the Food and Agriculture Organization of the United Nations (FAO), showed that although the intake of saturated fat in France was higher than in the United States (US), 108 grams (g) compared to 72 g per day, France had a 30%–40% lower risk of CHD. Over the years, studies suggest that one of the reasons the French have a lower rate of CHD, despite higher saturated fat intakes, may be related to their regular consumption of red wine.

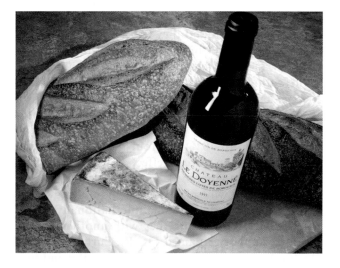

The French paradox refers to the low instance of obesity in France even though traditional meals include foods like wine, bread, and cheese. *(Jupiterimages)*

alcohol **consumption** may lower the risk of cognitive impairment in later life, but further research is needed.

Resveratrol has been linked to **cancer** prevention, but alcohol is associated with increased cancer risk, so wine should not be used as a cancer preventative.

Precautions

Individuals involved with activities that require attention, skill, or coordination, such as driving or operating machinery, should avoid alcoholic beverages. Alcohol has a depressant effect on the central nervous system and slows down brain function, which can affect judgment and emotions as well as behavior.

The 2011 Centers for Disease Control and Prevention (CDC) guidelines advise women who may become pregnant or are pregnant not to drink. Moderate drinking during pregnancy may result in behavioral or neurocognitive problems in children.

There is conflicting advice on moderate alcohol or no alcohol with breastfeeding. The American Academy of Pediatricians still recommends avoiding alcohol while breast-feeding. Alcohol can be passed on to the baby through the milk, which can affect the baby's feeding, sleeping or digestion. Heavy alcohol intakes have also been shown to reduce lactation. The National Childbirth Trust and the Association of Breastfeeding Mothers in UK advocate similar advice. The recommendation is to allow sufficient time between drinking and breast-feeding so the mother can fully metabolize the alcohol.

Individuals taking prescription and over-the-counter medications also need to be aware of the potential interactions any of their medications may have with alcohol and should consult a doctor.

Risks

Higher intakes of alcohol levels seem to offset the benefits of moderate drinking on CHD, by increasing risk of death from many other diseases.

Excessive intake of any kind of alcohol increases the risk of cancer of the mouth, esophagus, stomach, liver, breast and colon. The Cancer Prevention Study in 2002 found that one drink or less in postmenopausal women increased the risk of death from breast cancer by 30%. They did not find an increased risk in premenopausal women.

Excessive alcohol can increase blood pressure, which increases the risk for CHD. Cutting back to moderate drinking can lower systolic blood pressure by up to 10 mmHg.

According to a U.S. study published in 2005, older men who drink more than the daily recommendations of alcohol may be more likely to suffer from a stroke.

Triglycerides are a type of fat found in the bloodstream and in fat tissue. High levels are associated with an increased risk of CHD, and the liver produces more triglycerides with excess alcohol, **sugar**, and calories.

The risk of cirrhosis seems connected more with alcohol abuse than moderate use. Excessive drinkers will develop fatty liver, the first stage of alcoholic liver disease, but this can disappear when alcohol is reduced to moderate levels. Continued excessive alcohol can lead to alcoholic hepatitis or cirrhosis and liver failure.

Heavy alcohol use for ten years or more is the usual cause of Chronic Pancreatitis. Acute pancreatitis with severe abdominal pain can occur before this and will settle if drinking is discontinued.

Research and general acceptance

There has never been a controlled clinical trial testing the effect of alcohol, but there is agreement that while drinking too much of any kind of alcohol is not healthy, moderate alcohol intakes may have some health benefits. As such, a number of medical associations including the European Society of Cardiology, The National Institute on Alcohol Abuse and Alcoholism, **Academy of Nutrition and Dietetics**, American Heart Association, Royal College of Physicians, and British Heart Foundation have the recommendation for alcohol as, "If you use alcohol, do so in moderation." Recommendations on how many drinks per day equate to moderation differs from country to country. In the United States, moderation is defined as up to one drink per day for women and up to two drinks per day for men. In the United Kingdom, moderation is defined as not exceeding 2–3 units for women and 3–4 units for men.

Drs. Malcolm Law and Nicholas Wald, British specialists in preventive medicine at St. Bartholomew's and the Royal London School of Medicine and Dentistry and Dr. Marion Nestle, chairwoman of the department of nutrition at New York University, have put forward another explanation for the French diet and health. They argue that it is related to France's history of lower animal fat intakes rather than their consumption of red wine. Up to 1970, the French ate less animal fat and had significantly lower blood cholesterol levels than the British. French habits appear to be changing however, as they are eating more meat and fast foods and their consumption of animal fat is similar to those in Britain. The 1999 National Survey on Individual Food in France by the Research Center for the Study and Monitoring of Living Standards shows that between 1950 and 1980 the consumption of meat fat and oils doubled and alcohol intake halved. The rate of **obesity** in France has also increased from 8% in 1997 to 12%, and over 40% of the French are now considered overweight, not far off the 50% figure for the British and Americans. Scientists believe it takes

---

QUESTIONS TO ASK YOUR DOCTOR

- What does moderate drinking mean?
- How much wine should I be drinking?
- What health problems are associated with drinking?
- Can I drink when I am pregnant?
- What does one unit of alcohol include?
- How can I tell if I am getting the right nutrients?
- What tests are needed for a thorough assessment?
- What tests or evaluation techniques can you perform to see if my diet and nutritional choices promote a healthy condition?
- What kind of fitness program should I follow?
- Can you recommend a nutritionist or dietitian to assist me with making good food choices?

---

approximately 25–35 years for increased fat intake to translate into heart disease so it may be only a matter of time before France faces the obesity epidemics and CHD rates that began in America and Britain nearly 20 years ago.

The role of nutrition in CHD is also being explored in association with the **Mediterranean diet**. Foods associated with the Mediterranean diet include fish, poultry, vegetables, fruits, breads, potatoes, cereals, nuts, beans, and whole grains. Food is generally fresh, not processed. Olive oil is used more often than other fats such as butter, dairy products such as yogurt and cheese are usually low or reduced fat, and low to moderate amounts of red meat are consumed (usually lean red meats). Wine is consumed in low to moderate amounts, usually with meals. Individuals in the Mediterranean regions also adhere to daily physical activity, while paying attention to the daily intake of nutritional food.

Low animal-fat content of the Mediterranean diet, high consumption of whole cereals and vegetables, and the regular use of olive oil, have been shown to help in lowering serum cholesterol levels and blood pressure, both classic risk factors of CHD. Researchers and epidemiologists continue to compare and contrast the French paradox and Mediterranean diet to look for common links and associations in lowering risks for CHD.

Resources

BOOKS

Counihan, Carole., and Penny Van Esternik, eds. *Food and Culture*. 3rd ed. New York: Routledge, 2012.

Giesler, Beth. *Resveratrol: Unleashing the Benefits of Red Wine*. Summertown, TN: Healthy Living Publications, 2011.

Guiliano, Mireille. *French Women Don't Get Fat: The Secret of Eating for Pleasure*. New York: Random House, 2007.

Lewis, Perdue. *The French Paradox and Beyond: Living Longer with Wine and the Mediterranean Lifestyle*. Renaissance Publishing, 2011.

Mayle, Peter. *A Year in Provence*. New York: Random House, 2010.

PERIODICALS

Boffetta, P., and L. Garefinkel. "Alcohol Drinking among men Enrolled in an American Cancer Society Prospective Study." *Epidemiology* 1, no. 5 (1990): 42–48.

Corder, R., et al. "Red Wine Procyanidins and Vascular health." *Nature* 444 (November 2006): 566.

Doll, R., et al. "Mortality in Relation to Consumption of Alcohol: 13 Years' Observations on Male British Doctors" *British Medical Journal* 309 (Oct. 8, 1994): 911–18.

Feigelson H "Alcohol Consumption Increases The Risk Of Fatal Breast Cancer" *Cancer Causes and Control* December 2002.

Gunzerath, L., et al. "National Institute on Alcohol Abuse and Alcoholism Report on Moderate Drinking." *Alcoholism: Clinical & Experimental Research* 28, no. 6 (2004): 829–47.

Keys, A. "Coronary Heart Disease in Seven Countries." *Circulation* 41, suppl. I (1970): I-1–I-211.

Law, M., and N. Wald. "Why Heart Disease Mortality is Low in France: The Time Lag Explanation." *British Medical Journal* 318, no. 7196 (1999): 1471–80.

McElduff, P., and A.J. Dobson. "How Much Alcohol and How Often? Population Based Case-Control Study of Alcohol Consumption and Risk of a mAjor Coronary Event Prospective Study." *British Medical Journal* 314, no. 7088 (1997): 1159–64.

Mukamal, K.J., et al. "Alcohol and Risk for Ischemic Stroke in Men: The Role of Drinking Patterns and Usual Beverage." *Annals of Internal Medicine* 142, no. 1 (2005): 11–19.

Neafsey, Edward J., and Michael A. Collins. "Moderate Alcohol Consumption and Cognitive Risk." *Neuropsychiatric Disease and Treatment* 7 (August 11, 2011): 465–84. http://dx.doi.org/10.2147/NDT.S23159 (accessed September 28, 2012).

Thun, M.J., et al. "Alcohol Consumption and Mortality among Middle-Aged and Elderly U.S. Adults." *New England Journal of Medicine* 337, no. 24 (1997): 1705–14.

WEBSITES

American Cancer Society. "Alcohol Use and Cancer." http://www.cancer.org/Cancer/CancerCauses/Dietand PhysicalActivity/alcohol-use-and-cancer (accessed September 28, 2012).

Higdon, Jane, and Victoria J. Drake. "Resveratrol." Linus Pauling Institute, Oregon State University. http://lpi. oregonstate.edu/infocenter/phytochemicals/resveratrol (accessed September 28, 2012).

ORGANIZATIONS

Academy of Nutrition and Dietetics, 120 South Riverside Plz., Ste. 2000, Chicago, IL 60606-6995, (312) 899-0040, (800) 877-1600, amacmunn@eatright.org, http://www.eatright.org.

American Cancer Society, 250 Williams St. NW, Atlanta, GA 30303, (800) 227-2345, http://www.cancer.org.

American Heart Association, 7272 Greenville Ave., Dallas, TX 75231, (800) 242-8721, http://www.americanheart.org.

British Heart Foundation, Greater London House, 180 Hampstead Rd., London, United Kingom NW1 7AW, +44 20 7554 0000, http://www.bhf.org.uk.

National Heart, Lung, and Blood Institute, PO Box 30105, Bethesda, MD 20824-0105, (301) 592-8573, TTY: (240) 629-3255, Fax: (240) 629-3246, nhlbiinfo @nhlbi.nih.gov, http://www.nhlbi.nih.gov.

Tracy J. Parker, RD.
Laura Jean Cataldo, RN, EdD

Frozen-food diet

Definition

Frozen-food diets rely on packaged frozen foods for weight loss and weight control that are based on standardized portions, as well as for convenience and saving time.

Origins

A frozen-food diet was first introduced in *Good Housekeeping* magazine in September of 1998. In October of 2005 *Good Housekeeping* debuted a new frozen-food diet that consisted entirely of microwaveable meals. The new plan, based on research performed at the Department of Food Science and Human Nutrition at the University of Illinois at Champaign-Urbana, promised slightly increased weight loss and even less preparation time than the original diet.

Other frozen-food diets have also been developed. Nutrition expert Joy Bauer prepared a nine-day meal plan for the American Frozen Food Institute (AFFI) that consists entirely of frozen foods. Commercial frozen-food diets that are home-delivered weekly are

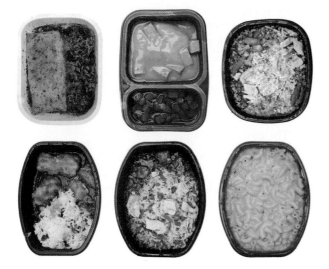

Frozen dinners. *(© Brooke Becker/shutterstock.com)*

also available. One such diet was devised by Dr. Caroline J. Cederquist, a board-certified physician in bariatrics, the medical specialty of weight management.

Description

The original Good Housekeeping diet

The original *Good Housekeeping* frozen-food diet consists of seven days of menus. However any meal can be switched for the same meal on a different day. It is a 1,400-calorie per day diet and the plan calls for 45 minutes of exercise four to five days per week. Brand-name products may be substituted with similar foods having the same number of **calories**. Spices, garlic, lemon, **soy** sauce, and vinegar are permitted.

BREAKFASTS. The day one breakfast consists of:

- one-half cup of Post 100% Bran or Kellogg's Bran Buds or three-quarters cup Kellogg's All Bran Original or Complete Bran Flakes
- one cup of fat-free milk
- 100 calories of fruit

The day two breakfast is:

- three frozen low-fat Aunt Jemima pancakes (150 calories) or two frozen low-fat Eggo Homestyle waffles (180 calories), with one-third cup of frozen unsweetened berries
- one cup of fat-free milk

The day three breakfast is:

- one frozen single-serving Weight Watchers Smart Ones English muffin sandwich with ham and cheese

(210 calories) or one frozen Swift Premium Morning Maker ham, egg, and cheese sandwich (250 calories)

- one 50-calorie fruit or 4 oz. (118 mL) of calcium-fortified orange juice

The day four breakfast consists of:

- one-half of a 3 oz. (85-g) frozen Lender's Big'n Crusty bagel (230 calories) with 1 oz. (28 g) of light Jarlsberg or reduced-fat cheddar cheese, broiled, or one Thomas's English muffin (110 calories)
- one cup of calcium-fortified orange juice

The day five breakfast is the same as day two except that 6 oz. (177 mL) of calcium-fortified orange juice may be substituted for the milk. The day six breakfast is the same as day one. The day seven breakfast is:

- one-half of a frozen Lender's Big'n Crusty toasted bagel with one teaspoon of light butter or margarine or one Thomas's English muffin (110 calories)
- one cup of fat-free Dannon yogurt
- one 50-calorie fruit

LUNCHES. The day one lunch is:

- one frozen Celentano Great Choice Low Fat Stuffed Shells, Manicotti, or Lasagna (250 calories) or one Healthy Choice Manicotti with Three Cheeses frozen entree (260 calories)
- two cups of loosely packed ready-to-eat salad greens with two tablespoons of fat-free Italian dressing or balsamic, rice, or raspberry vinegar
- two breadsticks
- one cup of fat-free milk

The day two lunch consists of:

- one frozen Old El Paso Bean & Cheese Burrito with two tablespoons of salsa or one Weight Watchers Smart Ones Santa Fe Style Rice & Beans frozen entree (290 calories)
- one 50-calorie fruit
- one cup of fat-free milk

The day three lunch is:

- a chicken sandwich made with three one-quarter-inch-thick slices of leftover chicken breast from the day one dinner or ten deli-thin slices of chicken breast, lettuce, sliced tomato, and one tablespoon of light mayonnaise or honey mustard, on two slices of whole-wheat bread
- one 50-calorie fruit
- one cup of fat-free milk

The day four lunch consists of:

- one frozen Lean Pockets Chicken Parmesan, Turkey, or Ham with Cheddar stuffed sandwich (280 calories) or one Ken & Robert's Truly Amazing Veggie Pocket, Oriental or Broccoli & Cheddar (250 calories)

- two cups of salad as for day 1
- one 50-calorie fruit
- one cup of fat-free milk

The day five lunch is:

- a tuna and bean salad made from three cups of ready-to-eat, loosely packed salad greens, 1 oz. (28 g) of crumbled reduced-fat feta cheese, one-third cup of canned drained red kidney beans, 2 oz. (56 g) of water-packed canned tuna, drained and flaked, and 2 tablespoons of fat-free Italian dressing or flavored vinegar
- three breadsticks
- a 100-calorie fruit

The day six lunch is:

- one frozen Stouffer's Lean Cuisine Swedish Meatballs with Pasta or Three Bean Chili with Rice (250–280 calories) or one frozen Lean Pockets stuffed sandwich (250 calories) or one Healthy Choice Chicken Enchilada Suiza frozen entree (270 calories)
- one small sliced tomato with two teaspoons of flavored vinegar
- one cup of fat-free milk

The day seven lunch consists of:

- one whole-wheat mini pita stuffed with one frozen Tyson or Banquet fat-free chicken-breast pattie (80–100 calories), diced tomatoes, 1 oz. (28 g) of crumbled reduced-fat feta cheese, and a splash of red-wine vinegar
- a 100-calorie fruit
- one cup of fat-free milk

DINNERS. Several of the dinner selections make three or four servings and the serving sizes can be increased for other family members. The day one dinner is:

- one-half of a fully cooked rotisserie chicken breast without the skin, about 4.5 oz. (130 g)
- two-thirds of a cup of Ore-Ida mashed potatoes cooked with one-third cup of low-fat milk
- one-third cup of heated fat-free chicken gravy from a jar
- one cup of steamed chopped frozen broccoli
- one 50-calorie fruit

The day two dinner consists of:

- frozen Master Choice Four Cheeses Gourmet pizza or Tombstone Oven Rising Crust Three Cheese

pizza, topped with a single layer of two cups of frozen chopped broccoli or spinach; makes four to six servings of 320 calories each; for one person, one-half cup of Stouffer's Lean Cuisine Cheese French Bread Pizza and one-half cup of vegetables

- two cups of the day one lunch salad
- one 50-calorie fruit

The day three dinner is:

- shrimp and couscous: one-half cup of frozen peas and carrots and 3 oz. (85 g) of peeled, raw, frozen shrimp (about eight medium shrimp) and one-half cup of chicken broth, heated to boiling, and one-third cup of couscous and some hot pepper sauce; or for one person, frozen Healthy Choice Herb Baked Fish (340 calories) or Chicken Francesca frozen meal (330 calories)
- a 100-calorie fruit

The day four dinner is:

- one 9 oz. (250 g) package of frozen Tyson Chicken Breast Strips with Rib Meat (90 calories per serving) and the frozen sauce from one Green Giant Create a Meal! Sweet & Sour Stir Fry (130 calories per serving), stir-fried with rice, and the frozen vegetables and pineapple, for three one-quarter-cup servings, with three-quarters cup of cooked rice per serving; for 1 person, frozen Healthy Choice Sweet and Sour Chicken (360 calories)
- two breadsticks
- one 50-calorie fruit

The day five dinner consists of:

- five Mrs. T's Pierogies Potato and Cheddar Pasta Pockets (300 calories), with one-third cup of salsa and two tablespoons of fat-free sour cream, or three Golden Potato Blintzes (270 calories)
- one cup of cooked frozen green beans
- one 50-calorie fruit

The day six dinner is:

- one whole-wheat mini pita pocket stuffed with one frozen Boca Burger—Chef Max's Favorite (110 calories), lettuce, tomato, onion, and one tablespoon of ketchup, or one frozen low-fat veggie burger
- 4 oz. (110 g) of baked frozen french fries (20–23 fries)
- one 100-calorie fruit

The day seven dinner is:

- one 6 oz. (170-g) individually frozen fish fillet, not breaded or flavored, sprinkled with one tablespoon of grated parmesan cheese, two teaspoons of dried bread crumbs, paprika, salt, pepper, and two teaspoons of olive oil, and baked at 500°F (260°C) for about seven minutes

- two cups of frozen country-style hash browns, cooked by the fat-free method (128 calories)
- one cup of cooked sliced zucchini

SNACKS. Snacks can be eaten at any time of day. The day one snacks are:

- one Dole Fruit Juice Bar (45 calories) or one 50-calorie fruit
- four reduced-fat Triscuits (65 calories) with 1 oz. (28 g) of light Jarlsberg or reduced-fat cheddar cheese
- one dill pickle

The day two snacks are:

- one Starbucks Ice Cream Mocha Frappuccino blended coffee bar (120 calories) or a Quaker Chewy granola bar (about 110 calories)
- one 50-calorie fruit
- eight raw baby carrots

The day three snacks include:

- one cup of fat-free Dannon yogurt (110 calories)
- one Dole fruit juice bar or one 50-calorie fruit
- 15 raw baby carrots

The day four snacks are:

- one Dole Fruit Juice Bar or one 50-calorie fruit
- one-half of a 3 oz. (85-g) frozen Lender's Big'n Crusty toasted bagel with one teaspoon of jam or preserves
- one dill pickle

The day five snacks include:

- four reduced-fat Triscuits (65 calories) with 1 oz. (28 g) of light Jarlsberg or reduced-fat cheddar cheese
- one frozen Haagen-Dazs sorbet bar (80 calories) or Betty Crocker Healthy Temptations ice-cream sandwich (80 calories)
- one dill pickle

The day six snacks are the same as for day two. The day seven snacks are:

- one-half of a 3 oz. (85-g) frozen Lender's Big'n Crusty toasted bagel with one teaspoon of jam or preserves
- one frozen Haagen-Dazs sorbet bar or Betty Crocker Healthy Temptations ice-cream sandwich
- one dill pickle

FRUITS. The 50-calorie fruit choices are:

- one-half cup of unsweetened applesauce
- three apricots

- one cup of blackberries
- one-quarter of a medium cantaloupe or one-half cup of cubes
- one-half of a medium grapefruit
- one cup of honeydew melon cubes
- one medium nectarine
- one large peach or two-thirds cup of frozen, unsweetened peaches
- one-half cup of juice-packed canned peaches, pears, or fruit cocktail
- two one-half-inch-thick slices of fresh pineapple or three-quarters cup of cubes
- one large plum
- two tablespoons of raisins
- one cup of fresh raspberries or two-thirds cup of frozen, unsweetened raspberries
- eight medium strawberries or two-thirds cup of frozen, unsweetened strawberries
- one medium tangerine

The 100-calorie fruits are:

- one large apple
- three dried apricot halves
- one cup blueberries
- one medium banana
- one cup (21) cherries
- three-quarters cup (28) grapes
- two medium kiwifruit
- one large orange
- three dried peach halves
- one medium pear
- two-thirds cup of juice-packed canned pineapple
- two and one-half cups of watermelon cubes

The new Good Housekeeping diet

The more recent *Good Housekeeping* frozen-food diet relies on strict portion control for weight loss. The diet consists of 28 microwaveable frozen meals and supplemental foods that follow strict nutritional criteria. It includes calorie-free beverages and a daily multivitamin/multimineral supplement.

BREAKFAST. The frozen-food diet breakfast consists of:

- one cup of fat-free milk or 6 oz. (170 g) of light yogurt
- three-quarters cup of Kashi GoLean or three-quarters cup of Cheerios or Wheaties mixed with one-quarter cup All-Bran Extra Fiber
- one serving of fruit

the rest of the family. Some frozen-food diets are designed for people with diabetes, without simple sugars that could rapidly increase blood-sugar levels. Frozen-food diets may be difficult for vegetarians to follow.

Benefits

In addition to being quick and convenient, frozen-food diets are intended to be well-balanced, low in fat and calories, and to provide the necessary **vitamins** and **minerals**. They supply a variety of different foods. The meals in the original *Good Housekeeping* frozen-food diet take less than 10 minutes to prepare and enables the dieter to lose 1 lb. (0.45 kg) per week. The meals in the newer *Good Housekeeping* frozen-food diet take 9 minutes or less to prepare and enable the dieter to lose about 1.5 lb. (0.7 kg) per week or 20 lb. (9 kg) in just over three months. Commercial frozen-food diets make weight-loss claims of an average of 2–3 lb. (0.9–1.4 kg) per week.

Frozen foods avoid spoilage problems associated with fresh foods, particularly those that are harvested, transported long distances, and stored before they reach the consumer. Frozen foods also require fewer trips to the grocery store.

Precautions

Frozen food, particularly frozen meals and entrées, can be very expensive compared to buying fresh or canned food and preparing meals, although frozen fruits and vegetables may be less expensive than fresh produce. Frozen-food diets also require a significant amount of frozen storage capacity. Recommended choices, such as those in the *Good Housekeeping* frozen-food diets, may be biased toward advertisers or corporate sponsors.

Like many processed foods, frozen foods—especially frozen diet foods—contain various chemicals that some believe may be harmful. Frozen diet foods often contain monosodium glutamate (MSG), flavorings, and hydrolyzed vegetable protein. In large quantities glutamate may be damaging to the brain and nervous system.

Risks

Frozen food is considered to be safe. Freezing inhibits the growth of some pathogens and reduces the risk of **food contamination**. However the thawing and refreezing of frozen foods may pose a risk. Frozen foods can remain too long in the freezer and can suffer from freezer burn and the formation of ice crystals.

Research and general acceptance

Research

In the 1990s the U.S. Food and Drug Administration declared frozen fruits and vegetables to be as nutritious as fresh produce and, in some cases, more nutritious.

The 2003 University of Illinois research study found that women who ate frozen main courses for lunch and dinner for an eight-week period lost an average of 12 lb. (5.4 kg). In contrast the women who followed a diet that was equivalent in calories to the frozen-food diet, but which required them to plan and cook meals, lost an average of only 8 lb. (3.6 kg). According to LeaAnn Carson, a research dietitian and one of the study's authors, the results suggest that women who prepare their own food actually consume more calories because they do not accurately measure the ingredients, whereas the portion sizes of the frozen-food entrées are strictly controlled.

According to Cederquist, medical research has shown that a diet that varies the number of daily calories slightly is preferable to one that strictly adheres to a set number of calories. Varying the caloric intake prevents the body's **metabolism** from adjusting to the set point and making it progressively harder to lose more weight and maintain the weight loss.

General acceptance

Frozen foods are a huge industry and frozen dinners and entrées constitute the largest category of frozen foods. Consumer demand for frozen meals grew steadily in the first years of the twenty-first century. The average American eats six frozen meals per month. In a survey reported by the AFFI, frozen-food products were among the top three food items that Americans did not want to live without. A poll conducted by the Tupperware Corporation found that on an average trip to the supermarket 94% of American shoppers sometimes purchase frozen food and 30% always buy some frozen food.

Surveys conducted in 2006 under the auspices of the AFFI found that the majority of American shoppers believe that frozen foods have many of the same good qualities as fresh foods and retain the same or more nutrients as foods that have not been frozen. Consumers generally believe that in recent years frozen foods have significantly improved in taste, variety, and ease of preparation. In general they also believe that frozen foods are safer than prepared refrigerated foods.

Resources

BOOKS

Blaylock, Russell L. *Excitotoxins: The Taste That Kills.* Santa Fe, NM: Health Press, 1998.

Fogle, Jared and Anthony Bruno. *Jared the Subway Guy: Winning Through Losing: 13 Lessons for Turning Your Life Around.* New York: St. Martin's Press, 2006.

PERIODICALS

Hammock, Delia A. "The Frozen-Food Diet: Quick Meals, Quick Results—Lose Six Pounds This Month With Our Yummy (Microwavable) Meals." *Good Housekeeping* 241 (October 2005): 231–35.

Mermelstein, Shari, and Carol Wapner. "The Frozen Food Diet." *Good Housekeeping* 237 (September 1998): 119–21.

WEBSITES

American Frozen Food Institute. "Frozen Food Buyer's Guide." http://frozenfoodindustrybuyersguide.com (accessed October 2, 2012).

"The Best Frozen Foods for Women." *Good Morning America*, August 20, 2007. http://abcnews.go.com/GMA/Diet/story?id=3498307&page=1#.UGtU4q7bT9Q (accessed October 2, 2012).

Jibrin, Janis. "A Frozen Food Guide." *Good Housekeeping*. http://www.goodhousekeeping.com/health/nutrition/nutrition-frozen-food-jibrin-0506 (accessed October 2, 2012).

ORGANIZATIONS

U.S. Food and Drug Administration, 10903 New Hampshire Ave., Silver Spring, MD 20993-0002, (888) INFO-FDA (463-6332), http://www.fda.gov.

Margaret Alic, PhD

Fructose intolerance

Definition

Fructose intolerance is a condition where the body has difficult digesting fructose and fructose-containing foods. It is treated by complete elimination of fructose and sucrose from the diet.

Sugars and sweeteners	
Tolerated	**Not tolerated**
Aspartame	Agave syrup
Barley malt syrup	Baker's sugar
Birch sugar (if pure)	Beet sugar
Corn starch	Brown rice syrup
Corn sugar	Brown sugar
Dextrin	Cane sugar
Erythitol (if pure)	Carob powder
Glucose	Corn syrup
Glucose polymers	Date sugar
Neotame	Dulcitol
Saccharin	Fruit juice sweeteners
	Grape syrup
	Gur
	Honey
	Maple syrup
	Molasses
	Polydextrose
	Sorbitol
	Stevia
	Turbinado
	Wasanbon

List prepared by the HFI laboratory at Boston University.
(Table by GGS Information Services. © 2013 Cengage Learning.)

Demographics

There are two types of fructose intolerances. The first, hereditary fructose intolerance (HFI), also known as fructosemia or fructose aldolase B deficiency, is a rare genetic disease. It affects the **metabolism** of fructose due to the absence of aldolase B, the enzyme that breaks fructose down in the body. As a result, fructose accumulates in the liver, kidney, and small intestine, and the body is unable to convert its energy storage material (glycogen) into glucose. If left untreated, blood sugar levels fall, resulting in hypoglycemia, and there is also formation of harmful substances that damage the liver. HFI is difficult to diagnose so its incidence rate is not known, but it is believed to be quite rare (between 1 in 12,000 to 1 in 58,000). Since it is inherited, it lasts for life—there is no cure.

The second type of fructose intolerance is dietary fructose intolerance (DFI), also called fructose malabsorption. DFI is quite common—according to the U.S. National Library of Medicine's Genetics Home Reference center, fructose malabsorption may affect up to 40% of people in the Western hemisphere. Its exact incidence is also difficult to evaluate since many people show no symptoms at all and its cause is not precisely known. It seems to be caused by the lack of special cells (epithelial cells) on the surface of the intestine usually aid in digestion. As a result, the body is not able to absorb fructose efficiently.

which are difficult to miss. In many young infants, the age of onset of symptoms leads to the diagnosis. Genetic counseling may be of value to prospective parents with a family history of fructose intolerance. Other tests that may be run include a blood sugar test, kidney function tests, liver function tests, a uric acid blood test, and urinalysis.

Treatment

Although having different causes, both HFI and DFI are treated by dietary adjustments. Complete elimination of fructose and sucrose from the diet is the only effective treatment for HFI. As for DFI, treatment also involves a fructose-free diet, with the treating physician allowing some concessions in mild cases. A strict fructose-free diet involves exclusion of any beverage or food containing fructose, sucrose, or sorbitol. Some patients may find a threshold level where they can eat some fructose without getting symptoms. Close dietary monitoring is important for good outcomes and should include at least semiannual visits to a biochemical geneticist (for HFI) and monthly meetings with a registered dietitian.

Nutrition and dietary concerns

Eating out is one of the most challenging parts of maintaining a fructose-free diet. This is because restaurant employees have little time to check food contents from the labels of the ingredients used by the kitchen to prepare menus. Some suggestions for eating at restaurants include:

• Be as clear and explicit as possible when talking with the waiting staff. Explain fructose intolerance in brief terms and order only foods that cannot have sugars and specify how they should be prepared. For example, an acceptable meal might include a steak, broiled on a piece of aluminum foil with no seasonings at all; a baked potato with butter; a lettuce-only salad with a small slice of lemon and oil on the side; plain steamed spinach; and coffee, tea, or milk.

• The person who knows the ingredients in the food is the person who prepares it, such as the chef or the cook, so it may be best to request to speak to that person directly.

• Be careful of soups. Many soups in restaurants are canned. Ask to read the label if possible. If the soup is made at the restaurant, it may also contain ingredients not compatible with a fructose-free diet.

• Whether grilled or broiled, seasoning is routinely used in meat preparation, so it is important to specify no seasonings. The chef will know if a sauce has fructose-containing ingredients. Canned sauces are

also used in many restaurants, so request to check the ingredient list, if possible.

• Non-dairy products are often used in restaurants and may contain intolerable ingredients. Three frequently used non-dairy products in restaurants are non-dairy creamer, non-dairy potato topping, and non-dairy whipped topping. Ask to read their labels, if possible.

Sugar is often an ingredient in foods that the consumer is not aware of, and not only in restaurants. High fructose corn syrup (HFCS) is present in products such as soft drinks, fruit drinks, sports drinks, baked goods, candies, jams, yogurts, condiments, canned and packaged foods, and other prepared and sweetened foods. Also, potatoes may provide a significant amount of fructose if prepared in a certain way. For this reason, the guidance of a registered dietitian is required in the treatment of fructose intolerance.

Prognosis

Absolute elimination of fructose and glucose from the diet produces good outcomes in most people with fructose intolerance. Medical researchers unanimously agree that symptoms can improve in dietary fructose intolerance patients willing to adhere to a low fructose diet. Research performed at the University of Innsbruck in Austria showed that fructose and sorbitol-reduced diets in subjects with fructose malabsorption did not only reduce gastrointestinal symptoms but also improved mood and early signs of depression. Improvement of the signs of depression were more pronounced in females than in males. For a rapidly diagnosed and treated infant, the outcome for a normal state of health is excellent. In the absence of substantial liver damage, life expectancy is normal.

Prevention

There is no known prevention for fructose intolerance.

Resources

BOOKS

Cornblath, M., Schwartz, R. *Disorders of Carbohydrate Metabolism in Infancy.* Cambridge, MA: Blackwell Scientific Publications, 1991.

Gazzola, A. *Living with Food Intolerance.* London, UK: Sheldon Press, 2006.

Smith, J. *Living With Dietary Fructose Intolerance: A Guide to Managing your Life With this New Diagnosis.* Charleston, SC: BookSurge Publishing, 2006.

PERIODICALS

Gijsbers, C., C. Kneepkens, and H. Büller. "Lactose and Fructose Malabsorption in Children with Recurrent Abdominal Pain: Results of Double-Blinded Testing." *Acta Paediatrica* 101, no. 9 (2012): e411–15. http://dx. doi.org/10.1111/j.1651-2227.2012.02721.x (accessed August 15, 2012).

Latulippe, M.E., and S.M. Skoog. "Fructose Malabsorption and Intolerance: Effects of Fructose with and without Simultaneous Glucose Ingestion." *Critical Reviews in Food Science and Nutrition* 51, no. 7 (2011): 583–92.

WEBSITES

American Gastroenterological Association. "Understanding Food Allergies and Intolerances." http://www.gastro. org/patient-center/diet-medications/food-allergies-fructose-intolerance-and-lactose-intolerance (accessed August 15, 2012).

Genetics Home Reference. "Hereditary Fructose Intolerance." Lister Hill National Center for Biomedical Communications, U.S. National Library of Medicine. http://ghr.nlm.nih.gov/condition/hereditary-fructose-intolerance (accessed August 15, 2012).

HFI Laboratory at Boston University. "HFI Treatment." http://www.bu.edu/aldolase/HFI/treatment/index. html (accessed August 15, 2012).

MedlinePlus. "Hereditary Fructose Intolerance." U.S. National Library of Medicine, National Institutes of Health. http://www.nlm.nih.gov/medlineplus/ency/ article/000359.htm (accessed August 15, 2012).

ORGANIZATIONS

American Gastroenterological Association, 4930 Del Ray Ave., Bethesda, MD 20814, (301) 654-2055, Fax: (301) 654-5920, member@gastro.org, http://www.gastro.org.

HFI Laboratory, Boston University, 24 Cummington St., Department of Biology, Boston, MA 02215, http://www. bu.edu/aldolase/HFI.

Monique Laberge, PhD

Fruitarian diet

Definition

A fruitarian diet is a strict form of a vegetarian diet that is generally limited to eating fresh fruits.

Origins

The fruitarian diet has been around for hundreds of years. In his writings, artist, scientist, and inventor Leonardo da Vinci (1452–1519) indicated he was a fruitarian. Despite the popular view that early humans were primarily meat-eaters, there is some scientific evidence to indicate that they ate a diet consisting primarily of fruits, nuts, and berries. Some religious scholars argue that the original fruitarians were Adam and Eve in the Garden of Eden. There are a number of historical references to a fruitarian diet in the 1800s and 1900s. In much of the historical documentation, people who became fruitarians switched to a more accepted diet after a few months or years, often renouncing the diet. Indian spiritual and political leader Mahatma Gandhi (1869–1948) was a fruitarian for six months in the early 1900s before going back to a vegetarian diet.

Description

A fruitarian diet, also called a fructarian diet, is a form of vegan diet that is generally limited to eating fruits. The definition of what is a fruit often varies among fruitarians (also called fructarians or frugivores). Some adhere to a strict interpretation, consuming only fruits from plants and trees. Some fruitarians include berries in their diet, others broaden the definition to include nuts and seeds, while others include some food that is commonly thought of as vegetables, including peppers, tomatoes, cucumbers, and avocados. A fourth type of fruitarian includes grains in the diet. One definition of a fruitarian is someone who has a diet comprised of more than 50% fruit. The website Beyond Vegetarianism defines a fruitarian diet as one containing at least 75% fruit (which includes grains and nuts) and the remainder of the diet being raw vegan foods other than fruits. Most fruitarians consume raw, fresh fruit over canned, frozen, or processed fruit. A few fruitarians also consume green leafy vegetables, root vegetables, or both in their diet.

Fruitarians can choose from seven basic fruit groups:

• Acid fruits: citrus, pineapples, strawberries, pomegranates, kiwi, cranberries, and sour apples.

- Subacid fruits: sweet apples, sweet cherries, raspberries, blackberries, blueberries, peaches, pears, cherimoyas, papayas, figs, apricots, and mangos.
- Sweet fruits: bananas, grapes, melons, and persimmons.
- Nuts: pecans, almonds, Brazil, cashews, walnuts, macadamias, pistachios, pine nuts, hazelnuts, beechnuts, and hickory.
- Seeds: sunflower, sesame, squash, and pumpkin.
- Dried fruits: dates, figs, apricots, apples, raisins, cherries, prunes, bananas, and cranberries.
- Oily fruits: avocados, coconuts, and olives.

Many fruitarians believe that the quality of fruit available in most commercial supermarkets is poor. This is due to hybridization, chemical fertilization, chemical pesticides, and harvesting before the fruit is at the peak of ripeness. They suggest buying certified organic fruit, preferably heirloom, often found at farmers' markets and health food stores.

Fruitarian and author David Wolfe says it is best to eat one type of fruit at a time and wait 45 minutes before another type of fruit is eaten. The Fruitarian Foundation recommends waiting at least 90 minutes between fruit types. If a person still is hungry after eating one type of fruit, they should eat more of the same type of fruit until their hunger is satisfied. People on the diet should eat only when hungry and then eat as much as they want until their hunger is satisfied. Those on a diet where only one type of fruit is eaten at a time will know when they have eaten enough, according to Wolfe. Their appetite will turn off and they will suddenly feel like they have eaten too much. Once satiated they will not gain the same satisfaction from the fruit. This is a signal from the body to stop eating, Wolfe states. The signal to stop eating is not as strong in people who eat more than one type of fruit at the same time. For a person who eats only fruit, there is no need to drink water. All the water the body needs is contained in the fruits. People whose diet is less than 100% fruit should supplement it with water. Some fruitarians fast one day a week. People fasting must drink a normal amount of water, usually 8–10 eight-ounce glasses a day.

One-day meal plan

The following is a typical one-day meal plan from the Fruitarian Foundation for a fruitarian diet:

- Early morning (6–9 a.m.): The juice of three to five lemons immediately upon waking, raisins, and an unlimited amount of melon or melon juice.

- Midmorning (9 a.m. to 12 p.m.): An unlimited amount of apples, pineapple, figs, pears, grapes, yellow plums, lima beans, kiwi, and cucumber.
- Noon (12–3 p.m.): Oranges or tangerines, peaches, apricots, and papayas in any amount desired.
- Midafternoon (3–6 p.m.): Mangoes, cherries, strawberries, red plums, persimmons, pomegranates, watermelon, and tomatoes.
- Evening 6–9 p.m.): Grapes, blackberries, and raspberries.
- Late evening (9 p.m. to 12 a.m.): Mango, cherries, strawberries, red plums, persimmons, pomegranates, watermelon, and tomatoes.

Items that can be eaten at any time are bananas, coconuts, organic olives, ripe avocados, any type of raw nuts, and lemon juice. The only items that should be consumed from midnight to 3 a.m., if desired, are four to six passion fruits, a small amount of water (if needed), and lemon juice.

Many people on a fruitarian diet give up the diet after a few months or several years because they find it too difficult to maintain. The problems include intense obsessions with food, social isolation, psychological problems, and frequent hunger. Because of these reasons and others, many people instead adopt a high-fruit diet composed of 50%–75% fruit. The rest of the diet contains vegetables, including beans for **protein**. In some cases, the diet is still one of only raw (uncooked and unprocessed) foods while in other cases, it may include some cooked foods, such as potatoes.

Social implications

Most websites about fruitarianism emphasize that there are social concerns associated with a fruitarian diet. Much of this is because many fruitarians adopt the diet as part of a larger philosophical shift that is outside the mainstream of Western society. This includes animal rights and environmental activism, New Age spiritualism, meditation, and pacifism. In the United States, becoming or being a fruitarian or vegetarian is often seen as both a social and political statement. This can sometimes lead to conflict with family, friends, and even society at large.

Function

There are as many reasons for being a fruitarian as there are variations of the fruitarian diet. One reason is the opposition to killing animals for food, another is opposition to consuming any products that come from animals. Other reasons include opposition to killing any plant for food, health benefits, environmental concerns, and spiritual beliefs. The primary function of a fruitarian diet is to promote health and energy. Once someone adopts a fruit diet, they become physically, mentally, emotionally, and spiritually healthier, according to the Fruitarian Foundation. The Foundation's philosophy states that fruitarians develop a fine-tuned body and experience few or no headaches, develop a greater resistance to illness, pain, and aging, and need less sleep. "The proper application of fruitarian dietary and lifestyle is calculated to allow the human to produce healthy offspring, live more than 100 years of age, be free of all disease, and only 'mature' while not aging, as most people think of it, and die a natural death in their sleep," according to a statement on the Foundation's website. "Man cannot eat of everything and maintain his good health. Man was created to eat of the fruits of the trees."

Benefits

The benefits of a fruitarian diet are mostly promoted by people on the diet, rather than scientific research. These benefits supposedly include increased mental power and clarity, creativity, happiness, energy, confidence, self-esteem, and concentration. Physical health benefits, according to the Fruitarian Foundation, include preventing and curing **cancer**, **constipation**, insomnia, depression, and digestive problems, weight loss, wound healing, strengthening the immune system, reducing or eliminating menstruation, increasing sexual vitality, improvements in the health and appearance of skin, hair, eyes, and nails, improving muscle coordination, and the ability to control addictions to alcohol, drugs, and tobacco. The U.S. Department of Agriculture (USDA) recommends that fruit be included in daily meal planning, but as part of a balanced diet that includes protein, vegetables, grains, and dairy. There is no scientific evidence to support any of the claims regarding the benefits of a fruitarian diet, including that eating a fruit-only diet can cure a disease.

Precautions

To get all of the **vitamins**, **minerals**, and nutrients that a body needs, a fruitarian must eat a wide variety of fruit and in many cases, large quantities. Very little protein can be obtained from fruit. To obtain the necessary amounts, fruitarians must include in their diet fruits and nuts that are highest in protein, including avocados, nuts, and dates. Still, it will be difficult to get the amount of protein the body needs on a daily basis. Vitamin, mineral, and other nutritional supplements can be taken to ensure that a person is getting the recommended amounts. However, this does not fit

into the nature-only philosophy of many fruitarians. Doctors strongly recommend that women who are pregnant or nursing not be on a fruitarian diet. Doctors also say children should not be on a fruitarian diet because their bodies require extra nutrients to sustain normal growth along with mental and physical development.

Risks

There are many risks associated with a fruitarian diet and the risks grow as the degree of fruitarianism increases. That is, a person whose diet is 75% fruit is likely to have more health issues that a person on a diet consisting of 50% fruit. There are serious risks associated with the diet for people with diabetes, since fruit has a high **sugar** content. People with diabetes and **insulin** resistance syndrome should not go on an all-fruit diet. There are also the risks of serious nutritional deficiencies, including **vitamin B$_{12}$**, **calcium**, **iron**, **zinc**, omega-3 and omega-6 amino acids, and protein. There is also the risk of severe weight loss, which can lead to anorexia and other health problems.

In 2001, a husband and wife from Surrey, England, were convicted of child cruelty in the death of their nine-year-old daughter. A pediatrician had

QUESTIONS TO ASK YOUR DOCTOR

- What are the risks of a fruitarian diet?
- Is this diet safe for me?
- What dietary changes, if any, would you recommend for me?
- What changes in my eating regimen would you recommend?
- How can I tell if I am getting the right nutrients?
- What symptoms or adverse effects are important enough that I should seek immediate treatment?

testified in court that the infant, who died from a chest infection caused by **malnutrition**, was not developing properly because the mother's breast milk was nutritionally deficient. The couple ate a diet of only raw vegetables, fruits, and nuts.

Research and general acceptance

There is little, if any, scientific research that supports fruitarianism as a healthy lifestyle, especially long-term, unless foods such as beans, green vegetables, **soy**, and **whole grains** are included in the diet. However, there is much scientific documentation on the benefits of a vegetarian diet. There is general and widespread disapproval of an all-fruit diet by the medical, scientific, fitness, and vegetarian communities. Many people experience positive results after initially going on a fruitarian diet, but over time develop health problems, including emaciation, constant hunger, weakness, and fatigue.

Resources

BOOKS

Carrington, Hereward. *The Fruitarian Diet.* Kila, MT: Kessinger Publishing, 2010.

Davis, Brenda, Vesanto Melina, and Rynn Berry. *Becoming Raw: The Essential Guide to Raw Vegan Diets.* Summertown, TN: Book Publishing Company, 2010.

Duyff, Roberta Larson. *American Dietetic Association Complete Food and Nutrition Guide.* 4th ed. New York: Wiley, 2012.

Mangels, Reed, Virginia Messina, and Mark Messina. *The Dietitian's Guide to Vegetarian Diets.* 3rd ed. Sudbury, MA: Jones & Bartlett Learning, 2010.

Morse, Joseph Stephen Breese. *The Evolution Diet: What and How We Were Designed to Eat.* 2nd ed. Seattle: Code Publishing, 2008.

PERIODICALS

Graff, Jackie. "The Benefits of Raw Food." *New Life Journal* (May 2006): 13–15.

Kiser, Sherry. "Avocado Lovers: Dig In! New Reasons and New Ways To Enjoy This Creamy, Rich Disease Fighter." *Prevention* (June 2002): 152–53.

Lofshult, Diane. "Focus on Fruit: Think Outside the Fruit Bowl for New Ways To Enjoy Nature's Sweetness." *Diabetes Forecast* (June 2006): 51–53.

———. "Tempting Young Adults With Fruit." *IDEA Fitness Journal* (February 2007): 67.

Mangels, Reed. "Raw Food Diets Have Positives and Negatives." *Vegetarian Journal* (May–June 2006): 12.

Sare, Chris. "Color Code: Looks Can Be Revealing When It Comes to the Shade of Veggies." *Muscle & Fitness* (July 2004): 248–49.

Walker, Vrinda. "Attitudes, Practices, and Beliefs of Individuals Consuming a Raw Foods Diet." *Vegetarian Journal* (Jul–Aug 2006): 27–29.

WEBSITES

"Beyond Vegetarianism." http://www.beyondveg.com (accessed August 25, 2012).

Ken R. Wells
Laura Jean Cataldo, RN, EdD

G

Gallstones

Definition

Gallstones are solid material that forms in the gallbladder or bile ducts. They are made of cholesterol, bilirubin, and **calcium** and range in size from a grain of sand to a golf ball. A single stone may be present, or they may exist in large numbers. Gallstones are also called choleliths.

Description

The gallbladder is a sac-like organ that lies on the right side of the abdomen underneath the liver. The liver makes bile that is then stored in the gallbladder. Bile is a yellowish-green fluid that helps digest **fats** and dissolve cholesterol. It contains bile salts, fats, proteins, cholesterol, and bilirubin. When a person eats a meal containing fat, the gallbladder contracts, and bile flows along the common bile duct, past the pancreatic duct that leads to the pancreas, and into the upper part of the small intestine (the duodenum) where it helps break down fat.

Gallstones form when some of the material in bile solidifies. At first, the solid particles are small and may form a semi-solid sludge in the gallbladder. Gradually particles come together to form larger solid masses. As many as 20% of Americans have gallstones, and most do not know it. These are called asymptomatic gallstones, and they do not need treatment. Sometimes the stones are incidentally discovered during imaging tests (e.g., x rays, computed tomography [CT] scans) being done for other purposes. Whether gallstones cause symptoms depends on their size and number and whether they move out of the gallbladder and block the common bile duct or the pancreatic duct.

Gallstones are categorized by their composition, not their shape or size. Cholesterol gallstones are the most common type of gallstone found in people in Western industrialized countries. In the United States, about 80% of gallstones are of this type. They are made of hardened cholesterol with small amounts of other substances. Pigment gallstones are black or dark brown stones made primarily of calcium and bilirubin. About 15%–20% of gallstones are pigment stones. Primary bile duct stones are a third type of stone. These form directly in the bile duct instead of in the gallbladder, and they are rare.

Demographics

Each year 1%–3% of Americans develop symptoms of gallstone disease. People of Northern European ancestry, Hispanics, and Native Americans are more likely to develop gallstone disease than African-Americans or Asians. Women are two to three times more likely than men to develop gallstones. The lifetime risk of a woman developing gallstones is 50%, but only 30% for a man. This difference is thought to be related to the effect of estrogen, a female hormone, on increasing the production of cholesterol.

Gallbladder surgery is one of the most commonly performed abdominal surgeries in the United States. About half a million gallbladder operations are done each year. Gallstones are uncommon in children, and when present are usually related to disorders present at birth (congenital disorders). The risk of developing gallstones increases with age. They are most common in people over age 60.

Causes and symptoms

Researchers are not exactly sure why some people develop gallstones and others do not. One thought is that gallstones are more likely to develop when the gallbladder contracts infrequently or sluggishly and does not empty completely. Twin studies also suggest that heredity plays a moderate role in who develops gallstones.

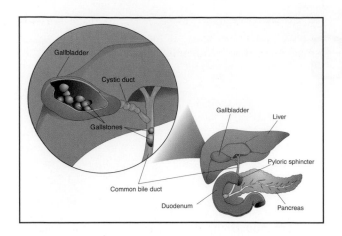

Gallstones in the gallbladder and the common bile duct.
(Illustration by Electronic Illustrators Group. © 2013 Cengage Learning.)

What researchers do know is that certain factors increase the risk of developing cholesterol gallstones. These include:

• overweight or obesity. The rate of gallstone formation increases with increasing weight. A body mass index (BMI) of 18.5–24.9 is considered normal weight and a BMI of 25.0–29.9 is overweight. A BMI of 30 and above is obese. A woman with a BMI of 32 has about a three times greater risk of developing gallstones than a woman with a BMI of 25.

• Too much cholesterol. If the liver makes too much cholesterol, it may not stay dissolved in bile, but may crystallize out and form a solid. The amount of cholesterol in bile is not related to the amount of cholesterol in blood, and cholesterol-lowering drugs do not affect the amount of cholesterol the liver makes. A diet high in fats and cholesterol also increases the risk of gallstones.

• Female gender, pregnancy, and estrogen drugs. The female hormone estrogen causes the liver to make more cholesterol. Women of reproductive age have higher levels of estrogen, which may explain why more women develop gallstones than men. In addition, oral contraceptives (birth control pills) contain estrogen, and until recently, many women took drugs containing estrogen to combat hot flashes and other symptoms of menopause. Gallstone formation also increases during pregnancy, a time of increased estrogen levels.

• Severe dieting. Losing weight rapidly—three or more pounds a week—increases the likelihood of developing gallstones. About one-quarter of people who go on very low-calorie diets (800 calories daily under medical supervision) and stay on them for several months develop gallstones. One-third of these people have symptoms severe enough to need gallbladder surgery. About one-third of people who have weight-loss surgery (bariatric surgery) also develop gallstones, usually in the first few months after surgery. Experts believe that somehow this surgery triggers gallstone formation.

• Weight cycling. People who repeatedly lose and gain back 10 lb. (4.5 kg) are more likely to develop gallstones.

• Bariatric surgery. People who have weight-loss surgery are at increased risk of developing gallstones.

The chance of developing pigment gallstones is increased in individuals who have diseases such as sickle-cell anemia, where there is an unusually high rate of red blood cell turnover. Bilirubin is the main component of pigment gallstones, and these diseases increase the amount of bilirubin formed in the liver.

Many people with gallstones never have any symptoms. Symptoms tend to occur when a gallstone moves out of the gallbladder and irritates or blocks the common bile duct or the entrance to the pancreatic duct. Sometimes symptoms come and go, as when stones irritating the bile duct move into the much larger small intestine.

Symptoms can include the following:

• sudden pain in the upper right part of the abdomen that lasts anywhere from 15 minutes to several hours and does not go away with changes in position

• pain radiating up into the back or right shoulder blade

• nausea and vomiting

• fever

• jaundice, a yellowing of the skin and whites of the eyes

Pain can occur frequently or at long intervals. Jaundice and fever are signs of advanced gallstone disease and infection. Sudden intense pain, especially if accompanied by high fever, nausea, vomiting, jaundice, and dark urine are signs of a medical emergency. Medical care should be sought immediately. Untreated bile duct blockages can lead to perforation of the bile duct, infection, and death.

Diagnosis

Diagnosis is made based on a physical examination and imaging studies. Ultrasound is the least invasive and often the most effective way to locate gallstones. Other imaging studies, such as plain x rays and CT scans, may also be used. However, these diagnostic tools may fail to locate gallstones in the bile duct.

KEY TERMS

Bile—A greenish-yellow digestive fluid produced by the liver and stored in the gallbladder. It is released into the small intestine where it helps digest fat, and then is removed from the body in feces.

Bilirubin—A yellow pigment that is the end result of hemoglobin breakdown. This pigment is metabolized in the liver and excreted from the body through the bile. Bloodstream levels are normally low; however, extensive red cell destruction leads to excessive bilirubin formation and jaundice.

Cholesterol—A waxy substance made by the liver and also acquired through diet. High levels in the blood may increase the risk of cardiovascular disease.

Pancreas—A gland near the liver and stomach that secretes digestive fluid into the intestine and the hormone insulin into the bloodstream.

Perforation—A hole in the wall of an organ in the body.

Other diagnostic tests can be used to better locate gallstones in the bile duct. A radionuclide scan, also called cholescintigraphy or HIDA scan, uses a small amount of radioactive tracer material that is injected into a vein. A machine locates the radioactive tracer as it moves through the body and in this way can tell if a stone is blocking the entrance or exit to the gallbladder or the common bile duct. Endoscopic retrograde cholangiopancreatography (ERCP) is an endoscopic procedure use to locate, and sometimes remove, gallstones from the bile and pancreatic ducts. In this procedure, a thin tube called an endoscope is passed down the throat, through the stomach, and into the first part of the small intestine. Air and dye are then injected, which allows the physician to see the place where the bile duct empties into the small intestine. If stones are present, a special tool may be inserted through the endoscope to remove them.

Treatment

By far, the most common and most successful treatment for gallstone disease is surgical removal of the gallbladder, an operation called a cholecystectomy. Removing the gallbladder has little effect on digestion. Bile simply goes directly from the liver to the small intestine instead of being stored. The difference is that the intestine receives a continuous flow of bile rather than receiving it only when it is needed. In about 1% of people, this continuous flow of bile causes mild diarrhea.

Most gallbladder surgery can be done laparoscopically. This means that surgery is done through a small cut in the abdomen instead of opening the entire abdominal cavity. A thin instrument called a laparoscope that contains a miniature video camera and a light is inserted through the cut. The surgeon uses the image from the video camera to insert small instruments through the incision and remove the gallbladder. Recovery from laparoscopic gallbladder surgery often takes only a few days.

If the gallbladder or pancreas is infected, or if there is scarring from previous surgeries, open gallbladder surgery is necessary. This involves making a large incision in the abdomen. Recovery time usually involves 5–7 days in the hospital and several weeks at home.

Some people are not healthy enough to undergo surgery. In this case, treatment options include a medication called ursodiol (Actigall) that helps dissolve cholesterol stones. However, the dissolving process can take 6–18 months. Sometimes this drug is given to people who are on medically supervised very-low-calorie diets for fast weight loss to help prevent them from developing gallstones. The other nonsurgical treatment option is sound wave therapy (extracorporeal shock wave lithotripsy). High-frequency sound waves are aimed at the gallstones to shatter them into smaller pieces. The pieces are then dissolved by the ursodiol or may pass into the small intestine without causing pain. With nonsurgical treatment, gallstones often reoccur. When the patient is healthy enough for surgery, gallbladder removal is usually the preferred option.

Nutrition and dietary concerns

Once recovery from surgery is complete, individuals who have had their gallbladder removed can return to a normal healthy diet. High-fat foods are more likely to cause gas and diarrhea and should be limited or avoided; products containing **caffeine** or dairy may also cause stomach problems. To help alleviate discomfort, patients should slowly increase their **fiber** consumption and avoid fried or other fatty foods.

Prognosis

Gallbladder surgery is quite safe, although all surgery carries risk of infection, reaction to anesthesia, and unintentional damage to other tissue. Once the gallbladder is removed, no more gallstones can form. Most complications from gallstones arise when treatment is delayed and the pancreas or gallbladder becomes infected. This is a serious, potentially fatal, complication because infection can spread rapidly and overwhelm the body. Gallstone disease is responsible

QUESTIONS TO ASK YOUR DOCTOR

- If I have only occasional pain from gallstones, should I consider surgery?
- What are my surgical options?
- Would less invasive non-surgical treatment eliminate my gallstones?
- What are the side effects of medication used to dissolve gallstones?

for about 10,000 deaths in the United States each year, of which only a few hundred are caused by surgical complications. The vast majority are caused by gallstone disease that has caused infection.

Prevention

The formation of gallstones cannot be prevented. However maintaining a healthy weight, exercising regularly, and eating a diet high in **whole grains** and fresh fruit and vegetables and low in fat and cholesterol decrease the chance that gallstones will develop.

Resources

PERIODICALS

Stokes, C.S., M. Krawczyk, and F. Lammert. "Gallstones: Environment, Lifestyle and Genes." *Digestive Diseases* 29, no. 2 (2011): 191–201.

Walcher, T., et al. "The Effect of Alcohol, Tobacco and Caffeine Consumption and Vegetarian Diet on Gallstone Prevalence." *European Journal of Gastroenterology & Hepatology* 22, no. 11 (2010): 1345–51.

OTHER

American Gastroenterological Association. "Understanding Gallstones." http://www.gastro.org/patient-center/digestive-conditions/AGAPatientBrochure_Gallstones.pdf (accessed August 9, 2012).

WEBSITES

MedlinePlus. "Gallstones." U.S. National Library of Medicine, National Institutes of Health. http://www.nlm.nih.gov/medlineplus/gallstones.html (accessed August 9, 2012).

National Institute of Diabetes and Digestive and Kidney Diseases (NIDDK). "Dieting and Gallstones." Weight-Control Information Network. http://win.niddk.nih.gov/publications/gallstones.htm (accessed August 9, 2012).

Nelson, Jennifer, and Katherine Zeratsky. "What's OK to Eat After Gallbladder Removal?" MayoClinic.com. http://www.mayoclinic.com/health/gallbladder-removal-diet/MY01815 (accessed August 9, 2012).

ORGANIZATIONS

American College of Gastroenterology (ACG), 6400 Goldsboro Rd., Ste. 450, Bethesda, MD 20817, (301) 263-9000, info@acg.gi.org, http://www.acg.gi.org.

American Gastroenterological Association (AGA), 4930 Del Ray Ave., Bethesda, MD 20814, (301) 654-2055, Fax: (301) 654-5920, http://www.gastro.org.

National Digestive Diseases Information Clearinghouse (NDDIC), 2 Information Way, Bethesda, MD 20892-3570, (800) 891-5389, TTY: (866) 569-1162, Fax: (703) 738-4929, info@niddk.nih.gov, http://digestive.niddk.nih.gov.

Tish Davidson, AM

Gastric bypass *see* **Bariatric surgery**

Gastroesophageal reflux disease (GERD)

Definition

Gastroesophageal reflux disease, or GERD, occurs when gastric juice from the stomach backs up into the bottom of the esophagus and causes irritation, inflammation, or erosion of the cells lining the esophagus. GERD is sometimes called acid reflux disease.

Description

The esophagus carries food from the mouth to the stomach. A ring of strong muscle called the lower esophageal sphincter (LES) is located at the spot where the esophagus enters the stomach. The LES relaxes and opens when a person swallows, allowing food to enter the stomach. The LES stays closed in healthy people the rest of the time, preventing the contents of the stomach from backing up into the esophagus. In people with GERD, the LES is weak and opens at inappropriate times, allowing a backwash of acidic stomach contents into the bottom part of the esophagus.

The stomach makes hydrochloric acid that is needed to digest food and help kill bacteria and other foreign organisms that are accidentally consumed with food. The cells lining the stomach secrete a thick layer of mucus that protects them from damage by stomach acid. The cells lining the esophagus do not secrete mucus, so when the LES opens and the acid mixture from the stomach come into contact with them, they become first irritated, then later inflamed, and finally eroded. The individual often feels this damage as

---

Gastroesophageal reflux disease (GERD) relief

Diet and lifestyle modifications:

- Eat smaller but more frequent meals
- Avoid common triggers (including tomato sauces, fried or spicy foods, alcohol, and caffeinated beverages)
- Lose excess weight
- Sleep with the head elevated
- Avoid eating before bed

Over-the-counter medications:

- Antacids (Tums*, Rolaids)
- OTC acid blockers (Pepcid AC, Prilosec OTC)

Prescription medications:

- Proton pump inhibitors (Nexium, Prevacid)
- Pro-motility drugs (Propulsid)
- Prescription-strength antacids (Carafate)
- Prescription-strength H2 blockers (Zantac, Tagamet)

*Drug names are provided as examples but are not meant to be recommendations or wholly representative of the treatments available.

SOURCE: The American College of Gastroenterology, "Heartburn or Gastroesophageal Reflux Disease (GERD)." Available online at: http://www.acg.gi.org/patients/women/whatisgerd.asp (accessed August 19, 2010).

(Table by PreMediaGlobal. © 2013 Cengage Learning.)

heartburn. Heartburn is a pain or burning behind the breastbone. GERD is diagnosed when the stomach acid comes in contact with the esophagus at least twice a week on a regular basis.

Demographics

Acid reflux or heartburn is extremely common. About 7% of Americans have heartburn every day. Reports suggest that between 25% and 40% of Americans have heartburn at least once a month, although not everyone who has heartburn has GERD, and not everyone who has GERD has heartburn. The exact number of people with GERD is difficult to determine, as many people never see a doctor and self-treat symptoms with over-the-counter medications.

People of any race or age can develop GERD, including infants and children, but the disease is most common among people over age 50, pregnant women, and people who are overweight or obese. The condition is often overlooked in infants and children and is likely to be underdiagnosed in this group.

Causes and symptoms

GERD is caused by stomach acid coming in contact with cells of the esophagus. The most common cause for this is weakening of the LES. Hiatal hernia is thought to increase the likelihood of developing GERD. The diaphragm is a sheet of muscle that divides the chest cavity from the abdominal cavity. With a hiatal hernia, a tear develops in the diaphragm and a portion of the stomach protrudes through the hole and up into the chest cavity. Hiatal hernias are very common, especially in people over age 50, and usually do not cause health problems or need treatment. However, the diaphragm gives support to the LES. When it is torn, this support is weakened, and the LES closes less tightly. The relationship between hiatal hernia and GERD is somewhat controversial. Many people with a hiatal hernia do not have heartburn, and some people who do not have a hiatal hernia do have heartburn.

Certain lifestyle choices increase the likelihood of developing GERD. These include:

- smoking
- alcohol consumption
- obesity
- pregnancy
- poor posture
- eating large meals shortly before bedtime

Certain foods also increase the likelihood of developing GERD. These foods include:

- greasy or fried foods
- citrus fruits or juices (e.g., oranges, grapefruit)
- caffeinated beverages (e.g., coffee, colas)
- garlic and onions
- tomato-based foods (e.g., spaghetti sauce, chili)
- chocolate
- foods flavored with mint
- garlic and onions
- spicy foods
- wine, beer, and distilled spirits

Symptoms

The most common symptom of GERD is heartburn. Heartburn is a sharp pain in the center of the chest that can spread to the neck and last for up to two hours. The pain can be substantial enough to be confused with angina or a heart attack. Note that if there is any question about whether the pain is caused by a heart attack, the individual should seek medical attention immediately. Heartburn pain does not get worse with physical activity, but often worsens when bending over or lying down. As noted above, heartburn is extremely common. Almost everyone experiences it at some time, usually after eating an unusually large or spicy meal.

GERD also has less typical symptoms. Some people regurgitate or involuntarily bring up the contents of the stomach into the mouth. This causes a bitter taste, and if it occurs often enough can erode tooth enamel.

Other less typical symptoms are wheezing, shortness of breath, increased incidence of asthma, and a persistent dry cough. GERD can also cause the person's voice to sound hoarse. Hoarseness is usually worse in the morning. These symptoms are caused by the contents of the stomach approaching or entering the airways.

Some people have difficulty swallowing or feel as if the food they have eaten is stuck behind their breastbone. This symptom can also be caused by a narrowing of the esophagus where it enters the stomach.

The most common symptoms of GERD in infants and children are repeated non-projectile vomiting (spitting up), persistent coughing, and wheezing.

Diagnosis

Often GERD is tentatively diagnosed based on the patient reporting heartburn twice or more a week on a regular basis. Normally the physician will suggest lifestyle changes, and if there is no improvement will order more extensive tests.

An upper GI series, sometimes called a barium swallow, includes x rays of the esophagus, stomach, and upper part of the intestine. Often the patient drinks a solution of barium to improve contrast on the x rays. These x rays help rule out abnormalities such as a narrowing of the esophagus (esophageal stricture) and **ulcers**.

An upper endoscopy is a diagnostic procedure that allows the physician to see the lining of the esophagus and stomach. It is performed in a doctor's office or an outpatient clinic under light sedation. A tube called an endoscope is inserted down the throat. At the end of the endoscope is a tiny camera that allows the doctor to see if there is damage to the cells lining the esophagus. During this procedure, the doctor may also remove small tissue samples (a biopsy) from the esophagus in order to look for abnormal cells under the microscope.

Occasionally 24-hour pH monitoring is necessary. The pH scale measures the strength of acids. In this test, a tube put down the esophagus measures how much stomach acid backs up into the esophagus. Monitoring usually for continues for 24 hours.

GERD is categorized according to the degree of damage to the esophagus.

- Grade I: redness and irritation of the esophagus
- Grade II: some non-adjacent spots of erosion of esophageal cells
- Grade III: increased and continuous patches of erosion
- Grade IV: Barrett's esophagus, a precancerous condition in which normal cells are replaced by abnormal ones.

Treatment

The goals of treating GERD are to eliminate heartburn and other symptoms, heal damage to the esophagus, and prevent return of symptoms. Treatment proceeds in four stages: lifestyle changes, over-the-counter remedies, prescription drug therapy, and surgery.

Lifestyle changes are the easiest and least expensive approach to treating GERD. They bring relief to many people. Recommended lifestyle changes include:

- quitting smoking
- if overweight, losing weight
- avoiding drinking alcoholic beverages
- avoiding foods likely to cause heartburn
- avoiding eating at least three hours before going to bed
- elevating the head of the bed about four inches on blocks or using a sloped piece of foam under the mattress to raise the head six or more inches

When lifestyle changes are not enough to relieve symptoms within a few weeks, the next step is to use over-the-counter medications. Antacids, such as Alka-Seltzer, Maalox, Rolaids, or Tums, reduce the acidity of liquid already in the stomach. Many antacids contain aluminum and **magnesium**. They should not be taken regularly for long periods because these **minerals** may disrupt the chemical balance in the body.

Drugs known as H2 blockers help reduce the production of acid in the stomach. H2 blockers that are available without a prescription include cimetidine (Tagamet), ranitidine (Zantac), and nizatidine (Axid). Some of these are also available in higher strengths with a doctor's prescription. H2 blockers are most effective when taken about an hour before meals. They do not affect acid already in the stomach.

Proton pump inhibitors use a different chemical mechanism to block acid production by the stomach.

They are more effective than H2 blockers and are used when H2 blockers fail. Some are available in over-the-counter strengths, while others require a prescription. Common proton pump inhibitors include omeprazole (Prilosec), lansoprazole (Prevacid), rabeprazole (Aciphex), esomeprazole (Nexium), omeprazole/sodium bicarbonate (Zegerid), and pantoprazole (Protonix).

Surgery is the most drastic treatment for GERD. It is used when all other treatments fail and symptoms remain. The most common surgical operation to correct GERD is called fundoplication. This surgery is done laparoscopically; the entire abdomen does not need to be opened. A small slit is made in the abdomen and a camera guides the surgeon who manipulates small instruments through this slit to wrap the top of the stomach (the fundus) like a cuff around the bottom of the esophagus. This provides additional support for the LES, and is initially successful in stopping GERD about 92% of the time. Long-term success rates are variable. Laparoscopic fundoplication usually requires a hospital stay of 1–3 days and takes about 2–3 weeks for complete recovery.

In 2012, the United States Food and Drug Administration (FDA) approved a device for treatment of chronic GERD called the LINX Reflux Management System. The LINX system involves the laparoscopic placement of a flexible band around the esophagus just above the stomach to create a natural barrier to reflux. The band is made of titanium beads with magnetic cores. When a person swallows, the magnetic bond holding the beads together is broken and allows the sphincter to open so that food and liquid can pass into the stomach. When swallowing is complete, the magnetic forces in the beads pull the band back together, creating a barrier between the stomach and the esophagus.

Nutrition and dietary concerns

Nutritional concerns related to GERD involve lifestyle changes designed to reduce or eliminate heartburn. These dietary changes are likely to have other beneficial health effects as well. Foods to avoid include:

- alcoholic beverages
- coffee, tea, and caffeinated soft drinks
- fatty or fried foods
- acidic foods such as citrus fruit or juice and tomato-based foods
- chocolate or foods with mint flavorings
- highly spiced foods

QUESTIONS TO ASK YOUR DOCTOR

- What is the best treatment for occasional heartburn?
- How can I tell the difference between severe heartburn and a heart attack?
- What is the difference between H2 blocker drugs and proton pump inhibitor drugs? Would one type of drug be less likely to interact with the other medications I am taking?
- Are over-the-counter medications as effective as prescription medications for the treatment of GERD?
- Under what circumstances should I consider surgical treatment for my GERD?
- Are you familiar with the LINX Reflux Management System, and would it be an option for me?

Prognosis

About 80% of people get relief from GERD through lifestyle changes and medication, although relapses are common. H2-blockers successfully treat 50%–60% of people with grade I or grade II GERD. Most people not helped by H2 blockers can be healed by 6–8 weeks of treatment with proton pump inhibitor drugs. Of the 20% of people not helped by medication, 92% improve with fundoplication surgery.

The most serious complication of GERD is Barrett's esophagus. In this disease, normal cells lining the esophagus are replaced with abnormal cells. About 30% of people with Barrett's esophagus go on to develop **cancer** of the esophagus. Those at highest risk are white men.

Other long-term complications of GERD include narrowing or scarring of the base of the esophagus, a condition called peptic stricture. This can cause difficulty swallowing. In addition, people with GERD can be more prone to ear infections and laryngitis. GERD may also worsen asthma.

As of 2012, there was some concern that people (especially older individuals) who remained on proton pump inhibitors for long periods (months, years) may be more susceptible to infection by the bacterium *Clostridium difficile*, which may cause pneumonia or severe diarrhea. Proton pump inhibitors also have the potential to interact with some common drugs including blood thinners such as Coumadin (warfarin), benzodiazepine anti-anxiety drugs such as diazepam (Valium), and disulfiram (Antabuse) used to treat alcohol abuse. These side effects and drug interactions remain under study.

Prevention

Prevention of GERD is very similar to the lifestyle changes suggested in the initial stage of treatment—stop smoking, lose weight, reduce or eliminate **alcohol consumption**, and avoid foods likely to cause heartburn.

Resources

BOOKS

Burns, David L., and Neeral Shah *100 Questions & Answers About Gastroesophageal Reflux Disease (GERD): A Lahey Clinic Guide*. Sudbury, MA: Jones and Bartlett Publishers, 2007.

Wyler, Susan, and Jorge Rodriguez. *The Acid Reflux Solution: A Cookbook and Lifestyle Guide for Healing Heartburn Naturally*. Berkeley, CA: Ten Speed Press, 2012.

OTHER

Consumer Health Reports. "Drugs to Treat Heartburn and Stomach Acid Reflux: The Proton Pump Inhibitors." *Best Buy Drugs*. Consumer Report, May 2010. http://www.consumerreports.org/health/resources/pdf/best-buy-drugs/PPIsUpdate-FINAL.pdf (accessed September 7, 2012).

WEBSITES

MedlinePlus. "GERD." U.S. National Library of Medicine, National Institutes of Health. http://www.nlm.nih.gov/medlineplus/gerd.html (accessed August 8, 2012).

National Institute of Diabetes and Digestive and Kidney Diseases (NIDDK). "Heartburn, Gastroesophageal Reflux (GER), and Gastroesophageal Reflux Disease (GERD)." National Digestive Diseases Information Clearinghouse. http://digestive.niddk.nih.gov/ddiseases/pubs/gerd/index.aspx (accessed August 8, 2012).

Patti, Marco. "Gastroesophageal Reflux Disease." Medscape Reference. http://emedicine.medscape.com/article/176595-overview (accessed August 8, 2012).

ORGANIZATIONS

American College of Gastroenterology (ACG), 6400 Goldsboro Rd., Ste. 450, Bethesda, MD 20817, (301) 263-9000, info@acg.gi.org, http://www.acg.gi.org.

American Gastroenterological Association (AGA), 4930 Del Ray Ave., Bethesda, MD 20814, (301) 654-2055, Fax: (301) 654-5920, http://www.gastro.org.

International Foundation for Functional Gastrointestinal Disorders, PO Box 170864, MilwaukeeWI 53217-8076, (888) 964-2001 USA only, (414) 964-1799, Fax: (414) 964-7176, iffgd@iffgd.org, http://www.iffgd.org.

National Digestive Diseases Information Clearinghouse (NDDIC), 2 Information Way, Bethesda, MD 20892-3570, (800) 891-5389, TTY: (866) 569-1162, Fax: (703) 738-4929, info@niddk.nih.gov, http://digestive.niddk.nih.gov.

Tish Davidson, AM

Genetically modified organisms (GMOs) *see* **Bioengineered foods**

GenoType diet *see* **Blood type diet**

Gestational diabetes

Definition

Gestational diabetes is an abnormal increase in blood sugar (glucose) levels that occurs during pregnancy in some women. Unlike other types of diabetes, gestational diabetes first appears during pregnancy and then disappears after the woman gives birth.

Demographics

Studies have found that in the United States between 3% and 10% of women experience diabetes during pregnancy. Ninety percent of these women develop gestational diabetes, about 8% have pre-existing type 2 (**insulin** resistant) diabetes, and about 1% have pre-existing type 1 (insulin deficiency) diabetes.

Race and ethnicity strongly affect the rate of development of gestational diabetes. Only about 1.4%–2% of Caucasian women develop gestational diabetes, while as many as 15% of Native American women from tribes in the Southwest United States develop the disorder. Between 5% and 8% of Hispanic Americans, African Americans, and Asian Americans develop gestational diabetes. If a woman experiences gestational diabetes, the chance of her developing it again in future pregnancies is as high as 68%.

Description

Carbohydrates (sugars and starches) found in foods such as sweets, potatoes, pasta, and breads, are broken down during digestion into glucose, a simple sugar that circulates in the blood and is used by cells for energy. The level of glucose changes depending on what food and how much of it a person eats. The level usually is highest about two hours after a meal. However, in order for the body to remain healthy, blood glucose levels must stay stable with certain narrow limits. In healthy people, the hormone insulin regulates the blood glucose level by controlling how much glucose enters cells. Once in cells, glucose either is used to meet the immediate energy needs of the cell or stored in liver, muscle, or fat cells for later release when blood glucose levels are low. In people with diabetes, this regulatory mechanism does not function correctly, and glucose builds up in the blood, a condition called hyperglycemia.

There are three types of diabetes. In type 1 diabetes, the pancreas, a digestive system organ, does not make any insulin or does not make enough insulin to properly regulate blood glucose levels. People with type 1 diabetes must control their blood glucose through diet, exercise, and most importantly, through the regular injection of synthetic or animal insulin.

In type 2 diabetes, the pancreas makes enough insulin, but cells become unresponsive to it, a condition called insulin resistance. As a result, adequate amounts of glucose cannot enter these cells, and glucose builds up in the blood. Many people with type 2 diabetes can control their blood glucose level through diet and exercise. Others must take supplemental insulin either by mouth (orally) or by injection.

In gestational diabetes, the pancreas makes insulin, but the placenta, which allows the fetus to obtain nourishment, produces hormones (e.g., estrogens, progesterone, and chorionic somatomammotropin) that increase the insulin resistance of cells. These hormones are at their highest levels during the third trimester of pregnancy. Their presence reduces the amount of glucose that can enter cells, so that more remains in the blood and hyperglycemia occurs. Most pregnant women do not develop gestational diabetes because the pancreas produces additional quantities of insulin (as much as 50% more than normal in the third trimester) in order to compensate for insulin resistance caused by pregnancy hormones. However, when a woman's pancreas cannot produce enough extra insulin, blood levels of glucose stay abnormally high, and the woman develops gestational diabetes.

Risk factors

Women at risk for gestational diabetes include those who:

- are overweight
- have a family history of diabetes
- have previously given birth to a very large, heavy baby
- have previously had a baby who was stillborn, or born with a birth defect
- have an unusually large amount of amniotic fluid (the cushioning fluid within the uterus that surrounds the developing fetus)

- are over 30 years of age
- belong to an ethnic group known to experience higher rates of gestational diabetes
- have a history of gestational diabetes during a pregnancy

Causes and symptoms

Since increasing levels of pregnancy hormones cause gestational diabetes, it develops late in pregnancy when pregnancy hormones are at their highest levels. Often women with gestational diabetes have few symptoms. However, leaving gestational diabetes undiagnosed and untreated is risky to the developing fetus. Left untreated, the mother's blood glucose levels will remain consistently high, and these same high levels will occur in the blood of the fetus. The fetal pancreas responds to the high glucose levels by secreting large amounts of insulin. This insulin allows the fetal cells to take in excess glucose that is converted into fat and stored. This conversion process uses oxygen that may be needed for other fetal processes. Low oxygen levels can lead to an increased risk of heart, breathing, and vision problems. Increased fat storage causes many babies born to women with gestational diabetes to be unusually large, often large enough to cause more difficult deliveries that may require the use of forceps, suction, or cesarean section.

Furthermore, when the baby is born, it will have an abnormally high level of insulin in the blood. After birth, when the mother and baby are no longer attached to each other via the placenta and umbilical cord, the baby will no longer be receiving the mother's high level of blood glucose. The infant's high level of insulin, however, will quickly use up the glucose circulating in the infant's bloodstream. The baby is then at risk for having a dangerously low level of blood glucose, a condition called hypoglycemia. When this occurs, it is easily resolved by giving the baby glucose from an external source.

Diagnosis

Since gestational diabetes often exists with no symptoms detectable by the mother, and since its existence puts the developing baby at risk for developmental abnormalities, screening for the disorder is a routine part of pregnancy care. This screening usually is done between the 26th and 28th week of pregnancy. At this point in the pregnancy, the placental hormones have reached a sufficient level to cause insulin resistance. Screening for gestational diabetes involves the pregnant woman drinking a special solution that contains exactly 50 grams of glucose. An hour later, the woman's blood is drawn and tested for its glucose level. A level of less than 140 mg/dL is considered normal.

Treatment

Treatment for gestational diabetes depends on the severity of the diabetes. Mild forms can be treated with changes in diet. Women may be put on strict, detailed diets, and instructed to stay within a certain range of carbohydrate intake. Exercise sometimes is used to help reduce blood glucose levels. Women often are asked to regularly measure their blood glucose level. This is done by pricking the finger with a needle called a lancet, putting a drop of blood on a special type of paper, and feeding the paper into a meter that analyzes and reports the blood glucose level. Self-monitoring of blood glucose helps to manage gestational diabetes and prevent complications. When diet and exercise do not keep blood glucose levels within an acceptable range, a woman may need to take regular shots of insulin.

Prognosis

Prognosis for women with gestational diabetes and their infants is generally good. Almost all such women have blood glucose levels that return to normal after the birth of their baby. However, research has shown that nearly half of these women who have gestational diabetes will develop type 2 diabetes within 15 years.

Pregnant women who have type 1 or type 2 diabetes that is poorly controlled have 4–8 times the chance of having a baby born with a birth defect than women who do not have diabetes. The risk is much lower for babies born to women who develop gestational diabetes because their fetus is exposed to high glucose levels for a much shorter time and only near the end of pregnancy after most organs are already formed. However, the child of a mother with gestational diabetes has a greater-than-normal chance of developing diabetes sometime in adulthood. A woman who has had gestational diabetes during one pregnancy has about a 68% chance of having it again during any subsequent pregnancies. Women who had gestational diabetes usually have their blood glucose levels tested at the post-partum checkup or after stopping **breastfeeding**.

Prevention

There is no known way to prevent gestational diabetes since it is caused by the effects of normal hormones of pregnancy. However, the effects of insulin resistance can be best handled through careful attention to diet, avoiding becoming overweight throughout life, participating in reasonable exercise, and avoiding smoking.

KEY TERMS

Glucose—A simple sugar that is the final product of the breakdown of carbohydrates.

Glycemic index—A ranking from 1–100 of how much carbohydrate-containing foods raise blood sugar levels within two hours after being eaten. Foods with a glycemic index of 50 or lower are considered "good."

Hormone—A chemical messenger that is produced by one type of cell and travels through the blood-stream to change the metabolism of a different type of cell.

Insulin—A hormone produced by the pancreas that is central to the processing of sugars and carbohydrates in the diet.

Placenta—An organ that is attached to the inside wall of the mother's uterus and to the fetus via the umbilical cord. The placenta allows oxygen and nutrients from the mother's bloodstream to pass into the unborn baby.

Type 1 diabetes—A chronic immune system disorder in which the pancreas does not produce sufficient amounts of insulin, a hormone that enables cells to use glucose for energy. It must be treated with insulin injections.

Type 2 diabetes—Formerly called adult-onset diabetes. In this form of diabetes, the pancreas either does not make enough insulin or cells become insulin resistant and do not use insulin efficiently.

Resources

BOOKS

American College of Obstetricians and Gynecologists, Women's, Health Care Physicians. *Your Pregnancy and Childbirth: Month to Month.* 5th ed. Washington, DC: American College of Obstetricians and Gynecologists, 2010.

Harms, Roger W. *Mayo Clinic Guide to a Healthy Pregnancy.* Rochester, MN: Mayo Clinic, 2004.

Roizen, Michael F., and Mehmet C. Oz. *YOU: Having a Baby: The Owner's Manual to a Happy and Healthy Pregnancy.* New York: Free Press, 2009.

OTHER

American Congress of Obstetricians and Gynecologists. "FAQ: Gestational Diabetes." http://www.acog.org/~/media/For Patients/faq177.pdf (accessed September 21, 2012).

WEBSITES

MedlinePlus. "Diabetes and Pregnancy." U.S. National Library of Medicine, National Institutes of Health. http://www.nlm.nih.gov/medlineplus/diabetesandpregnancy.html (accessed September 21, 2012).

National Diabetes Information Clearinghouse (NDIC). "What I Need To Know about Gestational Diabetes." National Institute of Diabetes and Digestive and Kidney Diseases (NIDDK). http://diabetes.niddk.nih.gov/dm/pubs/gestational (accessed September 21, 2012).

Office on Women's Health. "Pregnancy: Pregnancy Complications." U.S. Department of Health and Human Services. http://www.womenshealth.gov/faq/prenatal-care.cfm (accessed September 21, 2012).

ORGANIZATIONS

American Congress of Obstetricians and Gynecologists, PO Box 96920, Washington, DC 20090-6920, (202) 638-5577, http://www.acog.org.

American Diabetes Association, 1701 North Beauregard St., Alexandria, VA 22311, (800) DIABETES (342-2383), askADA@diabetes.org, http://www.diabetes.org.

American Pregnancy Association, 1425 Greenway Dr., Ste. 440, Irving, TX 75038, (972) 550-0140, Fax: (972) 550 0800, Questions@AmericanPregnancy.org, http://www.americanpregnancy.org.

National Diabetes Education Program, One Diabetes Way, Bethesda, MD 20814-9692, (301) 496-3583, http://www.ndep.nih.gov.

National Diabetes Information Clearinghouse, 1 Information Way, Bethesda, MD 20892-3560, (800) 860-8747, TTY: (866) 569-1162, Fax: (703) 738-4929, ndic@info.niddk.nih.gov, http://diabetes.niddk.nih.gov.

Office on Women's Health, Department of Health and Human Services, 200 Independence Ave. SW, Rm. 712E, Washington, DC 20201, (202) 690-7650, Fax: (202) 205-2631, http://www.womenshealth.gov.

Rosalyn Carson-DeWitt, MD
Tish Davidson, AM

GFCF diet *see* **Casein-free diet; Gluten-free diet**

Giardiasis

Definition

Giardiasis is a communicable gastrointestinal disease characterized by acute diarrhea. It is caused by a parasite, *Giardia lamblia*, also known as *Giardia intestinalis*. Giardiasis is the most common water-borne infection of the human intestine worldwide, affecting as many as 200 million people each year. According to the Centers for Disease Control and Prevention (CDC), there were 90 major community outbreaks of giardiasis in the United States between 1964 and 1984, and 34 major outbreaks since 1985.

The organism that causes giardiasis, *G. lamblia*, is a protozoan, a single-celled organism formerly classified as a member of the animal kingdom. It is a pear-shaped parasite with four flagella, which are long whip-like extensions of the cell that allow the organism to move. It was first seen under a microscope by the Dutch lens maker Antony van Leeuwenhoek in the seventeenth century. *G. lamblia* was found in human stool samples in 1859 by a Czech physician named Lambl, but was not identified as the cause of giardiasis until the 1970s. It was given its present name in 1915 to honor Alfred Giard, a French biologist, as well as Dr. Lambl.

Origins

Dietary treatment of patients with giardiasis has been a gradual process, dependent on better understanding of the causes of the disease as well as the development of nutritionally adequate rehydration solutions and anti-infective medications. A large part of dietary therapy for giardiasis, in fact, consists of measures to prevent the spread of the disease, not just to treat the symptoms after they appear.

Description

Life cycle of G. lamblia

In order to understand the symptoms, treatment, and prevention of giardiasis, it is helpful to understand the life cycle of *G. lamblia*. The parasite that causes giardiasis has a simple two-stage life cycle that does not require an intermediate host; it can be spread directly among human beings. The cycle begins when a person swallows as few as 10 to 15 cysts of *G. lamblia*. The cyst is a protective shell that the organism forms around itself that enables it to survive outside a human or animal host. The cysts of *G. lamblia* are smooth-walled and oval in shape, about 8–12 micrometers long and 5–15 micrometers wide. They are hardy and can survive for several months in cold water. They usually enter the human body through the mouth. The cysts may be transferred to the mouth directly from unwashed hands that have touched fecal matter containing cysts, or through having oral sex with an infected person. They may also enter the mouth through eating food or swallowing liquids contaminated by fecal matter containing *G. lamblia* cysts. *G. lamblia* is not, however, transmitted through blood.

Once inside the body, the cysts pass through the digestive tract until they reach the small intestine. Each cyst then opens—often within five minutes after arrival—and releases two trophozoites, which are the active feeding stage of the parasite. The trophozoites multiply rapidly, reproducing every 9 to 12 hours. They may remain free within the central cavity (lumen) of the small intestine or attach themselves to the mucous tissue lining the intestine by a sucking disk located on their ventral surface. It is the trophozoites that cause the violent diarrhea, nausea, intestinal gas, and cramping associated with giardiasis. However, researchers do not know the exact reason for the symptoms; some think that the parasites compete with the host for nutrients, while others think that they affect the host's immune system, cause damage to the tissues lining the intestine, or block the functioning of the intestinal mucosa by their sheer numbers.

As the trophozoites are carried toward the colon, they begin to secrete proteins to form the walls of a new cyst. Within the next 24 hours, the trophozoite completes the construction of its cyst and is shed into the outside environment through the person's feces.

Symptoms

About 15% of people who swallow cysts are asymptomatic. These cases are usually detected only if the person's stool is tested during a community outbreak. They are significant, however, because people carrying the cysts in their digestive tract, known as carriers, can still transmit giardiasis to others even if they do not develop the symptoms of the illness. It is estimated that between 30% and 60% of children in daycare centers and adults on Native American reservations are carriers of *G. lamblia*. Some domestic and wild animals can also be carriers of *G. lamblia*, dogs and beavers being the most common animal reservoirs.

Of the patients who have symptoms, 90% develop acute diarrhea within 7 to 10 days of ingesting the cysts; and 70%–75% have abdominal cramps, bloating, vomiting, and flatulence (the passage of intestinal gas). A small percentage of patients develop symptoms within three days of swallowing the cysts, including violent diarrhea, extremely foul-smelling intestinal gas, severe vomiting, fever, and headache. Most patients lose their appetite, and 50% lose weight—an average of ten pounds in adults. Without treatment, these symptoms can last for as long as seven weeks or even longer.

Between 20% and 40% of adults with giardiasis develop a temporary difficulty with digesting lactose, a **sugar** found in milk or milk products. This condition is called lactose intolerance and may last for a month or so after treatment with anti-parasite medications for giardiasis. Having lactose intolerance does not mean that the person has become reinfected.

There is no universal pattern to recovery from giardiasis. It is rarely fatal except in severely dehydrated and malnourished children, but may develop into chronic forms—malabsorption syndrome in adults and failure to thrive in children. Chronic giardiasis in adults is characterized by episodes of diarrhea that come and go, alternating with periods of **constipation** and normal bowel movements. Other symptoms of chronic giardiasis in adults include:

- Ongoing weight loss apart from intentional weight reduction.
- Steatorrhea. Steatorrhea is the medical term for the passage of large amounts of fat or greasy-looking material in the stool.
- Discomfort in the stomach or abdomen that is worse after a meal.
- Persistent bad breath or burping that smells like sulfur.
- Ongoing bloating, flatulence, or abdominal cramping.
- Recurrent headaches.
- Malaise (general feeling of sickness), fatigue, or weakness.

The symptoms of chronic giardiasis in children include:

- Failure to grow and gain weight at a normal rate for the child's age and sex.
- Recurrent episodes of pale, frothy, foul-smelling diarrhea.
- Loss of appetite.
- Abdominal pain and vomiting.
- Nutritional deficiencies caused by the inability to absorb nutrients in food.

Demographics

In the United States and other developed countries, giardiasis is most likely to affect children, particularly children in daycare centers. About 20%–25% of the children in daycare centers are infected with giardiasis even though they may not be symptomatic. Most of the community outbreaks in the United States since the 1980s, in fact, began in daycare centers.

Older adolescents and adults are more likely to be infected with giardiasis while hiking or traveling abroad. *G. lamblia* is a common cause of so-called **traveler's diarrhea**, although it is not the only organism that causes it. Giardiasis acquired its nickname of "beaver fever" because backpackers and hikers who drink water from or swim in streams close to beaver colonies are likely to ingest *G. lamblia* cysts shed into the water by infected animals. The CDC reports that as many as 80% of water samples from lakes, streams, and ponds in the United States contain *G. lamblia* cysts.

Outbreaks of giardiasis are most likely to occur in Canada and the United States during warmer weather, particularly in summer and fall. Race does not appear to be a factor in contracting giardiasis; however, males in all age groups are about 1.2 times more likely than females to develop the disease.

Risk factors

Some people are at increased risk of contracting giardiasis because of their location or lifestyle:

- Parents of infected small children.
- Employees (and their family members) of daycare centers in which some of the children are not yet toilet-trained.
- Employees (and their family members) of nursing homes or other custodial facilities.
- Male homosexuals, particularly those with several or many partners.
- People who swim in or boat on rivers, lakes, streams, or other bodies of water liable to contamination by fecal matter. The greatest risk of infection comes from accidentally swallowing a mouthful of water while swimming, diving, rafting, or water skiing.
- People who depend on well water for their household drinking supply.

Some people are at increased risk of a severe case of giardiasis because they have other health problems:

- an impaired immune system
- Crohn's disease, cystic fibrosis, or other diseases that weaken the intestines
- malnutrition
- recent surgery on the stomach or taking medications to lower stomach acid secretion (stomach acid kills *G. lamblia*)

Treatment

Most people with giardiasis can be diagnosed and treated by their primary care physician. Diagnosis is usually done by examining stool samples under a microscope for the characteristic cysts and trophozoites of *G. lamblia* (both forms of the organism may appear in the stool); by enzyme-linked immunosorbent assay (ELISA) tests; or by an Entero-test. The Entero-test, also called the string test, consists of a gelatin capsule containing a nylon string attached to a weight. The patient tapes one end of the string to the inside of the cheek and swallows the capsule. The string is left in place for four to six hours or overnight while the patient is fasting; it is then removed and the mucus on the string is examined for trophozoites.

Patients suspected of having chronic giardiasis may be referred to a gastroenterologist, who is a doctor with special training in digestive disorders. In some cases, the doctor may need to examine the patient's small intestine through an endoscope or remove a sample of tissue from the lining of the patient's intestine to make sure that the patient's symptoms are caused by a parasite and not by some other disorder.

Medications

Giardiasis is most commonly treated with one of the following drugs, which cause the death of the disease organisms:

- Metronidazole (Flagyl). The most common drug given to treat giardiasis. Adults are usually given three doses per day over a 5-day period, while children are usually given a 10 day course.
- Furazolidone (Furoxone). Some doctors prefer to treat children with this drug because it is available in a liquid form.
- Nitazoxanide (Alinia). This drug is also preferred for treating children because it causes fewer adverse effects in younger patients.
- Tinidazole (Tindamax). Tinidazole is a relatively new anti-infective drug; it was approved by the Food and Drug Administration (FDA) only in 2004. It has the advantage of requiring only one dose of 2000 mg for treatment of giardiasis rather than several days of repeated doses.
- Paromomycin (Humatin). Paramomycin is the only drug effective against *G. lamblia* that is considered safe to give pregnant women.

Some herbalists and naturopaths recommend barberry (*Berberis vulgaris*) as an anti-infective agent in treating giardiasis.

Children or adults who are carrying cysts are sometimes given anti-infective drugs even if they are not symptomatic, in order to lower the risk of transmission to other children in a daycare center or other family members.

Resources

BOOKS

"Giardiasis." Chapter 185, Section 14 in the *Merck Manual of Diagnosis and Treatment*. 18th ed. Edited by Mark H. Beers and Robert Berkow. Whitehouse Station, NJ: Merck, 2007.

Surawicz, Christina M., and Blanca Ochoa. *Diarrheal Diseases*. Bethesda, MD: American College of Gastroenterology (ACG), 2007.

PERIODICALS

Gavagan, Thomas, and Lisa Brodyaga. "Medical Care for Immigrants and Refugees." *American Family Physician* 57 (March 1, 1998): 1061–68.

Kucik, Corry Jeb, Gary L. Martin, and Brett V. Sortor. "Common Intestinal Parasites." *American Family Physician* 69 (March 1, 2004): 1161–68.

Rana, S.V., D.K. Bhasin, and V.K. Vinayak. "Lactose Hydrogen Breath Test in *Giardia lamblia*-positive Patients." *Digestive Diseases and Sciences* 50 (February 2005): 259–61.

WEBSITES

American Academy of Family Physicians. "Giardiasis." http://familydoctor.org/familydoctor/en/diseases-conditions/giardiasis.html (accessed October 2, 2012).

Centers for Disease Control and Prevention. "Parasites—Giardia." http://www.cdc.gov/parasites/giardia (accessed October 2, 2012).

Mukherjee, Sandeep. "Giardiasis." Medscape Reference. http://emedicine.medscape.com/article/176718-overview (accessed October 2, 2012).

Nemours Foundation. "Giardiasis." KidsHealth.org. http://kidshealth.org/parent/infections/stomach/giardiasis.html (accessed October 2, 2012).

PubMed Health. "Giardia infection." U.S. National Library of Medicine. http://www.ncbi.nlm.nih.gov/pubmedhealth/PMH0001333 (accessed October 2, 2012).

ORGANIZATIONS

American Academy of Family Physicians, 11400 Tomahawk Creek Pkwy., Leawood, KS 66211-2680, (913) 906-6000, (800) 274-2237, Fax: (913) 906-6075, http://www.aafp.org.

Centers for Disease Control and Prevention, 1600 Clifton Rd. NE, Atlanta, GA 30333, (800) CDC-INFO (232-4636), TTY: (888) 232-6348, cdcinfo@cdc.gov, http://www.cdc.gov.

U.S. Food and Drug Administration, 10903 New Hampshire Ave., Silver Spring, MD 20993-0002, (888) INFO-FDA (463-6332), http://www.fda.gov.

World Health Organization, Avenue Appia 20, 1211 Geneva 27, Switzerland, +4122791-2111, Fax: +4122791-3111, info@who.int, http://www.who.int.

Rebecca J. Frey, PhD

Ginkgo biloba

Definition

Ginkgo biloba is an herbal dietary supplement made from the leaves of the tree *Ginkgo biloba*.

Purpose

Ginkgo biloba, sometimes called *bai guo*, has been used in Traditional Chinese Medicine (TCM) for about 5,000 years to treat memory loss, mood, nerve, circulatory and many other health problems. Ginkgo biloba often is combined with **ginseng** to boost memory, improve the quality of life, and increase a sense of well being. The effectiveness of some TCM uses of ginkgo, such as relieving pain caused by clogged arteries in the leg (claudication), treating Alzheimer's disease, and improving blood flow to the brain have been evaluated in well-designed studies and are generally accepted by practitioners of conventional medicine. Many other TCM uses of ginkgo biloba are currently being investigated.

Description

Ginkgo biloba is the last existing member of an ancient family of trees. The fossil record shows that ginkgo trees existed 200 million years ago. *Ginkgo biloba* is native to China, Japan, and Korea. The tree was introduced to North America in the 1700s. Ginkgo trees grow to a height of 65–115 ft (20–35 m). They are extremely resistant to disease and insect damage and can live for several hundred years. Female trees produce bad-smelling fruit-like bodies the size of an apricot that contains seeds. Herbal practitioners sometimes use the seeds in treatment. The much cleaner male ginkgo is a popular tree for urban landscaping.

The fan-shaped leaves of the ginkgo are used for medicinal purposes. About twenty different

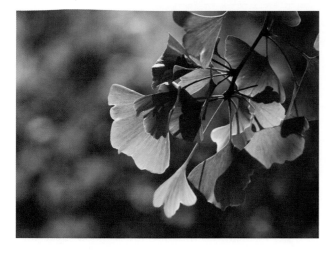

Ginkgo biloba leaves. *(© iStockphoto.com/etiennema)*

compounds have been identified in ginkgo leaves, but the medically active ingredients appear to be flavonoids and terpenoids. Flavonoids are **antioxidants** that help lower the level of free radicals in the body. Terpenoids are thought to protect nerves from damage, reduce inflammation, and decrease blood clotting.

In the United States, *Ginkgo biloba* is cultivated and the leaves are harvested and dried, then often used to make a standardized extract that contains 24%–25% flavonoids and 6% terpenoids. U. S. law does not require the standardization of **dietary supplements**, so consumers should read all labels carefully. Ginkgo biloba is often sold as capsules and tablets. Dry and liquid ginkgo extract is added to other herbal remedies as well as teas, energy or health bars, and similar products. An injectable form of ginkgo biloba extract that was available in Europe has been withdrawn from the market because of adverse side effects. Most well-designed studies have been done using a total of 80 240 mg of 50:1 standardized extract divided into 2 or 3 doses daily and taken by mouth.

Regulation of ginkgo biloba sales

Ginkgo biloba is one of the top selling herbal remedies in the United States and is even more popular in Europe. Under the 1994 Dietary Supplement Health and Education Act (DSHEA), the sale of ginkgo biloba is regulated by the U.S. Food and Drug Administration (FDA) as a dietary supplement. At the time the act was passed, legislators felt because many dietary supplements such as ginkgo biloba come from natural sources and have been used for hundreds of years by practitioners of complementary and alternative medicine (CAM), supplements did not need to

be regulated as rigorously as prescription and over-the-counter drugs used in conventional medicine.

The DSHEA regulates ginkgo biloba in the same way that food is regulated. Like food manufacturers, manufacturers of herbal products containing ginkgo biloba do not have to prove that they are either safe or effective before they can be sold to the public. This differs from conventional pharmaceutical drugs, which must undergo extensive human testing to prove their safety and effectiveness before they can be marketed. Also unlike conventional drugs, the label for a dietary supplement such as ginkgo biloba does not have to contain any statements about possible side effects. All herbal supplements sold in the United States must show the scientific name of the herb on the label.

Health claims

Ginkgo biloba is one of the most promising traditional herbs investigated by Western medicine. The National Center for Complementary and Alternative Medicine (NCCAM), a government organization within the National Institutes of Health, is sponsoring clinical trials to determine safety and effectiveness of ginkgo biloba as a treatment for more than a dozen diseases and disorders. Individuals interested in participating in a clinical trial at no charge can find a list of open trials at http://www.clinicaltrials.gov.

Some health claims for ginkgo biloba have already been evaluated in large, well-controlled studies that satisfy the proof of safety and effectiveness demanded by conventional medicine. There is good evidence that ginkgo biloba can cause short-term improvement in mental function in people with Alzheimer's disease. In a well-designed study, ginkgo biloba was as effective as the prescription drug donepezil (Aricept) in slowing the development of dementia in people with mild to moderate Alzheimer's. Ginkgo biloba has also been shown to be effective in improving blood flow to the brain and in treating certain other dementias. The effect of ginkgo biloba on memory in healthy young adults and in people with age-related memory impairment is inconsistent, but strong enough to continue to study the effects of the herb in these populations.

In other rigorous studies, ginkgo biloba has improved symptoms of claudication. Claudication is leg pain that occurs during walking when insufficient oxygen reaches the leg muscles. It is usually caused by blocked arteries in the leg. Ginkgo biloba's ability to reduce blood clotting ("thin the blood") is thought to account for improving symptoms in people with claudication. However, exercise and prescription medication were more effective in reducing leg pain due to claudication than ginkgo biloba alone. Ginkgo biloba has also been used, especially in Europe, to treat Raynaud's disease. Raynaud's disease causes the extremities of the body to feel cold in response to stress or cool temperatures. During an attack of Raynaud's disease, the blood vessels to the affected area narrow and blood flow is reduced.

Several health claims for ginkgo biloba center on treating disorders of the eye, including glaucoma, age-related macular degeneration, and type 2 diabetes-related retinopathy. Ginkgo appears to increase blood flow to the eye, but additional studies need to be done to evaluate its effectiveness in helping to treat these disorders.

The terpenoids in ginkgo biloba are thought to help prevent nerve damage. Because of this, ginkgo has been suggested as a treatment for tinnitus (ringing of the ears), multiple sclerosis, cochlear deafness, and Huntington's disease. Results of studies so far are inconsistent, and additional research is needed to determine the usefulness of ginkgo in nerve disorders.

Some researchers have suggested that ginkgo biloba is useful in treating depression, seasonal affective disorder, premenstrual syndrome, altitude sickness, vertigo (dizziness), premenstrual syndrome (PMS), gastric **cancer**, side effects of anti-cancer drugs, and pulmonary interstitial fibrosis, as well as generally improving quality of live and sense of well being. Further studies need to be done to evaluate these health claims.

Precautions

Ginkgo biloba seeds contain toxins that can cause vomiting, seizures, loss of consciousness, and death, especially in young children. Ginkgo biloba seeds are not safe and should be avoided.

Extracts of the leaf of *Ginkgo biloba* are generally safe and cause few side effects when taken at recommended doses for up to six months. People who are planning to have surgery should stop taking ginkgo biloba at least two days before their operation because of the risk of increased bleeding. The safety of ginkgo biloba in children and pregnant and **breastfeeding** women is still being studied.

Interactions

Ginkgo biloba has blood-thinning properties and is likely to increase the blood-thinning and anticoagulant effects of medicines such as warfarin (Coumadin),

clopidogrel (Plavix), aspirin, and nonsteroidal anti-inflammatory drugs (e.g., Advil, Motrin). Individuals taking these drugs should not begin taking ginkgo biloba without consulting their health care provider.

Ginkgo biloba may also interact with mono-amine-oxidase inhibitors (MAOIs) used to treat certain kinds of depression and mental illness. Examples of MAOIs include isocarboxazid (Marplan), phenelzine (Nardil) and tranylcypromine (Parnate). Individuals taking MAOIs along with ginkgo biloba may experience increased effects from the MAOI.

Some reports suggest that ginkgo biloba lowers blood sugar levels. Individuals who are taking **insulin** or other medications that also lower blood sugar, and those with type 2 diabetes, should consult their health care provider before starting to take ginkgo biloba.

Complications

Serious side effects of ginkgo biloba are rare. The most common mild side effects are headache, dizziness, nausea, diarrhea, increased restlessness, and racing heart. Increased bleeding may occur. Allergic reactions to ginkgo are possible, but uncommon. In severe rare cases, the skin blisters and sloughs off, a condition called Stevens-Johnson syndrome. People who are allergic to sumac, mango rind, cashews, poison oak, and poison ivy are at slightly higher risk to have an allergic reaction to ginkgo biloba.

Parental concerns

Parents should be aware that the safe dose of many herbal supplements has not been established for children. Accidental overdose may occur if children are give adult herbal supplements.

Resources

BOOKS

Cass, Hyla, and Jim English. *Basic Health Publications User's Guide to Ginkgo Biloba*. North Bergen, NJ: Basic Health Publications, 2002.

Fragakis, Allison. *The Health Professional's Guide to Popular Dietary Supplements* Chicago: American Dietetic Association, 2003.

PDR for Herbal Medicines. 3rd ed. Montvale, NJ: Thompson Healthcare, 2004.

Pierce, Andrea. *The American Pharmaceutical Association Practical Guide to Natural Medicines*. New York: William Morrow, 1999.

Tracy, Timothy S. and Richard L. Kingston, eds. *Herbal Products: Toxicology and Clinical Pharmacology*. Totowa, NJ, Humana Press, 2007.

Wildman, Robert E. C., ed. *Handbook of Nutraceuticals and Functional Foods*. 2nd ed. Boca Raton, FL: CRC/Taylor & Francis, 2007.

PERIODICALS

Akhondzadeh, S. and S. H. Abbasi. "Herbal Medicine in the Treatment of Alzheimer's Disease." *American Journal of Alzheimer's Disease and Other Dementias* 21, no. 2 (Mar–Apr 2006): 113–18.

Brinkley, Tina E. "Effect of *Ginkgo Biloba* on Blood Pressure and Incidence of Hypertension in Elderly Men and Women." *American Journal of Hypertension* 23, no. 5 (2010): 528–33.

Dugoua, J.J., et al. "Safety and Efficacy of Ginkgo (Ginkgo Biloba) During Pregnancy and Lactation." *Canadian Journal of Clinical Pharmacology* 13, no. 3 (Fall 2006): e277–84.

Oh, S M. and K H. Chung. "Antiestrogenic Activities of Ginkgo Biloba Extracts." *Steroid Biochemistry and Molecular Biology* 100, nos. 4–5 (August 2006): 167–76.

Sierpina, Victor S., Bernd Wollschlaeger, and Mark Blumenthal. "Ginkgo Biloba." *American Academy of Family Physicians* 68, (September 1, 2003): 923–26.

WEBSITES

Mayo Clinic staff. "Ginkgo Biloba." MayoClinic.com. http://www.mayoclinic.com/health/triglycerides/CL00015 (accessed October 2, 2012).

MedlinePlus. "Ginkgo." U.S. National Library of Medicine, National Institutes of Health. http://www.nlm.nih.gov/medlineplus/druginfo/natural/333.html (accessed October 2, 2012).

National Center for Complementary and Alternative Medicine. "Ginkgo." National Institutes of Health. http://nccam.nih.gov/health/ginkgo (accessed October 2, 2012).

University of Maryland Medical Center. "Ginkgo Biloba." http://www.umm.edu/altmed/articles/ginkgo-biloba-000247.htm (accessed October 2, 2012).

ORGANIZATIONS

American Association of Acupuncture and Oriental Medicine, PO Box 162340, Sacramento, CA 95816, Fax: (916) 443-4766, (866) 455-7999, http://www.aaaomonline.org.

American Botanical Council, PO Box 14435, Austin, TX 78723, (512) 926-4900, Fax: (512) 926-2345, (800) 373-7105, http://abc.herbalgram.org.

National Center for Complementary and Alternative Medicine Clearinghouse, PO Box 7923, Gaithersburg, MD 20898, (888) 644-6226, Fax: (866) 464-3616, info@nccam.nih.gov, http://nccam.nih.gov.

Natural Standard, One Davis Square, Somerville, MA 02144, (617) 591-3300, Fax: (617) 591-3399, questions@naturalstandard.com, http://naturalstandard.com.

Office of Dietary Supplements, National Institutes of Health, 6100 Executive Blvd., Rm. 3B01, MSC 7517, Bethesda, MD 20892-7517, (301) 435-2920, Fax: (301) 480-1845, ods@nih.gov, http://ods.od.nih.gov.

Tish Davidson, A.M.

Ginseng

Definition

Ginseng refers to two closely related herbs of the genus *Panax*. Asian ginseng (*P. ginseng*) and American ginseng (*P. quinquefolius*) have traditionally been used for healing. Asian ginseng is also known as Korean red ginseng, Chinese ginseng, Japanese ginseng, ginseng radix, ninjin, sang, and ren shen. American ginseng is also known as Canadian ginseng, North American ginseng, Ontario ginseng, Wisconsin ginseng, red berry, sang, and ren shen. Siberian ginseng (*Eleutherococcus senticosus*) is a plant with different properties that belongs to a completely different genus. Ginseng in this entry refers only to Asian and American ginseng of the genus *Panax*.

Purpose

Ginseng has been used for about 2,000 years in Traditional Chinese Medicine (TCM) to boost energy, hasten recovery from illness or injury, reduce stress, improve mental and physical performance (including sexual performance) and to treat several dozen different infections, gastrointestinal disorders, circulatory problems, and conditions as diverse as burns, cancers, diabetes, migraine headaches, and weight loss. The genus name *Panax* means "heal all," and ginseng is considered by herbalists to be an almost universal remedy. Most of these traditional uses of ginseng have not yet been substantiated by conventional medicine, however encouraging results from some well-designed, controlled human studies strongly suggest that ginseng may improve mental performance and have other health benefits.

Description

Ginseng is a perennial herb that grows in cool, damp, shady forests. Asian ginseng is native to Northern China and today is grown as a cash crop in China, Korea, Japan, and Russia. American ginseng once grew wild from the Appalachian Mountains to Minnesota. Today it is cultivated mainly in Wisconsin and in the Canadian provinces of Ontario and British Columbia. Most cultivated ginseng from North America is exported to Asia. In both Asia and North

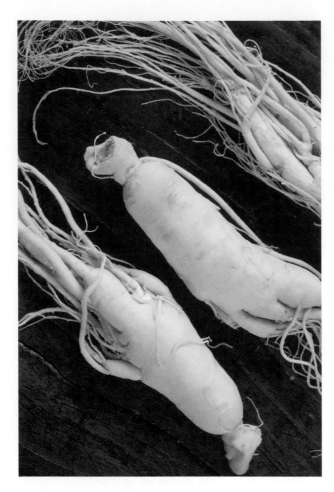

Ginseng root. (© iStockPhoto.com/yungshu chao)

America, wild ginseng is threatened with extinction from over harvesting. In the United States, a government permit is usually required to export wild ginseng. High-quality wild ginseng is very expensive. Illegal harvesting of wild ginseng from public lands is an ongoing law enforcement problem for the United States Fish and Wildlife Service.

Ginseng is a slow-growing plant that reaches a height of 12–30 in. and produces red berries. Only the root is used for medicinal purposes. Ginseng is difficult to cultivate. Plants must grow 4–6 years before the roots can be harvested. Ginseng roots are forked and twisted, looking somewhat like a miniature human body. They are occasionally used fresh but more often are dried and ground or powdered. The root can be soaked to make an extract or tincture. Ground ginseng can be added to tea and powered ginseng put into capsules. Ginseng extract can be added to products as diverse as chewing gum and soft drinks. Ginseng is sold under dozens of different brand names. It is often found in multi-herb remedies

sold under a huge variety of names. The active ingredients in ginseng are thought to be more than 20 compounds called ginsenosides. Some manufacturers standardize the amount of ginsenosides in their product while others do not. Standardized products usually contain 4% ginsenosides.

Regulation of ginseng sales

In the United States, ginseng is regulated by the Food and Drug Administration (FDA) as a dietary supplement under the 1994 Dietary Supplement Health and Education Act (DSHEA). At the time the act was passed, legislators felt because many **dietary supplements** such as ginseng come from natural sources and have been used for hundreds of years by practitioners of complementary and alternative medicine (CAM), these supplements did not need to be regulated as rigorously as prescription and over-the-counter drugs used in conventional medicine.

The DSHEA regulates ginseng in the same way that food is regulated. Like food manufacturers, manufacturers of herbal products containing ginseng do not have to prove that they are either safe or effective before they can be sold to the public. This differs from conventional pharmaceutical drugs, which must undergo extensive human testing to prove their safety and effectiveness before they can be marketed. Also unlike conventional drugs, the label for a dietary supplement such as ginseng does not have to contain any statements about possible side effects. All herbal supplements sold in the United States must show the scientific name of the herb on the label. Consumers should look for ginseng of the *Panax* variety. Sometimes less expensive herbs such as Siberian "ginseng" are substituted for true ginseng.

Health claims

Dozens of health claims are made for ginseng, many based on traditional or folk use of the herb. These claims are difficult to substantiate in ways that satisfy conventional medicine for several reasons including:

• The amount and strength of ginseng in dietary supplements is not standardized and a wide range of doses are used in different studies.

• Ginseng is often one of several herbs contained in herbal remedies, making it difficult to tell if the effects are due to ginseng or another herb.

• Many studies done on ginseng are poorly designed so that it is impossible to show a direct link between cause and effect, or they poorly reported, making analysis of the results difficult.

- Many rigorous and well-designed human studies have a small sample size.
- Many studies are sponsored by ginseng growers, manufacturers, or importers who have a financial interest in obtaining positive results.

Despite these drawbacks, there is enough evidence that ginseng provides health benefits that the National Center for Complementary and Alternative Medicine (NCCAM), a government organization within the National Institutes of Health, is sponsoring clinical trials to determine safety and effectiveness of ginseng as a treatment for several diseases and disorders. Individuals interested in participating in a clinical trial at no charge can find a list of open trials at http://www.clinicaltrials.gov.

Some health claims for ginseng appear more promising than others. There is good evidence that ginseng can cause short-term improvement in mental performance in both healthy young adults and elderly ill adults. Not enough information is available to determine if long-term gains also occur, but the results have been promising enough that ginseng is being studied in patients with Alzheimer's disease and other dementias. Along with improved mental performance, some studies have shown that ginseng improves the sense of well being and quality of life. Results of these studies are mixed, with some finding improvements and others finding no change. The situation is complicated by the fact that different studies define and measure "well being" and "quality of life" in different ways. In general, people with the worst quality of life report the most improvement.

Many claims are made that ginseng boosts the immune system, thus helping to prevent disease and promote a more rapid recovery from illness and injury. Some studies also claim that ginseng boosts the effect of antibiotics and improves the body's response to influenza vaccines. Some studies of patients with diseases that cause a low white cell count (white cells are a part of the immune system) show that white cell count increases with high doses of ginsenosides. Better studies are needed before the effect of ginseng on the immune system can be determined.

There is good evidence that ginseng lowers blood sugar in people with type 2 (non-insulin dependent) diabetes. The effect of ginseng on blood sugar in people with type 1 (**insulin** dependent) diabetes has not been studied enough to produce any definite findings.

Ginseng has been promoted as a preventative and/or cure for **cancer**. According the American Cancer Society in 2007, "There is no reliable scientific evidence that ginseng is effective in preventing or treating cancer in humans." However, controversial evidence from some studies done in Asia suggests the possibility that ginseng powder or extract may prevent some cancers. More and better studies are needed to clarify these results.

Some studies have reported that ginseng improves stamina and athletic performance and decreases fatigue, while other studies find no effect. There are so many other lifestyle variables in most of these studies that it is difficult to separate the effect of ginseng from other factors.

Studies of the effect of ginseng on the circulatory system are mixed. Some studies find that ginseng lowers blood pressure and in combination with other herbs prevents coronary artery disease and possibly congestive heart failure. Other studies find no effect, or that the effect is apparent only at very high, and possibly unsafe, doses. The effect of ginseng on the circulatory system continues to be investigated.

Many other health claims are made for herbal mixtures that contain ginseng. These claims are extremely difficult to evaluate because of the number of variables, including the strength of the mixture, the effects of the different herbs, and potential interactions among other herbs. Until much more is known about the chemical properties and active ingredients of common medicinal herbs, it is almost impossible to evaluate these mixtures in a way that satisfies the demands of conventional medicine.

Precautions

Ginseng is generally safe and causes few side effects when taken at recommended doses. The generally recommended dose is 100–200 mg of standardized ginseng extract containing 4% ginsenosides once or twice daily. The safety of ginseng in children and pregnant and **breastfeeding** women has not been studied. Pregnant and breastfeeding women should be aware that some tinctures of ginseng contain high levels of alcohol. Some herbalists recommend that individuals take ginseng for 2–3 weeks and then take a break of 1–2 weeks before beginning the herb again.

Independent laboratory analyses have repeatedly found that many products labeled as ginseng contain little or none of the herb. True ginseng is expensive, and unscrupulous manufacturers often substitute low-cost herbs for ginseng. Another problem is that some ginseng products have been found to be contaminated with pesticides and other chemicals that can cause serious side effects.

Interactions

Ginseng appears to interact with blood-thinning and anti-coagulant medicines such as warfarin (Coumadin), clopidogrel (Plavix), aspirin, and nonsteroidal anti-inflammatory drugs (e.g., Advil, Motrin). Individuals taking these drugs should not begin taking ginseng without consulting their health care provider.

Because ginseng lowers blood sugar levels, individuals who are taking insulin or other medications that also lower blood sugar, and those with type 2 diabetes, should be monitored for low blood sugar if they begin taking ginseng. Adjustments are needed in their other medications.

Ginseng may also interact with monoamine-oxidase inhibitors (MAOIs) used to treat certain kinds of depression and mental illness. Examples of MAOIs include isocarboxazid (Marplan), phenelzine (Nardil) and tranylcypromine (Parnate). Individuals taking MAOIs with ginseng may develop headache, tremors, increased anxiety, restlessness, sleeplessness, and mania.

Preliminary evidence suggests that ginseng may interact with certain blood pressure and heart medications. The herb may also interfere with the way the liver processes other drugs and herbs. Before beginning to take a supplement containing ginseng, individuals should review their current medications with their health care provider to determine any possible interactions.

Complications

Serious side effects of ginseng are rare. The most common side effects are increased restlessness, insomnia, nausea, diarrhea, and rash. Allergic reactions are possible, but uncommon. Some of the more serious side effects reported are thought to be the result of contamination with pesticides, heavy metals, or other chemicals rather than a side effect caused by ginseng.

Parental concerns

Parents should be aware that the safe dose of many herbal supplements has not been established for children. Accidental overdose may occur if children are give adult herbal supplements.

Resources

BOOKS

Court, William E. *Ginseng: The Genus Panax.* Australia: Harwood Academic, 2000.

Dasgupta, Amitava, and Catherine A. Hammett-Stabler, editors. *Herbal Supplements: Efficacy, Toxicity,* *Interactions with Western Drugs, and Effects on Clinical Laboratory Tests.* Hoboken, NJ: Wiley, 2011.

Fragakis, Allison. *The Health Professional's Guide to Popular Dietary Supplements.* Chicago: American Dietetic Association, 2007.

Johanssen, Kristin. *Ginseng Dreams: The Secret World of America's Most Valuable Plant.* Lexington, KY: University Press of Kentucky, 2006.

PDR for Herbal Medicines. Montvale, NJ: Thompson, 2007.

Sutton, Amy L, editor. *Complementary and Alternative Medicine Sourcebook.* Detroit: Omnigraphics, 2010.

Tracy, Timothy S. and Richard L. Kingston, eds. *Herbal Products: Toxicology and Clinical Pharmacology.* Totowa, NJ, Humana Press, 2007.

Wildman, Robert E.C., ed. *Handbook of Nutraceuticals and Functional Foods.* 2nd ed. Boca Raton, FL: CRC/Taylor & Francis, 2007.

PERIODICALS

Dougherty, Ursula, et al. "American Ginseng Suppresses Western Diet-Promoted Tumorigenesis in Model of Inflammation-Associated Colon Cancer: Role of EGFR." *BMC Complementary & Alternative Medicine* 11 (November 11, 2011): 111. http://dx.crossref.org/10.1186%2F1472-6882-11-111 (accessed October 2, 2012).

Kaneko, Hitoshi, and Kozo Nakanish. "Proof of the Mysterious Efficacy of Ginseng: Basic and Clinical Trials: Clinical Effects of Medical Ginseng, Korean Red Ginseng: Specifically, Its Anti-stress Action for Prevention of Disease." *Journal of Pharmacological Sciences* 95 (2004): 158–62.

Kiefer, David, and Traci Pantuso. "Panax Ginseng." *American Family Physician* 68 (October 15, 2003): 1539–42.

WEBSITES

American Cancer Society. "Ginseng." http://www.cancer.org/Treatment/TreatmentsandSideEffects/ComplementaryandAlternativeMedicine/HerbsVitaminsandMinerals/ginseng (accessed October 2, 2012).

MedlinePlus. "Ginseng, Panax." U.S. National Library of Medicine, National Institutes of Health. http://www.nlm.nih.gov/medlineplus/druginfo/natural/1000.html (accessed October 2, 2012).

———. "Ginseng, Siberian." U.S. National Library of Medicine, National Institutes of Health. http://www.nlm.nih.gov/medlineplus/druginfo/natural/985.html (accessed October 2, 2012).

National Center for Complementary and Alternative Medicine. "Ginseng." National Institutes of Health. http://nccam.nih.gov/health/asianginseng (accessed October 2, 2012).

ORGANIZATIONS

American Association of Acupuncture and Oriental Medicine, PO Box 162340, Sacramento, CA 95816, Fax: (916) 443-4766, (866) 455-7999, http://www.aaaomonline.org.

American Botanical Council, PO Box 14435, Austin, TX 78723, (512) 926-4900, Fax: (512) 926-2345, (800) 373-7105, http://abc.herbalgram.org.

National Center for Complementary and Alternative Medicine Clearinghouse, PO Box 7923, Gaithersburg, MD 20898, (888) 644-6226, Fax: (866) 464-3616, info@nccam.nih.gov, http://nccam.nih.gov.

Natural Standard, One Davis Square, Somerville, MA 02144, (617) 591-3300, Fax: (617) 591-3399, questions@naturalstandard.com, http://naturalstandard.com.

Office of Dietary Supplements, National Institutes of Health, 6100 Executive Blvd., Rm. 3B01, MSC 7517, Bethesda, MD 20892-7517, (301) 435-2920, Fax: (301) 480-1845, ods@nih.gov, http://ods.od.nih.gov.

Tish Davidson, A.M.

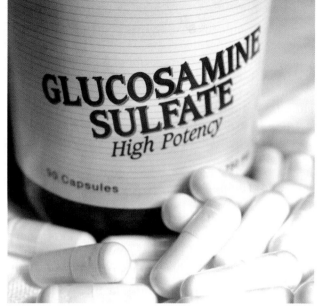

Glucosamine sulfate capsules. (© Envision/Corbis)

Glucosamine

Definition

Glucosamine is a natural compound found in the human body; more specifically, it is an amino monosaccharide (a nitrogen-containing **sugar**). It is thought to play a role in cartilage formation and repair and may also have anti-inflammatory capabilities. It is sold as a nutritional or dietary supplement in three forms: glucosamine hydrochloride (glucosamine HCl), glucosamine sulfate, and N-acetyl-glucosamine (NAG). Within medical studies, most of the research has been done on the first two, particularly glucosamine sulfate.

Purpose

When taken as an oral supplement, glucosamine is sometimes used in the treatment of osteoarthritis. Osteoarthritis is considered to be the most common type of arthritis. According to the U.S. Centers for Disease Control and Prevention (CDC), at least 26.9 million people in the United States annually suffer with osteoarthritis, and that number is considered to be a low estimate. Also called degenerative joint disease, osteoarthritis is caused by deterioration or loss of cartilage in one or more joints of the body. The symptoms of the condition range from mild pain and stiffness, to complete loss of use of the joint, and it may or may not have an identifiable cause; people aged 60 years or older often develop osteoarthritis.

Unlike the less common rheumatoid arthritis, osteoarthritis is not marked by inflammation. While osteoarthritis is commonly associated with being overweight, cartilage deterioration can be caused by excessive wear and tear on the joints, which may be due to excessive physical exercise or exertion. Many athletes take glucosamine supplements to help prevent cartilage damage.

The use of glucosamine in osteoarthritis therapy seems to be considered generally safe among medical professionals. However, it is not completely accepted within the medical community as being effective for osteoarthritis treatment and is considered an alternative medicine treatment. In the United States, the Food and Drug Administration (FDA) has not approved the use of glucosamine for medical use in humans. It is classified as a dietary supplement, so FDA approval is not needed as long as companies do not advertise it as a treatment for a medical condition. In Europe, however, glucosamine sulfate is approved as a medical drug.

Besides osteoarthritis, glucosamine is also used to relieve symptoms of leg pain, rheumatoid arthritis, chronic venous insufficiency, diabetes and related conditions, **inflammatory bowel disease** (such as ulcerative colitis and **Crohn's disease**), and temporomandibular joint (TMJ) disorders. Scientific results show some positive evidence for the effective use of glucosamine with osteoarthritis, specifically osteoarthritis of the knee; however, the scientific evidence is much more unclear for the other diseases.

Description

Glucosamine is also known as 2-amino-2-deoxy-glucose, 2-amino-2-deoxy-beta-D-glucopyranose, and chitosamine. The chemical symbol for glucosamine is $C_6H_{13}NO_5$. Glucosamine is taken from animal tissue, specifically from the shells of crabs, lobsters, and shrimp. Within these shellfish, glucosamine is made naturally in the form of glucosamine-6-phosphate, which eventually makes glycosaminoglycans, among other substances. Since glucosamine-6-phosphate helps to regulate the production of joint cartilage and glycosaminoglycans are a major component of cartilage, glucosamine may help to rebuild cartilage and treat arthritis. Whether these glucosamine processes could be involved in human arthritis remains undecided in the medical community. Not all medical professionals believe glucosamine is effective.

The two most commonly sold forms of glucosamine are glucosamine sulfate and glucosamine hydrochloride. Glucosamine is often sold in combination with other supplements, such as chondroitin sulfate (a sulfated glycosaminoglycan composed of a chain of alternating sugars) and methylsulfonylmethane (MSM, an organic sulfur compound within the chemical class of sulfones). Glucosamine is found in various forms when sold commercially, including capsules (500 mg, 550 mg, 750 mg, and 1,000 mg), liquid (500 mg per five mL), tablets (340 mg, 500 mg, and 1,000 mg), and powder.

When glucosamine is taken orally into the body (as a pill), according to conclusions from scientifically based animal studies, it is absorbed into the small intestine. It then travels into the liver where most of it is metabolized. Based on these studies, some of it does apparently go to the cartilage; however, it is not known how much is actually transmitted to the joints. It is primarily removed from the body through urine.

In 2002, the National Institutes of Health sponsored a large, multi-institutional clinical trial to test the effects of chondroitin sulfate, glucosamine, and the combination of the two on knee osteoarthritis. (Chondroitin is a carbohydrate that is a component of cartilage. It is thought to help promote water retention and elasticity in cartilage and help prevent enzymes from destroying cartilage.) The study was one of the largest of its kind to date with respect to research into the two substances.

The four-year study, known as the Glucosamine/Chondroitin Arthritis Intervention Trial (GAIT), involved almost 1,600 participants and 16 research facilities. It was funded by the National Center for Complementary and Alternative Medicine and the National Institute of Arthritis and Musculoskeletal and Skin Diseases. The lead researcher in the study was Daniel O. Clegg from the University of Utah, School of Medicine (Salt Lake City). Five different treatments were given daily for 24 weeks: glucosamine alone (1,500 mg), chondroitin sulfate alone (1,200 mg), glucosamine and chondroitin sulfate combined (same doses), a placebo, or celecoxib (Celebrex®), an FDA-approved osteoarthritis drug (200 mg).

The study found that patients taking glucosamine, chondroitin sulfate, or a combination of the two had no significant decrease in mild osteoarthritis symptoms when compared to taking a placebo. Patients who took celecoxib had the most significant decrease in the severity of their symptoms. However, glucosamine and chondroitin sulfate together did seem to help people with moderate-to-severe pain, as compared to a placebo.

Since then, other studies have been conducted on the efficacy of glucosamine, chondroitin, and their combination, including two follow-up GAIT studies. The first, concluded in 2008, had participants in the original GAIT study continue taking supplements for a total of two years. The goal was to assess the progression of cartilage deterioration. Although those taking only glucosamine showed the least amount of cartilage loss after two years, the researchers noted no significant differences in taking glucosamine supplements, prescription medications, or a placebo.

Another study, published in the September 2010 issue of the *British Journal of Medicine*, analyzed ten published trials to determine if glucosamine, chondroitin, or a combination of the two, helped to relieve pain. A total of 3,803 patients, with painful symptoms from hip or knee osteoarthritis, had participated in the studies. Dr. Peter Jüni and his colleagues at the University of Bern (Switzerland) found glucosamine, chondroitin, and their combination to not reduce joint pain or slow cartilage loss when compared to placebo.

Subsequently, the Jüni-led meta-analysis study was questioned as to the reliability of its data. Glucosamine is one of the most common non-mineral, non-vitamin **dietary supplements** used by adults. However, precaution should be used when taking it, because its level of effectiveness and safeness are not completely understood. Still, several medical organizations recommend glucosamine. For instance, the OsteoArthritis Research Society International (OARSI) states that "glucosamine and chondroitin sulphate may be effective in providing symptomatic pain relief in patients with knee osteoarthritis."

Recommended dosage

According to the Mayo Clinic, many studies suggest that adults (18 years or older) can take 500 milligrams (0.5 grams) of glucosamine sulfate by mouth three times daily, or 1,500 milligrams (1.5 grams) once daily. Other studies recommend a dose of 2,000 milligrams (2 grams) each day. A small number of studies have suggested 500 milligrams (0.5 grams) of glucosamine hydrochloride three times a day. Medical studies have yet to recommend any amount of glucosamine for children less than the age of 18 years. In fact, research involving children has shown a relationship between methylsulfonylmethane (MSM), which is often included with products containing glucosamine, and autism; however, it is not yet known whether that relationship is positive or negative.

Precautions

A person can overdose on glucosamine. The amount of glucosamine varies with the supplemental form. Pure glucosamine hydrochloride is at a concentration of about 83% in the glucosamine base; pure glucosamine sulfate is approximately 65%, and pure N-acetyl glucosamine is around 75%.

If deciding to take glucosamine, consumers should take it for at least six to eight weeks. It generally takes this amount of time before any noticeable effects are felt. If a reduction of symptoms is not noticed at the end of this period of time, the Arthritis Foundation states that glucosamine will probably not help.

The Arthritis Foundation recommends that consumers using glucosamine buy from established companies, because they can more easily be held accountable for their products. The Foundation also advises consumers to read product labels carefully, ask the pharmacist questions when necessary, and consult with their doctor before taking glucosamine. Glucosamine should not be used as a replacement for any prescription medicines already being taken without consent from the prescribing physician.

Since glucosamine is not approved by the FDA, a product's safety and formulation is determined solely by the manufacturer. Quality and content may vary among manufacturers. Tests have been performed by ConsumerLab.com, a leading provider of independent tests for nutritional and health products and services. Technicians at the laboratory report that the majority of companies manufacturing glucosamine for consumer use provide at least 90% of the amount of glucosamine stated on the label.

KEY TERMS

Arthritis—A condition causing often serious pain, swelling, or stiffness in one or more of the joints.

Cartilage—Elastic tissue found in many parts of the body, such as the ear, nose, and throat.

Chondroitin—A compound that makes up a part of cartilage; also available as a dietary supplement that is frequently used to reduce the symptoms of arthritis and other similar conditions.

Colitis—Inflammation of the colon (large bowel).

Inflammatory bowel disease—A disease of the bowel that causes inflammation.

Osteoarthritis—A type of arthritis characterized by the steady loss of joint cartilage; usually found in people who are middle aged or older.

Rheumatoid arthritis—A chronic disease located in the joints, which frequently causes swelling, stiffness, and weakness; it can lead to damage and eventually destruction of the joints.

Temporomandibular joint disorders—Abbreviated TMJD, TMD, or TMJ syndrome, a group of disorders that cause acute or chronic inflammation of the temporomandibular joint, which connects the skull and the mandible.

Ulcerative colitis—A type of colitis characterized by inflammation of the walls of the bowel (part of the intestines), along with the formation of ulcers; usually results in permanent bowel damage.

Medical research has not been comprehensive enough to know whether it is safe for pregnant or **breastfeeding** women to take glucosamine. Until more is known in the scientific community, most medical professionals do not recommend taking glucosamine during pregnancy or while breastfeeding.

Interactions

The use of alcohol, tranquilizers, sedatives, anti-convulsant drugs, anti-anxiety drugs, muscle relaxants, and/or antihistamine medicines may intensify the drowsiness side effect sometimes felt with glucosamine, adversely affecting the user's concentration.

Glucosamine is derived from the shells of shellfish, such as shrimp, lobster, and crab. People with shellfish allergies or **iodine** hypersensitivity may not want to take glucosamine. It is important to note that people with shellfish allergies are usually allergic to the

QUESTIONS TO ASK YOUR DOCTOR

- Will glucosamine help to relieve my condition?
- What dose should I take?
- How long will it take for glucosamine to start working?
- Should I take a higher dose if the initial dose does not help?
- How should I take the medicine? What time of day should I take it? Do I take it with or without food?
- Will it adversely interact with any of my other medicines?
- Are there any foods, other medicines, or herbal products that I should avoid with glucosamine?
- What are the possible side effects of glucosamine?

skin (**protein**) of shellfish, and not to the actual shells (chitin). According to a 2004 article from the *Journal of Allergy and Clinical Immunology*, most people with shellfish allergies can safely take glucosamine. In 2012, the MedlinePlus website stated that no allergic reactions had been reported in people with allergies to shellfish taking glucosamine. However, it is always wise to ask a physician before taking any new medicines. According to the U.S. National Institutes of Health (NIH), throat swelling may occur if glucosamine reacts negatively in people with shellfish allergies.

Glucosamine taken above the recommended dosages could decrease the effectiveness of **insulin** or other such drugs that control blood sugar levels in diabetes. According to the NIH, some studies show a connection while other studies do not; however, it is considered a possible risk by the medical community.

Complications

Clinical studies have consistently showed that glucosamine is safe when used as directed. However, according to the NIH, possible side effects may include drowsiness, headache, upset stomach, insomnia, skin reactions, light sensitivity, and nail toughening. Rare symptoms include abdominal pain, appetite loss, vomiting, nausea, intestinal gas, **heartburn**, and diarrhea.

People who are overweight or have diabetes or liver disease should check their blood sugar levels more frequently when taking glucosamine because it is an amino sugar.

Reports from the NIH suggest that glucosamine may also increase the risk of bleeding, especially when taking aspirin, blood thinners, anti-platelet drugs, and non-steroidal anti-inflammatory drugs. If taking blood-thinning medication or daily aspirin therapy, blood clotting time should be tested frequently.

People with asthma should be cautious before taking glucosamine. The use of glucosamine has been possibly linked to an increase in the frequency and severity of asthma attacks. However, there are not yet any concrete studies that show that glucosamine could cause an asthma episode; patients should always consult with their doctors before taking any new drugs or supplements, including glucosamine.

Parental concerns

According to the NIH, there is no scientific evidence to show that glucosamine should be given to children. Methylsulfonylmethane (MSM), which is sometimes packaged with glucosamine, has been shown to have a relationship with autism, but whether that association is preventive or causal is not yet known. In general, the effects of glucosamine supplements on a growing child or developing baby, or even on a child with osteoarthritis, are not yet known. For that reason, glucosamine is not recommended for, and should not be taken by, children.

Resources

BOOKS

Bagchi, Debasis, Hiroyoshi Moriyama, and Siba P. Raychaudhuri, eds. *Arthritis: Pathophysiology, Prevention, and Therapeutics.* Boca Raton, FL: CRB Press/Taylor & Francis, 2011.

Dunford, Marie, and J. Andrew Doyle. *Nutrition for Sport and Exercise.* 2nd ed. Belmont, CA: Wadsworth, Cengage Learning, 2012.

Imboden, John B., David B. Hellmann, and John H. Stone, eds. *Current Rheumatology Diagnosis and Treatment.* New York: Lange Medical Books/McGraw-Hill, 2004.

Sutton, Amy L., ed. *Complementary and Alternative Medicine Sourcebook.* Detroit: Omnigraphics, 2010.

PERIODICALS

Castell, L. M., et al. "A–Z of Nutritional Supplements: Dietary Supplements, Sports Nutrition Foods and Ergogenic Aids for Health and Performance (Part 9)." *British Journal of Sports Medicine* 44, no. 8 (2010): 609–11. http://dx.doi.org/10.1136/bjsm.2010.074625 (accessed August 3, 2012).

Clegg, Daniel O., et al. "Glucosamine, Chondroitin Sulfate, and the Two in Combination for Painful Knee Osteoarthritis." *New England Journal of Medicine* 354 (February 23, 2006): 795–808. http://dx.doi.org/10.1056/NEJMoa052771 (accessed August 3, 2012).

Jüni, Peter, et al. "Effects of Glucosamine, Chondroitin, or Placebo in Patients with Osteoarthritis of Hip or Knee: Network Meta-Analysis." *British Journal of Medicine* 341 (September 16, 2010): 4675. http://dx.doi.org/10.1136/bmj.c4675 (accessed August 3, 2012).

Maughan, R. L., P. L. Greenhaff, and P. Hespel. "Dietary Supplements for Athletes: Emerging Trends and Recurring Themes." *Journal of Sports Sciences* 29, supp. 1 (2011): S57–S66. http://dx.doi.org/10.1080/02640414.2011.587446 (accessed August 3, 2012).

Ostojic, S. M., et al. "Glucosamine Administration in Athletes: Effects on Recovery of Acute Knee Injury." *Research in Sports Medicine* 15, no. 2 (2007): 113–24.

Towheed, Tanvecr, et al. "Glucosamine Therapy for Treating Osteoarthritis." *Cochrane Database of Systematic Reviews* 2009, issue 2, art. no.: CD002946. http://dx.doi.org/10.1002/14651858.CD002946.pub2 (accessed August 3, 2012).

Zhang, W., et al. "OARSI Recommendations for the Management of Hip and Knee Osteoarthritis, Part II: OARSI Evidence-Based, Expert Consensus Guidelines." *Osteoarthritis and Cartilage* 16, no. 2 (2008): 137–62. http://dx.doi.org/10.1016/j.joca.2007.12.013 (accessed August 3, 2012).

WEBSITES

Brown, Andrew M. "Glucosamine Supplements for Arthritis Do Not Work, New Study Shows." *Health and Lifestyle* (blog), *The Telegraph*, September 17, 2010. http://blogs.telegraph.co.uk/news/andrewmcfbrown/100053833/glucosamine-supplements-for-arthritis-do-not-work-new-study-shows (accessed August 3, 2012).

Mayo Clinic staff. "Glucosamine: Dosing." MayoClinic.com. http://www.mayoclinic.com/health/glucosamine/NS_patient-glucosamine/DSECTION=dosing (accessed August 3, 2012).

MedlinePlus. "Glucosamine Sulfate." U.S. National Library of Medicine, National Institutes of Health. http://www.nlm.nih.gov/medlineplus/druginfo/natural/807.html (accessed August 3, 2012).

National Center for Complementary and Alternative Medicine. "Glucosamine/Chondroitin Arthritis Intervention Trial (GAIT)." U.S. National Institutes of Health. http://nccam.nih.gov/research/results/gait (accessed August 3, 2012).

ORGANIZATIONS

Arthritis Foundation, PO Box 7669, Atlanta, GA 30357, (800) 283-7800, oarsi@oarsi.org, http://www.arthritis.org.

National Center for Complementary and Alternative Medicine Clearinghouse, PO Box 7923, Gaithersburg, MD 20898, (888) 644-6226, Fax: (866) 464-3616, info@nccam.nih.gov, http://nccam.nih.gov.

Osteoarthritis Research Society International, 15000 Commerce Pkwy, Ste. C, Mt. Laurel, NJ 08054, (856) 439-1385, Fax: (856) 439-0525, oarsi@oarsi.org, http://www.oarsi.org.

William Arthur Atkins

Gluten-free, casein-free diet *see* **Casein-free diet**

Gluten-free diet

Definition

A gluten-free diet is a diet that is completely free of gluten, a generic name for a type of storage **protein** found in certain grains. A gluten-free diet is the prescribed medical treatment for people with gluten intolerance diseases such as **celiac disease** (also referred to as celiac sprue).

Origins

Guidelines for a gluten-free diet were developed by dietitians for several organizations associated with celiac disease and dermatitis herpetiformis, including the Gluten Intolerance Group, the Celiac Sprue Association, and the Celiac Disease Foundation. The **Academy of Nutrition and Dietetics** (formerly the American Dietetic Association) also sponsored the development of a gluten-free diet through a cooperative effort of expert dietitians in celiac disease in Canada and the United States.

Description

Gluten-free diets are used to treat and manage gluten intolerance diseases, including celiac disease and dermatitis herpetiformis. Celiac disease is a genetically inherited, chronic digestive disease. People with celiac disease develop an inflammatory immune system response to gluten that results in damage to parts of the small intestine responsible for the absorption of nutrients.

Celiac and related diseases

Celiac disease affects about 1% of people in the United States. Another million Europeans are affected. The highest rate of celiac disease is thought to be in Ireland and Finland, and celiac disease is most prevalent among people of Northern European ancestry, where wheat is a staple food. It is found infrequently among

Gluten-free diet

Ingredients/foods to avoid	May contain gluten	Foods allowed
Barley	Baking powder	Amaranth
Bran (wheat or oat)	Beans, baked	Beans, dried, unprocessed
Bulgur	Bouillon cubes	Buckwheat
Cake meal	Candy	Cassava
Couscous	Cheese sauces and spreads	Cheese, aged
Emulsifier	Chips, potato and tortilla	Corn
Farina	Chocolate drinks and mixes	Eggs, unprocessed
Flavoring	Coffee substitutes	Fish, unprocessed
Flour (enriched, durum, graham, semolina)	Cold cuts	Flax
Gluten	Communion wafers	Fruits and juices, fresh, frozen, or canned
Hydrolyzed plant protein	Corn cakes, popped	Herbs and spices, pure
Kamut	Egg substitutes, dried eggs	Ketchup
Malt and malt flavoring	French fries	Legumes
Matzo meal	Fruit pie fillings	Meats, unprocessed
Oatmeal and oat bran	Fruit-flavored drinks	Milk
Oats, rolled	Fruits, dried	Millet
Rye	Gravy	Mustard
Semolina	Hot dogs and other processed meats	Nuts, unprocessed, and nut flours
Seitan	Matzo	Olives
Soy	Mayonnaise	Pickles, plain
Soy sauce (including solids)	Milk drinks	Potatoes and sweet potatoes
Spelt	Nuts, dry roasted	Quinoa
Stabilizer	Peanut butter	Rice, wild rice, Indian rice
Starch, modified, or modified food starch	Pudding mixes	Sago
Triticale	Rice, brown	Seeds, unprocessed
Vegetable gum	Rice crackers and cakes	Soy flour
Vegetable protein	Rice mixes	Soy sauce, gluten-free
Vinegar, malt	Salad dressings	Sorghum
Wheat	Sauces	Tapioca
Wheat berries	Seasoning mixes	Tomato paste
Wheat bran	Sour cream	Vegetables without gluten-containing additives
Wheat, cracked	Soy nuts	Vinegar, apple cider and distilled white
Wheat germ	Syrup	Yucca
Wheat protein and hydrolyzed wheat protein	Teas, flavored and herbal	
Wheat starch	Turkey, self-basting	
Whole wheat	Vegetables in sauces	
	Yogurt, flavored or frozen	

(Table by PreMediaGlobal. © 2013 Cengage Learning.)

people of Chinese and Japanese heritage and individuals with an African-Caribbean background, where wheat is less widely consumed. Incidence of celiac disease has been increasing in India and the Middle East, but the rate is still considered low.

Some individuals with celiac disease also develop dermatitis herpetiformis, an itchy and blistering skin condition. Dermatitis herpetiformis is often a complication of gluten sensitivity. Approximately 20% of individuals with celiac disease have dermatitis herpetiformis, but about 90% of individuals with dermatitis herpetiformis have a gluten sensitivity, indicated by intestinal damage found on endoscopy.

When a person with celiac disease or gluten sensitivity consumes gluten, the villi of the small intestine—where absorption of key nutrients takes place—become damaged, resulting in nutrients passing through the digestive system without being absorbed.

Symptoms include gastrointestinal distress and eventually **malnutrition**. In infancy, celiac disease can cause failure to thrive, diarrhea, abdominal distention, developmental delay, and, in some infants, severe malnutrition.

After infancy, the symptoms of celiac disease are less dramatic. Older children may be short statured or exhibit dental enamel defects. Adult women are diagnosed with celiac disease about twice as often as men. Symptoms of celiac disease include diarrhea and/or **constipation**, intestinal gas, fatty and foul-smelling stools, bloating, nausea, vomiting, skin irritation, weight loss, anemia, neurological effects (including seizures and possibly migraine headaches), fatigue, and concentration and memory problems. In some cases, there may be intestinal damage without significant gastrointestinal symptoms. To control symptoms of gluten intolerance, affected individuals must completely avoid foods that contain gluten.

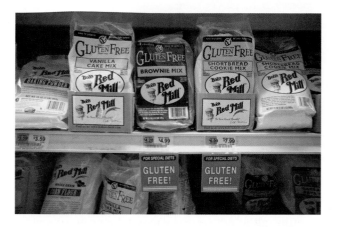

Gluten-free baking mixes. (© Richard Levine/Alamy)

Celiac disease is diagnosed by blood tests for certain antibodies and a small intestine biopsy. A positive small intestine biopsy, followed by an improvement in health after following a gluten-free diet, is confirmation of celiac disease. Since celiac disease is an inherited autoimmune disease, screening of family members is recommended. The chances of developing symptoms of gluten-sensitivity increases to 10%–20% in individuals who have a first-degree relative (parent, sibling, child) with celiac disease. Celiac disease is also associated with other autoimmune syndromes such as type 1 diabetes.

Gluten sensitivity

Some individuals may exhibit gluten sensitivity with less obvious gastrointestinal symptoms, but intestinal damage is still seen in a small intestine biopsy. As of 2012, gluten sensitivity was thought by many physicians to be a spectrum disorder, with celiac disease being considered the highest level of gluten intolerance. A less intense response to gluten is difficult to diagnose, but it may be confirmed by having the patient follow a gluten-free diet, followed by reintroduction of gluten-containing foods, to evaluate any health changes associated with the elimination or reduction of gluten from the diet. Some individuals with gluten sensitivity are able to tolerate a low-gluten diet under the supervision of a physician or dietitian. There is no standard agreement on the appropriate level of gluten intake for individuals exhibiting gluten sensitivity, so a method of trial and error is often necessary.

Gluten-free diet

The foods of concern for individuals with, or susceptible to, celiac disease are the grains that contain the storage proteins prolamin and glutelin (commonly referred to as glutens in wheat), including all varieties of wheat (e.g., durum, spelt, kamut), barley (where the storage proteins are called hordiens), rye (where the storage proteins are called secalins), and any crossbred hybrids (e.g., triticale).

In addition to gluten-containing grains, gluten can be found in a large variety of foods, including:

- soups
- salad dressings
- processed foods
- candy
- imitation bacon and seafood
- marinades
- processed luncheon meats
- sauces and gravies
- self-basting poultry
- soy sauce or soy sauce solids
- thickeners
- communion wafers
- natural flavorings

Unidentified starches, binders, and fillers in medications, supplements, or **vitamins**, as well as adhesives in stamps and stickers, can also be unsuspected sources of gluten. Playdough, which contains wheat, can be harmful if hands are put on or in the mouth after contact or hands are not washed after play.

OATS. Pure, uncontaminated oats eaten in moderation (about one cup cooked daily) may be safe for individuals with celiac disease. However, oats can become cross-contaminated with grains containing gluten during growth, harvest, transport, storage, or processing. Some individuals with celiac disease who introduce oats to their diet may experience abdominal discomfort, gas, and stool changes until they become accustomed to the increased **fiber** levels from the oats. Others with celiac disease may exhibit a hypersensitivity to oats and should avoid their consumption. Individuals with celiac disease should consult their healthcare provider or a registered dietitian before including oats in their diet and should have their antibody levels monitored regularly.

ALCOHOL. Most beers are brewed with barley or wheat, and thus they should not be consumed by a person following a gluten-free diet. Sorghum and buckwheat beers are available but are considered a specialty product. Most distilled forms of alcohol are gluten-free, unless additives and colorings containing gluten have been added. Wines are also usually gluten-free.

GLUTEN-FREE FOODS. Some grains and starches that are allowed in a gluten-free diet include rice, corn, **soy**, potato (and sweet potato), tapioca, and beans. Lesser-known gluten-free grains include garfava, sorghum, quinoa, millet, arrowroot, amaranth, teff, nut flours, and buckwheat—though some commercial buckwheat products are mixtures of wheat and buckwheat flours and should be avoided. Other foods that are allowed include fruits; vegetables; cow's milk; aged cheeses; unprocessed meats, poultry, and fish; eggs; dried beans; and nuts and seeds.

Many companies produce gluten-free counterparts to foods that ordinarily contain gluten, such as baking mixes and cereals. Gluten-free foods can be found in health food stores, through mail-order sources, and in some supermarkets. Cookbooks are available to help in food preparation. Many food manufacturers maintain lists of gluten-free products. A dietitian should be consulted to develop and monitor a gluten-free diet.

Gluten-free certification

Several organizations have established gluten-free certification programs to help consumers with celiac disease find gluten-free products. The U.S. Food and Drug Administration (FDA) allows manufacturers to label foods as gluten free if they contain less than 20 parts-per-million (ppm) of gluten, the level considered safe for people with celiac disease to consume. Most certification programs, however, set their limits at 10 ppm or less. Certification generally includes ingredient review, on-site inspection, product testing, and ongoing compliance, which is assessed by annual review. Certifying organizations include the Gluten-Free Certification Organization (GFCO), the Celiac Sprue Association (CSA), and the National Foundation for Celiac Awareness. Approved products display the logo or seal of the certifying organization on their packaging.

Function

Gluten-free diets are used by individuals who are sensitive to gluten to prevent damage to their small intestines and to prevent serious complications such as gastrointestinal cancers, iron-deficiency anemia, and decreased bone mineral density. The gluten-free diet is recognized by the medical community as the recommended treatment for individuals exhibiting gluten sensitivity.

Gluten-free diets may also be useful in treating other conditions. Research continues on the benefits of a gluten-free diet for individuals with multiple sclerosis and other autoimmune disorders, as well as for individuals with autism spectrum disorders, attention deficit **hyperactivity** disorder (ADHD), and some behavioral problems.

Benefits

A gluten-free diet has been shown to greatly reduce the risk for **cancer** and overall mortality for individuals with symptomatic celiac disease.

For many people with celiac disease, following a gluten-free diet will stop the symptoms of the disease and result in improved health, usually within several months, although recovery may take up to one year. However, the health of some people with extensive damage to their small intestine may not improve. Refractory celiac disease (RCD), a type of celiac disease that fails to respond to treatment, is a rare syndrome with a poor prognosis. RCD is defined by malabsorption due to gluten-related intestinal damage after initial or subsequent failure of a strict gluten-free diet and after exclusion of any other disease or disorder mimicking celiac disease. Other treatments may be necessary to treat RCD, such as the use of corticosteroids and immunosuppressant drugs, but data on their effectiveness is lacking.

Precautions

Gluten-free recommendations can be difficult to follow. An individual following a gluten-free diet must read labels every time a food item is purchased or consumed. It is recommended that an affected person keeps the diet simple at the beginning by eating fresh fruits and vegetables, milk, unprocessed protein foods such as fresh beef, pork, poultry, fish, and eggs, natural nuts, seeds, and vegetable oils without additives.

Sometimes it may not be obvious that a product contains gluten. Ingredients that may contain hidden sources of gluten include unidentified starch, modified food starch, hydrolyzed vegetable or plant protein (HVP or HPP), texturized vegetable protein (TVP), and binders, fillers, and extenders. In addition, manufacturers can change ingredients at any time, and a product may no longer be gluten-free. Ingredients may be verified by contacting a manufacturer and specifying the ingredient and lot number of a food item. If a person cannot verify ingredients in a food product or if the ingredient list is unavailable, the food should not be eaten to avoid the damage to the small intestine that occurs every time gluten is consumed.

Some seemingly gluten-free foods may still contain gluten by way of cross-contamination, even if gluten is not indicated on the ingredient list. For example, a conveyer belt may be dusted with a gluten-containing material to prevent foods from sticking, which may contaminate the finished food product.

Risks

A gluten-free diet is difficult to follow, and continued health problems usually are associated with problems adhering to the diet. A person can exhibit celiac-related symptoms for months after even a very small intake of gluten. Individuals with gluten-sensitivity who do not treat their disease are at a higher risk for gastrointestinal T-cell lymphoma and other gastrointestinal cancers. However, the maintenance of a long-term gluten-free state reduces the risk of lymphoma to the level seen in the general population. Other complications of gluten sensitivity include decreased mineral bone density and **iron** deficiency. Individuals with celiac disease and dermatitis herpetiformis must maintain a gluten-free diet for the rest of their lives, as the diseases cannot be cured.

Individuals are more likely to adhere to the diet if a dietitian and support groups are involved. If a person is not responding well to a gluten-free diet, the doctor may:

- investigate whether the initial diagnosis of celiac disease was correct
- check for other conditions that can be causing symptoms, such as pancreatic insufficiency, irritable bowel syndrome, bacterial overgrowth, lymphocytic colitis, T-cell lymphoma, fructose intolerance, or tropical sprue
- refer the person to a dietitian to check for errors in the diet or for compliance with the diet

To monitor dietary adherence to the gluten-free diet, the dietitian will examine the person's dietary history and habits. Blood tests will be conducted to see if gluten antibody levels have returned to normal levels. If there is clinical concern that a person is not adhering to the gluten-free diet or that the diet is not effective, a biopsy of the small intestine may be conducted.

Gluten-free diets are complex, and it cannot be assumed that chefs in restaurants or others who prepare food (including friends and family) are aware of all of the potential sources for gluten contamination. Education of family and friends is important in accomplishing a lifestyle change. In restaurants, simple dishes without sauces should be ordered, and customers should inquire whether grain products are prepared with the same equipment or utensils used to prepare other foods. Although a food may meet the standards required to be labeled gluten-free, it may be

---

KEY TERMS

Anemia—A condition in which there are too few red blood cells, too many abnormal red blood cells, or too little iron-containing hemoglobin for normal oxygen transport in the body.

Attention deficit hyperactivity disorder (ADHD)—A learning and behavioral disorder characterized by difficulty in sustaining attention, impulsive behavior, and excessive activity.

Autoimmunity—A condition in which the body's immune system produces antibodies in response to its own tissues or blood components instead of foreign particles or microorganisms.

Corticosteroids—Medication that acts like a type of hormone (cortisol) produced by the adrenal gland of the body. As a drug, a corticosteroid (sometimes just called steroid) provides extra cortisol, which helps treat infection or trauma to the body.

Immunosuppressant—Any agent that decreases the immune response of an individual.

Osteomalacia—A softening of bones caused by a lack of vitamin D and/or calcium in the diet.

Osteoporosis—A condition more common in older individuals in which bones decrease in density and become fragile and more likely to break. It can be caused by lack of vitamin D and/or calcium in the diet.

Type 1 diabetes—A chronic immune system disorder in which the pancreas does not produce sufficient amounts of insulin, a hormone that enables cells to use glucose (sugar) for energy. Formerly called juvenile diabetes, it must be treated with insulin injections and is sometimes referred to as insulin-dependent diabetes.

---

contaminated with gluten by the way in which it was prepared or stored. Other potential challenges associated with following a gluten-free diet include travel, where dietary needs may be difficult to accommodate; finding gluten-free foods, especially those of good quality; determining whether foods are gluten-free; not being invited out or not wanting to go out because of the diet; and maintaining a gluten-free diet when in the hospital, although a clinical dietitian should be able to assist in accommodating dietary needs.

As with any restrictive diet, a gluten-free diet has potential for nutritional inadequacy. Individuals who are sensitive to gluten are at increased risk for osteoporosis and osteomalacia due to malabsorption of **calcium** and **vitamin D**. Calcium and vitamin D supplementation along with strict adherence to a gluten-free diet usually results in remineralization of the skeleton. However, iron or other vitamin deficiencies may also be present and must be treated appropriately. The consumption of gluten-free, fiber-rich foods (e.g., brown rice, fruits, and vegetables) and adequate fluid intake is recommended to assist in the prevention of constipation.

Women with untreated celiac disease often exhibit a history of miscarriages, anemia, low-birthweight babies, and unfavorable pregnancy outcomes. It is suggested that testing for celiac disease be included in the battery of tests prescribed for pregnant women. Celiac disease is considerably more common than most of the diseases for which pregnant women are routinely screened.

Research and general acceptance

The National Institutes of Health has noted that the strict definition of a gluten-free diet remains controversial due to the lack of an accurate method to detect gluten in food products and the lack of scientific evidence for what constitutes a safe amount of gluten ingestion. No international agreement has yet been developed on how much gluten a person with gluten sensitivity can tolerate, and this amount likely falls on a spectrum for individual people. Research is ongoing to better identify levels that are acceptable, and health professionals involved in the therapy of celiac disease should keep up-to-date on the latest research. On January 23, 2007, the FDA proposed to set a standard of 20 parts per million as the maximum acceptable level of gluten allowed for a product to be labeled as gluten-free. Labeling is voluntary. European standards for labeling a food gluten-free are more strict than those in the United States.

In addition, a new enzyme that was being developed for commercial food processing has been found to break down gluten molecules quickly and almost completely. The enzyme is made from *Aspergillus niger*, a common fungus that is the source of other food grade enzymes already being manufactured for human consumption. Fritz Koning of Leiden University Medical Center in the Netherlands was leading the research as of early 2012. He stated that if the enzyme proves itself in clinical trials to eliminate the need for a gluten-free diet, it could be mass produced at a reasonable cost.

Resources

BOOKS

Brown, Marlisa. *Gluten-Free, Hassle Free: A Simple, Sane, Dietitian-Approved Program for Eating Your Way Back to Health*. New York: Demos Medical Publishing, 2010.

Bryan, Dale-Marie. *Living With Celiac Disease*. Minneapolis, MN: ABDO, 2012.

Case, Shelley. *Gluten-Free Diet: A Comprehensive Resource Guide*, rev. ed. Regina, Saskatchewan, Canada: Case Nutrition Consulting, 2010.

Dahlstrom, Carol Field. *Gluten-Free Made Simple: Easy Everyday Meals That Everyone Can Enjoy*. New York: St. Martin&s Griffin, 2011.

PERIODICALS

Dewar, D. H., et al. "Celiac Disease: Management of Persistent Symptoms in Patients on a Gluten-Free Diet." *World Journal of Gastroenterology* 18, no. 12 (2012): 1348–56.

Kabbani, T. A., et al. "Body Mass Index and the Risk of Obesity in Coeliac Disease Treated with the Gluten-Free Diet." *Alimentary Pharmacology & Therapeutics* 35, no. 6 (2012): 723–29. http://dx.doi.org/10.1111/j.1365-2036.2012.05001.x (accessed August 30, 2012).

Tanpowpong, P., et al. "Predictors of Gluten Avoidance and Implementation of a Gluten-Free Diet in Children and Adolescents without Confirmed Celiac Disease." *Journal of Pediatrics* (April 9, 2012): e-pub ahead of print. http://dx.doi.org/10.1016/j.jpeds.2012.02.049 (accessed August 30, 2012).

Virtal, Lauri J., Katri Kaukinen, and Pekka Collin. "Incidence and Prevalence of Diagnosed Coeliac Disease in Finland: Results of Effective Case Finding In Adults." *Scandinavian Journal of Gastroenterology* 44, no. 8 (2009): 933–38. http://dx.doi.org/10.1080/00365520903030795 (accessed August 30, 2012).

WEBSITES

Celiac Disease Foundation. "Gluten-Free Diet." http://www.celiac.org/index.php?option=com_content&view=article&id=138&Itemid=240 (accessed August 30, 2012).

Celiac Sprue Association. "CSA Recognition Seal Program Requirements." http://www.csaceliacs.info/csa_recog nition_seal_program_requirements.jsp (accessed August 30, 2012).

———. "Defining 'Gluten-Free.'" http://www.csaceliacs.info/ defining_the_term_glutenfree.jsp (accessed August 30, 2012).

———. "The Scoop on Oats." http://www.csaceliacs.info/ the_scoop_on_oats.jsp (accessed August 30, 2012).

Gluten-Free Certification Organization. "Certified Gluten-Free Companies/Products." http:// www.gluten.net/gfco/certified.aspx (accessed August 30, 2012).

Mayo Clinic staff. "Gluten-Free Diet: What's Allowed, What's Not." MayoClinic.com. http://www.mayoclinic. com/health/gluten-free-diet/MY01140 (accessed August 30, 2012).

MedlinePlus. "Celiac Disease." U.S. National Library of Medicine, National Institutes of Health. http:// www.nlm.nih.gov/medlineplus/celiacdisease.html (accessed August 30, 2012).

National Foundation for Celiac Awareness. "Gluten-Free Product Certification." http://www.celiaccentral.org/ gluten-free-certification (accessed Aubust 30, 2012).

National Institute of Arthritis and Musculoskeletal and Skin Diseases. "What People With Celiac Disease Need to Know About Osteoporosis." NIH Osteoporosis and Related Bone Diseases National Resource Center. http://www.niams.nih.gov/health_info/bone/osteopo rosis/conditions_behaviors/celiac.asp (accessed August 30, 2012).

National Institute of Diabetes and Digestive and Kidney Diseases. "Celiac Disease." National Digestive Diseases Information Clearinghouse. http://digestive.nidd-k.nih.gov/ddiseases/pubs/celiac (accessed August 30, 2012).

New York Times. "Genetic Testing for Celiac Disease." Consults: Experts on the Frontlines of Medicine (blog), January 13, 2010. http://consults.blogs.nytimes.com/ 2010/01/13/genetic-testing-for-celiac-disease (accessed August 30, 2012).

Storrs, Carina. "Will a Gluten-Free Diet Improve Your Health?" Health.com. April 5, 2011. http:// www.health.com/health/article/0,,20479423,00.html (accessed August 30, 2012).

U.S. Food and Drug Administration. "A Glimpse at 'Gluten-Free' Food Labeling." http://www.fda.gov/ ForConsumers/ConsumerUpdates/ucm265212.htm (accessed August 30, 2012).

ORGANIZATIONS

Academy of Nutrition and Dietetics, 120 S Riverside Plz., Ste. 2000, Chicago, IL 60606-6995, (800) 877-1600, http://www.eatright.org.

Celiac Disease Foundation, 20350 Ventura Boulevard, Ste. 240, Woodland Hills, CA 91364, (818) 716-1513, Fax: (818) 267-5577, cdf@celiac.org, http:// www.celiac.org.

Celiac Sprue Association, PO Box 31700, Omaha, NE 68131, (402) 558-0600, (877) CSA-4-CSA (272-4272), celiacs@csaceliacs.org, http://www. csaceliacs.info.

Gluten Intolerance Group, 31214 124th Ave. SE, Auburn, WA 98092, (253) 833-6655, Fax: (253) 833-6675, info@gluten.net, http://www.gluten.net.

National Foundation for Celiac Awareness (NFCA), 124 S. Maple St., Ambler, PA 19002, (215) 325-1306, Fax: (215) 643-1707, info@celiaccentral.org, http:// www.celiaccentral.org.

U.S. Food and Drug Administration, 10903 New Hampshire Ave., Silver Spring, MD 20993-0002, (888) INFO-FDA (463-6332), http://www.fda.gov.

Judith L. Sims
Tish Davidson, AM

Glycemic index diets

Definition

Glycemic index diets rank **carbohydrates** based on their ability to affect blood glucose (sugar) levels. These diets generally consider foods high in carbohydrates, such as bread, sugar, and pasta, as "bad," and low carbohydrate foods, such as meat, fish, and dairy products, as "good."

Origins

Low-glycemic diet concepts were first developed in the 1960s and were originally designed for individuals with diabetes. At that time, the prevailing medical attitude was that a diet emphasizing well-balanced foods while paying special attention to carbohydrates (carbs) and avoiding carbohydrate-rich foods helped to control blood sugar and **insulin** levels. This came after a number of medical studies linked eating foods high in carbohydrates with elevated blood glucose levels in people with diabetes. In the 1980s, researchers developed the glycemic index (GI).

Before 1981, carbohydrates were classified as simple or complex. Simple carbohydrates include fructose (fruit sugar), sucrose (table sugar), and lactose (milk sugar). Complex carbohydrates are also composed of sugars but the sugar molecules are strung together to form longer and more complex chains. Foods high in complex carbohydrates include vegetables (e.g., potatoes), **whole grains**, and beans. In 1981, researchers David Jenkins and Thomas Wolever of the University of Toronto Department of Nutritional Sciences

Glycemic index values of common food items

Food	Glycemic index (glucose = 100)	Serving size	Glycemic load (per serving)
Beans			
Baked beans*	40	150 g	6
Black beans	30	150 g	7
Beverages			
Apple juice, unsweetened*	44	250 mL (8.5 oz)	30
Coca Cola®*	63	250 mL (8.5 oz)	16
Orange juice, unsweetened	50	250 mL (8.5 oz)	12
Breads			
Bagel, white, frozen	72	70 g	25
Corn tortilla	52	50 g	12
Whole wheat bread*	71	30 g	9
Wonder™ bread*	73	30 g	10
Cereals			
Cornflakes™*	93	30 g	23
Instant oatmeal*	83	250 g	30
Oatmeal*	55	250 g	13
Raisin Bran™ (Kellogg's)	61	30 g	12
Fruits			
Apple*	39	120 g	6
Banana, ripe	62	120 g	16
Grapes*	59	120 g	11
Orange*	40	120 g	4
Watermelon	72	120 g	4
Nuts			
Cashews, salted	27	50 g	3
Peanuts*	7	50 g	0
Rice and pasta			
Macaroni*	47	180 g	23
Spaghetti, white, boiled 20 min*	58	180 g	26
White rice*	89	150 g	43
Snacks			
Graham crackers	74	25 g	14
Microwave popcorn, plain*	55	20 g	6
Rice cakes*	82	25 g	17
Vegetables			
Baked russet potato*	111	150 g	33
Green peas*	51	80 g	4
Sweet potato*	70	150 g	22

*Numbers are averages

SOURCE: Harvard Medical School, "Glycemic index and glycemic load for 100+ foods." Original data from Atkinson, Fiona S., Kaye Foster-Powell, and Jennie C. Brand-Miller, "International Tables of Glycemic Index and Glycemic Load Values: 2008," *Diabetes Care* 31, no. 12 (December 2008): 2281–83.

(Table by PreMediaGlobal. © 2013 Cengage Learning.)

developed the glycemic index (GI). They published a study suggesting that using the glycemic index of foods was a more accurate way of classifying carbohydrates than the simple and complex system.

Since 1981, dozens of low-carb diets and diet books using the glycemic index have come out. Among the more popular glycemic index-inspired diets are the Sugar Busters Diet, **Zone Diet**, Protein Power Diet, Suzanne Somers diet, and **South Beach Diet**.

In 1997, epidemiologist and nutritionist Walter Willett of the Harvard School of Public Health developed the glycemic load as a more accurate way of rating carbohydrates compared to the glycemic index. This is because the glycemic load factors in the amount of a food eaten, whereas the glycemic index

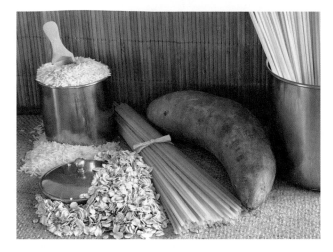

Foods with medium and low rankings on the glycemic index.
(Sandra Caldwell/Shutterstock.com)

does not. The glycemic load of a particular food is determined by multiplying the amount of net carbohydrates in a serving by the glycemic index and dividing that number by 100. Net carbohydrates are determined by taking the amount of total carbohydrates and subtracting the amount of dietary **fiber**. For example, popcorn has a glycemic index of 72, which is considered high. However, a serving of two cups has 10 net carbs because of its high fiber content, for a glycemic load of seven, which is considered low.

Description

Glycemic index (GI) diets vary in the specifics but most have one simple rule: people can eat as much food as they want providing the foods have a low glycemic index ranking. Most foods that are rated high on the glycemic index contain high levels of carbohydrates. Some people with diabetes use the GI as a guide in selecting foods and planning meals. The GI ranks foods based on their effects on elevating blood sugar levels. Foods with a high GI tend to increase blood glucose levels higher and faster than foods with a low GI value. The GI is not a measure of a food's calorie content or nutritional value.

The Glycemic Index

The GI is a ranking of carbohydrate foods that individuals with diabetes can use to manage their disease. The ranking is based on the rate at which carbohydrates affect blood glucose levels relative to pure glucose or white bread. Generally, the glycemic index is calculated by measuring blood glucose levels following the ingestion of a carbohydrate. This blood glucose value is compared to the blood glucose value

acquired following an equal carbohydrate dose of glucose or white bread. Glucose is absorbed into the bloodstream faster than any other carbohydrate, and is thus given the value of 100. Other carbohydrates are given a number relative to glucose. The lower the GI of a food, the slower the rate with which it is absorbed into the bloodstream.

A number of factors influence the digestion and absorption rate of food, including ripeness, particle size, the nature of the starch, the degree of processing and preparation, the commercial brand, and the characteristics of the individual consuming the food. These factors naturally affect each food's glycemic index rank. In addition, differences exist in various glycemic indices of foods due to the choice of reference food, the timing of blood sampling, or the computational method used to calculate the glycemic index.

The glycemic index measures the quality rather than the quantity of carbohydrates found in food. Quality refers to how quickly blood sugar levels are raised following eating. The GI is a standard. It is determined by having ten or more healthy people eat a measured quantity of a digestible carb, usually white bread. The rise in their blood glucose level is measured for the next two hours. The rise is assigned an index value of 100. Other foods are compared to the standard in order to arrive at their ratings. The higher the GI number, the faster blood sugar increases when that particular food is eaten. A high GI is considered to be 70 and greater, a medium GI is 56–69, and a low GI value is 55 or less. A related value is glycemic load (GL). Glycemic load is calculated as follows: GL = GI x the amount of available carbohydrate in a 100 g serving/100. In general, low-carb diets recommend a glycemic load of 80 or less. A high glycemic load is considered to be 120 or more.

The following is the GI for a few common foods:

- cornflakes, 83
- grapefruit, 25
- watermelon, 72
- sugar, 64
- potato chips, 56
- white bread, 70
- sourdough bread, 54
- macaroni, 46
- baked red potato, 93
- french fries, 75

The GI is not a straightforward formula when it comes to reducing blood sugar levels. Various factors affect the GI value of a specific food, such as how the food is prepared (boiled, baked, sautéed, or fried, for example) and what other foods are consumed with it.

The following foods are acceptable on a low-glycemic index diet:

- cornflakes
- oats, barley, and bran cereals
- citrus fruits to slow emptying of the stomach
- a variety of vegetables, especially salad vegetables
- wild rice or brown rice instead of white rice
- whole grain breads
- al dente whole grain pastas
- reduced sugar desserts

Function

Glycemic index diets have two separate functions. The first is to help individuals with diabetes or insulin resistance syndrome maintain normal and steady blood glucose levels. The second is to aid in weight loss.

The objectives of insulin management in diabetic patients are to reduce hyperglycemia, prevent hypoglycemic episodes, and reduce the risk of complications. For people with diabetes, the glycemic index is a useful tool in planning meals to achieve and maintain control of blood glucose. Foods with a low-glycemic index release sugar gradually into the bloodstream, producing minimal fluctuations in blood glucose. High GI foods, however, are absorbed quickly into the bloodstream, causing an escalation in blood glucose levels and increasing the possibility of hyperglycemia. The body compensates for the rise in blood sugar levels with an accompanying increase in insulin, which within a few hours can cause hypoglycemia. As a result,

awareness of the glycemic indices of food assists in preventing large variances in blood glucose levels.

Athletes may also use GI diets to prepare for athletic competitions or to recover from training. Low GI is often favored before an event, while higher GI aids in the replenishment of glycogen stores.

Benefits

There is conflicting scientific research on the benefits of a low-glycemic index diet for both people with diabetes and people trying to lose weight. Glycemic index diets may help people with diabetes maintain constant levels of blood glucose. By consuming more fruits and vegetables and whole grains rather than processed foods, low-glycemic diets encourage higher fiber consumption.

Experts disagree regarding the use of the glycemic index in athletes' diets and in exercise performance. Research published in the January 2010 issue of *Sports Medicine* found that eating a low-glycemic meal prior to prolonged exercise may have some merit, though this effect may be minimized if carbohydrates are consumed during the activity. Regardless, a low-GI pre-event meal may be beneficial for athletes who respond negatively to carbohydrate-rich foods prior to exercise or who cannot consume carbohydrates during competition. Athletes are advised to consume carbohydrates of moderate-to-high GI during prolonged exercise to maximize performance, approximately one gram per minute of exercise. Following exercise, moderate-to-high GI foods enhance glycogen storage.

Precautions

If an individual has health concerns, a low-glycemic index diet should be undertaken only under the supervision of a doctor. Doctor supervision of the GI diet is not necessary when the individual is healthy and disease-free. People with diabetes should consult an endocrinologist, who may recommend discussing the diet with a diabetes dietitian.

Risks

Eating a diet based solely on the glycemic index of foods can lead to overeating and a weight gain rather than loss. No emphasis is placed on total calorie intake or on the amount of saturated fat content. By basing one's diet on glycemic index alone, it is still possible to eat excess **calories** and to gain weight.

QUESTIONS TO ASK YOUR DOCTOR

- Do you believe eating a low-glycemic index diet will help me control my diabetes? Why or why not?
- Have you found that eating a low-glycemic index diet helps people like me lose weight?
- Is this a diet my whole family can follow safely? Is it safe for children?
- What precautions should I take if I go on this diet?
- Can you recommend a dietitian experienced in developing low-glycemic index diets?

Research and general acceptance

There is mixed acceptance of glycemic index diets by the medical community. Some studies have shown GI diets can be effective in controlling blood sugar levels in people with diabetes and in helping people lose weight. Other studies have contradicted these findings. No major studies or research has shown that GI diets are harmful to a person's health. The **American Diabetes Association** has adopted a position that there is not enough conclusive evidence to recommend the general use of a low-GI diet for people with diabetes. Not all physicians and endocrinologists (medical specialists who treat disorders of the glands, including diabetes) subscribe to the Association's position.

Resources

BOOKS

Beale, Lucy and Julie Alles. *The Complete Idiot's Guide to Glycemic Index Snacks.* New York: Alpha, 2011.

Raffetto. Meri B. *The Glycemic Index Diet for Dummies.* Indianapolis, IN: Wiley Pub., 2009.

Smith, LeeAnn. *The Everything Glycemic Index Cookbook.* 2nd ed. Avon, MA: Adams Media, 2010.

PERIODICALS

Foster-Powell, Kaye, Susanna H. A. Holt, and Janette C. Brand-Miller. "International Table of Glycemic Index and Glycemic Load Values: 2002." *American Society for Clinical Nutrition* 76, no. 1 (2002): 5–56. http://www.ajcn.org/content/76/1/5.full (accessed August 9, 2012).

O'Reilly, John, Stephen Wong, and Yajun Chen. "Glycaemic Index, Glycaemic Load and Exercise Performance." *Sports Medicine* 40, no. 1 (January 2010): 27–39. http://dx.doi.org/10.2165/11319660-000000000-00000 (accessed August 9, 2012).

WEBSITES

Harvard Health Publications. "Glycemic Index and Glycemic Load for 100+ Foods." Harvard Medical School. http://www.health.harvard.edu/newsweek/Glycemic_index_and_glycemic_load_for_100_foods.htm (accessed August 9, 2012).

Harvard School of Public Health. "Carbohydrates and the Glycemic Index," *Carbohydrates: Good Carbs Guide the Way.* The Nutrition Source, Department of Nutrition, Harvard University. http://www.hsph.harvard.edu/nutritionsource/what-should-you-eat/carbohydrates-full-story/index.html#glycemic-index (accessed August 9, 2012).

Higdon, Jane, and Victoria J. Drake. "Glycemic Index and Glycemic Load." Linus Pauling Institute Micronutrient Information Center, Oregon State University. http://lpi.oregonstate.edu/infocenter/foods/grains/gigl.html (accessed August 9, 2012)

Mayo Clinic staff. Glycemic Index Diet: What's Behind The Claims. MayoClinic.com. August 24, 2011. http://www.mayoclinic.com/health/glycemic-index-diet/MY00770 (accessed August 9, 2012).

MedlinePlus. Carbohydrates. February 8, 2012http://www.nlm.nih.gov/medlineplus/carbohydrates.html (accessed August 9, 2012).

University of Sydney. *Glycemic Index.* http://www.glycemicindex.com (accessed August 9, 2012).

ORGANIZATIONS

Academy of Nutrition and Dietetics, 120 South Riverside Plz., Ste. 2000, Chicago, IL 60606-6995, (312) 899-0040, (800) 877-1600, amacmunn@eatright.org, http://www.eatright.org.

American Diabetes Association, 1701 North Beauregard St., Alexandria, VA 22311, (800) DIABETES (342-2383), askADA@diabetes.org, http://www.diabetes.org.

Center for Food Safety and Applied Nutrition (CFSAN), U.S. Food and Drug Administration, 5100 Paint Branch Pkwy., College Park, MD 20740, (888) SAFEFOOD (723-3366), consumer@fda.gov, http://www.fda.gov/Food/default.htm.

National Diabetes Education Program, One Diabetes Way, Bethesda, MD 20814-9692, (301) 496-3583, http://www.ndep.nih.gov.

Ken Wells, AM
Tish Davidson, AM

GMOs *see* Bioengineered foods

Gout diet

Definition

A gout diet is a nutritional routine that includes eating foods low in purines to help reduce the occurrence and severity of gout attacks. Gout is a form of arthritis with symptoms of sudden and severe pain, redness, and tenderness in joints.

Origins

Physicians have known that there is an association between gout and diet for at least 2,000 years. It is the oldest known type of arthritis and was described by the Greek physician Hippocrates 2,500 years ago. It subsequently became known as the disease of kings due to its association with eating rich foods and **alcohol consumption**, a lifestyle to which only the wealthy had access. The association between gout and the production of uric acid has been known since the 1800s. In his 1861 medical book, *Gunn's New Domestic Physician: Home Book of Health*, American physician John Gunn describes gout as, "a peculiar disease, somewhat resembling rheumatism, affecting the joints, most generally those of the foot or toes." Gunn writes that the cause of gout is excess uric acid in the blood. That description is generally accurate today, although much more is known about gout, including how it develops, what causes it, and how it can be treated.

It wasn't until the 1960s that researchers developed an accurate understanding of the biochemistry of uric acid production in the human body. With this understanding came effective medical and dietetic therapy for the condition. In the 1800s, a rudimentary gout diet was developed that recommended avoidance of "rich foods," generally defined as cream and other high-fat dairy products, and alcoholic beverages. In the 1960s and 1970s, as more become known about gout and uric acid production, the diet was revised and refined. Experts encouraged avoiding high-fat and high-protein foods, alcohol, coffee, and soft drinks, along with anchovies, asparagus, legumes, mushrooms, meat, animal organ meat such as heart and liver, and shellfish.

Description

A gout diet is low in purines (a group of compounds that occur in DNA), especially those from red meat and seafood. Traditionally, doctors have recommended that people avoid or limit eating foods high in purines. Foods that are highest in purines include sardines, mackerel, organ meats (such as

---

Gout

Gout risk factors

- Family history of the disease
- Male
- Overweight
- Excessive alcohol use
- Purine-rich diet
- Enzyme defect that makes it difficult for the body to break down purines
- Exposure to lead in the environment
- Organ transplant recipient
- Use of medicines such as diuretics, aspirin, cyclosporine, or levodopa
- Use of niacin (vitamin) supplements

Signs of gout

- Hyperuricemia
- Presence of uric acid crystals in joint fluid
- More than one attack of acute arthritis
- Arthritis that develops in a day, producing a swollen, red, and warm joint
- Attack of arthritis in only one joint, often the toe, ankle, or knee

SOURCE: National Institute of Arthritis and Musculoskeletal and Skin Diseases, National Institutes of Health, U.S. Department of Health and Human Services.

(Table by PreMediaGlobal. © 2013 Cengage Learning.)

---

brains, kidneys, and liver), scallops, mussels, goose, caviar, and yeast extract. Foods that are high in purines that can be eaten in moderation include: crab, shrimp, red meat, poultry, trout, legumes, beans, lentils, peas, asparagus, cauliflower, mushrooms, spinach, wheat germ, and bran. There are no restrictions on eating foods low in purines, including dairy products, nuts, eggs, pasta, non-whole grain breads and cereals, chocolate, and **fats** (such as butter, margarine, and cooking oils). Medical research released in 2004–2006 suggests that vegetarian diets high in purines from vegetables and **soy** products are less likely to lead to gout than diets containing meat and seafood.

By eating less meat, poultry, and seafood while taking in more low-fat or non-fat dairy products, men can cut their chances of getting gout by 50%, according to the results of a 12-year study of nearly 50,000 men who had no history of gout. The study is the most definitive and comprehensive research done on gout. It was conducted by rheumatologist Hyon K. Choi and his colleagues at Massachusetts General Hospital in Boston. The study followed men aged 40–75 years. During the study, the men, all healthcare professionals, were quizzed periodically on how much of 130 foods and beverages they had eaten along with questions on weight, medications they had taken, and their medical condition. At the end of the study, 730 (about 2%) of the men had developed gout.

The study found that men with the highest consumption of seafood were 51% more likely to develop gout than those who consumed the least amount of seafood. It also found that men with the highest consumption of beef, pork, and lamb had a 41% higher incidence of gout than those who ate the least amount of these meats. Men who had the highest consumption of low-fat dairy products had a 42% lower rate of developing gout compared to those who consumed the least amount of dairy products. Vegetables that are high in purines that were previously associated with an increased risk for developing gout were found not to increase the risk of getting the disease. These vegetables include peas, beans, mushrooms, cauliflower, asparagus, and spinach.

The study also looked at the role alcohol consumption plays in gout. The risk of gout increased by 30% with the consumption of one drink a day, compared to people who did not drink alcohol at all. Two drinks a day increased the risk to 50%, and three drinks a day increased the risk by 100%. There were some differences in the types of alcohol consumed. Two glasses of wine a day did not increase the risk of gout at all when compared to men who drank no wine. Alcohol other than beer or wine increased the risk by 15% per serving. Beer increased the risk by 49 % per serving. Researchers are uncertain why the risk of gout varies depending on the type of alcohol consumed. Some suggest that other non-alcoholic ingredients in beer that are not found in wine or spirits may be responsible for increased risk of gout.

What is gout?

Gout, also called gouty arthritis, is a painful but treatable form of arthritis that affects up to five million Americans, primarily men over the age of 40. The disease is characterized by sudden and severe pain, redness, swelling, heat, stiffness, and inflammation in one or more joints. It most commonly affects the big toe first. Subsequent attacks of gout, usually limited to a single joint at a time, can occur in the instep, ankles, heels of the feet and hands, knees, wrists, fingers, and elbows.

Gout is caused by needle-like crystals of uric acid, a substance that results from the metabolic breakdown of purines, which are found in many foods and are part of normal human tissue. Uric acid is normally dissolved in the blood and filtered through the kidneys into the urine. If uric acid production is increased by the body or it is not sufficiently eliminated from the kidneys, it can build up in the blood, resulting in a condition called hyperuricemia (high uric acid). This

can lead to gout. High amounts of uric acid can also collect in the kidneys, causing kidney stones.

General dietary guidelines

People with gout should consult their doctors about developing individualized meal plans. Diets should take into account all aspects of medical nutrition therapy, especially for people with heart disease, high blood pressure, or diabetes. General **dietary guidelines** for people with gout include:

- Limit protein consumption from meat and replace it with low-fat or nonfat dairy products and soy products, such as soybeans and tofu.
- Consume dairy products low in fat rather than those high in fat.
- Since carbohydrates help increase the excretion of uric acid, carbohydrates should be about 50% of total calories consumed. To accomplish this, people should eat six to ten servings a day of breads, pasta, cereals, and other starchy foods, and five servings of fruits and vegetables daily.
- Fat consumption should be limited to 30% of total calories consumed.
- Cholesterol intake should be limited to 300 milligrams (mg) per day.
- Maintaining a healthy body weight is essential.
- Alcohol, especially beer, should be avoided.
- It is important to stay hydrated by drinking eight to ten 8 oz. glasses of fluids, preferably water, every day.

Regular physical activity can also help with weight loss or maintenance, as well as support overall health.

Dietary management of gout is centered around reducing uric acid in the body and managing conditions that often occur in people with gout, including diabetes, **obesity**, high cholesterol, high blood pressure, and atherosclerosis (hardening of the arteries). A diet of foods low in purines is recommended for most people with gout, although it is not possible to completely eliminate purines from the diet. The Arthritis Foundation recommends that people with gout learn by trial and error which foods cause problems and what their personal limits of these foods are.

Laura Rall, a nutrition researcher at Tufts University in Boston, advocates the trial and error method of developing a gout diet. She suggests: "Begin by eliminating foods in the high-purine category, while reducing your intake of foods in the moderate-purine category. If you don't have gout attacks after trying this, you may add more foods from the moderate category, or occasionally try a food from the high category. Using these guidelines, you may be able to determine a safe level of purine consumption and enjoy some of your favorite foods without experiencing (gout) attacks."

Function

The function of a gout diet is to lower uric acid levels in the blood by eating less meat that is high in purines, which increase uric acid levels in the blood. Uric acid is a waste product formed as purines break down in the body. By reducing uric acid levels in the blood, people with gout usually experience a decrease in pain and swelling in joints afflicted with the disease. Without treatment, gout can lead to joint damage and disability. Gout is also associated with an increased risk of heart disease and kidney disease, according to the American College of Rheumatology.

Benefits

The main benefit of a gout diet is a decrease in the pain, tenderness, swelling, redness, warmth, and inflammation of joints associated with the condition, and prevention of joint damage and disability. It also improves the quality of life in gout sufferers by helping prevent repeat attacks.

Precautions

The gout diet is designed for people who have gout or who may be prone to developing gout since it can be inherited. People who do not have gout or have no predisposition to the condition do not need to be on the diet. There are no precautions associated with the diet. However, since the diet recommends a severe curtailment or elimination of meat and seafood from the diet, people on or planning to go on the diet should consult a dietitian in addition to their physician or rheumatologist. People who eliminate meat and seafood from their diets should make sure they are getting adequate **protein** and other nutrients found in meat. This may include adding vitamin, mineral, and other nutritional supplements to the diet, similar to those taken by non-vegan vegetarians. These may include **iron**, **calcium**, **zinc**, **vitamin D**, **riboflavin**, vitamin B-12, **vitamin A**, **iodine**, and omega-3 and omega-6 amino acids derived from non-fish sources, such as **flaxseed** oil, evening primrose oil, and borage oil.

Risks

There are no known risks associated with a gout diet.

QUESTIONS TO ASK YOUR DOCTOR

- What are the risk factors for developing gout?
- Is there a reason for me to consider a gout diet if the disease has occurred previously in my family?
- Can you give me a diet that helps to prevent gout, or do I need to see a specialist about developing a personalized diet?
- Is gout a life-threatening disease? If not, what are the worst long-term consequences I can expect to experience from the disease?
- Are there ways of treating gout other than with dietary adjustments?

Research and general acceptance

There is general acceptance among health care professionals of the low-purine diet for people with gout or those who have a family history of the disease.

Resources

BOOKS

Coleman, Laura A. *Nutrition and Rheumatic Disease.* Totowa, NJ: Humana Press, 2008.

Craggs-Hinton, Christine. *Coping With Gout: Overcoming Common Problems.* 2nd rev. ed. London: Sheldon Press, 2010.

Emmerson, Bryan. *Getting Rid of Gout.* New York: Oxford University Press, 2003.

Konshin, Victor. *Beating Gout: A Sufferer's Guide to Living Pain Free.* Williamsville, NY: Ayerware, 2009.

Tugwell, Peter, et al., eds. *Evidence-Based Rheumatology.* London: BMJ Books, 2004.

PERIODICALS

Choi, Hyon, et al. "Purine-Rich Foods, Dairy and Protein Intake, and the Risk of Gout in Men." *New England Journal of Medicine* 350, no. 11 (2004): 1093–1103.

Dalbeth, N., and K. Palmano. "Effects of Dairy Intake on Hyperuricemia and Gout." *Current Rheumatology Reports* 13, no. 2 (2011): 132–137.

Krishnan, Eswar, et al. "Gout and the Risk Of Acute Myocardial Infarction." *Arthritis & Rheumatism* 54, no. 8 (2006): 2688–2696.

Zimmet, P. Z., et al. "International Study Backs Diet For Treating Gout." *Environmental Nutrition* 29, no. 8 (August 2006): 3.

WEBSITES

American Academy of Family Physicians. "Low-Purine Diet." FamilyDoctor.org. http://familydoctor.org/

familydoctor/en/prevention-wellness/food-nutrition/weight-loss/low-purine-diet.html (accessed August 9, 2012).

Mayo Clinic staff. "Gout Diet." MayoClinic.com. http://www.mayoclinic.com/health/gout-diet/MY01137 (accessed August 9, 2012).

ORGANIZATIONS

Academy of Nutrition and Dietetics, 120 South Riverside Plaza, Ste. 2000, Chicago, IL 60605, (800) 877-1600, http://www.eatright.org.

American College of Rheumatology, 2200 Lake Blvd., NE, Atlanta, GA 30319, (404) 633-3777, http://www.rheumatology.org.

Arthritis Foundation, PO Box 7669, Atlanta, GA 30357-0669, (800) 568-4045, http://www.arthritis.org.

National Institute of Arthritis and Musculoskeletal and Skin Diseases, National Institutes of Health, 1 AMS Circle, Bethesda, MD 20892-3675, (301) 495-4484, NIAMSinfo@mail.nih.gov, http://www.niams.nih.gov.

Ken R. Wells

Grapefruit diet

Definition

There are several diets or approaches to dieting that have been referred to as the "grapefruit diet." The first two are **fad diets** that have been circulating via chain letters, photocopies, faxes, and e-mail since the 1930s. The third form might be better described as the regular use of grapefruit or grapefruit juice as part of a general approach to weight reduction. It received considerable attention following the 2004 publication of a study conducted at the Scripps Clinic in California.

Origins

According to the Academy of Nutrition and Dietetics, the fad type of grapefruit diet began in the 1930s, when it was also known as the **Hollywood diet**. There were two regimens, a 7-day and a 21-day version, both of which were very low-calorie diets or VLCDs. The dieter consumed little except black coffee and half a grapefruit at each meal, with small amounts of salad and lean meat. This Depression-era version of the "Hollywood diet" was quite different from the current version, which amounts to a 24- or 48-hour juice fast intended to detoxify the dieter's body as well as promote rapid weight loss.

In the 1940s, the VLCD grapefruit diet reappeared under the name of the Mayo Clinic Diet—a name that has also been attached to several other so-called mono diets, one based on eggs and the other on meat. The Mayo Clinic has issued a disclaimer regarding the use of its name in connection with the grapefruit diet as well as other fad diets that have used the clinic's name. It is also possible that the VLCD form of the grapefruit diet may have influenced Herman Tarnower's first version of the **Scarsdale diet** in the 1960s. The original mimeographed diet sheet that the doctor gave his overweight cardiology patients specified 18 servings of grapefruit—14 at breakfast and 4 for dessert in the evenings—over the two-week period of the diet, and some of his patients referred to the Scarsdale diet informally as a grapefruit diet.

The VLCD grapefruit diet has also been recommended since the 1970s as a detoxification diet. Some writers recommend taking apple cider vinegar along with the grapefruit in order to "flush the system of impurities." The fact that the **fiber** in grapefruit speeds up the passage of foods through the intestine and eases **constipation** is another reason why some advocates of **detoxification diets** design their regimens around grapefruit.

The high-protein version of the grapefruit diet began to circulate at some point during the 1970s and has reappeared at various intervals since then. It is the variation most commonly found on Internet sites that post fad diets. Some forms of this diet claim that it works because grapefruit supposedly contains special "fat-burning" enzymes.

The term grapefruit diet has also been used by journalists since 2004 to refer to the findings of a 12-week research study conducted at the Scripps Clinic in California in 2003. The term diet is a bit of a misnomer, because the study was designed to measure the effectiveness of grapefruit and grapefruit products in treating **insulin** resistance as well as lowering weight in 91 overweight subjects who were not otherwise trying to diet. The study received considerable publicity and revived interest in incorporating grapefruit into nutritionally sound weight reduction diets. Its use of grapefruit in capsule form as well as fresh grapefruit, however, also prompted the development of several new lines of over-the-counter "miracle diet aids."

Description

Very low-calorie grapefruit diet plan

The basic menu plan is the same for each day of the week:

- Breakfast: 1/2 grapefruit + 2 slices of bacon + 2 boiled eggs + black coffee (no sugar) or unsweetened tea.
- Lunch: 1/2 grapefruit + 1 cup of salad with low-calorie dressing + 8 ounces of lean chicken or water-packed tuna fish + black coffee (no sugar) or unsweetened tea.
- Dinner: 1/2 grapefruit + as much salad with low-calorie dressing as desired + 8 ounces of lean chicken, lean beef, or fish + black coffee (no sugar) or unsweetened tea
- No snacks are allowed, and the only seasonings permitted for the meat or fish are herbs; no soy sauce, mustard, catsup, or other condiments are allowed.

The dieter is supposed to follow this diet for 12 days, then take two days off, and repeat the two-week cycle indefinitely.

High-protein grapefruit diet plan

This version of the grapefruit diet has been described as "just plain weird" because it comes with a curious set of rules as well as lists of foods that the dieter may or may not have. It also promises a weight loss of 52 pounds over 2-1/2 months.

"The Rules":
- Drink eight 8-ounce glasses of water every day (64 ounces total).
- Eat until you are full.
- Eat the minimum of each food listed at each meal.
- Do not eliminate any item from the diet, especially the bacon at breakfast and the salads. These combinations of food burn the fat; omitting one part of the combination will cause the whole thing not to work.
- The grapefruit or fruit juice is important because it acts as a catalyst that starts the burning process. Do not add to or reduce the amount of grapefruit or juice.
- Cut down on coffee because it affects the insulin balance that hinders the burning process. Try to limit intake to one cup of coffee at meal time.
- Do not eat between meals.
- Frying food in butter and using generous amounts of butter on the vegetables is permitted.
- Do not eat desserts, bread, white vegetables, or sweet potatoes.
- It is okay to eat double or triple helpings of meat, salad, or vegetables.
- Stay on the diet 12 days, then stop the diet for 2 days and repeat.

The daily diet plan:
- Breakfast: Either 1/2 grapefruit or 8 ounces of unsweetened fruit juice (any fruit) + 2 eggs any style + 2 slices of bacon.
- Lunch: Either 1/2 grapefruit or 8 ounces of unsweetened fruit juice (any fruit) + salad with any dressing + meat any style and any amount.
- Dinner: Either 1/2 grapefruit or 8 ounces of unsweetened fruit juice (any fruit) + salad with any dressing or a red or green vegetable cooked in butter or spices + meat or fish any style cooked any way + coffee or tea (1 cup).
- Bedtime snack: 8 ounces of tomato juice or skim milk.

Foods the dieter may eat: red onions, bell peppers, broccoli, radishes, cucumbers, carrots, green onions, leaf spinach, cabbage, tomatoes, green beans, lettuce, chili (no beans), mayonnaise, any cheese, hot dogs, cole slaw, salad dressing, dried nuts, dill pickles.

Foods the dieter may *not* eat: white onions, potatoes, celery, peas, cereal, corn, starchy vegetables, potato chips, peanut butter, pasta, corn chips, jelly or jam, sweet pickles, pretzels, fruit, low-fat or diet salad dressings.

2004 grapefruit research diet

The 91 subjects in this 12-week study were randomly assigned to four groups: one group received a placebo capsule plus 7 ounces of apple juice before each meal, the second group received grapefruit capsules plus 7 ounces of apple juice, the third group received 8 ounces of grapefruit juice plus a placebo capsule, and the fourth group received one-half of a fresh grapefruit plus a placebo capsule. At the end of the 12 weeks, the subjects in the three groups that had received some form of grapefruit had lost significantly greater amounts of weight than those in the group that had received only the placebo, with those who received the fresh grapefruit losing the most weight. The patients were not asked to make any other changes in their food intake, but they were required to take 30-minute walks three times a week.

Grapefruit diet capsules

Some Internet websites sell grapefruit pills or capsules with the claim that they will help people lose weight. The "grapefruit pectin diet tablets" are said to "help release fat deposits" that the dieter already carries on the stomach and hips. "They can also prevent new fat from penetrating the cells by redirecting it to the muscles where it is burned off, thereby eliminating fat deposits." The pills contain 200 mg of grapefruit pectin, plus cellulose and fiber. Given the high fiber content of these pills, it is most likely that they simply speed up the dieter's digestion and elimination.

The Grapefruit Solution Natural Diet, based on a book published in 2004, makes use of capsules that contain "pure, organic whole grapefruit. ... Five years of study and research has gone into developing and perfecting the technique of taking whole grapefruit and converting it into concentrated power while retaining all the benefits of the entire grapefruit." In addition to the capsules, however, this diet does emphasize the importance of exercise as well as a balanced diet of complex **carbohydrates** and **protein** foods.

Function

The fad versions of the grapefruit diet are intended for rapid weight loss. They are usually recommended as a good way to lose weight after holiday-related overeating or to fit into a special outfit for an important occasion. Several of the versions available on the Internet, however, claim that the grapefruit diet can be used for weight maintenance or for long-term nutrition on a twelve-days-on, two-days-off schedule.

The 2004 research version of the diet is intended to assess the effectiveness of grapefruit in counteracting **metabolic syndrome** (a group of risk factors for heart disease related to insulin resistance) as well as its usefulness in weight reduction diets. Preliminary results indicate that regular inclusion of grapefruit in the diet is effective in helping patients lose weight at a moderate rate and in improving their response to insulin.

Benefits

The fad versions of the grapefruit diet should be avoided in spite of their promises of rapid weight loss. The VLCD version does not allow enough **calories** to supply the daily energy needs of even a moderately active adult and is nutritionally unbalanced. The high-protein version is highly unlikely to help anyone lose weight, since its allowance of "meat any style and any amount" and "double or triple helpings" of meat and vegetables could easily encourage overeating.

Using grapefruit as an adjunct to a balanced weight-reduction diet by eating half a grapefruit before meals, however, appears to be helpful in reducing hunger **cravings**. It also contributes fiber and **vitamins** to the dieter's daily intake.

Precautions

General precautions

A general precaution for anyone seeking to lose weight is to consult a physician before trying any specific diet. This precaution is particularly important for adolescents, women who are pregnant or nursing, people with kidney or liver disorders, people with **eating disorders**, anyone who has had recent surgery, and anyone who needs to lose more than 30 pounds.

Drug interactions

Grapefruit contains certain compounds that interact with various types of medications in the digestive tract (it does not, however, affect drugs taken by injection). Although apple juice and orange juice may also interact with some prescription drugs, grapefruit contains three compounds known as naringin, bergamottin, and dihydroxybergamottin, which inhibit a family of enzymes in the intestine known as the cytochrome P450 system—in particular an enzyme called CYP3A4. CYP3A4 metabolizes many drugs; when it is inhibited by grapefruit juice, it increases the potency of a medicine by allowing more of it to enter the bloodstream. This effect of grapefruit juice was first discovered in 1989 by a group of researchers in Ontario who were studying the effects of alcohol on a blood pressure drug called Plendil. The scientists needed a liquid that would hide the taste of alcohol from their test subjects, and used grapefruit juice to do so. They were surprised to discover that the blood levels of the blood pressure drug went up in the subjects who received grapefruit juice alone as well as those who received a mixture of grapefruit juice and alcohol. Most interactions between grapefruit juice and prescription drugs do not have serious consequences, but others are potentially fatal.

Here is a list of families of medications known to interact with grapefruit juice. Readers should consult their doctor or a pharmacist if they are taking a specific medication that belongs to any of these groups:

- calcium channel antagonists (given to treat high blood pressure)
- immunosuppressants (given to control autoimmune diseases)
- statins (given to reduce blood cholesterol levels)
- HIV protease inhibitors (given to treat HIV infection)
- antihistamines (given to treat seasonal allergies)
- antiarrhythmics (given to control irregular heartbeat)
- sedatives, sleep medications, and benzodiazepine tranquilizers

KEY TERMS

Cytochromes—Complex proteins within cell membranes that carry out electron transport. Grapefruit juice interferes with the functioning of an enzyme belonging to the cytochrome P-450 group.

Glycemic index (GI)—A system devised at the University of Toronto in 1981 that ranks carbohydrates in individual foods on a gram-for-gram basis in regard to their effect on blood glucose levels in the first two hours after a meal. There are two commonly used GIs, one based on pure glucose as the reference standard and the other based on white bread.

Insulin resistance—A condition in which normal amounts of insulin in a person's blood are not adequate to produce an insulin response from fat, muscle, and liver cells. Insulin resistance is often a precursor of type 2 (adult-onset) diabetes.

Lycopene—A plant pigment that appears red in natural light and is responsible for the red color of tomatoes. Grapefruit is rich in lycopene, which is a powerful antioxidant and is thought to slow skin aging and may help to protect against chronic diseases such as heart disease and cancer.

Metabolic syndrome—A group of risk factors related to insulin resistance and associated with an increased risk of heart disease. Patients with any three of the following five factors are defined as having metabolic syndrome: waist circumference over 102 cm (41 in) for men and 88 cm (34.6 in) for women; high triglyceride levels in the blood; low

levels of HDL cholesterol; high blood pressure or the use of blood pressure medications; and impaired levels of fasting blood glucose (higher than 110 mg/dL).

Mono diet—A type of detoxification diet based on the use of only one food or beverage. Some versions of the grapefruit diet are essentially mono diets.

Pectin—A water-soluble heterosaccharide (complex molecule composed of a sugar molecule and a non-sugar component) found in the cell walls of higher plants. It is used primarily as a gelling agent in making jams and jellies, but can also be taken by mouth as a form of plant fiber to relieve constipation.

Placebo—An inert or medically inactive substance, often formulated to look like a pill or capsule, administered to subjects as part of clinical research trials to determine the effectiveness of a drug or treatment. Placebo comes from the Latin and means "I shall please," because the name was first given to sugar pills dispensed by some doctors to satisfy some patients' demands for drugs they didn't need.

Pomelo—A large pear-shaped citrus fruit with a thick rind that was crossed with the sweet orange in the West Indies to produce the modern grapefruit.

Very low-calorie diet (VLCD)—A term used by registered dietitians to classify weight-reduction diets that allow around 800 or fewer calories a day. Some versions of the grapefruit diet are VLCDs.

- birth control pills
- selective serotonin reuptake inhibitors (given to treat depression)
- drugs given for male impotence
- some anti-migraine drugs

In addition, people who are using herbal teas, other Western herbal preparations, or herbal compounds associated with Ayurveda or traditional Chinese medicine should consult their doctor or a pharmacist before beginning a grapefruit diet, as the chemicals in herbs can interact with grapefruit as well as with prescription medications.

Risks

The risks of using the fad versions of the grapefruit diet include nutritional imbalance (for both versions) and weight gain (for the high-protein version).

The researcher who designed and conducted the Scripps Clinic trial has specifically warned people against the fad grapefruit diets, saying that both are unhealthy.

The risk of a severe interaction between grapefruit and prescription drugs can be minimized by checking with a physician or pharmacist before adding large amounts of grapefruit or grapefruit juice to the diet.

Research and general acceptance

Basic nutritional information about grapefruit

Unlike some other fruits, such as apples, grapes, and lemons, that have figured in mono diets, grapefruit is a relatively new addition to the human table. It was not known to the ancient world and was first

QUESTIONS TO ASK YOUR DOCTOR

- Are any of my prescription medications known to interact with grapefruit?
- What is your opinion of the Scripps Clinic study?
- Are there any health risks that you know of related to adding grapefruit to a well-balanced weight reduction diet?

encountered by Europeans in the 1750s on the island of Barbados in the West Indies. Grapefruit (*Citrus paradisi*) developed as a hybrid of the pomelo (*Citrus maxima*), a large citrus fruit with a sour taste, and the sweet orange (*Citrus sinensis*). It is not known whether the hybridization occurred spontaneously in the citrus groves on the island or was carried out by native fruit growers.

The grapefruit was originally called the *shattuck* or *shaddock* until the 1820s. The name came from a Captain Shaddock, a seventeenth-century Englishman who had brought the first pomelo seeds to Barbados in 1693. In 1823 the new hybrid was brought to Florida by a Frenchman named Odette Philippe; it was first cultivated only as an ornamental plant. By the 1880s, however, grapefruit were being shipped from Florida to New York and Philadelphia. It was not until the 1940s that improved methods of packaging and faster transportation made grapefruit a household favorite in the Northeast as well as in Florida and the Southwest. In 2007, the United States produced 41% of the world's grapefruit.

According to the U.S. Department of Agriculture (USDA), half a standard grapefruit (4 inches in diameter) weighs 128 grams, 116 of which are water. It contains 41 calories, 10.3 grams of carbohydrates (1.4 grams of fiber and 8.93 grams of fruit sugars), 0.81 grams of protein, and less than 0.13 grams of total fat. Grapefruit are rich in **vitamin C** (44 mg), **vitamin A** (1187 IU), lycopene (1453 mcg in red and pink varieties), and potassium (178 mg). Apart from concern about drug interactions, grapefruit is considered a healthful fruit to include in a well-balanced diet. Its high vitamin C content helps to protect against scurvy, while the lycopene contained in red and pink varieties is an antioxidant thought to slow down the aging of skin and connective tissue. Lycopene may

also be important in preventing chronic diseases such as heart disease and prostate cancer. In addition, the fiber content of grapefruit is helpful in preventing constipation.

Evaluations of grapefruit in weight reduction diets

Grapefruit is considered a good food choice for people watching their weight because it is relatively filling thanks to its fiber content. It also has a low glycemic index (GI), which is a measurement of the rate at which carbohydrates in the food affect a person's blood glucose level within two hours after eating the food. Foods with low GI scores break down slowly in the digestive tract and thus prevent sudden changes in the blood sugar level—an important consideration for people with metabolic syndrome or type 2 diabetes and possibly for those watching their weight for other reasons. Grapefruit has a GI of 25 (pure sugar is 100), which is lower than the GI scores of apples (40), oranges (51), and bananas (51).

According to the research team at Scripps Clinic, it is not yet known why grapefruit appears to improve insulin response in overweight people or why it assists weight loss. Ongoing research may help to answer this question, but one finding at least is clear: grapefruit does not contain any miracle fat-burning enzymes.

Resources

BOOKS

Dunford, Randall Earl *The Grapefruit and Apple Cider Vinegar Combo Diet.* McKinney, TX: The Magni Company, 2002.

Scales, Mary Josephine. *Diets in a Nutshell: A Definitive Guide on Diets from A to Z.* Clifton, VA: Apex Publishers, 2005.

Thompson, Daryl L., and M. Joseph Ahrens. *The Grapefruit Solution: Lower Your Cholesterol, Lose Weight, and Achieve Optimal Health with Nature's Wonder Fruit.* n.p.: Linx Corporation, 2004.

PERIODICALS

Bakalar, Nicholas. "Experts Reveal the Secret Powers of Grapefruit Juice." *New York Times*, March 21, 2006.

Cunningham, E., and W. Marcason. "Is It Possible to Burn Calories by Eating Grapefruit or Vinegar?" *Journal of the American Dietetic Association* 101 (October 2001): 1198.

Fujioka, K., F. Greenway, J. Sheard, and Y. Ying. "The Effects of Grapefruit on Weight and Insulin Resistance: Relationship to the Metabolic Syndrome." *Journal of Medicinal Food* 9 (Spring 2006): 49–54.

"Grapefruit and Weight Loss." *Medical News Today* (January 24, 2004). http://www.medicalnewstoday.com/releases/5495.php (accessed October 2, 2012).

WEBSITES

Academy of Nutrition and Dietetics. "Fad Diet Timeline." http://www.eatright.org/nnm/games/timeline/index.html (accessed August 10, 2012).

Callahan, Maureen. "The Grapefruit Diet." Health.com. http://www.health.com/health/article/0,,20410196,00.html (accessed September 22, 2012).

Rebecca J. Frey, PhD

Greek and Middle Eastern diet

Definition

The "Mediterranean diet" gained much recognition and worldwide interest in the 1990s as a model for healthful eating habits. The diet is based on the traditional dietary patterns of Crete, a Greek island, and other parts of Greece and southern Italy. The diet has become a popular area of study due to observations made in 1960 of low incidences of chronic disease and high life-expectancy rates attributed to the populations who consumed a traditional **Mediterranean diet**. This healthful diet model goes far beyond the use of particular ingredients and recipes. It attains its full meaning in the context of climate, geography, customs, and the way of life of Mediterranean peoples.

Origins

The Mediterranean Basin

In efforts to understand the Mediterranean diet, it is necessary to first learn about the many countries that border the Mediterranean Sea. The diet is closely tied geographically to areas of olive oil cultivation in the Mediterranean Basin. It can be defined by diets of the early 1960s in Greece, southern Italy and other Mediterranean regions in which olive oil was the principal source of dietary fat. The olive remains the most typical Mediterranean tree because it has adapted to the regional climate of long, very hot, dry summers and mild, damp winters.

The lands surrounding the Mediterranean Sea contain some of the oldest cultures on Earth. Greece, as well as other countries of Europe, North Africa, and some Middle Eastern nations, played a central role in the expansion of empires and cross-cultural exchanges over the centuries. Over 2,000 years ago trade by means of sea routes allowed Greek, Roman, Phoenician, Carthaginian, Arab, and Oriental products and traditions to intermix, resulting in mutual enrichment and an evolution of what is now incorporated into the Mediterranean diet. However, many different diets exist throughout the Mediterranean region, and there is no such thing as just one Mediterranean diet. Variations of this diet have traditionally existed in the North African countries of Morocco and Tunisia, parts of Turkey, and other Middle Eastern countries such as Lebanon and Syria.

Culture

Mediterranean and Middle Eastern culture is centered on a strong patriarchal family. This has lessened in recent years, but family ties are still strong. Customs and family traditions influence nutrition greatly.

Food is an integral part of family celebrations, special days of honor, and festivals. In the Middle Eastern nation of Israel, kosher dietary laws concerning the selection, preparation, and eating of food remains influential in Jewish life. The Jewish laws of *kashrut*, or keeping kosher, determines which foods are kosher and which are non-kosher. Many ancient practices and rituals, handed down from generation to generation, are observed.

Many people from Mediterranean and Middle Eastern cultures observe Islam and Eastern Orthodox religions, which influence the kinds of food chosen and how the foods are combined. Fasting from sunrise to sunset is a Muslim religious obligation practiced during the sacred month of Ramadan. Muslims do not eat any form of pork, or any meat that has been slaughtered without mentioning God's name. Muslims cannot drink alcoholic beverages or foods flavored with alcohol—which differs from Greek and other Mediterranean cultures, where wine is a large part of the diet. Dairy product consumption is rising in the Middle East but must be imported due to the dry climate.

Description

Traditional eating habits

Traditional eating habits of Mediterranean countries, and those countries along the basin, include olives, fish, lamb, wheat, rice, chick peas and other legumes, pistachios, dates, cheese, and yogurt. Bread typically accompanies each meal.

Halal (Halaal) food products	Haram (Haraam) food products (not halal)	Mashbooh (questionable or cautionary ingredients)
Milk and eggs from halal animals (cows, sheep, camels, goats)	Pork and pork by-products	Animal fat or proteins
Honey	Animals improperly slaughtered or dead before slaughtering	Antioxidants
Fish and most seafood	Alcohol and intoxicants	Cheese
Vegetables that are not intoxicants	Carnivorous animals, birds of prey, and land animals without external ears	Emulsifiers
Fresh or dried fruits		Enzymes
Legumes and nuts	Blood and blood by-products	Flavorings
Grains such as wheat, rice, rye, barley, and oats	Foods contaminated with any of the above products	Gelatin
		Glycerin
		Vitamins
		Whey

SOURCE: Islamic Food and Nutrition Council of America, http://www.ifanca.org.

(Table by PreMediaGlobal. © 2013 Cengage Learning.)

Traditional food consumption includes the following:

Dairy products. Most dairy products are eaten in fermented forms, such as yogurt and cheese. Whole milk is used in desserts and puddings. Feta cheese, traditionally made of sheep or goat's milk, is the most commonly consumed cheese.

Meats. Lamb is the most widely eaten meat. Pork is eaten only by Christians, not by Muslims or Jews. Many Middle Easterners will not combine dairy products or shellfish with the meal. Kosher beef, kosher poultry, lox (brine-cured cold-smoked salmon, much of which is slightly saltier than other smoked salmon), and sardines are also common foods. Legumes such as black beans, chick peas (garbanzo beans), lentils, navy beans, fava beans, and red beans are used in many dishes.

Breads and Cereals. Some form of wheat or rice accompanies each meal. Pita and matzoh (unleavened bread) are common. Filo dough, which is used to make baklava, is also used in many dishes.

Fruits. Fruits tend to be eaten as dessert or as snacks. Fresh fruit is preferred. Fruits made into jams and compotes (a cooked preparation of fruit in syrup) are eaten if fresh fruit is not available. Lemons and concentrated lemon juice are commonly used for flavoring.

Vegetables. Potatoes and eggplant are the most commonly consumed vegetables. Fruit and vegetables are preferred raw or mixed in a salad. Vegetables are often stuffed with rice or meats. Green and black olives are present in many dishes, and olive oil is most frequently used in food preparation.

Food preparation and storage

Grilling, frying, grinding, and stewing are the most common ways of preparing meats in countries bordering the Mediterranean Basin. A whole, roasted lamb or leg of lamb is a special dish prepared for festive gatherings. Spices and seasonings are essential in the preparation of Middle Eastern dishes. Common spices and herbs include dill, garlic, mint, cinnamon, oregano, parsley, leek, and pepper.

Function

Today, the Mediterranean region is characterized by a high increase in modernization. The traditional diet of the Mediterranean region has been affected by modernization, particularly in the area of agricultural production for trade. The countries of North Africa and the Middle East struggle the most with modernization problems. This has led to an increase in the dependence on costly food imports from outside the region. While the Greek economy remains rooted in agriculture and the government places a strong emphasis on agricultural reforms, Middle Eastern nations face constraints such as high rates of urbanization, leading to the loss of vital agricultural land.

Modernization has created significant changes in food consumption patterns in the countries of the Mediterranean region. The factors affecting the traditional dietary customs of the region are economy, environment, society and culture, disasters (e.g., war, drought), the expansion of food industries, and advertising campaigns promoting certain foods (e.g., soda, candy bars). Fast-food restaurant chains are also altering traditional diets. The expansion of fast food has resulted in the population consuming processed foods such as sweets and snack foods, which were never a part of their nutritional sustenance.

Benefits

The wide use of olive oil in food preparation throughout the Mediterranean region contributes to a diet high in monounsaturated fatty acids. Research

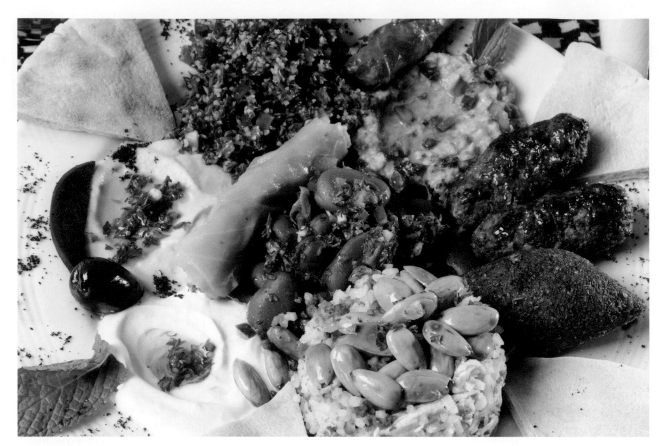

Lebanese meal including hummus, pita bread, tabouli, grape leaves, rice, and lamb. *(karam Miri/Shutterstock.com)*

has shown that a Mediterranean diet is generally healthful, and a diet that derives much of its fat from olive oil and other products containing monounsaturated **fats** may lower low-density lipoprotein (LDL) cholesterol levels (often referred to as "bad" cholesterol). Olive oil also contains **antioxidants** that may help prevent artery clogging.

The Mediterranean diet offers a practical and effective strategy that is relatively easy to adopt and more likely to be successful over the long term than most heart-healthy nutrition plans. In April 2001, the American Heart Association (AHA) published a science advisory stating that some components of the Mediterranean diet may be beneficial when used in conjunction with the association's traditional diets for the prevention and treatment of cardiovascular disease.

In the Mediterranean diet, not all fat is regarded as bad, however. In fact, the focus of the diet is not to limit total fat consumption, but rather to make wise choices about the type of fat in the diet. The Mediterranean diet is low in saturated fat, which is found mostly in meat and dairy products, vegetable oils such as coconut and palm oils (tropical oils), and butter. The diet views two types of protective fats, **omega-3 fatty acids** and monounsaturated fats, as healthful and places no restrictions on their consumption. Omega-3 fatty acids are found in fatty fish (e.g., sardines, salmon, fresh tuna) and in some plant sources (e.g., walnuts, flax seeds, hemp, rapeseed, **soy**, and green leafy vegetables). Monounsaturated fat is abundant in olive oil, nuts, and avocados.

Precautions

Many Middle Eastern nations, such as Turkey, Syria, and Lebanon, have predominantly Muslim populations. Eating *halal* is obligatory for every Muslim. *Halal* is an Arabic word meaning "lawful" or "permitted," and refers to Islamic law regarding the diet. Animals such as cows, sheep, goats, deer, moose, chickens, ducks, and game birds are *halal*, but they must be *zabihah* (slaughtered according to Islamic method) in order to be suitable for consumption. Halal foods are those that are:

KEY TERMS

Antioxidant—A molecule that prevents oxidation. In the body antioxidants attach to other molecules called free radicals and prevent the free radicals from causing damage to cell walls, DNA, and other parts of the cell.

Fatty acids—Molecules rich in carbon and hydrogen; a component of fats.

Lactose intolerance—Inability to digest lactose, or milk sugar.

Saturated fat—A fat with the maximum possible number of hydrogens; more difficult to break down than unsaturated fats.

Trans fat—A type of fat thought to increase the risk of heart disease.

- free from any component or ingredient taken or extracted from an unlawful animal or ingredient that muslims are prohibited from consuming
- processed, manufactured, prepared, or stored with apparatus, equipment and/or machinery that has been cleansed according to Islamic law
- free from contamination when prepared or processed with anything considered unclean

Risks

Because the Mediterranean diet emphasizes eating whole, natural foods and is generally low in *trans* fats, which are thought to contribute to heart disease. These fats are found in hard margarine and deep-fried and processed snacks and food, including fast food and commercially baked products. They are similar to saturated fats and are known to raise levels of LDL cholesterol. Eating a diet incorporating the traditional foods of the Mediterranean, such as a variety of fruits and vegetables, has been shown to decrease the risk of heart disease. Five important dietary factors may contribute to the cardioprotective effect of this eating pattern. These are the inclusion of fish rich in omega-3 fatty acids, olive oil, nuts, and moderate amounts of alcohol, and the exclusion of *trans* fatty acids.

Research and general acceptance

Many common characteristics exist among the countries along the Mediterranean Basin, but each country has adapted to the geography and developed its own customs. The common core, however, can be seen in the diets of these countries. It is important to remember that the Mediterranean diet emphasizes eating whole, unprocessed foods that are extremely low in harmful LDL cholesterol. Recent studies indicate that the use of natural, monounsaturated oils such as olive oil, a balanced intake of vegetables and fish, and a low intake of red meats provides a natural defense against cardiovascular disease. Although more research is needed, the Mediterranean way of eating is potentially an ideal diet to improve the health of people by warding off illnesses.

Resources

BOOKS

Bender, David A. *A Dictionary of Food and Nutrition.* New York: Oxford University Press, 2009.

Counihan, Carole., and Penny Van Esternik, eds. *Food and Culture.* 3rd ed. New York: Routledge, 2012.

Larsen, Laura, ed. *Diet and Nutrition Sourcebook.* 4th ed. Detroit, MI: Omnigraphics Inc, 2011.

Simopoulos, A. P., and F. Visoli. "Mediterranean Diets." In *World Review of Nutrition and Dietetics*, vol. 87. Switzerland: Karger Publishers, 2000.

Spiller, G. A., and B. Bruce. *The Mediterranean Diet: Constituents and Health Promotion.* Boca Raton, FL: CRC Press, 2002.

Zacharias, Eric. *The Mediterranean Diet: A Clinician's Guide for Patient Care.* New York: Springer, 2012.

PERIODICALS

Mehio, Sibai A., et al. "Nutrition Transition and Cardiovascular Disease Risk Factors in Middle East and North Africa Countries: Reviewing the Evidence." *Annals of Nutrition & Metabolism* 57, nos. 3–4 (2010): 193–203.

Musaiger, Abdulrahman O., and Hazzaa M Al-Hazzaa. "Prevalence and Risk Factors Associated with Nutrition-Related Noncommunicable Diseases in the Eastern Mediterranean Region." *International Journal of General Medicine* 5 (February 29, 2012): 199–217. http://dx.doi.org/10.2147/IJGM.S29663 (accessed September 28, 2012).

WEBSITES

Oldways. "Mediterranean Diet & Pyramid." http://www.oldwayspt.org/resources/heritage-pyramids/mediterranean-diet-pyramid (accessed September 28, 2012).

ORGANIZATIONS

Academy of Nutrition and Dietetics, 120 South Riverside Plz., Ste. 2000, Chicago, IL 60606-6995, (312) 899-0040, (800) 877-1600, amacmunn@eatright.org, http://www.eatright.org.

American Heart Association, 7272 Greenville Ave., Dallas, TX 75231, (800) 242-8721, http://www.americanheart.org.

cardiovascular disease (e.g., heart attack, stroke) but just as likely to die of cancer as non-tea drinkers.

There are many difficulties associated with studying the role of green tea in the development of cancer in human populations. These include:

• The amount and strength of green tea and green tea extract are not standardized, and a wide range of doses are used in different studies.

• Many studies done on green tea are poorly designed or poorly reported, so it is difficult to show a direct link between cause and effect.

• Many human studies have a small sample size.

• Cancer takes a long time to develop, making it difficult to follow study participants and determine outcomes.

• Many studies are sponsored by tea growers, manufacturers, or importers who have a financial interest in obtaining positive results.

Despite these drawbacks, the possibility that EGCG and other antioxidants in green tea can slow or prevent cancer is strong enough that many research studies are being supported by government health agencies around the world. However, the official position of the American Cancer Society states, "While the results of lab studies have been promising, at this time there is no conclusive evidence that green tea can help prevent or treat any specific type of cancer in humans."

WEIGHT LOSS. Some studies in mice have shown that the polyphenols in green tea lower the level of blood glucose (sugar), lipids (fats), and cholesterol and reduce the amount of body fat deposited under the skin. Other studies have shown that green tea increases body **metabolism**. However, these results have not been rigorously duplicated in humans. Although green tea may be good food for dieters when used in conjunction with a calorie-reduced diet and increased exercise, it is not a "magic bullet" that will cause weight loss by itself.

MENTAL PERFORMANCE. Any effects of green tea on mental alertness and performance are most likely due to the effects of caffeine and caffeine-like compounds found in green tea. Caffeine is a drug classified as a stimulant, or a psychoactive drug. It acts on the central nervous system, helping the body to be more alert and less drowsy.

CARDIOVASCULAR DISEASE. Claims have been made that green tea decreases cholesterol and fats in the blood. This is thought to reduce the risk of clogged arteries and help prevent heart attack and stroke. There is not enough reliable evidence to determine if

these claims are true. One large study done in Japan did show improved cardiovascular health in individuals that used green tea, but these individuals tended to be thinner than the average American and also had other dietary differences. It is not clear how the Japanese results might apply to other populations.

OTHER HEALTH CLAIMS. The tannins in green tea have an astringent or drying effect. One folk remedy to stop the bleeding where a tooth has been extracted is to bite down on a used tea bag. Tannins in green tea may also be responsible for helping to control diarrhea. Caffeine may provide additional benefits, including longer life and improved memory, though most caffeine studies are done on coffee, not tea.

Recommended dosage

According to the American Cancer Society (ACS), the amount of green tea consumed daily varies widely. The ACS also mentions that the amount of green tea needed for beneficial effects has not been medically proven. In the past and today, the typical amount of green tea consumed in drink form in Asian countries is three cups or more daily. It is usually brewed using one to two teaspoons of dried tea in one cup of boiling water. Three capsules of green tea extract per day is a common recommended dosage for supplements, according to the ACS. However, the benefit from taking such a dosage is unclear in the scientific community.

Precautions

Green tea has been safely used for thousands of years. The FDA includes tea on their list of "generally recognized as safe" substances. However, some precautions exist with green tea. Most negative effects are attributable to the caffeine content. Some individuals are sensitive to caffeine. Children and pregnant and **breastfeeding** women may want to avoid the effects of caffeine by choosing naturally decaffeinated green tea. People with heart disease, fibrocystic breasts, birth defects, reproductive issues, or stomach **ulcers** may wish to reduce or eliminate caffeine from their diet.

Anyone wishing to reduce their intake of caffeine may wish to drink green tea rather than coffee or black tea. Green tea contains less caffeine than black tea and significantly less caffeine than coffee. Prepared green tea drinks may, however, contain added amounts of caffeine. Often, prepared green tea energy drinks have a very high caffeine content. Always read product labels before consuming such drinks. Caffeine in any type of drink or product may make individuals more prone to nervousness or restlessness and may cause difficulty sleeping.

Interactions

Adverse interactions can exist between some of the substances within green tea (such as caffeine, tannin, and EGCG) and various drugs. Some of these interactions include:

- Adenosine. Caffeine may reduce the effects of adenosine, a medication used for irregular heart rhythm.
- Atropine and codeine. Tannin may reduce the absorption of atropine and codeine.
- Benzodiazepines. Caffeine within green tea can reduce sedative effects in benzodiazepine medications used to treat anxiety, such as lorazepam and diazepam.
- Beta blockers. Caffeine in green tea can increase blood pressure in people taking beta blockers to treat high blood pressure and heart disease, such as propranolol and metoprolol.
- Beta-lactam antibiotics. Green tea may increase the effectiveness of beta-lactam antibiotics by reducing bacterial resistance.
- Blood-thinning medications. Vitamin K in green tea can make blood-thinning medications, such as warfarin and aspirin, ineffective.
- Boronic acid-based proteasome inhibitors. EGCG may reduce the therapeutic effect of boronic acid-based proteasome inhibitors, such as bortezomib.
- Chemotherapy drugs. Green tea may increase the effectiveness of some chemotherapy medications, such as doxorubicin and tamoxifen.
- Clozapine. The antipsychotic effects of clozapine may be reduced if taken within 40 minutes of using green tea.
- Ephedrine. Taking green tea and ephedrine together may cause agitation, insomnia, weight loss, or tremors.
- Lithium. The level of lithium in the bloodstream can be reduced when used with green tea; lithium is used to treat manic/depression.
- Monoamine oxidase inhibitors (MAOIs). Green tea may increase blood pressure if taken with MAOIs, which are used to treat depression.
- Oral contraceptives. The use of caffeine in green tea and oral contraceptives may increase the stimulating effects of caffeine.
- Phenylpropanolamine. The use of green tea and phenylpropanolamine, often found in over-the-counter and prescription cough and cold medications and

weight loss products, may cause mania and a dramatic increase in blood pressure.

Other drugs that may be affected by green tea include anticoagulants/antiplatelets, **iron** supplements, verapamil, irinotecan, cytochrome P450 3A4 substrates, and UGT (Uridine 5'-diphospho-glucuronosyltransferase) substrates. Consumers should consult with a trusted medical professional before using green tea along with any drug or herb.

Complications

Green tea is generally safe, and complications are few even when large amounts of tea are drunk. The safety of green tea extract has not been established. Individuals with hypersensitivity to caffeine or who use large amounts of green tea may develop caffeine-related insomnia or upset stomach. The tannin in green tea may contribute to iron deficiency in individuals with low amounts of iron in their diet. For this reason, tea should not be drunk with meals.

KEY TERMS

Antioxidant—A substance that decreases the oxidation process within the body or within food.

Cholesterol—With chemical formula $C_{27}H_{45}OH$, a solid compound within the blood, made by the liver, found in all animal cells, and important to the health of the body.

Deoxyribonucleic acid (DNA)—The substance that contains the genetic information of any organism except a few viruses.

Extract—The substance left over from a gas, liquid, or solid compound after some type of chemical or industrial process is applied to it.

Free radical—A highly reactive atom or molecule containing an unpaired electron.

Insomnia—Often chronic inability or difficulty falling asleep or remaining asleep.

Polyphenol—Any organic chemical, whether it is natural, synthetic, or a combination of the two, that is characterized by the presence of large multiples of phenol structures.

Tannin—A type of brown or yellowish-colored polyphenolic compound, found naturally in plants and synthetically, that binds to proteins and some other organic compounds.

Description

Although there are a number of plant-based oils used in cooking that contain monounsaturated fats, such as olive oil, peanut oil, **flaxseed** oil, and sesame oil, the Hamptons diet claims to be based on a "secret ingredient"—macadamia nut oil from Australia. Macadamia nuts are produced by an evergreen tree, *Macadamia integrifolia*, that is native to the rain forests of Queensland and New South Wales in Australia.

The Hamptons diet uses macadamia nut oil not only for cooking, but also in salad dressings and marinades. Pescatore claims that macadamia nut oil is "the most monounsaturated oil on the planet." Macadamia nut oil contains 84% monounsaturated fats, 3.5% polyunsaturated fats, 12.5% saturated fats, and no cholesterol.

In addition to the "secret ingredient," the Hamptons diet is distinctive for the use of food lists defined by how much weight the dieter needs to lose. **Calories** and portion sizes are not emphasized; the dieter is expected to divide the recipes into portions according to the number of servings indicated by each recipe. The basic menu plans, however, provide between 1,000 and 1,200 calories per day. There are three food groups, labeled A, B, and C:

- A group: Foods on this list are for people who need to lose more than 10 pounds. These dieters are limited to between 23 and 26 grams of carbohydrates per day.
- B group: For dieters with less than 10 pounds to lose. They may select foods from both the A and B lists, which allow 40 to 43 grams of carbohydrates per day.
- C group: Foods on this list are slowly added to the meal plans as the dieter reaches his or her weight loss goal and begins a maintenance diet. Foods in this group provide up to 65 grams of carbohydrates per day.

Function

The Hamptons diet is essentially a low-carbohydrate diet intended to promote a moderate rate of weight loss in otherwise healthy people. It is not intended to treat any chronic medical conditions or disorders.

Benefits

The Hamptons diet promotes gradual weight loss and encourages eating a balanced range of foods. It allows dieters complex **carbohydrates** (including whole-grain breads and fresh fruit), discourages the use of processed foods, and distinguishes between healthy and unhealthy sources of fat in the diet. Its preference for such lean sources of **protein** as chicken and fish rather than the higher–saturated fat items

---

KEY TERMS

Macadamia nut—A hard-shelled nut resembling a filbert, produced by an evergreen tree native to Australia and cultivated extensively in Hawaii. The nut is named for John Macadam, an Australian chemist.

Monounsaturated fat—A fat or fatty acid with only one double-bonded carbon atom in its molecule. The most common monounsaturated fats are palmitoleic acid and oleic acid. They are found naturally in such foods as nuts and avocados; oleic acid is the main component of olive oil.

***Trans* fatty acid**—A type of unsaturated fatty acid that occurs naturally in small quantities in meat and dairy products; however, the largest single source of *trans* fatty acids in the modern diet is partially hydrogenated plant oil, used in the processing of fast foods and many snack foods.

---

such as bacon and steaks is also in its favor. In addition, some people like the fact that the Hamptons diet allows moderate amounts of alcohol and the kinds of flavorful foods featured in the Mediterranean diet. The gourmet-quality recipes in this diet may also be useful to dieters who want to cook for a family or for guests without having to prepare two separate meals.

Precautions

Although the Hamptons diet is not a very low-calorie diet (VLCD), it is always advisable for people who need to lose 30 pounds or more; are pregnant or nursing; are below the age of 18; or have such chronic disorders as diabetes, kidney disease, or liver disease to check with a physician before starting a weight-reduction diet.

The Hamptons diet has been criticized for its inadequate allowances of **fiber**, **vitamin C**, **calcium**, **folate**, **vitamin D**, and **vitamin E**. The diet is also high in fat, which provides as much as 70% of the calories in some menu plans, particularly those that call for cream cheese, bacon, and heavy whipping cream. The Hamptons diet does not focus on high saturated fat intake. Therefore, the cream cheese, bacon, and heavy whipping cream are generally only recommended in moderation.

A frequent criticism of the Hamptons diet from those who have tried it is that the recipe ingredients are often costly and hard to find. Many of the ingredients

QUESTIONS TO ASK YOUR DOCTOR

- What have your other patients liked and disliked about the Hamptons diet?
- What feedback have your patients given you regarding the recipes?
- What is your opinion of the author's emphasis on macadamia oil?
- What is your opinion of low-carbohydrate diets? What about diets that emphasize certain types of fat?

called for in the recipes would be unfamiliar to anyone except a professional chef, and some are quite costly. For example, the macadamia nut oil recommended by Dr. Pescatore costs about $10 for a bottle containing 8.5 ounces (slightly more than a cup), or $20 for a bottle containing 16.9 ounces (slightly more than a pint). In addition, the diet recommends organic, not just fresh, ingredients, which are almost always more expensive than nonorganic produce or meats. It is perhaps not surprising that the Hamptons diet has spawned a Hamptons Diet Market website, where the dieter may purchase the "uniquely healthy products from the Hamptons world of wellness" online.

Another potential drawback of the Hamptons diet for many people is that many of the recipes require advance preparation, as much as a day ahead of eating the dish. Others are time-consuming to cook or assemble apart from the time required for advance preparation.

Risks

The relatively high fat content of some of the recipes formulated for the Hamptons diet may be worrisome for dieters; however, only saturated and *trans* fats pose risks for heart health. Monounsaturated and polyunsaturated fats, including omega-3 fatty acids, may actually promote heart health.

Research and general acceptance

The Hamptons diet has been featured primarily in celebrity, fashion, and homemaking magazines rather than in clinical studies. There have been no clinical trials of the Hamptons diet reported in mainstream research journals. Pescatore is involved in two groups listed on his website, presumably to establish his credentials as a researcher. He is the president of the International and American Association of Clinical Nutritionists (IAACN) and a member of the American College for the Advancement of Medicine.

Like the **Scarsdale diet**, some of the appeal of the Hamptons diet comes from its name, which is shared with a group of villages in Long Island, New York. The Hamptons is typically viewed as a luxurious and expensive location.

Resources

BOOKS

Pescatore, Fred. *The Allergy and Asthma Cure: A Complete 8-Step Nutritional Program.* New York: J. Wiley, 2003.

———. *Feed Your Kids Well: How to Help Your Child Lose Weight and Get Healthy.* New York: J. Wiley, 1998.

———. *The Hamptons Diet: Lose Weight Quickly and Safely with the Doctor's Delicious Meal Plans.* Hoboken, NJ: J. Wiley, 2004.

———. *Thin for Good: The One Low-Carb Diet That Will Finally Work for You.* New York: J. Wiley, 2000.

Pescatore, Fred, and Jeff Harter. *The Hamptons Diet Cookbook: Enjoy the Hamptons Lifestyle Wherever You Live.* Hoboken, NJ: J. Wiley, 2006.

Scales, Mary Josephine. *Diets in a Nutshell: A Definitive Guide on Diets from A to Z.* Clifton, VA: Apex Publishers, 2005.

PERIODICALS

Cohen, Deborah. "Latest Spin on Atkins Calls for 'Oil Change.'" *Forbes*, March 18, 2004.

Fishman, Steve. "The Diet Martyr." *New York Magazine*, March 15, 2004. http://nymag.com/nymetro/news/people/features/n_10035 (accessed October 2, 2012).

WEBSITES

Callahan, Maureen. "The Hamptons Diet." Health.com. http://www.health.com/health/article/0,,20410195,00.html (accessed October 2, 2012).

"The Hamptons Diet (official website)." http://www.hamptonsdiet.com/hamptonsdiet (accessed October 2, 2012).

"A Truly Tasteful Way to Losing Weight." *Today*, May 21, 2004. http://today.msnbc.msn.com/id/5023897#.UGtYVK7bT9Q (accessed October 2, 2012).

Rebecca J. Frey, PhD

Hawaiian diet *see* **Pacific Islander American diet**

Hay diet

Definition

The Hay diet is named for the New York physician who created a plan that prohibited the consumption of starches and proteins during the same meal. William Howard Hay began developing the food-combining diet in 1904 to treat himself for medical conditions including a dilated heart. He lost 50 pounds (22.7 kilograms) in approximately three months and recovered from the conditions.

Origins

When William Howard Hay (1866–1940) graduated from New York University Medical College in 1891, he practiced medicine and specialized in surgery. That changed 16 years later when his own medical troubles led him to research the connection between diet and health. Hay then weighed 225 pounds (102 kilograms) and had high blood pressure

and Bright's Disease, a kidney condition. Hay discovered that his heart was dilated while running to catch a train.

The dilated heart caused by weakened heart muscles meant that his blood could not pump efficiently. Hay knew from treating patients that his future did not "look overlong or very bright," according to his 1929 book *Health via Food*. The title described Hay's health theories, his condition, and treatment.

Hay diagnosed the causes of his conditions as the "very familiar trinity of troubles" that then ranked as the primary cause of death: the combination of high blood pressure, kidney disease, and dilated heart.

Hay wrote that his legs had swelled, and he slept seated because he was afraid he would drown in his fluids if he slept lying down. He wasn't able to lose the weight through exercise and what he thought was a proper diet. Hay wrote that the dilated heart made his prospects bleak. He knew from treating patients

Food combining guidelines

Food groups	Foods	Combine with	Do not combine	Exceptions
Acid fruits	Grapefruit, oranges, lemons, limes, pineapples, pomegranates, tomatoes	Sub-acid fruit and nuts and seeds	Sweet fruit and other food groups	Tomatoes can be eaten with low and non-starchy vegetables and avocado
Sub-acid fruits	Apples, apricots, berries, grapes, kiwi, mango, nectarines, papaya, peaches, pears, plums, strawberries	Acid or sweet fruits, not both, and nuts and seeds	Other food groups	
Sweet fruits	Bananas, coconut, dates, dried fruits, prunes, raisins	Sub-acid fruits, and nuts and seeds	Acid fruit and other food groups	
Melons	Cantaloupe, honeydew, watermelon	Eat alone	All groups	
Protein	Meat, poultry, fish, eggs, dairy, dry beans/peas, nuts & seeds, peanuts, soy beans, soy products, tofu	Low and non-starchy vegetables	Other proteins, fats, carbohydrates and starches, and fruits	Drink milk alone
Low and non-starchy vegetables	Asparagus, artichokes, green beans, beets, broccoli, cabbage, cauliflower, cucumber, eggplant, garlic, lettuce, celery, carrots, onions, parsley, peas, peppers, turnips, mushrooms, zucchini	Protein, fats, carbohydrates, and starches	Fruits	
Carbohydrates and starches	Bread, pasta, grains/cereals, potatoes, pumpkin, winter squashes, yams	Low and non-starchy vegetables and fats	Fruits and protein	
Fats	Avocado, olives, coconut, butter, cream, and olive, avocado, flax, sesame, and canola oils	Low and non-starchy vegetables, carbohydrates and starches, and protein	Protein, fruits	Avocado can be eaten with fruits

(Table by GGS Information Services. © 2013 Cengage Learning.)

that there was no medical treatment for a dilated heart. He advised them to prepare for the "final hop-off" (death). With that diagnosis applied to himself, Hay looked at his life to evaluate his own situation. He described himself as a "strong man of splendid heredity," so Hay looked at his eating habits.

Plain food of the American table

After graduating from medical school, Hay ate at hotels, boarding houses, and restaurants for 11 years. He then married, and his wife prepared meals for the following five years. As a married man, Hay wrote that he could control what he ate. However, his food preferences were formed during his years of "public eating."

At home, each of Hay's meals consisted of meat or other concentrated **protein**. He usually combined this with white bread and generally ate a potato of some form. Hay described this meal as the "plain food of the American table." His meal ended with pastries and two to three cups of coffee that he sweetened with **sugar** and cream.

Hay's eating habits weren't unusual. Meat and potatoes were long part of a traditional American meal. In addition, Americans during the early 1800s tended to eat large meals. Excess weight was regarded as a sign of prosperity. That perspective began to change later in the century, with a range of weight-loss solutions proposed during the 1890s.

Dr. Edward Hooker Dewey's plan involved skipping breakfast. Horace Fletcher, a businessman, created a plan after he couldn't get life insurance because of his weight. He lost 40 pounds (18.1 kilograms) by slowly chewing his food until it liquefied. He then swallowed it. The slow-chewing technique became known as "Fletcherism."

Developing a new diet

Hay started his special diet by eliminating two meals and eating only vegetables for the third. He stopped drinking coffee, but continued to smoke cigarettes and drink alcohol. Hay wrote that his craving for coffee ended in two weeks. Several months later, he gave up smoking. By the third month, Hay weighed 175 pounds (79.4 kilograms).

Hay considered that a normal weight. He spent the next four years researching diet and exercise, examining those issues from the conventional and alternative perspectives. His research included studying the work of Ivan Petrovich Pavlov, the Russian physiologist known for his research involving dogs.

Pavlov's studies of the digestion process of dogs indicated that it took about two hours to digest starches and four hours to digest proteins. However, it could take 13 hours to digest a mixture of protein and starch.

Hay's research led to a diet based on the theory that health was affected by the chemical process of digestion. The body uses an alkaline digestive process for **carbohydrates**, the group that Hay classified as consisting of starchy foods and sweet things. The digestion of proteins involved acid. If carbohydrates and proteins were consumed at the same time, the alkaline process was interrupted by the acid process. Combining incompatible foods caused acidosis, the accumulation of excess acid in body fluids. Hay linked the combination of foods to medical conditions like Bright's disease and diabetes. The wrong combinations "drained vitality" and caused people to gain weight.

Hay maintained that the solution was to eat proteins at one meal and carbohydrates at another. He classified fruits with acids. Hay labeled vegetables in the neutral category that could be consumed with either group. He also advocated the daily administration of an enema to cleanse the colon.

The Hay diet was credited with curing the doctor. He pointed out in *Health via Food* that the book was written 24 years after his bleak diagnosis. Hay said that after changing his eating habits that his blood pressure was lower, the swelling caused by fluid was gone, and he could run quickly and at a distance.

He gave up his traditional medical practice, surgery, and administering drugs. He believed that his eating plan was more beneficial. Hay introduced his diet in 1911 and spent the rest of his life promoting it. He lectured in the United States and Canada and wrote books. *The Medical Millennium* was published in 1927, followed by *Health via Food* in 1929 and *A New Health Era* in 1939.

In addition to writing diet books, Hay used the diet to treats patients at sanatoriums. He worked as the medical director of the East Aurora Sun Diet and Health Sanatorium in New York state from 1927 through 1932. He then founded the Pocono Haven Sanatorium Hotel in Mount Pocono, Pennsylvania. He served as its director until he died in a traffic accident in 1940.

Hay's eating plan was the forerunner of late twentieth century food-combining diets including Stephen's Twiggs' Kensington Diet and Judy Mazel's New **Beverly Hills Diet**.

Description

William Howard Hay evaluated health theories and weight-loss methods while developing his plan. When he concluded that proper food combination was the solution to improved health, he saw some benefits in Fletcherism. The slow-chewing method could aid in the digestion of incompatible foods in some cases, Hay wrote in *Health via Food*. Bread could be chewed into a liquid, but the process wasn't effective with foods like cheese.

Exercise did not provide the answer, Hay said. He pointed out that farmers who were physically active were diagnosed with some of the same conditions that less sedentary people were. Hay concluded that the solution was a lifetime of his diet and a daily enema. Hay regarded the enema as vital to providing relief to the colon and eliminating the toxins produced by a poor diet. He pointed out that some patients were constipated for two weeks because of their poor eating habits.

Hay also maintained that fresh air provided a benefit, especially when people slept. However, the Hay diet was the foundation of his treatment. The plan, which scheduled when food was consumed, generally consisted of one food group per meal. Foods were classified as Proteins, Starches, and Neutral Foods that could be combined with proteins or starches. *Health via Food* included a month-long schedule of suitable meals. It gave the public a guide to follow. For the contemporary reader, the diet plan offers a perspective on the Hay diet and the eating habits of those times. Although food items were limited, people could eat as much as they wanted.

The Hay diet menus for the summer included the following meal recommendations:

- A Friday plan began with a breakfast of orange juice and milk. Lunch was tomato bullion, a baked onion, a tomato-and-cucumber salad with mayonnaise dressing, and apricots for dessert. Dinner was broiled fish or steak, steamed chicory, steamed carrots, and a salad of shredded cabbage, onions, and radishes. Mayonnaise dressing was allowed, and dessert consisted of lemon ice.

- A Saturday plan started with a breakfast of whole-wheat muffins, honey, butter, and black coffee. Lunch was cream of carrot soup, steamed celery, and a salad of pineapples, pears, and grapes. Salad was served with mayonnaise dressing. Dessert was lemon fluff. Dinner was broiled lamb chops, steamed cauliflower, steamed kale, and a salad of grapefruit

and sauerkraut with mayonnaise dressing. The dessert was fresh peaches with unsweetened cream.

The contemporary Hay diet

Contemporary versions of the Hay diet no longer recommend a daily enema. The eating plan still follows Hay's classification of foods into three categories, along with the rules about how the foods are combined at mealtime. The diet consists primarily of fruits and vegetables, and dieters are advised to wait at least four hours before consuming a meal from an incompatible category.

Some versions of the Hay diet recommend eating small portions of proteins, starches, and **fats**. There is also an emphasis on eating whole-grain products and unprocessed starches. Some plans allow alcoholic beverages; others prohibit processed foods with ingredients such as refined sugar, margarine, and white flour.

The Hay diet meal plan is based on the categories of Proteins, Starches, and Neutral Foods. Proteins and Neutral Foods may be combined, and Neutral Foods may be combined with Starches. The combination of Proteins and Starches should be avoided.

The Protein category consists of:

- Meat, poultry, fish, eggs, and dairy products including milk, cheese, and yogurt. Milk should be avoided with meat, but combines well with fruit.
- Beans including lentils, pinto beans, kidney beans, soy beans, garbanzo beans (chickpeas), haricot beans, and lima beans.
- The majority of fruits. In this category are apples, apricots, berries, cherries, currants, gooseberries, grapefruit, grapes, guavas, kiwis, lemons, limes, lychees, mangoes, nectarines, oranges, passionfruit, pears, pineapples, prunes, raspberries, strawberries, and tangerines. Melons are in this category but should be consumed separately.
- Beverages allowed are red wine, white wine, and cider.

In the Neutral Foods category are:

- All vegetables except those in the Starches category.
- All nuts except peanuts.
- Fats including butter, cream, egg yolks, and olive oil.
- Beverages in this category are whisky and gin.

In the Starches category are:

- Cereal, bread, rice, and products made from flour and whole-grains such as wheat, oats, corn, and barley.
- Starchy vegetables such as potatoes, sweet potatoes, pumpkins, and Jerusalem artichokes.
- Sweet fruits such as raisins, dates, figs, sweet grapes, and ripe bananas. Extremely ripe fruit is not allowed because the sugar content is higher.
- Beverages in this category are beer and ale.

Function

Hay created his meal plan to treat medical problems associated with **obesity**. He claimed that a change in eating habits rather than medication was beneficial in the treatment of conditions such as cardiac disease, kidney disease, and kidney disorders.

QUESTIONS TO ASK YOUR DOCTOR

- How much weight do I need to lose?
- Will the Hay diet's food-combining rules help me to lose weight more quickly?
- Does the Hay diet help to improve conditions like diabetes or indigestion?
- Is there another diet that will better help me reach my goals?
- Should I avoid certain foods because of medications I'm taking or because of a health condition?
- What are the risks of this diet?

In contemporary times, the Hay diet is used as a weight-loss plan by the general public and people interested in alternative treatments. Advocates of natural health maintain that the plan reverses conditions such as arthritis, indigestion, **constipation**, and flatulence. The Hay diet is also regarded as a natural method for providing relief to people diagnosed with asthma and allergies.

Benefits

Hay wrote in *Health via Food* that he saw "the comeback of thousands of patients" who followed his regimen. The Hay diet features some nutritional principles endorsed by organizations including the U.S. Department of Agriculture (USDA), the Academy of Nutrition and Dietetics, and the medical community. Their recommendations call for eating lean meat and poultry and a variety of fruits and vegetables.

Those recommendations are also found in the Hay diet. People who follow those recommendations and fill up on fruits and vegetables will lose weight. Those are low-calorie foods that are rich in **fiber**. Whole-grain products also contain fiber. Eating high-fiber food produces the sense of fullness more quickly than the consumption of foods with fat does.

Precautions

Although there are some nutritional aspects of the Hay diet, there are some flaws. The diet does not include serving sizes, and portion control is an important aspect of maintaining a healthy weight. In addition, people may miss out on **vitamins** and nutrients by restricting food groups to one meal per day.

Risks

Although the consumption of fruits and vegetables will help to relieve constipation, people should not rely solely on the Hay diet to treat conditions such as heart disease, arthritis, allergies, and asthma. People diagnosed with those conditions may need medication and should consult their physician before undertaking the Hay diet or any weight-loss plan.

Research and general acceptance

Food-combining diets are generally not supported by the medical community and are not supported by clinical evidence.

Resources

PERIODICALS

Blonz, Ed. "Logic Behind Call to Avoid Certain Food Combinations is Faulty." *The San Diego Union Tribune*, Sept. 14, 2005. http://www.signonsandiego.com/uniontrib/20050914/news_lz1f14focus.html (accessed October 2, 2012).

OTHER

Hay, William Howard. "Health via Food." http://www.soilandhealth.org/02/0201hyglibcat/020165.hay.pdf (accessed October 2, 2012).

WEBSITES

Clarke, Jane. "Sorry, but Food Combining is Just a Silly Fad!" *UK Daily Mail* Online, January 2008. http://www.dailymail.co.uk/debate/columnists/article-509672/Sorry-food-combining-just-silly-fad.html (accessed October 2, 2012).

Liz Swain

Healthy People 2020

Definition

Healthy People 2020 is a large-scale public health initiative of the U.S. Department of Health and Human Services (HHS). Healthy People 2020 is based on the accomplishments of four previous Healthy People initiatives: *Healthy People: The Surgeon General's Report on Health Promotion and Disease Prevention* issued in 1979, *Healthy People 1990: Promoting Health/Preventing Disease: Objectives for the Nation, Healthy People 2000: National Health Promotion and Disease Prevention Objectives*, and *Healthy People 2010: Objectives for Improving Health*. Each initiative lasts one decade, and the year in the title is followed by the vision for that initiative. The vision for Healthy People 2020 is "A Society in Which All People Live Long, Healthy Lives."

Purpose

The Healthy People initiative is grounded in the principle that setting national objectives and monitoring progress can motivate action and improve health. Throughout the United States, health departments at the city, county, and state levels use the Healthy People program as a way to track the effectiveness of local health initiatives.

Healthy People is a systematic, science-based approach to improving the health of all Americans. It is based on the premise that clear objectives and scientifically based benchmarks for tracking progress will both motivate and focus public health activities. Healthy People's objectives are broad-based and designed to promote healthy practices among individuals and institutions to improve disease prevention. Each new Healthy People initiative utilizes public health data from the previous decade to identify emerging public-health priorities and to realign strategies, research, and resources to address those priorities.

Overarching public health goals

Healthy People promotes collaborations across various professional sectors and administrative levels. Its objectives, targets, and generated data have become important strategic management tools for various public and private agencies and organizations at the federal, state, and local levels. Of particular importance is Healthy People's focus on measuring progress toward health objectives within specific populations. Each Healthy People initiative formulates broad or overarching public health goals.

HEALTHY PEOPLE 2000 GOALS. The goals of Healthy People 2000 were to:

- increase the healthy lifespan of Americans
- reduce health disparities among Americans
- achieve universal access to preventive health services

HEALTHY PEOPLE 2010 GOALS. The goals of Healthy People 2010 were to:

- increase the years and quality of healthy life for Americans
- eliminate health disparities among different segments of the population by 2010 and eliminate remaining racial disparities in health care utilization and outcomes

HEALTHY PEOPLE 2020 GOALS. The goals of Healthy People 2020 are to:

- attain high-quality, longer lives free of preventable disease, disability, injury, and premature death
- achieve health equity, eliminate disparities, and improve the health of all groups
- create social and physical environments that promote good health for all
- promote quality of life, healthy development, and healthy behaviors across all life stages

Description

Healthy People was launched in 1979 by HHS's Office of Disease Prevention and Health Promotion. Each successive Healthy People initiative sets 10-year objectives within priority or focus areas. The federal government awards millions of dollars in grants to state and community programs based on these objectives. The Healthy People objectives are required to be of significance, easily understandable, and actionable. They must also be measurable by available high-quality data and be comparable to the objectives and achievements of previous Healthy People initiatives.

Healthy People initiatives collect data, monitor and assess outcomes, and evaluate the successes and failures of health improvement programs and activities nationwide according to specified health indicators. The National Center for Health Statistics (NCHS), within the Centers for Disease Control and Prevention (CDC), is responsible for tracking progress toward objectives. NCHS works with HHS to update data as it becomes available. Progress reviews are also done periodically by topic area. Throughout the years 2010–2020, HHS will monitor the direction that the initiative moves from the baselines set at the beginning of the decade.

Healthy People 2000

"Healthy People 2000: National Health Promotion and Disease Prevention Objectives" was released in September 1990. It consisted of 376 objectives in 22 priority areas, for a total of 319 primary objectives, since some were duplicated in different priority areas.

Healthy People 2000 health-status indicators included total deaths and specific causes of death such as **cancer**, cardiovascular disease, and motor-vehicle crashes. Other indicators included the incidences of various infectious and sexually transmitted diseases, prenatal care, births to adolescents, low-birth-weight newborns, childhood poverty, and poor air quality.

Priority data requirements for Healthy People 2000 included data on immunizations, water quality, pap tests and mammograms, and cigarette smoking and alcohol misuse. There was also a need for data on medical insurance coverage, access to primary care and dental services, and the incidences of people who are overweight or suffering from **hypertension** (high blood pressure), hypercholesterolemia (high blood cholesterol), hepatitis B, high blood lead levels in young children, childhood tooth decay, and child abuse and neglect.

HEALTHY PEOPLE 2000 RESULTS. *Healthy People 2000 Final Review* was released in October 2001. The targets for reducing deaths from **coronary heart disease** and cancer were surpassed. Health disparities were reduced for more than one-half of the special populations identified as being at increased risk. Sixty-eight objectives (21%) were met. Another 129 objectives (41%) progressed toward their targets. Thirty-five objectives (11%) showed mixed results. Seven objectives (2%) showed no change. Forty-seven objectives (15%) moved away from their targets. Assessments could not be obtained for 32 objectives (10%).

Healthy People 2010

Healthy People 2010, launched in January 2000, consisted of 467 objectives in 28 focus areas. Healthy People 2010's leading health indicators were a select set of objectives chosen based on their ability to motivate action, their relevance as broad public health issues, and the availability of data for measuring progress. These included physical activity, tobacco use, responsible sexual behavior, injury and violence, immunization, overweight and **obesity**, substance abuse, mental health, environmental quality, and access to health care.

HEALTHY PEOPLE 2010 RESULTS. The data sets for Healthy People 2010 were collected from more than 190 different sources. HHS released the assessment of Healthy People 2010 objectives on October 6, 2011, in a report titled *Healthy People 2010 Final Review*. The report indicated that Americans met or were moving toward meeting 71% of 2010 targets, including those associated with reducing deaths from coronary heart disease and stroke. However, health disparities had not changed for approximately 80% of the health objectives and increased for an additional 13%. In addition, obesity rates increased in all age groups.

Among the promising data was that the United States met the Healthy People objectives of reducing cholesterol levels, while making minor strides toward reducing smoking rates. As a result, according to the National Vital Statistics System, the nation experienced a major drop in deaths from heart disease and strokes over the previous decade. Furthermore, the overall life expectancy continued to rise and several objectives that tracked mental health status, treatment, and services met their 2010 targets.

Although life expectancy was on the upswing, the rising obesity rates could later cause a reduction in the life expectancy because obesity also leads to conditions such as heart disease. The 2010 final review showed dramatic rises in obesity in every age group:

- 54.5% in children ages 6–11
- 63.6% in adolescents ages 12–19
- 48% in adults

The 2010 Final Review also described changes to be made for the Healthy People 2020 initiative. These included revising wording and definitions of the objectives for food and nutrient consumption. This was done so that they were applicable to the *2010 Dietary Guidelines for Americans* (DGA) issued by HHS and the U.S. Department of Agriculture (USDA).

When the 2010 Final Review was released, HHS noted that reducing health disparities and curbing obesity were top priorities for both the administration of President Barack Obama and the department. HHS actions included working with government and private sector partners to improve outcomes across all racial and economic groups. In addition, HHS:

- launched the *HHS Action Plan to Reduce Health Disparities* in April 2011 to promote integrated approaches, evidence-based programs, and best practices to reduce health disparities
- was working to tackle obesity by partnering with the National Prevention Council to implement the National Prevention Strategy's goal of increasing the number of Americans who are healthy at every stage of life
- was working with First Lady Michelle Obama's "Let's Move!" campaign to increase physical activity and encourage increased access to healthy foods

Healthy People 2020

Drawing upon findings from the earlier Healthy People initiatives, experts from many federal agencies prepared draft objectives for Healthy People 2020. The objectives were made available for public comment so that Healthy People 2020 would reflect the needs and priorities of all Americans. Public comment was received during a series of nine regional meetings across the country, on a public comment website, during a public meeting of the advisory committee, and through a request for public comment published in the *Federal Register*.

After the public-comment period, the draft objectives were reviewed by the Federal Interagency Workgroup (FIW). The working group included representatives from HHS agencies and the U.S. Departments of Agriculture (USDA), Education (ED), Housing and Urban Development (HUD), Justice (DOJ), Interior (DOI), and Veterans Affairs (VA), as well as the Environmental Protection Agency (EPA).

HHS invited agencies and organizations that supported Healthy People 2020 goals to join the Healthy People Consortium. Members across the nation were committed to achieving Healthy People 2020 goals and objectives. Enrollment in the consortium was ongoing, and consortium members included colleges, universities, private businesses, and religious organizations.

Launched on December 2, 2010, Healthy People 2020 contains 42 topic areas with nearly 600 objectives that encompass 1,200 measures. A smaller set of Healthy People 2020 objectives, called Leading Health Indicators, was selected to communicate high-priority health issues and actions that could be taken to address them. The Healthy People 2020 Leading Health Indicators place renewed emphasis on overcoming those challenges as HHS tracks progress over the course of the decade. The indicators are used to assess the health of the nation, facilitate collaboration across sectors, and motivate action at the national, state, and community levels.

NEW FOCUS AREAS. Thirteen new focus areas were identified for Healthy People 2020:

- early and middle childhood
- adolescent health
- older adults
- lesbian, gay, bisexual, and transgender health
- blood disorders and blood safety
- healthcare-associated infections
- sleep health
- dementias, including Alzheimer's disease
- health-related quality of life and well-being
- preparedness
- social determinants of health
- genomics
- global health

OBJECTIVES. Many objectives focus on interventions that are designed to reduce or eliminate illness, disability, and premature death among individuals and communities. Other objectives focus on broader issues such as:

- eliminating health disparities
- addressing social determinants of health

- improving access to quality health care
- strengthening public health services
- improving the availability and dissemination of health-related information

Nutrition, physical activity, and obesity

Nutrition, physical activity, and obesity are leading health indicator topics in Healthy People 2020. Proper nutrition, physical activity, and a healthy body weight are essential to overall health and well-being. Together, they can help decrease the risk of developing serious health conditions such as high blood pressure, high cholesterol, diabetes, heart disease, stroke, and cancer. A healthy diet, regular exercise, and a healthy weight are also crucial to managing health conditions so they do not worsen over time.

Many Americans do not eat a healthy diet and are not physically active at the levels needed to maintain proper health. According to Healthy People 2020, fewer than one in three adults and an even lower proportion of adolescents eat the recommended amount of vegetables each day. In addition, 81.6% of adults and 81.8% of adolescents do not get the recommended amount of physical activity.

Because of these behaviors, the United States has experienced a dramatic increase in obesity. Approximately one in three adults and one in six children and adolescents are obese. Obesity-related conditions include heart disease, stroke, and type 2 diabetes. These conditions are among the leading causes of death in the United States, according to the initiative.

The Healthy People 2020 nutrition and weight status objectives are attempting to change those trends by increasing the number of Americans who eat healthier foods and exercise. Objectives in this area are defined by a target for improvement to be reached by 2020. This is a measurable goal, such as increasing the percentage of people who exercise. The target is measured in relation to a baseline, which is a percentage from the previous decade. The four priority objectives are:

- Adults who meet current federal physical activity guidelines for aerobic physical activity and for muscle-strengthening activity. The target is for 20.1% of adults to meet the standards. The baseline is that 18.2% of adults met the objectives for aerobic physical activity and for muscle-strengthening activity in 2008.
- Adults who are obese. The objective is to reduce the proportion of adults considered obese. The target is 30.6%. The baseline is 34.0% of people age 20 and

older who were obese in the years 2005 through 2008. Age was adjusted to the year 2000 standard population.

- Children and adolescents who are obese. The objective is to reduce the proportion of children and adolescents between the ages of 2 and 19 who are considered obese. The target is 14.6%, with a baseline of 16.2% of children and adolescents who were obese in the years 2005 through 2008.
- Total daily vegetable intake for people age 2 and older. The objective is to increase consumption of total vegetables, referring to all vegetables and not just those in a specific category, such as green vegetables. The target of vegetables or their equivalents is 1.1 cup (8.8 oz. or 0.25 kg) of vegetables per 1,000 calories consumed each day. The baseline is 0.8 cups (6.3 oz. or 0.18 kg) of total vegetables per 1,000 calories consumed during the years 2001 through 2004.

Other nutrition-related objectives in Healthy People 2020 include:

- Increase the amount of fruits consumed each day by people age 2 and older. The target is 0.9 cups (7.8 oz. or 0.22 kg) per 1,000 calories consumed. The baseline is 0.5 cups (3.9 oz. or 0.11 kg) of fruits per 1,000 calories consumed.
- Increase the daily intake of dark green vegetables, orange vegetables, and legumes by people age 2 and older. The target is 0.3 cups (2.5 oz. or 0.07 kg) of vegetables or equivalents per 1,000 calories. The baseline is 0.1 cups (0.7 oz. or 0.02 kg).
- Increase the contribution of whole grains to the diets of the population age 2 and older. The daily target is 0.7 oz. (0.02 kg) of whole grains per 1,000 calories. The baseline is 0.3 oz. (8.50 g) of whole grains per 1,000 calories.
- Reduce consumption of calories from solid fats. The target is solid fats representing 16.7% of daily calorie intake. The baseline is 18.9% of solid fats consumed in total daily calories.
- Reduce consumption of calories from added sugars, those sugars added to products rather than those that occur naturally in foods. The target is added sugars representing 10.8% of daily calorie intake. The baseline is 15.7% of added sugars consumed in total daily calories.
- Reduce consumption of sodium from sources including food, dietary supplements and antacids, drinking water, and salt used at the table. The daily target is 2,300 mg; the baseline is 3,641 mg.

KEY TERMS

Cholesterol—A fat-soluble steroid alcohol (sterol) found in animal fats and oils and produced in the body from saturated fats. Cholesterol is required to produce vitamin D and various hormones and for the formation of cell membranes; however, high cholesterol levels contribute to the development of cardiovascular disease.

Health disparities—Differences in health, health care, and/or health outcomes among different racial and ethnic groups, genders, and geographical locations within a single population.

Hypertension—High blood pressure.

National Center for Health Statistics (NCHS)—The division within the U.S. Centers for Disease Control and Prevention (CDC) that compiles, analyzes, and disseminates health statistics for the nation.

Obesity—More than 20% over an individual's ideal weight for height and age or having a body mass index (BMI) of 30 or greater.

Overweight—A body mass index (BMI) between 25 and 30.

• Increase consumption of calcium from foods, dietary supplements and antacids, and drinking water. The daily target is 1,300 mg; the baseline is 1,118 mg.

Parental concerns

The primary concern for parents is whether their children are meeting the standards identified in the Healthy People objectives. Parents should examine the Healthy 2020 goals in terms of whether their children are eating enough fruits, vegetables, and other healthy foods. Parents should also implement nutritious eating plans and physical activities for themselves and their children.

Resources

BOOKS

Institute of Medicine, Committee on Leading Health Indicators for Healthy People 2020. *Leading Health Indicators for Healthy People 2020: Letter Report.* Washington, DC: National Academies Press, 2011.

Institute of Medicine, Division of Health Promotion and Disease Prevention, Committee on Leading Health Indicators for Healthy People 2010. *Leading Health Indicators for Healthy People 2010, Final Report.* Washington, DC: National Academy of Sciences, 1999.

Stoto, Michael A., Ruth A. Behrens, and Connie Rosemont. *Healthy People 2000: Citizens Chart the Course.* Washington, DC: National Academy Press, 1990.

U.S. Department of Health and Human Services. *Healthy People 2010: Understanding and Improving Health.* 2nd ed. Washington, DC: U.S. Department of Health and Human Services, 2000.

———. *Tracking Healthy People 2010.* Washington, DC: U.S. Department of Health and Human Services, 2000.

U.S. Public Health Service. *Healthy People 2000: National Health Promotion and Disease Prevention Objectives: Full Report, with Commentary.* Washington, DC: U.S. Department of Health and Human Services, Public Health Service, 1991.

PERIODICALS

"Are You Better than Average?" *Consumer Reports on Health* 23, no. 1 (January 2011): 1.

Bellamy, Gail R., Jane Nelson Bolin, and Larry D. Gamm. "Rural Healthy People 2010, 2020, and Beyond: The Need Goes On." *Family and Community Health* 34, no. 2 (April–June 2011): 182–88.

Dye, Bruce A., and Gina Thornton-Evans. "Trends in Oral Health by Poverty Status as Measured by Healthy People 2010 Objectives." *Public Health Reports* 125, no. 5 (November/December 2010): 817–30.

Hurley, Dan. "Obesity Reaches Epidemic Proportions." *Discover* 32, no. 1 (January/February 2011): 30.

Koh, Howard K. "A 2020 Vision for Healthy People." *New England Journal of Medicine* 362, no. 18 (May 6, 2010): 1653–56.

Krisberg, Kim. "Healthy People 2020 Tackling Social Determinants of Health." *Nation's Health* 38, no. 10 (December 2008/January 2009): 1–25.

Rachid, Nafisa. "Health Care." *Network Journal* 18, no. 2 (February 2011): 10–12.

"Report Shows U.S. Women Fail to Meet Health Goals." *Policy & Practice* 69, no. 2 (April 2011): 43.

Slade-Sawyer, Penelope. "Healthy People 2020 Inspires People to Improve Health of Communities." *Nation's Health* 41, no. 4 (May/June 2011): 515.

Sondik, E. J., et al. "Progress Toward the Healthy People 2010 Goals and Objectives." *Annual Review of Public Health* 31 (2010): 271–81.

Thompson, Dennis. "To Get Americans Healthier, U.S. Targets the Heart." *HealthDay Consumer News Service* (April 22, 2011).

OTHER

Centers for Disease Control and Prevention. "Healthy People 2010 Final Review." http://www.cdc.gov/nchs/data/hpdata2010/hp2010_final_review.pdf (accessed September 5, 2012).

WEBSITES

Centers for Disease Control and Prevention. "Data2010… The Healthy People 2010 Database." CDC Wonder. http://wonder.cdc.gov/data2010 (accessed September 5, 2012).

Centers for Disease Control and Prevention. "Healthy People 2010." http://www.cdc.gov/nchs/healthy_people/hp2010.htm (accessed September 5, 2012).

Centers for Disease Control and Prevention and National Center for Health Statistics. "Healthy People 2000." http://www.cdc.gov/nchs/healthy_people/hp2000.htm (accessed September 5, 2012).

"Let's Move!" http://www.letsmove.gov (accessed September 5, 2012).

U.S. Department of Agriculture. "MyPlate." Choose MyPlate.gov. http://www.choosemyplate.gov (accessed September 5, 2012).

U.S. Department of Agriculture and U.S. Department of Health and Human Services. *Dietary Guidelines for Americans, 2010.* 7th ed. Washington, DC: U.S. Government Printing Office, December 2010. http://health.gov/dietaryguidelines (accessed February 22, 2012).

U.S. Department of Health and Human Services. "Healthy People 2020." http://www.healthypeople.gov/2020/default.aspx (accessed September 5, 2012).

———. "Nutrition, Physical Activity, and Obesity." http://www.healthypeople.gov/2020/LHI/nutrition.aspx (accessed September 5, 2012).

ORGANIZATIONS

Centers for Disease Control and Prevention, 1600 Clifton Rd. NE, Atlanta, GA 30333, (800) CDC-INFO (232-4636), TTY: (888) 232-6348, cdcinfo@cdc.gov, http://www.cdc.gov.

Office of Disease Prevention and Health Promotion, PO Box 1133, Washington, DC 20852, (301) 565-4167, (800) 336-4797, healthypeople@nhic.org, http://www.healthypeople.gov.

U.S. Department of Health and Human Services, 200 Independence Ave. SW, Washington, DC 20201, (877) 696-6775, http://www.hhs.gov.

Margaret Alic, PhD
Liz Swain

Heart disease *see* **Coronary heart disease**

Heartburn

Definition

Heartburn is a burning sensation in the chest that can extend to the neck, throat, and face; it is worsened by bending or lying down. It is the primary symptom of gastroesophageal reflux, which is the movement of stomach acid into the esophagus. On rare occasions, it is due to gastritis (stomach lining inflammation).

Description

More than one-third of the population is afflicted by heartburn, with about one-tenth afflicted daily. Infrequent heartburn is usually without serious consequences, but chronic or frequent heartburn (recurring more than twice per week) can have severe consequences. Accordingly, early management is important.

Understanding heartburn depends on understanding the structure and action of the esophagus. The esophagus is a tube connecting the throat to the stomach. It is about 10 in. (25 cm) long in adults, lined with squamous (plate-like) epithelial cells, coated with mucus, and surrounded by muscles that push food to the stomach by sequential waves of contraction (peristalsis). The lower esophageal sphincter (LES) is a thick band of muscles that encircles the esophagus just above the uppermost part of the stomach. This sphincter is usually tightly closed and normally opens only when food passes from the esophagus into the stomach. Thus, the contents of the stomach are normally kept from moving back into the esophagus.

The stomach has a thick mucous coating that protects it from the strong acid it secretes into its interior when food is present, but the much thinner esophageal coating does not provide protection against acid. Thus, if the LES opens inappropriately or fails to close completely, and stomach contents leak into the esophagus, the esophagus can be burned by acid. The resulting burning sensation is called heartburn.

Occasional heartburn has no serious long-lasting effects, but repeated episodes of gastroesophageal reflux can ultimately lead to esophageal inflammation (esophagitis) and other damage. If episodes occur more frequently than twice a week, and the esophagus is repeatedly subjected to acid and digestive enzymes from the stomach, ulcerations, scarring, and thickening of the esophagus walls can result. This thickening of the esophagus wall causes a narrowing of the interior of the esophagus. Such narrowing affects swallowing and peristaltic movements. Repeated irritation can also result in changes in the types of cells that line the esophagus. The condition associated with these changes is termed Barrett's syndrome and can lead to esophageal **cancer**.

Causes and symptoms

Causes

A number of different factors may contribute to LES malfunction with its consequent gastroesophageal acid reflux:

- The eating of large meals that distend the stomach can cause the LES to open inappropriately.

- Lying down within two to three hours of eating can cause the LES to open.
- Obesity, pregnancy, and tight clothing can impair the ability of the LES to stay closed by putting pressure on the abdomen.
- Certain drugs, notably nicotine, alcohol, diazepam (Valium), meperidine (Demerol), theophylline, morphine, prostaglandins, calcium channel blockers, nitrate heart medications, anticholinergic and adrenergic drugs (drugs that limit nerve reactions), including dopamine, can relax the LES.
- Progesterone is thought to relax the LES.
- Greasy foods and some other foods such as chocolate, coffee, and peppermint can relax the LES.
- Paralysis and scleroderma can cause the LES to malfunction.
- Hiatal hernia may also cause heartburn according to some gastroenterologists. (Hiatal hernia is a protrusion of part of the stomach through the diaphragm to a position next to the esophagus.)

Symptoms

Heartburn itself is a symptom. Other symptoms also caused by gastroesophageal reflux can be associated with heartburn. Often heartburn sufferers salivate excessively or regurgitate stomach contents into their mouths, leaving a sour or bitter taste. Frequent gastroesophageal reflux leads to additional complications including difficult or painful swallowing, sore throat, hoarseness, coughing, laryngitis, wheezing, asthma, pneumonia, gingivitis, bad breath, and earache.

Diagnosis

Gastroenterologists and internists are best equipped to diagnose and treat gastroesophageal reflux. Diagnosis is usually based solely on patient histories that report heartburn and other related symptoms. Additional diagnostic procedures can confirm the diagnosis and assess damage to the esophagus, as well as monitor healing progress. The following diagnostic procedures are appropriate for anyone who has frequent, chronic, or difficult-to-treat heartburn or any of the complicating symptoms.

X rays taken after a patient swallows a barium suspension can reveal esophageal narrowing, ulcerations, or a reflux episode as it occurs. However, this procedure cannot detect the structural changes associated with different degrees of esophagitis. This diagnostic procedure has traditionally been called the "upper GI series" or "barium swallow" and costs about $250.00.

Esophagoscopy is a newer procedure that uses a thin flexible tube to view the inside of the esophagus directly. It should be done by a gastroenterologist or gastrointestinal endoscopist and costs about $700. It gives an accurate picture of any damage present and gives the physician the ability to distinguish between different degrees of esophagitis.

Other tests may also be used. They include pressure measurements of the LES; measurements of esophageal acidity (pH), usually throughout a 24-hour period; and microscopic examination of biopsied tissue from the esophageal wall (to inspect esophageal cell structure for Barrett's syndrome and malignancies).

Newer technology allows for continuous monitoring of pH levels to help determine the cause. A tiny wireless capsule can be delivered to the lining of the esophagus through a catheter and data recorder on a device the size of a pager that is clipped to the patient's belt or purse for 48 hours. The capsule eventually sloughs off and passes harmlessly through the gastrointestinal tract in seven to 10 days.

Note: A burning sensation in the chest is usually heartburn and is not associated with the heart. However, chest pain that radiates into the arms and is not accompanied by regurgitation is a warning of a possible serious heart problem. Anyone with these symptoms should contact a doctor immediately.

Treatment

Drugs

Occasional heartburn is probably best treated with over-the-counter antacids. These products go straight to the esophagus and immediately begin to decrease acidity. However, they should not be used as the sole treatment for heartburn sufferers who either have two or more episodes per week or who suffer for periods of more than three weeks. There is a risk of kidney damage and other metabolic changes.

H2 blockers (histamine receptor blockers, such as Pepcid AC, Zantac, Tagamet) decrease stomach acid production and are effective against heartburn. H2 blocker treatment also allows healing of esophageal damage but is not very effective when there is a high degree of damage. It takes 30–45 minutes for these drugs to take effect, so they must be taken prior to an episode. Thus, they should be taken daily, usually two to four times per day for several weeks. Six to 12 weeks of standard-dose treatment relieves symptoms in about one-half the patients. Higher doses relieve symptoms in a greater fraction of the population, but at least 25% of heartburn sufferers are not helped by H2 blockers.

Proton-pump inhibitors also inhibit acid production by the stomach, but are much more effective than H2 blockers for some people. They are also more effective in aiding the healing process. Esophagitis is healed in about 90% of the patients undergoing proton-pump inhibitor treatment.

The long-term effects of inhibiting stomach acid production are unknown. Without the antiseptic effects of a consistently acidic stomach environment, users of H2 blockers or proton-pump inhibitors may become more susceptible to bacterial and viral infection. Absorption of some drugs is also lowered by this less-acidic environment.

Prokinetic agents (also known as motility drugs) act on the LES, stimulating it to close more tightly, thereby keeping stomach contents out of the esophagus. It is not known how effectively these drugs promote healing. Some of the early motility drugs had serious neurological side effects, but a newer drug, cisapride, seems to act only on digestive system nerve connections.

Surgery

Fundoplication, a surgical procedure to increase pressure on the LES by stretching and wrapping the upper part of the stomach around the sphincter, is a treatment of last resort. About 10% of heartburn sufferers undergo this procedure. It is not always effective and its effectiveness may decrease over time, especially several years after surgery. Dr. Robert Marks and his colleagues at the University of Alabama reported in 1997 on the long-term outcome of this procedure. They found that 64% of the patients in their study who had fundoplication between 1992 and 1995 still suffered from heartburn and reported an impaired quality of life after the surgery.

However, laparoscopy (an examination of the interior of the abdomen by means of the laparoscope) now provides hope for better outcomes. Fundoplication performed with a laparoscope is less invasive. Five small incisions are required instead of one large incision. Patients recover faster, and it is likely that studies will show they suffer from fewer surgical complications.

Nutrition and dietary concerns

Prevention, as outlined below, is a primary feature for heartburn management in alternative medicine and traditional medicine. Dietary adjustments can eliminate many causes of heartburn.

Herbal remedies include bananas, aloe vera gel, chamomile (*Matricaria recutita*), ginger (*Zingiber officinale*), and citrus juices, but there is little agreement here. For example, ginger, which seems to help some people, is claimed by other practitioners to *cause* heartburn and is

---

KEY TERMS

Barrett's syndrome—Also called Barrett's esophagus or Barrett's epithelia, this is a condition where the squamous epithelial cells that normally line the esophagus are replaced by thicker columnar epithelial cells.

Digestive enzymes—Molecules that catalyze the breakdown of large molecules (usually food) into smaller molecules.

Esophagitis—Inflammation of the esophagus.

Fundoplication—A surgical procedure that increases pressure on the LES by stretching and wrapping the upper part of the stomach around the sphincter.

Gastroesophageal reflux—The flow of stomach contents into the esophagus.

Hiatal hernia—A protrusion of part of the stomach through the diaphragm to a position next to the esophagus.

Metabolic—Refers to the chemical reactions in living things.

Mucus—Thick, viscous, gel-like material that functions to moisten and protect inner body surfaces.

Peristalsis—A sequence of muscle contractions that progressively squeeze one small section of the digestive tract and then the next to push food along the tract, similar to pushing toothpaste out of its tube.

Scleroderma—An autoimmune disease with many consequences, including esophageal wall thickening.

Squamous epithelial cells—Thin, flat cells found in layers or sheets covering surfaces such as skin and the linings of blood vessels and esophagus.

Ulceration—An open break in surface tissue.

---

thought to relax the LES. There are also many recommendations to *avoid* citrus juices, which are themselves acidic. Licorice (*Glycyrrhiza uralensis*) can help relieve the symptoms of heartburn by reestablishing balance in the acid output of the stomach.

Several homeopathic remedies are useful in treating heartburn symptoms. Among those most often recommended are *Nux vomica, Carbo vegetabilis*, and *Arsenicum album*. Acupressure and acupuncture may also be helpful in treating heartburn.

Sodium bicarbonate (baking soda) is an inexpensive alternative to use as an antacid. It reduces esophageal acidity immediately, but its effect is not long-lasting and should not be used by people on sodium-restricted diets.

Prognosis

The prognosis for people who get heartburn only occasionally or people without esophageal damage is excellent. The prognosis for people with esophageal damage who become involved in a treatment program that promotes healing is also excellent. The prognosis for anyone with esophageal cancer is very poor. There is a strong likelihood of a painful illness and a less than 5% chance of surviving more than five years.

Prevention

Given the lack of completely satisfactory treatments for heartburn or its consequences and the lack of a cure for esophageal cancer, prevention is of the utmost importance. Proponents of traditional *and* alternative medicine agree that people disposed to heartburn should:

• Avoid eating large meals.

• Avoid alcohol, caffeine, fatty foods, fried foods, hot or spicy foods, chocolate, peppermint, and nicotine.

• Avoid drugs known to contribute to heartburn, such as nitrates (heart medications such as Isonate and Nitrocap), calcium channel blockers (e.g., Cardizem and Procardia), and anticholinergic drugs (e.g., Probanthine and Bentyl), and check with their doctors about any drugs they are taking.

• Avoid clothing that fits tightly around the abdomen.

• Control body weight.

• Wait about three hours after eating before going to bed or lying down.

• Elevate the head of the bed 6–9 inches to alleviate heartburn at night. This can be done with bricks under the bed or with a wedge designed for this purpose.

Preventing heartburn's switch to cancer begins with preventing heartburn in the first place. A study in Great Britain in 2004 also looked at using a combination of aspirin and an anti-ulcer drug to try to prevent Barrett's esophagus from forming in patients with long-term heartburn. Aspirin has been found in previous studies to reduce cases of esophageal cancer. However, since one of its side effects is an increased risk of stomach **ulcers**, the researchers were including an effective anti-ulcer drug for participants.

Resources

PERIODICALS

"Aspirin Trial Launched to Block Heartburn's Switch to Cancer." *Drug Week* (January 23, 2004): 188.

Bealfsky, Peter C., and William Halsey. "An Endoscopic View of a Wireless pH–Monitoring Capsule." *Ear, Nose and Throat Journal* (April 2003): 254.

Olafsdottir, Linda Bjork, et al. "Natural History of Heartburn: A 10-year Population-Based Study." *World Journal of Gastroenterology* 17, no. 5 (2011): 639–45.

Orlando, Roy, Sherry Liu, and Marta Illueca. "Relationship between Esomeprazole Dose and Timing to Heartburn Resolution in Selected Patients with Gastroesophageal Reflux Disease." *Clinical and Experimental Gastroenterology* 3 (September 2010): 117–25.

Savarino, E., et al. "Functional Heartburn Has More in Common with Functional Dyspepsia Than with Non-Erosive Reflux Disease." *Gut* 58, no. 9 (2011): 1185–91.

WEBSITES

International Foundation for Functional Gastrointestinal Disorders. "When Is Simple Heartburn Not So Simple?" http://www.iffgd.org/site/news-events/press-releases/2007-1118-when-is-simple-heartburn-not-so-simple (accessed October 2, 2012).

Mayo Clinic staff. "Heartburn." MayoClinic.com. http://www.mayoclinic.com/health/heartburn-gerd/DS00095 (accessed October 2, 2012).

MedlinePlus. "Heartburn." U.S. National Library of Medicine, National Institutes of Health. http://www.nlm.nih.gov/medlineplus/heartburn.html (accessed October 2, 2012).

ORGANIZATIONS

American College of Gastroenterology (ACG), PO Box 3099, Alexandria, VA 22302, (800) HRT-BURN (478-2876), https://www.healthtouch.com.

American Gastroenterological Association, 4930 Del Ray Ave., Bethesda, MD 20814, (301) 654-2055, Fax: (301) 654-5920, member@gastro.org, http://www.gastro.org.

American Society for Gastrointestinal Endoscopy, 1520 Kensington Rd., Ste. 202, Oak Brook, IL 60523, (866) 353-2743, http://www.asge.org.

International Foundation for Functional Gastrointestinal Disorders, PO Box 170864, Milwaukee, WI 53217, (414) 964-1799, (888) 964-2001, Fax: (414) 964-7176, iffgd@iffgd.org, http://www.iffgd.org.

National Digestive Diseases Information Clearinghouse, 2 Information Way, Bethesda, MD 20892–3570, (800) 891–5389, TTY: (866) 569–1162, Fax: (703) 738–4929, nddic@info.niddk.nih.gov, http://www.digestive.niddk.nih.gov.

Lorraine Lica, PhD
Teresa G. Odle

Heart-healthy diets

Definition

A heart-healthy diet is an eating plan designed to keep blood cholesterol low and prevent the risk of cardiovascular (heart) disease. This is usually achieved

Healthy heart diets

	NHLBI heart healthy diet guidelines	Therapeutic Lifestyle Changes (TLC) diet guidelines	American Heart Association diet and lifestyle guidelines
Saturated fat	8%–10% of the day's total calories	Less than 7% of the day's total calories	Less than 7% of the day's total calories
Total fat	30% or less of the day's total calories	25%–35% or less of the day's total calories	25%–35% or less of the day's total calories
Dietary cholesterol	Less than 300 milligrams a day	Less than 200 milligrams a day	Less than 300 milligrams a day
Sodium	Less than 2,400 milligrams a day	Less than 2,400 milligrams a day	Less than 1,500 milligrams a day
Calories	Enough calories to achieve or maintain a healthy weight and reduce blood cholesterol level	Enough calories to achieve or maintain a healthy weight and reduce blood cholesterol level	Number of calories based on age, gender, height, weight, and physical activity level, and whether trying to lose, gain, or maintain weight

(Table by PreMediaGlobal. © 2013 Cengage Learning.)

by eating foods that are low in saturated fat, *trans* fat, total fat, cholesterol, and **sodium**.

Origins

The original Healthy Heart diet arose out of ongoing nutrition research by organizations including the U.S. Department of Agriculture (USDA) and the American Heart Association (AHA). The USDA first issued dietary recommendations for Americans in an 1894 Farmer's Bulletin, according to the 1996 USDA report *Dietary Recommendations and How They Have Changed Over Time*. The recommendations came from W. O. Atwater, first director of the USDA's Office of Experiment Stations. He proposed a diet for American men based on **protein, carbohydrates**, fat, and mineral matter. In a 1902 Farmer's Bulletin, he warned about the danger of a diet consisting of too much protein or fuel ingredients (carbohydrates and fat). In 1941, the USDA first issued the recommended dietary allowances (RDAs). The allowances covered areas like calorie intake and nine essential nutrients: protein, **iron, calcium, vitamins** A and D, **thiamin, riboflavin, niacin**, and ascorbic acid (**Vitamin C**). The USDA also released national food guides during the 1940s. The guides provided a foundation diet with recommendations for foods that contained the majority of nutrients. The guide was modified in 1956 with recommended minimum portions from food groups that the USDA called the "Big Four": milk, meats, fruits and vegetables, and grain products.

The guides remained in effect until the 1970s, when an increasing amount of research showed a relationship between the overconsumption of fat, saturated fat, cholesterol, and sodium, and the risk of chronic diseases, such as heart disease and stroke. In 1979, the USDA guide included the Big Four and a fifth category

that included **fats**, sweets, and alcoholic beverages. The following year, the USDA and the U.S. Department of Health and Human Services (HHS) issued the first edition of the *Dietary Guidelines for Americans*. The USDA and HHS update the federal guidelines every five years. *Dietary Guidelines for Americans 2010* features more specific recommendations for adults and children in response to the growing concern in the United States with being overweight and obese.

The National Heart, Lung, and Blood Institute (NHLBI), part of the National Institutes of Health (NIH), is one source of information for the **dietary guidelines**. The institute developed both the Healthy Heart diet and the Therapeutic Lifestyle Changes diet (**TLC diet**), which are aimed at keeping cholesterol low and promoting overall health. The American Heart Association (AHA) is a nonprofit organization also concerned with educating the public about the relationship between diet and heart health. The organization's public education activities include issuing nutritional guidelines that are periodically revised. They reflect current scientific thinking on the importance of diet and exercise in preventing heart disease, a combination endorsed by the medical community and public health organizations.

Description

Heart-healthy diets share fundamental elements about how to prevent heart disease. The process starts with an understanding of why some foods should be avoided and others are beneficial to the heart. The first step is for the person to be aware of how food affects heart health.

An internal delivery system

The heart is a muscle, and the body's muscles require a steady supply of oxygen and nutrients. This supply is brought to the heart by blood in the coronary arteries. Heart-healthy diets are designed to keep the coronary arteries open for the delivery of oxygen and nutrients. When the arteries become narrow or clogged, the heart will not receive enough blood. This blockage causes coronary heart diseases. If the heart does not receive enough of the blood containing oxygen, the person feels a chest pain, which is known as angina. If the coronary artery is totally blocked off and no blood reaches the heart, the person experiences a heart attack.

The narrowing or clogging of the arteries is known as atherosclerosis. The blockages are caused by deposits of cholesterol and fat. Cholesterol is a soft, waxy substance that is similar to fats (lipids). Cholesterol occurs naturally and is found throughout the body in the bloodstream and cells.

Cholesterol's functions

Cholesterol is used by the body to produce **Vitamin D**, hormones, and the bile acids that dissolve food, according to the NHLBI. However, the body does not need much cholesterol to perform those functions, and the extra cholesterol is deposited in the arteries.

Cholesterol and fats do not dissolve in the bloodstream and are moved through the body by lipoproteins. These are a combination of a lipid (fat) surrounded by a protein, according to the AHA. Total cholesterol consists of low-density lipoprotein (LDL), high-density lipoprotein (HDL), and very low-density lipoprotein (VLDL).

VLDL carries **triglycerides**, a form of blood fat that could affect the heart. LDL is known as "bad" cholesterol, and HDL is known as "good" cholesterol. HDL may help the body by clearing fat from the blood and removing extra cholesterol, according to the AHA.

The body produces LDL and receives more of it from food. When foods rich in cholesterol and some fats are consumed, the body creates more LDL. The **dietary cholesterol** comes from animal products, such as meat. Also contributing to the LDL build-up are foods that are high in **trans fats** and saturated fats.

Fat facts

Food contains three types of fats that should be monitored on a heart-healthy diet:

• Saturated fat is the popular term for saturated fatty acid. Saturated fat tends to raise cholesterol levels and is found in meat, poultry, whole-milk dairy products (including cheese and butter), cocoa butter, lard, and tropical vegetable oils (such as coconut and palms oils). Saturated fat remains solid at room temperature.

• *Trans* fat is a type of vegetable oil that was processed to make the liquid more solid. The process, called hydrogenation, produces hydrogenated and partially hydrogenated vegetable oils. These oils are found in stick margarine, vegetable shortening, commercial fried food, and baked goods (such as cookies and crackers).

• Unsaturated fats include polyunsaturated fats and monounsaturated fats. Polyunsaturated fats are found in fish, walnuts, corn oil, and safflower oil. Monounsaturated fats are found in avocados, olives, olive oil, canola oil, and peanut oil.

Saturated and *trans* fats contribute to high LDL cholesterol and an increased risk of heart disease. Unsaturated fats, on the other hand, promote higher levels of HDL cholesterol and help keep overall cholesterol in check. The AHA recommends limiting total fat intake to 25%–35% of daily calorie intake, with no more than 7% coming from saturated fats and less than 1% from *trans* fats. The majority of fats should come from poly- and monounsaturated sources.

Sodium

Sodium and salt are sometimes used interchangeably in information about heart-healthy diets. The AHA recommends that people consume less than 2,300 milligrams (mg) of salt per day. This amounts to about 1 teaspoon of salt. Some organizations recommend a slightly higher amount of less than 2,400 mg. The recommended amount is for healthy people and may be lower for people with some health conditions.

The diets of most Americans contain too much salt, and processed foods are generally the source of this sodium. A diet high in salt tends to raise blood pressure, and this could lead to heart disease, stroke, and kidney damage.

Reducing the amount of sodium in a diet will lower blood pressure and aid in reaching healthy cholesterol levels. In addition, foods high in potassium (such as bananas, dates, dried apricots, prunes, raisins, and avocados) counteract some of the effect of sodium on blood pressure, according to the USDA guidelines.

Creating a heart-healthy diet

The U.S. federal government and the AHA are among the organizations that provide recommendations for a healthy lifestyle. The recommendations frequently parallel those of the NHLBI's Healthy Heart diet, a plan that emphasizes the consumption of less fat, less cholesterol, and less sodium. There is also agreement that diets should include fiber-rich foods like fruits, vegetables, and whole-grain products.

Guidelines also focus on the importance of regular physical activity to prevent or lower the risk of conditions such as heart disease. Generally, people are advised to exercise at least 30 minutes most days of the week. While some recommendations are designed for healthy people, the guidelines also apply to a heart-healthy diet. There may be more specific instructions in plans to lower cholesterol levels.

DIETARY GUIDELINES FOR AMERICANS 2010. *Nutrition and Your Health: Dietary Guidelines for Americans* defines a healthy eating plan as one that:

- emphasizes fruits, vegetables, whole grains, and fat-free or low-fat milk and milk products
- includes lean meats, poultry, fish, beans, eggs, and nuts
- is low in saturated fats, *trans* fats, cholesterol, salt, and added sugars
- lists that total fat intake should be between 20%–35% of the daily calories consumed

On February 31, 2011, the USDA and the HHS announced the 2010 *Dietary Guidelines for Americans*. The 2010 release is the seventh edition of the dietary guidelines. The new version of the guidelines was developed to help combat the increasing **obesity** problem in the United States, and focuses on providing recommendations that are easy for busy people to put into practice in their daily lives.

Some additional guidelines added in 2010 include:

- Enjoy your food, but eat less.
- Avoid oversized portions.
- Make half your plate fruits and vegetables
- Drink water instead of sugary drinks.
- Switch to fat-free or low-fat milk.

The 2010 guidelines also include a wide variety of other recommendations. The two overarching themes of the recommendations are maintaining calorie balance over time to achieve and sustain a healthy weight and consuming nutrient-dense foods and beverages. The full text of the recommendations, as well as a variety of interactive tools and other helpful nutrition information, can be found online at http://health.gov/dietaryguidelines/2010.asp.

People can create a diet following these guidelines by using online tools like the USDA's ChooseMyPlate (formerly MyPyramid) plan and calculators on the NHLBI pages for the Heart Healthy and TLC diets. Some Internet sites produce an individualized plan with specific calorie amounts, recommended foods, serving portions, and a system to track physical activity.

AMERICAN HEART ASSOCIATION DIET AND LIFESTYLE RECOMMENDATIONS. The AHA's plan starts with the person determining how many **calories** are needed to maintain a healthy weight. People are advised not to eat more calories than they burn through activity. They should create a meal plan that includes:

- a variety of vegetables and fruits and unrefined, whole-grain foods
- fish at least twice a week, including oily fish such as salmon, trout, and, which herring, which contain long-chain omega-3 fatty acids (these acids may help reduce the risk of fatal coronary disease)
- lean meats and poultry without skin (and prepared without added saturated or *trans* fats)
- less than 300 milligrams (0.3 grams) of cholesterol each day
- no more than a moderate amount of alcohol, with one drink per day for women and two drinks per day for men
- fat-free, 1% fat, or low-fat dairy products
- food containing little or no salt

The association advises the public to cut back on:

- foods containing hydrogenated or partially hydrogenated vegetable oils to reduce *trans* fat in their diets
- foods high in dietary cholesterol
- beverages and foods with added sugars

The association certifies grocery products that meet the organization's standards. Certification on packaging is indicated by a red heart with a white check mark. Products with that symbol meet association criteria for recommended amounts of saturated fat and cholesterol for healthy people above the age of 2. The standard certification designation is based on one serving that contains 1 gram or less of saturated fat, 20 milligrams or less of cholesterol, and 480 milligrams or less of sodium. The whole-grains certification is issued to foods containing those quantities and an amount of whole-grain at a proportion of 51% by weight with reference to the amount customarily consumed.

THE NHLBI HEART HEALTHY DIET. The NHLBI recommends that meal planning for the Healthy Heart diet be based on these guidelines:

- A person should eat just enough calories to achieve or maintain a healthy weight and reduce blood cholesterol level—a doctor or registered dietitian can determine what a reasonable calorie level is.

• Saturated fat should account for 8%–10% of the day's total calories.

• Total fat should be 30% or less of the day's total calories.

• Dietary cholesterol should be limited to less than 300 milligrams (0.3 grams) per day.

• Sodium intake should be limited to 2,400 milligrams (2.4 grams) a day.

The NHLBI website features heart-healthy diet guidelines and an online tool to create a personal eating plan. The online activity starts with the person providing information about height, weight, gender, age, and level of physical activity. This action generates a recommendation for a daily calorie allowance. That allowance is used to determine the percentage of total fat and saturated fat permitted at that calorie level. The consumer then receives prompts to select food choices for three meals and a snack.

As information is received, the person sees the amounts of calories, fats, cholesterol, and sodium that would be consumed. After the final entry is made, the nutritional information is totaled. The total is compared with the recommended amounts. Along with that data are recommendations on how to modify the meal plan to lower fat and cholesterol consumption.

THE TLC DIET. The Therapeutic Lifestyles Changes (TLC) diet helps to lower the cholesterol of people who have a heart disease or are at risk of developing one. The TLC section of the NHLBI contains online tools similar to those for the Healthy Heart diet. The guidelines for the low-saturated fat, low-cholesterol TLC diet are:

• The person should eat just enough calories to achieve or maintain a healthy weight and reduce the blood cholesterol level.

• Saturated fat should account for less than 7% of the daily total calorie total.

• Fat consumed should amount to no more than 25%–35% of the day's total calories.

• The person should eat less than 200 milligrams (0.2 grams) of dietary cholesterol per day.

• Sodium intake should be limited to 2,400 milligrams (2.4 grams) per day.

Function

Heart-healthy diets help reduce the risk of cardiac disease. This is achieved by the consumption of foods that keep total cholesterol and LDL cholesterol at healthy levels. A heart-healthy diet may involve lowering cholesterol levels by reducing the amount of foods high in cholesterol, fat, and sodium. At the

---

---

same time, people should work to increase HDL levels through diet and exercise.

A heart-healthy diet is a lifelong process that starts with education about the effects of food on the heart. People on this diet learn to make wise food choices, relying on information including the nutritional labels on processed food. The labels provide information about the calories, fats, sodium, and **sugar** in a single serving of the product.

Benefits

Heart-healthy diets are intended to help people lower their cholesterol levels and reduce their risks of cardiovascular disease. Heart-healthy diets can be preventive and, since they employ basic principles of healthy eating, are considered safe for people ages 2 and older to follow. Parents who place their children on heart-healthy diets not only help them with physical health but also give their children the basics for a lifetime of healthy habits.

The NHLBI Healthy Heart diet and other formal diets can also be used as weight loss plans to help obese and overweight people shed excess pounds. Obesity is a risk factor for heart disease, as are diabetes and high blood pressure. People diagnosed with these conditions will benefit from a following a heart-healthy diet in addition to the treatments recommended by their doctors.

Because heredity is a risk factor for heart disease and high cholesterol, people with a family history of either condition may wish to follow a heart-healthy diet. The NHLBI defines a person at higher risk of developing heart disease as someone with a father or brother diagnosed with this condition before the age of 55 or someone with a mother or sister with this condition diagnosed before the age of 65.

Furthermore, cholesterol levels rise as a person ages. The level rises in men at age 45 and older. For women, the increase is generally seen at age 55 and older, according to NHLBI.

Precautions

Heart-healthy diets are safe for people ages 2 and older. However, some people may need to consult their doctor before eating some foods, such as fish. In 2004, the United States Food and Drug Administration and the Environmental Protection Agency warned pregnant women and nursing mothers to limit their consumption of fish and shellfish to 12 ounces (340.2 grams) per week. The warning was issued because of the risk that toxins in seafood would cause developmental problems in babies and children. Furthermore, women who are pregnant or nursing should not eat shark, marlin, and swordfish because of the high mercury content in these fish.

Risks

When following a heart-healthy diet, people need to be aware of the nutritional content of the foods they consume. They need to evaluate that information and make wise food choices. For example, the AHA points out that nuts and seeds are cholesterol-free sources of protein and a source of unsaturated fat. However, nuts and seeds are high in calories. Furthermore, frozen meals that are low in calories and fat should be examined for their sodium content.

Nuts, seeds, and frozen foods can be part of a heart-healthy diet. However, people need to observe nutritional recommendations for daily fat, sodium, and calorie allowances. Otherwise, their diet will aggravate a condition, such as high blood pressure or obesity.

Research and general acceptance

More than a century ago, W. O. Atwater of the USDA cautioned about the dangers of overeating. His warning proved accurate. Cardiovascular disease

(CVD) has been the leading cause of death in the United States in each year since 1900, with the exception of 1918, according to the American Heart Association's *Heart Disease and Stroke Statistics—2012 Update*. The AHA compiles the statistical report annually in conjunction with government agencies.

According to the 2012 report, CVD accounted for 32.8% (811,940) of all 2,471,984 deaths in 2008, or about 1 of every 3 deaths in the United States. In addition, over 2,200 Americans die of CVD each day, which is an average of 1 death every 39 seconds. About 150,000 Americans who died from CVD in 2008 were 65 years of age or older. In 2008, 33% of deaths due to CVD occurred before the age of 75 years, well before the average life expectancy of 77.9 years.

By the 1970s, research showed the link between chronic diseases, like heart disease and stroke, and a diet high in fat, saturated fat, cholesterol, and sodium. Research since then has affirmed the connection between poor diet and increased risk of disease.

During those years, Americans ate more of the foods that put them at risk for heart disease. The average calorie consumption rose 16% between 1970 and 2003, according to the USDA figures cited in the AHA report. In 2008, according to the report, 149,399,999 American adults were overweight or obese (excessively overweight). This represented 67.3% of the adult population. Of those people, 33.7% were obese. The AHA report indicated that being in a particular race, ethnic group, or gender did not matter when it came to being overweight or obese. Among children 2 to 19 years of age, 31.7% were overweight or obese, or 23.6 million. Of that number, 12.6 million were obese (16.9%).

Being obese increases the risk of early mortality. It is also associated with the development of **diabetes mellitus**, **coronary heart disease**, stroke, heart failure, asthma, **cancer**, **hypertension**, degenerative joint disease, and many other diseases and conditions. Increase in caloric intake in the United States has been shown to be concentrated to greater carbohydrate intake, especially of starches, refined grains, and sugars. The AHA reports that this increase is also due to larger portion sizes, more calories eaten per meal, increased consumption of sugar-sweetened beverages, more snacks, increased consumption of commercially prepared meals (especially fast-foods), and additional higher energy-density (high-calorie) foods. Federal agencies and organizations are responding with a range of programs to promote the benefits of heart-healthy diets.

Resources

BOOKS

American Heart Association. *American Heart Association No-Fad Diet: A Personal Plan for Healthy Weight Loss.* 2nd ed. New York: Clarkson Potter, 2011.

OTHER

Davis, Carole, and Etta Sallow. "Dietary Recommendations and How They Have Changed Over Time." In *America's Eating Habits: Changes and Consequences*, edited by Elizabeth Frazao. U.S. Department of Agriculture, Economic Research Service, Food and Rural Economics Division, Agriculture Information Bulletin no. 750, May 1999. http://www.ers.usda.gov/publications/aib-agricultural-information-bulletin/aib750.aspx (accessed August 23, 2012).

WEBSITES

American Heart Association. "Diet and Lifestyle Recommendations." http://www.heart.org/HEARTORG/GettingHealthy/Diet-and-Lifestyle-Recommendations_UCM_305855_Article.jsp (accessed August 3, 2012).

———. "Heart and Stroke Statistics (2012)." http://www.heart.org/HEARTORG/General/Heart-and-Stroke-Association-Statistics_UCM_319064_SubHomePage.jsp (accessed August 3 2012).

———. "Lifestyle Changes." http://www.heart.org/HEARTORG/Conditions/HeartAttack/PreventionTreatmentofHeartAttack/Lifestyle-Changes_UCM_303934_Article.jsp (accessed August 3, 2012).

———. "Nutrition Center." http://www.heart.org/HEARTORG/GettingHealthy/NutritionCenter/Nutrition-Center_UCM_001188_SubHomePage.jsp (accessed August 3, 2012).

Centers for Disease Control and Prevention, National Center for Chronic Disease Prevention and Health Promotion. "Obesity: Halting the Epidemic by Making Health Easier." http://www.cdc.gov/chronicdisease/resources/publications/aag/obesity.htm (accessed August 3, 2012).

ChooseMyPlate.gov. U.S. Department of Agriculture. http://www.choosemyplate.gov (accessed August 3, 2012).

Mayo Clinic staff. "Heart-Healthy Diet: 8 Steps to Prevent Heart Disease." MayoClinic.com. http://www.mayoclinic.com/health/heart-healthy-diet/NU00196 (accessed August 3, 2012).

MedlinePlus. "Diets." U.S. National Library of Medicine, National Institutes of Health. http://www.nlm.nih.gov/medlineplus/diets.html (accessed August 3, 2012).

National Heart, Lung, and Blood Institute. "Healthy Weight Tools." National Institutes of Health. http://www.nhlbi.nih.gov/health/public/heart/obesity/lose_wt/tools.htm (accessed August 3, 2012).

———. "Reduce Salt and Sodium in Your Diet." http://www.nhlbi.nih.gov/hbp/prevent/sodium/sodium.htm (accessed August 3, 2012).

U.S. Department of Agriculture. "Food and Nutrition." http://www.usda.gov/wps/portal/usda/usdahome?navid=FOOD_NUTRITION&navtype=SU (accessed August 3, 2012).

U.S. Department of Agriculture and U.S. Department of Health and Human Services. *Dietary Guidelines for Americans, 2010.* 7th ed. Washington, DC: U.S. Government Printing Office, December 2010. http://health.gov/dietaryguidelines (accessed February 22, 2012).

ORGANIZATIONS

Academy of Nutrition and Dietetics, 120 South Riverside Plz., Ste. 2000, Chicago, IL 60606-6995, (312) 899-0040, (800) 877-1600, amacmunn@eatright.org, http://www.eatright.org.

American Heart Association, 7272 Greenville Ave., Dallas, TX 75231, (800) 242-8721, http://www.americanheart.org.

National Heart, Lung, and Blood Institute, PO Box 30105, Bethesda, MD 20824-0105, (301) 592-8573, TTY: (240) 629-3255, Fax: (240) 629-3246, nhlbiinfo@nhlbi.nih.gov, http://www.nhlbi.nih.gov.

Liz Swain
Tish Davidson, AM

Hemorrhoids

Definition

Hemorrhoids, also called piles, refers to a condition in which the veins around the anus or rectum are swollen and inflamed. Dietary adjustments are known to help relieve hemorrhoids.

Origins

Ten million people in the United States have hemorrhoids, leading to a prevalence greater than 4%. Up to a third of these people require medical treatment, resulting in 1.5 million prescriptions per year. The peak age for hemorrhoids is 45–65 years. The term hemorrhoid is usually related to symptoms caused by hemorrhoids. Hemorrhoids can occur in healthy individuals. It is when they become enlarged, inflamed, or prolapsed that most people refer to the condition as hemorrhoids. They are rarely a serious risk to health and result from too much pressure on the hemorrhoidal veins in the rectum. The strain of **constipation**, diarrhea, or pregnancy can cause the veins to swell. Other factors such as **obesity** and liver disease can also increase pressure and cause hemorrhoids. There are three types of hemorrhoids:

- Internal hemorrhoids: Internal hemorrhoids cannot be seen; they are inside the anus. Straining or irritation from passing stool can injure a hemorrhoid's delicate surface and cause bleeding. Because internal anal membranes lack pain-sensitive nerve endings, these hemorrhoids usually do not cause discomfort.
- External hemorrhoids: These hemorrhoids are under the skin around the anus and tend to be painful. Sometimes blood may collect in an external hemorrhoid and form a clot, causing severe pain, swelling and inflammation. When irritated, external hemorrhoids can itch or bleed.
- Prolapsed hemorrhoids: These are internal hemorrhoids that are so distended that they are pushed outside the anus.

In the absence of complications, treatment usually involves over-the-counter corticosteroid creams that can reduce the pain and swelling of hemorrhoids and bathing in tubs with warm water to ease painful perianal conditions. Another important step in treating hemorrhoids is to relieve anal pressure and straining. This can often be done by controlling constipation with a **high-fiber diet**.

Description

Foods that are high in **fiber** have been shown to help in the treatment of constipation and hemorrhoids. The American Academy of Family Physicians recommends the following simple **dietary guidelines** to prevent or lower hemorrhoids symptoms:

- Eat at least 4.5 cups of fruits and vegetables each day.
- Replace white bread with whole-grain breads and cereals.
- Eat bran cereal for breakfast.
- Add 1/4 cup of wheat bran (Miller's bran) to foods such as cooked cereal or applesauce or meat loaf.

(This advice is contrary to other experts and organizations, who advise against this practice as it can make constipation worse.)

- Eat cooked beans each week.

In its most recent public health recommendations for dietary fiber, the National Academy of Sciences established an adequate intake (AI) level of 38 g of total daily fiber for males 19–50 years of age and 25 g for women in this same age range. The following foods are excellent sources of dietary fiber and can be included as part of a hemorrhoid diet:

- cinnamon, ground, 2 tsp (2.5 g)
- turnip greens, cooked, 1 cup (5.0 g)
- basil, dried, ground, 2 tsp (1.2 g)
- coriander seeds, 2 tsp (1.4 g)
- oregano, dried, ground, 2 tsp (1.3 g)
- raspberries, 1 cup (8.3 g)
- thyme, dried, ground, 2 tsp (1.1 g)
- mustard greens, boiled, 1 cup (2.8 g)
- rosemary, dried, 2 tsp (0.9 g)
- romaine lettuce, 2 cups (1.9 g)
- cauliflower, boiled, 1 cup (3.4 g)
- collard greens, boiled, 1 cup (5.3 g)
- broccoli, steamed, 1 cup (4.7 g)
- cloves, dried, ground, 2 tsp (1.5 g)
- celery, raw, 1 cup (2.0 g)
- swiss chard, boiled, 1 cup (3.7 g)
- cabbage, shredded, boiled, 1 cup (3.5 g)
- spinach, boiled, 1 cup (4.3 g)
- chili pepper, dried, 2 tsp (2.6 g)
- black pepper, 2 tsp (1.1 g)
- fennel, raw, sliced, 1 cup (2.7 g)
- green beans, boiled, 1 cup (4.0 g)
- eggplant, cooked, 1 cup (2.5 g)
- cayenne pepper, dried, 2 tsp (1.0 g)
- cranberries, 1/2 cup (2.0 g)
- strawberries, 1 cup (3.3 g)
- bell peppers, red, raw, 1 cup (1.8 g)
- winter squash, baked, 1 cup (5.7 g)
- kale, boiled, 1 cup (2.6 g)
- split peas, cooked, 1 cup (16.3 g)
- summer squash, cooked, 1 cup (2.5 g)
- carrots, raw, 1 cup (3.7 g)
- lentils, cooked, 1 cup (15.6 g)
- Brussels sprouts, boiled, 1 cup (4.1 g)
- asparagus, boiled, 1 cup (2.9 g)
- black beans, cooked, 1 cup (15.0 g)

which is a type of marketing plan that uses direct marketing along with franchisers and/or independent contractors to sell its products. According to the company's website, "Herbalife's innovative products have been developed by scientists, doctors and nutritionists with your personal wellness goals in mind."

Herbalife is headquartered in Los Angeles, California, with more than 5,000 employees worldwide. The company is part of the nutrition and skin care products industry. It sells a wide range of herbal, botanical, and other health-based products including Male Factor 1000, 21-Day Herbal Cleansing, Nite-Works, HeartBar, Shapeworks, MentalBalance, Health & Fitness Bulk & Muscle Program, Derma-jetics skin care products, Cell-U-Loss supplement, and Nature's Raw Guyana. Herbalife sells products in 84 countries, and has annual retail sales of $3 billion. Over two million (qualified and unqualified) independent distributors are associated with the company.

Purpose

According to information contained in the Herbalife website, the company sells its products to consumers so they can manage and control their weight, add nutritional supplements to their diets, and provide personal care items to their daily body regimen. Weight management and weight-loss products include **protein** snacks, enhancers for energy support, enhancers for appetite support, and enhancers for digestive support. Nutritional supplements sold by the company include herbs, **minerals**, and **vitamins**. Some of its nutritional supplements are devoted to specific body parts such as the heart and digestive system, and on certain physical and mental conditions such as stress, energy/fitness, and aging. Its personal care products emphasize nutritional and herbal ingredients such as aloe vera and **vitamin C**, and deal with such matters as skin essentials and skin revitalizers, anti-aging, body essentials, hair essentials, and fragrances.

The Herbalife mission, according to its website, is to "change people's lives by providing the best business opportunity in direct selling and the best nutrition and weight management products in the world." The company states that it provides safe weight control products that supplement a balanced low-calorie diet and a regular exercise program. Its weight management and nutritional products use macronutrient and micronutrient food formulas. **Macronutrients** include **carbohydrates**, **fats**, and proteins, which together provide most of the energy needed by humans. Micronutrients are essential elements (minerals and vitamins) that are needed in minute quantities for a healthy body. Such essential elements include **chromium**, cobalt, **copper**, **iron**, **manganese**, **molybdenum**, **selenium**, and **zinc**.

As part of their advertising and marketing strategy, Herbalife relies on testimonials from health professionals. Customer testimonials also appear on the company's website.

Description

The company was incorporated in 1979, but essentially started operations in February 1980 when its first distributor, Mark Hughes, began selling Herbalife products from the trunk of his automobile. As his customers tried and liked the products, Hughes's business quickly grew. He rented an office and a warehouse in the Beverly Hills, California area, and soon developed a network of distributors.

Within two years, the company had grown to over two million dollars in sales through its distributorships in the United States and its sole distributor in Canada. Vehicles all over the United States were seen with the company's slogan: "Lose weight now, ask me how!" At this time, the Herbalife plan recommended only one meal each day, which was supplemented with protein powders and nutritional pills.

By 1985, Herbalife was listed on *INC.* magazine's fastest growing private companies. Its five-year profits from 1980 to 1985 went from $386,000 to $423 million. More than 700,000 distributors in the United States, Canada, the United Kingdom, and Australia had total gross sales of about $500 million.

In 1994, Hughes started the Herbalife Family Foundation in order to help children worldwide. In 1996, Herbalife reached one billion dollars in sales. However, four years later, Hughes died from an overdose of alcohol and doxepin (a psychoactive drug with antidepressant and anti-anxiety properties).

Today, signs posted on telephone poles, fences, mailboxes, newsstands, vehicle windshields, and other public structures and locations state such slogans as: "Lose Weight Now—Ask Me How," "Have a Computer?—Work from Home," and "Lose 30 lbs in 30 days!" These and other advertising means are often seen promoting a way for people to earn cash. When people call the toll-free number or browse the listed website they are directed to Herbalife.

Precautions

Historically, there has been controversy with Herbalife due to the way the company operates its business. This controversy, specifically, has been directed to potentially dangerous ingredients in some products, perceived inaccurate marketing claims, and unconventional distribution methods. Company supporters stress that Herbalife is a profitable and reputable business that is a member of the New York Stock Exchange (NYSE). Critics state that the company is run like a pyramid scheme, its independent distributors use improper customer methods, and the company has poor organization and management of distributors.

Some of the early products sold by Herbalife consisted of ma huang (*Ephedra sinica*). The herb contained ephedrine (EPH), which is one of the active ingredients in the plant genus *Ephedra*. Ephedrine was used widely as an appetite suppressant, asthma and hay fever aid, decongestant and cold reliever, and hypotension treatment. Eventually, Herbalife eliminated ephedrine after consumers complained of adverse reactions and its insurance premiums were increased. The U.S. Food and Drug Administration (FDA) banned the sale of all ephedra-containing supplements beginning on April 12, 2004.

In 1981, the FDA began receiving complaints from Herbalife consumers with symptoms of **constipation**, diarrhea, headaches, and nausea from various products. Initially, Herbalife officials informed distributors to tell customers that such symptoms were the result of the removal of poisons and toxins from the body by the use of such products. The FDA acted against Herbalife in 1982 for making claims that its Herbal-Aloe drink helped to treat bowel, kidney, and stomach **ulcers**, and that its Herbalife Formula–2 should be used to treat bursitis, **cancer**, herpes, and impotence. Consequently, the FDA required the company to eliminate the ingredients of mandrake and poke.

The Canadian Department of Justice filed numerous criminal charges against Herbalife for false medical claims and misleading advertising practices in 1984. The California Department of Health, California Attorney General, and FDA brought a civil lawsuit against the company in 1985. The company was charged with misleading consumers, making improper product claims, and operating an illegal "endless-chain" scheme. Herbalife reached an out-of-court settlement by paying $850,000 in costs, fees, and penalties.

In 1986, Herbalife expanded into other countries, including Israel, Japan, Mexico, and New Zealand, after U.S. and Canadian sales declined due to negative news stories. In order to raise cash, the company merged with a Utah-based public company, and called itself Herbalife International.

In 2001, the U.S. Federal Trade Commission (FTC) provided to interested parties, in response to the Freedom of Information Act (FOIA), numerous customer complains against Herbalife International. The customer complaints arc listed in the FTC website at http://www.ftc.gov/foia/herbalife.pdf.

Still later, the company was cited by the U.S. Securities and Exchange Commission (SEC) for numerous violations involving its business practices. Herbalife officials promised to fix their managerial problems. In 2006, the company reported to the SEC that it now annually re-qualifies distributors as a way to better manage its independent contractors.

Complications

Information gleaned from various sources indicate that it is often difficult for Herbalife distributors to make a profit. Initially, they must pay large amounts of money to become a distributor. For example, according to interviews and research performed by Rob Cockcrham (whose website is considered a well-known anti-scam site for Herbalife) between March and July 2002, potential distributors must purchase an informational packet for $36 and, later, an International Business Packet for $195. After completing a distributor's application, the new independent distributor receives a catalog, order forms, sales and marketing manuals, product samples, and other such literature.

The distributor then signs up for Herbalife Advantage Program, which costs $80 each month for informational brochures and Web pages that describe products. In addition, the company recommends that distributors buy a Herbalife diet and skin product website for $315 and a Herbalife business promotion website, also for $315. Furthermore, Gold and Platinum E-Commerce Business Packages cost between $952.90 and $1,994.22.

There are many websites on the Internet that advertise Herbalife products, both on the corporate and individual distributor levels. Distributors, according to Herbalife, can earn up to $250,000 annually. However, the average earning per distributor is estimated at only around $1,500. As independent contractors, distributors do not earn salaries nor benefits from the company.

Parental concerns

Herbalife, as do many other companies, sells products that are not under FDA regulatory protection. The FDA, under the Department of Health and

Human Services, is responsible for the regulation of foods, drugs, **dietary supplements**, biological medical products, blood products, medical devices, radiation-emitting devices, veterinary products, and cosmetics. With respect to dietary supplements, the FDA, under the Dietary Supplement Health and Education Act of 1994, can only take action against manufacturers if their dietary supplements are proven unsafe. Manufacturers can legally claim their products have health benefits; however, they cannot claim these products diagnose, treat, cure, or prevent disease.

Cosmetics are regulated by the FDA's Center for Food Safety and Applied Nutrition. Cosmetics are generally not approved before they reach the marketplace. However, color added to cosmetics must be FDA approved before being sold. The FDA does regulate cosmetic labeling. According to the FDA, cosmetics that have not been thoroughly tested must advise so on their labels.

Network marketing, or multi-level marketing, is legal in most U.S. states under the stipulation that a company's sales force receives earnings from customers other than relatives. In the Herbalife network marketing plan, new distributors buy products up front at 25% off the retail price. Once a distributor buys $2,000 to $4,000 of products, the distributor becomes a supervisor, at which time they get 50% off the retail price. Distributors also become supervisors by bringing other distributors into the network. Distributors then get a percentage of each recruit's sales, generally about 8%. As supervisors increase in rank, they gain the potential to earn more money. This pyramiding of earnings often is criticized as being a pyramid scheme.

In addition, Herbalife sponsors many sporting events that are especially attractive to children and young adults. For instance, the company is a regular sponsor of AVP Pro Beach Volleyball, at times being the event's Official Nutritional Advisor. It has also been (or still is) the sponsor of the JPMorgan Chase Open WTA tennis tournament, the Los Angeles Galaxy, the Tour of California bicycle road race, the Michelob Ultra London Triathlon, the Nautica Malibu Triathlon, and the Thai Airways International Laguna Phuket Triathlon. Parents need to be especially concerned that children do not think that Herbalife products are safe to use based solely on sponsorship in such events.

Before parents give children any unregulated FDA products such as nutritional supplements—whether it be from Herbalife or any other company—they should consult their family doctor. Any company or individual can make, market, and sell nutritional supplements without adhering to quality control requirements

KEY TERMS

Botanical—Relating to plants.

Doxepin—A psychoactive drug characterized with helping treat depression and anxiety.

Macronutrient—Any carbohydrate, fat, or protein.

Micronutrient—Essential elements needed for human life such as minerals and vitamins.

Pyramid scheme—A fraudulent act in which perpetrator(s) recruit other people to pay money to those above them in a structured hierarchy with the expectation that they will get a portion of that money.

from the FDA. They also are not required to perform research to prove the safety or effectiveness of such products. Only products under FDA regulation are required by their manufacturers to perform such activities.

In addition, parents need to be aware that some medical conditions may be adversely affected when used with unregulated products. Even though a product is advertised as being natural, this does not mean it is necessarily safe to use in all situations and with all people. Also, since nutritional supplements are not regulated by the FDA, there is little way to determine if each dosage is identical in quantity and quality with the advertised labeling. In fact, in 2004, the Commission for Scientific Medicine and Mental Health (CSMMH) formally requested that the FDA require manufacturers of herbal remedies and dietary supplements to insert label warnings on products that have been associated with adverse health reactions in consumers.

Resources

BOOKS

Hendler, Sheldon, and David Rorvik. *PDR for Nutritional Supplements.* 2nd ed. Montvale, NJ: Physician's Desk Reference, 2008.

Skidmore-Roth, Linda. *Mosby's Handbook of Herbs and Natural Supplements.* St. Louis, MO: Mosby, 2006.

Talbott, Shawn M. *The Health Professional's Guide to Dietary Supplements.* Philadelphia, PA: Lippincott Williams and Wilkins, 2007.

PERIODICALS

Appelhans, K., et al. "Revisiting Acute Liver Injury Associated with Herbalife Products." *World Journal of Hepatology* 3, no. 10 (2011): 275–77.

WEBSITES

"About Herbalife." http://company.herbalife.com (accessed October 2, 2012).

ORGANIZATIONS

Center for Food Safety and Applied Nutrition (CFSAN), U.S. Food and Drug Administration, 5100 Paint Branch Pkwy., College Park, MD 20740, (888) SAFE-FOOD (723-3366), consumer@fda.gov, http://www.fda.gov/Food/default.htm.

U.S. Food and Drug Administration, 10903 New Hampshire Ave., Silver Spring, MD 20993-0002, (888) INFO-FDA (463-6332), http://www.fda.gov.

William Arthur Atkins

High blood pressure *see* **Hypertension**
High cholesterol *see* **Dietary cholesterol**

High-fat, low-carb diets

Definition

High-fat, low-carb diets promote a high intake of **protein** and fat while severely restricting **carbohydrates**. These diets are based on the premise that high-carbohydrate consumption increases levels of **insulin** in the blood. Insulin is a hormone that helps the body covert food into energy in the form of glucose or **sugar**. High insulin levels have been linked to medical conditions such as type 2 diabetes, cardiovascular disease, and **obesity**.

Origins

The earliest recognized publication of a high-fat, low-carb diet was William Banting's *Letter on Corpulence*, published in 1863, in which Banting reported weight loss and improved health by following a low-carbohydrate diet prescribed by his doctor, William Harvey. Banting suffered from obesity and hearing loss caused by fat compressing his inner ear. After following a low-carb diet, he lost weight and his hearing improved.

In the 1920s, the Epilepsy Center at Johns Hopkins Hospital began to use a high-fat/moderate-protein/low-carbohydrate diet called the ketogenic diet to treat children with intractable, or hard to control, seizures. The Johns Hopkins Epilepsy Center continues to use a modified version of this diet program. Also in the 1920s, explorer Vilhjalmur Stefansson lived for many years with the Inuit people of arctic Canada. Cultures that have historically followed high-fat, low-carb diets, such as that of the Inuit Eskimos, tend to live long, healthy lives and have provided the basis for some of the earliest studies on low-carbohydrate diets. Stefansson's diet consisted exclusively of meat and fish. Since it was a virtually carbohydrate-free diet and high in fat, it was expected that his health would suffer, but upon his return home, his physician (Dr. Clarence Lieb) found him in good health. Lieb was able to duplicate these results later in a yearlong controlled study.

One of the most popular and well-known of high-fat, low-carb diets is the **Atkins diet**, first published in 1972 by cardiologist Robert Atkins. Another example is the **Paleo diet**, based on the Paleolithic way of eating.

Description

Low-carbohydrate diets are based on the premise that weight gain and obesity are tied to inefficient or unhealthy insulin cycles. When consumed, carbohydrates in food are converted to glucose in the body. Glucose raises blood sugar levels and stimulates the body to produce the hormone insulin. Insulin is a hormone that helps the body transport glucose from the bloodstream to cells, where it is used for energy. Any excess glucose is stored in the form of glycogen in the muscles and liver. These glycogen stores are used as fuel by the body when glucose is not available. If the stores are not used, however, they are converted to fat. High-fat, low-carb diets aim to avoid these spikes in blood sugar and reduce the amount of glycogen stored in the body. These diets rely on ketones, which are the products of the incomplete breakdown of fat used for energy when carbohydrates are not available. These diets claim that ketone **metabolism** is a very efficient form of energy production that does not involve the production of insulin, and that the combination of ketone metabolism (ketosis) and the stable insulin levels created in the absence of carbohydrates will lead to rapid weight loss.

High-fat, low-carb diets vary in the number of grams of carbohydrates recommended to be consumed each day. Most diet plans include three or more phases or stages. The earliest stages allow the fewest grams of carbohydrate to be eaten per day and typically last for two weeks. The middle stage is considered the weight-loss stage, and carbohydrate grams are slightly increased and then maintained at that level until the desired weight loss is achieved. During the final phases, carbohydrates are gradually increased until weight loss stops or weight gain begins. At this point, the dieter reduces the amount of carbohydrates consumed until weight has stabilized.

Most low-carb diet plans consider the "optimal" range of carbohydrates to be between 25 and 45 grams per day. This number may vary based on the diet plan and individual—some people on low-carb diets are able to eat up to 100 grams each day.

Carbohydrate counts are determined by counting the number of grams per serving for each meal, minus the food's "net carbs." The net carbs are the total number of carbohydrates found in the food minus the number of grams of **fiber** (per serving). While insoluble fiber is technically a form of carbohydrate, it is not absorbed by the body and does not raise blood insulin levels, so it is not included in the overall carbohydrate count. Soluble fiber does have a modest effect on insulin and blood sugar, but this is not included in the total count. Sugar alcohol is another substance that can be subtracted from the net carbs. It is a chemically altered carbohydrate that adds sweetness to foods but is metabolized more slowly than sugar and is not as readily absorbed.

Glycemic index

Many high-fat, low-carb diets recognize that not all carbohydrates cause spikes in blood sugar levels. Some carbohydrates digest more slowly than others, causing a gradual rise in blood sugar after eating. The glycemic index is a system used to rank carbohydrates and other foods according to the effect they have on blood sugar, based on a scale of 0–100. Foods with higher glycemic index ratings break down quickly and cause a sharp rise in blood sugar. When blood sugar rises quickly, the body produces a surge of insulin to lower the amount of glucose in the blood. Foods with lower glycemic index ratings break down more slowly. They cause a more gradual rise in blood sugar, which means that less insulin will be needed. Lower blood sugar and insulin levels have been shown to prevent or treat type 2 diabetes and heart disease. Lower-glycemic foods are also thought to help with weight loss by promoting satiety, or a feeling of fullness.

Foods that have a high glycemic index rating include white bread, white rice, white potatoes, beer, corn products, and products containing refined sugars. Foods with moderate glycemic index ratings include whole grain breads and pastas, brown rice, sweet potatoes, green peas, many fruits (especially when eaten alone), and yogurt. Low glycemic index foods include rye grain; nuts; legumes, such as black beans and lentils; green vegetables; apricots; and cherries.

Foods that are high in fiber tend to have lower glycemic index numbers, because fiber takes longer to digest. Studies have shown that **fats** like olive oil and acidic products like vinegar can also slow digestion and keep blood sugar from rising too quickly. The glycemic index can be used along with a high-fat, low-carb diet to help choose which carbohydrates can be eaten with the least effect on blood sugar.

Examples of high-fat, low-carb diets

PROTEIN POWER. Developed by doctors Michael and Mary Dan Eades, this diet plan emphasizes adequate protein consumption and limiting carbs to between 20 to 40 grams per day during the initial phase. Consumption is increased to 50 grams per day during the middle phase, and once ideal weight is achieved, consumption is maintained at between 70 to 130 grams per day. Fat is considered neutral, but the authors admit that excessive fat consumption will make weight loss difficult.

EAT FAT, GET THIN. Created by Dr. Barry Groves, this plan allows up to 60 grams of carbohydrate per day until ideal weight is reached. The dieter is then advised to gradually increase the grams of carbohydrates consumed until weight loss stops. Unlimited amounts of meat, fish, poultry, cheese, and eggs are allowed. Sugar, most grains, and breads are eliminated. Fruits are allowed, except for those highest in sugar, such as grapes and bananas. All vegetables are allowed except starchy vegetables (such as potatoes), and green leafy vegetables are encouraged.

LIFE WITHOUT BREAD. Dr. Wolfgang Lutz was an early proponent of high-fat, low-carb eating, and his plan deals primarily with the purported health benefits of the diet. He recommends a carbohydrate limit of no more than 72 grams per day and encourages unlimited meat, non-starchy vegetables, cheese, and natural fats. He advises moderation when eating nuts and other dairy products.

THE DIET CURE. Dr. Julia Ross's plan advises eating 20 grams of protein at each meal and limiting carbohydrates to 20 grams per meal. The plan is called "undieting" and stresses the importance of breakfast, avoiding hunger, and avoiding white flour, sugar, and refined products.

NEANDERTHIN. Nutritionist Ray Audette believes that modern technology and overly processed food are to blame for the obesity epidemic. His Neanderthin plan advises people to eat foods as close to their natural state (raw) as possible. The diet forbids all grains, all beans, all dairy products, and sugar.

THE STONE AGE DIET. In one of the earliest books espousing the benefits of high-fat, low-carb diets, author Richard Mackarness warns against refined sugar, encourages high consumption of fat and protein, and recommends restricting carbohydrates to 60 or fewer grams per day.

THE CARBOHYDRATE ADDICT'S DIET. Authors Richard and Rachel Heller created this plan for people who crave carbohydrates and either consume too many or have a metabolic disorder that causes them to produce too much insulin in response to carbohydrates. The **Carbohydrate Addict's diet** plan includes two low-carb meals a day and one reward meal that allows more carbohydrates. This reward meal must include a large salad to start; must include equal portions of protein, vegetables, and carbohydrates; and must be eaten within a one-hour period. The plan does not count carbohydrate grams; instead, it provides a list of "Craving-Reducing Foods" that are allowed throughout the day.

Function

Most experts agree that high-fat, low-carb diets do cause weight loss, at least initially. The high-protein intake and strict limitation of carbohydrates causes the human body to rid itself of the water stored with glycogen. This rapid loss of fluid causes an initial loss of weight. Ketosis may also cause loss of appetite, resulting in lowered caloric intakes.

Benefits

Current literature indicates that low-carbohydrate dietary meal plans are more effective for short-term weight loss (e.g., six months) than high-carbohydrate diets, but little is known about their long-term influence on chronic disease risk. High-protein diets are associated with satiety, which makes it easier to follow the meal plan for longer periods of time. In one study of overweight men with **hyperlipidemia**, a low-carb, **high-protein diet** was no more effective at lowering blood glucose, insulin, glycolated hemoglobin, and insulin resistance than was a low-fat, high-carb diet. However, this diet was superior at lowering blood lipids (fats). Other studies on high-protein/low-carb diets show similar effects on lipids, but the long-term effects are not known.

Precautions

Anyone interested in following a high-fat, low-carb diet should first talk it over with their physician or other healthcare professional. Patients taking medication for a chronic condition—such as diabetes or hypertension—may require a dosage reduction if a significant amount of weight is lost. A large change in dietary intake may also alter the availability of **vitamins** such as **vitamin K**; therefore, the monitoring of patients receiving anticoagulation therapy is important both before and during the dietary changes. However, no

---

KEY TERMS

Diabetes—A condition in which the body either does not make or cannot respond to the hormone insulin. As a result, the body cannot use glucose (sugar).

Hyperlipidemia—Elevation of lipid levels (fats) in the bloodstream. These lipids include cholesterol, cholesterol compounds, phospholipids, and triglycerides, all carried in the blood as part of large molecules called lipoproteins.

Insulin—A hormone made in the pancreas that is essential for the metabolism of carbohydrates, lipids, and proteins, and that regulates blood sugar levels.

Ketones—Chemicals produced by fat breakdown.

Ketosis—An abnormal increase in the number of ketones in the body, produced when the liver breaks down fat into fatty acids and ketone bodies. Ketosis is a common side effect of low-carbohydrate diets. If continued for a long period of time, ketosis can cause serious damage to the kidneys and liver.

Macronutrient—A nutrient needed in large quantities (protein, carbohydrate, and fat).

Metabolism—The chemical process in the body that converts food into energy.

---

changes in medication levels should be made without the consent of the prescribing physician, and patients with diabetes should not make changes to their diet without first discussing them with a physician.

Ketosis can place significant strain on the kidneys and liver. The kidneys also separate wastes and protein in the bloodstream. Since high-fat, low-carb diets are typically high in protein, they can result in damage to already impaired kidneys. Individuals with liver or kidney disease should not attempt high-fat, low-carb diets because of the risk of kidney failure. A diet high in fats may be harmful to individuals with advanced coronary artery disease or gout. These conditions may be worsened by the increased fat consumption.

This diet is not recommended for women who are pregnant or nursing.

Risks

When restricting carbohydrates, fiber intake also decreases. Insufficient fiber intake can cause **constipation** and may increase the risk of developing diverticulitis, hemorrhoids, and certain types of **cancer**. A high-protein diet has been associated with a higher risk for kidney stones and may also be associated with **calcium** loss, which could result in osteoporosis over time.

The human body does not actually need carbohydrates to survive, but it does need the many vitamins and **minerals** found in carbohydrate-containing foods, such as fruits, vegetables, and **whole grains**. Nutritional deficiencies can occur when certain foods or food groups are restricted or eliminated, and people following high-fat, low-carb or similar diets should meet with their physician or a registered dietitian (RD) to ensure that they are consuming adequate nutrients.

Medical professionals have expressed concerns over the long-term adherence to diets high in saturated fat. The American Heart Association advises against following any diet plan that encourages increased fat consumption and a reduced consumption of a variety of fruits and vegetables, with the concern that these types of diets will lead to increased risk of **coronary heart disease**, stroke, and cancer.

Reports of individuals experiencing ketosis after following a high-fat, low-carb diet are isolated, and many doctors argue that in individuals with normal kidney and liver function, high-fat, low-carb diets will not cause this condition. At least two long-term studies with significant numbers of participants reported no cases of metabolic acidosis (ketosis). Drinking plenty of water will help flush ketones out of the body and regulate bowel movements.

Research and general acceptance

Most carbohydrate-restricted diets tend to encourage consumption of animal products, which may increase the risk of chronic conditions, such as type 2 diabetes. Red and processed meat contain several components that may elevate a person's risk. Heme **iron**, found in meat, can generate reactive hydroxyl radicals from less-reactive ones, such as hydrogen peroxide. Iron deposition in the muscle, liver, and pancreas may cause focal tissue and ß cell damage, which disrupts insulin signaling. Both the Iowa Women's Health and Nurses' Health studies reported positive associations between heme iron intake and type 2 diabetes. Nitrites and nitrates, found in processed meat; their intestinal metabolites nitrosamines; and byproducts formed when grilling meat have also been found to be risk factors for insulin resistance and diabetes in animal studies. In small, randomized trials, individuals with high proportions of saturated fat intake, found in animal products—as opposed to mono- and polyunsaturated fatty acids,

found in plants, fish, and nuts—have been found to have greater insulin resistance and higher type 2 diabetes risk.

Although incompletely understood, the mechanisms responsible for the increased risk may involve changes in cell membrane fluidity, glucose transporter function, and gene expression. In other studies, both unprocessed and processed red meat intakes were positively associated with an increase in type 2 diabetes. One study of over 40,000 participants, published in the *American Journal of Clinical Nutrition*, found that a low-carbohydrate diet high in animal protein and fat was positively associated with the risk of type 2 diabetes in men. Researchers stated that obtaining protein and fat from foods other than red and processed meats—such as chicken, fish, eggs, dairy, legumes, and nuts—may help decrease this risk.

In randomized, controlled studies, both high-protein and low-glycemic index diets usually showed an increase in percentage of body fat lost when compared to high-carbohydrate diets. However, high-carbohydrate, low-glycemic diets have been associated with decreased risk of heart disease. The most promising diet composition based on clinical research includes increased protein through sources like chicken, fish, eggs, low or nonfat dairy, legumes, nuts, and seeds; fat consumption of no more than 30% of total caloric intake, favoring polyunsaturated fats; and carbohydrate intake of between 40%–50% of total **calories**, focusing on the consumption of low-glycemic foods.

In a study of 43,396 Swedish women aged 30–49, published June 2012 in *BMJ*, reduced carbohydrate or increased protein intake was associated with a significantly increased rate of cardiovascular disease. The study data expressed an additional four to five cases of cardiovascular disease per ten thousand women per year compared with those who did not regularly eat a low-carbohydrate, high-protein diet. The study authors expressed that dietary factors associated with the increase in cardiovascular risk could be equivalent to a daily decrease of 20 grams of carbohydrates (equivalent to a small bread roll) and a daily increase of 5 grams of protein (equivalent to one boiled egg).

The modest short-term benefits of high-fat, low-carb diets for weight loss have made these diets appealing, but further research is needed on the long-term effects.

Resources

BOOKS

Allan, Christian, and Wolfgang Lutz. *Life Without Bread: How a Low-Carbohydrate Diet Can Save Your Life.* New York: McGraw-Hill, 2000.

Atkins, Robert. *Atkins New Diet Revolution.* New York: Avon Books, 1992.

Audette, Ray. *Neanderthin: Eat Like a Caveman to Achieve a Lean, Strong, Healthy Body.* New York: St. Martin's Press, 1999.

Eades, Michael, and Mary Eades. *Protein Power.* New York: Bantam Books, 1996.

———. *The 30-Day Low-Carb Solution.* Hoboken, NJ: John Wiley & Sons, Inc, 2003.

Groves, Barry. *Eat Fat Get Thin!* London: Vermillion, 2000.

Heller, Rachel, and Richard Heller. *The Carbohydrate Addict's Diet: The Lifelong Solution to Yo-Yo Dieting.* New York: Signet, 1993.

Ross, Julia. *The Diet Cure: The 8-Step Program to Rebalance Your Body Chemistry and End Food Cravings, Weight Problems, and Mood Swings—Now.* New York: Viking Penguin, 1999.

Schwarzbein, Diana, and Nancy Deville. *The Schwarzbein Principle: The Truth about Losing Weight, Being Healthy and Feeling Younger.* Deerfield Beach, FL: Health Communications, Inc., 1999.

Voegtlin, Walter. *The Stone Age Diet.* New York: Vantage Press, 1975.

PERIODICALS

Chen, T.S., et al. "A Life-Threatening Complication of Atkins Diet." *Lancet* 367 (2006): 958.

Dansinger, M.L., et al. "Comparison of the Atkins, Ornish, Weight Watchers, and Zone Diets for Weight Loss and Heart Disease Risk Reduction: A Randomized Trial." *JAMA* 293 (Jan 2005): 43–53.

de Koning, L., et al. "Low-Carbohydrate Diet Scores and Risk of Type 2 Diabetes in Men." *American Journal of Clinical Nutrition* 93, no. 4 (2011): 844–50.

Friedman, A.L., et al. "Comparative Effects of Low-Carbohydrate High-Protein Versus Low-Fat Diets on the Kidney." *Clinical Journal of the American Society of Nephrology* 7, no. 7 (2012): 1103–11.

Gögebakan O., et al. "Effects of Weight Loss and Long-Term Weight Maintenance with Diets Varying in Protein and Glycemic Index on Cardiovascular Risk Factors: The Diet, Obesity, and Genes (DiOGenes) Study: A Randomized, Controlled Trial." *American Journal of Clinical Nutrition* 86, no. 2 (2007): 276–84.

Lagiou, Pagona. "Low Carbohydrate-High Protein Diet and Incidence of Cardiovascular Diseases in Swedish Women: Prospective Cohort Study." *BMJ* 344 (June 26, 2012). http://dx.doi.org/10.1136/bmj.e4026 (accessed September 10, 2012).

Lieb, C.W. "The Effects on Human Beings of a Twelve-Months Exclusive Meat Diet." *JAMA* 93, no. 1 (1929): 20–22.

McAuley, K.A., et al. "Comparison of High-Fat and High-Protein Diets with a High-Carbohydrate Diet in Insulin-Resistant Obese Women." *Diabetologia* 48, no. 1 (2005): 8–16.

McMillan-Price, J., et al. "Comparison of 4 Diets of Varying Glycemic Load on Weight Loss and Cardiovascular Risk Reduction in Overweight and Obese Young Adults: A Randomized Controlled Trial." *Archives of Internal Medicine* 166, no. 14 (2006): 1466–75.

Pan, A., et al. "Red Meat Consumption and Risk of Type 2 Diabetes: 3 Cohorts of US Adults and an Updated Meta-Analysis." *American Journal of Clinical Nutrition* 94, no. 4 (2011): 1088–96.

ORGANIZATIONS

Academy of Nutrition and Dietetics, 120 S Riverside Plz., Ste. 2000, Chicago, IL 60606, (312) 899-0040, (800) 877-1600, amacmunn@eatright.org, http://www.eatright.org.

American Heart Association, 7272 Greenville Ave., Dallas, TX 75231, (800) 242-8721, http://www.americanheart.org.

Deborah L. Nurmi, MS
Megan Porter, RD

High-fiber diet

Definition

A high-fiber diet is a diet in which an individual consumes foods that meet or exceed the dietary reference intake (DRI) for dietary **fiber** set by the U.S. Institute of Medicine (IOM) of the National Academy of Sciences.

Origins

No single person developed the high-fiber diet. Over the years, researchers have compared the rate of various chronic diseases in populations that had high-fiber diets with those that had lower dietary fiber intake. They found, for example, that native Africans who ate a high-fiber, plant-based diet were

Food sources of fiber

Soluble fiber	Insoluble fiber
Apples	Apples (with skin)
Bananas	Barley
Black beans	Bran and bran cereals
Black-eyed peas	Brown rice
Blackberries	Bulgur
Blueberries	Carrots
Broccoli	Cauliflower
Brussels sprouts	Celery
Chickpeas	Couscous, whole wheat
Citrus fruit (oranges, grapefruit)	Cucumbers
Kidney beans	Green beans
Lentils	Pears (with skin)
Navy beans	Tomatoes
Northern beans	Vegetables, raw
Nuts and seeds	Wheat bran
Oat bran	Whole grain cereals
Oatmeal and foods made with oats	Whole grains
Peaches	Whole wheat breads
Pears	Whole wheat pasta
Peas, dried	Zucchini
Pinto beans	
Plums	
Prunes	
Strawberries	

(Table by GGS Information Services. © 2013 Cengage Learning.)

rarely bothered by **constipation**. However, in industrialized countries where a lot of animal products are consumed, constipation is common. Observations like this encouraged researchers to look at other roles that dietary fiber might play in health. From their findings came a consensus that a high-fiber diet is a healthy diet. This is reflected in the U.S. Department of Agriculture's (USDA) *Dietary Guidelines for Americans*, which encourages people to eat more high-fiber foods such as **whole grains**.

Description

Dietary fiber refers to a group of indigestible carbohydrate-based compounds found in plants. There are two types relevant to human health: insoluble fiber and soluble fiber. Soluble fiber is found in many vegetables and fruits, including carrots, apples, pears, and citrus fruits. Other sources include legumes, barley, oats, and oat bran. Soluble fiber helps to slow digestion so that a person fills full for a longer period of time. This sense of fullness, known as satiety, helps with appetite control and weight loss. Soluble fiber also helps to decrease cholesterol levels, which lowers the risk for heart disease.

Insoluble fiber is found in whole-grain foods, bran, brown rice, and raw vegetables. This fiber, known as roughage, helps move food waste through the digestive system by adding bulk. The increased

bulk causes the walls of the intestine to contract rhythmically (peristalsis) so that waste moves through the large intestine more rapidly. In the colon, most of the water in digested food is reabsorbed into the body, and then the solid waste is eliminated. By passing through the colon more rapidly, less water is reabsorbed from the waste. The stool remains soft and moist and is easy to expel without straining, preventing constipation.

Recommended intake

The U.S. Institute of Medicine (IOM) of the National Academy of Sciences has set **dietary reference intakes (DRIs)** for fiber based on research data that applies to American and Canadian populations. **DRIs** provide nutrition guidance to both health professionals and consumers. The recommendations for fiber are as follows:

- children ages 1–3: 19 grams
- children ages 4–8: 25 grams
- boys ages 9–13: 31 grams
- men ages 14–50: 38 grams
- men 51 and older: 30 grams
- girls ages 9–18: 26 grams
- adult women ages 19–50: 25 grams
- women 51 and older: 21 grams
- pregnant women: 28 grams
- breastfeeding women: 29 grams

Function

The average American consumes only 14 grams of fiber each day, despite extensive research that shows that higher levels of fiber provide increased health benefits. The purpose of a high-fiber diet is to encourage people to eat more fiber in order to receive those health benefits. The high-fiber diet is not designed specifically to be a weight-loss diet, although weight loss may occur as a side effect of the diet.

Benefits

Perhaps the most important health benefit of a high-fiber diet is its potential to protect against heart disease. Multiple large, well-designed studies have shown that soluble fiber can lower blood cholesterol levels. High levels of cholesterol can lead to the build up of plaque, a hard, waxy substance, on the walls of arteries. This can block blood flow and result in stroke or heart attack. The mechanism for lowering cholesterol appears to be connected to the fact that cholesterol binds with soluble fiber in the intestine and can then be eliminated from the body or bile acids. Soluble fiber in oats and oat products appears to be more

KEY TERMS

Adequate intake (AI)—Recommendations for vitamins and minerals that are established when there is not enough evidence to determine a recommended dietary allowance (RDA).

Cholesterol—A waxy substance made by the liver and also acquired through diet. High levels in the blood may increase the risk of cardiovascular disease.

Constipation—Either having fewer than three bowel movements a week or having difficulty passing stools that are often hard, small, and dry.

Diverticular disorders—Disorders that involve the development of diverticula, small pouches in the muscular wall of the large intestine.

effective in lowering cholesterol than soluble fiber from other grains. This finding has been accepted by the American Heart Association, which recommends a high-fiber diet to maintain or improve heart health.

A high-fiber diet can prevent digestive system problems such as constipation, **hemorrhoids**, and diverticulitis by keeping stool soft and easy to expel. Hemorrhoids are swollen veins around the anus caused by straining to eliminate stool. Diverticulitis is a disease in which sections of the intestine bulge out to form pockets (called diverticuli) that can collect food and become infected. Increased bulk and moisture from dietary fiber helps materials move more easily through the intestine and not become trapped in these pockets.

Claims have been made that a diet high in fiber might reduce the risk of colon **cancer**. The theory is that fiber speeds up the elimination of waste from the colon, decreasing the time that cells lining the intestinal wall are exposed to potential cancer-causing agents. A study completed in the mid-2000s followed 80,000 nurses for 16 years and found no relationship between dietary fiber and colon cancer. More research remains to be done in this area.

Precautions

Fiber should be increased in the diet gradually. If fiber intake increases too suddenly, abdominal pain, gas, and diarrhea may result. When eating a high-fiber diet, it is important to drink at least eight glasses (64 oz. or 2 L) of water or other fluids daily. People whose fluid intake must be restricted for medical reasons should avoid a high-fiber diet.

Risks

Few risks are associated with a high-fiber diet in healthy individuals. However, in people with gastrointestinal disorders such as **irritable bowel syndrome** or **inflammatory bowel disease**, a high-fiber diet may irritate the bowel and worsen their symptoms. Likewise, people who have had a surgical weight-loss procedure may be unable to tolerate a high-fiber diet. Adding bran fiber to foods is not recommended due to the risk of poor intakes of some **vitamins** that bind with phytates or oxalates in many high-fiber foods.

Research and general acceptance

Many large, well-designed, long-term studies have been done on the health effects of a diet high in fiber. It is almost universally accepted that health benefits result when individuals meet fiber requirements for their age group. This concept is so well accepted that it has become the official position of the National Institutes of Health and other U.S. government agencies charged with improving the health of the nation.

One contested benefit is fiber's role in the prevention of diverticular disease. Since the 1960s, doctors have advocated a high-fiber diet to prevent the formation of pouches in the digestive system known as diverticula. When many pouches form on the wall of the large intestine, the condition is known as diverticulosis. The presence of these pouches could lead to diverticulitis, a condition where a diverticulum (one pouch) or diverticula in the digestive tract become inflamed or infected. Complications of diverticulitis include infection and bleeding.

A 2012 study of more than 2,100 people between the ages of 30 and 80, conducted by the University of North Carolina, indicated that individuals who consumed the lowest amount of fiber were 30% less likely to develop the pouches than people with the greatest fiber intake. Further research is needed, however, and there are still many benefits to including fiber in the diet.

Resources

BOOKS

Spiller, Gene A. and Monica Spiller. *What's with Fiber?* Laguna Beach, CA: Basic Health Publications, 2005.

Watson, Brenda and Leonard Smith. *The Fiber35 Diet: Nature's Weight Loss Secret*. New York: Free Press, 2007.

PERIODICALS

Anderson, J.W., et al. "Health Benefits of Dietary Fiber." *Nutrition Reviews* 67, no. 4 (2009): 188–205.

Clemens, R., et al. "Filling America's Fiber Intake Gap: Summary of a Roundtable to Probe Realistic Solutions with a Focus on Grain-Based Foods." *Journal of Nutrition* 142, no. 7 (2012): 1390S–401S.

Ho, K.S., et al. "Stopping or Reducing Dietary Fiber Intake Reduces Constipation and its Associated Symptoms." *World Journal of Gastroenterology* 18, no. 33 (2012): 4593–96.

Slavin, J.L. "Position of the American Dietetic Association: Health Implications of Dietary Fiber." *Journal of the American Dietetic Association* 108, no. 10 (2008): 1716–31.

WEBSITES

American Academy of Family Physicians "Fiber: How to Increase the Amount in Your Diet." FamilyDoctor.org. http://familydoctor.org/familydoctor/en/prevention-wellness/food-nutrition/nutrients/fiber-how-to-increase-the-amount-in-your-diet.html (accessed September 27, 2012).

"Diets High in Fiber Won't Protect Against Diverticulosis." UNC (University of North Carolina) Health Care. http://news.unchealthcare.org/news/2012/january/diets-high-in-fiber-wont-protect-against-diverticulosis (accessed September 27, 2012).

Mayo Clinic staff. "Dietary Fiber: Essential for a Healthy Diet." MayoClinic.com. http://www.mayoclinic.com/health/fiber/NU00033 (accessed September 27, 2012).

MedlinePlus. "Dietary Fiber." U.S. National Library of Medicine, National Institutes of Health. http://www.nlm.nih.gov/medlineplus/dietaryfiber.html (accessed September 27, 2012).

University of California San Francisco (UCSF) Medical Center. "Increasing Fiber Intake." http://www.ucsfhealth.org/education/increasing_fiber_intake/index.html (accessed September 27, 2012).

U.S. Department of Agriculture, National Agricultural Library. "DRI Tables." Food and Nutrition Information Center. http://fnic.nal.usda.gov/dietary-guidance/dietary-reference-intakes/dri-tables (accessed August 16, 2012).

U.S. Department of Agriculture and U.S. Department of Health and Human Services. *Dietary Guidelines for Americans, 2010.* 7th ed. Washington, DC: U.S. Government Printing Office, December 2010. http://health.gov/dietary guidelines (accessed February 22, 2012).

ORGANIZATIONS

Academy of Nutrition and Dietetics, 120 South Riverside Plz., Ste. 2000, Chicago, IL 60606-6995, (312) 899-0040, (800) 877-1600, amacmunn@eatright.org, http://www.eatright.org.

Center for Nutrition Policy and Promotion, U.S. Department of Agriculture, 3101 Park Center Drive, 10th Fl., Alexandria, VA 22302, (703) 305-7600, Fax: (703) 305-3300, support@cnpp.usda.gov, http://www.cnpp.usda.gov.

Dietitians of Canada, 480 University Ave., Ste. 604, Toronto, Canada, Ontario M5G 1V2, (416) 596-0857, Fax: (416) 596-0603, centralinfo@dietitians.ca, http://www.dietitians.ca.

National Digestive Diseases Information Clearinghouse, 2 Information Way, Bethesda, MD 20892–3570, (800) 891–5389, TTY: (866) 569–1162, Fax: (703) 738–4929, nddic@info.niddk.nih.gov, http://www.digestive.niddk.nih.gov.

U.S. Department of Agriculture, 1400 Independence Ave. SW, Washington, DC 20250, (202) 720-2791, http://www.usda.gov.

Tish Davidson, AM

High-protein diet

Definition

Protein, along with **fats** and **carbohydrates**, is one of the three **macronutrients**, which are the nutrients that provide energy (as **calories**). Protein contains approximately 4 calories per gram. The composition of a high-protein diet can be determined as an absolute amount of the protein, usually in grams per day; as a percentage of a person's total energy needs per day; or as the amount of protein ingested per kg of a person's body weight. In general, the recommended dietary

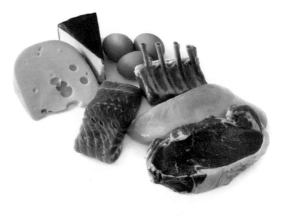

Examples of high-protein foods include cheese, eggs, fish, meat, and poultry. (© Istockphoto.com/Robyn Mackenzie)

allowance (RDA) for protein is 10%–35% of a person's daily calories, or about 0.8 grams (g) per kilogram (kg) of body weight for a healthy adult. A high-protein diet would be one based on the upper levels of these recommendations or would surpass them.

Origins

High-protein diets have been popular off and on since the 1960s. In the 1960s, Dr. Maxwell Stillman of the Stillman Diet was one of the first to advocate a high-protein, no-carbohydrate, **low-fat diet** for fast weight loss. In the 1990s, diet books promoting high-protein diets began to appear on bestseller lists. The most popular of these was the **Atkins Diet**. Other high-protein diets include the **Zone Diet**, Protein Power, and Sugar Busters. These diets were slightly modified from the Stillman Diet to include some carbohydrates and encouraged high-protein diets for weight loss and/or for bodybuilding.

In the medical field, a high-protein, high-calorie diet is needed for certain medical conditions such **cancer**, **AIDS**, severe burns, failure to thrive, **malnutrition**, following a surgery or illness, sarcopenia, traumatic brain injury, and other diseases that increase a person's need for protein and/or calories. High-protein, high-caloric diets may also be followed by competitive athletes, who have higher protein and energy requirements than the general public. According to the Agriculture Research Service of the U.S. Department of Agriculture (USDA), in 2009–10 (the most recent data available), most adults aged 20 and older consumed approximately 15% of their daily calories as protein.

Description

All human protein is made from about 20 different small molecules called amino acids. Out of these 20 amino acids, 9 are essential in adults. They are considered essential because the body cannot make them (or make a sufficient amount) from other nutrients. If they are not obtained from the diet, the body will begin to break down its own protein to obtain them.

Both animals and plants provide sources of protein. Animal protein has a higher biological value than most plants because it is a complete protein. Complete proteins contain all nine essential amino acids. Animal proteins include meat, poultry, fish, egg whites, and dairy products.

Plant proteins typically have a lower biological value because most are incomplete proteins that do not contain all nine essential amino acids. Some plants are better sources of protein than others because they lack only one or two essential amino acids. Better plant proteins include dried beans and bean products such as tofu (made from soybeans), nuts, and grains such as corn and quinoa; quinoa is one of the few grains that serves as a complete protein. Incomplete proteins can be combined in one meal to form complete proteins, such as red beans with rice or corn tortillas with beans.

The requirements for protein in individuals requiring higher amounts of protein and calories varies. Protein intake is usually increased from 0.8 g of protein per kg (2.2 lb.) of body weight to 1–2 g per kg of body weight. Higher intakes are often used for children. High-protein diets for weight loss recommend that between 35% (Atkins) and 64% (Stillman) of daily calories come from protein. This is equivalent to about 2.2–4.4 g per kg (1–2 g per lb.).

Extra amino acids are not stored in the body. Instead, they are split apart by enzymes. The part containing nitrogen is excreted by the kidneys in urine, while the remainder is either converted into glucose (a simple sugar) and used for energy or stored as glycogen, a compound that can later be reconverted into glucose or converted to fat and stored for later use.

Function

High-protein diets as medical treatment

In certain medical disorders, a person's metabolic rate is increased, and breakdown of tissue (tissue catabolism) predominates over building of tissue (anabolism). Continued catabolism, usually of protein, impairs a person's capacity to recover from the illness, surgery, or trauma. A high-protein, high-calorie diet is used to promote the positive intake of nitrogen from protein since many aspects of the patient's recovery are dependent on active protein synthesis. For example, healing of traumatic or surgical wounds, rebuilding damaged tissue, replacement of red blood cells from blood loss, replacing lost plasma protein, and immune response to infection are all processes of synthesis of new protein, making increased protein intake necessary to recovery.

High-protein diets for weight loss

For people who want to lose weight, they take in higher quantities of protein but must restrict their total intake of calories, usually carbohydrates. This promotes a fast initial weight loss, but most of the loss comes from losing water weight. The reason for this is that the body is driven into a state called ketosis. The body prefers to break down carbohydrates into glucose and use that glucose for energy. When the body is starved of carbohydrates, it begins converting fat into glucose. The process of converting fat into glucose releases water molecules that then leave the body as urine.

KEY TERMS

Amino acid—Molecules that are the basic building blocks of proteins.

B-complex vitamins—A group of water-soluble vitamins that often work together in the body. These include thiamin (B_1), riboflavin (B_2), niacin (B_3), pantothenic acid (B_5), pyridoxine (B_6), biotin (B_7 or vitamin H), folate/folic acid (B_9), and cobalamin (B_{12}).

Dietary fiber—Also known as roughage or bulk. Insoluble fiber moves through the digestive system almost undigested and gives bulk to stools. Soluble fiber dissolves in water and helps keep stools soft.

Enzyme—A protein that changes the rate of a chemical reaction within the body without being depleted in the reaction.

Essential amino acid—An amino acid that is necessary for health but that cannot be made by the body and must be acquired through diet.

Glucose—A simple sugar that results from the breakdown of carbohydrates and, under some conditions, proteins and fats. Glucose circulates in the blood and is the main source of energy for the body.

Glycogen—A compound produced when the level of glucose (sugar) in the blood is too high. Glycogen is stored in the liver and muscles for release when blood glucose levels are too low.

Mineral—An inorganic substance found in the earth that is necessary in small quantities for the body to maintain health. Examples: zinc, copper, iron.

Osteoporosis—A condition found in older individuals in which bones decrease in density and become fragile and more likely to break. It can be caused by lack of vitamin D and/or calcium in the diet.

Quinoa—A high-protein grain native to South America (pronounced keen-wah).

Vitamin—A nutrient that the body needs in small amounts to remain healthy but that the body cannot manufacture for itself and must acquire through diet.

Dieters wish to burn fat, but when fat is burned exclusively, molecules called ketones build up in the blood. Ketones are part of the body's defense against starvation. They suppress appetite and can also cause bad breath. If the body is deprived of carbohydrates for a long time, these ketones accumulate and can result in metabolic imbalances that cause serious harm to the kidneys and other organs.

Benefits

High-protein diets as medical treatment

Medical patients who are in a catabolic state may lose up to 40 g of nitrogen in their urine each day, equivalent to approximately 1 kg of muscle. Depletion of lean body mass occurs rapidly. Many other systems are affected in this hypermetabolic state, and if left untreated it can result in malnutrition or eventually death. A high-protein, high-calorie diet supports the body's need for more nitrogen in the form of protein and more calories to promote quick healing and strengthening of the immune system.

High-protein diets for weight loss

High-protein, low-calorie diets offer fast weight loss. The Stillman Diet claims that an individual can lose up to 30 lb. (13.5 kg) in 28 days. Popular high-protein diets also claim health benefits—the Zone diet

claims to improve physical and mental performance, prevent chronic cardiovascular diseases, improve immune system functioning, decrease signs of aging, and increase longevity, but there is little scientific evidence that supports these claims. Rapid weight loss does occur with high-protein, low-calorie diets, but much of the loss comes from losing water. This weight soon returns when the dieter goes off the diet.

Precautions

High-protein diets can be high in saturated fats. Saturated fats are primarily found in animal fats, including dairy. They are considered "bad" fats because they raise the level of LDL cholesterol ("bad" cholesterol) in the blood. High LDL cholesterol levels have been associated with an increased risk of heart disease.

High-protein diets may also restrict calories by severely restricting carbohydrates. Whole-grain carbohydrates are a significant source of B-complex **vitamins**. There are groups of people who require extra protein—rapidly growing adolescents, pregnant and nursing women, bodybuilders, endurance athletes, and some cancer patients—but protein should be increased as part of a well-balanced diet, without restricting other nutrients.

The risk of kidney damage is greater in individuals with poor kidney function who choose a high-protein diet. High-protein diets place an extra workload on the kidneys due to the high excretion of nitrogen. Although this is usually not a problem for healthy kidneys, it can cause more damage in kidneys whose functioning is already reduced.

Risks

People with medical conditions or recent trauma or illness should not attempt a high-protein, high-calorie diet by themselves without the advice and monitoring of a medical professional, such as a doctor or registered dietitian.

Virtually all high-protein diets for weight loss recommend that dieters take some sort of vitamin or mineral supplement. Diets that severely restrict carbohydrates tend to be lower in vitamins, **minerals**, and dietary **fiber**. High-protein diets also increase the amount of **calcium** excreted by the kidney. This increases the loss of calcium from bone and can lead to osteoporosis. It also increases the risk of kidney stones, which are more likely to form when large amounts of calcium are present. Cholesterol levels can increase on high-protein diets that encourage high consumption of animal protein due to the resulting increased intake of saturated fats. Finally, if the body reaches a state of ketosis, the ketones that accumulate make the body more acidic, which can cause major damage to various organs.

Research and general acceptance

The use of high-protein, high-calorie diets in the medical field is well accepted for certain medical conditions.

High-protein diets for weight loss purposes have received a lot of criticism, even though several studies have shown that the Atkins diet is not as problematic as was originally thought. Dietitians tend to find high-protein diets, especially high-protein, high saturated fat, and severely carbohydrate-restricted diets, to be unhealthy, unbalanced, and generally unnecessary. High-protein diets such as the Zone Diet and the Atkins Diet, however, remain fairly popular. Bodybuilders, weightlifters, and other people wishing to gain muscle mass also favor high-protein diets. The Mayo Clinic does not necessarily endorse high-protein diets but acknowledges that high-protein diets are probably not harmful to healthy individuals with good kidney function, at least in the short term (no longer than six months). The American Heart Association does not recommend these diets (for weight loss), as many of them restrict healthy foods and do not allow for a large enough variety of foods to meet the

---

QUESTIONS TO ASK YOUR DOCTOR

- Is a high-protein diet better for me than a regular calorie-reduced diet?
- Does this diet pose any health risks for me that I should be aware of?
- Do I have any special dietary needs that this diet might not meet?
- Do I need to take a dietary supplement while I am on this diet?
- What are my risk factors for cardiovascular disease and how will this diet affect them?
- How long can I stay on this diet?
- Are there any symptoms that should signal me to stop this diet?

---

nutritional requirements of a well-balanced diet. Increased saturated fat intake may increase the risk of cardiovascular disease, although some reviews of the literature have questioned whether saturated fat is to blame or if other fatty acids in combination with saturated fat contribute to the increased risk.

Resources

BOOKS

Eades, Michael R. and Mary Dan Eades. *The Protein Power Lifeplan.* New York: Warner Books, 2000.

PERIODICALS

American Heart Association Science Advisory. "Dietary Protein and Weight Reduction." *Circulation* 104 (2001): 1869–74.

de Oliveira Otto, Marcia C., et al. "Dietary Intake of Saturated Fat by Food Source and Incident Cardiovascular Disease: the Multi-Ethnic Study of Atherosclerosis." *American Journal of Clinical Nutrition* 96, no. 2 (2012): 397–404. http://dx.doi.org/10.3945/ajcn.112.037770 (accessed August 20, 2012).

Friedman, Allon N., et al. "Comparative Effects of Low-Carbohydrate High-Protein Versus Low-Fat Diets on the Kidney." *Clinical Journal of the American Society of Nephrology* 7, no. 7 (2012): 1103–11.

Lagiou, Pagona, et al. "Low Carbohydrate-High Protein Diet and Incidence of Cardiovascular Diseases in Swedish Women: Prospective Cohort Study." *BMJ* 344 (June 26, 2012). http://dx.doi.org/10.1136/bmj.e4026 (accessed August 20, 2012).

Larsson, Susanna C., Jarmo Virtamo, and Alicja Wolka. "Dietary Protein Intake and Risk of Stroke in Women." *Atherosclerosis* (July 24, 2012): e-pub ahead of print.

http://dx.doi.org/10.1016/j.atherosclerosis.2012.07.009 (accessed August 20, 2012).

Merino, Jordi, et al. "Negative Effect of a Low-Carbohydrate, High-Protein, High-Fat Diet on Small Peripheral Artery Reactivity in Patients with Increased Cardiovascular Risk." *British Journal of Nutrition* (July 31, 2012): e-pub ahead of print. http://dx.doi.org/10.1017/S0007114512003091 (accessed August 20, 2012).

WEBSITES

American Heart Association. "High-Protein Diets." http://www.heart.org/HEARTORG/GettingHealthy/NutritionCenter/High-Protein-Diets_UCM_305989_Article.jsp (accessed August 20, 2012).

HealthDay News. "Atkins-Type Diets Look Kidney-Friendly: Study." MedlinePlus, May 31, 2012. http://www.nlm.nih.gov/medlineplus/news/fullstory_125767.html (accessed August 20, 2012).

MedlinePlus. "Protein in Diet." U.S. National Library of Medicine, National Institutes of Health. http://www.nlm.nih.gov/medlineplus/ency/article/002467.htm (accessed August 20, 2012).

USDA Agricultural Research Service. "Table 1, Nutrient Intakes from Food, by Gender and Age." *What We Eat in America*, National Health and Nutrition Examination Survey 2009–2010. http://www.ars.usda.gov/Services/docs.htm?docid = 18349 (accessed August 20, 2012).

Zeratsky, Katherine. "Are High-Protein Diets Safe for Weight Loss?" MayoClinic.com. http://www.mayoclinic.com/health/high-protein-diets/AN00847 (accessed August 20, 2012).

ORGANIZATIONS

Academy of Nutrition and Dietetics, 120 South Riverside Plz., Ste. 2000, Chicago, IL 60606-6995, (312) 899-0040, (800) 877-1600, amacmunn@eatright.org, http://www.eatright.org.

Agricultural Research Service, U.S. Department of Agriculture, Jamie L. Whitten Bldg., 1400 Independence Ave. SW, Washington, DC 20250, http://www.ars.usda.gov.

American Heart Association, 7272 Greenville Ave., Dallas, TX 75231, (800) 242-8721, http://www.americanheart.org.

Tish Davidson, AM
Megan Porter, RD

Hilton Head metabolism diet

Definition

The Hilton Head **metabolism** diet was created by Peter M. Miller, PhD, who believes that a dieter's metabolism can be increased by eating five small meals a day and getting the correct amount and type exercise. This increase in metabolism will help allow the dieter to lose weight.

Origins

The Hilton Head metabolism diet was created by Peter M. Miller. Miller was born on October 5, 1942. He attended the University of Maryland, from which he received a bachelor's degree in psychology in 1964. He then attended the University of South Carolina, from which he received a master's degree in 1966 and a doctoral degree in 1968, both in psychology. He was a professor in the Department of Psychiatry and Behavioral Sciences, and in the College of Graduate studies, at the Medical University of South Carolina, and since 2008 has taught in the College of Dental Medicine. He is also the education coordinator of the Alcohol Research Center at the same institution.

Miller's writings on a variety of subjects have been published in many scholarly journals. In addition to publishing studies looking at saturated fat intake, **binge eating**, and weight loss intervention programs, he also studies alcoholism and other addiction behaviors. He is the editor of the journals *Addictive Behaviors* and *Eating Behaviors* and is on the editorial board of many other journals. He is board certified in clinical psychology.

In 1979, Miller founded what is now known as the Hilton Head Health Institute on Hilton Head Island in South Carolina. The institute is a weight loss and lifestyle modification retreat and spa where dieters can go to lose weight and learn new health and wellness skills. The Hilton Head metabolism diet was created by Miller using information and insights that he gained through helping dieters at the institute. Miller was the executive director of the institute until 2000.

The Hilton Head metabolism diet first appeared as a book of the same in 1983. The book was extremely popular and since then Miller has published additional books targeted at specific groups, including *The Hilton Head Over-35 Diet* and *The Hilton Head Diet for Children and Teenagers*. In 1996 he published an updated version of his original book, called *The New Hilton Head Metabolism Diet*.

Description

The Hilton Head metabolism diet aims to increase a dieter's base metabolic rate. By doing this its intent is to not only help the dieter lose weight while on the diet, but to make weight maintenance easier for the dieter in the future. Miller says that 70% of the **calories** that a person burns each day are burned through metabolic processes, and only the other 30% are burned through exercise and activity. Metabolic activity is all of the processes that are required to support life, such as the processes necessary for temperature regulation, digestion, making new cells, breaking down products for use by the body, and creating proteins and other necessary substances. All of these processes require energy that is acquired each day from food. If not enough food is eaten to supply the body's energy needs, the body looks for energy elsewhere, such as in the form of stored fat.

Miller believes that because such a large percentage of caloric expenditure comes from metabolic activity, weight loss can be achieved more effectively through increased metabolism than through increased exercise alone. This diet is intended to help dieters raise their metabolic rates leading to increased calorie usage, which in turn can lead to weight loss through the burning of fat stores as energy.

An important aspect of this diet is that Miller provides psychological and emotional help to dieters who may have been struggling for many years with their weight, and who may feel uncomfortable or ashamed about their weight or appearance. He tells dieters that it is not their fault that they are overweight, and that they should not allow others to put them down. He says that although overweight people do not usually have metabolisms that are abnormal, they do often have metabolisms that are slow compared to the metabolisms of thinner people. This is why it is so important for overweight people to change their metabolism if they are going to lose weight, and keep it off.

The diet plan consists of a six-week weight-loss phase followed by a two-week weight-maintenance phase. This eight-week plan can be repeated as many times as necessary until the desired weight loss has been achieved. Miller suggests that at first dieters aim to lose 10% of their body weight, especially very overweight dieters, because it is through this first amount of weight loss that the greatest health benefits are often seen.

Miller provides meal plans and recipes to go along with this diet. During the weight loss phase the dieter is limited to what amounts to about 1,000 calories per day. On the weekends, however, the dieter is allowed an increased caloric consumption, usually about 200 to 250 more calories each day than during the week. During the weight maintenance phase the dieter is allowed a number of calories based on various personal needs.

The diet provides meal plans that are generally low in fat, usually fewer than 15 to 20 grams per day, and that include many different fruits and vegetables. The diet also includes **carbohydrates** and lean meats. Miller recommends that at least five eight-ounce glasses of water or other liquids be drank each day

while on the diet. Although the dieter has many drink choices, no caffeinated beverages are allowed, and low- or no-calorie drinks are recommended.

The Hilton Head metabolism diet recommends that dieters walk for 20 minutes, two times each day. Three times each week a set of strength training exercises should be done in place of one of the walks. Miller also recommends that dieters may want to take a multivitamin and a **calcium** supplement while on this diet.

Function

The Hilton Head metabolism diet is intended to help dieters lose weight by increasing their base metabolic rate. The six weeks of weight loss followed by two weeks of weight maintenance can be repeated as many times as necessary for the desired amount of weight loss to be achieved.

It is intended to also be a lifestyle changing plan that provides recommendations for exercise and information to help dieters who might be feeling upset about their weight. A long-lasting purpose of this diet is that the increase in the dieter's metabolism is supposed to make weight control easier in the future.

Benefits

There are many benefits to weight loss and increased fitness. There are many diseases and conditions for which **obesity** if considered a risk factor,

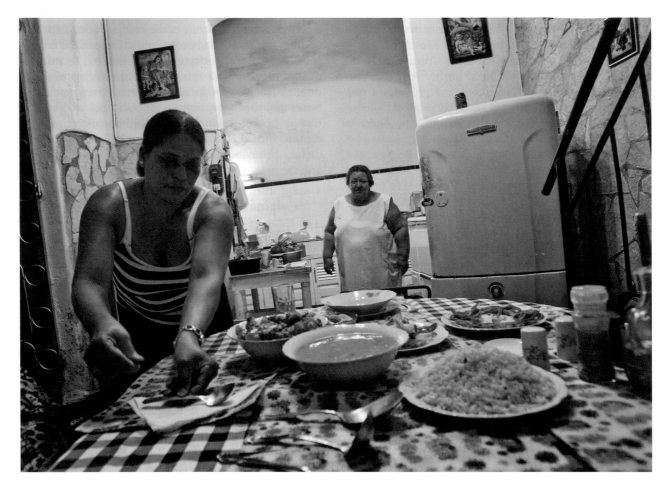

Woman cooking a traditional Cuban meal for guests. *(Patrick Farrell/Miami Herald/MCT via Getty Images)*

Description

Characteristics of the Hispanic diet

Information about what Hispanics in the United States eat has been compiled through national surveys conducted by the U.S. Department of Agriculture (USDA). Among the highlights of these data are that Hispanics tend to eat more rice, but less pasta and ready-to-eat cereals, than their non-Hispanic white counterparts. With the exception of tomatoes, Hispanics are also less likely to consume vegetables, although they have a slightly higher consumption of fruits. Compared to non-Hispanic whites, Hispanics are more than twice as likely to drink whole milk, but much less likely to drink low-fat or skim milk. Hispanics are also more likely to eat beef, but less likely to eat processed meats such as hot dogs, sausage, and luncheon meats. Hispanics are more likely to eat eggs and legumes than non-Hispanic whites, and less likely to consume **fats** and oils or sugars and candy.

Analysis of the macronutrient content of the diet reveals that Hispanics, especially Mexican Americans, have a lower intake of total fat and a higher intake of dietary **fiber** compared to non-Hispanic white populations, with much of the dietary fiber coming from legumes. In general, Mexican Americans and other Hispanic subgroups are low in many of the same micronutrients as the general population, with intakes of **vitamin E**, **calcium**, and **zinc** falling below recommended daily allowances.

Function

Acculturation and the Hispanic Diet

Just as Hispanics have altered American cuisine, American culture has also altered the diet of Hispanic Americans. As with many other immigrant groups in the United States, the lifestyle of Hispanic Americans is undergoing a transition away from one based on the traditional values and customs of their ancestry, as they begin to adopt the values and behaviors of their adopted country. With regard to health behaviors, this process of acculturation is typically characterized by a more sedentary lifestyle and a change in dietary patterns. The effects of acculturation on the Hispanic diet are illustrated in national dietary survey data that show that Hispanic Americans who continue to use Spanish as a primary language eat somewhat more healthful diets than those who use English as a primary language. These healthier eating behaviors include lower consumption of fat, saturated fat, and cholesterol. Additional analysis of survey data reveals that these dietary differences do not appear to be the result of greater nutritional knowledge or greater awareness of food-disease relationships.

Benefits

The degradation of diet quality that occurs as Hispanic Americans become acculturated into the mainstream U.S. population occurs in the context of improvements in, rather than degradation of, economic status. For example, first-generation Mexican American women, despite being of lower socioeconomic status than second-generation Mexican American or non-Hispanic white women, tend to have higher intakes of **protein**, **vitamins** A and C, folic acid, and calcium than these other groups. The diets of second-generation Mexican American women more closely resemble those of non-Hispanic white women of similar socioeconomic status.

Precautions

The process of acculturation and the changing nature of the Hispanic diet has serious implications for the state of Hispanic health. The prevalence of type 2 **diabetes mellitus** is two to three times higher in Hispanic Americans than in non-Hispanic whites, affecting an estimated 10% of adults over the age of 20 and 25%–30% of adults over age 50. The prevalence of the disease is especially high among Mexican Americans. Diabetes, a disease characterized by high levels of glucose in the blood, is a major cause of death and disability in the United States. Compared to non-diabetic individuals, those with the disease are also at two to four times higher risk of developing cardiovascular disease, the leading cause of death in the country. Accompanying this increased risk of diabetes among Hispanics is a marked increase in the risk of **obesity**.

Risks

Much of the increased risk of diabetes experienced by Hispanic Americans is believed to be attributable to the changing lifestyle that accompanies the acculturation process, including the changing quality of the Hispanic diet and the adoption of more sedentary habits. These trends are occurring across all segments of the

KEY TERMS

Cholesterol—A waxy substance made by the liver and also acquired through diet. High levels in the blood may increase the risk of cardiovascular disease.

Diabetes—A condition in which the body either does not make or cannot respond to the hormone insulin. As a result, the body cannot use glucose (sugar).

Glucose—A simple sugar that results from the breakdown of carbohydrates. Glucose circulates in the blood and is the main source of energy for the body.

Macronutrient—A nutrient needed in large quantities.

Saturated fat—Fats found in animal products and in coconut and palm oils. They are more difficult to break down than unsaturated fats and contribute to high cholesterol.

Hispanic population, although the extent of the changes are more pronounced in some subgroups (e.g., Mexican Americans in large urban areas) than in others. Although Hispanic Americans generally smoke less than their non-Hispanic white counterparts, the direction of Hispanic health is also threatened by an increasing frequency of cigarette smoking, particularly among younger segments of the population.

Research and general acceptance

Approaches for improving the health of Hispanics need to be broad-based and need to consider the complexities of a variety of lifestyle factors. Nutrition education programs aimed at improving the quality of the Hispanic diet are currently based on a combination of preserving some elements of the traditional Hispanic diet—including a reliance on beans, rice, and tortillas—and a change in others—such as reduced consumption of high-fat dairy products and using less fat in cooking.

Resources

BOOKS

Bender, David A. *A Dictionary of Food and Nutrition*. New York: Oxford University Press, 2009.

Counihan, Carole, and Penny Van Esternik, eds. *Food and Culture*. 3rd ed. New York: Routledge, 2012.

Cramer, Janet M., and Lynn M. Walters. *Food as Communication/Communication as Food*. New York: Peter Lang Publishing, 2011.

Larsen, Laura, ed. *Diet and Nutrition Sourcebook*. 4th ed. Detroit: Omnigraphics Inc, 2011.

PERIODICALS

Arandia, G., et al. "Diet and Acculturation Among His-panic/Latino Older Adults in the United States: A Review of Literature and Recommendations." *Journal of Nutrition in Gerontology and Geriatrics* 31, no. 1 (2012): 16–37.

Ashida, S., A.V. Wilkinson, and L.M. Koehly. "Social Influence and Motivation to Change Health Behaviors among Mexican-Origin Adults: Implications for Diet and Physical Activity." *American Journal of Health Promotion* 26, no. 3 (2012): 176–79.

Flores, G., J. Maldonado, and P. Durán. "Making Tortillas Without Lard: Latino Parents' Perspectives on Healthy Eating, Physical Activity, And Weight-Management Strategies for Overweight Latino Children." *Journal of the Academy of Nutrition and Dietetics* 112, no. 1 (2012): 81–89.

Liu, J.H., et al. "Generation and Acculturation Status are Associated with Dietary Intake and Body Weight in Mexican American Adolescents." *Journal of Nutrition* 142, no. 2 (2012): 298–305.

OTHER

Ennis, Sharon R., Merarys R'os-Vargas, and Nora G. Albert. "The Hispanic Population: 2010." *2010 Census Briefs*. Washington, DC: U.S. Census Bureau, 2011. http://www.census.gov/prod/cen2010/briefs/c2010br-04.pdf (accessed September 7, 2012).

U.S. Department of Agriculture, Agricultural Research Service. "Nutrient Intakes from Food: Mean Amounts Consumed per Individual, by Race/Ethnicity and Age, in the United States, 2009–2010." *What We Eat in America*, National Health and Nutrition Examination Survey (NHNES), 2009–2010. http://www.ars.usda.gov/SP2UserFiles/Place/12355000/pdf/0910/Table_2_NIN_RAC_09.pdf (accessed September 7, 2012).

WEBSITES

Oldways. "Latino Diet & Health." http://www.oldwayspt.org/resources/heritage-pyramids/latino-diet-pyramid/latino-diet-health (accessed September 7, 2012).

ORGANIZATIONS

Centers for Disease Control and Prevention, 1600 Clifton Rd. NE, Atlanta, GA 30333, (800) CDC-INFO (232-4636), TTY: (888) 232-6348, cdcinfo@cdc.gov, http://www.cdc.gov.

Office of Minority Health & Health Equity (OMHHE), U.S. Centers for Disease Control and Prevention (CDC), Mail Stop K-77, 4770 Buford Hwy, Atlanta, GA 30341, (770) 488-8343, Fax: (770) 488-8140, OMHHE@cdc.gov, http://www.cdc.gov/minorityhealth/index.html.

World Health Organization, Avenue Appia 20, 1211 Geneva 27, Switzerland, +41 22 791-2111, Fax: +41 22 791-3111, info@who.int, http://www.who.int.

Braxton D. Mitchell
Laura Jean Cataldo, RN, EdD

HIV diet *see* **AIDS/HIV diet and nutrition**

Hollywood diet

Definition

The Hollywood diet products are intended to produce extreme weight loss in a very short time. The Hollywood diet 30 Day Miracle Program is intended to allow dieters to lose weight over the course of a month by using various Hollywood diet products combined with healthy living strategies.

Origins

The Hollywood diet products were created by Jamie Kabler. He is a self-proclaimed "diet counselor to the stars." According to the Hollywood diet website, Kabler invented the Hollywood 48 Hour Miracle Diet after visiting a European health spa. He was at the spa to help him manage his own weight, and afterward decided that he wanted to help people lose weight and detoxify their bodies by creating a product that everyone could afford. The Hollywood 48 Hour Diet was first available in December of 1997. According to its website, more than 10 million people have used the product since then. The Hollywood 48 Hour Miracle Diet was the first of the Hollywood Diet products, but since that time the line has been expanded to include the Hollywood 24 Hour Miracle Diet, the Hollywood Daily Miracle Diet Drink Mix Meal Replacement, and various **dietary supplements**.

Description

The Hollywood 48 Hour Miracle Diet is probably the best known of the various Hollywood products. It is an orange-colored drink that is intended to be a complete food replacement for a 48 hour period. Dieters are instructed to shake the bottle well and then mix four ounces of the drink with four ounces of water (bottled water is recommended) and sip this mixture over the course of four hours. This is to be repeated four times each day. The dieter is instructed to drink eight glasses of water each day while on this diet.

For the two days that the dieter is following the Hollywood 48 Hour Miracle Diet, the drink mixture and water are all that the dieter is allowed to consume. The dieter cannot eat or drink anything else. This restriction even includes drinks that have no **calories**, such as diet sodas and chewing gum. During this time the dieter is told that for optimal results he or she cannot have any **caffeine** or alcohol while on the diet, and cannot smoke.

The Hollywood 24 Hour Miracle Diet is largely the same as the 48 Hour formulation, except that it is intended only for one day use. The same restrictions about food, caffeine, and alcohol intake apply, as does the ban on smoking. The website recommends that dieters use one version of the diet or the other at least one time per month, and says that many people choose to do the 48 Hour Diet once a week.

Both Hollywood diet formulations are made mainly of fruit juice concentrates. They do contain a significant number of **vitamins**. The 24-hour version of the diet contains 100% of the daily recommended value of vitamins A, B$_6$, B$_{12}$, C, D, and E, as well as **thiamin**, **riboflavin**, **niacin**, folic acid, and **pantothenic acid** in each four-ounce serving. The 48-hour formulation contains 75% of the daily required value of these vitamins and nutrients. Both formulations contain 25 grams of **carbohydrates**, 20 milligrams of **sodium**, 22 grams of **sugar**, and no **protein** in each four-ounce serving.

Each four-ounce serving of the Hollywood diet contains 100 calories. This means that if a dieter follows the diet's instructions and drinks four four-ounce servings over the course of the day, he or she will be ingesting 400 calories. Because no other food or drink products are allowed during this diet, this means that anyone following it will only consume 400 calories per day. This qualifies the diet as a very low-calorie diet. Very low-calorie diets are usually used to treat extremely obese patients with more than 30% excess body fat, and are only administered under the supervision of a doctor or other trained medical professional. If either Hollywood diet formulation were to be used regularly or for an extended period of time, this would be considered a traditional very low-calorie diet and would require medical supervision.

The Hollywood diet website also includes an alternative diet plan that is more comprehensive than either the 48 or 24 Hour diets. This diet plan is called the 30 Day Miracle Program. It suggests that this program be followed to help the dieter maintain the positive results achieved during the 48 or 24 Hour Diets.

The first step of the 30 Day Miracle Program is for the dieter to do the 24 or 48 Hour Diet. After this diet is finished, and the dieter returns to eating solid foods, the second step is to replace one meal per day with another Hollywood Product, the Hollywood Daily Miracle Diet Drink Mix Meal Replacement. It is suggested that the dieter replace dinner for the most successful outcome. The dieter is also encouraged to avoid foods that are high in fat or salt or contain sugar, and to avoid dairy products, red meat, and diet sodas.

The diet also recommends that the dieter take another Hollywood product, Hollywood Meta Miracle,

twice each day. This product is supposed to be able to help dieters not feel hungry, boost their **metabolism**, and give them more energy. The other supplement recommended by the diet is the Hollywood Mega Miracle 75 nutritional supplement. The diet instructs that it be taken twice every day. This product supposedly contains 75 different nutrients needed by the body for good health.

The diet also suggests that dieters eat a healthy breakfast and lunch, do not eat after 6 p.m. each day, and eat fruits and vegetables as snacks. The diet recommends that a dieter take a brisk walk for 30 minutes or more each day. The final instruction of the diet is to repeat either the Hollywood 48 Hour Diet or the Hollywood 24 Hour diet on a regular basis. Once a month or each weekend are suggested.

Function

The Hollywood 48 Hour Miracle Diet and Hollywood 24 Hour Miracle Diet are intended to produce large amounts of weight loss in very short times. The 48 hour diet claims that dieters can lose up to 10 pounds in just two days. The 24 hour diet claims that dieters can lose up to 5 pounds in just one day. These diets suggest that they be repeated often until the desired weight loss has been achieved. These diets also claim that they will detoxify the body and rejuvenate the dieter. The 30 Day Miracle Diet is intended to provide more long-term weight loss over a period of one moth. The amount of weight that dieters can expect to lose during that time period is not specified.

The Hollywood 48 and 24 Hour Diets are not intended to be lifestyle changing diets. They do not provide recommendations for exercise, and they do not provide the dieter with any other forms of healthy lifestyle support, such as stress reduction techniques. The 30 Day Miracle Diet encompasses the 48 and 24 Hour products, but is intended to be a lifestyle program for more long-term weight loss. It does provide healthy eating and exercise recommendations for the dieter to follow during the course of the diet.

Benefits

The Hollywood 24 and 48 Hour diets do contain fruit products and many vitamins and **minerals** that are part of a balanced diet. Drinking the diet product instead of a higher-calorie, sugary drink such as soda may have some health benefits. Used as a diet, however, the benefits are unclear. The dieter may lose weight on the diet, but it is likely to return quickly after the diet is stopped if old eating habits are resumed. There may be some psychological benefit to quick weight loss but this is likely to be undone if the weight is regained.

The 30 Day Miracle Program may have some benefits. The suggestions for helping dieters maintain the weight loss achieved by the 24 or 48 Hour Diets follow many guidelines for healthy eating and moderate exercise. Following these suggestions, such as avoiding sugar, red meat, and fatty foods, are more likely than the 24 and 48 hour diets to result in moderate, sustainable weight loss. Weight loss can have many health benefits if achieved through healthy eating and exercise. **Obesity** is a risk factor for many diseases and conditions, such as type 2 diabetes and heart disease. Weight loss can reduce this risk. Following the diet's recommendation for 30 minutes or more per day of brisk walking may also have health benefits. Regular exercise has been shown to reduce the risk of cardiovascular disease.

Precautions

The Hollywood 24 and 48 Hour Diets specify that they should not be undertaken by pregnant or **breast-feeding** women, nor by people with diabetes, people who are taking medication, or people with any other medical conditions. People without any of these conditions should also be extremely cautious about beginning this diet because of its very low calorie content. Anyone thinking of beginning this or any other diet should consult a physician or other medical professional.

Risks

Although the 24 and 48 Hour diets may provide many essential vitamins and minerals, there are many substances necessary for good health that they do not provide. They do not provide significant amounts of protein or fat. Protein is a very important part of a

healthy diet, and some fat is required for the body to function properly. The 24 and 48 Hour diets also do not contain other nutrients that are important for good health. This means that dieters who follow these diet plans have a high risk of nutrient deficiencies. Dieters considering this diet should consult a doctor about an appropriate multivitamin or supplement to help reduce this risk. Vitamins and supplements have their own associated risks and are not regulated by the U.S. Food and Drug Administration in the same way as medicines.

There may be some negative side effects from following the 24 or 48 Hour diets. Some dieters who have tried them reported intestinal cramping, light headedness, and generally not feeling well. The website suggests that the first time a dieter try these products it be done on a day off or a weekend.

Repeating this diet frequently or for an extended period could have serious consequences. Very low-calorie diets can have many negative side effects. For extremely obese people these risks of side effects can be reduced by proper medical supervision, and may be outweighed by the benefit of significant weight loss. Very low-calorie diets are usually only prescribed for people who are suffering serious medical consequences from obesity. Very low-calorie diets can result in many different side effects including **gallstones** and cardiovascular problems. Very low-calorie diets are not appropriate for people who are not extremely obese, and are never appropriate without medical supervision.

Research and general acceptance

There have been no significant scientific studies of Hollywood 24 or 48 Hour Diets, or any of the other

Hollywood products. The use of very low-calorie starvation-type diets is generally accepted to be negative to health. Some people do advocate the use of juice fasting as a way to detoxify the body, but this is extremely controversial, and there is no research on the Hollywood diets being safe or effective for this kind of use. It is generally recommended that for safe, effective, long-term weight loss and maintenance, dieters follow a reduced-calorie diet full of fruits and vegetables and get regular exercise.

Resources

BOOKS

Downing, Frank, and O. Bardoff. *The Hollywood Emergency Diet*. Montclair, NJ: Millburn Book Corp, 1979.

Larsen, Laura, ed. *Diet and Nutrition Sourcebook*. Detroit, MI: Omnigraphics, 2011.

Willis, Alicia P., ed. *Diet Therapy Research Trends*. New York: Nova Science, 2007.

PERIODICALS

Larhammar, Dan. "Fakes and Fraud in Commercial Diets." *Scandinavian Journal of Food and Nutrition* (June 2005): 78–80.

WEBSITES

Hollywood Diet official website. http://www.hollywood diet.com (accessed October 2, 2012).

Helen M. Davidson

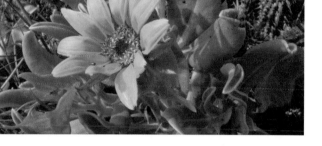

Flowering hoodia plant. *(© Anthony Bannister/Gallo Images/ Corbis)*

Hoodia

Definition

Hoodia is a genus of desert plants containing 13 species. One species, *Hoodia gondonii*, is marketed in the United States as a weight-loss supplement. In this entry, hoodia refers only to *Hoodia gondonii*.

Purpose

Marketers of hoodia claim that it suppresses the appetite so that individuals eat less and lose weight. Claims that hoodia is a safe and effective weight-loss supplement are highly controversial.

Description

Hoodia is a succulent desert plant that looks like a cactus. Its upright stem bears sharp spines and large pinkish flowers. The plant takes 4–6 years to mature and can reach a height of 3 ft. (1 m). When eaten, chemicals in the stem are said to prevent the body from feeling hungry.

Hoodia grows wild in the very dry Kalahari and Namib Deserts of South Africa, Botswana, and Namibia. For many years, the San Bushmen who live this region have eaten hoodia to dull their appetite on long trips through the desert. Hoodia is an endangered species. It is protected by both international and national laws in the countries where it grows wild. A special license is required to harvest the plant from the wild and export it.

The politics of hoodia

In the 1970s, the South African Council for Scientific and Industrial Research (CSIR) began a program to investigate bush foods, including hoodia. As part of this program, scientists isolated from hoodia an appetite suppressant ingredient that they called P57. In 1996, CSIR licensed P57 to Phytopharm, a

British Company that produces functional foods whose active ingredients come from plants with traditional medicinal uses. Because hoodia is rare and endangered, Phytopharm began the difficult task of cultivating the plant on farms in Africa. Meanwhile, Phytopharm partnered with Pfizer, a large, traditional international pharmaceutical company, to work on ways to extract and purify P57 from plants or to make it synthetically in the laboratory.

In 2002, a lawyer representing the San threatened to sue the CSIR for "bio-piracy" of hoodia. The threat of legal action resulted in an agreement that the San, a poor and marginalized ethnic group in South Africa, would share in the profits of marketing any products that contained hoodia. That same year, Pfizer ended its relationship with Phytopharm and P57. Although Pfizer scientists had been able to make synthetic P57, the company felt it was too difficult and too expensive to manufacture in the large amounts needed to produce a commercial weight-loss supplement. In addition, Pfizer's research suggested that the compound might rapidly be inactivated in the body and that it had negative side effects on the liver.

In 2003, with Pfizer out of the picture, Phytopharm decided to market products containing natural hoodia and continued their efforts to grow hoodia on plantations in South Africa. At the same time, they reached an agreement with Unilever, a consumer products company, to find ways to add hoodia to various Unilever foods and beverages. These new products were expected to reach the market in 2008.

Meanwhile, in 2004, hoodia received high profile media coverage when *60 Minutes* reporter Leslie Stahl visited a South African hoodia plantation, ate some of the plant, and declared on television that it had kept her from feeling hungry all day without any side effects. Stahl's report stimulated interest among the public in hoodia as a diet aid. Hoodia supplements began to be advertised heavily, especially over the Internet.

Health claims

Manufacturers of products containing hoodia claim that it reduces or eliminates the desire to eat and drink by tricking the brain into believing that the body does not need food and water. This claim is made only for *Hoodia gondonii* and not the other 12 species of hoodia. Hoodia/P57 is available primarily in capsules of various strengths, and can also be added to foods such as diet bars, diet shakes, and lollipops.

Hoodia is considered a dietary supplement in the United States. The Food and Drug Administration (FDA) regulates **dietary supplements** under the 1994 Dietary Supplement Health and Education Act (DSHEA). At the time the act was passed, legislators felt that because many dietary supplements like hoodia come from natural plant sources and have been used for hundreds of years in herbal and folk healing, these products did not need to be as rigorously regulated as prescription and over-the-counter drugs used in conventional medicine.

Under the terms of DSHEA, hoodia is regulated in the same way that food is regulated. Like food manufacturers, manufacturers of products containing hoodia do not have to prove that the products are either safe or effective before they can be sold to the public. Instead, the burden of proof falls on the FDA to show that the supplement is either unsafe or ineffective before the supplement can be restricted or banned. Information about a dietary supplement's safety and effectiveness is normally gathered only after people using the product develop health problems or complain that the product does not work.

Hoodia is a relative newcomer to the world of diet supplements and has not been well studied in humans. The claim that hoodia helps people to lose weight is controversial because:

• The amount and strength of hoodia in dietary supplements is not standardized and a wide range of doses is used.
• Few animal studies have been done on hoodia, and it is not possible to verify that hoodia will have the same effect in humans as it does in laboratory animals.
• The only human studies have a very small sample size.
• The results of human studies have not been published in peer-reviewed journals or duplicated by independent scientists.
• Most hoodia studies have sponsored by Phytopharm and others who have a financial interest in obtaining positive results.

One hoodia study done at Brown University Medical School injected P57 directly into the brain of rats. The rats did eat less and lose weight. However, humans take hoodia by mouth in much smaller quantities, so the results of the rat study are not necessarily going to be seen in humans. Other human studies have had fewer than 10 participants who have taken hoodia only for short periods.

The future of hoodia

In the United States, dietary supplements are required to be clearly labeled with the word "supplement." In

KEY TERMS

Conventional medicine—Mainstream or Western pharmaceutical-based medicine practiced by medical doctors, doctors of osteopathy, and other licensed health care professionals.

Dietary supplement—A product, such as a vitamin, mineral, herb, amino acid, or enzyme, that is intended to be consumed in addition to an individual's diet with the expectation that it will improve health.

Functional food—Also called nutraceuticals, these products are marketed as having health benefits or disease-preventing qualities beyond their basic supply of energy and nutrients. Often these health benefits come in the form of added herbs, minerals, vitamins, etc.

Succulent—Plants with large, fleshy leaves, stems, and roots capable of storing a lot of water. These plants grow in dry environments.

addition, the label must show the volume or weight of the contents; the serving size; a list of dietary ingredients and nondietary ingredients (e.g., artificial color, binders, fillers, flavorings); the name of the manufacturer, packer, or distributor; and directions for use. If the supplement is an herb, such as hoodia, the label must contain its scientific name.

Real *Hoodia gondonii* is expensive and in very short supply. Several independent laboratories have tested products claiming to contain hoodia. About half the products contained no hoodia at all and others contained much less than the label claimed. The lack of hoodia in weight-loss products claiming to contain the herb has lead to lawsuits. New Jersey and California have both sued the manufacturers of TrimSpa's X32 hoodia product that was marketed by the now-deceased celebrity spokesperson Anna Nicole Smith. Other lawsuits are likely to follow as investigations prove that other hoodia weight-loss products contain no real hoodia. Many Web sites promoting hoodia appear to contain false testimonials and inaccurate or false information about scientific results of hoodia studies. In March 2006, the independent *Consumer Reports* magazine investigated hoodia supplements and declared that it could not recommend hoodia as a weight-loss product.

Precautions

Consumers have no way of telling by looking at or tasting the product whether it actually contains

hoodia. In addition, very little is known about the safety of hoodia when used on a daily basis for an extended time, nor has any standard dosage been developed. It is true that the San have used this herb for many years to curb hunger. However, they use hoodia only occasionally and for short periods.

Interactions

Not enough is know about hoodia to know if or how it interacts with drugs or other herbs.

Complications

Very little is known about the long-term effects of hoodia use. There are some anecdotal stories about people using hoodia forgetting to drink and suffering complications of **dehydration**.

Parental concerns

Parents should be aware that the safe dose of many herbal supplements has not been established for children. Accidental overdose may occur if children are give adult herbal supplements.

Resources

BOOKS

Fragakis, Allison. *The Health Professional's Guide to Popular Dietary Supplements*. Chicago: American Dietetic Association, 2003

Wildman, Robert E.C., ed. *Handbook of Nutraceuticals and Functional Foods*. 2nd ed. Boca Raton, FL: CRC/Taylor & Francis, 2007.

PERIODICALS

Duewald, Mary. "An Appetite Killer for a Killer Appetite? Not Yet." *New York Times*, April 19, 2005.

Khalsa, K.P.S. "Halt Hunger With Hoodia?" *Better Nutrition* 69, no. 1 (January 31, 2007): 26.

WEBSITES

Adams, Mike. "Consumer Alert: Hoodia Gordonii Weight Loss Pills Scam Exposed by Independent Ingestigation." News Target, March 26, 2005. http://www.newstarget.com/006016.html (accessed October 3, 2012).

Leung, Rebecca. "African Plant May Help Fight Fat." *60 Minutes*, November 21, 2004. http://www.cbsnews.com/stories/2004/11/18/60minutes/main656458.shtml (accessed October 3, 2012).

Mayo Clinic staff. "Is Hoodia an Effective Appetite Suppressant?" MayoClinic.com. http://www.mayoclinic.com/health/hoodia/AN01182 (accessed October 3, 2012).

National Center for Alternative and Complementary Medicine. "Hoodia." National Institutes of Health. http://nccam.nih.gov/health/hoodia (accessed October 2, 2012).

ORGANIZATIONS

National Center for Complementary and Alternative Medicine Clearinghouse, PO Box 7923, Gaithersburg, MD 20898, (888) 644-6226, Fax: (866) 464-3616, info@nccam.nih.gov, http://nccam.nih.gov.

U.S. Food and Drug Administration, 10903 New Hampshire Ave., Silver Spring, MD 20993-0002, (888) INFO-FDA (463-6332), http://www.fda.gov.

Tish Davidson, A.M.

Hormone-free foods

Definition

The phrases "hormone free" or "no hormones" are used to describe beef or milk that has been produced without the use of additional natural or synthetic sex steroids or **protein** growth hormones. The use of these phrases in **food labeling** is regulated by the U.S. Department of Agriculture (USDA) in the United States and by Health Canada in Canada. Some controversy surrounds the use of hormones in animal husbandry, primarily in regard to possible side effects of these drugs on humans and the environment and also whether or not certain types of food labeling and advertising are intended to influence consumer choice.

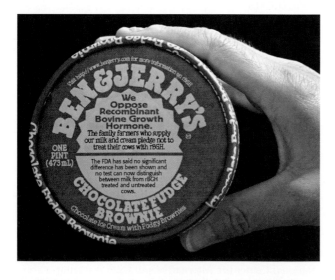

Ben & Jerry's ice cream uses milk from cows that have not been given recombinant bovine growth hormone (rGBH). *(AP Photo/Toby Talbot)*

Purpose

There are several reasons for using hormones in beef and milk production, including to:

- ensure that the animal uses its feed efficiently and absorbs the nutrients contained in the food
- produce leaner, better-quality meat
- allow steers (castrated male animals) to continue growing after castration; young male beef cattle are castrated to prevent rough or dangerous behavior and to control bleeding
- reduce costs for consumers, as well as farmers or ranchers, due to increased production; a lactating cow treated with recombinant bovine somatotropin (rbST) will produce on average 7–8 more pounds of milk per day than an untreated cow
- reduce the impact of animal husbandry on the environment—a study carried out at Cornell University in 2008 reported that the use of hormones in milk production reduced the use of food and water, the amount of cropland needed to produce the milk, the amount of waste products, and the use of fossil fuels compared with equivalent milk production from cows that had not been treated with hormones.

The major reasons for not using hormones in beef or milk production are international trade and consumer preference. The European Union (EU) began to ban beef produced from hormone-treated cattle in 1988, but the United States and Canada opposed the ban and raised duties on EU imports. In 2012, an agreement was reached, with the EU agreeing to import quotas of untreated beef from Canada and the United States.

In the case of milk, consumer concerns about the possible side effects of milk produced from cows treated with rbST has led to a controversy about the use of "hormone free" in milk labeling. Some dairy farmers maintain that the use of "hormone free" or "no hormones" labeling is a scare tactic intended to influence consumers to choose some brands of milk over others. A study carried out by the **Academy of Nutrition and Dietetics** (formerly the American Dietetic Association) in 2008 reported that "[milk] label claims were not related to any meaningful differences in the milk compositional variables measured."

Description

The use of "hormone free" is somewhat of a misnomer, as the milk and other body tissues of all mammals contain hormones. For example, the production of human breast milk requires the interaction of at least six different hormones, some of which are passed on in the mother's milk to the nursing infant. The same is true of lactating dogs, cats, mice, goats, and sheep. Similarly, the meat from cattle raised for beef production contains small amounts of sex hormones. Some researchers prefer the terms *endogenous* and *exogenous* to distinguish the two types of hormones; endogenous hormones are produced inside the animal's body, and exogenous hormones are administered from the outside.

Hormones in beef production

The use of exogenous hormones in beef production dates back to the late 1930s, and it was practiced in over 20 countries until the EU ban of 1988. There are six steroid hormones used to increase muscle tissue in beef cattle—three naturally occurring chemicals (estradiol, progesterone, and testosterone), and three synthetic (melengestrol acetate, trenbolone acetate, and zeranol). These hormones are administered to cattle either in their feed or through implants (pellets) inserted under the skin of the ear. The animal's ear is removed at the time of slaughter to prevent the implant from entering the human food supply.

Hormones in milk production

The use of hormones in dairy farming was less widespread until the 1990s, when Monsanto developed a process for producing recombinant bovine somatotropin, or rbST, through genetic engineering; prior to this, the hormone could be produced only from the cadavers of cows, which were in limited supply. The product, which is also called artificial growth hormone, was approved by the FDA in 1993 after lengthy testing and was first used in commercial milk production in 1994. The synthetic hormone, sold under the trade name Posilac, was used in about one-third of the nine million dairy cattle in the United States in 2010. Its use is banned in Canada, Australia, New Zealand, and the European Union; however, none of the major countries that allow the import and sale of U.S. dairy products have restrictions on milk or dairy products from cows supplemented with rbST, and none of them require special labeling of such products.

Posilac is a protein hormone rather than a steroid hormone. Posilac is given by injection about 60 days into a cow's lactation period. Cows usually begin their lactation period with only a moderate rate of lactation, with the rate rising until it reaches a peak about 70 days after the start of lactation. It then declines gradually until the cow is dry. The rise and fall in milk production levels are related in part to the number of milk-producing cells in the cow's udder. These cells are gradually lost during the phase of decline in lactation and do not regrow until the cow's next

lactation period. Posilac works by sustaining the number of milk-producing cells in the udder, which is the reason for its being given shortly before the cow's milk production reaches its peak. The hormone is sold in packages of single-dose injections to reduce the risk of accidental overdose.

Hormones in other animals

The USDA specifies that foods cannot be labeled as hormone free if they are produced from animals that cannot be legally treated with hormones—primarily pork and poultry. The USDA states, "Hormones are not allowed in raising hogs or poultry. Therefore, the claim 'no hormones added' cannot be used on the labels of pork or poultry unless it is followed by a statement that says 'federal regulations prohibit the use of hormones…' The term 'no hormones administered' may be approved for use on the label of beef products if sufficient documentation is provided to the Agency by the producer showing no hormones have been used in raising the animals."

Precautions

Consumers should research information from reliable sources about the controversies concerning the use of hormones in beef and milk production, and then decide for themselves whether they prefer hormone-free food products. These products often cost more than milk or meat obtained from hormone-treated animals because production costs are higher.

Consumers who are concerned about the possible health effects of food products from hormone-treated animals can look for foods that are certified as organic (produced without the administration of antibiotics as well as hormones). As the ADA notes, however, "all foods [produced and sold in the United States] are covered under U.S. **food safety** laws and regulations, regardless of production method."

Complications

Consumer controversies over the use of exogenous hormones in beef and dairy cattle have focused on two major concerns: increased **cancer** risk and early puberty.

Cancer

Some observers have expressed concern that consuming milk or meat from hormone-treated animals increases a person's risk of developing cancer, specifically prostate or breast cancer; however, there is no evidence that such a risk exists. The greatest sources of estrogen, progesterone, and testosterone in humans are the human body itself and the use of oral contraceptives or hormone replacement therapy (in menopausal women). As of 2012, alcohol was the only known dietary factor directly associated with an increased risk of breast cancer.

In addition, natural hormones used to treat cattle are destroyed in the human digestive tract; less than 10% of the hormones found in beef after slaughter are absorbed by the human body during digestion. Even direct injections of bovine growth hormone into humans do not affect the human body; this fact was discovered in the 1950s when some researchers used injections of bovine growth hormone in attempting to treat children who were deficient in human growth hormone.

Health Canada has established minimum residue levels (MRLs) for the safe use of the synthetic hormones melengestrol acetate, trenbolone acetate, and zeranol in beef cattle. There are no MRLs for the natural hormones.

Effects on puberty

A series of so-called hormone scandals in Italy in the late 1970s and early 1980s led to questions about the safety of hormone-treated milk and meat in terms of the premature onset of puberty. Doctors investigating a cluster of cases of early puberty and abnormal breast enlargement in schoolchildren in northern Italy inquired whether growth hormones used (illegally) in cattle used to produce luncheon meat were responsible for these cases. Although it is true that the average age of children at puberty has continued to decline in the developed countries since surveys of adolescent development were first taken in the 1940s, there is no evidence that food products from hormone-treated animals are responsible for this drop in age. The factors most clearly related to the lowered age at puberty in both boys and girls are improved nutrition in the West since World War II, and the increase in the numbers of overweight and obese children.

Research & general acceptance

There is no conclusive evidence that meat or milk produced from animals treated with exogenous hormones is less safe or less nutritious than hormone-free products. The ADA stated in 2008 that "A study of milk quality among conventional (without and with use of recombinant bovine somatotropin [rbST]) and organic varieties showed no biologically significant differences in quality, nutrients and hormones, although conventional milk had statistically lower bacterial counts."

Research into potential links between milk from cows treated with rbST and breast cancer will

KEY TERMS

Animal husbandry—Also called animal science, the practice of breeding and raising livestock (including poultry) for meat and other food products.

Bovine—Referring to domestic cattle.

Endogenous—Something produced inside an organism (or other system).

Exogenous—Something introduced into an organism or other system from an outside source.

Hormone—A chemical released by one or more cells that affects cells in other parts of the organism. Some hormones can be made synthetically.

Mammal—Any animal belonging to the large class of warm-blooded vertebrates whose young are fed with milk secreted by the mammary glands of the female.

Maximum residue limit (MRL)—The maximum amount of a drug residue that can be allowed to remain in a food product at the time of human consumption.

Organic—In the context of animal husbandry, a label applied to meat or milk produced from animals that have not been treated with either antibiotics or hormones and that have not been exposed to chemical fertilizers or pesticides.

Recombinant bovine somatotropin (rbST)—An artificial growth hormone produced by recombinant DNA technology, given to lactating cows to increase milk production. It is marketed under the trade name Posilac.

Steers—Castrated male beef cattle.

continue, as it is known that breast cancer takes decades to develop and Posilac has only been used to increase milk production in the United States since 1994.

Resources

BOOKS

Goldstein, Myrna Chandler, and Mark A. Goldstein. *Controversies in Food and Nutrition*. Westport, CT: Greenwood Press, 2002.

Redman, Nina E. *Food Safety: A Reference Handbook*. 2nd ed. Santa Barbara, CA: ABC-CLIO, 2007.

PERIODICALS

Capper, J.L., et al. "The Environmental Impact of Recombinant Bovine Somatotropin (rbST) Use in Dairy Production." *Proceedings of the National Academy of Sciences of the United States of America* 105 (July 15, 2008): 9668–73.

Danby, F. W. "Comparing rbST-free, Organic, and Conventional Milk." *Journal of the American Dietetic Association* 108 (December 2008): 1991.

Vicini, J., et al. "Survey of Retail Milk Composition as Affected by Label Claims Regarding Farm-Management Practices." *Journal of the American Dietetic Association* 108 (July 2008): 1198–1203.

Zepeda, L., et al. "Consumer Risk Perceptions toward Agricultural Biotechnology, Self-Protection, and Food Demand: The Case of Milk in the United States." *Risk Analysis* 23 (October 2003): 973–84.

OTHER

Canadian Cattlemen's Association (CCA) and Beef Information Centre (BIC). "Understanding Use of Antibiotic and Hormonal Substances in Beef Cattle." *Nutrition Perspective* (June 2003). http://www.afac.ab.ca/current/bichormones.pdf.

Raymond, Richard, et al. "Recombinant Bovine Somatotropin (rbST): A Safety Assessment." July 14, 2009. http://www.ads.uga.edu/documents/rbSTExpert Paper-6.26.09-FINAL.pdf.

WEBSITES

American Cancer Society. "What are the Risk Factors for Breast Cancer?" http://www.cancer.org/Cancer/Breast Cancer/DetailedGuide/breast-cancer-risk-factors (accessed June 20, 2012).

Reilhac, Gilbert. "Vote Ends EU-U.S. Hormone-Treated Beef Row." Reuters, March 14, 2012. http://www.reuters.com/article/2012/03/14/eu-trade-beef-idUSL5E8EE50620120314 (accessed June 20, 2012).

U.S. Department of Agriculture (USDA) Food Safety and Inspection Service (FSIS). "Beef. . .from Farm to Table." http://www.fsis.usda.gov/Factsheets/Beef_-from_Farm_to_Table/index.asp (accessed June 20, 2012).

———. "Food Labeling: Meat and Poultry Labeling Terms." http://www.fsis.usda.gov/Fact_Sheets/Meat_&_Poultry_Labeling_Terms/index.asp (accessed June 20, 2012).

U.S. Department of Agriculture (USDA) Foreign Agricultural Service (FAS). "The U.S.-EU Hormone Dispute." http://www.fas.usda.gov./itp/policy/hormone.html (accessed June 20, 2012).

U.S. Food and Drug Administration (FDA). "Report on the Food and Drug Administration's Review of the Safety of Recombinant Bovine Somatotropin (updated April 2009)." http://www.fda.gov/AnimalVeterinary/SafetyHealth/ProductSafetyInformation/ucm130321.htm (accessed June 20, 2012).

———. "Steroid Hormone Implants Used for Growth in Food-Producing Animals." http://www.fda.gov/AnimalVeterinary/SafetyHealth/ProductSafetyInformation/ucm055436.htm (accessed June 20, 2012).

U.S. Food and Drug Administration (FDA). "Voluntary Labeling of Milk and Milk Products from Cows That Have Not Been Treated with Recombinant Bovine Somatotropin: Interim Guidance." http://www.fda.gov/Food/GuidanceComplianceRegulatoryInformation/GuidanceDocuments/FoodLabelingNutrition/ucm059036.htm (accessed June 20, 2012).

ORGANIZATIONS

Academy of Nutrition and Dietetics, 120 South Riverside Plz., Ste. 2000, Chicago, IL 60606-6995, (312) 899-0040, (800) 877-1600, amacmunn@eatright.org, http://www.eatright.org.

Food and Agriculture Organization of the United Nations (FAO), Viale delle Terme di Caracalla, Rome, Italy 00153, +39 06 57051, Fax: +39 06 570 53152, FAO-HQ@fao.org, http://www.fao.org.

Food Safety and Inspection Service (FSIS), U.S. Department of Agriculture (USDA), 1400 Independence Ave. SW, Washington, DC 20250-3700, (888) 674-6854 (USDA Meat and Poultry Consumer Hotline), MPHotline. fsis@usda.gov, http://www.fsis.usda.gov.

Health Canada, Address Locator 0900C2, Ottawa, Ontario, Canada K1A 0K9, (613) 957-2991, (866) 225-0709, TTY: (800) 267-1245, Fax: (613) 941-5366, info@hc-sc.gc.ca, http://www.hc-sc.gc.ca/contact/index-eng.php.

U.S. Food and Drug Administration, 10903 New Hampshire Ave., Silver Spring, MD 20993-0002, (888) INFO-FDA (463-6332), http://www.fda.gov.

Rebecca J. Frey, PhD

Human immunodeficiency virus (HIV) diet *see* **AIDS/HIV diet and nutrition**

Hydration

Definition

Hydration refers to the human body's ability to take in and maintain a steady level of water in its tissues and organs down to the cellular level. It describes a condition of fluid balance (water homeostasis) when adequate fluid levels are maintained. An imbalance caused by too little fluid intake results in **dehydration**. It is also possible for people to become overhydrated from excessive fluid intake; this condition is sometimes called water intoxication. Overhydration can lead to hyponatremia, a condition in which the level of **sodium** in the blood plasma is too low. Severe hyponatremia can result in neurological symptoms, including swelling of brain tissue, seizures, and in some cases, death.

- acute or chronic illnesses that affect normal eating and drinking habits
- mental confusion or communication problems
- difficulty swallowing

Water intoxication

Risk factors for water intoxication (overhydration) include:

- Drinking too much water during or after exercise without replacing electrolytes lost through sweating. This imbalance can lead to hyponatremia, or abnormally low levels of sodium in the body. Athletes or workers who notice salt stains or rings on their clothing should drink sports drinks, as well as plain water, to maintain hydration. Some doctors, however, recommend a 50/50 balance between plain water and sports drinks. While some sports drinks do contain high levels of glucose (sugar) and electrolytes, any beverage that contains more than 8% carbohydrates will be absorbed more slowly through the digestive tract than fluids with lower levels of glucose and electrolytes. Mixing or combining the sports drink with plain water speeds up the body's absorption of the glucose and electrolytes.

- Misinformation about the amount of water needed for adequate hydration during exercise or heavy work. Some athletes—particularly marathon runners—interpret guidelines about fluid intake during long periods of exercise to mean that they should drink as much water as their stomachs could tolerate, leading to hyponatremia. Medical personnel at marathon races are trained to immediately suspect water intoxication when runners collapse or show signs of mental confusion. Wilderness hikers are another group at increased risk of overhydration as a result of misinformation about the amount of fluid that they need.

- Small body mass. Infants, particularly those below nine months of age, can easily take in too much fluid when offered it because their overall body mass is so small.

- Cholera or severe gastroenteritis leading to dehydration through diarrhea. Attempting to replace fluid loss with water alone increases the risk of water intoxication. Oral rehydration solution, which is designed to restore electrolyte balance as well as replace lost fluid, is the treatment of choice for patients with cholera or other diarrheal diseases.

- Drug or alcohol intoxication. People who consume large amounts of alcohol or drugs, such as MDMA (medically known as 3,4-Methylenedioxymethamphetamine and commonly called ecstasy), may drink large amounts of water to replace fluid lost

during their "high" and fail to replace lost electrolytes as well.

- Water-drinking contests. Some fraternity hazing rituals used to include forcing pledges to drink large amounts of water in a short time period. Several deaths each year are regularly reported at various U.S. colleges and universities due to these hazing rituals.

- Psychiatric conditions. There is a psychiatric disorder known as psychogenic polydipsia, in which patients drink water in sufficient amounts to lead to hyponatremia and seizures. The condition is often associated with schizophrenia but has also been reported in patients with developmental disorders.

Results

The results of adequate hydration are basic good health, rapid recovery from any diarrheal disease, and enjoyment of athletic activity without risk of dehydration and eventual heat-related illness.

QUESTIONS TO ASK YOUR DOCTOR

- How much fluid should I take in per day given my age, activity level, and geographical location?
- How can I tell if I am adequately hydrated?
- What are the health risks of dehydration?
- What are the health risks of overhydration?

Health care team roles

A family doctor can order a yearly urine and blood test for people who do not need to monitor their level of hydration closely. Athletes and those who perform heavy labor outdoors in hot weather may wish to consult a nutritionist or specialist in sports medicine to evaluate their need for closer monitoring of hydration levels or an individual plan for maintaining adequate hydration.

Caregiver concerns

Caregiver concerns include monitoring the fluid intake of elderly patients to make sure it is adequate and monitoring the fluid intake of infants to make sure they are not overhydrated.

Resources

BOOKS

Dunford, Marie. *Fundamentals of Sport and Exercise Nutrition.* Champaign, IL: Human Kinetics, 2010.

Isaac, Jeff. *Outward Bound Wilderness First-Aid Handbook*, rev. and upd. Guilford, CT: Falcon Guides, 2008.

Knoop, Kevin J., et al., eds. *Atlas of Emergency Medicine.* 3rd ed. New York: McGraw-Hill Professional, 2009.

Micheli, Lyle J., ed. *Encyclopedia of Sports Medicine.* Thousand Oaks, CA: SAGE, 2011.

Moorman III, Claude T., and Donald T. Kirkendall, eds. *Praeger Handbook of Sports Medicine and Athlete Health.* Santa Barbara, CA: Praeger, 2011.

Rich, Brent E., and Mitchell K. Pratte. *Tarascon Sports Medicine Pocketbook.* Sudbury, MA: Jones and Bartlett Publishers, 2010.

Smolin, Lori A., and Mary B. Grosvenor. *Nutrition for Sports and Exercise.* New York: Chelsea House, 2010.

PERIODICALS

American College of Sports Medicine (ACSM). "American College of Sports Medicine Position Stand: Exercise and Fluid Replacement." *Medicine and Science in Sports and Exercise* 39 (February 2007): 377–90.

Dalal, S., et al. "Is There a Role for Hydration at the End of Life?" *Current Opinion in Supportive and Palliative Care* 3 (March 2009): 72–78.

Dundas, B., et al. "Psychogenic Polydipsia Review: Etiology, Differential, and Treatment." *Current Psychiatry Reports* 9 (June 2007): 236–41.

Montain, S.J. "Hydration Recommendations for Sport 2008." *Current Sports Medicine Reports* 7 (July–August 2008): 187–192.

Noakes, T.D. "Hydration in the Marathon: Using Thirst to Gauge Safe Fluid Replacement." *Sports Medicine* 37 (April–May 2007): 463–66.

Rogers, I.R., and T. Hew-Butler. "Exercise-Associated Hyponatremia: Overzealous Fluid Consumption." *Wilderness and Environmental Medicine* 20 (Summer 2009): 139–43.

Wotton, K., et al. "Prevalence, Risk Factors, and Strategies to Prevent Dehydration in Older Adults." *Contemporary Nurse* 31 (December 2008): 44–56.

WEBSITES

American College of Sports Medicine. "Heat and Hydration: Important Concerns for Outdoor Workouts." http://www.acsm.org/about-acsm/media-room/acsm-in-the-news/2011/08/01/heat-and-hydration-important-concerns-for-outdoor-workouts (accessed August 23, 2012).

American Council on Exercise. "Fit Facts: Healthy Hydration." http://www.acefitness.org/fitfacts/fitfacts_display.aspx?itemid=173 (accessed August 5, 2012).

Johnston, Brian D., and Paul L. Liebert. "Overview of Exercise." *Merck Manual for Health Care Professionals.* http://www.merckmanuals.com/professional/special_subjects/exercise/overview_of_exercise.html (accessed August 23, 2012).

Mayo Clinic staff. "Water: How Much Should You Drink Every Day?" MayoClinic.com. http://www.mayoclinic.com/health/water/NU00283 (accessed August 23, 2012).

ORGANIZATIONS

American College of Sports Medicine, 401 W Michigan St., Indianapolis, IN 46202, (317) 637-9200, Fax: (317) 634-7817, http://www.acsm.org.

American Council on Exercise, 4851 Paramount Dr., San Diego, CA 92123, (858) 576-6500, Fax: (858) 576-6564, (888) 825-3636, support@acefitness.org, http://www.acefitness.org.

Centers for Disease Control and Prevention, 1600 Clifton Rd. NE, Atlanta, GA 30333, (800) CDC-INFO (232-4636), TTY: (888) 232-6348, cdcinfo@cdc.gov, http://www.cdc.gov.

World Health Organization, Avenue Appia 20, 1211 Geneva 27, Switzerland, +41 22 791-2111, Fax: +41 22 791-3111, info@who.int, http://www.who.int.

Rebecca J. Frey, PhD
William A. Atkins, BB, BS, MBA

Hyperactivity

Definition

Hyperactivity is behavior characterized by overactivity, impulsivity, distractibility, and decreased attention span. Though it has not been scientifically proven, many people believe that children are more likely to be hyperactive if they eat higher amounts of **sugar**.

Demographics

Hyperactive children vary from 3%–15% of all children. As of 2012, the U.S. Centers for Disease Control and Prevention (CDC) reported that 9.5% of children had ever been diagnosed with attention deficit hyperactivity disorder (ADHD) in the United States. American sugar consumption hit a record high in 1999, at an average of 155 pounds per person annually. Data indicates that this amount had decreased slightly by 2012. The U.S. Department of Agriculture (USDA) stated in 2000 that the average American, who consumes about 2,000 **calories** per day, can healthfully eat up to 10 teaspoons (40 g) of added sugars if he or she eats a healthful diet containing all the recommended servings of fruits, dairy products, and other foods. However, sugar is added to seemingly all food products, making it difficult to stay within the recommended range.

Description

Hyperactive children tend to be overly energetic and have constant difficulty paying attention. Normal activity levels in children vary with their age. It is appropriate for a toddler to have a shorter attention span than an older child. Attention levels may also vary depending on the child's interest in the activity. Hyperactive children are those whose activity level is consistently higher than expected for their age group.

Names for added sugars that appear on food labels

- Brown sugar
- Corn sweetener
- Corn syrup
- Corn syrup frutose
- Dextrose
- Fructose
- Fruit juice concentrates
- Galactose
- Glucose
- High-fructose corn syrup
- Honey
- Invert sugar
- Lactose
- Maltose
- Malt syrup
- Molasses
- Raw sugar
- Sucrose
- Sugar
- Syrup

(Table by GGS Information Services. © 2013 Cengage Learning.)

The hyperactivity-sugar controversy arose due to numerous claims made by parents after observing hyperactivity in children who ate foods containing sugar or **artificial sweeteners**, such as aspartame. However, most researchers hold to the belief that the effects of sugar on children are negligible, with several studies reporting that sugar does not cause hyperactivity in children.

From a physiological point of view, however, sugar should affect children's activity, simply because it can enter the bloodstream quickly, producing rapid changes in blood glucose levels and triggering adrenaline. Adrenaline is the substance produced by the body when it falls under stress, providing a short-term energy boost to cope with the stressor. A 1995 study by pediatric researchers at Yale University confirmed that sugar did affect adrenaline when ingested. In the study, healthy children were given large doses of sugar on an empty stomach; within a few hours, their bodies released large amounts of adrenaline, which induced shakiness, anxiety, excitement, and concentration problems. These reactions were observed only in children, and an examination of their brain waves revealed significant changes in their ability to pay attention. However, no direct link was established with dietary sugar, since the study involved the ingestion of large amounts of sugar on an empty stomach.

Causes and symptoms

The causes of hyperactivity can include:

- attention deficit hyperactivity disorder (ADHD), a condition characterized by inattentiveness, overactivity, and impulsivity
- stress or other emotional disorders, which may prompt hyperactivity as a response (often with aggressive behavior)
- brain or central nervous system disorders for which hyperactivity is a symptom, such as schizophrenia, bipolar disorder, obsessive-compulsive disorder, panic disorder, borderline personality disorder, autism, pervasive developmental disorders, and Tourette syndrome
- hyperthyroidism, a condition caused by the effects of too much thyroid hormone on tissues of the body; common symptoms include palpitations, nervousness, and hyperactivity
- high levels of lead exposure, which can lead to hyperactivity in children

Food additives and artificial colorings

A widely publicized study conducted by Dr. Ben Feingold in the early 1970s suggested that allergies to certain foods and **food additives** caused the characteristic hyperactivity of ADHD children. Although some children may have adverse reactions to certain foods that can affect their behavior (for example, a rash might temporarily cause a child to be distracted from other tasks), follow-up studies have uncovered no link between **food allergies** and ADHD.

Controversy continues regarding the subject of food additives (especially synthetic colorings and dyes) with respect to hyperactivity. In the United States, food manufactures can use nine different dyes in food, 90% of which are made up of dyes Red 40, Yellow 5, and Yellow 6. Some food manufactures in Europe have done away with food dye in their products; however, this practice has not yet occurred in the United States.

The U.S. Food and Drug Administration (FDA) notes that they have not found a cause and effect relationship between dyes and hyperactivity in children. On its website, the FDA states that "food and color additives are strictly studied, regulated and monitored. Federal regulations require evidence that each substance is safe at its intended level of use before it may be added to foods. Furthermore, all additives are subject to ongoing safety review as scientific understanding and methods of testing continue to improve. Consumers should feel safe about the foods they eat."

Continued studies are needed to further examine hyperactivity in children who consume food with and without artificial coloring. Future studies may yield new and beneficial results shedding light and a better understanding on this subject.

Diagnosis

It can be difficult to distinguish between hyperactivity and the normal activity level of a child. Because adults are rarely as active as small children, a child may be normally active for his or her age but deemed hyperactive by caregivers.

A medical evaluation will reveal whether hyperactivity is due to neurological disorders or hyperthyroidism. In the case of ADHD, the American Academy of Pediatrics (AAP) has issued guidelines for pediatricians to clarify the issue. Child psychologists can also determine whether the hyperactivity has an underlying emotional origin. The following tests may be used to evaluate hyperactivity:

- parent and teacher questionnaires
- psychological evaluation of the child and of the family
- developmental, mental, nutritional, physical, and psychosocial examinations

---

KEY TERMS

Adrenaline—The substance made by the body when under stress, which provides a short-term energy boost and increases heart and respiration rates.

Dietary fiber—Also known as roughage or bulk. Insoluble fiber moves through the digestive system almost undigested and gives bulk to stools. Soluble fiber dissolves in water and helps keep stools soft.

Obese—Having a body mass index (BMI) greater than the 95th percentile for age for children aged 2–20.

Treatment

If the hyperactivity is related to an underlying neurological or psychological cause, treatment of the condition will result in improvement. For hyperactivity unrelated to a medical condition, the following measures can help:

- limit stimulation in the child's environment
- provide instruction on an individual basis
- ensure that the child gets enough sleep

Nutrition and dietary concerns

Children need plenty of **fiber** in their diet to keep adrenaline levels as steady as possible throughout the day. Fiber is found in whole-grain products, such as whole-grain bread, brown rice, high-fiber cereals, fresh and dried fruits, vegetables, and beans. It is also recommended to limit the amount of processed sugars that children eat as much as possible. High-sugar foods tend to have fewer **vitamins** and **minerals**, and should be replaced by more nutritious foods. Processed foods that are high in sugar can cause tooth decay and contribute to **obesity**. It has also been established that the brain of a child may be more sensitive than the adult brain to the effect of low blood sugar, causing children to be more prone to sugar **cravings**. Since sugar enters the bloodstream quickly, its effects can be reduced if it is consumed along with other nutrients, such as fat and **protein**. As a rule, sweet desserts consumed after mixed meals that include protein, fat, complex **carbohydrates**, and fiber are preferable to eating sweet snacks between meals. Besides sugars, many sodas also contain **caffeine**, a stimulant that contributes to hyperactivity. These soft drinks should be avoided and replaced by water, juices, and caffeine-free drinks.

Some good selections for an afternoon snack include:

- raw vegetables, such as carrots, celery, or tomatoes, with a low-fat dip or chopped avocado
- fresh fruit
- peanut butter on whole-wheat bread
- cold chicken and a glass of milk
- a hardboiled egg on oatmeal bread
- half of a grilled cheese sandwich
- yogurt
- a bagel or muffin and a glass of milk
- a bowl of cereal with milk

Therapy

Drug therapy is not recommended for hyperactivity that has no medical cause. Medications prescribed for ADHD that decrease hyperactivity, such as Concerta and Ritalin, may have adverse side effects and should only be considered if the ADHD diagnosis has been established.

Massage and relaxation therapies are starting to be considered beneficial in lowering hyperactivity. Studies performed on hyperactive adolescents have shown improved mood and a reduction in hyperactivity in students undergoing massage therapy for ten consecutive school days.

Other measures effective in reducing hyperactivity include choosing schools that can provide a structured classroom environment and teaching relaxation techniques at home. For instance, children might be taught to have periods of "quiet time" so that they can learn how to calm themselves.

Prognosis

There is no cure for hyperactivity, but with practice it can be controlled.

Prevention

While there is no proven way to prevent hyperactivity, early identification may help prevent the development of ADHD and other developmental disorders.

Resources

BOOKS

Brown, Richard P., and Patricia L. Gerber. *Non-Drug Treatments for ADHD: New Options for Kids, Adults, and Clinicians.* New York: W.W. Norton & Company, 2012.

Dorfman, Kelly. *What's Eating Your Child?: The Hidden Connection Between Food and Childhood Ailments.* New York: Workman, 2011.

Smith, Matthew. *An Alternative History of Hyperactivity: Food Additives and the Feingold Diet.* Critical Issues in Health and Medicine. Piscataway, NJ: Rutgers University Press, 2011.

PERIODICALS

Blunden, Sarah Lee, Catherine M. Milte, and Natalie Sinn. "Diet and Sleep In Children With Attention Deficit Hyperactivity Disorder." *Journal of Child Health Care* 15, no. 1 (March 2011): 14–24.

Johnson, Richard J., et al. "Attention-Deficit/Hyperactivity Disorder: Is It Time to Reappraise the Role of Sugar Consumption?" *Postgraduate Medicine* 123, no. 5 (September 2011): 39–49.

Jones, Timothy W., et al. "Enhanced Adrenomedullary Response and Increased Susceptibility to Neuroglycopenia: Mechanisms Underlying the Adverse Effects of Sugar Ingestion in Healthy Children." *The Journal of Pediatrics* 126, no. 2 (1995): 171–77.

Kim, Y., and H. Chang. "Correlation between Attention Deficit Hyperactivity Disorder and Sugar Consumption, Quality of Diet, and Dietary Behavior in School Children." 5, no. 3 (2011): 236–45.

McCann, Donna, et al. "Food Additives and Hyperactive Behaviour in 3-Year-Old and 8/9-Year-Old Children in the Community: A Randomised, Double-Blinded, Placebo-Controlled Trial." *The Lancet* 370, no. 9598 (2007): 1560–67. http://dx.doi.org/10.1016/S0140-6736(07)61306-3 (accessed September 12, 2012).

WEBSITES

MedlinePlus. "Hyperactivity and Sugar." U.S. National Library of Medicine, National Institutes of Health. http://www.nlm.nih.gov/medlineplus/ency/article/002426.htm (accessed September 12, 2012).

U.S. Food and Drug Administration. "Food Ingredients and Colors." http://www.fda.gov/food/

foodingredientspackaging/ucm094211.htm (accessed September 12, 2012.

Wilson, Philip. "Sugar Makes Children Hyperactive—and Other Medical Myths." *Consumer Reports*, January 9, 2009. http://news.consumerreports.org/health/2009/01/medical-myths.html (accessed September 12, 2012).

ORGANIZATIONS

American Academy of Pediatrics (AAP), 141 Northwest Point Blvd., Elk Grove Village, IL 60007, (847) 434-4000, (800) 433-9016, Fax: (847) 434-8000, http://www.aap.org.

Attention Deficit Disorder Association, PO Box 7557, Wilmington, DE 19803, (800) 939-1019, info@adda.org, http://www.add.org.

Children and Adults with Attention Deficit Disorder (CHADD), 8181 Professional Pl., Ste. 150, Landover, MD 20785, (301) 306-7070, Fax: (301) 306-7090, (800) 233-4050, http://www.chadd.org.

Monique Laberge, PhD
Laura Jean Cataldo, RN, EdD

Hyperlipidemia

Definition

Hyperlipidemia, also known as hyperlipoproteinemia or dyslipidemia, is an elevation of lipid levels (**fats**) in the bloodstream. These lipids include cholesterol, cholesterol compounds, phospholipids, and **triglycerides**, all carried in the blood as part of large molecules called lipoproteins.

Description

Hyperlipidemia affects the way lipids are produced, used, carried in the blood, or disposed of by the body. There are three types of hyperlipidemias:

- Hyperlipoproteinemia: elevated levels of lipoproteins in the blood;
- Hypercholesterolemia: high cholesterol levels in the blood;
- Hypertriglyceridemia: high triglyceride levels in the blood.

It has been shown that people with a hyperlipidemia disorder are more likely to develop heart disease. For example, the normal body makes enough cholesterol for its needs. But when there is too much cholesterol, it accumulates in arteries, which can lead to their narrowing (atherosclerosis) and to heart disease or stroke.

Cholesterol levels

Able to control

What you eat. Certain foods have types of fat that raise your cholesterol level.

- Saturated fat raises your low-density lipoprotein (LDL) cholesterol level more than anything else in your diet.
- *Trans* fatty acids (*trans* fats) are made when vegetable oil is hydrogenated to harden it. *Trans* fatty acids raise cholesterol levels.
- Cholesterol is found in foods that come from animal sources, for example, egg yolks, meat, and cheese.

Weight. Being overweight tends to increase your LDL level, lower your high-density lipoprotein (HDL) level, and increase your total cholesterol level.

Activity level. Lack of regular exercise can lead to weight gain, which could raise your LDL cholesterol level. Regular exercise can help you lose weight and lower your LDL level. It can also help you raise your HDL level.

Unable to control

Heredity. High blood cholesterol can run in families. An inherited genetic condition (familial hypercholesterolemia) results in very high LDL cholesterol levels. It begins at birth, and may result in a heart attack at an early age.

Age and sex. Starting at puberty, men have lower levels of HDL than women. As women and men get older, their LDL cholesterol levels rise. Younger women have lower LDL cholesterol levels than men, but after age 55, women have higher levels than men.

SOURCE: National Heart, Lung and Blood Institute, National Institutes of Health, U.S. Department of Health and Human Services

More information available online at http://www.nhlbi.nih.gov/health/health-topics/topics/hbc/causes.html. *(Table by GGS Information Services. © 2013 Cengage Learning.)*

The lipoproteins present in blood plasma that transport lipids belong to the following major groups:

- Very high-density lipoprotein (VHDL). VHDL consists of proteins and a high concentration of free fatty acids.
- High-density lipoprotein (HDL). HDL helps remove fat from the body by binding with it in the bloodstream and carrying it back to the liver for excretion in the bile and disposal. A high level of HDL may lower chances of developing heart disease or stroke.
- Intermediate-density lipoprotein (IDL). IDLs are formed during the degradation of very low-density lipoproteins; some are cleared rapidly into the liver and some are broken down to low-density lipoproteins.
- Low-density lipoproteins (LDL). LDL transports cholesterol to extrahepatic tissues (outside the liver). A high LDL level may increase chances of developing heart disease.
- Very low-density lipoprotein (VLDL). VLDLs carry triglycerides from the intestine and liver to fatty

(adipose) and muscle tissues; they contain primarily triglycerides. A high VLDL level can cause the buildup of cholesterol in arteries and increase the risk of heart disease and stroke.

- Chylomicrons. Proteins that transport cholesterol and triglycerides from the small intestine to tissues after meals.

Generally speaking, LDL levels should be low, and HDL levels high. This is why HDL is often called the "good cholesterol" and LDL the "bad cholesterol."

Demographics

According to the Centers for Disease Control and Prevention (CDC), approximately 13.4% of the adult population has high blood cholesterol in the United States. Anyone can develop high cholesterol, including children. It has been shown to represent a major risk factor for heart disease, the leading cause of death in the country. In 2009, there were 96 million visits to doctors' offices that included a cholesterol test being done or ordered. Among African Americans, about 27.7% of women and 34.4% of men have high LDL cholesterol. Among Mexican Americans, about 31.6% of women and 41.9% of men have high LDL cholesterol. Among whites, 32% of women and 30.5% of men have high LDL cholesterol. In 2010, 68% of adults reported that they had their cholesterol checked within the previous 5 years, according to data from CDC's Behavioral Risk Factor Surveillance System.

Symptoms

Hyperlipidemia by itself does not cause symptoms, so people are generally not aware that their lipid levels are too high.

Diagnosis

Simple blood tests are done to check blood lipid levels. The National Cholesterol Education Program recommends that people be tested every 5 years after age 20. A lipoprotein test, also called a fasting lipid test, is commonly performed as part of a routine medical examination. The test measures lipid levels and usually reports on four groups:

- Total cholesterol (normal: 100–199 mg/dL)
- LDL (normal: less than 100 mg/dL)
- HDL (normal: 40–59 mg/dL)
- Triglycerides (normal: less than 150 mg/dL)

A total cholesterol value greater than 200 mg/dL is indicative of a greater risk for heart disease. However, LDL levels are a better predictor of heart disease,

and they determine how your high cholesterol should be treated.

Treatment

Treatment depends on lipid levels, the presence of risk factors for heart disease, and general health. When lipid levels are not balanced, the goal is to bring them under control, and this is done by changing dietary habits. Hyperlipidemia is first treated by modifying eating habits accordingly:

- Reduce saturated fat intake to 7% of the daily intake of calories.
- Reduce total fat intake to 25%–35% of the daily intake of calories.
- Limit the dietary cholesterol to less than 200 mg per day.
- Ensure the intake of 20–30 g a day of soluble fiber.
- Ensure the intake of plant sterols at 2–3 g daily.

If dietary changes do not correct the hyperlipidemia, a course of drug therapy may be indicated. In the Unites States, men older than age 35 and postmenopausal women are generally candidates for lipid-lowering medications.

Nutrition and dietary concerns

To treat hyperlipidemia, a diet low in total fat, saturated fat, and cholesterol is recommended, along with reducing or avoiding alcohol intake. The American Heart Association (AHA) endorses the following dietary recommendations for people with high blood cholesterol:

- Total fat: 25% of total calories
- Saturated fat: less than 7% total calories
- Polyunsaturated fat: up to 10% total calories
- Monounsaturated fat: up to 20% total calories
- Carbohydrates: 50%–60% total calories
- Protein: ~15% total calories
- Cholesterol: less than 200 mg/dL
- Plant sterols: 2 g
- Soluble fiber such as psyllium: 10–25 g

Categories of appropriate foods include:

- Lean meat/fish: less than 5 oz./day
- Eggs: less than 2 yolks per week (whites unlimited)
- Low-fat dairy products (1% fat): 2–3 servings/day
- Grains, especially whole grains: 6–8 servings/day
- Vegetables: 3–5 servings/day
- Fruits: 2–5 servings/day

These recommendations translate into the following practical **dietary guidelines**:

- Select only the leanest meats, poultry, fish, and shellfish. Choose chicken and turkey without skin or remove skin before eating. Some fish, like cod, have less saturated fat than either chicken or meat.

- Limit goose and duck. They are high in saturated fat, even with the skin removed.

- Some chicken and turkey hot dogs are lower in saturated fat and total fat than pork and beef hot dogs. There are also lean beef hot dogs and vegetarian (tofu) franks that are low in fat and saturated fat.

- Dry peas, beans, and tofu can be used as meat substitutes that are low in saturated fat and cholesterol. Dry peas and beans also have a lot of fiber, which can help to lower blood cholesterol.

- Egg yolks are high in dietary cholesterol. A yolk contains about 213 mg. They should be limited to no more than 2 per week, including the egg yolks in baked goods and processed foods. Egg whites have no cholesterol, and can be substituted for whole eggs in recipes.

- Like high-fat meats, regular dairy foods that contain fat, such as whole milk, cheese, and ice cream, are also high in saturated fat and cholesterol. However, dairy products are an important source of nutrients, and the diet should include 2 to 3 servings per day of low-fat or nonfat dairy products.

- When shopping for hard cheeses, select ones that are fat free, reduced fat, or part skim.

- Select frozen desserts that are lower in saturated fat, such as ice milk, low-fat frozen yogurt, low-fat frozen dairy desserts, sorbets, and popsicles.

- Saturated fats should be replaced with unsaturated fats. Select liquid vegetable oils that are high in unsaturated fats, such as canola, corn, olive, peanut, safflower, sesame, soybean, and sunflower oils.

- Limit butter, lard, and solid shortenings. They are high in saturated fat and cholesterol.

- Select light or nonfat mayonnaise and salad dressings.

- Fruits and vegetables are very low in saturated fat and total fat, and have no cholesterol. Fruits and vegetables should be eaten as snacks, desserts, salads, side dishes, and main dishes.

- Breads, cereals, rice, pasta, grains, dry beans, and peas are high in starch and fiber and low in saturated fat and calories. They also have no dietary cholesterol, except for some bakery breads and sweet bread products made with high-fat, high-cholesterol milk, butter, and eggs.

- Select whole-grain breads and rolls whenever possible. They have more fiber than white breads.

- Most dry cereals are low in fat. Limit high-fat granola, muesli, and cereal products made with coconut oil and nuts, which increases the saturated fat content.

- Limit sweet baked goods that are made with saturated fat from butter, eggs, and whole milk such as croissants, pastries, muffins, biscuits, butter rolls, and doughnuts.

- Snacks such as cheese crackers and some chips are often high in saturated fat and cholesterol. Select low-fat ones such as bagels, bread sticks, cereals without added sugar, frozen grapes or banana slices, dried fruit, non-oil baked tortilla chips, popcorn, or pretzels.

Therapy

Generally, drug therapy is considered when:

- LDL cholesterol is 190 mg/dL or higher
- LDL cholesterol is 160 mg/dL or higher and there is one risk factor for heart disease
- LDL cholesterol is 130 mg/dL or higher and there are two risk factors for heart disease or diabetes
- LDL cholesterol is 100 mg/dL or higher and there is heart disease
- LDL cholesterol is greater than 70 mg/dL and there is recent heart disease along with diabetes, smoking, high blood pressure, high triglycerides, low HDL, or obesity

There are several types of drugs available to help lower blood cholesterol levels, and they work in different ways. Some are better at lowering LDL cholesterol, some are good at lowering triglycerides, and others help raise HDL cholesterol. Lipid-lowering medications include:

- statin drugs, such as lovastatin, which prevent the liver from manufacturing cholesterol
- bile acid resins, such as cholestyramine and colestipol, which prevent the body from reabsorbing the cholesterol present in bile
- fibrates, such as bezafibrate, fenofibrate, or gemfibrozil, which are particularly effective in treating high triglyceride levels
- niacin (vitamin B_3)

Prognosis

Prognosis depends on the presence of any additional risk factors for heart disease, such as diabetes, high blood pressure, being male and over age 45 or

KEY TERMS

Adipose—Tissue that contains fat cells.

Artery—A blood vessel that carries blood from the heart to the body.

Atherosclerosis—Clogging, narrowing, and hardening of the large arteries and medium-sized blood vessels. Atherosclerosis can lead to stroke, heart attack, eye problems, and kidney problems.

Bile—A digestive juice secreted by the liver and stored in the gallbladder that helps in the digestion of fats.

Blood plasma—The pale yellowish, protein-containing fluid portion of the blood in which cells are suspended. Blood plasma is 92% water, 7% protein, and 1% minerals.

Cholesterol—Soft, waxy substance found among the lipids present in the bloodstream and in all cells of the body.

Extrahepatic—Originating or occurring outside the liver.

Fatty acid—Any of a large group of monobasic acids, especially those found in animal and vegetable fats and oils, having the general formula CnH.

Heart attack—A heart attack occurs when blood flow to the heart muscle is interrupted. This deprives the heart muscle of oxygen, causing tissue damage or tissue death.

Lipids—Group of chemicals, usually fats, that do not dissolve in water, but dissolve in ether.

Lipoproteins—Proteins present in blood plasma. The five major families are: chylomicrons, very low-density lipoproteins (VLDL), intermediate-density lipoproteins (IDL), low-density lipoproteins (LDL), and high-density lipoproteins (HDL).

Phospholipid—Any phosphorous-containing lipid, such as lecithin and cephalin, composed mainly of fatty acids, a phosphate group, and a simple organic molecule.

Plant sterols—Plant sterols are present naturally in small quantities in many fruits, vegetables, nuts, seeds, cereals, legumes, vegetable oils, and other plant sources.

Psyllium—Psyllium husk comes from the crushed seeds of the Plantago ovata plant, an herb native to parts of Asia, the Mediterranean, and North Africa. Similar to oats and wheat, psyllium is rich in soluble fiber and has been used as a gentle bulk-forming laxative for constipation.

Saturated fat—A type of fat that comes from animals and that is solid at room temperature.

Sterols—Any of a group of predominantly unsaturated solid alcohols of the steroid group.

Stroke—The sudden death of some brain cells due to a lack of oxygen when the blood flow to the brain is impaired by blockage or rupture of an artery to the brain.

Triglyceride—The storage form of fat consisting of three fatty acids and glycerol. Triglycerides are used by the body to store energy.

Unsaturated fat—A type of fat derived from plant and some animal sources, especially fish, that is liquid at room temperature.

Whole-grain foods—A grain is considered whole when all three parts—bran, germ, and endosperm—are present. Common whole-grain foods include wild rice, brown rice, whole-wheat breads and cookies, oatmeal, whole oats, barley, whole rye, bulgar, and popcorn.

female and over age 55, having a first-degree female relative diagnosed with heart disease before age 65, or a first-degree male relative diagnosed before age 55 and with **obesity**. Outcome is also highly related to early diagnosis and treatment and compliance with therapy.

Prevention

Hyperlipidemia can be prevented by keeping a healthy diet, maintaining a normal weight, and being physically active. Everyone can take steps to maintain proper cholesterol levels. The most important are to eat foods that are low in saturated fat, to exercise regularly, to lose weight if overweight, and to get routine medical examinations and cholesterol tests.

Resources

BOOKS

American Heart Association. *American Heart Association Low-Fat, Low-Cholesterol Cookbook, 3rd Edition: Delicious Recipes to Help Lower Your Cholesterol.* New York: Clarkson Potter, 2005.

Durrington, P.N. *Hyperlipidemia (Fast Facts).* Albuquerque, NM: Health Press, 2005.

Freeman, M.W., and C.E. Junge. *Harvard Medical School Guide to Lowering Your Cholesterol.* New York: McGraw-Hill, 2005.

Kowalski, R.E. *The New 8-Week Cholesterol Cure: The Ultimate Program for Preventing Heart Disease.* New York: Collins, 2002.

Lipski, E. *Digestive Wellness.* New York: McGraw-Hill, 2004.

McGowan, M.P. *50 Ways to Lower Cholesterol.* New York: McGraw-Hill, 2002.

PERIODICALS

Shah, Nilay D., et al. "Comparative Effectiveness of Guidelines for the Management of Hyperlipidemia and Hypertension for Type 2 Diabetes Patients." *PLoS [Public Library of Science] One* 6, no. 1 (2011): e16170. http://dx.doi.org/10.1371/journal.pone.0016170 (accessed October 2, 2012).

WEBSITES

American Heart Association. "Hyperlipidemia." http://www.heart.org/HEARTORG/Conditions/Cholesterol/AboutCholesterol/Hyperlipidemia_UCM_434965_Article.jsp (accessed October 2, 2012).

Centers for Disease Control and Prevention. "Cholesterol: Facts." http://www.cdc.gov/cholesterol/facts.htm (accessed October 29, 2012).

ORGANIZATIONS

American Heart Association, 7272 Greenville Ave., Dallas, TX 75231, (800) 242-8721, http://www.americanheart.org.

British Heart Foundation, Greater London House, 180 Hampstead Rd., London, United Kingom NW1 7AW, +44 20 7554 0000, http://www.bhf.org.uk.

Centers for Disease Control and Prevention, Division for Heart Disease and Stroke Prevention, 4770 Buford Hwy NE, Mail Stop F-72, Atlanta, GA 30341-3717, (800) CDC-INFO (232-4636), TTY: (800) 232-6348, Fax: (770) 488-8151, cdcinfo@cdc.gov, http://www.cdc.gov/dhdsp.

National Heart, Lung, and Blood Institute, PO Box 30105, Bethesda, MD 20824-0105, (301) 592-8573, TTY: (240) 629-3255, Fax: (240) 629-3246, nhlbiinfo@nhlbi.nih.gov, http://www.nhlbi.nih.gov.

Monique Laberge, PhD

Hypertension

Definition

Hypertension is the medical term for high blood pressure. Each time the heart beats, it forces blood into the arteries. Blood pressure is the force created when blood moving through the body's arteries pushes against the artery walls. Arteries are the blood vessels

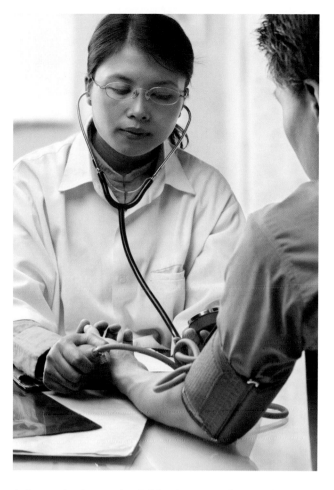

A doctor checks a patient's blood pressure levels. *(OtnaYdur/Shutterstock.com)*

that carry blood from the heart throughout the body. Though many factors contribute to hypertension, diet plays a major role in controlling blood pressure levels.

Demographics

According to the American Heart Association (AHA), nearly one in three adults (31.3%) have been diagnosed with high blood pressure, or about 76.4 million people 20 years or older in the United States. Of these, 79.6% know they have the disease, 47.8% have it controlled, and 70.9% are under current treatment. However, 52.2% do not have it controlled, and often they are not aware they have high blood pressure because there are no real symptoms. The AHA reported that in 2008, high blood pressure was the primary or contributing cause of 347,689 deaths in the United States.

African Americans are less likely to develop high blood pressure than Caucasian Americans. Men are more likely to develop the disease between the ages of 35 and 55, while women are more at risk for

Blood pressure category	Systolic mm Hg (upper#)		Diastolic mm Hg (lower#)
Normal	less than **120**	and	less than **80**
Prehypertension	**120 – 139**	or	**80 – 89**
High blood pressure (Hypertension) **stage 1**	**140 – 159**	or	**90 – 99**
High blood pressure (Hypertension) **stage 2**	**160** or higher	or	**100** or higher
Hypertensive crisis (emergency care needed)	Higher than **180**	or	Higher than **110**

(Table by Electronic Illustrators Group. © 2013 Cengage Learning.)

hypertension after menopause. In 2003, a report found that high blood pressure incidence was rising among children, most likely due to the increased number of overweight and obese children and adolescents. In 2011, the AHA reported that about 1 in 3 American children and teenagers were overweight or obese, and that this rise has led to the development of diseases in children that were previously seen only in adults, including high blood pressure, type 2 diabetes, and high cholesterol.

Description

Blood pressure is measured as it pushes against the inside of artery walls. The low blood pressure point, when the heart is at rest (between beats, when the heart is refilling with blood), is called diastolic pressure; the high blood pressure point, when the heart beats (contracts), is called systolic pressure. The number for the systolic pressure is larger than the number for the diastolic pressure. Blood pressure is measured in millimeters of mercury (mm Hg). The systolic reading is read and recorded first, and the diastolic pressure is read next. For example, if a person's high, or systolic, pressure is 118 and his or her low, or diastolic, pressure is 70, the blood pressure would be announced and recorded as 118/70 mm Hg, or "118 over 70." This would fall into the normal range, according to the AHA. The AHA's recommended blood pressure levels are less than 120 mm Hg for systolic pressure and less than 80 mm Hg for diastolic pressure.

If the systolic pressure rises to a level of 120–139 mm Hg or the diastolic pressure rises to a level of 80–89 mm Hg, a person is considered "prehypertensive." Stage 1 hypertension is defined as having a systolic

pressure of 140–159 mm Hg or a diastolic pressure of 90–99 mm Hg. Stage 2 is defined as having a systolic pressure of 160 mm Hg or higher or a diastolic pressure of 100 mm Hg or higher. If the systolic pressure raises above 180 mm Hg or the diastolic pressure goes above 110, the person is considered to be in hypertensive crisis and emergency care is needed. High blood pressure can have serious health consequences and is a major risk factor for stroke and heart attack.

Causes and symptoms

There is not a known primary cause of hypertension, and in many cases, the underlying cause cannot be determined. This is referred to as essential hypertension. If a specific cause has been found—usually kidney disease—the condition is referred to as secondary hypertension.

Several factors may be involved in the development of hypertension, including:

- chronic kidney disease
- adrenal and thyroid disorders
- too much sodium (salt) in the diet
- stress
- being overweight or obese (excessively overweight)
- smoking or using tobacco products
- no or little physical activity
- too much alcohol consumption (more than one drink for women or two drinks for men per day)
- older age
- genetics
- family history of high blood pressure

Symptoms are normally not present when blood pressure is high. Because of this, hypertension is often called "the silent killer." When symptoms do occur, they usually include:

- headache
- dizziness
- blurred vision
- nausea and/or vomiting
- chest pain
- shortness of breath

Diagnosis

Hypertension is usually diagnosed by taking a person's blood pressure with a blood pressure cuff, known as a sphygmomanometer. Machines are also available that take it automatically (even with home units). A regular annual physical examination is a good way to track blood pressure levels and overall health. The exam will generally include taking the patient's pulse rate, respiratory rate, body temperature, and weight. During the exam, the medical professional will inquire about past medical history, family medical conditions, medicine use, and other such pertinent information helpful in diagnosing hypertension, such as habits in smoking, **alcohol consumption**, lifestyle, exercise, drug use, and food consumption. Other checks performed during the exam include feeling for pulses on the extremities, such as ankles; touching the abdomen, especially the aorta; and examining the eyes.

Treatment

A hallmark of controlling high blood pressure is to eat foods rich in potassium and to avoid foods high in **sodium**. Diets like the **DASH diet** encourage eating more servings of fresh fruits and vegetables, which are naturally low in sodium. They also encourage keeping a check on total **calories**, fat, and **carbohydrates**. These diet strategies help keep weight at a healthy amount and help balance levels of sodium and other dietary **minerals**.

Though a **low-fat diet** is recommended as part of a healthy lifestyle, there is no direct link between fat, particularly saturated fat, and development of hypertension. However, **omega-3 fatty acids** may offer slight protective benefits; studies have shown minor reductions in blood pressure levels in people taking higher doses (more than 3 grams) of omega-3 fatty acids. Other studies have found conflicting results, however, so further research is needed. **Vitamins** B_6, C, D, and E may all also play roles in the prevention and treatment of hypertension, but studies are ongoing, and patients should consult with their physicians before taking any vitamins or other **dietary supplements**.

Patients with stage 1 hypertension may be advised to take antihypertensive medication. There are

numerous drugs available, and the choice of medication depends on the stage of hypertension, side effects, other medical conditions the patient may have, and other medicines the patient is taking. If treatment with a single medication fails to lower blood pressure to the desired level, a different drug may be tried or added to the first. Patients with more severe hypertension may initially be given a combination of drugs. Patients should never stop taking any medications without first checking with their physicians.

Nutrition and dietary concerns

Diet is an important part of controlling high blood pressure. A diet to control hypertension requires eating fewer overall calories, reducing salt, eating more potassium, reducing alcohol consumption, and eating lots of fruits and vegetables. Eating fewer calories and reducing fat, especially saturated fat, will help keep weight down. In addition, lowering weight to a normal range usually helps lower blood pressure. Salt is a well-known problem for people with high blood pressure, and much of the sodium that people eat comes from prepared and pre-packaged foods. Most diets for hypertension include decreasing use of table salt and of sodium in processed foods.

Potassium does the opposite of sodium and helps to lower blood pressure. Potassium is best obtained from foods rather than supplements. Foods rich in potassium include apricots, avocados, bananas, melons, kiwis, lima beans, oranges, prunes, dates, spinach, tomatoes, squash, potatoes, and **whole grains**. Fresh fruits and vegetables are low in sodium and rich in potassium and **fiber**, as well as other vitamins and minerals.

Plant proteins also may help lower blood pressure. Examples of plant proteins include **soy**, beans, peas, lentils, and nuts. Fresh produce is recommended over canned, since manufacturers may add sodium to help preserve canned products; the same is true for fish and poultry.

DASH diet

In the 1990s, scientists from the National Heart, Lung, and Blood Institute (NHLBI) conducted key studies to look at the effects of diet on blood pressure. These trials, called DASH (Dietary Approaches to Stop Hypertension), showed that an eating plan low in saturated fat, cholesterol, and total fat and high in fruits, vegetables, and low-fat dairy foods helped to lower blood pressure. DASH trials also followed the effects of a reduced-sodium diet on blood pressure. As a result, a comprehensive eating plan (the DASH diet) was developed with specific suggestions from each food group.

The DASH diet emphasizes lean meats, fish, chicken, low-fat dairy, fruits, vegetables, whole grains, legumes, nuts, and seeds. Vegetarian diets also may help keep blood pressure low, as may fiber and monounsaturated **fats**. The OmniHeart diet is similar to DASH but may emphasize a particular food group, such as **protein**, more. Other lifestyle changes, such as quitting cigarette smoking and increasing physical activity, are also recommended.

Eating plans, such as DASH or those suggested by a physician, must be followed carefully in order to work. Learning how to read food labels and to recognize hidden salt in prepared dishes is as important as pushing away the saltshaker at meals. People who begin the DASH eating plan may want to gradually work up to eating the recommended amount of fiber to prevent bloating and potential diarrhea. People with kidney trouble or heart failure should talk with their physicians before starting a diet that boosts potassium.

Therapy

It is important to involve a physician or registered dietitian in diet planning. Credible organizations, such as the American Heart Association, the Academy of Nutrition and Dietetics, or the National Heart, Lung, and Blood Institute, may also offer information on antihypertensive diets. People with high blood

---

QUESTIONS TO ASK YOUR DOCTOR

- How can I prevent high blood pressure?
- Can I reverse my hypertension if I eat better?
- What types of other lifestyle changes will also help me to lower my blood pressure?
- My parent had high blood pressure. Does that mean I will, too?

---

pressure should not rely on "fad" diets for quick weight loss or blood pressure fixes.

Prognosis

Though hypertension can be managed, it cannot be cured, and people with hypertension must work to control their blood pressure levels and keep them within normal ranges. The preferred way to do so is with careful monitoring of blood pressure and a combination of lifestyle and diet changes, as well as possible use of medications.

Prevention

Though excessive salt intake may be a trigger for high blood pressure, not everyone is sensitive to salt. Some people have high blood pressure for other reasons, such as heredity. Still, about one-half of people with high blood pressure are thought to be "salt sensitive," with high sodium intake resulting in raised blood pressure levels. Being overweight or obese are other factors affecting blood pressure, so developing dietary and lifestyle habits aimed at maintaining or losing weight are encouraged. Closely following a diet, such as DASH or one prescribed by a physician, to keep weight in the normal range will help control blood pressure. In addition, people who follow eating plans that consist of controlled portions, balanced intake from all food groups, and reduced sodium will enjoy other heart-healthy benefits, such as lower cholesterol.

Resources

BOOKS

Houston, Mark. *Handbook of Hypertension*. Hoboken, NJ: Wiley-Blackwell, 2009.

Moore, Thomas. *The DASH Diet for Hypertension*. New York: Simon & Schuster, 2011.

Rhoden, Chad, and Sarah Wiley Schein. *Bringing Down High Blood Pressure*. Lanham, MD: M. Evans, Rowman & Littlefield, 2010.

PERIODICALS

American Heart Association. "Heart Disease and Stroke Statistics—2012 Update." *Circulation* 125, no. 1 (2012): e2–e220. http://circ.ahajournals.org/content/125/1/e2 (accessed July 24, 2012).

Blumenthal, J.A., et al. "Effects of the DASH Diet Alone and in Combination with Exercise and Weight Loss on Blood Pressure and Cardiovascular Biomarkers in Men and Women with High Blood Pressure: The ENCORE Study." *Archives of Internal Medicine* 170, no. 2 (2010): 126–35.

Cabo, J., R. Alonso, and P. Mata. "Omega-3 Fatty Acids and Blood Pressure." *British Journal of Nutrition* 107, suppl. 2 (June 2012): S195–200.

Lin, Pao-Hwa, et al. "Blood Pressure-Lowering Mechanisms of the DASH Dietary Pattern." *Journal of Nutrition and Metabolism* (January 30, 2012): online only. http://dx.doi.org/10.1155/2012/472396 (accessed July 24, 2012).

Racine, E., et al. "The Effect of Medical Nutrition Therapy on Changes in Dietary Knowledge and DASH Diet Adherence in Older Adults with Cardiovascular Disease." *Journal of Nutrition, Health, and Aging* 15, no. 10 (2011): 868–76.

WEBSITES

American Heart Association. "High Blood Pressure." http://www.heart.org/HEARTORG/Conditions/HighBloodPressure/High-Blood-Pressure_UCM_002020_SubHomePage.jsp (accessed July 24, 2012).

———. "High Blood Pressure in Children." http://www.heart.org/HEARTORG/Conditions/HighBloodPressure/UnderstandYourRiskforHighBloodPressure/High-Blood-Pressure-in-Children_UCM_301868_Article.jsp (accessed July 24, 2012).

Cleveland Clinic. "High Blood Pressure and Nutrition." http://my.clevelandclinic.org/disorders/hypertension_high_blood_pressure/hic_high_blood_pressure_and_nutrition.aspx (accessed August 24, 2012).

German Institute for Quality and Efficiency in Health Care (IQWiG). "Hypertension: Does Losing Weight Reduce High Blood Pressure?" PubMed Health, U.S. National Library of Medicine. http://www.ncbi.nlm.nih.gov/pubmedhealth/PMH0005068 (accessed July 24, 2012).

Mayo Clinic staff. "DASH Diet: Healthy Eating to Lower Your Blood Pressure." Mayo Clinic. http://www.mayoclinic.com/health/dash-diet/HI00047 (accessed July 24, 2012).

National Heart, Lung, and Blood Institute. "Reduce Salt and Sodium in Your Diet." U.S. National Institutes of Health. http://www.nhlbi.nih.gov/hbp/prevent/sodium/sodium.htm (accessed July 24, 2012).

———. "Your Guide to Lowering High Blood Pressure." U.S. National Institutes of Health. http://www.nhlbi.nih.gov/hbp/index.html (accessed August 24, 2012).

ORGANIZATIONS

Academy of Nutrition and Dietetics, 120 South Riverside Plz., Ste. 2000, Chicago, IL 60606-6995, (312) 899-0040, (800) 877-1600, amacmunn@eatright.org, http://www.eatright.org.

American Heart Association, 7272 Greenville Ave., Dallas, TX 75231, (800) 242-8721, http://www.americanheart.org.

National Heart, Lung, and Blood Institute, PO Box 30105, Bethesda, MD 20824-0105, (301) 592-8573, TTY: (240) 629-3255, Fax: (240) 629-3246, nhlbiinfo@nhlbi.nih.gov, http://www.nhlbi.nih.gov.

Teresa G. Odle
William A. Atkins, BB, BS, MBA

Hypertriglyceridemia

Definition

Hypertriglyceridemia is an elevation of triglyceride levels in the bloodstream.

Origins

Hypertriglyceridemia is a condition characterized by elevated triglyceride levels. **Triglycerides** are the chemical form in which more than 90% of dietary fat and body fat exist. There are two sources of triglycerides: they are either obtained from the diet (dietary triglycerides) or manufactured by the body itself in the liver. They circulate constantly with all the lipoprotein carriers of the blood. The most important lipoproteins are:

- Very high-density lipoprotein (VHDL). VHDL consists of proteins and a high concentration of free fatty acids.
- High-density lipoprotein (HDL). HDL helps remove fat from the body by binding with it in the bloodstream

Possible causes of Hypertriglyceridemia

- Acute pancreatitis
- Certain medications
- Diabetes mellitus
- Excessive alcohol intake
- High-carbohydrate diet
- High-sugar diet
- Hypothyroidism
- Genetics
- Metabolic syndrome
- Nephrotic syndrome
- Obesity
- Pregnancy

(Table by GGS Information Services. © 2013 Cengage Learning.)

and carrying it back to the liver for excretion in the bile and disposal. A high level of HDL may lower chances of developing heart disease or stroke, which is why it is called the "good cholesterol."

- Intermediate-density lipoprotein (IDL). IDLs are formed during the degradation of very low-density lipoproteins; some are cleared rapidly into the liver and some are broken down to low-density lipoproteins.

- Low-density lipoprotein (LDL). LDL transports cholesterol to extrahepatic tissues (outside the liver). A high LDL level may increase chances of developing heart disease, which is why it is referred to as the "bad cholesterol."

- Very low-density lipoprotein (VLDL). VLDLs carry triglycerides from the intestine and liver to fatty (adipose) and muscle tissues; they contain primarily triglycerides. A high VLDL level can cause the buildup of cholesterol in arteries and increase the risk of heart disease and stroke.

- Chylomicrons. Proteins that transport cholesterol and triglycerides from the small intestine to tissues after meals.

A blood cholesterol test usually reports on both cholesterol and triglyceride levels. The American Heart Association endorses the National Cholesterol Education Program (NCEP), a division of the National Institutes of Health (NIH), and its guidelines for the detection of high cholesterol. The following are considered normal results:

- Total cholesterol (100–199 mg/dL)
- LDL (less than 100 mg/dL)
- HDL (40–59 mg/dL)
- Triglycerides (less than 150 mg/dL)

Hypertriglyceridemia is a common disorder in the United States. It is made worse by uncontrolled **diabetes mellitus**, **obesity**, cirrhosis of the liver, and sedentary habits, all of which are more common in industrialized countries than in developing nations. The condition generally occurs in people who have low-**protein** and high-carbohydrate diets, but also has genetic causes, which are not very well-defined. One inherited form is "familial hypertriglyceridemia," affecting about 1 out of 300 individuals in the United States. Hypertriglyceridemia can also result from a disorder of lipoprotein **metabolism** (dyslipidemia). Triglyceride levels increase gradually in men until about age 50 and then decline slightly. In women they continue to increase with age.

In 2001, the National Cholesterol Education Program (NCEP) released recommendations on triglyceride levels that should determine whether hypertriglyceridemia treatment is required or not:

- Normal: less than 150 mg/dL
- Borderline: 150–199 mg/dL
- High: 200–499 mg/dL
- Very high: higher than 500 mg/dL

In the Fredrickson classification of hyperlipidemias, the general term for elevated lipids in the blood, hypertriglyceridemia is classified as four different types:

- Type I: This is a rare disorder characterized by severe elevations in chylomicrons and extremely elevated triglyceride levels, always well above 1,000 mg/dL and reaching as high as 10,000 mg/dL or higher. Because chylomicrons contain cholesterol, blood cholesterol levels are also quite high.

- Type IIb: This is a mixed hyperlipidemia (high cholesterol and triglycerides) caused by elevations in both LDL and VLDL.

- Type III: This form is characterized by elevated total cholesterol and triglyceride levels. This type is easily confused with type IIb, but type III also features elevations in IDL.

- Type IV: This type is characterized by abnormal elevations of VLDL, with triglyceride levels almost always lower than 1,000 mg/dL. Blood cholesterol levels are normal.

When levels exceed 150 mg/dL, health care practitioners will recommend a diet aimed at lowering levels.

Description

Since there are different types of hypertriglyceridemia, often associated with other diseases or disorders (diabetes mellitus, obesity), diets need to be individually tailored. In general, people with hypertriglyceridemia are typically advised to lose weight and limit the consumption of processed foods, simple sugars, alcohol, and saturated **fats**. These fats are primarily found in animal foods, such as meat, eggs, and dairy products, and in tropical oils such as palm and coconut. Specific **dietary guidelines** include:

- Total fat intake should be restricted if weight loss is also required. If triglyceride levels are greater than 1,000 mg/dL, allowing no more than 10% of total calories from fat usually lowers levels quickly and significantly.

- If dietary intake of white flour products is significant, restricting simple carbohydrates and increasing dietary fiber can lower triglyceride levels substantially.

- Alcohol should be avoided or limited to no more than 1 standard alcoholic beverage per day.
- Omega-3 fatty acids, found mainly in fatty fish and some plant products such as flaxseed, have a significant effect on triglyceride levels. In large amounts (10 g daily or more), they lower triglycerides by 40% or more. Achieving this dose, however, requires supplements or eating very large amounts of fatty fish, such as sardines, herring, and mackerel.
- Refined sugars increase triglyceride levels, and people with elevated levels should accordingly lower their intake of sugar, sweets, and other sugar-containing foods.
- Individuals who consume a lot of tea and coffee should change to decaffeinated products, as eliminating caffeine has been shown to reduce triglyceride levels.
- Water-soluble fibers, such as pectin found in fruit, guar gum and other gums found in beans, and beta-glucan found in oats, may be particularly beneficial in lowering triglycerides.

Most foods contain several different types of fats, and some kinds are better for improving overall health. The four main types of fats are:

- Saturated fats: These fats consist of fatty acid chains that have no double bonds between the carbon atoms of the chain. They are called saturated because they are fully saturated with hydrogen atoms and cannot incorporate more. They are solid at room temperature and are most often of animal origin. Examples are butter, cheese, and lard.
- Monounsaturated fats: These are composed mostly of monounsaturated fatty acids, meaning molecules with one double-bonded carbon, with all the others carbons being single-bonded. They are liquid at room temperature. Examples are olive, peanut, and canola oil.
- Polyunsaturated fats: These fats are composed mostly of fatty acids, such as linoleic or linolenic acids, that have two or more double bonds in each molecule, as for example corn oil and safflower oil. They are also liquid at room temperature and can be further divided into the omega-6 and the omega-3 families. Fatty fish contains omega-3s, and they are also found in walnuts and some oils like soybean and rapeseed.
- *Trans* fatty acids. Unsaturated fats come in different chemical structures: a bent *cis* form or a straight *trans* form. When they adopt the trans form, they are called *trans* fatty acids. They are produced by the partial hydrogenation of vegetable oils and are present in hardened vegetable oils, most margarines, commercial baked foods, and many fried foods.

Unsaturated, monounsaturated, and polyunsaturated fats are considered better than others to lower the risk of heart disease since they lower the total and LDL cholesterol levels. **Omega-3 fatty acids** may be especially beneficial to the heart. They appear to decrease the risk of coronary artery disease and may also protect against irregular heartbeats and help lower blood pressure levels. Saturated and *trans* fats are considered less healthy because they can increase the risk of heart disease by increasing total and LDL cholesterol levels. Tips to limit fat in the diet are accordingly focused on reducing foods high in saturated and trans fats. For example, the Mayo Clinic offers the following:

- Cook with olive oil instead of butter.
- Use olive oil instead of vegetable oil in salad dressings and marinades. Use canola oil when baking.
- Sprinkle chopped nuts or sunflower seeds on salads instead of bacon bits.
- Snack on a small handful of nuts rather than potato chips or processed crackers.
- Add slices of avocado, rather than cheese, to sandwiches.
- Prepare fish such as salmon and mackerel, which contain monounsaturated and omega-3 fats, instead of meat one or two times a week.

Function

The function of a hypertriglyceridemia diet is to bring triglyceride levels back to normal recommended levels (less than 150 mg/dL).

Benefits

The benefits of normal triglyceride levels are numerous. Triglycerides carry fat-soluble **vitamins** A, D, E, and K to where they are required; help the synthesis of some hormones; and protect cell membranes. The fat tissues in which they are stored also cushion and protect organs such as the kidneys and provide thermal insulation.

Precautions

The National Heart, Lung, and Blood Institute (NHLBI), through its National Cholesterol Education Program (NCEP), recommends that the triglycerides of diabetic individuals be checked regularly. Diabetes can increase triglycerides significantly, especially when blood sugar is out of control. Healthy adults over 40 should get their triglycerides tested at least once a year, and more often if levels are high until they reach the desirable level.

KEY TERMS

Adipose—Tissue that contains fat cells.

Artery—A blood vessel that carries blood from the heart to the body.

Atherosclerosis—Clogging, narrowing, and hardening of the large arteries and medium-sized blood vessels. Atherosclerosis can lead to stroke, heart attack, eye problems, and kidney problems.

Blood plasma—The pale yellowish, protein-containing fluid portion of the blood in which cells are suspended. Blood plasma is 92% water, 7% protein, and 1% minerals.

Cholesterol—Soft, waxy substance found among the lipids present in the bloodstream and in all cells of the body.

Chylomicronemia—An excess of chylomicrons in the blood.

Chylomicrons—Intestinal triglycerides.

Cirrhosis—A life-threatening disease that scars liver tissue and damages its cells. It severely affects liver function, preventing it from removing toxins like alcohol and drugs from the blood.

Diabetes mellitus—A group of disorders in which there is a defect in the transfer of glucose (sugar) from the bloodstream into cells, leading to abnormally high levels of blood sugar (hyperglycemia).

Dyslipidemia—A disorder of lipoprotein metabolism, including lipoprotein overproduction or deficiency. Dyslipidemias may be manifested by elevation of the total cholesterol, the "bad" low-density lipoprotein (LDL) cholesterol and the triglyceride concentrations, and a decrease in the "good" high-density lipoprotein (HDL) cholesterol concentration in the blood.

Fatty acid—Any of a large group of monobasic acids, especially those found in animal and vegetable fats and oils, having the general formula CnH.

Fredrickson classification—A classification system of hyperlipidemias by ultracentrifugation followed by electrophoresis that uses plasma appearance, triglyceride values, and total cholesterol values. There are five types: I, II, III, IV, and V.

Heart attack—A heart attack occurs when blood flow to the heart muscle is interrupted. This deprives the heart muscle of oxygen, causing tissue damage or tissue death.

Hyperlipidemia—Elevation of lipid levels (fats) in the bloodstream. These lipids include cholesterol, cholesterol compounds, phospholipids, and triglycerides, all carried in the blood as part of large molecules called lipoproteins.

Lipids—Group of chemicals, usually fats, that do not dissolve in water, but dissolve in ether.

Metabolic syndrome X—Also called insulin resistance syndrome or prediabetic syndrome. The syndrome is closely associated with hypertriglyceridemia and with low HDL ("good") cholesterol.

Omega-3 fatty acids—Any of several polyunsaturated fatty acids found in leafy green vegetables, vegetable oils, and fish such as salmon and mackerel, capable of reducing serum cholesterol levels and having anticoagulant properties.

Triglycerides—Triglycerides are the chemical form in which most fat exists in food as well as in the body. They consist of three fatty acids and glycerol. Triglycerides are used by the body to store energy.

Unsaturated fat—A type of fat derived from plant and some animal sources, especially fish, that is liquid at room temperature.

Fat restriction should be carefully evaluated. When reducing fat intake results in a required weight loss, triglyceride levels usually improve. When they are severely elevated (1,000 mg/dL), a **low-fat diet** will decrease chylomicron and VLDL. However, when triglycerides are only moderately elevated, a low-fat diet will increase them and may also decrease HDL levels.

Risks

Triglycerides do not cause complications until elevations of 1,000 mg/dL or more are reached. There is a risk of chylomicronemia syndrome when levels are 800 mg/dL or higher. The syndrome causes recurrent episodes of abdominal pain that may be accompanied by nausea and vomiting. Extreme elevations of triglycerides, usually greater than 1,000 mg/dL, may cause an inflammation of the pancreas (pancreatitis). The pancreas is the organ that makes **insulin** and substances to help digest food, and pancreatitis is a serious disorder. People with hypertriglyceridemia are also at risk for fatty liver, the accumulation of fat in liver cells. Triglyceride levels of 4,000 mg/dL or higher may cause a

QUESTIONS TO ASK YOUR DOCTOR

- What causes hypertriglyceridemia?
- What type of hypertriglyceridemia do I have?
- Can it be cured?
- How is it treated?
- How serious is this condition?
- How effective is diet in controlling hypertriglyceridemia?
- What are some simple steps for reducing triglyceride levels in my diet?
- Are there foods that should be avoided?
- Are there foods that are recommended?
- Should I get help from a dietitian to prepare an eating plan?

condition known as lipemia retinalis, in which eye examination reveals retinal blood vessels that have a pale pink, milky appearance.

Women trying to become pregnant who have elevated triglycerides before conception may develop severe hypertriglyceridemia, with levels well above 1,000 mg/dL, and the associated risk of pancreatitis. These women require counseling for diet, exercise, and weight management before becoming pregnant and should be monitored closely during their pregnancies.

Research and general acceptance

Though it is unclear if elevated triglycerides independently contribute to cardiovascular disease, they have been associated with multiple conditions that contribute to diabetes and **metabolic syndrome** X. After much debate, consensus is emerging among medical experts that lowering elevated triglycerides is beneficial. For a long time, triglycerides were overshadowed by other blood lipids, especially by LDL, previously considered more important than triglycerides as a contributing factor to cardiovascular disease. In 1994, a study published in the American Heart Association's journal *Circulation* reported that LDL seemed to be masking arterial damage caused by triglyceride-rich VLDL and IDL. The study found that despite aggressive treatment of the LDL, patients with high triglyceride levels continued to suffer damage to arterial walls. Another report, in the *New England Journal of Medicine* HealthNews, described a Danish study involving 3,000 healthy men that concluded that the risk of having a first heart attack was twice as high in the men with the highest triglyceride levels, compared to those with the lowest levels. The connection between high triglycerides and heart disease is now established. However, some uncertainty remains concerning the relationship between triglycerides and HDL, the "good cholesterol." It has been observed that whenever triglycerides are increased, HDL cholesterol decreases. Researchers are still investigating whether the increased risk associated with high triglycerides is due to the triglycerides themselves, or to the associated reduction in HDL cholesterol and increase in LDL cholesterol.

The NCEP triglyceride recommendation of less than 150 mg/dL per day has been challenged by some. Cardiologists at the University of Maryland Medical Center have presented evidence that the recommended level may still represent a significant risk for heart disease. Their study suggests that less than 100 mg/dL would be more appropriate.

Resources

BOOKS

American Heart Association. *American Heart Association Low-Fat, Low-Cholesterol Cookbook, 3rd Edition: Delicious Recipes to Help Lower Your Cholesterol.* New York: Clarkson Potter, 2005.

Freeman, M.W., Junge, C.E. *Harvard Medical School Guide to Lowering Your Cholesterol.* New York: McGraw-Hill, 2005.

Kowalski, R.E. *The New 8-Week Cholesterol Cure: The Ultimate Program for Preventing Heart Disease.* New York: Collins, 2002.

Larson Duyff, R. *ADA Complete Food and Nutrition Guide.* 3rd ed. Chicago: American Dietetic Association, 2006.

McGowan, M.P. *50 Ways to Lower Cholesterol.* New York: McGraw-Hill, 2002.

Mierzejewski, A. *Bring Your Triglycerides Down Naturally: A Drug-Free Solution to High Blood Lipids.* Peterborough, ON: Full of Health Inc., 2006.

PERIODICALS

Oh, Robert C., and J. Brian Lanier. "Management of Hypertriglyceridemia." *American Family Physician* 75, no. 9 (2007): 1365–71.

Yuan, George, Khalid Z. Al-Shali, and Robert A. Hegele. "Hypertriglyceridemia: Its Etiology, Effects and Treatment." *Canadian Medical Association* 176, no. 8 (2007): 1113–1120.

WEBSITES

MedlinePlus. "Familial Hypertriglyceridemia." U.S. National Library of Medicine, National Institutes of Health. http://www.nlm.nih.gov/medlineplus/ency/article/000397.htm (accessed October 3, 2012).

University of Maryland Medical Center. "Study Finds 'Normal' Triglyceride Levels are Risky." http://www.umm.edu/news/releases/riskytrig.htm (accessed October 29, 2012).

ORGANIZATIONS

American Heart Association, 7272 Greenville Ave., Dallas, TX 75231, (800) 242-8721, http://www.americanheart.org.

British Heart Foundation, Greater London House, 180 Hampstead Rd., London, United Kingom NW1 7AW, +44 20 7554 0000, http://www.bhf.org.uk.

Centers for Disease Control and Prevention, Division for Heart Disease and Stroke Prevention, 4770 Buford Hwy NE, Mail Stop F-72, Atlanta, GA 30341-3717, (800) CDC-INFO (232-4636), TTY: (800) 232-6348, Fax: (770) 488-8151, cdcinfo@cdc.gov, http://www.cdc.gov/dhdsp.

Heart Foundation (Australia), 80 William St., Level 3, Sydney NSW, Australia 2011, +61 2 9219 2444, http://www.heartfoundation.org.au.

National Heart, Lung, and Blood Institute, PO Box 30105, Bethesda, MD 20824-0105, (301) 592-8573, (240) 629-3255, Fax: (240) 629-3246, nhlbiinfo@nhlbi.nih.gov, http://www.nhlbi.nih.gov.

Monique Laberge, PhD

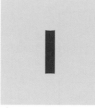

IBD *see* **Inflammatory bowel disease**
IBS *see* **Irritable bowel syndrome**
Indian diet *see* **Asian diet**

Infant nutrition

Definition

Children between the ages of birth and one year are considered infants. Infants grow very rapidly and have special nutritional requirements that are different from other age groups.

Purpose

Infant nutrition is designed to meet the special needs of very young children and to give them a healthy start in life. Children under one year old do not have fully mature organ systems. They need nutrition that is easy to digest and contains enough **calories**, **vitamins**, **minerals**, and other nutrients to allow them to grow and develop normally. Infants also need to receive the proper amount of fluids for their immature kidneys to process wastes. In addition, infant nutrition involves avoiding exposing infants to substances that are harmful to their growth and development.

Description

Infancy is a time of incredibly rapid growth and development. Ensuring that infants get the right kinds of nutrients in the right quantities and avoid the wrong kinds of substances gives them their best chance at a healthy start to life. Parents and caregivers are responsible for seeing that their infant's nutritional needs are met. Infant nutrition is so important that the U.S. Department of Agriculture (USDA) has developed the Women, Infants, and Children (WIC) program. This program provides free health and social service referrals, nutrition counseling, and vouchers for healthy foods to supplement the diet of pregnant and **breastfeeding** women, infants, and children up to the age of five who live in low-income households and are considered nutritionally at risk. In 2010, WIC served about 9.17 million people, including 2.17 million infants, 4.86 million children, and 2.14 million pregnant and nursing women.

Breastfeeding

Human milk is uniquely suited to meet the nutritional needs of newborns. Many health organizations, including the American Academy of Pediatrics (AAP), the American Medical Association (AMA), the **Academy of Nutrition and Dietetics** (formerly the American Dietetic Association), and the World Health Organization (WHO), support the position that breast milk is the best and most complete form of nutrition for infants. The AAP recommends that infants be exclusively breastfed for the first six months of life and that breastfeeding continue for at least 12 months.

Breastfeeding in the United States slowly increased in acceptance in the last decade of the twentieth century. In 1998, 64% of American mothers breastfed their babies for a short time after birth, but only 29% were still breastfeeding by the time their baby was 6 months old. One of the goals of Healthy People 2000, a set of health goals for the nation developed by the U.S. Department of Health and Human Services, was for 75% of American women to breastfeed their babies for a period immediately after birth and for 50% to breastfeed for the first six months of their infant's life. Women were divided into groups based on ethnicity, but none of the groups met the target. The next initiative, Healthy People 2010, eliminated the ethnic categories, but the goals stayed the same, with the addition of a third target: 75% to breastfeed for a period after birth, 50% to breastfeed for 6 months, and 25% to breastfeed for a full year.

Select recommended dietary allowances (RDA) and adequate intakes (AI) for infants

	0–6 months	6–12 months
Vitamins		
Folate (folic acid)*	65 µg	80 µg
Niacin*	2 mg	4 mg
Riboflavin (vitamin B$_2$)*	0.3 mg	0.4 mg
Thiamin (vitamin B$_1$)*	0.2 mg	0.3 mg
Vitamin A*	400 µg	500 µg
Vitamin B$_6$*	0.1 mg	0.3 mg
Vitamin B$_{12}$*	0.4 µg	0.5 µg
Vitamin C*	40 mg	50 mg
Vitamin D	10 µg	10 µg
Vitamin E*	4 mg	5 mg
Vitamin K*	2 µg	2.5 µg
Elements		
Calcium*	200 mg	260 mg
Fluoride*	0.01 mg	0.5 mg
Iron	0.27 mg*	11 mg
Magnesium*	30 mg	75 mg
Potassium*	0.4 g	0.7 g
Selenium*	15 µg	20 µg
Sodium*	0.12 g	0.37 g
Zinc	2 mg*	3 mg
Macronutrients		
Carbohydrates*	60 g	95 g
Fat*	31 g	30 g
Protein	9.1 g*	11 g
Water*	0.7 L	0.8 L

*Indicates Adequate Intake (no RDA has been established).
µg = microgram (mcg)

SOURCE: U.S. Department of Agriculture, National Agricultural Library, Food and Nutrition Information Center.

(Table by PreMediaGlobal. © 2013 Cengage Learning.)

ADVANTAGES OF BREASTFEEDING. Research comparing formula-fed and breastfed babies convincingly shows that both full-term and premature breastfed infants have certain advantages over formula-fed infants. One of the most important advantages conferred by breast milk is an increased resistance to infection.

Infants are born with immature immune systems that do not become fully functional for about two years. Since immune system cells make antibodies to fight infection, having incompletely developed immune systems leaves infants vulnerable to many bacterial and viral infections. However, nursing mothers have fully developed immune systems, and many of the antibodies and other components of the immune system are passed into breast milk. Nursing infants take in their mother's antibodies along with the other nutrients when they nurse. These antibodies survive passage through the infant's digestive system and are absorbed into the infant's blood, where they help protect against infection. Well-designed studies have repeatedly documented the fact that breastfed babies have fewer ear infections, bouts of diarrhea, respiratory infections, and cases of meningitis than formula-fed babies. Overall, the death rate of breastfed babies during the first year of life is lower than the death rate of formula-fed babies.

Another way that breastfeeding protects against infection is by helping prevent exposure to waterborne contaminants. In developing countries, water supplies are often contaminated with bacteria and chemicals. Using this water to mix formula increases the risk of the baby ingesting these pathogens and toxins. Breastfed babies are not exposed to this type of contamination.

Another advantage of breastfeeding is that infants are unlikely to gain excess weight. **Childhood obesity** is a major concern in the United States. Since mothers are unable to measure how much breast milk their baby consumes, they are less likely to encourage overfeeding. Research suggests that breastfed babies have a lower risk of developing type 2 diabetes. Other research suggests that the rate of other chronic diseases such as asthma, **celiac disease**, **inflammatory bowel disease**, and various allergies appears to be lower in breastfed babies than in babies fed with formula. Premature babies especially appear to benefit from reduced chronic disease as a result of breastfeeding.

Breastfeeding also provides benefits to the nursing mother. Breastfeeding is more economical than buying formula, even taking into account the extra food—about 500 calories daily—that the mother needs to eat when she is nursing. Since breastfed babies on average get sick less than formula-fed babies, the family is also likely to save money on doctor visits, medicine, and time off from work to care for a sick child.

The mother's health also benefits from breastfeeding. Nursing mothers tend to lose the weight they put on during pregnancy faster than mothers who do not nurse. The hormones that are released in the mother's body when her infant nurses also help her uterus contract and become closer to the size it was before pregnancy. Mothers who nurse their babies also seem to be less likely to develop breast, ovarian, or uterine **cancer** early in life. Finally, breastfeeding offers psychological benefits to the mother as she bonds with her baby and may reduce the chance of postpartum depression.

DISADVANTAGES OF BREASTFEEDING. Although breast milk is the best food for an infant, breastfeeding does have some disadvantages for the mother. Initially, babies breastfeed about every two to three hours. Some women find it exhausting to be available to the baby so frequently. When the infant is older, the mother may need to pump breast milk for her child to eat while she is away or at work. Fathers sometimes feel shut out during the early weeks of breastfeeding because of the close bond between mother and child. In addition, women who are breastfeeding must watch their diet carefully. Some foods or substances, such as **caffeine**, can pass into breast milk and cause the baby to be restless and irritable. Finally, some women simply find the idea of breastfeeding messy and distasteful, and resent the fact that they need to be available much of the time for feeding. For women who cannot or do not want to breastfeed, infant formula provides an adequate alternative.

Formula feeding

Although infant formula is not as perfect a food as breast milk for infants (it is harder for them to digest and is not a chemical replica of human milk), formula does provide all of the nutrients that babies need to grow up healthy. The U.S. Food and Drug Administration (FDA) regulates infant formula under the Federal Food, Drug, and Cosmetic Act (FFDCA). The FDA sets the minimum amounts of nutrients (29) that must be present in infant formula and sets maximum amounts for nine other nutrients. Some of these nutrients include vitamins A, D, E, and K, and **calcium**. Some formulas contain **iron**, while others do not.

Substances used in infant formulas must be foods on the FDA-approved "Generally Recognized as Safe" (GRAS) list. Facilities that manufacture infant formula are regularly inspected by the FDA and are required to keep process and distribution records for each batch of formula. Every container of formula must show an expiration or use-by date. The FDA must be informed of any changes made to the formula.

Infant formulas are either cow's milk based or **soy** based. Infants who show signs of lactose intolerance (colicky, restless, gassy, spitting up) usually do well on soy-based formula. Formula comes in three styles: ready-to-feed, concentrated liquid, and powder. Ready-to-feed formulas are the easiest to use and can be poured straight from the can into a bottle; however, they are also the most expensive. Concentrated liquids need to be mixed with an equal portion of water. Powder formulas, which also need to be mixed with water, are the least expensive and keep longer than the liquid varieties.

REASONS TO FORMULA FEED. Not every woman wants or is able to breastfeed. Aside from personal preference, women should use formula feed if they:

• are adoptive parents
• have HIV, active tuberculosis, or hepatitis C, which all can be passed on to their infants through breast milk

• use street drugs or abuse prescription medicines, which can pass to the infant and permanently damage a baby's health
• are taking chemotherapy drugs, certain mood stabilizers, migraine headache medications, or any other drugs that may pass into breast milk
• have alcoholism or are binge drinkers, as the alcohol will be present in their breast milk
• have difficult-to-control diabetes, as blood sugar levels may be even harder to control if breastfeeding
• are going to be separated from their baby for significant periods of time
• have had breast surgery that interferes with milk production
• are emotionally repelled by the idea of breastfeeding

A few babies are born with a genetic inborn error in **metabolism** that prevents them from digesting any mammalian milk. These babies must be fed soy-based formula in order to survive.

PROS AND CONS OF FORMULA FEEDING. Formula feeding has some definite advantages. Anyone, not just the mother, can feed the infant. This gives the mother more flexibility in her schedule and allows the father or other relatives to enjoy a special closeness with the baby that comes with feeding. Also, the mother does not need to be concerned about how her diet affects her baby, and she does not need to worry about breast milk leakage. Since formula is digested more slowly than breast milk, feedings are less frequent. Some women feel uncomfortable nursing in front of other people or find it difficult to locate places to nurse in private. Formula feeding eliminates this problem.

There are also disadvantages to formula feeding. Aside from the fact that formula is not an exact duplicate of breast milk and is harder to digest, it also costs more and requires more advance preparation. Bottles need to be washed, and the water used to mix formula, at least in the early months, needs to be boiled or be special bottled water suitable for infants. The Academy of General Dentistry warns that some public water supplies are fluoridated at levels too high for infants, and that fluorodosis of the primary (baby) teeth may result. Finally, formula must be refrigerated once it is mixed or a can is opened. It can only be kept about two days in the refrigerator, so waste is more likely to occur. Likewise, when traveling, bottles need to be refrigerated. Although most babies do not mind cold formula, many parents like to heat their child's bottles to body temperature, another inconvenience when traveling.

Required nutrients for infant formula

Nutrient	Minimum per 100 calories	Maximum per 100 calories
Protein (g)[1]	1.8 g	4.5 g
Fat	3.3 g 30% calories	6 g 54% calories
Essential fatty acids (linoleate)	300 mg 2.7% calories	
Vitamins		
A	250 IU (75 mcg)	750 IU (225 mcg)
D	40 IU	100 IU
K[2]	4 mcg	
E[3]	0.7 IU	
C (ascorbic acid)	8 mg	
B1 (thiamine)	40 mcg	
B2 (riboflavin)	60 mcg	
B6 (pyridoxine)[4]	35 mcg	
B12	0.15 mcg	
Niacin[5]	250 mcg	
Folic acid	4 mcg	
Pantothenic acid	300 mcg	
Biotin[6]	1.5 mcg	
Choline[6]	7 mg	
Inositol[6]	4 mg	
Minerals		
Calcium[7]	60 mg	
Phosphorus[7]	30 mg	
Magnesium	6 mg	
Iron	0.15 mg	3 mg
Iodine	5 mcg	75 mcg
Zinc	0.5 mg	
Copper	60 mcg	
Manganese	5 mcg	
Sodium	20 mcg	60 mcg
Potassium	80 mg	200 mg
Chloride	55 mg	150 mg

[1]Amounts apply to proteins with a biological quality equivalent to or better than that of casein. If the quality is less than that of casein, the minimum amount must be increased—e.g., formula containing protein with a biological quality of 75% of casein will need at least 2.4 grams of protein (1.8/0.75). All formulas must use a protein with a biological quality of at least 70% of casein's.
[2]Added vitamin K must be in the form of phylloquinone.
[3]Must be 0.7 IU per gram of linoleic acid.
[4]At least 15 mcg for each gram of protein (past the required 1.8 g).
[5]Includes niacin (nicotinic acid) and niacinamide (nicotinamide).
[6]Required only for non-milk-based infant formulas.
[7]The ratio of calcium to phosphorus in infant formula must be no less than 1.1 but not more than 2.0.

SOURCE: U.S. Food and Drug Administration.

Code of Federal Regulations Title 21, available online at http://www.accessdata.fda.gov/scripts/cdrh/cfdocs/cfCFR/CFRSearch.cfm?fr=107.100. *(Table by PreMediaGlobal. © 2013 Cengage Learning.)*

Transitioning to solid foods

When an infant is between four and six months old, most pediatricians recommend introducing the infant to some baby foods, but they do not need solid food before six months of age, particularly if breastfed. By this age, infants begin to have the muscle coordination to swallow stage one, or pureed, baby foods. If infants are force-fed early, some may rebel and develop feeding problems. Weaning of a breastfed infant depends on the preferences and needs of the mother and infant. Weaning gradually over weeks or months is easiest. When the infant is about seven months old, one feeding may be replaced by a bottle, and by ten months, the infant may be weaned to a cup. Thereafter, one or two feedings daily can be continued until the mother and child are ready to stop.

To determine an infant's tolerance, solid foods should be offered by spoon and introduced one food at a time. Stage one baby foods are essentially thick liquids, with stage two foods progressing in consistency and stage three foods introducing small pieces. Commercial baby foods with high **sodium** content, more than 200 mg/jar, should be avoided. If there is a family history of **food allergies**, some pediatricians recommend waiting until six months or older to add in additional foods.

The introduction of foods normally begins with a small amount of iron-fortified rice cereal or other single-grain cereal mixed into a slurry the consistency of thin gravy with formula or breast milk. The infant is then offered a small amount of cereal on a small spoon; it should never be offered in a bottle. It may take many attempts before the infant will eat the new food. After runny cereal is accepted, a thicker cereal can be offered. When the child eats this with ease, parents can begin feeding one new pureed food every week. Commercial baby food is available in jars or frozen. Baby food can also be made at home using a blender or food processor. Portions can be frozen in an ice cube tray and thawed as needed.

About the same time babies begin eating solid food, they are ready to take small sips of apple, grape, or pear juice (but not citrus juices) from a cup. Juice should not be served in a bottle. By the end of the first year, infants can eat a variety of ground or chopped soft foods that the rest of the family eats.

Foods that should not be fed to infants

Some foods are not appropriate for children during their first year. These include:

- Homemade formula. The nutrient requirements for infants are very specific, and even small excesses or deficits of a particular nutrient can permanently harm the child's development.
- Cow's milk. Plain cow's milk should not be offered before six months. After this, it can be introduced in

small amounts as part of weaning foods, but it should not be offered as the main drink before age one. The American Academy of Pediatrics advises that whole cow's milk should not be given to a child during the first year of life. The cow's milk used in some formulas has been altered to make it acceptable for infants.

- Honey. Honey can contains spores of the bacterium *Clostridium botulinum*. This bacterium causes a serious, potentially fatal disease called infant botulism. Older children and adults are not affected. *C. botulinum.* can also be found in maple syrup, corn syrup, and undercooked foods.

- Well-cooked eggs, fish, shellfish, and peanut butter. Opinions differ on how early to introduce these foods into the diet, as young children may be more prone to allergic reactions, especially during the first year.

- Orange, grapefruit, or other citrus juices. These often cause a painful diaper rash during the first year.

- Home-prepared spinach, collard greens, turnips, or beets. These may contain high levels of harmful nitrates from the soil. Jarred versions of these foods are okay.

- Raisins, whole grapes, hot dog rounds, hard candy, popcorn, raw carrots, nuts, and stringy meat. These and similar foods can cause choking, a major cause of accidental death in infants and toddlers.

Precautions

Mothers with certain health conditions or using certain drugs should not breastfeed. Women with chronic diseases should consult with their healthcare providers before breastfeeding.

Parents using concentrated liquid and powdered formulas must measure and mix formula accurately. Inaccurate measuring can harm the infant's growth and development. Water used in mixing formula must be free of pathogens, contaminants, and excessive levels of **fluoride**.

Interactions

Street drugs, many prescription and over-the-counter drugs, and alcohol can all pass into breast milk and have the potential to permanently harm an infant's growth and development. Pregnant or breastfeeding women should consult their healthcare providers before taking any drug or supplement. Caffeine also passes into breast milk. Some women find that even moderate amounts of coffee or caffeinated sodas cause their infants to become restless and irritable, while others find little effect. Breastfeeding women should monitor their caffeine intake and try to keep it to a minimum.

Complications

Many women have trouble getting newborn infants to latch on and begin breastfeeding. This can usually be overcome with the help of a lactation consultant or pediatric nurse. Breastfeeding can cause the mother to develop sore, infected nipples. This is usually a temporary condition and should not be a reason to stop breastfeeding.

Complications from bottle feeding tend to be related to the infant's difficulty with digesting formula. Some infants become gassy and colicky and may fuss, cry for long periods, and spit up cow's milk–based formula. A switch to soy-based formula, if approved by a healthcare professional, usually relieves this problem. Other complications of formula feeding are generally related to improper mixing of formula.

Parental concerns

Breastfeeding parents often are concerned about whether their baby is getting enough milk, since there is no way to directly measure how much milk a baby consumes when nursing. Newborns should have a minimum of six to eight wet diapers and four bowel movements per day during the first two weeks of life. As the child grows, these numbers will gradually decrease. In addition, a woman's breasts should feel hard and full (sometimes even painful) before nursing, and softer after nursing. Newborns nurse every two to three hours, and they should seem satisfied after nursing. The most definite sign that the baby is getting enough food is that he or she is gaining weight.

Infants grow in irregular spurts. They may eat hungrily for a few days and then eat little a few days later. Parents often worry about this, but it is a normal pattern.

QUESTIONS TO ASK YOUR DOCTOR

- Are there any medical reasons why I should not breastfeed?

- Is there a particular type of formula you recommend?

- If my baby is bottle fed, how many ounces of formula should he/she be drinking at every feeding?

- What are some signs that my formula-fed baby is full?

- What food should I introduce first after cereal?

- When is my infant ready for table food, or the same food that I am eating?

The transition to solid food is often a slow process. Infants eat very small amounts and often must be exposed to a new food multiple times before they will eat it willingly. Parents should avoid strictly feeding an infant only foods that they like, as the infant should be allowed to form his or her own taste preferences. Since childhood **obesity** is a major problem in the United States, parents and caregivers should avoid encouraging the infant to overeat.

Resources

BOOKS

Behan, Eileen. *The Baby Food Bible: A Complete Guide to Feeding Your Child, from Infancy On*. New York: Ballantine Books, 2008.

Dietz, William H., and Loraine Stern, eds. "What's Best for my Newborn?" In *Nutrition: What Every Parent Needs to Know*. 2nd ed. Elk Grove Village, IL: American Academy of Pediatrics, 2012.

Meek, Joan Younger, ed. *The American Academy of Pediatrics New Mother's Guide to Breastfeeding*. 2nd ed. New York: Bantam Books, 2011.

Samour, Patricia Q. and Kathy King, eds. *Pediatric Nutrition*. 4th ed. Sudbury, MA: Jones and Bartlett Learning, 2010.

PERIODICALS

American Academy of Pediatrics. "Breastfeeding and the Use of Human Milk (Policy Statement)." *Pediatrics* 129, no. 3 (2012): e827–41. http://dx.doi.org/10.1542/peds.2011-3552 (accessed September 12, 2012).

WEBSITES

American Academy of Pediatricians. "Breastfeeding Initiatives." http://www2.aap.org/breastfeeding (accessed September 12, 2012).

BabyCenter. "Baby Food Basics." http://www.babycenter.com/0_baby-food-basics_9194.bc (accessed September 12, 2012).

International Food Information Council. "Questions and Answers About the Nutritional Content of Processed Baby Food." FoodInsight.org. http://www.foodinsight.org/Resources/Detail.aspx?topic = Questions_and_Answers_About_the_Nutritional_Content_of_Processed_Baby_Food_ (accessed September 12, 2012).

March of Dimes. "Feeding Your Baby." http://www.marchofdimes.com/baby/feeding_babyfood.html (accessed September 12, 2012).

MedlinePlus. "Infant and Toddler Nutrition." U.S. National Library of Medicine, National Institutes of Health. http://www.nlm.nih.gov/medlineplus/infantandnewbornnutrition.html (accessed September 12, 2012).

ORGANIZATIONS

American Academy of Pediatrics, 141 NW Point Blvd., Elk Grove Village, IL 60007, (847) 434-4000, Fax: (847) 434-8000, http://www.aap.org.

La Leche League International, 957 N Plum Grove Rd., Schaumburg, IL 60173, (847) 519-7730, (800) 525-3243, Fax: (847) 969-0460, http://www.llli.org.

March of Dimes, 1275 Mamaroneck Ave., White Plains, NY 10605, (914) 997-4488, http://www.marchofdimes.com.

Women, Infants, and Children, Supplemental Food Programs Division, Food and Nutrition Service, USDA, 3101 Park Center Dr., Rm. 520, Alexandria, VA 22302, (202) 305-2746, Fax: (703) 305-2196, http://www.fns.usda.gov.

Tish Davidson, AM

Inflammatory bowel disease

Definition

Inflammatory bowel disease (IBD) refers to a group of inflammatory disorders of all or part of the digestive tract, including the small intestine and large intestine. The two main types of IBD are ulcerative colitis and **Crohn's disease**, which cause the intestines to become inflamed. Symptoms of IBD can be painful and debilitating, and in some instances lead to serious complications, including the need for surgery.

Description

Although ulcerative colitis and Crohn's disease have some features in common, there are some important differences.

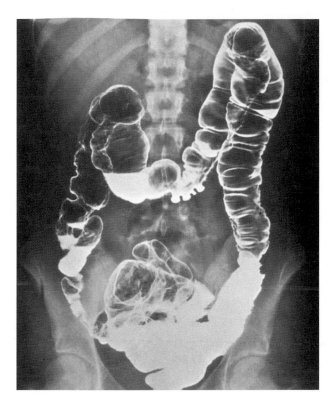

X ray showing Crohn's disease, a type of inflammatory bowel disease. *(© Medical-on-Line/Alamy)*

Crohn's disease

Crohn's disease (CD) involves ongoing (chronic) inflammation of the gastrointestinal tract, from the mouth to the anus, with ulceration and formation of fistulas and perianal abscesses. Five types are recognized, depending on the affected region:

- ileocolitis, the most common form, affects the lowest part of the small intestine (ileum) and the large intestine (colon)

- ileitis type affects the ileum

- gastroduodenal CD causes inflammation in the stomach and first part of the small intestine (duodenum)

- jejunoileitis causes spotty inflammation in the top half of the small intestine (jejunum)

- granulomatous CD colitis affects the large intestine

Ulcerative colitis

Ulcerative colitis typically involves continuous inflammation from the rectum to the entire colon. The disease usually begins in the rectal area and may eventually spread to the entire large intestine. Repeated inflammation thickens the wall of the intestine and rectum with scar tissue.

Demographics

More than 600,000 Americans are diagnosed every year with some type of inflammatory bowel disease. Ulcerative colitis may affect any age group, although peaks occur at ages 15–30 and 50–70. Crohn's disease may occur at any age, but it commonly affects people between ages 15 and 35. Risk factors include a family history of Crohn's disease, Jewish ancestry, and smoking tobacco products. Men and women appear to be at equal risk of developing IBD. According to the Crohn's and Colitis Foundation of America, two-thirds to three-quarters of patients with Crohn's disease will need bowel surgery at some time.

A large study conducted from 1976 to 2003 and published in 2012 in the journal *Gut* ("Geographical variation and incidence of inflammatory bowel disease among US women") found that women are less at risk for developing IBD if they live in a sunny climate. More than 238,000 women participated in the study, called the Nurses' Health Study. Data and medical records were collected on the participants at birth, at age 15 years, and at age 30 years.

The U.S. study, conducted by American gastroenterologist Hamed Khalilil (Massachusetts General Hospital, Boston) and fellow Massachusetts colleagues, concluded that women in southern climates, which receive more sunlight than northern ones, had a 52% lower risk of being diagnosed with Crohn's disease and a 38% lower risk of developing ulcerative colitis by age 30 when compared to women living in northern latitudes. The study results were in line with research done in Europe and suggest that sun exposure may play a role in IBD development, although further research is needed to examine this relationship.

Causes and symptoms

The exact causes of IBD are unknown. The disease may be caused by a germ or by an immune system problem. It is known that IBD is not contagious and it seems to be hereditary. In the case of ulcerative colitis, symptoms vary in severity and may start gradually or suddenly. They usually include all or some of the following:

- abdominal pain and cramps that usually disappear after a bowel movement
- constipation or difficulty passing stool
- diarrhea
- fever
- gastrointestinal bleeding
- gurgling or splashing sound heard over the intestine
- nausea and vomiting

- pain in the joints
- undesired weight loss

The exact cause of Crohn's disease is also unknown, but it has been linked to a problem with the body's immune system (autoimmune disease). The immune system helps protect the body from harmful foreign substances and pathogens. In patients with Crohn's disease, the immune system cannot distinguish between the body's own cells and foreign invaders. The result is an overactive immune response that leads to chronic inflammation. Since Crohn's disease can affect any part of the gastrointestinal tract, symptoms can vary greatly between affected individuals. The following may be observed:

- abdominal fullness and gas
- abdominal pain and cramps
- blood clotting problems
- constipation
- persistent diarrhea (usually watery)
- eye inflammation
- fatigue
- fever
- fistulas
- foul-smelling stools
- gastrointestinal bleeding
- gurgling or splashing sound heard over the intestine
- kidney stones
- loss of appetite
- pain in the joints
- rectal bleeding and bloody stools
- skin rash
- swollen gums
- undesired weight loss

Diagnosis

Based on a careful history of symptoms, the examining physician will be able to distinguish between Crohn's disease and ulcerative colitis. However, diagnosis can be difficult, because other diseases have IBD-like symptoms. For example, Crohn's disease, because it can affect various regions of the gastrointestinal tract, is commonly misdiagnosed as **celiac disease** or diverticulitis. To help ensure correct diagnoses, physicians may use additional tests such as:

- Barium enema with x rays. In this test, also called a "lower gastrointestinal (GI) series," an enema tube is inserted into the patient's rectum and a barium solution is allowed to flow in to improve the contrast of the x rays.

- Colonoscopy. This test allows the physician to look inside the colon using a colonoscope, a long, flexible tube that has a miniaturized color-TV camera at one end. It is inserted through the rectum into the colon and provides a view of the lining of the lower digestive tract on a television monitor.
- Complete blood count (CBC) test. This test measures the number of red and white blood cells, the amount of hemoglobin in the blood, the fraction of the blood composed of red blood cells (hematocrit), and the size of the red blood cells.
- C-reactive protein (CRP). CRP is a test that measures the amount of a protein in the blood that signals acute inflammation.
- Endoscopic ultrasound (EUS). Technique that uses sound waves to create a picture of the inside of the body. It uses a special endoscope that has an ultrasound device at the tip. It is placed in the gastrointestinal tract, close to the area of interest.
- Esophagogastroduodenoscopy (EGD). EGD is a technique used to look inside the esophagus, stomach, and duodenum. It uses an endoscope to investigate swallowing difficulties, nausea, vomiting, reflux, bleeding, indigestion, abdominal pain, or chest pain.
- Flexible sigmoidoscopy. This technique allows doctors to look at the inside of the large intestine from the rectum through the last part of the colon, called the sigmoid colon.
- Sedimentation rate (ESR). This test draws blood from a vein, usually from the inside of the elbow or the back of the hand. It measures the distance that red blood cells settle in unclotted blood toward the bottom of a specially marked test tube.
- Stool guaiac. This test finds hidden (occult) blood in the stool.

Treatment

The primary goal of IBD treatment is to control inflammation and reduce the symptoms of pain, diarrhea, and bleeding when present. Many types of medicine can reduce inflammation, including anti-inflammatory drugs such as sulfasalazine (Azulfidine), corticosteroids such as prednisone, and immune system suppressors such as azathioprine (Imuran) and mercaptopurine (Purinethol). An antibiotic, such as metronidazole (Flagyl), may also be helpful for destroying germs in the intestines, especially for Crohn's disease. Antidiarrheal medications, laxatives, or pain relievers may also be prescribed. If symptoms are severe, such as diarrhea, fever, or vomiting, hospitalization may be required to administer intravenous fluids and medicines.

In the case of severe ulcerative colitis that cannot be helped by medications, a type of surgery called bowel resection may be performed to remove a damaged part of the intestine or to drain an abscess. If a part of the bowel is removed, a procedure is done to connect the remaining two ends of the bowel (anastomosis). In very severe cases, removal of the entire large intestine (colectomy) is required. Bowel resections may also be performed for Crohn's disease patients.

Nutrition and dietary concerns

Diet is an essential component of IBD treatment and management. Eating a diet sufficient in energy and balanced in **macronutrients** and essential micronutrients is important to avoid **malnutrition** and weight loss. Foods that worsen diarrhea should also be avoided. People who experience blockage of the intestines may need to avoid raw fruits and vegetables. Those who have difficulty digesting lactose (a condition known as lactose intolerance) also need to avoid milk products, though calcium-fortified **soy** milk may be substituted. Drinking plenty of fluids (8–10 servings daily) will help to keep the body hydrated and prevent **constipation**.

Eating a **high-fiber diet** may help manage symptoms when IBD is under control ("in remission"). High-fiber foods include:

- whole grains (whole-grain breads, buns, bagels, and muffins; bran cereals, including oat bran, corn bran, and 100% bran and fiber cereal; shredded whole wheat; whole-wheat pastas; barley; popcorn; brown rice)
- fruits (dried fruits such as apricots, dates, prunes and raisins; berries such as blackberries, blueberries, raspberries, and strawberries; oranges; apple with skin; avocado; kiwi; mango; pear)
- vegetables (broccoli, spinach, kale, and other dark green leafy vegetables; dried peas and beans such as kidney beans, lima beans, black-eyed peas, chickpeas, and lentils)
- nuts and seeds (almonds, whole flaxseed, soynuts)

During an IBD attack, however, a high-fiber diet may worsen symptoms, while low-residue diets may help give the bowel a rest and minimize symptoms. A low-residue diet includes:

- grains that are not whole (enriched refined white bread, buns, bagels, and English muffins; plain cereals such as Kellogg's Corn Flakes, cream of wheat, Kellogg's Rice Krispies, or Kellogg's Special K; arrowroot cookies; tea biscuits; soda crackers; plain melba toast; white rice; refined pasta and noodles)

KEY TERMS

Celiac disease—A digestive disease that causes damage to the small intestine. It results from an inability to digest gluten found in wheat, rye, and barley.

Diverticulitis—Inflammation caused by protrusions (diverticula) within the lining of the intestines.

Fistula—An opening between two organs or between an organ and the skin, caused by genetics, injury, or disease.

Immune system—The integrated body system of organs, tissues, cells, and cell products (such as antibodies) that protects the body from foreign organisms or substances.

Rectum—The lower portion of the large intestine.

Sorbitol—An artificial sweetener present in many brands of chocolate, snacks, and candy.

- fruits and fruit juices (except berries, raisins or dried fruits, and prune juice); serve without skin
- vegetables (vegetable juices, potatoes [without skin], well-cooked alfalfa sprouts, beets, green or yellow beans, carrots, celery, cucumber, eggplant, lettuce, mushrooms, green or red peppers, squash, zucchini)
- meats (well-cooked and tender lean meats, fish, fresh eggs); a high-protein diet may help relieve symptoms

Foods that should be avoided during IBD flare-ups include:

- beans, lentils, peas, all nuts and seeds, and any foods that may contain seeds (such as yogurt)
- lactose-containing foods, if lactose intolerance is present; calcium-fortified soymilk may be substituted
- caffeine, alcohol, and sorbitol (an artificial sweetener), which may exacerbate IBD symptoms
- vegetables in the cabbage family (broccoli, cabbage, cauliflower, Brussels sprouts, kale)
- onions and chives
- hot or chili peppers
- carbonated drinks

During flare-ups, small frequent meals may be preferable. Fat intake should be reduced if part of the intestine has been surgically removed, because high fat foods usually cause diarrhea and gas for such patients. A daily multivitamin and mineral supplement may be needed to replace lost nutrients.

QUESTIONS TO ASK YOUR DOCTOR

- Where can I learn more about how to better live with inflammatory bowel disease?
- Is IBD reversible?
- Do I need to take any vitamins or supplements?
- What drug therapies are available for Crohn's disease and ulcerative colitis?

Some studies suggest that fish oil and flax seed oil may be helpful in managing IBD. Recent studies also suggest a role in the healing process for **probiotics** and prebiotics such as psyllium, a soluble **fiber** that comes from a plant called Plantago afra. These may also be helpful in helping the recovery of the intestines.

Therapy

The management of IBD depends on the type diagnosed, and pharmacologic and other therapies are tailored accordingly to individual cases, depending on severity and patient history. Therapeutic agents are carefully selected based on symptom severity and drug side effects. Since IBD is a chronic illness with an important and unpredictable impact on a person's life, effective therapy usually requires much more than the initial treatment of symptoms. Patient cooperation is crucial for improvement, as dietary and lifestyle changes have been shown to be beneficial. Whatever the symptoms, patients also need to get enough rest while learning to manage the stress in their lives, as intestinal problems tend to be worse in overly stressed people. The Crohn's and Colitis Foundation of America (CCFA) can provide patient information on IBD and support groups that can often help with the stress of dealing with IBD, with useful tips for finding the best treatment and coping with the disease.

Prognosis

The outcome of ulcerative colitis is variable. It may be dormant and then worsen over a period of years, or it may progress quickly. The risk of colon **cancer** increases after ulcerative colitis is diagnosed.

There is no cure for Crohn's disease, but it is not a deadly illness. Periods of improvement are often followed by flare-ups of symptoms. People with Crohn's disease have an increased risk of small bowel or colorectal cancer.

Prevention

IBD is not considered preventable, and once it occurs it is a lifelong disease. However, it is possible to prevent IBD secondary complications. For instance, depression is a common problem in people diagnosed with IBD. This may be the result of the underlying diagnosis or the medications used to treat the conditions. Specific information is available for patients and their families about ways to manage their condition and treatments and to help prevent developing depression as a result of the disease.

Resources

BOOKS

Bickston, Stephen J, and Richard S. Bloomfeld, eds. *Handbook of Inflammatory Bowel Disease*. Baltimore: Lippincott Williams & Wilkins/Wolters Kluwer Health, 2010.

Cohen, Russell D. *Inflammatory Bowel Disease: Diagnosis and Therapeutics*. New York: Humana Press, 2011.

Dubinsky, Marla C., and Sonia Friedman, eds. *Pocket Guide to IBD*. 2nd ed. Thorofare, NJ: SLACK, 2011.

Orchard, Timothy R., et al. *Inflammatory Bowel Disease: An Atlas of Investigation and Management*. Oxford; Ashland, OH: Clinical Pub., 2011.

Sklar, J. *The First Year: Crohn's Disease and Ulcerative Colitis: An Essential Guide for the Newly Diagnosed*. New York: Marlowe and Company, 2007.

PERIODICALS

Guagnozzi, D., and A.J. Lucendo. "Colorectal Cancer Surveillance in Patients with Inflammatory Bowel Disease: What is New?" *World Journal of Gastrointestinal Endoscopy* 4, no. 4 (2012): 108–16.

Khalili, Hamad, et al. "Geographical Variation and Incidence of Inflammatory Bowel Disease among U.S. Women." *Gut* (January 11, 2012): e-pub ahead of print. http://dx.doi.org/10.1136/gutjnl-2011-301574 (accessed April 27, 2012).

Lindfred, H., et al. "Self-Reported Health, Self-Management, and the Impact of Living with Inflammatory Bowel Disease during Adolescence." *Journal of Pediatric Nursing* 27, no. 3 (2012): 256–64.

WEBSITES

Centers for Disease Control and Prevention. "Inflammatory Bowel Disease." http://www.cdc.gov/ibd (accessed April 27, 2012).

Crohn's & Colitis Foundation of America. "Diet and Nutrition." http://www.ccfa.org/info/diet (accessed April 26, 2012).

———. "Maintenance Therapy." http://www.ccfa.org/info/treatment/maintenance (accessed April 26, 2012).

National Institute of Arthritis, Musculoskeletal and Skin Diseases. "What People with Inflammatory Bowel Disease Need to Know About Osteoporosis." NIH Osteoporosis and Related Bone Diseases National Resource Center. http://www.niams.nih.gov/Health_Info/Bone/Osteo

porosis/Conditions_Behaviors/inflammatory_bowel. asp (accessed April 27, 2012).

University of California San Francisco. "Nutrition Tips for Inflammatory Bowel Disease." http://www.ucsfhealth. org/education/nutrition_tips_for_inflammatory_bowel_ disease/index.html (accessed April 27, 2012).

ORGANIZATIONS

American Gastroenterological Association, 4930 Del Ray Ave., Bethesda, MD 20814, (301) 654-2055, (800) 877-1600, Fax: (301) 654-5920, member@gastro.org, http://www.gastro.org.

Crohn's and Colitis Foundation of America, 386 Park Ave. South, 17th Fl., New York, NY 10016, (800) 932-2423, info@ccfa.org, http://www.ccfa.org.

International Foundation for Functional Gastrointestinal Disorders, PO Box 170864, Milwaukee, WI 53217-8076, (414) 964-1799, Fax: (414) 964-7176, (888) 964-2001, iffgd@iffgd.org, http://www.iffgd.org.

National Institute of Diabetes and Digestive and Kidney Diseases, 31 Center Dr., MSC 2560, Bethesda, MD 20892-2560, (301) 496-3583, (800) 891-5389, http://www2.niddk.nih.gov.

Monique Laberge, PhD
William A. Atkins, BB, BS, MBA

Insulin

Definition

Insulin is a peptide hormone synthesized from amino acids in specialized cells (beta cells) within the pancreas of humans and other animals that regulates the **metabolism** of **carbohydrates** and **fats**. Insulin prompts cells in muscle, liver, and fat tissue to take up glucose from the blood and store it as a complex **sugar** (polysaccharide) called glycogen. The name of the hormone is derived from *insula*, the Latin word for island, because it is produced by specialized areas of tissue within the pancreas known as islets of Langerhans—named for the German anatomist who first identified them in 1869.

Insulin that is produced within the body of a human or other animal is called endogenous insulin to distinguish it from exogenous insulin, which is insulin derived from an outside source and given as a medication to treat diabetes in humans or other animals.

Purpose

Endogenous insulin serves a number of different purposes in human physiology. Insulin:

Brands of insulin

Rapid-acting
NovoLog or NovoRapid (insulin aspart)
Apidra (insulin glulisine)
Humalog (insulin lispro)

Short-acting
Humulin R (human recombinant)
Novolin R

Intermediate-acting
Humulin N (human recombinant)
Novolin N

Long-acting
Levemir (insulin detemir)
Lantus (insulin glargine)

Premixed
Humulin 70/30, Novolin 70/30 (NPH and regular)
Humalog Mix 75/25, Humalog Mix 50/50 (insulin lispro protamine suspension [intermediate] and insulin lispro [rapid])
NovoLog Mix 70/30 (insulin aspart protamine suspension [intermediate] and insulin aspart [rapid])

(Table by PreMediaGlobal. © 2013 Cengage Learning.)

- regulates blood sugar uptake and metabolism by forcing cells in the liver and in muscle tissue to absorb glucose from the blood and store it as glycogen
- enhances learning and memory, particularly verbal memory
- increases DNA replication and protein synthesis through its control of amino acid uptake
- decreases the conversion of lipids stored in fat cells to fatty acids in the blood, lowering blood fatty acid levels
- relaxes the muscle tone in the walls of arteries, increasing blood flow
- decreases the breakdown of protein in the body
- stimulates cells in the lining of the stomach to secrete hydrochloric acid to assist digestion

Exogenous insulin is used as a medication to treat **diabetes mellitus** in humans, cats, and dogs. All humans diagnosed with type 1 diabetes require treatment with exogenous insulin; about 40% of patients with type 2 diabetes require exogenous insulin as part of their therapy.

Description

Endogenous insulin

Endogenous human insulin is a hormone composed of a chain of 51 amino acids with a molecular weight of 5808 Da (dalton). It is formed from a precursor known as proinsulin, which is encoded by the much longer period of time, and insulin resistance plays a much larger role in the emergence of the disease.

Insulin produced by several other animal species is close enough to endogenous human insulin to be clinically effective in treating diabetes. Porcine (pig) insulin differs from human insulin by only one amino acid, and bovine (cattle) insulin by only three. Even shark insulin is close enough to human insulin to have been used for many years in Japan to treat diabetes.

Historical background

Diabetes mellitus has been recognized as a disease since 1500 BC, when it was described in an ancient Egyptian medical text as an illness characterized by excessive urine production. Indian physicians of the same period observed that the urine of a diabetic patient was sweet enough to attract ants. It was not until the nineteenth century, however, that the role of the pancreas in blood sugar regulation was identified and understood. Although Paul Langerhans had identified the islets in pancreatic tissue that now bear his name in 1869, he did not analyze their function. In 1889 the German physician Oskar Minkowski (1858–1931) established the relationship between the loss of pancreatic function and the symptoms of diabetes through experiments on dogs, but it was not until 1901 that an American medical student, Eugene Opie (1873–1971), identified the islets of Langerhans as the specific portion of pancreatic tissue whose destruction causes diabetes.

The next stage in finding a treatment for diabetes was isolating the substance secreted by the islets. Several scientists in Europe and the United States experimented with various types of pancreatic extracts, but their work was interrupted by World War I (1914–1918). In 1920, Frederick Banting (1891–1941), a Canadian physician, was studying one of Minkowski's papers and decided to try to extract the substance that was secreted by the islets of Langerhans. Working with Charles Best (1899–1978), Banting succeeded in isolating a substance that he called isletin—now known as insulin—from the pancreas of a dog, and tested it on another dog whose pancreas had been removed. When the second dog was able to survive on injections of the isletin, Banting and Best felt ready for a clinical trial in humans. Their first patient was Leonard Thompson, a 14-year-old Toronto boy who was dying of type 1 diabetes. Thompson was successfully treated with Banting and Best's extract in January 1922. By November 1922, research had progressed to the point that the drug firm of Eli Lilly and Company was able to produce large quantities of highly purified animal insulin for general distribution in

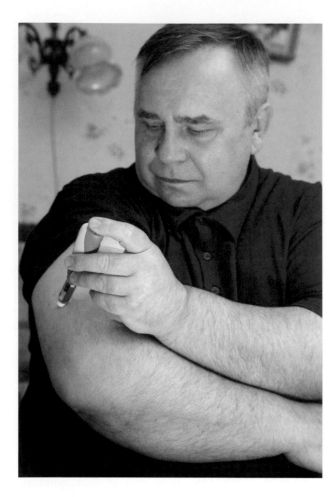

Man injecting himself with insulin. *(Vikulin/Shutterstock.com)*

INS gene and produced in the endoplasmic reticulum of the beta cells within the islets of Langerhans in the pancreas. Proinsulin contains 86 amino acids and is converted into mature insulin in a series of steps that involves the removal of 35 amino acids. Four amino acids are removed altogether; the remaining 31 are split off to form the C-peptide protein. The clinical significance of C-peptide is its use as a marker for testing endogenous insulin secretion.

The human pancreas contains between one and three million islets of Langerhans. The beta cells account for 65%–80% of all the cells within the islets. The beta cells store insulin as well as release it in response to a rise in blood glucose levels. If a person's blood glucose level rises rapidly, the beta cells can release stored insulin while producing more of the hormone at the same time. Type 1 diabetes results from the destruction or dysfunction of the beta cells by an autoimmune process that results partly from genetic susceptibility and partly from environmental triggers. In type 2 diabetes, however, the beta cells decline over a

Canada and the United States. Banting and Best shared the Nobel Prize in Physiology or Medicine in 1923.

All exogenous insulin that was used to treat people with diabetes was derived from animal sources from 1922 through the early 1960s. Although the amino acid sequence of human insulin was identified in the 1950s, the first synthetic insulins were not produced in laboratories until the 1960s. Humulin, the first commercially available biosynthetic human insulin, was not approved for use until 1982. As of 2012, however, the vast majority (70% worldwide) of people with diabetes were treated with synthetic insulins.

Types of exogenous insulin

Exogenous insulin used in the treatment of diabetes is either animal-derived or manufactured in a laboratory using recombinant DNA technology.

ANIMAL. Porcine and bovine insulins for human usage are no longer produced in the United States. A brand of porcine insulin called Vetsulin is still produced by Schering-Plough Animal Health, however, for treating diabetes in dogs and cats, and is approved by the FDA for this purpose. The FDA also permits the importation of animal-derived insulin from the United Kingdom for the small minority of humans whose diabetes is better controlled by animal insulin than by one of the biosynthetic forms.

SYNTHETIC. Synthetic insulins can be classified in several ways, most commonly by their activity in the body or by their method of production. There are three important measurements for the doctor to consider in prescribing an insulin: onset (the time required for the insulin to enter the bloodstream and start to lower the patient's blood sugar level), peak (the time period when the insulin is most effective), and duration (the total length of time the insulin continues to lower blood sugar). The National Institute of Diabetes and Digestive and Kidney Diseases (NIDDK) classifies insulins according to activity in the body as follows:

- Rapid-acting insulins have an onset of 15 minutes, peak at 30 minutes, and have a duration of 3–5 hours. Generic names include insulin aspart, insulin glulisine, and insulin lispro.
- Short-acting insulins have an onset of 30–60 minutes, peak at 2–4 hours, and have a duration of 5–8 hours. They are sometimes called regular insulins.
- Intermediate-acting insulins have an onset of 1–3 hours, peak at 8 hours, and have a duration of 12–16 hours. Their generic name is NPH, which stands for neutral protamine Hagedom, Hagedom being the

last name of the Danish chemist who devised their formula in 1936.

- Long-acting insulins have an onset of 1 hour, no peak, and a duration of 20–26 hours. Generic names include insulin detemir and insulin glargine.
- Premixed insulins consist of an intermediate-acting and a short- or rapid-acting insulin combined in a single compound, to eliminate the need for multiple injections of two different types of insulin. Premixed formulas include 70/30 and 50/50 NPH/regular insulin, 75/25 and 50/50 premixed insulin lispro protamine suspension (intermediate-acting) and insulin lispro (rapid-acting), and 70/30 premixed insulin aspart protamine suspension (intermediate-acting) and insulin aspart (rapid-acting).

Synthetic insulins are manufactured using recombinant DNA technology. The first such insulin, Humulin, was first marketed in 1982 by Eli Lilly, and is made by inserting human DNA into cells of *Escherichia coli* and allowing the cells to grow and reproduce normally. Novo Nordisk, a Danish company, uses a similar process to produce an insulin called NovoLog from yeast.

A newer category of synthetic insulin is called an insulin analogue—it is different from any insulin that occurs in nature, but it can still be used by the human body to control blood sugar levels. Insulin analogues are technically called insulin receptor ligands by the FDA. They have had their amino acid sequences altered by genetic engineering to alter their speed of onset and duration. There are two major types of insulin analogues: rapid-acting, intended to supply the bolus level of insulin required after a meal, and long-acting, intended to be released slowly in the bloodstream and supply the basal level of insulin for a full day. Rapid-acting insulin analogues include insulin aspart, insulin glulisine, and insulin lispro. Long-acting analogues include insulin detemir and insulin glargine.

Methods of administration

All insulins used to treat diabetes in humans must be injected subcutaneously (under the skin). An inhalable insulin called Exubera was developed and approved by the FDA in 2006, but it was withdrawn from the market in 2007 due to lack of acceptance. An intranasal insulin called Nasalin was in clinical trials as of 2012, but there was little information regarding its future availability. There is considerable interest in developing a form of insulin that could be taken by mouth, as many people with diabetes would prefer an oral insulin to repeated injections. The difficulty in formulating an oral insulin is that insulin itself is a protein that is broken down in the stomach during the digestive process. A Connecticut-based company called Biodel is attempting to develop a tablet containing insulin that would be placed under the tongue, where it would dissolve quickly and deliver insulin into the bloodstream through the oral mucosa. An Israeli company is working on a capsule that would protect the insulin during its passage through the stomach and enhance the absorption of the insulin when the capsule reaches the small intestine. Neither product, however, was available commercially as of 2012.

People with diabetes requiring insulin therapy have three options for administering the drug by subcutaneous injection: syringes with needles, repeat-use injection pens with needles, or insulin pumps. Insulin injection pens come in two types: some use cartridges that must be inserted into the pen, while others are prefilled with insulin and discarded when all the insulin has been used. To use the pen, the patient dials the correct amount of insulin to be delivered, and the pen injects the insulin into the skin through a needle in a manner similar to a syringe.

An insulin pump is a device consisting of a reservoir, controls, batteries, a processing module, and a tubing system that is inserted under the skin. It delivers rapid-acting insulin throughout the day through a catheter, eliminating the need for slower-acting insulins or periodic injections. Insulin pumps are, however, considerably more expensive than syringes, require a daylong stay in the hospital for training in the correct use of the pump, and can cause complications if the catheter is displaced or the insulin in the reservoir runs out.

Recommended dosage

The strength of insulin is measured by the number of units (U) per milliliter (mL). One unit equals 45.5 micrograms of pure crystalline insulin. Prior to 1973, insulins came in strengths ranging from 40 units/mL (U-40) to 100 units/mL (U-100). In 1973 the FDA standardized insulins sold in the United States to U-100 to reduce prescription and dosage errors. Most other countries adopted the U-100 standard, although some still dispense U-40 insulin.

The daily dosage varies widely from person to person, however. There is no universal standard dosage because of the number of different types of insulin available; their speed of onset and duration of action; the method of administration; the patient's height, age, sex, weight, and activity level; the type of diabetes requiring treatment; the body location chosen for injection; the nutritional composition of the patient's

meals; and a number of other factors. Type 1 diabetes usually requires a combination of a longer-acting insulin to maintain a basal blood sugar rate throughout the day plus a rapid-acting insulin to cover changes in the blood sugar level associated with meals; this second type of injection is called a bolus injection. Because balancing basal and bolus injections as well as learning to monitor blood sugar levels at home is quite complicated, the **American Diabetes Association** strongly recommends that people newly diagnosed with diabetes enroll in a diabetes education program in order to understand the complex details of insulin administration as well as other aspects of diabetes care.

Precautions

There are numerous precautions that patients must observe regarding insulin administration, storage, timing, and monitoring.

Insulin storage

All currently available insulins require careful storage. They are complex preparations that contain preservatives and other chemicals to adjust the acidity of the insulin (to prevent reactions at the injection site) as well as the actual drug. Insulin can be stored in the refrigerator, but can also be kept for as long as a month at room temperature to minimize the discomfort caused by injecting cold insulin. Insulin should never be kept in a freezer, exposed to direct sunlight or extreme heat or cold, or stored in the glove compartment of a car.

Insulin should never be used past the expiration date on the vial. In addition, vials of insulin should never be shaken but rubbed gently between the hands to make sure the insulin ingredients are mixed. Patients using regular or NPH insulin should examine the vial before each use to make sure that no clumps, crystals, or "frosting" are visible inside the vial. If any of these are found, the insulin should not be used.

Injection timing

With the exception of the long-acting insulins, which are designed to be injected only once a day, insulin injections are timed with respect to the patient's meals. To keep blood glucose at an acceptable level, an injection of regular insulin is given about 30 minutes before a meal, while a rapid-acting insulin can be given at the beginning of the meal. Type 1 diabetes usually requires three or four injections each day of different types of insulin. People with type 2 diabetes may need only a single injection of insulin per day, usually given at supper or bedtime; others, however, may need three or four injections per day to keep their blood sugar level under control.

Injection sites

Insulin is absorbed into the bloodstream at different speeds depending on the site on the body used for the injection. The abdomen is the most commonly used site because it allows the insulin to be absorbed rapidly. Other sites include the upper arms, where absorption is slower, and the thighs or buttocks, where absorption is very slow. Patients are advised to use the same general body area for each injection so that each dose of insulin is absorbed at the same speed; however, they should avoid using the exact same spot each time. The reason for moving the injection site from one dose to the next is to prevent the formation of lumps, pits, or fatty deposits beneath the skin; these deposits affect the body's absorption of insulin, and some patients may find them unsightly.

Other conditions and allergies

Some patients may develop allergies to the additives and preservatives used in the manufacture of synthetic insulins—particularly the intermediate- and long-acting formulations.

Insulin aspart and insulin glargine should not be used during pregnancy or lactation because they have not been studied in pregnant women. NPH and regular insulins are preferred for use during pregnancy. Because insulin is secreted in breast milk, blood glucose levels should be monitored in both mother and child during lactation.

Interactions

Patients should inform their doctor of all prescription and over-the-counter medications that they are presently using before starting insulin injections (and vice-versa). There are a large number of drugs that can interact with insulins. They include:

- beta blockers such as acebutolol, atenolol, betaxolol, esmolol, metoprolol, carteolol, nadolol, penbutolol, pindolol, propranolol, timolol, and bisoprolol (intensify the effects of insulin)
- MAO inhibitors (MAOIs) such as furazolidone, linezolid, phenelzine, selegiline, and tranylcypromine (intensify the effects of insulin)
- steroids such as prednisone and hydrocortisone (decrease the effectiveness of insulin)
- ACE inhibitors such as enalapril, captopril, lisinopril, quinapril, benazepril, and ramipril

- salicylates such as aspirin and bismuth subsalicylate (Pepto-Bismol)
- niacin
- the thiazide diuretics furosemide and hydrochlorothiazide (decrease the effectiveness of insulin)
- estrogens and oral contraceptives (decrease the effectiveness of insulin)
- isoniazid (decreases the effectiveness of insulin)
- octreotide
- cold and allergy drugs
- medications that contain alcohol or sugar

Tests

LABORATORY. There are several laboratory tests that are used to evaluate people for the presence of diabetes or the effectiveness of insulin therapy, including:

- Fasting insulin level. This test requires a blood sample taken after 8 hours of fasting. It is done to measure insulin resistance or to diagnose the presence of an insulinoma. A level of blood insulin higher than the upper level considered normal indicates the presence of insulin resistance or an insulin-secreting tumor in the pancreas.
- Glucose tolerance test. This test is done to see how quickly the patient's body uses sugar. The patient has one sample of blood drawn after fasting overnight and the second sample taken two hours after drinking a sugary liquid in the doctor's office or diagnostic laboratory. Blood sugar levels higher than normal but not high enough to indicate type 2 diabetes are considered a sign of prediabetes.
- C-peptide test. C-peptide is a protein formed during the transformation of proinsulin in the beta cells of the pancreas into mature insulin. The presence of C-peptide in a blood or urine sample indicates that the patient's pancreas is secreting insulin, and how much it is presently producing.
- Hemoglobin A1c test. This test measures how well a person's diabetes is being controlled. It measures the average level of blood glucose over a 6- to 12-week period. It is used together with home blood glucose monitoring to make adjustments in the patient's insulin dosage. The goal for people with diabetes is to keep the hemoglobin A1c level below 7%. Doctors recommend repeating this test every three months to make sure the blood glucose level is under good control.
- Fructosamine test. Fructosamine is a compound formed from blood serum proteins like albumin. It can be measured to assess control of diabetes in patients who have a blood disorder or other condition

KEY TERMS

Basal injection—An injection of a long-acting insulin or low level of continuous infusion from an insulin pump to cover the glucose output of the liver.

Beta cells—The specialized cells within the islets of Langerhans that secrete and store insulin. They represent 65%–80% of the tissue in the islets.

Bolus injection—A single injection of rapid-acting insulin given with a meal to cover the rise in blood sugar that occurs with digestion.

C-peptide—A protein that is produced in the body as part of the sequence of insulin production. It can be used to measure the amount of endogenous insulin secretion or to evaluate a person for insulin resistance.

Endogenous insulin—Insulin produced naturally within the human or animal body by the pancreas.

Exogenous insulin—Insulin produced by another animal or in the laboratory and delivered into the body to supplement insufficient secretion of endogenous insulin.

Glycogen—A polysaccharide (complex sugar) that functions as a form of energy storage in humans and other animals. Glycogen in humans is stored primarily in the liver and in muscle tissue, and is converted to glucose as the body requires it.

Hypoglycemia—Abnormally low level of blood glucose.

Insulin resistance—A state or condition in which a person's body tissues have a lowered level of response to insulin, a hormone secreted by the pancreas that helps to regulate the level of glucose (sugar) in the body.

Insulinoma—A pancreatic tumor that originates in the beta cells of the pancreas and secretes insulin. It is one potential cause of hypoglycemia.

Islets of Langerhans—The regions of the human pancreas that contain its insulin-producing cells. They were discovered in 1869 by Paul Langerhans (1847–1888), a German anatomist and biologist. The islets of Langerhans account for 1%–2% of the total tissue mass of the pancreas.

Lipoatrophy—Loss of fat or formation of a lump under the skin resulting from repeated injections of insulin in the same location.

Polycystic ovary syndrome (PCOS)—An endocrine disorder that develops in 3%–10% of premenopausal women as a result of the formation of cysts (small fluid-filled sacs) in the ovaries. Women with PCOS do not have normal menstrual periods, are often infertile, and may develop excess body hair or other indications of high levels of androgens (male sex hormones) in the blood.

Proinsulin—A precursor of human insulin that is synthesized in the beta cells of the pancreas and processed in a series of biochemical changes to form active insulin.

that makes the hemoglobin A1c test unusable. The test requires a blood sample drawn from a vein in the arm or from a fingerstick.

HOME GLUCOSE TESTING. In addition to laboratory tests that measure endogenous insulin secretion and blood glucose control, patients with diabetes should monitor their blood glucose levels at home. The traditional method of home monitoring involves the use of a glucometer, a small handheld battery-operated device that measures the level of blood glucose in a tiny amount of blood drawn from a fingerstick and placed on the end of a test strip inserted in the meter. Newer glucometers can calculate blood sugar averages over a two-week period, store information that can be uploaded onto a computer, or interpret blood sugar levels in blood drawn from sites other than the fingertip. People who take multiple injections of insulin each day or use an insulin pump are usually advised to check their blood sugar three times per day.

An alternative to the use of a glucometer is a continuous glucose monitoring (CGM) system. A typical system consists of a sensor worn under the skin that is replaced every few days, a link from the sensor to a (non-implanted) receiver that communicates with a receiver, and the receiver itself, which is worn like a pager. Traditional fingersticks are required from time to time to calibrate the CGM, however. In addition, CGM system readings lag about five minutes behind actual changes in blood glucose levels. For this reason, patients using a CGM system are advised to use a fingerstick blood glucose measurement to confirm an abnormal blood glucose CGM reading before taking corrective action.

Complications

Glucose control is essential to diabetes treatment. Abnormal levels can result in a wide range of complications.

Hypoglycemia

The most common complication of insulin use is hypoglycemia, or abnormally low blood sugar. It is a recurrent risk for diabetic patients receiving insulin therapy, particularly those with type 1 diabetes. Hypoglycemia can result from injecting too much insulin (measuring the dose incorrectly or misunderstanding the doctor's instruction), not eating enough food to raise blood sugar levels, lowering blood sugar levels through overexercise, or taking other medications that interact with insulin by increasing its effectiveness. In rare cases, hypoglycemia can result from an insulinoma, or a tumor in the pancreas that secretes excessive amounts of insulin.

The symptoms of hypoglycemia range from mild feelings of unease or irritability to yawning, mental confusion, nausea, hunger, tiredness, perspiration, headache, heart palpitations, numbness around the mouth, tremors, muscle weakness, and blurred vision. Severe hypoglycemia may include seizures, coma, and eventually permanent brain damage or death. It has been estimated that 2%–4% of deaths in people with type 1 diabetes result from hypoglycemia.

Mild hypoglycemia is treated by raising the blood sugar level through eating or drinking something sweet or sugary, often a piece of candy, a cookie, or orange juice. People with diabetes are typically advised to carry candy or a similar sweet or high-carbohydrate food with them at all times in case they experience the symptoms of hypoglycemia or their glucometer registers an abnormally low blood sugar level during home glucose testing. Severe diabetic hypoglycemia, sometimes called insulin shock, requires emergency hospital treatment. It is treated by intravenous administration of dextrose, a simple sugar, or glucagon, a peptide hormone that raises blood sugar levels.

Lipoatrophy

Lipoatrophy is the medical term for the formation of a pit, small dent, or lump beneath the skin caused by repeated injections of insulin into the same location. One of the potentially serious consequences of lipoatrophy is that the injured tissue may reject the insulin or slow down its absorption, thereby complicating blood glucose measurement and accurate assessment of the patient's current insulin dosage. Lipoatrophy can usually be prevented by rotating the site of insulin injections.

Infection

Because current insulins must be injected subcutaneously, infections can result from failure to cleanse

---

QUESTIONS TO ASK YOUR DOCTOR

- What should I know about proper storage of my insulin?
- How can I tell whether my insulin is no longer effective or safe to use?
- What type of glucometer would you recommend for home glucose monitoring?
- How can I best avoid hypoglycemia?
- What is your opinion of insulin pumps as a replacement for self-injection?

---

the skin before injection or from nonsterile needles. Patients are instructed to cleanse the injection site before each injection by swabbing the skin with a cotton ball moistened with rubbing alcohol, and to avoid reusing insulin syringes. Although the American Diabetes Association notes that syringes can be safely reused by some patients to save costs, those with weakened immune systems, chronic illnesses, or open wounds on the hands should not risk the dangers of infection from reused syringes.

Homicide

Although such cases are fortunately rare, there were at least 70 instances of murder (or suicide) documented worldwide as of 2012 that involved the administration of large amounts of insulin in order to produce insulin shock, coma, and eventual death in the victim. It is possible to kill people who do not have diabetes with high doses of insulin (as well as those with diabetes), although the lethal dose varies somewhat from person to person.

Parental concerns

Children diagnosed with either type 1 or type 2 diabetes will need instruction on the care and proper injection of their insulin as well as help from other family members in coping with the emotional impact of diabetes. Parents may need to monitor their child's compliance with insulin injections as well as with home glucose testing. The Nemours Foundation Diabetes Center (http://kidshealth.org/parent/centers/diabetes_center.html#cat20724) is an excellent resource for diabetes- and insulin-related issues in children.

Resources

BOOKS

Hinson, Joy, Peter Raven, and Shern Chew. *The Endocrine System: Basic Science and Clinical Conditions*, 2nd ed. New York: Churchill Livingstone/Elsevier, 2010.

Holt, Richard I.G., et al., eds. *Textbook of Diabetes*, 4th ed. Hoboken, NJ: Wiley-Blackwell, 2010.

Kaufman, Francine R., and Emily Westfall. *Insulin Pumps and Continuous Glucose Monitoring*. Alexandria, VA: American Diabetes Association, 2012.

Unger, Jeff. *Diabetes Management in Primary Care*, 2nd ed. Philadelphia, PA: Wolters Kluwer Health/Lippincott Williams and Wilkins, 2013.

PERIODICALS

Berenson, D.F., et al. "Insulin Analogs for the Treatment of Diabetes Mellitus: Therapeutic Applications of Protein Engineering." *Annals of the New York Academy of Sciences* 1243 (December 2011): E40–E54.

Blumer, I., et al. "Insulin-Pump Therapy for Type 1 Diabetes Mellitus." *New England Journal of Medicine* 367 (July 26, 2012): 383–384.

Donner, T., and M. Muñoz. "Update on Insulin Therapy for Type 2 Diabetes." *Journal of Clinical Endocrinology and Metabolism* 97 (May 2012): 1405–1413.

Frank, J., et al. "Performance of the CONTOUR® TS Blood Glucose Monitoring System." *Journal of Diabetes Science and Technology* 6 (January 1, 2011): 196–205.

Katz, M.L., et al. "Contemporary Rates of Severe Hypoglycaemia in Youth with Type 1 Diabetes: Variability by Insulin Regimen." *Diabetic Medicine* 29 (July 2012): 926–932.

King, A.B., et al. "How Much Do I Give? Dose Estimation Formulas for Once-Nightly Insulin Glargine and Pre-meal Insulin Lispro in Type 1 Diabetes Mellitus." *Endocrine Practice* 18 (May–June 2012): 382–386.

Marks, V. "Murder by Insulin: Suspected, Purported and Proven—A Review." *Drug Testing and Analysis* 1 (April 2009): 162–176.

Patterson, M.E., et al. "Hyperinsulinism Presenting in Childhood and Treatment by Conservative Pancreatectomy." *Endocrine Practice* 18 (May–June 2012): e52–e56.

Swelheim, H.T., et al. "Lipoatrophy in a Girl with Type 1 Diabetes: Beneficial Effects of Treatment with a Glucocorticoid Added to an Insulin Analog." *Diabetes Care* 35 (March 2012): e22.

Tamborlane, W.V., and K.A. Sykes. "Insulin Therapy in Children and Adolescents." *Endocrinology and Metabolism Clinics of North America* 41 (March 2012): 145–160.

WEBSITES

American Diabetes Association. "Blood Glucose Control." http://www.diabetes.org/living-with-diabetes/treatment-and-care/medication/insulin (accessed July 24, 2012).

———. "Insulin." http://www. diabetes.org/living-with-diabetes/treatment-and-care/blood-glucose-control (accessed September 28, 2012).

———. "Insulins Used in the United States." http://forecast.diabetes.org/files/images/InsulinChart_rev_12-20.pdf?utm_source=WWW&utm_medium=ContentPage&utm_content=Insulin-types&utm_campaign=DF (accessed July 24, 2012).

Lab Tests Online. "Insulin." http://labtestsonline.org/understanding/analytes/insulin/tab/glance (accessed July 24, 2012).

MedicineNet. "Insulin." http://www.medicinenet.com/insulin/article.htm (accessed July 24, 2012).

National Institute of Diabetes and Digestive and Kidney Diseases (NIDDK). "Types of Insulin." http://diabetes.niddk.nih.gov/dm/pubs/medicines_ez/insert_C.aspx (accessed July 24, 2012).

Nemours Foundation. "How to Give an Insulin Injection." http://kidshealth.org/parent/diabetes_center/meds_monitoring/injection_graphic.html#cat20724 (accessed July 26. 2012).

WebMD. "Types of Insulin for Diabetes Treatment." http://diabetes.webmd.com/diabetes-types-insulin (accessed July 25, 2012).

ORGANIZATIONS

American Diabetes Association, 1701 North Beauregard St., Alexandria, VA 22311, (800) 342-2383, AskADA@diabetes.org, http://www.diabetes.org.

Food and Drug Administration (FDA), 10903 New Hampshire Ave., Silver Spring, MD 20993, (888) INFO-FDA (463-6332), http://www.fda.gov/default.htm.

National Institute of Diabetes and Digestive and Kidney Diseases (NIDDK), Bldg. 31, Room 9A06, 31 Center Drive, MSC 2560, Bethesda, MD 20892-2560, (301) 496-3583, http://www2.niddk.nih.gov/Footer/Contact-NIDDK, http://www2.niddk.nih.gov.

Rebecca J. Frey, PhD

Intermittent fasting

Definition

Intermittent fasting (IF) is a name for a group of **calorie restriction** (CR) diets in which the dieter alternates between periods of fasting (usually understood to mean consumption of water or no-calorie beverages only) and non-fasting. IF is based on time periods rather than on meal plans, food lists, recipes, calorie counting, or similar features of most weight-loss diets. One common form of IF appears to be a two-day cycle in which 24 hours of fasting are followed by 24 hours of feeding. This pattern is alternately known as alternate-day fasting (ADF), every-other-day fasting (EOD), or every-other-day feeding (EODF). Other IF diets may divide each day into a period of fasting and a period of feeding, such as 20 hours of fasting/4 fours of feeding or 19 hours of fasting/5 hours of feeding. Another variation is to consume a very limited number of **calories** (usually 15% to 20% of normal intake) on "fasting" days rather than taking in no calories at all.

Origins

Intermittent fasting as a dietary regimen appears to have originated with laboratory experiments on animals (mice in most cases) in the 1940s, in which researchers discovered that calorie restriction (CR) in the form of intermittent fasting appeared to extend the animals' life spans. Calorie restriction without **malnutrition** has been shown to extend the median and maximum life spans in such different species as yeast, fish, and dogs as well as mice, but its effects in humans are not yet fully understood because of the length of the human lifespan in comparison to those of other animals.

IF seems to be practiced primarily by bodybuilders and athletes in developed countries, who may combine it with food cycling regimens of various types. Food cycling refers to the practice followed by some weight trainers of reversing the proportions of **fats** and **carbohydrates** in the diet according to the phase of the training schedule—usually high carbohydrate/low fat on training days and low carbohydrate/high fat on rest days.

Description

There is no single IF diet, but rather several different regimens. Some of the better-known IF regimens include 2 Meal, LeanGains, Fast-5, Eat Stop Eat, and the Warrior Diet.

2 Meal (IF Life)

The 2 Meal version of intermittent fasting has been popularized by Michael O'Donnell, a personal trainer and fitness coach who began to write about his approach in 2007 and refers to himself as "2 Meal Mike." The 2 Meal system, also called IF Life, is the easiest version of IF to tailor to an individual's preferences; O'Donnell describes it as "a simple way to eat less overall for weight loss." The "2 Meal" in the program's title refers to limiting one's eating to two meals a day. O'Donnell states that he rarely eats breakfast, has a late lunch, and then eats one other meal per day, usually in the early evening. Rather than specify an ideal length of time for fasting/feeding, O'Donnell

notes that his own daily feeding "window" can vary from 6 to 10 hours in length. While he advises beginners to start with set times for meals so that they do not have too many variables to adjust, he emphasizes that "less is more" and that "many ways can work" for people to benefit from the 2 Meal approach.

O'Donnell's claims for his version of IF are modest. He notes that no one diet plan works for everyone, and that such factors as **insulin** resistance, general level of activity, choice of foods and total calorie consumption, amount of rest and sleep, and the presence of any metabolic disorders can affect the rate of weight loss and success in weight maintenance. His overall advice is to avoid making intermittent fasting unduly complicated—the focus should be on enjoying life rather than worrying about the diet.

LeanGains

LeanGains is an IF program devised and popularized by Martin Berkhan, a Swedish personal trainer and magazine writer who maintains a blog about his dietary recommendations at http://www.lcangains.com. Berkhan, who holds an undergraduate degree in public health sciences and education, maintains that he became interested in IF when he found that the six-meals-a-day regimen often recommended for athletes didn't work for him either physically or psychologically; in particular, he noticed that his life had started to revolve around food: "The constant meal preparing, the obsessiveness about eating the perfect meals at the right time, and the way I sometimes made excuses not to participate in social gatherings in order to meet my calorie and macronutrient goals for the day." He experimented with intermittent fasting, noted the range of IF patterns reported in the literature, and settled on one that worked for him and his bodybuilding clients.

Berkhan's version of IF is based on a 16/8 daily pattern of fasting/eating rather than an alternate-day pattern. He and most of his clients eat three meals during the eight-hour feeding window: a pre-workout meal and two post-workout meals. Unlike O'Donnell, Berkhan has strong convictions about the proper balance of nutrients in the pre- and post-workout meals, stating that the pre-workout meal should be light (about 500 calories), with equal amounts of carbohydrates and proteins, as well as "some fat for taste." A typical pre-workout meal for Berkhan might include 5 ounces of lean meat, a potato or other vegetable, and a large apple. The post-workout meals should account for 80% of the day's calorie intake and be high in carbohydrates, moderate in **protein**, and low in fat. Berkhan states that he usually eats one post-workout meal immediately after the workout and the second meal about an hour before bedtime. Like most proponents of intermittent fasting, Berkhan notes that limiting one's total calorie consumption is still necessary to lose weight, and that IF will not work if people regard the eating window as an excuse to binge.

Fast-5

The Fast-5 approach to intermittent fasting was devised in the early 2000s by a physician named Bert Herring and his wife, also a physician. The Herrings published a 52-page book on their version of IF, which is available on their website: http://www.fast-5.com.

The Fast-5 program resembles O'Donnell's 2 Meal approach in that it is relatively flexible. It is based on a 19/5 daily pattern of fasting/eating, with all eating to be done within the five-hour window. During that five-hour period, the dieter is to eat as much as they want, so long as they are truly hungry. No liquids containing calories are to be consumed during the 19-hour fasting period, although the dieter may drink as much water or other calorie-free beverages as desired. The Herrings emphasize that any period of five consecutive hours is fine to use as the eating window, so that users can identify a time frame that works for them.

The Herrings outline two ways to start the Fast-5 program: a "cold turkey" approach, in which the dieter simply waits to eat until the chosen five-hour window, or a gradual adjustment approach, in which the timing of the eating window is pushed back by half an hour or an hour every day or every few days until the person reaches the desired time setting for the window. With regard to choice of foods, the Herrings recommend a variety of fruits and vegetables containing **fiber**; a variety of protein sources that include fish, eggs, and meat; and nuts or sunflower seeds—in short, "a balance of carbohydrate, fats, and protein."

The Herrings advise that people may not notice weight loss until they have used the Fast-5 approach for three or four weeks, and that they may find they are losing inches from the waistline before their scale registers a loss in weight. The Herrings refer to the initial three weeks as the adjustment period, and maintain that dieters using the Fast-5 approach should begin to lose about a pound per week after a month or longer on the program.

Eat Stop Eat

Eat Stop Eat is a version of intermittent fasting popularized by Brad Pilon, who blogs at http://bradpilon.com and is the author of two e-books, *Eat Stop Eat* (in two versions, one for men and one for women) and *The Zen of Nutrition*. Pilon's approach to IF consists of one or two 24-hour fasts per week, the day(s) chosen by the user. Pilon recommends that people choose days when they are not too busy. Exercise should be done when energy levels are highest, which will usually be toward the beginning of the fast. The fast usually begins on the evening before the fast day and ends 24 hours later on the following evening. During the fast, the dieter may drink any fluid that does not contain calories: coffee, unsweetened tea, water, club soda, diet soft drinks, and the like.

Pilon's program is advertised as costing $9.99 for a three-day trial period at http://eatstopeat.com, but there is an additional charge of $27 if the user decides to continue with the program.

Warrior Diet

The Warrior diet is sometimes loosely grouped together with other IF regimens because it is based on a daily cycle of overeating and undereating, but it differs from intermittent fasting in a number of important respects. Designed by Ori Hofmekler (1952–), a former member of the Israeli Defense Force (IDF), the Warrior diet is a total workout, fitness, and nutrition program; it is not primarily a weight-loss program. Second, the undereating phase of the Warrior diet is not really a fast; the dieter is allowed to consume light snacks of raw fruits or vegetables or a light protein food like yogurt for the 10 to 18 hours a day that constitute the undereating period. In addition, Hofmekler maintains that people do not need to count calories during the overeating period; they can basically eat as much food as they wish. This advice is quite different from that of most IF proponents, who state that the eating window in their various plans is not an excuse to binge, and that calories do count if the user wishes to lose weight. Third, the Warrior diet is accompanied by an intense and rigorous exercise program based on whole-body workouts that may last as long as 45 minutes.

The Warrior diet also differs from the IF plans described above in its rules about cooking and eating. Like Berkhan, Hofmekler believes in food cycling; dieters should alternate between high-fat and high-carbohydrate days in order to maximize the body's fat burning during exercise. Hofmekler advises people to avoid storing foods in plastic containers or purchasing foods wrapped or contained in plastic. He believes that only bottled water should be used for drinking and cooking and that supermarket foods contain "estrogenic compounds." Hofmekler's preoccupation with estrogens in the environment has no parallel in other IF regimens. Last, Hofmekler has a website called Defense Nutrition at http://www.defensenutrition.com, through which he markets a number of **dietary supplements** intended to help the body burn fat, detoxify, rid itself of estrogenic compounds, and maintain a normal hormonal balance. These products are quite expensive—$170 for a 30-day "protein support kit" as of 2012—which again sets the Warrior diet apart from other IF regimens.

Function

The function of intermittent fasting is to help otherwise healthy adults lose weight at a slow but steady rate while choosing foods that appeal to them and an overall fasting/feeding pattern that works for them as individuals. Berkhan also maintains that IF can be used by bodybuilders to increase lean muscle mass and/or decrease the proportion of body fat.

Benefits

In addition to a healthful rate of weight loss, proponents of IM maintain that it offers several additional benefits:

- The calorie restriction that occurs with IM has been shown to reduce inflammation, lower blood pressure and blood glucose levels, lower triglyceride and total cholesterol levels, and reduce body fat while sparing lean muscle tissue.
- The flexibility of IM relieves people of the emotional burdens of calorie counting, obsessions with meal planning and preparation, and feelings of deprivation related to "forbidden" foods. Most proponents of IM encourage people to have something they consider a pleasure or a "treat" during the feeding window.
- IM also allows people to adjust the timing of their feeding window for eating out, business trips, social events, and similar occasions, thus easing concerns about social isolation.
- Many users report increased mental energy and ability to concentrate because they are not constantly preoccupied with food or food preparation.
- Other users report less interest in sweets or processed foods and heightened enjoyment of natural flavors in foods.
- IF can easily accommodate people with food allergies who may need to avoid certain foods often included in conventional weight loss plans.
- IF is easy on the food budget because users do not have to spend money on exotic foods or cooking equipment, dietary supplements (with the exception of the Warrior diet), diet books, membership in a diet program, or similar expenses. They also usually find that they save money on food because they are eating less.

Precautions

Although Martin Berkhan claims that he has clients with diabetes who have successfully used his approach to IF, most IF proponents state that their programs are intended for otherwise healthy adults who need to lose weight; they are not intended for children or adolescents who are still growing, pregnant or lactating women, or anyone with a chronic disorder, including diabetes.

There are many difficulties to following an IF regimen. People with a history of **eating disorders**, stress, or anxiety disorders may find that the restrictions of IF can worsen these conditions. The diets can be hard to follow for an extended period of time, especially for people who live with others who do not practice IF. Some researchers are concerned that IF promotes **weight cycling** or yo-yo dieting, due to the extremes between eating nothing and eating anything.

Risks

Repeated fasting can result in nutrient deficiencies. People may feel fatigued during the fasting periods. Anyone interested in IF should first consult with their physician to help avoid any complications.

QUESTIONS TO ASK YOUR DOCTOR

- What is your opinion of intermittent fasting as a weight-loss regimen? As a general preventive health measure?

- Have any of your patients ever tried intermittent fasting? If so, did it work for them?

- In your opinion, are there any groups of people who should not try intermittent fasting?

- What do you think of claims that intermittent fasting can slow the aging process?

Research and general acceptance

Relatively little scientific research has been done on IF in humans, possibly because there are a number of different fasting/feeding patterns that identify themselves as intermittent fasting. Many of the writers in the field are personal trainers or bodybuilders rather than research scientists. The **Academy of Nutrition and Dietetics** had posted no reviews of IF, whether of the practice in general or of specific IF regimens, as of summer 2012. Of the nine clinical trials of IF registered with the National Institutes of Health in 2012, only one was a study of the effects of IF on weight loss; seven others were all studies of the effects of IF on drug uptake and **metabolism**. The ninth study, which was recruiting subjects, proposed to compare different patterns of meal frequency; specifically, the effects of IF compared to a three-meal- or six-meal-per-day eating pattern.

There are only a handful of published studies on IF in humans compared to those that used mice models. One study reported that IF does *not* appear to affect the metabolism of different nutrients in healthy subjects compared to control subjects on a normal diet. A British study stated in 2011 that IF is at least as effective as a daily calorie-restricted diet in weight management and insulin sensitivity in overweight women. A team of Israeli investigators suggested in 2010 that the beneficial effects reported by adults using an IF feeding regimen may be due in part to the way in which IF resets the body's circadian rhythm. Most registered dietitians maintain that much more research needs to be done on intermittent fasting in humans to gain a clearer understanding of its effects on the human body or the aging process, and the metabolic pathways or other reasons for those beneficial effects.

Resources

BOOKS

Herring, Bert W. *The Fast-5 Diet and the Fast-5 Lifestyle.* [No place of publication]: Fast-5 LLC, 2005.

Hofmekler, Ori. *Warrior Diet: Switch on Your Biological Powerhouse for High Energy, Explosive Strength, and a Leaner, Harder Body*, 2nd ed., revised and expanded. Berkeley, CA: Blue Snake Books, 2007.

Johnson, James B., and Donald R. Laub. *The Alternate-Day Diet: Turn on Your "Skinny Gene," Shed the Pounds, and Live a Longer and Healthier Life.* New York: Perigee, 2009.

Mattson, Mark P. *Diet-Brain Connections: Impact on Memory, Mood, Aging, and Disease.* Boston: Kluwer Academic Publishers, 2002.

PERIODICALS

Froy, O., and R. Miskin. "Effect of Feeding Regimens on Circadian Rhythms: Implications for Aging and Longevity." *Aging* (Albany, NY) 2 (December 11, 2010): 7–27.

Harvie, M.N., et al. "The Effects of Intermittent or Continuous Energy Restriction on Weight Loss and Metabolic Disease Risk Markers: A Randomized Trial in Young Overweight Women." *International Journal of Obesity* 35 (May 2011): 714–727.

Soeters, E.R., et al. "Intermittent Fasting Does Not Affect Whole-Body Glucose, Lipid, or Protein Metabolism." *American Journal of Clinical Nutrition* 80 (November 2009): 1244–1251.

WEBSITES

Falaro, Tony. "Intermittent Fasting—To Feast or Not to Feast: An Interview with Martin Berkhan." http://articles. elitefts.com/features/interviews/intermittent-fasting%E2 %80%94to-feast-or-not-to-feast-an-interview-with-martin-berkhan (accessed July 12, 2012).

Fast-5 Life. "Fast-5 Diet Summary." http://www.fast-five. com/content/summary (accessed July 12, 2012).

———. "Frequently Asked Questions about Fast-5." http:// www.fast-five.com/content/faq (accessed July 12, 2012).

The IF Life. "The Advantages of Using Intermittent Fasting/ Feeding (IF)." http://www.theiflife.com/advantages-intermittent-fasting-feeding (accessed July 12, 2012).

———. "Intermittent Fasting 101—How to Start Burning Fat." http://www.theiflife.com/intermittent-fasting-101-how-to-start-part-i (accessed July 12, 2012).

Introduction to the Warrior Diet. http://warriordiet.com/ content/view/24/35 (accessed July 14, 2012).

Neighmond, Patti. "Retune the Body with a Partial Fast." National Public Radio, *All Things Considered* (radio broadcast), November 21, 2007. http://www.npr.org/ templates/text/s.php?sId = 16513299&m = 1 (accessed September 28, 2012).

Peele, Leigh. "Martin Berkhan and Intermittent Fasting: Interview." http://www.leighpeele.com/martin-berkhan-and-intermittent-fasting-interview (accessed July 12, 2012).

Pilon, Brad. *Eat Blog Eat* (blog). http://bradpilon.com (accessed July 12, 2012).

ORGANIZATIONS

Academy of Nutrition and Dietetics, 120 South Riverside Plz., Ste. 2000, Chicago, IL 60606-6995, (312) 899-0040, (800) 877-1600, amacmunn@eatright.org, http://www.eatright.org.

National Institute on Aging (NIA), Building 31, Room 5C27, 31 Center Drive, MSC 2292, Bethesda, MD 20892, (800) 222-2225, niaic@nia.nih.gov, http://www.nia.nih.gov.

Rebecca J. Frey, PhD

Intuitive eating

Definition

Intuitive eating is a program based on the premise that the human body possesses innate knowledge of the best foods to eat and the most appropriate eating habits. Intuitive eating rejects the multitude of diets and dietary recommendations that flood the marketplace and create confusion among consumers. Rather than scientific explanations and rigid dietary requirements, intuitive eating emphasizes the psychological components of eating habits as important nutritional factors. Thus, the goal of an intuitive eating program is to rediscover and reconnect with the inherent wisdom of one's own body, using practices that facilitate this process.

Origins

The concept of intuitive eating was first developed in the 1990s by two California-based registered dietitians (RDs), Evelyn Tribole and Elyse Resch. Their book, *Intuitive Eating: A Recovery Book for the Chronic Dieter; Rediscover the Pleasures of Eating and Rebuild Your Body Image*, was first published in 1996. An updated edition, *Intuitive Eating: A Revolutionary Program That Works*, came out in 2003. The third edition, published in 2012, was extensively updated and expanded and included two new chapters: "Raising an Intuitive Eater: What Works with Kids and Teens," and a chapter on the science behind intuitive eating, including more than 25 scientific studies. Tribole and Resch have also produced an audio CD, *Intuitive Eating: A Practical Guide to Make Peace with Food, Free Yourself from Chronic Dieting, Reach Your Natural Weight* (2009).

Tribole is a nutrition counselor who, in addition to intuitive eating, specializes in **eating disorders** and **celiac disease**. Her other books include *Healthy Homestyle Cooking* (1994), *Healthy Homestyle Desserts* (1996), *Stealth Health: 100 Delicious Recipes and 1,000 Tips for Eating Right in Spite of Yourself* (2000), *More Healthy Homestyle Cooking* (2002), *Eating on the Run* (2003), and *The Ultimate Omega-3 Diet* (2007).

Resch is a nutritional therapist who specializes in eating disorders, in addition to intuitive eating. She is a certified child and adolescent **obesity** expert and a fellow of the **Academy of Nutrition and Dietetics**.

Tribole and Resch have promoted their intuitive eating philosophy and ideas through workshops, seminars, teleseminars, support groups, blogs, and an online community. They also train and certify intuitive eating counselors. As a result, intuitive eating programs have proliferated, and other dietitians have developed their own versions. Intuitive eating has come to be accepted by a range of nutrition and obesity experts.

Description

All diets, no matter how well-designed and well-intentioned, are based, to at least some degree, on short-term or long-term food deprivation. In contrast, intuitive eating programs draw on anti-diet movements that shun dieting and instead encourage people to accept their bodies as they are, rather than trying to change them, and to concentrate on improving self-image. However, intuitive eating programs also recognize that poor dietary habits, overweight, and obesity are major causes of chronic illness and disease. By integrating these two realities and recognizing the need to encourage the incorporation of healthy eating habits into daily lifestyles, intuitive eating emphasizes the roles that psychological patterns play in eating habits.

Although intuitive eating programs provide general recommendations, the focus is on a highly personalized approach, recognizing that people have a wide variety of dietary needs and preferences. Tribole and Resch have stressed the value of moving away from struggling with willpower and moving toward the freedom of self-empowerment, away from forced behaviors and toward behaviors that arise naturally from within.

Intuitive eating programs draw heavily from behavioral therapy and self-help movements. Intuitive eating trains people to distinguish between emotional **cravings**, which can lead to destructive eating habits, and physical cravings, which are valid nutritional needs. Learning to distinguish between authentic feelings of hunger and emotional cravings is a cornerstone of intuitive eating and helps people avoid overeating and bingeing.

Tribole and Resch have also stressed that their intuitive eating program is process-oriented rather than results-oriented. This means that both successes and setbacks are welcomed, accepted, and used as learning experiences. Borrowing from the language of behavioral therapy, their program focuses on becoming aware of one's eating habits by identifying and naming one's dominant "eating personalities." Common eating personalities that lead to problems include "the careful eater," "the professional dieter," "the distracted eater," and "the unconscious eater." People with these personalities may be obsessive or guilt-ridden with regard to food and eating. They may constantly be on some form of restrictive or difficult diet, without being aware of the reasons that they keep making poor food choices. Unconscious and distracted eaters may be unaware of what they just ate and how much, sometimes because they engage in other activities, such as watching television or reading, while they eat. By identifying and naming their eating personalities, people can begin to develop an awareness of how and why their natural and innate intuitive eating habits became lost or overshadowed. This allows people to reconnect with the part of their mind that knows how to eat, without guilt or compulsion, in order to fulfill the body's nutritional requirements.

Principles of intuitive eating

Reawakening the intuitive eater happens in stages. First, many people hit "diet rock bottom," realizing that dieting does not work for them and that their attempts to diet are fueled by guilt and poor **body image**. Next comes the "exploration" stage, in which people become increasingly aware of the emotions, cravings, and behaviors that they experience around food. This stage also entails releasing guilt feelings about foods or "making peace with foods," sorting out food likes and dislikes, learning to recognize feelings of hunger and fullness, and distinguishing between emotional and biological eating signals. The next stage is "crystallization," in which the principles of intuitive eating come to be practiced regularly. In the final stage, the "intuitive eater awakens," and intuitive eating patterns are internalized and become natural habits. At this point, people are able to "treasure the pleasure" of eating in a way that is emotionally and physically gratifying.

Tribole and Resch detail ten fundamental principles for establishing healthy and natural eating habits, and they recommend steps and practices for incorporating each principle into daily life.

- Their first principle, "Reject the Diet Mentality," means throwing out the diet books and giving up all diets and related habits such as calorie counting. It means recognizing that the advice and judgments of others are limited or irrelevant. It means giving up the hope that there is yet another diet out there that will lead to quick, easy, and permanent weight loss.

- Their second principle, "Honor Your Hunger," emphasizes paying close attention to biological hunger signals and reacting to them by eating without guilt, so as to not overeat because of excessive hunger. This principle helps build self-trust and conscious, moderate eating.

- The third principle, "Make Peace with Food," means giving oneself permission to eat whatever foods one truly enjoys and appreciates. Depriving oneself of favorite foods can lead to uncontrollable cravings, bingeing, and feelings of guilt.

- The fourth principle, "Challenge the Food Police," means paying close attention to how one internally judges oneself and one's food choices and challenging the unreasonable rules of dieting.

- The fifth principle, "Respect Your Fullness," involves listening to body signals and learning to detect when one is comfortably full, so as to avoid overeating. For example, this may involve pausing in the middle of a meal to appreciate the taste of the food and recognize feelings of satiety.

- The sixth principle, "Discover the Satisfaction Factor," means learning to take pleasure in eating and savoring the experience.

- The seventh principle, "Honor Your Feelings Without Using Food," means learning not to confuse biological signals with emotional signals. It means finding ways to comfort and nurture oneself and experience one's emotions without using food.

- The eighth principle, "Respect your Body," means overcoming a negative self-image.

- Principle nine, "Exercise—Feel the Difference," encourages people to simply become more active or adopt exercise programs that are easy and fun, learning to enjoy the feelings of well-being that come with exercise. Motivation to exercise should come from enjoying how it feels to move one's body and become more energized rather than from burning calories.

- Principle ten, "Honor Your Health," is what Tribole and Resch call "gentle nutrition." This means making food choices that are nutritious and pleasurable and that help people feel well and function well. Furthermore, healthy food choices evolve over time, and occasional missteps are a natural part of the process. The goal should never be to maintain a perfect diet.

Function

The limitations and failures of conventional weight-loss programs are well known. Despite the proliferation of diet plans and the many millions of people around the world following one plan or another, most dieters fail to lose weight and often continue to gain weight. More than one-third of adult Americans are obese, compared with only 15% in 1980. Approximately two-thirds of American adults are either overweight or obese. Furthermore, about 17% of American children and adolescents are obese, three times the prevalence in 1980. One-third are either overweight or obese, including almost 40% of African American and Hispanic children. Furthermore, many dieters experience what Tribole and Resch call the "diet backlash"—frequent dieting sometimes lead to eating disorders and unhealthy behaviors, including consumption of unhealthy foods, compulsive eating, bingeing, guilt, and self-loathing.

As evidence of unhealthy phenomena that can accompany dieting, Tribole and Resch cite a 1991 study in the *New England Journal of Medicine* by Dr. Leann Birch that examined the eating habits of children. The study concluded that children are naturally able to regulate their eating habits in a healthy manner, and that parental control over children's eating habits can be counterproductive. Other studies have indicated that children can develop eating disorders, such as anorexia and bulimia, as a result of parental pressure around dietary behaviors or negative self-image. Thus, children may possess innate dietary wisdom that can become obscured by social pressure and expectations. The philosophy behind intuitive eating holds that adults can recover this innate wisdom that may have become lost during childhood.

Benefits

Tribole and Resch, as well as other proponents, believe that intuitive eating represents a paradigm shift around food and eating. People are asked to perceive life and eating in a different way, to move away from guilt and negative self-image and toward a mindset based on acceptance and emotional awareness. The ultimate goal of intuitive eating programs is the reestablishment of a fundamental relationship with food—eating as a source of pleasure and satisfaction in daily life, rather than as a source of obsession and stress.

KEY TERMS

Anorexia—Anorexia nervosa; an eating disorder characterized by extreme weight loss, distorted body image, and fear of gaining weight.

Bingeing—Uncontrolled eating.

Bulimia—Bulimia nervosa; an eating disorder characterized by binges—eating a large amount of food in a short time—followed by purging behaviors, such as vomiting or using laxatives.

Eating disorders—Psychological disorders characterized by disturbances in eating patterns, abnormal attitudes toward food, and unhealthy efforts to control weight. Types of eating disorders include anorexia nervosa, binge eating disorder, and bulimia nervosa.

Obesity—An abnormal accumulation of body fat, usually 20% or more above ideal body weight or a body mass index (BMI) of 30.0 or above.

Overweight—A body mass index (BMI) between 25.0 and 30.0.

Registered dietitian (RD)—A health professional with at least a bachelor's degree in nutrition who has undergone practical training and is legally registered.

Precautions

An intuitive eating program is recommended as an adjunct treatment for individuals with eating disorders, such as anorexia and bulimia, that have their origins in psychological issues. Patients with eating disorders should first seek treatment from a qualified medical practitioner, counselor, or psychologist in conjunction with programs such as intuitive eating.

Research and general acceptance

Numerous studies have reported that the majority of long-term dieters either do not lose weight or do not successfully maintain their weight loss. Frequently, the weight lost by dieting is not only regained, additional weight is gained. Thus, there is ample evidence that most traditional diets do not work and that weight loss and weight maintenance require permanent changes in eating habits. A 2006 study published in the *American Journal of Health Education* concluded that intuitive eaters had lower obesity rates, increased pleasure in eating, and fewer dieting behaviors and food anxieties. A study published in 2011 in *The Journal of the American Dietetic Association* surveyed nutrition faculty members at American universities about their attitudes toward diet- and

QUESTIONS TO ASK YOUR DOCTOR

- Are you familiar with the concept of intuitive eating?
- Would you recommend that I try an intuitive eating program?
- Can you recommend an intuitive eating counselor?
- Should I seek treatment for an eating disorder?

non-diet-based weight-management strategies for overall health and well-being. The top three methods among the options presented were exercise (54%), eating competence (46%), and intuitive eating (39%). Eating competence is similar to intuitive eating in that competent eaters have positive attitudes toward food and eating, enjoy their food, and trust their bodies to signal hunger and satiety.

Resources

BOOKS

Bernard, Jane. *Am I Really Hungry? 6th Sense Diet: Intuitive Eating.* New York: Transitions, 2011.

Resch, Elyse, and Evelyn Tribole. *Intuitive Eating: A Practical Guide to Make Peace with Food, Free Yourself from Chronic Dieting, Reach Your Natural Weight* (audiobook). Boulder, CO: Sounds True, 2009.

Tribole, Evelyn, and Elyse Resch. *Intuitive Eating: A Revolutionary Program That Works.* 3rd ed. New York: St. Martin's Griffin, 2012.

PERIODICALS

Bacon, Linda, and Lucy Aphramor. "Weight Science: Evaluating the Evidence for a Paradigm Shift." *Nutrition Journal* 10, no. 1 (2011): 9.

Caldwell, Karen L., Michael J. Baime, and Ruth Q. Wolever. "Mindfulness Based Approaches to Obesity and Weight Loss Maintenance." *Journal of Mental Health Counseling* 34, no. 3 (July 2012): 269–82.

Gilmore, L., D.E. Clifford, and M. Neyman Morris. "Nutrition Faculty Attitudes and Teaching Methods of Diet and Non-Diet Approaches to Weight Management." *Journal of the American Dietetic Association* 111, no. 9, Supplement (September 2011): A39.

Heileson, J. L., and R. Cole. "Assessing Motivation for Eating and Intuitive Eating in Military Service Members." *Journal of the American Dietetic Association* 111, no. 9, Supplement (September 2011): A26.

Pietiläinen, K. H., et al. "Does Dieting Make You Fat? A Twin Study." *International Journal of Obesity* 36, no. 3 (March 2012): 456–64.

Rubin, Lisa R., and Julia R. Steinberg. "Self-Objectification and Pregnancy: Are Body Functionality Dimensions Protective?" *Sex Roles* 65, nos. 7–8 (October 2011) 606–18.

Smith, TeriSue, and Steven R. Hawks. "Intuitive Eating, Diet Composition, and the Meaning of Food in Healthy Weight Promotion." *American Journal of Health Education* 37, no. 3 (May/June 2006): 130–36.

Tylka, Tracy L., and Rachel M. Calogero. "Fiction, Fashion, and Function Finale: An Introduction and Conclusion to the Special Issue on Gendered Body Image, Part III." *Sex Roles* 65, nos. 7–8 (October 2011): 447–60.

WEBSITES

"IntuEating." Jane Bernard & Transitions Press. http://www.intueating.com (accessed September 9, 2012).

Tribole, Evelyn. "Can You Really Be Addicted to Food?" http://www.intuitiveeating.org/content/can-you-really-be-addicted-food (accessed September 6, 2012).

———. "Warning: Dieting Increases Your Risk of Gaining MORE Weight (an Update)." http://www.intuitiveeating.org/content/warning-dieting-increases-your-risk-gaining-more-weight-update (accessed September 6, 2012).

ORGANIZATIONS

Academy of Nutrition and Dietetics, 120 South Riverside Plaza, Ste. 2000, Chicago, IL 60606-6995, (312) 899-0040, (800) 877-1600, http://www.eatright.org.

Intuitive Eating, 1100 Quail, Ste. 111, Newport Beach, CA 92660, (949) 478-5016, Etribole@gmail.com, elyse@elyseresch.com, http://www.intuitiveeating.org.

National Association of Anorexia Nervosa & Associated Disorders, Inc., 800 East Diehl Road #160, Naperville, IL 60563, (630) 577-1330, anadhelp@anad.org, http://www.anad.org.

Douglas Dupler, MA
Margaret Alic, PhD

Intussusception

Definition

Intussusception is a medical emergency in which one portion of the intestine (bowel) slides or "telescopes" into another section of bowel, cutting off the blood supply and blocking the flow of materials through the digestive system.

Description

In the process of intussusception, one part of the intestine infolds into another section the intestine. The most common place for this to occur is at the junction where the end of the small intestine (the ileum) meets the large intestine (the colon). Here, the small intestine slides into the large intestine. Occasionally one part of the small intestine will slide into another part of the small intestine, but this is much less common.

Once the infolding begins, the blood supply to the intestines and the tissue (mesentery) that surrounds and holds them it in place is cut off. The intestines are a long tube. The infolding tissue creates an obstruction that blocks the passage of material through the intestine. The walls of the intestine and the surrounding tissue begin to swell, increasing the blockage. The intestine may bleed or rupture, and eventually gangrene develops as the tissue dies.

Demographics

Intussusception occurs most often in infants and toddlers. It is the leading cause of intestinal obstruction in children ages 3 months to 5 years. The highest rate of intussusception occurs in children ages 3 to 12 months. Two-thirds of cases occur before the child's first birthday. Intussusception is the leading cause of abdominal surgery in children age 5 and younger.

In infants, 3 boys develop intussusception for every 2 girls that do, but as children age, the rate changes sharply and the disorder becomes much more common in boys. By age 4, the boy:girl ration is 8:1. There is no difference in the rate of intussusception among races or ethnic groups. Internationally, although few statistics are available, the rate seems to be about the same as in the United States.

Adults can develop intussusception, but the condition is rare.

Causes and symptoms

The cause of most cases of intussusception cannot be identified (idiopathic intussusception). In general, researchers believe that uneven forces on the wall of the intestine start the process. In some cases, a spot called a lead point develops. This seems to be a heavy spot or pocket on the wall of the intestine that then "leads" the slide of one section of intestine into another. Some lead points develop around surgical scar tissue, tumors, polyps, collections of blood or fluid in the intestinal wall, or, in the case of cystic fibrosis, the accumulation of sticky mucus on the wall of the intestine. However, a lead point is identified in less than 12% of cases in children.

Another theory on why intussusception develops suggests that the process is set off by uncoordinated bowel contractions (peristalsis). Viral infection may also play a role. There is an association between recent

---

KEY TERMS

Gangrene—Death of body tissue due to a cutting off of the blood supply.

Idiopathic—Occurring from unknown causes.

Perforation—A hole in the wall of an organ in the body.

Polyp—A tissue growth that extends out into the hollow space of an organ such as the intestine or uterus.

Rectum—The last few inches of the large intestine.

---

viral infection and intussusception, but no clear cause and effect relationship has been determined. At one time, it appeared that vaccination for rotavirus, a virus that causes severe diarrhea in young children, increased the rate of intussusception. The vaccine in question was withdrawn from the U.S. market. Its replacement vaccine, RotaTeq, has been found in some studies to show a slight association with increased intussusception rates in certain populations, but there have been no definitive patterns, and the benefits far outweigh the risk.

Intussusception is a medical emergency. Symptoms of intussusception usually appear suddenly in an otherwise healthy child. The classic symptoms of intussusception are abdominal pain, vomiting, and passing reddish, jelly-like stools called "current jelly" stools. The jelly-like material comes from a shedding of mucus from the intestinal wall, and the red is from fresh blood. However, this constellation of three symptoms is present in only about 20% of children. About 50% of children have abdominal pain and current jelly stools without vomiting.

An infant with intussusception will appear healthy but may suddenly draw up his or her legs and scream or cry frantically in pain. The child may vomit. This is followed by a period when the pain disappears and the child appears normal. Painful episodes return, however, at roughly 10–20 minute intervals. The child may have loose watery stools at first. Over time, the stools become reddish and jelly-like. Eventually the child becomes lethargic between bouts of pain and may develop a swollen abdomen and fever. If left untreated, intussusception is fatal.

Adults can also experience intussusception, although the disorder is uncommon to rare. In adults, the cause is often an unsuspected tumor or polyp growing in the intestine. Symptoms often appear much more gradually in adults and may come and go over a long period. Adult symptoms of intussusception include changes in bowel frequency, urgent desire to have a bowel movement, abdominal cramps, pain in a single area of the abdomen, rectal bleeding, nausea, and vomiting. These symptoms resemble the symptoms of other gastrointestinal disorders, complicating diagnosis.

Diagnosis

Diagnosis is made on the basis of patient history and imaging studies. X-ray images of the abdominal region will show a mass or obstruction in the bowels. Computed tomography (CT) scans or ultrasound may be done in addition to x rays. If there is no sign that the bowel has torn (perforated) or ruptured, a contrast x ray is done on the large intestine. In a contrast colon x ray, a liquid containing barium is inserted through the rectum and into the colon. The barium contrasts with the surrounding tissue to provide clearer x-ray images of the affected area.

Treatment

With intussusception, diagnosis sometimes results in treatment. Forcing barium into the colon may reduce the intussusception as pressure from the barium pushes the infolded piece of bowel back out of the large intestine. This occurs in as many as 75% of cases. Sometimes the procedure needs to be repeated to get complete reversal of the infolding. When a barium enema provides effective treatment, the pain stops immediately and the child becomes dramatically better. The child is usually hospitalized for observation for about 18–24 hours. This precaution is taken because most recurrences of the intussusception occur within that time.

If the initial x rays show that the bowel has ruptured, has a perforation, or if massive infection is present (peritonitis), a barium enema cannot be used and emergency surgery is required. Surgery is also required if the barium enema is ineffective in reversing the blockage. About 25% of children require surgery. Recovery after surgery is usually complete and no complications are expected.

Nutrition and dietary concerns

Individuals whose intussusception is successfully treated without surgery can return to a normal diet immediately. Individuals who require surgery will initially be fed intravenously (IV), followed by a clear liquid diet, then progressing to soft foods until normal bowel function is established. At this time they can return to their regular diet.

Prognosis

Untreated intussusception is fatal, usually within 2–5 days. Death is caused by complications from gangrene and massive infection. Individuals who are successfully treated for intussusception usually recover without complications. Repeat intussusception can be as high as 10% in individuals whose intussusception is cleared by barium enema. Most of the time, if recurrence is going to occur, it happens within the first 24 hours, although a longer time frame is always possible.

Prevention

There is no way to prevent intussusception. However, prompt medical care can prevent death.

Resources

BOOKS

Lalani, Amina, and Suzan Schneeweiss, eds. *The Hospital for Sick Children Handbook of Pediatric Emergency Medicine.* Sudbury, MA: Jones & Bartlett Publishers, 2007.

PERIODICALS

Yakan, Savas, et al. "Intussusception in Adults: Clinical Characteristics, Diagnosis and Operative Strategies." *World Journal of Gastroenterology* 15, no. 16 (2009): 1985–1989.

WEBSITES

Children's Hospital of Wisconsin. "Intussusception." http://www.chw.org/display/PPF/DocID/22808/router.asp (accessed October 2, 2012).
Mayo Clinic staff. "Intussusception." MayoClinic.com. http://www.mayoclinic.com/health/intussusception/DS00798 (accessed October 2, 2012).
Neumors Foundation. "Intussusception." KidsHealth.org. http://kidshealth.org/parent/system/surgical/intussusception.html (accessed October 2, 2012).
World Health Organization. "Statement on Rotarix and Rotateq Vaccines and Intussusception." http://www.who.int/vaccine_safety/committee/topics/rotavirus/rotarix_and_rotateq/intussusception_sep2010/en/index.html (accessed October 24, 2012).

ORGANIZATIONS

American Academy of Family Physicians, 11400 Tomahawk Creek Pkwy., Leawood, KS 66211-2680, (913) 906-6000, (800) 274-2237, Fax: (913) 906-6075, http://www.aafp.org.
American Academy of Pediatrics (AAP), 141 Northwest Point Blvd., Elk Grove Village, IL 60007, (847) 434-4000, (800) 433-9016, Fax: (847) 434-8000, http://www.aap.org.
North American Society for Pediatric Gastroenterology, Hepatology, and Nutrition, PO Box 6, Flourtown, PA 19031, (215) 233-0808, Fax: (215) 233-3918, naspghan@naspghan.org, http://www.naspghan.org.

Tish Davidson, A.M.

Iodine

Definition

Iodine (I) is a non-metallic element that the body needs in very small (trace) amounts in order to remain healthy. It can only be acquired through diet. Deficiencies of iodine are a serious health problem in some parts of the world.

Purpose

Iodine is essential to the formation of the thyroid hormones triiodothyronine (T3) and thyroxine (T4). Thyroid hormones regulate many basic metabolic processes. Solutions containing iodine can be used on the skin as a disinfectant because iodine kills bacteria. It can also be used to purify water contaminated with bacteria. In medical settings, iodine is used in diagnostic radioisotope scanning and it has other industrial uses.

Description

The thyroid gland is located in the front of the neck just below the Adam's apple. It is part of a complex, tightly controlled feedback cycle that regulates basic aspects of **metabolism**, such as how fast the body burns **calories**, growth rate, and body temperature.

Under stimulation by thyroid stimulating hormone (TSH) produced by the pituitary gland, the thyroid produces two hormones, triiodothyronine (T3) and thyroxine (T4). The formation of one molecule of T3 requires three molecules of iodine, while formation of T4 requires four molecules of iodine. The body contains between 20 and 30 mg of iodine, 60% of which is stored in the thyroid. The remainder is found in the blood, muscles, and ovaries. Thyroid hormones are broken down in the liver and some of the iodine is recycled. The rest is lost to the body in urine.

Iodine is found in soil and in the ocean. The amount of iodine varies widely by location. In mountainous regions where heavy rain and snow cause erosion or in low-lying regions where regular flooding occurs, the soil is especially deficient in iodine. The mountains of the Himalayas, Andes, and Alps are all iodine-poor as is the Ganges river valley. The International Council for the Control of Iodine Deficiency Disorders (ICCIDD) estimates that 38% of the world's population, or about 2.2 billion people, live in areas where they are unlikely to get enough iodine without supplementation.

Iodine deficiency disorders (IDDs) create serious health problems. In the early 1900s, iodine deficiency was common in interior regions of the United States and Canada, as well as many other non-coastal regions of the world. In the 1920s, the United States began a voluntary program of adding iodine (in the form of potassium iodide) to salt. Salt was chosen because all races, cultures, and economic classes use it, its consumption is not seasonal, and it is inexpensive. Adding 77 mcg of iodine per gram of salt costs about $0.04 per year per person in the United States. About 50% of table salt sold in the United States contains iodine. It is labeled "iodized salt." All table salt sold in Canada is iodized. In most other countries iodine is added at lower concentrations ranging from 10–40 mcg/gram.

Normal iodine requirements

The United States Institute of Medicine (IOM) of the National Academy of Sciences has developed values called **dietary reference intakes (DRIs)** for **vitamins** and **minerals**. The **DRIs** consist of three sets of numbers. The recommended dietary allowance (RDA) defines the average daily amount of a nutrient needed to meet the health needs of 97%–98% of the population. The adequate intake (AI) is an estimate set when there is not

Iodine

Age	Recommended dietary allowance (mcg)	Tolerable upper intake level (mcg)
Children 0–6 mos.	110*	Not established
Children 7–12 mos.	130*	Not established
Children 1–3 yrs.	90	200
Children 4–8 yrs.	90	300
Children 9–13 yrs.	120	600
Adolescents 14–18 yrs.	150	900
Adults 19≤ yrs.	150	1,100
Pregnant women 18≥ yrs.	220	900
Pregnant women 19≤ yrs.	220	1,100
Breastfeeding women 18> yrs	290	900
Breastfeeding women 19≤yrs.	290	1,100

Food	Iodine (mcg)
Seaweed, dried, 1 g	up to 2,984
Cod, 3 oz.	99
Salt, iodized, ¼ tsp.	71
Milk, low-fat, 1 cup	56
White bread, enriched, 2 slices	45
Shrimp, 3 oz.	35
Egg, 1 large	24
Tuna, canned in oil, 3 oz.	17
Apple juice, 1 cup	7

AI = Adequate intake
mcg = microgram

SOURCE: U.S. Office of Dietary Supplements, National Institutes of Health.

(Table by PreMediaGlobal. © 2013 Cengage Learning.)

enough information to determine an RDA. The tolerable upper intake level (UL) is the average maximum amount that can be taken daily without risking negative side effects. The DRIs are calculated for children, adult men, adult women, pregnant women, and **breastfeeding** women.

The IOM has not set UL levels for iodine in children under one year old because of incomplete scientific information. RDAs for iodine are measured in micrograms (mcg). The following are the daily RDAs and AIs for iodine for healthy individuals (they are the same as the recommendations made by the World Health Organization [WHO]):

- children 0–6 months: AI 110 mcg; UL not available
- children 7–12 months: AI 130 mcg; UL not available
- children 1–3 years: RDA 90 mcg; UL 200 mcg
- children 4–8 years: RDA 90 mcg: UL 300 mcg
- children 9–13 years: RDA 120 mcg; UL 600 mcg
- adolescents 14–18 years: RDA 150 mcg; UL 900 mcg
- adults 19 years and older: RDA 150 mcg; UL 1,100 mcg
- pregnant women under age 19: RDA 220 mcg; UL 900 mcg
- pregnant women age 19 and older: RDA 220 mcg; UL 1,100 mcg
- breastfeeding women under age 19: RDA 290 mcg; UL 900 mcg
- breastfeeding women age 19 and older: RDA 290 mcg; UL 1,100 mcg

Sources of iodine

Iodine must be acquired from diet. Marine plants and animals, such as cod, haddock, and kelp (seaweed), are an especially good source of iodine because they are able to concentrate the iodine found in seawater. Freshwater fish are a less good source. Plants contain varying amounts of iodine depending on the soil in which they are grown.

In industrialized countries, feed for cattle, chickens, and other domestic animals is often fortified with iodine. Some of this iodine finds its way into animal products that humans eat—milk, eggs, and meat. In developing countries where feed is not enriched or cattle are raised on grass, these animal products do not serve as a source of iodine.

Commercially processed foods are often made with iodized salt. The iodine content of salt changes very little during processing. Sometimes an iodine-containing stabilizer is added to commercial bread dough. This increases the iodine content of bread. The stabilizer is used less often now than it was in the twentieth century. However, for many people, commercially processed foods are their main source of iodine. Iodine is also found in most multivitamin tablets.

Iodine can be absorbed through the skin from iodine-based disinfectant solutions. Automobile exhaust puts some iodine into the air, and this can be absorbed through the lungs. Neither of these provide significant amounts of iodine for most people.

The following list gives the approximate iodine content for some common foods:

- kelp, 1/4 cup wet: 415 mcg or more (amount is highly variable)
- salt, iodized, 1 g: 77 mcg; 1 teaspoon: 400 mcg
- haddock, 3 ounces: 104–145 mcg
- cod, 3 ounces: 99 mcg
- shrimp, 3 ounces: 21–37 mcg
- processed fish sticks: 17 mcg per piece
- tuna, canned, 3 ounces: 17 mcg
- milk, 1 cup: 55–60 mcg
- cottage cheese, 1/2 cup: 25–75 mcg
- egg, 1 large: 18–29 mcg
- turkey breast, cooked, 3 ounces: 34 mcg
- ground beef, cooked, 3 ounces: 8 mcg
- seaweed, dried, 1 ounce: up to 18,000 mcg

Iodine deficiency

Because of iodine supplementation, iodine deficiency is not a serious health problem in most industrialized countries, but it is in many developing countries. Internationally, about 2.2 billion people are at risk for IDDs. Women who do not get enough iodine have higher rates of infertility, miscarriages, pregnancy complications, and low birth weight babies than women who have adequate iodine intakes. However, iodine deficiency has its most damaging effects on the developing fetus.

Iodine deficiency is the leading cause of preventable intellectual disability worldwide. Children born to iodine-deficient mothers have a condition called cretinism. Cretinism involves severe and permanent brain damage. These children have intellectual and developmental disorders such as deafness, mutism, and inability to control muscle movements. Iodine deficiency in newborns and infants also results in abnormal brain development and intellectual disabilities.

The most visible sign of iodine deficiency in children, adolescents, and adults is the development of a goiter. A goiter is a lump near the throat that signals

KEY TERMS

Hormone—A chemical messenger produced by the body that is involved in regulating specific bodily functions such as growth, development, reproduction, metabolism, and mood.

Mineral—An inorganic substance found in the earth that is necessary in small quantities for the body to maintain health. Examples: zinc, copper, iron.

Pituitary gland—A small gland at the base of the brain that produces hormones that regulate many bodily functions.

an enlarged thyroid. When not enough iodine is available, the thyroid grows larger in a futile attempt to make more thyroid hormone. In adults, hard lumps may form inside the goiter. When iodine deficiency is pronounced enough for a goiter to develop, memory and language skills decline. In children IQ may be affected. Some of these effects can be reversed in children, but not adults, by increasing iodine intake. In adults with goiter, increasing iodine intake may send the thyroid into overdrive, causing it to produce too much thyroid hormone, a serious condition called hyperthyroidism. Other conditions can also cause the thyroid gland to produce too much or too little hormone. A urine test is used to determine if an individual is iodine deficient, and blood tests can check for other thyroid function problems.

Precautions

Pregnant and breastfeeding women must be especially careful to get enough iodine, since iodine deficiency has its greatest effect on the fetus and newborn. Vegans, who do not eat animal products and depend on **soy** for much of their **protein**, are at higher risk of iodine deficiency than the general population.

Interactions

Amiodarone (Cordarone), a drug used to prevent irregular heart rhythms, contains enough iodine that it may affect thyroid function.

Some foods contain substances called goitrogens that interfere with the body's ability to absorb or use iodine. These include broccoli, cabbage, cauliflower, and Brussels sprouts. Other foods that contain goitrogens are canola oil, soybeans, turnips, peanuts, and cassava. These foods should not cause iodine deficiency unless they are the mainstay of a very limited diet.

Selenium deficiency amplifies the effects of iodine deficiency. **Vitamin A** deficiency may amplify iodine deficiency.

Complications

Complications of iodine deficiency are discussed above. Iodine excess rarely is caused by diet, although an excess of thyroid hormones may result from other causes.

Parental concerns

In developed countries, parents should have few concerns about their healthy children getting enough iodine, so long as they use iodized table salt.

Resources

BOOKS

Food and Nutrition Board, Institute of Medicine, National Academy of Sciences. *Dietary Reference Intakes for Vitamin A, Vitamin K, Arsenic, Boron, Chromium, Copper, Iodine, Iron, Manganese, Molybdenum, Nickel, Silicon, Vanadium, and Zinc.* Washington, DC: National Academy Press, 2001, pp. 162–77.

Lieberman, Shari, and Nancy Bruning. *The Real Vitamin and Mineral Book: The Definitive Guide to Designing Your Personal Supplement Program.* 4th ed. New York: Avery, 2007.

WEBSITES

Higdon, Jane, and Victoria J. Drake. "Iodine." Linus Pauling Institute, Oregon State University. http://lpi. oregonstate.edu/infocenter/minerals/iodine (accessed October 3, 2012).

International Council for the Control of Iodine Deficiency Disorders. "Iodine Deficiency." http://www.iccidd.org/pages/iodine-deficiency.php (accessed October 3, 2012).

MedlinePlus. "Iodine." U.S. National Library of Medicine, National Institutes of Health. http://www.nlm.nih.gov/medlineplus/druginfo/natural/35.html (accessed October 3, 2012).

U.S. Department of Agriculture, National Agricultural Library. "DRI Tables." Food and Nutrition Information Center. http://fnic.nal.usda.gov/dietary-guidance/dietary-reference-intakes/dri-tables (accessed August 16, 2012).

ORGANIZATIONS

Food and Nutrition Information Center, National Agricultural Library, 10301 Baltimore Ave., Rm. 105, Beltsville, MD 20705, (301) 504-5414, Fax: (301) 504-6409, fnic@ars.usda.gov, http://fnic.nal.usda.gov.

Institute of Medicine, National Academy of Sciences, 500 Fifth St. NW, Washington, DC 20001, (202) 334-2352, iomwww@nas.edu, http://www.iom.edu.

International Council for the Control of Iodine Deficiency Disorders, PO Box 51030, 375 des Epinettes, Ottawa, Ontario, Canada K1E 3E0, http://www.iccidd.org.

U.S. Food and Drug Administration, 10903 New Hampshire Ave., Silver Spring, MD 20993-0002, (888) INFO-FDA (463-6332), http://www.fda.gov.

Helen Davidson

Irish diet *see* **Northern European diet**

Iron

Definition

Iron (Fe) is a metal essential to almost all bacteria, plants, and animals. In humans, iron is a component of the red pigment hemoglobin that gives red blood cells their color and allows the transport of oxygen throughout the body, conversion of nutrients into energy, production of new deoxyribonucleic acid (DNA, genetic material), and regulation of cell growth and cell differentiation. Without iron, life on earth would not exist. Humans must acquire all of the iron they need from diet (the body does not produce its own iron).

Purpose

Most iron in the body is used to transport oxygen. Oxygen is carried in red blood cells through the circulatory system to all cells in the body. Hemoglobin is the **protein** within red blood cells that makes this possible, and iron is at the center of the hemoglobin molecule. An average-size adult male has about 4 grams of iron in his body and an adult female has about 3.5 grams. Approximately two-thirds of this iron is in hemoglobin. Myoglobin, a protein in muscle, also contains iron. Myoglobin provides short-term storage for oxygen. When muscles do work, this oxygen is released to meet the increased metabolic needs of muscle cells.

Iron is found in every cell in the body, including brain cells. It is needed to synthesize adenosine triphosphate (ATP), the compound that supplies most of the energy for cellular **metabolism**. Iron is also used in enzyme reactions that create new DNA, and in this way it affects cell division and differentiation. Iron also is essential to other enzyme reactions that break down potentially harmful molecules formed when immune system cells attack bacteria.

Description

Plants absorb iron from the earth, and humans acquire iron through eating both plants and animals. In the stomach, acid in gastric juice acts on iron and

Iron

Age	Recommended dietary allowance (mg)	Tolerable upper intake level (mg)
Children 0–6 mos.	0.27	40
Children 7–12 mos.	11	40
Children 1–3 yrs.	7	40
Children 4–8 yrs.	10	40
Children 9–13 yrs.	8	40
Boys 14–18 yrs.	11	45
Girls 14–18 yrs.	15	45
Men 19–50 yrs.	8	45
Women 19–50 yrs.	18	45
Adults 51≤ yrs.	8	45
Pregnant women	27	45
Breastfeeding women 18≥ yrs.	10	45
Breastfeeding women 19≤ yrs.	9	45

Food	Heme iron (mg)
Chicken liver, cooked, 3 oz.	11.0
Oysters, canned, 3 oz.	5.7
Beef liver, cooked, 3 oz.	5.2
Turkey, dark meat, cooked, 3 oz.	2.0
Sirloin, cooked, 3 oz.	1.6
Tuna, light, canned, 3 oz.	1.3
Chicken, light meat, cooked, 3 oz.	0.9
Crab, Alaskan king, cooked, 3 oz.	0.7
Pork loin, cooked, 3 oz.	0.7
Shrimp, cooked, 4 large	0.3

Food	Nonheme iron (mg)
Cereal, 100% iron fortified, ¾ cup	18.0
Oatmeal, fortified, 1 packet	11.0
Soybeans, boiled, 1 cup	8.8
Beans, kidney, cooked, 1 cup	5.2
Beans, lima, cooked, 1 cup	4.5
Beans, black, cooked, 1 cup	3.6
Tofu, raw, ½ cup	3.4
Spinach, frozen, cooked, ½ cup	1.9
Raisins, ½ cup	1.6
Bread, whole wheat, 1 slice	0.7

mg = milligram

SOURCE: U.S. Department of Agriculture, National Agricultural Library, Food and Nutrition Information Center and U.S. Office of Dietary Supplements, National Institutes of Health.

(Table by PreMediaGlobal. © 2013 Cengage Learning.)

changes it into a form that the body can absorb. Absorption takes place mainly in the first part of the small intestine (the duodenum). Once iron is absorbed into the bloodstream, it binds to a protein called transferrin and is carried to all parts of the body, including the bone marrow where new red blood cells are made. Once in the cells, some iron is changed to ferritin, a protein that holds the iron in reserve. When too much iron is absorbed, there is not enough transferrin to bind all of it. Free iron can build up in cells and trigger activities that cause damage and create health problems. Too little iron, on the other hand, can interfere with the body's ability to get enough oxygen.

Sources of iron

The body has complex mechanisms to achieve iron balance by regulating iron absorption, reuse, and storage processes. Red blood cells live for about 120 days. When they die, most of the iron in hemoglobin is recycled in the liver and sent to the bone marrow, where it is reused in new red blood cells. As a result, humans lose only a small amount of iron daily.

Only about 10%–20% of the iron in food, or 1–2 mg for every 10 mg eaten, is absorbed into the bloodstream. Under normal conditions, when iron stores in the body are low, more iron is automatically absorbed. When stores are high, less is absorbed. Iron that is not absorbed enters cells that line the intestine. As these cells fill up with iron, they fall into the intestine and leave the body in waste.

The iron found in plant and animal foods comes in two forms, heme and nonheme, which are not equally available to the body. Heme iron comes from hemoglobin. It is found mainly in animal tissue. Red meat is an especially rich source of heme iron. Only trace amounts of heme iron are found in plants. Heme iron is in a form that is easier for humans to use. It is absorbed at a higher rate than nonheme iron, and its rate of absorption is less influenced by other foods that are simultaneously present in the digestive system.

The following list gives the approximate iron content for some common sources of heme iron:

- chicken liver, cooked, 3 ounces: 12.8 mg
- beef, cooked, 3 ounces: 3.2 mg
- turkey light meat, cooked, 3 ounces: 2.3 mg
- chicken dark meat, cooked, 3 ounces: 1.13 mg
- pork loin, cooked, 3 ounces: 0.8 mg
- oysters, 6 medium: 5.04 mg
- shrimp, cooked, 8 large: 1.36 mg
- tuna, light, canned, 3 ounces: 1.3 mg
- halibut, cooked, 3 ounces: 0.9 mg
- crab, cooked, 3 ounces: 0.8 mg

About 40%–45% of iron in animal tissue and functionally all of the iron in plants is nonheme iron. Nonheme iron is also the type of iron found in **dietary supplements** and added to iron-fortified foods. Nonheme iron is less easily used by humans; it must be changed in the digestive system before it can be absorbed. Only about 2%–10% of nonheme iron in food is absorbed, compared to 20%–25% of heme iron. In addition, the absorption of nonheme iron is strongly influenced by other substances present in the digestive system. The ability of the body to absorb nonheme iron is decreased by the simultaneous presence of tea, coffee, dairy products, phytic acid (a substance found in grains, dried beans, and rice), eggs, **soy** protein, and some chocolates. Absorption of nonheme iron is increased by the simultaneous presence of **vitamin C**, certain organic acids, and a small amount of meat, fish, or poultry, which boosts the absorption of nonheme iron as well as providing heme iron. Vegetarians and vegans should take into consideration the influence of other foods on iron absorption when planning meals.

The following list gives the approximate iron content for some common foods that contain nonheme iron:

- cereal, 100% iron fortified, 1 cup: 18 mg
- soybeans, boiled, 1 cup: 8.8 mg
- tofu, firm, 1/2 cup: 6.22 mg
- kidney beans, cooked, 1 cup: 5.2 mg
- lima beans, cooked, 1 cup: 4.5 mg
- pinto beans, cooked, 1 cup: 3.6 mg
- blackstrap molasses, 1 tablespoon: 3.5 mg
- raisins, small box, 1.5 ounces: .89 mg
- potato, medium with skin: 2.75 mg
- cashew nuts, 1 ounce: 1.70 mg
- whole wheat bread, 1 slice: 0.9 mg

Dietary requirements

The U.S. Institute of Medicine (IOM) of the National Academy of Sciences has developed recommended values for **vitamins** and **minerals** called **dietary reference intakes (DRIs)**. The **DRIs** consist of three sets of numbers: recommended dietary allowance (RDA), adequate intake (AI), and tolerable upper intake level (UL). The RDA defines the average daily amount of the nutrient needed to meet the health needs of 97%–98% of the population. AI is an estimate set when there is not enough information to determine an RDA. The UL is the average maximum amount that can be taken daily without risking negative side effects. The DRIs are calculated for children, adult men, adult women, pregnant women, and **breastfeeding** women.

Iron requirements vary substantially at different ages. Periods of rapid growth in children increase the need for iron. Women who menstruate need more iron because of blood loss during menstruation. Pregnancy puts high demands on the iron supply in the body because of increased production of red blood cells to supply the developing fetus. In 2001, the IOM set RDAs for iron based on preventing iron deficiency at each age. Iron passes into breast milk, and infants can meet their iron needs through breast milk or iron-fortified formula. RDAs and ULs for iron are measured in milligrams (mg).

The following list gives the daily RDAs, AIs, and ULs for iron for healthy individuals as established by the IOM.

- children 0–6 months: AI 0.27 mg; UL 40 mg
- children 7–12 months: RDA 11 mg; UL 40 mg
- children 1–3 years: RDA 7 mg; UL 40 mg
- children 4–8 years: RDA 10 mg; UL 40 mg
- children 9–13 years: RDA 8 mg; UL 40 mg
- boys 14–18 years: RDA 11 mg; UL 45 mg
- girls 14–18 years: RDA 15 mg; UL 45 mg
- men 19 and older: RDA 8 mg; UL 45 mg
- women 19–50: RDA 18 mg; UL 45 mg
- women 51 and older: RDA 8 mg; UL 45 mg
- men who smoke: RDA 25 mg; UL 45 mg
- pregnant women: RDA 27 mg; UL 45 mg
- breastfeeding women 18 years and younger: RDA 10 mg; UL 45 mg
- breastfeeding women 19 years and older: RDA 9 mg; 45 mg

Precautions

Pregnant women should consult their healthcare providers before the 15th week of pregnancy about the need for iron supplementation. They should not start taking an iron supplement on their own.

Men and women over age 55 are not at increased risk for iron deficiency and should take a multivitamin containing iron only on instruction from their healthcare provider.

People with kidney disease, liver damage, alcoholism, or **ulcers** should consult a healthcare professional before taking a supplement containing iron.

Interactions

Iron interacts with many drugs and nutritional supplements. General categories of substances that may affect the amount of iron that is absorbed include:

- medications that decrease stomach acidity (antacids), such as cimetidine (Tagamet), ranitidine (Zantac), omeprazole (Prilosec), and esomeprazole (Nexium)
- pancreatic enzyme supplements
- calcium supplements and dairy products
- vitamin C
- citric, malic, tartaric, and lactic acids
- copper

The presence of iron also alters the effectiveness of many prescription drugs. Individuals should review

---

their medications with a doctor or pharmacist when they begin taking an iron supplement to see if their other medications need adjustment.

Complications

Iron deficiency

The World Health Organization (WHO) considers iron deficiency to be the most widespread dietary disorder in the world. WHO estimates that up to 80% of the world's population is iron deficient and that up to 30% have iron deficiency anemia. The two main causes of iron deficiency are low dietary iron intake and excessive blood loss. Deficiency is less common in the United States, but women of childbearing age, young children, people with diseases that interfere with the absorption of iron (e.g., **Crohn's disease**, **celiac disease**), and people receiving kidney dialysis are most likely to be seriously iron deficient. Men in the United States rarely have low levels of iron because they tend to eat more meat than women and do not lose blood through menstruation.

The body is able to use stored iron to try and make up for an iron deficit, but over time, the amount of hemoglobin decreases and a condition called iron deficiency anemia develops. (This is only one type of anemia; other anemias have other causes.) Iron deficiency anemia decreases the amount of oxygen-reaching cells in the body. Symptoms of iron deficiency anemia include:

- lack of energy
- feelings of weakness (fatigue)
- frequently feeling cold

- increased infections
- irritability
- decreased work or school performance
- sore swollen tongue
- desire to eat dirt, clay, or other non-food substances (pica)

The preferred way to treat mild iron deficiency is through changes in diet. If these changes are ineffective, iron supplements may be used. Dietary supplements contain different formulations such as ferrous fumarate, ferrous sulfate, and ferrous gluconate. Iron in these different formulations is absorbed at different rates. Because too much iron can cause serious health problems, iron supplements should be taken under the supervision of a healthcare professional.

Iron excess

Iron overload caused by an inherited disorder is called hereditary hemochromatosis. This disorder affects as many as 1 in every 200 people of northern European descent. People affected by hereditary hemochromatosis have a genetic mutation that causes them to absorb iron from the intestine at a rate far higher than normal. The condition is treated by avoiding iron-rich foods and removing blood (usually through blood donation) from the individual on a regular basis.

People who have many blood transfusions can also develop iron overload, but by far the most common cause of excess iron is accidental poisoning. Over 20,000 children accidentally ingest iron each year in the United States, usually in the form of dietary supplements. Iron overdose is a medical emergency. Symptoms occurring within the first 12 hours include nausea, vomiting, abdominal pain, black stool, weakness, rapid pulse, low blood pressure, fever, difficulty breathing, and coma. If death does not occur within the first 12 hours, damage to the kidney, liver, cardiovascular system, and nervous system may appear within two days. Examples of long-term damage to survivors of iron poisoning include cirrhosis (liver damage), permanent central nervous system damage, and stomach problems.

Parental concerns

Parents should be aware that the RDA and UL for vitamins and minerals are much lower for children than for adults. Accidental overdose may occur if children take adult vitamins or dietary supplements. Parents should keep all dietary supplements away from children, just as they would other medicines.

QUESTIONS TO ASK YOUR DOCTOR

- How can I tell if I am iron deficient?
- Do I need an iron supplement if I choose to follow a vegan or vegetarian diet?
- If I have hereditary hemochromatosis, what is the chance that a child of mine will inherit the disorder?
- Why should I stop taking a supplement containing iron after I reach age 55?

Resources

BOOKS

Garrison, Cheryl D., ed. *The Iron Disorders Institute Guide to Anemia.* 2nd ed. Naperville, IL: Cumberland House, 2009.

———. *The Iron Disorders Institute Guide to Hemochromatosis.* 2nd ed. Naperville, IL: Cumberland House, 2009.

Mason, Pamela. *Dietary Supplements.* 5th ed. Chicago: Pharmaceutical Press, 2011.

Sarubin-Fragakis, Allison. *The Health Professional's Guide to Popular Dietary Supplements.* 3rd ed. Chicago: American Dietetic Association, 2007.

PERIODICALS

Bánhidy, F., et al. "Iron Deficiency Anemia: Pregnancy Outcomes With or Without Iron Supplementation." *Nutrition* 27, no. 1 (2011): 65–72.

Derbyshire, E. "Strategies to Improve Iron Status in Women at Risk of Developing Anaemia." *Nursing Standard* 26, no. 20 (2012): 51–57.

Iannotti, Lora L., et al. "Iron Supplementation in Early Childhood: Health Benefits and Risks." *American Journal of Clinical Nutrition* 84 (2006): 1261–76.

WEBSITES

Centers for Disease Control and Prevention. "Iron and Iron Deficiency." http://www.cdc.gov/nutrition/everyone/basics/vitamins/iron.html (accessed August 30, 2012).

Higdon, Jane. "Iron." Linus Pauling Institute, Oregon State University. http://lpi.oregonstate.edu/infocenter/minerals/iron (accessed August 30, 2012).

Iron Disorders Institute. "About Iron." http://www.irondisorders.org/about-iron (accessed August 30, 2012).

Mangels, Reed. "Iron in the Vegan Diet." Vegetarian Resource Group. http://www.vrg.org/nutrition/iron.htm (accessed August 30, 2012).

MedlinePlus. "Iron." U.S. National Library of Medicine, National Institutes of Health. http://www.nlm.nih.gov/medlineplus/druginfo/natural/912.html (accessed August 30, 2012).

National Heart, Lung, and Blood Institute. "What is Iron-Deficiency Anemia?" http://www.nhlbi.nih.gov/health/health-topics/topics/ida (accessed August 30, 2012).

Office of Dietary Supplements. "Dietary Supplement Fact Sheet: Iron." U.S. National Institutes of Health. http://ods.od.nih.gov/factsheets/iron (accessed August 30, 2012).

World Health Organization. "Micronutrient Deficiencies: Iron Deficiency Anaemia." http://www.who.int/nutrition/topics/ida/en/index.html (accessed August 30, 2012).

ORGANIZATIONS

Academy of Nutrition and Dietetics, 120 South Riverside Plz., Ste. 2000, Chicago, IL 60606-6995, (312) 899-0040, (800) 877-1600, amacmunn@eatright.org, http://www.eatright.org.

American Academy of Pediatrics, 141 Northwest Point Blvd., Elk Grove Village, IL 60007-1098, (847) 434-4000, Fax: (847) 434-8000, http://www.aap.org.

Iron Disorders Institute, PO Box 675, Taylors, SC 29687, (864) 292-1175, (888) 565-IRON (4766), Fax: (864) 292-1878, info@irondisorders.org, http://www.irondisorders.org.

National Heart, Lung, and Blood Institute, PO Box 30105, Bethesda, MD 20824-0105, (301) 592-8573, TTY: (240) 629-3255, Fax: (240) 629-3246, nhlbiinfo@nhlbi.nih.gov, http://www.nhlbi.nih.gov.

Office of Dietary Supplements, National Institutes of Health, 6100 Executive Blvd., Room 3B01, MSC 7517, Bethesda, MD 20892-7517, (301) 435-2920, Fax: (301) 480-1845, ods@nih.gov, http://ods.od.nih.gov.

World Health Organization, Avenue Appia 20, 1211 Geneva 27, Switzerland, +41 22 791-2111, Fax: +41 22 791-3111, info@who.int, http://www.who.int.

Tish Davidson, AM

Irradiated food

Definition

Irradiated foods are foods that have been exposed to a radiant energy source to kill harmful bacteria, insects, or parasites, or to delay spoilage, sprouting, or ripening.

Purpose

There are many reasons that foods are irradiated. The most common reason is for increased **food safety**. The Centers for Disease Control (CDC) estimates that there are about 76 million cases of foodborne illness each year in the United States, resulting in about 5,000 deaths annually. Irradiating foods can reduce the risk of many foodborne illnesses by killing the bacteria or pathogens responsible, or harming them to such an extent that they are not able to reproduce or cause disease. The National Aeronautics and Space Administration (NASA) exposes the food that astronauts eat while in space to a level of irradiation far higher than that approved for commercial use in order to reduce the risk that astronauts will develop illness while in space. Patients who have diseases that severely impair the functioning of the immune system are often fed irradiated foods to decrease the risk that they will develop a serious disease.

Irradiation can also be used to destroy insects and other pests that may be present on produce. When

Foods permitted to be irradiated under FDA regulations (21 CFR 179.26)

Food	Purpose	Dose
Fresh, non-heated processed pork	Control of *Trichinella spiralis*	0.3 kGy min. to 1 kGy max.
Fresh foods	Growth and maturation inhibition	1 kGy max.
Foods	Arthropod disinfection	1 kGy max.
Dry or dehydrated enzyme preparations	Microbial disinfection	10 kGy max.
Dry or dehydrated spices/seasonings	Microbial disinfection	30 kGy max.
Fresh or frozen, uncooked poultry products	Pathogen control	3 kGy max.
Frozen packaged meats (solely NASA)	Sterilization	44 kGy min.
Refrigerated uncooked meat products	Pathogen control	4.5 kGy max.
Frozen uncooked meat products	Pathogen control	7 kGy max.
Fresh shell eggs	Control of *Salmonella*	3.0 kGy max.
Seeds for sprouting	Control of microbial pathogens	8.0 kGy max.
Fresh or frozen molluscan shellfish	Control of *Vibrio* species and other foodborne pathogens	5.5 kGy max.
Fresh iceberg lettuce and fresh spinach	Control of food-borne pathogens, and extension of shelf-life	4.0 kGy max.

kGy = kiloGray

SOURCE: U.S. Food and Drug Administration.

Available online at http://www.fda.gov/Food/FoodIngredientsPackaging/IrradiatedFoodPackaging/ucm074734.htm. *(Table by PreMediaGlobal. © 2013 Cengage Learning.)*

produce is shipped from Hawaii to the mainland United States, it must be fumigated to kill any insects or insect eggs that might be present so that they do not spread to the mainland. Irradiating this produce is sometimes used as an alternative to fumigation, as it does not leave a residue of chemicals on the produce in the way that fumigation can.

Some fruits and vegetables can be kept fresh longer by the use of low to moderate levels of irradiation. When exposed to low levels of radiation, potatoes, onions, and other vegetables do not sprout as quickly. Strawberries and other berries can benefit from irradiation as well, as irradiation can significantly delay the growth of mold. Strawberries stay fresh from 3–5 days when they are not irradiated or treated in any way, but can stay fresh and unspoiled for up to three weeks after being irradiated.

Description

Irradiated foods are foods that have been exposed to ionizing radiation. Ions are electrically charged particles, and ionizing radiation is radiation that produces these charged particles. Nonionizing radiation is produced by microwaves, television and radio waves, and visible light. Ionizing radiation is higher in power than these types of radiation, although it is in the same spectrum. The kinds of ionizing radiation used for food irradiation include gamma rays, beams of high-energy electrons, and x rays.

When foods are irradiated, they are exposed to the source of the ionizing radiation for a short time. This radiation produces short-lived compounds that damage the deoxyribonucleic acid (DNA) of living organisms, such as bacteria that are in the food. Because DNA makes up the genes that contain the instructions that tell an organism how to grow and reproduce, once the DNA is damaged the organism cannot do this correctly and will die.

The amount of radiation required to irradiate foods depends on the type and thickness of the food product and the types of organisms that are present. The larger the DNA of the organism, generally the less radiation is required to irradiate it. Insects and parasites have the larger DNA and require the lowest levels of radiation, while bacteria generally require slightly more, and viruses have very small amounts of DNA and require very high levels of radiation. Most parasites, insects, and bacteria can be eliminated at levels of radiation approved for commercial use, but many viruses cannot.

Irradiating foods does not make the foods radioactive in any way. Irradiation done using beams of

high-energy electrons or x rays does not even use any radioactive material. Irradiation done using gamma rays involves exposure of the food to a radioactive substance, usually cobalt 60 or cesium 137, for a short period. The radioactivity of this substance is not in any way transferred to the food that is exposed to it.

Precautions

Irradiation is not a substitute for safe food handling practices. Although irradiation kills or disables many pathogenic organisms, these organisms can be reintroduced to the foods if cross contamination occurs. In addition, not every pathogen is completely destroyed by irradiation, and leaving foods such as raw meat out at room temperature can allow these pathogens to reproduce to significant levels. Irradiation should be viewed as an extra step to help ensure that the food supply is safe, not as a replacement for food safety practices that are already in place.

Interactions

Irradiated foods are not expected to interact with any other foods, medicines, or products.

Complications

There are no complications expected from consuming irradiated foods. Some concerned groups have expressed fears that the long-term effects of eating irradiated foods are unknown. However, many different scientific studies have examined the effects on both animals and humans of consuming irradiated foods. There has not been any evidence that irradiated foods are harmful in either the short or long term. One study even examined many generations of animals fed irradiated foods and found no harmful effects. Irradiating food is accepted as a safe practice and is endorsed by many organizations including the World Health

QUESTIONS TO ASK YOUR DOCTOR

- What are the risks of handling irradiated food?
- Is eating irradiated food safe for me?
- How can I tell if I am getting the right nutrients?
- What symptoms or adverse effects are important enough that I should seek immediate treatment?

Organization, the CDC, the U.S. Food and Drug Administration (FDA), and the American Medical Association.

Parental concerns

Some parents may have concerns that the vitamin and nutrient content of irradiated foods may be reduced compared to the content of the same foods that have not been irradiated. For most **vitamins**, **minerals**, and nutrients this is not the case. Studies have shown that the levels of most vitamins in irradiated foods are not significantly different from the levels in foods that have not been irradiated. Some vitamins, however, such as thiamin (vitamin B_1), have been found to be sensitive to irradiation. The extent to which such vitamins are destroyed depends greatly on the type of food being irradiated. Thiamin was found to be decreased by 50% in a water solution that was exposed to radiation, but only decreased by 5% in a dried egg exposed to the same level of radiation. Many vitamins, like thiamin, that are sensitive to irradiation are as sensitive, or even more sensitive, to heat, and are broken down at least as much by the process of canning or heat treatments. Therefore, although levels of some vitamins may be decreased in irradiated foods compared to fresh foods, the levels of these vitamins may be higher in irradiated foods than in comparable canned or otherwise sterilized foods.

Resources

BOOKS

Bender, David A. *A Dictionary of Food and Nutrition*. New York: Oxford University Press, 2009.

Larsen, Laura, ed. *Diet and Nutrition Sourcebook*. 4th ed. Detroit, MI: Omnigraphics, 2011.

Rodrigues, Sueli, and Fabiano Andre Narciso Fernandes, eds. *Advances in Fruit Processing Technologies*. Boca Raton, FL: CRC Press, 2012.

Sommers, Christopher H, and Xuetong Fan, eds. *Food Irradiation Research and Technology*. 2nd ed. New York: Wiley-Blackwell, 2012.

WEBSITES

Organic Consumers Association. "Information on Food Irradiation." http://www.organicconsumers.org/irradlink.cfm (accessed August 30, 2012).

ORGANIZATIONS

Centers for Disease Control, 1600 Clifton Rd., Atlanta, GA 30333, (800) 311-3435, http://www.cdc.gov.

U.S. Department of Agriculture, 1400 Independence Avenue SW, Washington, DC 20250, http://www.usda.gov.

U.S. Food and Drug Administration, 10903 New Hampshire Ave., Silver Spring, MD 20993, (888) 463-6332, http://www.fda.gov.

World Health Organization, Avenue Appia 20, Geneva, Switzerland, +41 22 791-2222, http://www.who.int/en.

Tish Davidson, AM
Laura Jean Cataldo, RN, EdD

Irritable bowel syndrome

Definition

Irritable bowel syndrome (IBS) is an idiopathic functional gastrointestinal disorder. The bowel appears normal but does not function correctly, and the reason for this is unknown. IBS is also called spastic colon, mucous colitis, and irritable colon, among others.

Demographics

Between 9% and 20% of the world's population—more than 50 million people—are thought to be affected by IBS. Because of this high percentage, IBS is considered one of the most common medical disorders. According to the U.S. National Library of Medicine, approximately one out of every six people in the United States had symptoms of IBS in 2011. U.S. physicians report that up to 3.5 million visits to the doctor occur annually, which equates to about $21 billion in medical expenses, missed work, and other related costs.

The disorder appears to be most common in Western countries. However, poor access to medical care, different cultural attitudes toward illness, and the fact that the disorder is neither life threatening nor contagious and does not have to be reported to any central authority makes it difficult to tell what the actual rates are in developing countries. In Western countries, estimates of the number of people with IBS range from 9%–23% of the population.

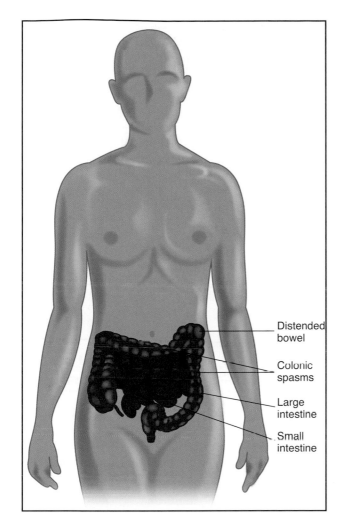

Symptoms of irritable bowel syndrome (IBS) include distended bowel and colonic spasms. *(Illustration by Electronic Illustrators Group. © 2013 Cengage Learning.)*

IBS occurs in both children and adults. About 14% of high school students and 6% of middle school students report IBS symptoms. In these groups, IBS accounts for 4%–5% of all absences from school. In about half of all people who have the disorder, symptoms begin before age 35, and 30% say that their symptoms began in childhood. Most other people with IBS develop symptoms between ages 35 and 50. Women are two to three times more likely to have IBS than are men, and IBS in women is more likely to occur during menstruation, with more discomfort during premenstrual and postovulatory periods.

Description

Irritable bowel syndrome is not a life-threatening disorder and does not progress to a more serious disorder, but it is the cause of about one in every ten

doctor visits in the United States. Its symptoms, although not medically serious, are varied, changeable, and intrusive enough to impact an individual's quality of life. IBS causes people to miss school or work and to avoid certain activities, and it interferes with personal relationships.

IBS involves both the large intestine (colon) and the small intestine. Symptoms include pain, cramping, and either **constipation**, diarrhea, or alternating periods of both. It is not contagious, is not strictly inherited, and despite the discomfort, the bowel is structurally normal—no infection, no tumors or polyps, and no abnormalities in the cells lining the intestinal wall.

IBS should not to be confused with **inflammatory bowel disease** (IBD). Inflammatory bowel diseases such as **Crohn's disease** and ulcerative colitis cause changes in the cells lining the wall of the intestine. These cell abnormalities can be seen in samples (biopsies) taken from the wall of the intestine. In a person who has IBS, the cells in samples taken from the lining of the intestine look normal. Inflammatory bowel diseases increase the risk of developing intestinal cancers; IBS does not.

Causes and symptoms

The cause of IBS is unknown. Some researchers believe that the bowel of people with IBS is inappropriately sensitive and overreacts to normal things such as the passage of food and stress. Other researchers suggest that there is a flaw in the way the brain and the gut interact. Some scientists suggest that an earlier infection predisposes some people to develop IBS. Others have found that there are abnormal numbers of receptors for the neurotransmitter serotonin in the gastrointestinal tract of people with IBS. Low doses of some antidepressant drugs that affect serotonin levels have been found to improve IBS symptoms in some people.

Whatever the cause, symptoms of IBS include pain or discomfort in the abdomen; feeling bloated (fullness) or having a lot of gas; diarrhea, constipation, or alternating periods of both; and mucus in the stool. The symptoms come and go, being present for a few days each month or lasting for around three months. They range from mild to severe (though most people have mild symptoms) and can change in a single individual over time. The impact of symptoms can also range from mild to severe, and the intensity of symptoms can also change over time. Symptoms are usually reduced or relieved by a bowel movement.

Although outside factors are not thought to cause IBS, certain things can trigger IBS symptoms. Triggers vary from person to person. Possible triggers include:

- Food. Different foods are triggers for different people. Some common trigger foods are dairy products, sorbitol (a sweetener used in sugar-free products), caffeine, chocolate, and alcohol.
- Stress. Stress from any source often triggers or worsens symptoms in people with IBS.
- Illness. Other gastrointestinal illnesses caused by bacteria or viruses can trigger symptoms.
- Menstruation. Women seem to have more severe symptoms when they are menstruating, suggesting that changing hormone levels may affect symptoms.

Diagnosis

There are no tests for IBS. It is often diagnosed by ruling out other disorders with similar symptoms, such as ulcerative colitis. When other possible diseases have been eliminated through medical testing, then IBS is diagnosed.

Another approach to diagnosis is to use what is known as the Rome criteria for diagnosis. Following the Rome criteria, IBS is diagnosed if the symptoms of abdominal pain, diarrhea and/or constipation are present for at least 12 weeks (the weeks do not have to be consecutive) and several of the following conditions are met:

- changes in the frequency of bowel movements
- changes in the consistency of the stool
- straining to empty the bowels or a feeling of urgency to empty the bowels
- frequently feeling that the bowel is not completely empty
- mucus in the stool
- bloating
- reduction in symptoms after a bowel movement

Often these two approaches to diagnosis are combined, and the physician may initially perform a sigmoidoscopy or a colonoscopy to look at the inside of the bowel. In these procedures, a tube called an endoscope is inserted through the rectum and into the colon. At the end of the endoscope is a tiny camera that allows the doctor to see if there is damage to the cells lining the digestive tract. During this procedure, the doctor also removes small tissue samples (biopsies) in order to look for abnormal cells under the microscope. This can eliminate inflammatory bowel syndrome as the cause of symptoms.

The doctor may also do a lactose intolerance test. Lactose is a **sugar** found in milk. People who lack the enzyme to break down this sugar have symptoms similar to those of irritable bowel syndrome. Lactose intolerance is common, and a lactose intolerance test can confirm or eliminate lactose as the source of the symptoms.

The doctor may also do a blood test to determine if symptoms are caused by early or mild **celiac disease**. People with celiac disease are sensitive to gluten, a **protein** found in wheat, barley, rye, and the products made from these grains. Eating foods containing gluten often causes symptoms similar to IBS in people with celiac disease.

Note that blood in the stool, vomiting, fever, and diarrhea that awakens a person at night are not symptoms of IBS. Individuals with these symptoms should see a doctor.

Treatment

Because no functional problems can be found in people with IBS, family members and even some healthcare providers may be inclined to dismiss symptoms as psychological. Finding a doctor with whom the patient can establish good communication and feel comfortable is an important first step in treatment.

Treatment of IBS is aimed at relieving symptoms and falls into three categories: lifestyle adjustments, coping skills, and drug therapy.

Traditional

Lifestyle adjustments include:

- increasing fiber in the diet
- keeping a food diary to learn which foods are trigger foods and then avoiding them
- drinking at least six glasses of water daily to help prevent constipation
- getting regular exercise
- eating meals at regular times and not skipping meals
- avoiding large meals

Learning new coping skills may involve psychotherapy (talk therapy) or professional counseling to help resolve problems that are causing stress or learning techniques to cope with stress. Some of these coping techniques include biofeedback, yoga, massage, meditation, deep breathing exercises, progressive relaxation exercises, and hypnosis.

Drugs

Drug therapy depends on specific symptoms. Over-the-counter antidiarrheal products such as loperamide (Imodium) and diphenoxylate (Lomotil) can improve bowel movements and reduce the impact of IBS on daily activities. In addition, bile acid–binding agents, such as cholestyramine (Questran), help to reduce bile acids from building up in the colon, which slows the passage of stool and relieves diarrhea.

Over-the-counter laxatives can be helpful in treating constipation but must be used sparingly, because regular use creates bowel dependence. Bulk-forming or fiber-supplement laxatives are generally considered the safest type of laxative. Some common brand names of fiber-supplement laxatives are Metamucil, Citrucel, Fiberall, Konsyl, and Serutan. These must be taken with water. They provide extra **fiber** that absorbs water and helps keep the stool soft. The extra bulk also helps move materials through the colon. Lubiprostone (Amitiza) is also used for constipation by helping to increase the fluid levels in the intestines, which allows the stool to pass easier.

Stool softeners help prevent stool from drying out. They are recommended for people who should not strain to have a bowel movement, such as people recovering from abdominal surgeries or childbirth. Brand names include Colace and Surfak. Stimulant laxatives, such as Dulcolax, Senokot, Correctol, and Purge, increase the rhythmic contractions of the colon and help to move the material along faster. They also help to reduce irritation within the lining of the intestines.

Lubricants add grease to the stool so that it moves more easily through the colon. Mineral oil is the most common lubricant. Saline laxatives such as Milk of Magnesia draw water from the body into the colon to help soften and move the stool.

Two prescription drugs are available to treat IBS, but both have restrictions regarding their use. Alosetron (Lotronex) is used to treat sensitivity of the abdomen (as part of the symptoms of IBS). In the United States, alosetron was temporarily withdrawn from the market because of serious side effects, including four deaths. It was later reapproved by the U.S. Food and Drug Administration (FDA), but with limitations. The drug can only be prescribed by doctors enrolled in a special program, and it should only be used for cases of severe diarrhea-type IBS that have failed to respond to all other treatments. The drug is only approved for use in women.

Lubiprostone (Amitiza) is used to treat constipation-type IBS in both men and women. Lubiprostone causes

KEY TERMS

Celiac disease—A digestive disease that causes damage to the small intestine. It results from the inability to digest gluten found in wheat, rye, and barley.

Colonoscopy—A medical examination of the large bowel and the distal part of the small bowel with the use of a tiny CCD (charged-couple device) camera or an optical fiber camera attached to the end of a flexible tube.

Gluten—A combination of two proteins found in some cereal grains, such as wheat.

Neurotransmitters—Chemicals that carry nerve impulses from one cell to another. Abnormal levels of specific neurotransmitters could make the bowel more reactive.

Serotonin—A neurotransmitter derived from the amino acid tryptophan, widely found within the tissues of the body; its chemical formula is $C_{10}H_{12}N_2O$.

Sigmoidoscopy—A minimally invasive examination of the large intestine, going from the rectum to the last portion of the colon.

the small intestine to secrete additional fluids, which helps stool pass more easily. Like alosetron, lubiprostone is only to be used in severe cases and when all other treatment types have failed.

Tegaserod (Zelnorm), previously prescribed for severe constipation, was withdrawn from the U.S. market at the request of the FDA in March 2007 because of serious heart-related side effects.

Some people with IBS have seen their symptoms improve when treated with low levels of tricyclic antidepressants that target serotonin levels in the brain. The dosage of these drugs is lower than that used to treat depression. Serotonin is a neurotransmitter that some researchers think plays a role in IBS. Newer selective serotonin reuptake inhibitor (SSRI) antidepressants seem to be less effective. People whose symptoms do not improve with lifestyle changes may want to talk to their doctor about this option and should also seek treatment for any accompanying depression or anxiety.

Nutrition and dietary concerns

The main dietary concern of people with constipation-type IBS is increasing the amount of

QUESTIONS TO ASK YOUR DOCTOR

- Where can I learn more about how to live better with irritable bowel syndrome?

- Can I reverse my health problems if I live a lifestyle more suitable to IBS?

- What type of nutritional supplementation should I take with irritable bowel syndrome?

- Will less stress help me eliminate or reduce the occurrence of IBS?

fiber in the diet. Insoluble fiber helps material move through the large intestine faster so that the body reabsorbs less water and the stool remains softer. Soluble fiber dissolves in water and forms a gel that keeps the stool soft. Good sources of fiber include apples with skin, dried beans, pears with skin, brown rice, oatmeal, and popcorn.

Prognosis

Every year, the symptoms of about 10% of people with IBS spontaneously disappear. The reason for this is not understood. For most people, however, IBS is a chronic disorder that lasts for a lifetime. Symptoms are erratic and changeable; there are periods where symptoms improve and periods when symptoms worsen. For some people, the symptoms of IBS can adversely affect activities of daily life, such as going to school or work, attending social events, taking vacations, or running errands. IBS is not considered a symptom of any other disorder, and it does not cause permanent harm to the intestines or develop into more serious diseases.

Prevention

Since the cause of IBS is unknown, the disorder cannot be prevented.

Resources

BOOKS

Dahlman, David. *Why Doesn't My Doctor Know This? Conquering Irritable Bowel Syndrome, Inflammatory Bowel Disease, Crohn's Disease, and Colitis.* Garden City, NJ: Morgan James Publishing, 2008.

Newman, Alvin. *The Essential IBS Book: Understanding and Managing Irritable Bowel Syndrome & Functional Dyspepsia.* Toronto: Robert Rose, 2011.

Nicol, Rosemary. *Irritable Bowel Syndrome: A Natural Approach.* Berkeley, CA: Ulysses Press, 2007.

Talley, Nicholas J. *Conquering Irritable Bowel Syndrome: A Guide to Liberating Those Suffering with Chronic Stomach or Bowel Problems.* Hamilton, Ontario: BC Decker, 2006.

U.S. Department of Health and Human Services. *Irritable Bowel Syndrome in Children.* Bethesda, MD: National Institutes of Health, 2008.

PERIODICALS

Aragon, G., et al. "Probiotic Therapy for Irritable Bowel Syndrome." *Gastroenterology & Hepatology* 6, no. 1 (2010): 39–44.

McKenzie, Y.A., et al. "British Dietetic Association Evidence-Based Guidelines for the Dietary Management of Irritable Bowel Syndrome in Adults." *Journal of Human Nutrition and Dietetics* (April 2012): e-pub ahead of print. http://dx.doi.org/10.1111/j.1365-277X.2012.01242.x (accessed May 1, 2012).

Ostgaard, H., et al. "Diet and Effects of Diet Management on Quality of Life and Symptoms in Patients with Irritable Bowel Syndrome." *Molecular Medicine Reports* 5, no. 6 (2012): 1382–90. http://dx.doi.org/10.3892/mmr.2012.843 (accessed May 1, 2012).

Trinkley, K.E., and M.C. Nahata. "Treatment of Irritable Bowel Syndrome." *Journal of Clinical Pharmacy and Therapeutics* 36, no. 3 (2011): 275–82. http://dx.doi.org/10.1111/j.1365-2710.2010.01177.x (accessed May 1, 2012).

WEBSITES

International Foundation for Functional Gastrointestinal Disorders. "Learn About IBS: Frequently Asked Questions." http://www.aboutibs.org/site/about-ibs/faq (accessed May 1, 2012).

Mayo Clinic staff. "Irritable Bowel Syndrome." MayoClinic.com. http://www.mayoclinic.com/health/irritable-bowel-syndrome/DS00106 (accessed May 1, 2012).

MedlinePlus. "Irritable Bowel Syndrome." U.S. National Library of Medicine, National Institutes of Health. http://www.nlm.nih.gov/medlineplus/irritablebowelsyndrome.html (accessed May 1, 2012).

National Digestive Diseases Information Clearinghouse (NDDIC). "Irritable Bowel Syndrome." U.S. National Institute of Diabetes and Digestive and Kidney Diseases (NIDDK), National Institutes of Health. http://digestive.niddk.nih.gov/ddiseases/pubs/ibs (accessed May 1, 2012).

ORGANIZATIONS

American College of Gastroenterology, 6400 Goldsboro Rd., Ste. 450, Bethesda, MD 20817, (301) 263-9000, http://www.acg.gi.org.

American Gastroenterological Association, 4930 Del Ray Ave., Bethesda, MD 20814, (301) 654-2055, (800) 877-1600, Fax: (301) 654-5920, member@gastro.org, http://www.gastro.org.

International Foundation for Functional Gastrointestinal Disorders, PO Box 170864, Milwaukee, WI

53217-8076, (414) 964-1799, (888) 964-2001, Fax: (414) 964-7176, iffgd@iffgd.org, http://www.iffgd.org.

Irritable Bowel Syndrome Self Help and Support Group, 24 Dixwell Ave., #118, New Haven, CT 06511, (203) 424-0660, http://www.ibsgroup.org.

National Institute of Diabetes and Digestive and Kidney Diseases, 31 Center Dr., MSC 2560, Bethesda, MD 20892-2560, (301) 496-3583, (800) 891-5389, http://www2.niddk.nih.gov.

Tish Davidson, AM
William A. Atkins, BB, BS, MBA

Irritable bowel syndrome diet

Definition

The **irritable bowel syndrome** diet is a set of recommendations designed to reduce the symptoms that are common with irritable bowel syndrome (IBS), including **constipation** and diarrhea. It is not a diet designed for weight loss.

Origins

No specific person or organization originated the irritable bowel syndrome diet. Instead, it has developed out of research, observations, and trial and error by gastroenterologists and their patients with IBS.

Description

Irritable bowel syndrome is a disorder in which the intestine (bowel) appears normal but does not function correctly. The disorder is very common, but its cause is not known. At least 15% of people in the United States are thought to have symptoms of IBS, ranging from mild and annoying to severe and life altering.

The main symptoms of IBS are pain or discomfort in the abdomen, bloating, and having a lot of gas (flatulence), diarrhea, constipation, or alternating periods of both diarrhea and constipation. Symptoms come and go and can vary in severity in a single individual over time. Although a person's diet does not cause IBS, certain foods can trigger symptoms. These foods differ from person to person. Common food triggers include alcohol, dairy products, beverages that contain **caffeine**, and the **artificial sweeteners** sorbitol and mannitol. The IBS diet is designed to avoid foods that will trigger symptoms and encourages the consumption of foods that help reduce diarrhea, constipation, and gas.

General aspects of the IBS diet include:

- reducing or eliminating foods that may make diarrhea worse, such as alcohol, artificial sweeteners, caffeine, fatty foods, foods high in sugar, gas-producing foods (such as beans, broccoli, and cabbage), and dairy products (such as milk, yogurt, and cheese)
- reducing constipation by adding fiber to the diet, drinking plenty of water, and getting regular exercise
- keeping a daily food journal of what is eaten and whether symptoms become noticeable after eating
- eating slowly and having meals in a relaxing environment

Function

The function of the irritable bowel syndrome diet is to give individuals more control over the symptoms of IBS, thus improving quality of life. The challenge of this diet is twofold. First, constipation and diarrhea are opposite in their effect, yet they can appear in the same individual as part of the same disorder. Constipation occurs when food stays in the large intestine (colon) too long. Too much water is reabsorbed into the body, and the stool (waste) in the large intestine becomes hard, dry, and difficult or painful to eliminate. With diarrhea, food moves too quickly through the large intestine, and not enough water is reabsorbed. Stools are loose and watery, and the individual may feel extreme urgency to have a bowel movement.

The second challenge to this diet is that individuals with IBS may respond to the same foods in different ways. The IBS diet is not a list of "must eat" and "must not eat" foods; rather, it includes suggested foods personalized through trial and error. Keeping a food journal often helps people with IBS to pinpoint which foods are beneficial and which worsen symptoms.

High-fiber/low-fat IBS diet

Dietary **fiber** is the collective name for a group of indigestible carbohydrate-based compounds found in plants. They are the materials that give plants their rigidity and structure. The IBS diet is a high-fiber/low-fat diet. The role of fiber, also called roughage or bulk, is crucial in controlling the quality of stool in the colon, and reducing fat consumption is both healthful and avoids counteracting the actions of fiber.

Two types of dietary fiber are important to human health: insoluble fiber and soluble fiber. Insoluble fiber is fiber that moves through the digestive system essentially unchanged. It is not digested by the body, and it does not provide energy (**calories**). Insoluble fiber provides bulk to stool, which helps it move through the large intestine. It also traps water, which helps the stool remain soft and easy to eliminate.

Soluble fiber (also called prebiotic or viscous fiber) is modified within the body and is readily fermented in the colon and converted into gases and physiologically active byproducts. Soluble fiber dissolves in water to form a gel-like substance. This gel helps keep stool soft.

Studies find that the average American eats only 5–14 grams of fiber daily, but the recommended amounts are much higher. The U.S. Institute of Medicine (IOM) of the National Academy of Sciences has issued the following daily adequate intakes (AI) for fiber:

- men aged 9–13: 31 grams
- men aged 14–50: 38 grams
- men aged 51 and older: 30 grams
- women aged 9–18: 26 grams
- women aged 19–50: 25 grams
- women aged 51 and older: 21 grams
- children aged 0–1 not determined
- children aged 1–3: 19 grams
- children aged 4–8: 25 grams

To follow the IBS diet, individuals should gradually increase their consumption of fiber to meet or exceed the AI. Foods that are high in insoluble fiber include:

- whole grains (whole-wheat bread, wheat bran, brown rice, whole-wheat pasta, bran and bran breakfast cereals, barley, bulgar, couscous)
- vegetables (carrots, cucumbers, celery, onions, zucchini)
- fruits (apples with skin, berries, bananas)

Good sources of soluble fiber include:

- oatmeal and foods made with oats
- legumes (beans, peas, lentils)
- fruits (apples, pears, prunes, plums), citrus fruits (lemons, oranges, limes, grapefruit)
- vegetables (carrots, broccoli, Brussels sprouts)

As of 2012, the FDA required nutritional food labels to include the total amount of dietary fiber per serving; however, the FDA did not require that fiber be broken down into amounts of soluble and insoluble fiber.

People with IBS who have trouble consuming enough fiber may wish to ask their doctors about bulk-forming laxatives or fiber supplements. These supplements are considered safe but should not be used for long periods unless directed by a doctor,

because the colon will become dependent on them to move stool. Some common brand names of fiber supplements are Metamucil, Citrucel, Fiberall, Konsyl, and Serutan. These must be taken with water. Fiber supplements provide extra fiber that absorbs intestinal water and helps keep stool soft. The extra bulk also helps move materials through the colon.

Low-residue/low-fat IBS diet

For some people, the high-fiber/low-fat diet helps control both constipation and diarrhea. For others, high-fiber foods trigger diarrhea. These individuals may wish to try a low-fiber/low-residue diet. This diet substitutes cooked fruits and vegetables for raw ones and reduces the amount of whole-grain products. The low-fiber diet also includes a variety of low-fat foods.

Some foods that help control diarrhea include:

- applesauce
- low-fat mashed potatoes
- grated apples without the skin
- avocado
- cream of rice
- smooth peanut butter
- tapioca

Other tips to help control diarrhea include:

- consume food and drink at room temperature rather than at hot temperatures
- drink liquids between meals rather than with meals
- limit dairy products
- rest after meals (this slows down the digestive process)

Because symptoms and triggers for IBS vary greatly, these diets are considered starting points for individuals to develop their own lists of foods that control their individual symptoms. Keeping a food journal that records what was eaten and what caused symptoms can help speed the development of a personalized effective IBS diet.

Benefits

In addition to controlling symptoms, the IBS high-fiber/low-fat diet has several other benefits, including lower cholesterol levels, reduced risk of type 2 diabetes and diverticulitis, and potential weight loss (the increased bulk of high-fiber foods helps people feel full faster, so they may eat less).

KEY TERMS

Cholesterol—A waxy substance made by the liver and also acquired through diet. High levels in the blood may increase the risk of cardiovascular disease.

Constipation—Abnormally delayed or infrequent passage of feces. It may be either functional (related to failure to move the bowels) or organic (caused by another disease or disorder).

Diabetes—A condition in which the body either does not produce or appropriately respond to the hormone insulin. As a result, the body cannot use glucose (sugar). There are two types, type 1 (insulin dependent) and type 2 (non-insulin dependent).

Diarrhea—Thin, watery feces discharged from the anus during bowel movements, often frequently and excessively.

Diverticulitis—Protrusions on the lining of the large intestine, which often cause inflammation, abdominal pain, fever, and constipation.

Prebiotic—A non-digestible carbohydrate that helps grow beneficial microorganisms in the large intestine.

Viscous—Any liquid with a thick consistency.

Precautions

The IBS diet is safe for anyone, although it may not control the symptoms of IBS for every individual. Symptoms may worsen while the individual is experimenting with personalizing his or her food plan.

Risks

The amount of fiber in the diet should be increased gradually. Increasing fiber too rapidly can result in abdominal pain and large amounts of gas. Individuals who do not drink enough water on a **high-fiber diet** may develop abdominal pain and constipation.

Research and general acceptance

The IBS diet is accepted as healthy and helpful in controlling the symptoms of IBS by almost all gastroenterologists. High-fiber diets are endorsed as having health benefits by the American Heart Association, the **Academy of Nutrition and Dietetics**, the U.S. Department of Health and Human Services, and many individual healthcare organizations.

Resources

BOOKS

Holt, Susanna. *Eat Well, Live Well with IBS: High-Fibre Recipes and Tips*. North Vancouver, British Columbia, Canada: Whitecap, 2007.

Knoff, Laura J. *The Whole-Food Guide to Overcoming Irritable Bowel Syndrome: Strategies & Recipes for Eating Well with IBS, Indigestion & Other Digestive Disorders*. Oakland, CA: New Harbinger, 2010.

Koff, Ashley. *Recipes for IBS: Great-Tasting Recipes and Tips Customized for Your Symptoms*. Beverly, MA: Fair Winds Press, 2007.

PERIODICALS

Heizer, William D., Susannah Southern, and Susan McGovern. "The Role of Diet in Symptoms of Irritable Bowel Syndrome in Adults: A Narrative Review." *Journal of the Academy of Nutrition and Dietetics* 109, no. 7 (2009): 1204–14. http://dx.doi.org/10.1016/j.jada.2009.04.012 (accessed August 30, 2012).

Williams, Lauren, and Joanne Slavin. "Dietary Fiber and Other Alternative Therapies and Irritable Bowel Syndrome." *Topics in Clinical Nutrition* 24, no. 3 (2009): 262–71.

WEBSITES

Cleveland Clinic. "Foods to Choose if You Have Mixed Irritable Bowel Syndrome." http://www.clevelandclinic.org/health/health-info/docs/4000/4060.asp?index=13096 (accessed August 30, 2012).

Harvard School of Public Health. "Fiber: Start Roughing It!" Nutrition Source, Department of Nutrition, Harvard University. http://www.hsph.harvard.edu/nutritionsource/index.html (accessed August 30, 2012).

International Foundation for Functional Gastrointestinal Disorders. "IBS Diet." aboutIBS.org. http://www.aboutibs.org/site/about-ibs/management/ibs-diet (accessed August 30, 2012).

Mayo Clinic staff. "High-Fiber Foods." MayoClinic.com. http://www.mayoclinic.com/health/high-fiber-foods/NU00582 (accessed August 30, 2012).

University of Pittsburgh Medical Center. "Irritable Bowel Syndrome Diet." http://www.upmc.com/HealthAtoZ/patienteducation/G/Pages/irritablebowelsyndromediet.aspx (accessed August 30, 2012).

U.S. Food and Drug Administration. "Nutrition Labeling; Questions G1 through P8." *Guidance for Industry: A Food Labeling Guide*. http://www.fda.gov/Food/GuidanceComplianceRegulatoryInformation/

GuidanceDocuments/FoodLabelingNutrition/Food LabelingGuide/default.htm (accessed August 30, 2012).

ORGANIZATIONS

American College of Gastroenterology, 6400 Goldsboro Rd., Ste. 450, Bethesda, MD 20817, (301) 263-9000, http://www.acg.gi.org.

American Gastroenterological Association, 4930 Del Ray Ave., Bethesda, MD 20814, (301) 654-2055, Fax: (301) 654-5920, (800) 877-1600, member@gastro.org, http://www.gastro.org.

International Foundation for Functional Gastrointestinal Disorders, PO Box 170864, Milwaukee, WI 53217-8076, (414) 964-1799, Fax: (414) 964-7176, (888) 964-2001, iffgd@iffgd.org, http://www.iffgd.org.

Irritable Bowel Syndrome Self Help and Support Group, 24 Dixwell Ave. #118, New Haven, CT 06511, (203) 424-0660, http://www.ibsgroup.org.

National Institute of Diabetes and Digestive and Kidney Diseases, 31 Center Dr., MSC 2560, Bethesda, MD 20892-2560, (301) 496-3583, (800) 891-5389, http://www2.niddk.nih.gov.

Monique Laberge, PhD
William A. Atkins, BB, BS, MBA

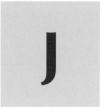

Japanese diet *see* **Asian diet**

Jenny Craig diet

Definition

Jenny Craig is a calorie-based, three-stage lifestyle weight-loss program that incorporates pre-packaged food, transition to regular food, and long-term weight maintenance.

Origins

Jenny Craig and her husband Sid Craig founded the Jenny Craig Weight Management Program in Australia in 1983. The program has since expanded to the United States, Canada, New Zealand, and Puerto Rico and offers both a center-based program and an at-home program. Craig, who has no training as a nutritionist, based her program on her own successful experience with personalized weight loss. The program has a medical advisory board consisting of at least one physician, nutritionist, and behaviorist. Pre-packaged meals are planned by a registered dietitian.

Description

The Jenny Craig program is a three-stage program. In the first stage, dieters eat only Jenny Craig pre-packaged foods that are supplemented with approved fruits, vegetables, and non-fat dairy products. These meals contain 50%–60% **carbohydrates**, 20%–25% **protein**, and 20%–25% **fats**, and contain between 1,200 and 2,500 **calories** daily. This generally is in line with the federal *Dietary Guidelines for Americans* published by the U.S. Department of Agriculture. Vegetarian options are available. However, no other food is permitted during the first stage of the program, which can make eating away from home

difficult. The pre-packaged meals are intended to model healthy eating and portion control. A personalized exercise program supplemented by optional workout videos and workout equipment encourage the dieter to become more active.

Once dieters have used the pre-packaged meals to become familiar with healthy foods and correct portion sizes, they move to the second stage of the program in which written material supported by consultants teach techniques for healthy meal planning, cooking, and eating out. This stage of the program is designed to develop lifelong habits of moderation and good food choices. The consultant also addresses behavioral issues such as handling stress and emotional triggers for eating.

The final stage of the Jenny Craig program is a maintenance stage. Dieters move into this stage when their weight-loss goal is met. This final stage is designed to keep weight off for life.

Dieters can join the Jenny Craig program in one of two ways. Jenny Craig Weight Loss Centers are physical locations that the dieter visits weekly for individual consultations with a Jenny Craig counselor. Unlike some other center-based weight-loss programs (e.g., **Weight Watchers**), Jenny Craig centers do not offer group meetings. The philosophy behind the Jenny Craig program is one-on-one weight loss help.

Dieters who live too far from a Jenny Craig center or who do not wish to attend one can join Jenny Direct. This is a complete at-home weight-loss program. In the Jenny Direct program, pre-packaged meals and weight-loss literature are delivered to the dieter's home. The dieter is supported by online tools accessed through the Jenny Craig website and a required private 15-minute telephone consultation with a Jenny Craig consultant once a week. Consultants do not have formal training in nutrition.

To join either Jenny Craig program, one must first talk to a consultant by telephone. Several different levels of Jenny Craig membership provide different benefits. Jenny Craig advertises heavily and often has special membership discounts. All programs require that the dieter buy Jenny Craig food.

The Jenny TuneUp is targeted at people who have fewer than 20 lb. (10 kg) to lose. It is an entry-level program with a lower enrollment fee. JennyOnTrack is a six-month program, and Jenny Rewards is a long-term program. Jenny Craig does not reveal the enrollment costs of the OnTrack and Rewards programs on its website, but they amount to several hundred dollars plus the cost of food. Lifetime memberships are available, as are programs for 13–17-year-olds and **breast-feeding** women. All Jenny Craig advertising is geared toward getting the dieter to call a toll-free telephone number for additional information.

Function

The stated goals of the Jenny Craig program are to help dieters:

• develop a healthy relationship with food

• live an active lifestyle

• achieve a balanced approach to living

Dieters are supported in reaching these goals by a 24-hour, 7-day-a-week customer care telephone line, personalized meals and activity plans, one-on-one consultant support, online e-tools, and weight-loss manuals. By achieving these goals, dieters learn to eat healthy foods in appropriate portions, incorporate exercise into their daily routine, and nurture their mental and physical well-being.

Benefits

Jenny Craig promises dieters that if they follow her program, they will lose 1–2 pounds or 1% of their body weight weekly. Once the weight-loss goal is met, a maintenance program is designed to solidify lifestyle changes and keep the weight off. Jenny Craig does not make any claims about the percentage of people who successfully kept weight off for an extended period.

The Jenny Craig program appeals to dieters who want low-calorie meals without having to weigh and measure their food or dieters who do not want to attend group weight-loss programs. They may also be a good solution for single people who do not want to cook; however, dieters with families may find that the pre-packaged approach is less convenient if they still have to cook for family members.

• Are their other diet programs that would better meet my goals?

• Do I have any special dietary needs that this diet might not meet?

• At what level of intensity is it appropriate for me to begin exercising?

• Do you have any experience with the long-term success of this diet?

• If one of your family members wanted to go on a diet, would you recommend this one?

Precautions

Jenny Craig is a diet and exercise program that meets the basic nutritional needs of most people. As with all diet and exercise programs, individuals should check with their healthcare provider to make sure the program is suitable for them.

Risks

Meals on the Jenny Craig plan fall within the federal *Dietary Guidelines for Americans*, and **dietary supplements** provided with the pre-packaged meals ensure that the dieter is getting an adequate supply of **vitamins** and **minerals**. The greatest risk to this diet program is that people do not learn how to shop and prepare healthy meals on their own. They lose weight eating the pre-packaged meals, but when they transition to the next stage of the diet, they go back to their old eating habits and gain the weight back. This type of **weight cycling** or yo-yo dieting can cause potential health problems.

Research and general acceptance

The main client complaint about the Jenny Craig program is cost. Prepackaged food can cost around $500 per month in addition to steep enrollment fees and optional extras such as exercise videos and equipment. Some clients complain that the Jenny Craig personal consultants do not have any formal training in nutrition and are more like sales people than counselors. Clients also criticize the taste and selection of meals. There is no way try Jenny Craig meals before committing to the program.

Generally, registered dietitians agree that the dietitian-planned pre-packaged meals provide adequate nutrition for a low-calorie diet, but question whether clients will become bored with pre-packaged foods. They praise the level of support the program offers through their online site and telephone contacts, but question whether the program prepares dieters to go back to preparing regular food once the first stage of the program is completed.

The Jenny Craig website offers many testimonials and inspiring success stories but is thin on results from independently conducted research studies. One preliminary study that looked at weight loss, triglyceride levels (an indication of the amount of fats in the blood) and carotenoid levels (an indication of vegetable intake) was paid for by Jenny Craig and performed by a former Jenny Craig advisory board member.

Resources

BOOKS

Craig, Jenny. *The Jenny Craig Story: How One Woman Changes Millions of Lives.* Hoboken, NJ: John Wiley & Sons, 2004.

———. *Jenny Craig's Simple Pleasures: Recipes to Nourish Body and Soul.* Birmingham, AL: Oxmoor House, 1998.

———. *Jenny Craig Diabetes Cookbook: Easy Homestyle Recipes for Healthy Living.* Birmingham, AL: Oxmoor House, 1997.

WEBSITES

"Jenny Craig Diet." U.S. News & World Report: Health. http://health.usnews.com/best-diet/jenny-craig-diet (accessed October 3, 2012).

Jenny Craig official website. http://www.jennycraig.com (accessed October 3, 2012).

"Jenny Craig: What It Is." WebMD.com. http://www.webmd.com/diet/jenny-craig-what-it-is (accessed October 3, 2012).

U.S. Department of Agriculture and U.S. Department of Health and Human Services. *Dietary Guidelines for Americans, 2010.* 7th ed. Washington, DC: U.S. Government Printing Office, December 2010. http://health.gov/dietaryguidelines (accessed September 27, 2012).

Tish Davidson, A.M.

▌Jillian Michaels diet

Definition

The Jillian Michaels diet focuses on self, science, and sweat to help dieters achieve weight loss, toning, and increased health and fitness.

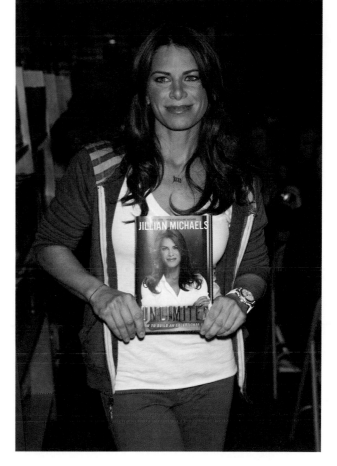

Fitness trainer Jillian Michaels. *(DFree/Shutterstock.com)*

Origins

Jillian Michaels is best known as one of the stars of the popular television program *The Biggest Loser*. *The Biggest Loser* airs on NBC, and pits two teams of significantly overweight individuals against each other to see who can lose the most weight. Jillian Michaels is a strength trainer and life coach for one of the teams of contestants. The strategies that she uses on the show to help her contestants lose weight are some of the techniques that inspired her diet and exercise program.

In addition to being a television personality, Jillian Michaels is also the co-owner of the Sky Sport and Spa fitness club in Beverly Hills, California. She is certified by two programs that certify personal trainers, the National Exercise and Sports Trainers Association and the American Fitness Association of America. She has been doing martial arts since the age of 14 and is experienced in Muay Thai and Akarui-Do, two forms of martial arts. She has achieved the status of black belt in Akarui-Do.

Michaels believes that she brings a special understanding to people struggling with their weight because she has not always been fit herself. She has said that at one time she was 50 pounds overweight. She used her own experiences becoming fit and healthy to design a program that would help other people reach their weight and fitness goals.

Description

Jillian Michaels's diet begins with a very basic premise: for weight loss to occur, **calories** going out have to be greater than calories coming in. Calories out include all calories lost through basic day-to-day activities and the calories burned providing energy to the body's cells during the day. This baseline caloric use is added to the number of calories that are burned during exercise. Calories in include all calories from any food and drink consumed during the day. To lose weight the calories out need to be greater than the calories coming in. This way fat will be broken down to provide the additional calories needed by the body.

The diet can be customized to allow a dieter to determine how many calories should be consumed each day based on how many calories are being expended during the day generally, how many are being used through exercise, and what a person's specific weight-loss goals are. A pound of fat is comprised of about 3,500 calories. That means that to lose a pound each week a dieter would have to use up 3,500 more calories than are taken in that week. Spread evenly throughout the week, this means that each day 500 more calories should be used than are taken in. So if a dieter calculates that he or she is using 2,000 calories a day, that person should consume 1,500 each day to lose one pound per week.

Jillian Michaels breaks her diet down into three parts: self, science, and sweat. Each of these parts comprises one of the parts she feels is important for successful, long-term weight loss and better health. Her diet provides information, recommendations, and opportunities for the dieter to customize their program in each of these areas.

By "self" Michaels means all of the psychological and emotional issues and problems associated with eating, bad habits, and being overweight. She shares many of her own insights that she gained from when she was overweight, and ways that she managed to overcome her own problems.

Michaels focuses largely on ways to change problem behaviors. Problem behaviors include any kind of eating behaviors that stem from reasons other than hunger or necessary nutrition. These include eating when a person feels stressed or upset instead of when they are hungry. Michaels believes that it is important to identify and change these problem behaviors, because these are often the reasons that people have difficulty controlling their calorie intake. She provides suggestions for ways to change these behaviors and offers alternative ways to deal with the underlying issues, such as stress. She also deals with issues like the emotional aspects of being overweight. Throughout all of her diet and exercise programs she provides inspiration to help dieters overcome any setbacks and find the inner force to keep going and meet their goals.

The science portion refers to information about basic nutrition and how the body uses food and calories. Michaels believes that the reason many diets do not work for most people is that they are general and are not designed to meet the individual needs of a dieter. To this end, she believes that there are three different ways that people metabolize food, and that a diet cannot be successful unless it is specifically designed for a dieter's metabolic type. The three types she identifies are fast oxidizers, slow oxidizers, and balanced oxidizers.

Michaels believes that dieters with different metabolic types need different combinations of **fats**, **protein**, and carbohydrates to make their meals the most efficient. Fast oxidizers change the **carbohydrates** in their food to energy very quickly, and thus tend to have spikes of blood sugar right after meals. Because of this, Michaels says that people who are fast oxidizers should eat meals that have higher levels of protein and fats, which are converted to energy more slowly, and lower amounts of carbohydrates, so that the energy levels are more stable during the periods after and between meals.

Slow oxidizers are the opposite of fast oxidizers, and they have metabolisms that break down carbohydrates into energy very slowly. Michaels suggests that slow oxidizers should eat meals that contain large percentages of carbohydrates and lower amounts of fats and proteins. Balanced oxidizers should eat balanced amounts of all three (fats, proteins, and carbohydrates). This is because their **metabolism** converts food neither very quickly nor very slowly. Michaels provides a detailed quiz to determine what kind of metabolizer a dieter is so that menus can be customized effectively.

The sweat part refers to exercise. Michaels believes that not only is exercise the most effective way to increase the number of calories going out, but that in addition to the calories used during the actual exercise, the average number of calories burnt during regular daily activities increases as overall fitness and muscle mass increases.

Michaels believes in a balanced combination of cardiovascular exercises and strength training. She suggests exercising for 60 minutes a day, with five minutes at the beginning and the end being used for stretching, warm up and cool down, and 50 minutes being used for the rigorous exercise. She provides many different exercises and routines that can be customized for the fitness level of the dieter. She also provides information about how muscles work, what the main muscle groups are, and which exercises are best for training which areas of the body. Her exercises and routines draw from many different areas of fitness such as Pilates, yoga, kickboxing, weight lifting, and traditional aerobics. Her exercises are designed to be done at home, and she says that there is no need to join a gym.

Function

Jillian Michaels's diet and exercise program is intended to allow people to lose weight, become more fit, and achieve better overall health and well-being. She also intends it to give people the ability to feel better and more empowered in their daily lives as they take control of their weight, appearance, and health.

Benefits

There are many benefits to losing weight and being fit. The benefits of weight loss can be very significant, and are even greater for people who are the most obese. People who are obese are at higher risk of diabetes, heart disease, and many other diseases and disorders. The risk and severity of these disorders is generally greater the more obese a person is. Weight loss, if achieved at a moderate pace through a healthy diet and regular exercise, can reduce the risk of these and many other obesity-related diseases. Increased exercise can also reduce the risk of cardiovascular and other diseases.

Precautions

Anyone thinking of beginning a new diet and exercise regimen should consult a medical practitioner. Requirements of calories, fat, and nutrients can differ significantly from person to person, depending on gender, age, weight, and many other factors such as the presence of any diseases or conditions. Pregnant or **breastfeeding** women should be especially cautious because deficiencies of **vitamins** or **minerals** can have a significant negative impact on a baby. Exercising too strenuously can cause injury, and exercise should be

---

KEY TERMS

Dietary supplement—A product, such as a vitamin, mineral, herb, amino acid, or enzyme, that is intended to be consumed in addition to an individual's diet with the expectation that it will improve health.

Mineral—An inorganic substance found in the earth that is necessary in small quantities for the body to maintain health. Examples: zinc, copper, iron.

Obese—More than 20% over an individual's ideal weight for height and age or having a body mass index (BMI) of 30 or greater.

Vitamin—A nutrient that the body needs in small amounts to remain healthy but that the body cannot manufacture for itself and must acquire through diet.

---

started gradually until the dieter knows what level of intensity is appropriate. It is important to remember that the contestants on *The Biggest Loser* work out for several hours a day and adhere to very strict diets, so although they usually lose a lot of weight in a relatively short amount of time, this will not necessarily be the result for all dieters. Contestants on the show are closely monitored by physicians and other professionals and their diet and exercise plans are specifically tailored to their dietary needs and levels of fitness.

Risks

With any diet or exercise plan there are some risks. It is often difficult to get enough of some vitamins and minerals when eating a limited diet. Anyone beginning a diet may want to consult their physician about whether taking a vitamin or supplement might help them reduce this risk. Injuries can occur during exercise, such as strained or sprained muscles, and proper warm-up and cool-down procedures should be followed to minimize these risks. It is often best to begin with light or moderate exercise and increase the intensity slowly over weeks or months to minimize the risk of serious injury that could occur if strenuous exercise is begun suddenly and the body is not sufficiently prepared.

Research and general acceptance

Jillian Michaels's diet has not been the subject of any significant scholarly research. It is the diet followed by many of the contestants on NBC's *The Biggest Loser*. Sometimes contestants have problems with obesity-related diseases and conditions when they begin the show, such as diabetes, sleep apnea, and high cholesterol levels. By the end of the show, when

---

large amounts of weight have been lost and better fitness has been achieved, some contestants either no longer suffer from these conditions or have reduced symptoms, and some are even able to discontinue many of their medications. These results do not necessarily represent what is likely to occur for a person following the more general form of the diet on their own at home. These results also do not necessarily result from this specific diet, but are more likely the result of the weight loss achieved through reduced caloric intake and increased exercise. There is also no reported scientific evidence to suggest that people can be fast or slow oxidizers; the terms and quiz were created by Jillian Michaels.

Although this diet has not been studied specifically, limiting caloric intake and eating a diet low in fats and carbohydrates and high in vegetable and plant products is generally accepted as a healthy diet for most people. The U.S. Centers for Disease Control and Prevention recommends a minimum of 30 minutes per day of light to moderate exercise for healthy adults. Following Michaels's fitness and exercise program would exceed these minimum recommendation.

Resources

BOOKS

Larsen, Laura, ed. *Diet and Nutrition Sourcebook*. Detroit, MI: Omnigraphics, 2011.

Michaels, Jillian. *Making the Cut: The 30-Day Diet and Fitness Plan For the Strongest, Sexiest You*. New York: Crown, 2007.

————. *Unlimited: A Three-Step Plan for Achieving Your Dreams*. New York: Crown, 2012.

————. *Winning by Losing: Drop the Weight, Change Your Life*. New York: Collins, 2005.

Willis, Alicia P., ed. *Diet Therapy Research Trends*. New York: Nova Science, 2007.

WEBSITES

"Jillian Michaels' Diet." EveryDiet.org. http://www.everydiet.org/diet/jillian-michaels-diet (accessed October 3, 2012).

Jillian Michaels official website. http://www.jillianmichaels.com (accessed October 3, 2012).

Helen Davidson

Juice fasts

Definition

Juice fasts, sometimes called juice therapy, are short-term dietary practices—typically one to three days in length—during which a person voluntarily consumes only fruit, vegetable, or other plant juices; their extracts; or fruit teas.

Origins

Juice fasts can be traced back over 5,500 years to an annual ritual of bodily detoxification and spiritual preparation known as *pancha karma*, which is part of the practice of Ayurvedic medicine in India. Ayurveda is a traditional system of health care that dates back to about 3500 BCE, and its name is Sanskrit for "science of long life." *Pancha karma* is undergone for disease prevention, which in Ayurvedic practice requires spiritual renewal and the breaking of negative emotional patterns as well as physical purification. It has three phases: a preparation phase, in which the person eliminates sweets, caffeinated drinks, and processed foods from the diet and spends more time meditating and taking walks in natural surroundings; the cleansing phase, which includes bloodletting, emesis (forced vomiting), nasal cleansing, and the use of enemas and laxatives as well as a very restricted diet; and a rejuvenation phase, in which solid foods are gradually reintroduced to the diet. It is not unusual for people to experience spiritual and psychological changes during this third phase. In addition to *pancha karma*, contemporary Ayurvedic practice recommends juice fasts for colitis and other ailments of the digestive tract. Ayurvedic medicine is a system that emphasizes the prevention of disease by identifying and treating imbalances within the body rather than making diagnoses of

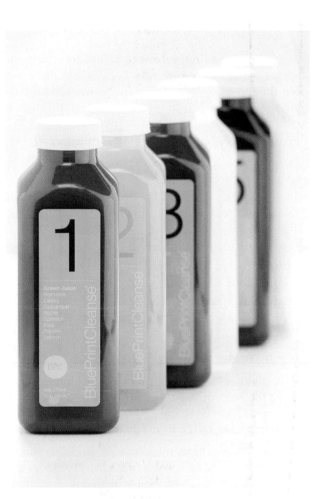

Example of a commercial juice cleanse. (© Istockphoto.com/ Nicole S. Young)

existing illnesses in the usual Western fashion. Juice fasts are therefore regarded as a way of restoring balance within the person's physical constitution rather than as "treatments for illness" in the Western sense.

The second major influence on the popularity of juice fasts in Canada and the United States is naturopathy, which is an approach to health care that developed out of the natural healing movement in Germany and North America in the late nineteenth century. Naturopaths of the twenty-first century use a variety of techniques in treating patients, including hydrotherapy, spinal manipulation, and physical therapy, as well as nutritional and dietary advice. Like Ayurveda, naturopathy emphasizes prevention of disease and recommends noninvasive treatments that rely on the body's own self-healing powers. Juice fasts are an important part of naturopathic dietary therapy.

The third factor that has contributed to interest in juice fasts is that fasting is used in nearly every religion

of the world, including Christianity, Judaism, Buddhism, and Islam. Many of history's great spiritual leaders fasted for mental and spiritual clarity, including Jesus, Buddha, and Mohammed. In one of the famous political acts of the last century, the Indian leader Mahatma Gandhi fasted for 21 days to promote peace.

Description

A juice fast can be done for several reasons: to cleanse the body of heavy metals and other chemical toxins; as a practice related to Ayurvedic medicine; as the first step in the treatment of colitis, arthritis, depression, **cancer**, HIV infection, or other diseases; for weight reduction; as part of a vegetarian, fruitarian, or vegan lifestyle; or as a part of a general program of eliminating other unhealthy habits such as smoking, drinking large amounts of alcohol or caffeinated beverages, and overeating. Some people drink large amounts of freshly extracted fruit or vegetable juices as part of their regular diet without necessarily fasting, a practice known as "juicing."

Many people who undergo juice fasts combine them with massage therapy or the use of laxatives and enemas to completely relax the body and cleanse the digestive tract.

Preparation

Most practitioners of juice fasting recommend restricting it to the warmer months of the year, or traveling to a spa in a warm climate for a wintertime juice fast. Most people undergo juice fasting only once or twice a year; however, some undergo a one-day juice fast every week, or a two-day fast once a month.

Beginning 7 to 10 days before the fast, the person should reduce intake of or eliminate entirely all stimulants (coffee, tea, cocoa, and cola drinks), alcoholic beverages, animal meats, fish, eggs and dairy products, **sugar**, and wheat. The diet during this preparation period should consist entirely of organic fruits, vegetables, and beans.

Making and consuming the juice

The dieter is instructed to drink between 32 and 64 ounces of juice per day, with 6 glasses of warm filtered water in addition. Some therapists recommend one or more cups of herbal tea each day in addition to the juice and water. The juice should be made in a juicer from fresh organic produce; prepackaged juices should not be used, because they are pasteurized to retard spoilage. The heat required for pasteurization destroys some of the **vitamins** and enzymes in the fruit. If organic fruits and vegetables are unavailable, ordinary supermarket produce may be used, provided it is peeled or washed in a special produce cleaner (available at health food stores) to remove pesticide residue. A combination of fruits and vegetables is recommended rather than fruit or vegetable juice alone. The juice should be consumed within half an hour of processing in the juicer, because the natural enzymes in the fruits or vegetables begin to break down the other nutrients in the juice after that time. It should not be refrigerated.

There are a number of recipe books for combining fruit and vegetable juices to make the fast as tasty as possible. Fruits and vegetables that are commonly recommended in these books for juicing include:

- Greens: parsley, beet greens, kale, chard, celery, spinach, dandelion greens
- Cruciferous vegetables: broccoli, cabbage, Brussels sprouts
- Root vegetables: carrots, beets, sweet potatoes
- Fruits: grapes, apples, watermelon, pineapple, cranberries, strawberries, peaches, some citrus fruits
- Herbs: fennel, yucca, spearmint, peppermint, basil, ginger, garlic
- Wheatgrass and bean sprouts
- Aloe vera gel: sometimes taken orally as part of a juice fast for treatment of arthritis

Bowel care

An important part of juice fasting is the use of laxatives or enemas to cleanse the lower digestive tract, because the juice will not supply enough **fiber** to keep the bowels moving. Since many practitioners believe that juice fasts are necessary to detoxify the body, the removal of wastes is considered essential to prevent the toxins in the digestive tract from being reabsorbed into the bloodstream. Some juice therapists recommend mixtures of slippery elm or other herbs to cleanse the colon; others prefer saltwater laxatives, enemas, or colonics for cleansing the bowel. A colonic is a procedure in which a large amount of water, sometimes as much as 20 gallons, is infused into the colon through the rectum a few pints at a time. It differs from an enema in that much more fluid is used, and a colonic is infused into the colon, whereas an enema infuses water or a cleansing solution into the rectum only. Mainstream physicians do not recommend colonics, on the grounds that they are unnecessary, based on a nineteenth-century misunderstanding of the process of digestion, and very often uncomfortable for the patient. In some cases, they pose serious risks to health.

Breaking the fast

People should not return to solid foods immediately at the end of a juice fast, because the intestines need time to readjust to grains and other solid foods. One sequence of breaking the juice fast through a gradual return to a full diet is as follows:

- Day 1: Two pieces of fruit, each divided in half.
- Day 2: Steamed non-starchy vegetables, such as spinach or zucchini.
- Day 3: Green salads and brown rice. Rice and other solid foods should be thoroughly chewed to assist digestion.
- Day 4: Organic yogurt and eggs.
- Day 5: Chicken, fish, red meat (if a normal part of the diet), or tofu.
- Day 6: Beans and grains other than rice.
- Day 7: All other foods.

Function

As has been mentioned, people may undergo juice fasting for one or more of the following reasons:

Spiritual or religious practice

Some people find a juice fast to be useful as part of a general religious or spiritual retreat. The first stage of an Ayurvedic *pancha karma* includes extra time given to meditation and nature walks as well as gradual exclusion of stimulants and solid foods from the diet. Those who undertake a juice fast in order to wean themselves from smoking, drugs, or a food addiction are also often looking for spiritual as well as physical release from the habit they are struggling to break. Many people report relief from emotional stress as a side benefit of juice fasting.

Weight loss

Many people turn to juice fasts for quick weight loss. However, during a juice fast, if a person drinks an abundance of **calories** from the fruit and vegetable juices, they will not lose weight. Most experts recommend a combination of reducing calories, choosing healthy and nutritious foods, and engaging in regular physical activity as the best method of weight loss.

Detoxification

Naturopaths frequently recommend juice fasting as a way of ridding the body of various toxins, which they identify as coming from several sources:

- Heavy metals. These include such substances as cadmium, arsenic, nickel, aluminum, chromium, mercury, vanadium, strontium, antimony, cobalt, and lead, which are used in various manufacturing processes and some medical procedures and are also present in batteries, electronic equipment, coins, cookware, food containers, and other common household items.

- Toxic chemicals taken directly into the digestive tract, through alcoholic beverages, pesticide residues on supermarket produce, additives in processed foods, or drugs of abuse, or chemicals taken into the respiratory tract through breathing household solvents (nail polish remover, spot or stain removers containing benzene, etc.).

- Toxins in the digestive tract produced by yeast and other microorganisms. Ridding the body of this group of toxins is frequently cited as a reason for combining laxatives or enemas with a juice fast. Again, it should be noted that mainstream physicians dispute the notion that normal digestion produces toxic substances in the colon that must be removed by a laxative or enema.

- Ammonia, urea, and other breakdown products of protein metabolism. Naturopaths often recommend a vegetarian lifestyle as well as periodic juice fasts in order to minimize the production of these byproducts of meat and dairy product consumption.

Treatment of specific illnesses

Juice fasting is sometimes recommended by non-medical professionals for the treatment of specific diseases and disorders, most commonly arthritis, autoimmune disorders, and depression, but it has also been claimed to be an effective treatment for severe infections (including AIDS), multiple sclerosis, and cancer. One theory that is sometimes advanced to explain the healing power of juice fasting is that the energy that the body would normally use digesting heavy or high-protein meals is instead directed to its natural self-healing capacity. The medical profession *does not* recommend juice fasting as a means of disease treatment, especially for such chronic conditions.

Benefits

The benefits of juice fasting may include immediate weight loss in some people. Mainstream medical research also indicates that juice fasts are useful in providing a period of rest for the digestive tract for patients with **irritable bowel syndrome** or other functional disorders of the intestines. Juice fasts have sometimes been helpful in identifying **food allergies**. As solid foods are gradually reintroduced after the fast, some people discover that they have a previously unsuspected allergy to one or more foods. Some people also feel that they broke free of their **cravings** for certain foods during the period of abstinence from those foods. Enlightenment through fasts is sometimes claimed to occur for those who fast for spiritual reasons.

Precautions

In general, anyone considering a juice fast should consult a health professional beforehand. Some groups of people, however, should not undertake a juice fast:

- pregnant or lactating women

- children

- people with diabetes, hypoglycemia, anorexia or bulimia nervosa, kidney or liver disease, gout, asthma, impaired immune function, epilepsy, cancer, terminal illness, active infections, AIDS, anemia, malnutrition, or ulcerative colitis

- people who are underweight

- people who have increased energy needs, such as those who have recently undergone surgery or treatment for severe burns

People taking prescription medications should consult their primary care physician before a juice fast, as the bioavailability of some drugs is affected by fasting. In addition, grapefruit, apple, orange, pomegranate, and other juices should *not* be used for a juice fast because the juices of these fruits may increase the blood levels of prescription medications in the body.

Juice fasts should not be extended beyond three or four days without medical supervision, as longer fasts can lead to poor intake of nutrients such as **protein** and **calcium** and could lead to deficiencies or toxic levels of some vitamins/minerals. In addition, anyone who feels faint or dizzy, develops an abnormal heart rhythm, feels nauseated or vomits, or has signs of low blood pressure, should discontinue the fast and consult their doctor at once.

On the economic side, juice fasting is a potentially expensive form of dietary therapy. Readers interested in juice fasts at home or in juicing as a dietary addition should be prepared to pay between $60 and $200 for a juicer or juice extractor—although some deluxe models are marketed for as much as $2,000. The chief difference is that juice extractors remove the fruit or vegetable pulp from the juice (and are difficult to clean), while juicers generally leave the pulp in the juice. In addition to the cost of the machine and the fruits or vegetables

KEY TERMS

Ayurveda—The traditional system of natural medicine that originated in India around 3500 BCE. Its name is Sanskrit for "science of long life." Juice fasts can be traced back to Ayurvedic practice.

Bioavailability—The rate at which a substance or chemical is absorbed into the body or made available for a specific physiological process. Juice fasting sometimes affects the bioavailability of prescription medications.

Colonic—Sometimes called colonic hydrotherapy, a colonic is a procedure similar to an enema in which the patient's colon is irrigated (washed out) with large amounts of water. Some people undergoing a juice fast have one or more colonics to remove fecal matter remaining in the intestines during their fast; however, this procedure is discouraged by mainstream physicians because of its potential risks to health.

Detoxification diets—A group of diets that are followed in order to purify the body of heavy metals, toxic chemicals, harmful microbes, waste products of digestion, and other substances thought to be harmful. Juice fasts are one type of detoxification diet.

Diverticulitis—Inflammation of small pouches (diverticula) that can form in the weakened muscular wall of the large intestine.

Fruitarian—A vegetarian who eats only plant-based products, such as fruits, seeds, and nuts, that can be obtained without killing the plant. Many fruitarians make occasional use of juice fasts.

Naturopathy—A system of disease treatment that emphasizes natural means of health care, such as natural foods, dietary adjustments, massage and manipulation, and electrotherapy, rather than conventional drugs and surgery. Naturopaths (practitioners of naturopathy) often recommend juice fasts as a way of cleansing the body.

Pancha karma—An intensive one- to two-week ritual of detoxification practiced in Ayurvedic medicine that includes enemas, bloodletting, and nasal irrigation as well as fasting.

Pasteurization—A process for partial sterilization of milk or juice by raising the liquid to a temperature that destroys disease organisms without changing the basic taste or appearance. Pasteurized fruit or vegetable juices are considered unsuitable for juice fasts on the grounds that pasteurization destroys important nutrients in the juices.

Spa—A hotel or resort for relaxation or health- and fitness-related activities. Some people undergoing a juice fast do so at a spa in order to combine the fast with colonics, massage therapy, or other practices associated with juice fasts. The English word *spa* comes from the name of a famous health resort in Belgium.

Vegan—A vegetarian who excludes all animal products from the diet, including those that can be obtained without killing the animal. Vegans are also known as strict vegetarians. Some vegans practice juice fasting.

to be juiced, people on a juice fast will usually need to purchase laxatives or enemas for cleansing the bowel.

Risks

For a child, undergoing a juice fast for longer than 1–3 days can result in negative health consequences and even death. An infant should never be placed on a fast of any type for any length of time.

The major risks to health from juice fasts include metabolic crises in patients with undiagnosed diabetes or hypoglycemia; dizziness or fainting due to sudden lowering of blood pressure; diarrhea, which may result in **dehydration** and an imbalance of **electrolytes** in the body; and protein or calcium deficiencies, which may occur from unsupervised long-term juice fasts.

Minor side effects include headaches, fatigue, **constipation**, acne, bad breath, and increased body odor.

Juice fasters who undergo colonics are at risk of contracting an infection from improperly sterilized colonic equipment; of serious illness or death from electrolyte imbalances in the blood; or of serious illness or death resulting from perforation of the intestinal wall by improperly inserted equipment. Colonics can also worsen the symptoms of ulcerative colitis.

Research and general acceptance

Many diseases, such as high blood pressure, cardiovascular disease, and type 2 diabetes, may be prevented with a diet high in fruits and vegetables and decreased consumption of red meats, processed meats, and saturated **fats**. During a juice fast, research shows that a person may lend protection to their cardiovascular system by increasing the intake of rich antioxidant fruits and vegetables by increasing total antioxidant status and by decreasing lipid per-oxidation, thus decreasing overall cardiovascular risk, but the benefit is short-term if consumption of the fruits and vegetables decreases. **Liquid diets** are often recommended to people with diverticulitis during flare ups.

Juice fasts as a specific dietary practice to treat medical disorders have not received much attention from mainstream medical practitioners or researchers; however, they have received some evaluation within clinical studies of Ayurveda and naturopathy as alternative medical systems. Part of the difficulty is that Ayurveda and naturopathy do not lend themselves easily to the scientific method used in medical research.

There have been two studies conducted in Germany in 2005 and 2006 that have reported on the benefits of juice fasting in general lifestyle adjustment and in treating functional bowel disorders. In the United States, the National Center for Complementary and Alternative Medicine (NCCAM) has carried out clinical trials of two specific plants that are often used in juice fasts, aloe vera (*Aloe barbadensis*) and cranberry (*Vaccinium macrocarpon*). Cranberry juice is still being studied for its possible usefulness in preventing urinary tract infections in women. With regard to aloe vera, NCCAM warns that the gel from the plant has a laxative effect that causes cramps and diarrhea in some people, and may inhibit the absorption of prescription drugs.

Juice fasts as a treatment for AIDS and other severe diseases, however, have come under severe criticism from mainstream physicians. Physician Stephen Barrett summarizes his critique of juicing by saying, "The enzymes in plants help regulate the metabolic function of plants. When ingested, they do not act as enzymes within the human body, because they are digested rather than absorbed intact into the body.... Sensible eating, which is not difficult to do, furnishes an adequate nutrient supply.... Since the fiber in fruits and vegetables is an important part of a balanced diet, there is no reason to remove it while making juice. There's nothing wrong with including extracted juices in a diet that is adequate in fiber. But promoting them as alternatives to whole foods or as powerful healing agents is irresponsible."

QUESTIONS TO ASK YOUR DOCTOR

- What are the potential health risks of a juice fast, if any, for me as an individual?
- What are the potential benefits, if any, for a person of my age, gender, and lifestyle in taking a periodic juice fast?
- Will juice fasting help my digestive disorder when it flares up?
- Will any fruit or vegetable juices interact with the medications that I am currently taking?
- I would like to do a juice fast, but can I do this safely while controlling my chronic disease(s)?
- Are there any specific types of juice that you would or would not recommend, and why?
- I want to fast to gain control over my attitude toward eating. Would it be safe for me to lose a few pounds by fasting and would any of my medication dosages need to change?

Resources

BOOKS

Cabot, Sandra. *The Juice Fasting Bible*. Ulysses Press, 2007.

Canole, Drew. *Juicing Recipies for Vitality and Health*. FitLife TV, 2012.

Estante, Rheba. *Juice Fasting: Reboot Your Body*. Hyperink, 2012.

Meyerowitz, Steve. *Juice Fasting and Detoxification: Use the Healing Power of Fresh Juice to Feel Young and Look Great*. 6th ed. Great Barrington, MA: Sproutman Publications, 1999.

Pelletier, Kenneth R. *The Best Alternative Medicine*. Chapter 7, "Naturopathic Medicine," and Chapter 10, "Ayurvedic Medicine and Yoga." New York: Fireside Books, 2002.

PERIODICALS

"The Juice Craze." *Consumer Reports* 57 (1992): 747–51.

Michalsen, A., et al. "Incorporation of Fasting Therapy in an Integrative Medicine Ward: Evaluation of Outcome, Safety, and Effects on Lifestyle Adherence in a Large Prospective Cohort Study." *Journal of Alternative and Complementary Medicine* 11 (August 2005): 601–607.

Mishra, L., B.B. Singh, and S. Dagenais. "Healthcare and Disease Management in Ayurveda." *Alternative Therapies in Health and Medicine* 7 (March 2001): 44–50.

Potter A.S., et al. "Drinking Carrot Juice Increases Total Antioxidant Status and Decreases Lipid Peroxidation in Adults." *Nutrition Journal* 24, no. 10 (2011): 96.

WEBSITES

Barrett, Stephen. "Juicing." http://www.quackwatch.org/01 QuackeryRelatedTopics/juicing.html (accessed September 23, 2012).

National Center for Complementary and Alternative Medicine (NCCAM). "Herbs at a Glance: Aloe Vera." http://nccam.nih.gov/health/aloevera (accessed September 23, 2012).

———. "Herbs at a Glance: Cranberry." http://nccam.nih.gov/health/cranberry (accessed September 23, 2012).

Newman, Judith. "The Juice Cleanse: A Strange and Green Journey." *New York Times*, October 27, 2010. http://www.nytimes.com/2010/10/28/fashion/28Cleanse.html (accessed September 27, 2012).

"Panchakarma: Purifying the Body." Chopra Center. http://www.chopra.com/namaste/panchakarma (accessed September 27, 2012).

ORGANIZATIONS

American Association of Naturopathic Physicians (AANP), 818 18th St. NW, Ste. 250, Washington, DC 20006, (866) 538-2267, member.services@naturopathic.org, http://www.naturopathic.org.

American Vegan Society (AVS), 56 Dinshah Lane, PO Box 369, Malaga, NJ 08328, (856) 694-2887, http://www.americanvegan.org/index.htm.

National Center for Complementary and Alternative Medicine Clearinghouse, PO Box 7923, Gaithersburg, MD 20898, (888) 644-6226, Fax: (866) 464-3616, info@nccam.nih.gov, http://nccam.nih.gov.

National Institute of Ayurvedic Medicine (NIAM), 584 Milltown Rd., Brewster, NY 10509, (845) 278-8700, http://niam.com.

North American Vegetarian Society (NAVS), PO Box 72, Dolgeville, NY 13329, (518) 568-7970, http://www.navs-online.org.

Rebecca J. Frey, PhD

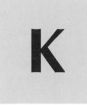

Ketogenic diets

Definition

Ketogenic diets are a group of high-fat, moderate-protein, and very low-carbohydrate diets given to treat some children and adolescents with epilepsy, and some adults with epilepsy and other diseases. The name *ketogenic* refers to the increased production of ketone bodies as a result of this special diet. Ketone bodies are three compounds that are formed during the **metabolism** of **fats** and are ordinarily excreted in the urine. An abnormally high level of ketone bodies is called ketosis, and this condition is the goal of the ketogenic diet. It is thought that ketosis helps to control the frequency and severity of epileptic seizures, even though the reasons for this effect are not fully understood.

Origins

It has been known since Biblical times that some people with epilepsy were helped by prolonged periods of fasting, with good results. In earlier periods of history, children were kept on clear liquids for as long as two or three weeks until their seizures improved. This type of fasting, however, was obviously not sustainable as a long-term treatment. In 1921, a doctor at the Mayo Clinic named R. M. Wilder devised a diet for patients with epilepsy that was intended to mimic the biochemical changes that take place during fasting—ketosis, acidosis, and **dehydration**. Dr. Wilder's ketogenic diet provided 10–15 grams of **carbohydrates** per day, 1 gram of **protein** for each kilogram of the patient's body weight, and the remaining **calories** from fat. The calorie level was 75% of the normal daily allowance for the patient's weight, and fluids were restricted to 80%. Wilder's diet is almost identical to the protocol used at Johns Hopkins.

Until the late 1930s, the Mayo Clinic ketogenic diet was used to treat adults as well as

children with epilepsy. In 1938, however, the first anticonvulsant drug—phenytoin (Dilantin)—was introduced, and was quickly followed by others. After these medications were introduced, people were less interested in the ketogenic diet; many doctors considered it unnecessary or too much trouble. The number of hospitals that used it as therapy fell off sharply, while many practitioners regarded it as a "holistic" or even "alternative" treatment for epilepsy.

Interest in the ketogenic diet was reawakened in the mid-1990s, when the father of a two-year-old with seizures that had not responded to any medications or surgical procedures read about the diet in medical textbooks. He started his son on the ketogenic diet with very good results; the child stopped having seizures and was able to discontinue his medications. The father then established the Charlie Foundation, which continues to provide information and guidance about the ketogenic diet to parents, dietitians, and other health care professionals. Since 1994, the diet has been generally accepted by doctors; it is used in about 40 countries around the world for the treatment of childhood epilepsy. The costs of the diet are reimbursed by most insurance carriers in the United States.

Description

Classic ketogenic diet (Johns Hopkins protocol)

The ketogenic diet used at the Johns Hopkins Pediatric Epilepsy Center is commonly considered the standard or classic form of this diet. Its usual protocol for children between the ages of 3 and 12 provides a ratio of 4 parts fat to 1 part protein and carbohydrate combined. Infants, toddlers, and adolescents are usually started on a 3:1 ratio. Individual patients may require ratios ranging from 2.5:1 to 5:1; these ratios are worked out by fine-tuning the diet once the child has been started on it.

Potential side effects of the Classic Ketogenic Diet
Abnormally high levels of blood lipids after discontinuing the diet
Decreased bone density
Dehydration
Growth retardation caused by protein deficiency
Inflammation of the pancreas
Kidney stones or gallstones
More frequent infections due to a weakened immune system
Nausea, vomiting, or constipation
Protein deficiency, causing growth retardation
Menstrual irregularities
Vitamin and mineral deficiency

(Table by GGS Information Services. © 2013 Cengage Learning.)

PREPARATION. The most important aspect of preparation for the ketogenic diet is deciding whether it will benefit the child. Most doctors prefer not to use it if the child is taking medications that are effective in controlling seizures without producing severe side effects. If, however, the child has tried two or more anticonvulsants without success, or is having serious side effects from the drugs, the ketogenic diet offers a chance to have a more normal life. It helps if the child is not a fussy eater and is willing to try foods that he or she might not ordinarily choose. The child also must be capable of self-control, as eating only a few cookie crumbs or anything else containing **sugar** (including toothpaste and other oral care products) can break the effect of the diet and possibly bring on a seizure.

Another important aspect of preparation is commitment on the part of the entire family. It takes considerable time and care to measure food portions, test the child's urine at home, watch for possible side effects, and keep a balance between the needs of the epileptic child and the food preferences of other family members. Parties and holiday meals may require some advice from a dietitian so that the child can have a treat that will not break the diet and will allow him or her to enjoy the meal or party with other friends or family members.

INITIAL FAST. The classic ketogenic diet begins with placing the child on a 24- to 48-hour fast followed by a stay of several days as a hospital inpatient, so that his or her body fluids can be measured and possible side effects monitored. The reason for the fast is to force the body to exhaust its glucose supply and begin burning stored fat for energy. The foods that are given after the fast are intended to keep the process of fat burning going by providing slightly fewer calories than the body needs and providing 80% of those calories in the form of fat.

Prior to coming to the hospital, the child's food records are kept over a three-day period so that the doctors will know the average daily calorie intake in order to tailor the special diet to the child's growth needs. The goal is to maintain the child's **body mass index** at the 50th percentile. The amount of protein in the diet is based on the child's age, kidney function, and stress factors. While the child is in the hospital, the parents are given a four-day educational program to help them understand the diet and give them practice in preparing meals as well as monitoring the child.

The Johns Hopkins schedule for the child's hospital stay is as follows:

- Sunday (night before admission): Child begins fasting at home in the evening.
- Day 1 (Monday): Child is admitted to the hospital. Fasting continues, fluid intake is restricted, and blood glucose is monitored every 6 hours.
- Day 2 (Tuesday): Child is given "eggnog" for dinner (1/3 of the maintenance calorie allotment for dinner); blood glucose checks are discontinued. The parents are asked to start checking the child's urine ketone levels. Ketone levels should be between 80 and 160 mg/dL when the diet is working properly.
- Day 3 (Wednesday): Breakfast and lunch are given as eggnog (1/3 of the maintenance calorie allotment for those meals); dinner (more eggnog) is increased to 2/3 maintenance level.
- Day 4 (Thursday): Breakfast and lunch are given at 2/3 maintenance level; dinner is the child's first full ketogenic meal (not eggnog).
- Day 5 (Friday): After a full ketogenic breakfast, the child's prescriptions are reviewed, follow-up is arranged, and the child is discharged from the hospital.

Some hospital programs do not require fasting to initiate the child's diet. Follow-ups for most children take place at three-month intervals, although infants may be seen monthly. Children must take multivitamins and mineral supplements (particularly **calcium**) while on the ketogenic diet. Anticonvulsant medications are usually continued for the first few months of the diet, but may be given in lower dosages if the child responds well to the diet, or even discontinued altogether.

SAMPLE MENUS. A typical day's menu for a child on the standard 4:1 ratio diet, allowing 1,500 calories per day, is as follows:

- Breakfast: egg with bacon, made with heavy whipping cream and butter, plus an apple
- Snack: peanut butter mixed with butter
- Lunch: tuna salad made with celery, mayonnaise, and heavy whipping cream, served with lettuce

- Snack: keto yogurt (made with heavy whipping cream, sour cream, strawberries, and artificial sweetener)
- Dinner: cheeseburger with lettuce and green beans
- Snack: keto custard (heavy whipping cream, egg, and pure unsweetened vanilla flavoring)

Resources are available to help parents and dietitians devise menus that will take the individual child's food preferences into account as well as keep the meal selections within the correct nutritional ratio.

TAPERING AND TERMINATION. The ketogenic diet is a long-term diet but is not intended for indefinite use in children. Most children who respond favorably to it remain on it about two years. The diet must not be stopped abruptly, however; most doctors recommend that parents slowly start to add regular foods to the child's menu to see whether the seizures are still controlled.

Sanggye Paik Hospital diet

The Sanggye Paik Hospital diet is a version of the ketogenic diet developed in Korea for the treatment of Asian children, whose diets typically contain much less fat than the diets of Western children. The Sanggye Paik protocol does not require an introductory fast and introduces high-fat foods to the patient's diet gradually, although it uses the same 4:1 ratio of fats to protein and carbohydrates as the Johns Hopkins protocol. It is reported to have the same proportion of successes in patients as the Johns Hopkins ketogenic diet.

Modified Atkins diet

In 2002, the Johns Hopkins treatment center initiated a case series of six children and adults who used a modified version of the **Atkins diet** to control seizures rather than the classic 4:1 ketogenic diet. These patients were not admitted to the hospital; did not have to fast at the beginning of the diet; did not have their calories, protein, or fluid intake restricted; were limited to 10 grams of carbohydrates per day; and were encouraged to eat foods rich in fats. Half the patients showed a marked reduction in seizures.

Based on this initial success, the Johns Hopkins doctors drew up a modified Atkins diet protocol for a group of 20 children, as follows:

- A carbohydrate counting guide is given to the patient's family.
- Carbohydrate intake is limited to 10 g per day for the first month.

- A generous intake of fats in the form of mayonnaise, butter, oils, heavy cream, etc., is encouraged, although precise amounts are not defined.
- Clear carbohydrate-free fluids and calories are unrestricted.
- The patient is given a low-carbohydrate multivitamin and a calcium supplement.
- Ketones in the urine are checked twice a week and weight once a week.
- Low-carbohydrate store-bought products (shakes, snack bars, etc.) are discouraged for at least the first month.
- The patient is given a complete blood test and metabolic workup every three months.

Of the 20 patients, two-thirds had a significant reduction in seizures, 9 were able to reduce medication dosages, and none developed kidney stones.

Function

The function of ketogenic diets is therapeutic—improved control of seizures in children, adolescents, and some adults with epilepsy; treatment of some other rare metabolic disorders; and slowed progression of such other diseases as amyotrophic lateral sclerosis.

Benefits

The benefits of the ketogenic diet are improved seizure control without the need for large doses of anticonvulsant drugs with their associated side effects. Patients who respond well to the diet are able to lead nearly normal lives.

Patients with amyotrophic lateral sclerosis or other disorders being treated experimentally with a ketogenic diet may benefit by having their disease progress at a slower rate even when a cure is not possible.

Precautions

The most important precaution to note is that the ketogenic diet is *not* a do-it-yourself nutritional regimen. It is a serious form of therapy and requires careful medical supervision as well as parental monitoring. Patients on the diet must be followed by an experienced treatment team, usually based in a specialized epilepsy treatment center. Even though the diet may seem like a more "natural" way to control seizures than taking medications, it is based on a highly unnatural selection of foods and forces the body to obtain its necessary energy in an unusual way.

Another important precaution is preventing the child from accidentally ingesting sugar in over-the-counter medications, toothpastes, mouthwashes, or similar products. A list of sugar-free products can be found in PDF format on the Charlie Foundation website.

Risks

Success rate

Not all patients respond to the ketogenic diet. According to the Johns Hopkins treatment center, about half the children who begin the classic ketogenic diet will have at least a 50% reduction in seizures within 6 months. Half of that group will show greater than 90% improvement, with about 15% completely seizure-free. Many families are able to taper or completely eliminate the use of anticonvulsant medications.

As of the early 2000s, there is no way to predict ahead of time whether a child will respond to the diet. It is recommended that the child follow the diet for a period of 2–6 months before deciding that it isn't working. Ineffectiveness is the single most common reason for discontinuing the diet, although some people discontinue it because they cannot tolerate the foods allowed even after fine-tuning, or because of side effects. The Johns Hopkins program reports that about half the children who begin the ketogenic diet in their treatment center are still using it a year later.

Side effects

Because the 4:1 ketogenic diet is an unnatural way to obtain nutrition, it has some potential side effects. Reported adverse effects in patients using the classic ketogenic diet include:

• Growth retardation caused by protein deficiency.
• Vitamin and mineral deficiencies.
• Nausea, vomiting, or constipation.
• Abnormally high levels of blood lipids after discontinuation of the diet.
• Kidney stones or gallstones. Parents are taught to monitor the child's urine for blood as well as ketone levels, because blood in the urine is often an early sign of kidney stone formation.
• More frequent infections due to a weakened immune system.
• Inflammation of the pancreas.
• Dehydration.
• Decreased bone density.
• Menstrual irregularities (in adolescent and adult females).

KEY TERMS

Amyotrophic lateral sclerosis (ALS)—A rare progressive and eventually fatal disease affecting the nerve cells that control movement. It is also known as Lou Gehrig's disease. There is some evidence that the ketogenic diet can slow the progression of ALS.

Anticonvulsant—A drug given to prevent or control seizures.

Double-blind study—A study in which neither the researchers nor the subjects know the identity of the people in the experimental and control groups during the course of the research.

Ketone bodies—A group of three compounds (acetoacetic acid, acetone, and beta-hydroxybutyric acid) that are formed in an intermediate stage of fat metabolism and excreted in the urine. Measuring the level of ketone bodies in the urine of a patient on the ketogenic diet is the primary way of assessing the diet's effectiveness.

Ketosis—An abnormally high level of ketone bodies in the blood or urine, produced when the body begins to burn fat for energy instead of glucose (sugar).

Longitudinal study—A clinical study in which the researchers follow the same group of patients over a period of time. Most studies of the ketogenic diet have been longitudinal studies.

Research and general acceptance

The 4:1 ketogenic diet was the subject of a number of longitudinal studies in the years immediately following Dr. Wilder's initial case report in 1921. Although research lagged in the years after World War II, there has been a significant burst of interest in the diet since the 1990s, with over 200 articles published in the period between 1996 and 2006. As of late 2012, the National Institutes of Health (NIH) was recruiting subjects for two clinical studies of the effectiveness of the modified Atkins diet in the management of epilepsy. The National Institute of Neurological Disorders and Stroke (NINDS) is conducting ongoing research on the biochemical effects of the ketogenic diet; scientists are hoping that they might be able to eventually formulate a medication that will have the same effectiveness as the diet itself without the potential side effects.

Another area of recent research is the use of the ketogenic diet in the treatment of other disorders. It appears to be beneficial in the treatment of patients with glucose transporter defects (genetically transmitted disorders in which glucose in the blood cannot cross the blood-brain barrier) and a few other inborn metabolic disorders. In 2006, a group of researchers at Mount Sinai School of Medicine in New York reported that the diet showed promise in slowing the progression of amyotrophic lateral sclerosis, a progressive and fatal disease of the nerve cells that control movement.

Resources

BOOKS

"Carbohydrate Metabolism Disorders." Chapter 296, Section 19 in the *Merck Manual of Diagnosis and Treatment*, 18th ed. Edited by Mark H. Beers and Robert Berkow. Whitehouse Station, NJ: Merck, 2007.

Freeman, John M., et al. *The Ketogenic Diet: A Treatment for Children and Others with Epilepsy*. 4th ed. New York: Demos, 2007.

"Seizure Disorders." Chapter 214, Section 16 in the *Merck Manual of Diagnosis and Treatment*, 18th ed. Edited by Mark H. Beers and Robert Berkow. Whitehouse Station, NJ: Merck, 2007.

PERIODICALS

Coppola, G., et al. "The Ketogenic Diet in Children, Adolescents and Young Adults with Refractory Epilepsy: An Italian Multicentric Experience." *Epilepsy Research* 48 (February 2002): 221–27.

Freeman, J.M., E.H. Kossoff, and A.L. Hartman. "The Ketogenic Diet: One Decade Later." *Pediatrics* 119 (March 2007): 535–43.

Hartman, A.L., and E.P. Vining. "Clinical Aspects of the Ketogenic Diet." *Epilepsia* 48 (January 2007): 31–42.

Hussain, T.A., et al. "Effect of Low-Calorie Versus Low-Carbohydrate Ketogenic Diet in Type 2 Diabetes." *Nutrition* 28, no. 10 (2012): 1016–21.

Johnston, Carol S., et al. "Ketogenic Low-Carbohydrate Diets Have No Metabolic Advantage over Nonketogenic Low-Carbohydrate Diets." *American Journal of Clinical Nutrition* 83, no. 5 (2006): 1055–61.

Kang, H.C., and H.D. Kim. "Diet Therapy in Refractory Pediatric Epilepsy: Increased Efficacy and Tolerability." *Epileptic Disorders* 8 (December 2006): 309–16.

Kang, H.C., et al. "Use of a Modified Atkins Diet in Intractable Childhood Epilepsy." *Epilepsia* 48 (January 2007): 182–86.

Paoli, A., et al. "Ketogenic Diet Does Not Affect Strength Performance in Elite Artistic Gymnasts." *Journal of the International Society of Sports Nutrition* 9, no. 1 (2012): 34.

Stafstrom, C.E., and J.M. Rho. "The Ketogenic Diet as a Treatment Paradigm for Diverse Neurological Disorders." *Frontiers in Pharmacology* 3 (April 9, 2012): 59.

Turner, Zahava, and Eric H. Kossoff. "The Ketogenic and Atkins Diets: Recipes for Seizure Control." *Practical Gastroenterology* (June 2006): 53–64.

Zhao, Z., et al. "A Ketogenic Diet as a Potential Novel Therapeutic Intervention in Amyotrophic Lateral Sclerosis." *BMC Neuroscience* 7 (April 3, 2006): 29.

WEBSITES

The Charlie Foundation to Help Cure Pediatric Epilepsy. "Ketogenic Diet." http://www.charliefoundation.org/faq/ketogenic-diet.html (accessed October 3, 2012).

Epilepsy Foundation. "Ketogenic Diet." http://www.epilepsyfoundation.org/aboutepilepsy/treatment/ketogenicdiet/index.cfm (accessed October 3, 2012).

National Institute of Neurological Disorders and Stroke (NINDS). "Curing Epilepsy: The Promise of Research." National Institutes of Health. http://www.ninds.nih.gov/disorders/epilepsy/epilepsy_research.htm (accessed October 3, 2012).

ORGANIZATIONS

The Charlie Foundation To Help Cure Pediatric Epilepsy, 515 Ocean Ave. #602N, Santa Monica, CA 90402, (310) 393-2347, ketoman@aol.com, http://www.charliefoundation.org.

Epilepsy Foundation, 8301 Professional Place, Landover, MD 20785-7223, (800) 332-1000, (866) 748-8008 (Spanish), ContactUs@efa.org, http://www.epilepsyfoundation.org.

NIH Neurological Institute, PO Box 5801, Bethesda, MD 20824, (301) 496-5751, TTY: (301) 468-5981, (800) 352-9424, http://www.ninds.nih.gov.

Rebecca J. Frey, PhD

Kidney diet *see* **Renal nutrition**

Kids' diets *see* **Children's diets**

Korean diet *see* **Asian diet**

L

LA Weight Loss program

Definition

The LA Weight Loss program is a diet plan based around weight loss centers. The centers offer counseling, personalized weight-loss planning, and exercise guidelines.

Origins

The LA Weight Loss Centers company was founded by Vahan Karian in 1989. It was founded as a privately held company and remains so today. The company grew very quickly; in 1994 there were 18 LA Weight Loss Centers and by 2006 there were more than 800. It claims to be one of the fastest growing weight-management companies in the world. The company is headquartered in Horsham, Pennsylvania.

Description

LA Weight Loss Centers can be found throughout the United States, and they also have centers in Canada, Australia, Puerto Rico, and Costa Rica. These centers are the basis for the LA Weight Loss program. The centers provide one-on-one counseling and work with dieters to develop personalized meal plans and customized exercise guidelines. Counselors at the centers also provide emotional and motivational support.

The LA Weight Loss program involves helping dieters learn to use regular foods, available at their normal supermarket, to create healthy meals. Dieters have the option of purchasing special LA Weight Loss foods, but the company says this is not a necessary part of the program. Counselors at the LA Weight Loss Centers teach dieters about nutrition and how to eat a balanced diet. Dieters are also taught how to choose healthy nutritious foods, even when eating at their favorite restaurants. Counselors also help to develop an exercise program for each individual dieter.

The first step to the LA Weight Loss plan is an individual meeting with one of the counselors at an LA Weight Loss Center. In that meeting dieters determine their current health status and their weight-loss goals. Together with a counselor, they also then build a plan for attaining those goals. After the initial meeting, dieters can call anytime they need encouragement or want to set up another meeting to review their progress.

In addition to the weight-loss centers, the company offers an online version of their weight-loss plan called "LA at Home." The online version is based on the same principles as the center-based plan. Dieters can receive online counseling that will design a personalized weight-loss plan and provide ongoing support. Online tools are available to help with planning meals, choosing restaurants, and ordering foods, and also allows dieters to track their progress. Dieters who join the online program can also submit their favorite recipes to the "LA Chef" and receive instructions on how to create a healthier version of their favorite foods. Through the website, dieters can also purchase LA Weight Loss food products.

One of the hallmarks of the LA Weight Loss Program has been celebrity endorsements. In television and print commercials, as well as through their website and other promotional materials, celebrities have partnered with the company and promoted its message. The list of celebrities to do this includes actress Whoopi Goldberg, actor Steve Harvey, Philadelphia Eagles Coach Andy Reid, Chicago Bears Coach Mike Ditka, and former NFL greats Ron Jaworski, Jim Kelly, Joe Greene, Ed Jones, and Dan Dierdorf.

Separate from their regular weight-loss plan, LA Weight Loss Centers offer "The Man Plan," which is aimed at men. Marketing materials for the plan feature famous sports figures who say they've lost weight using the plan. It is intended to satisfy a larger appetite, using foods like pizza, hot dogs, and potatoes. Men can use the plan by going into one of the LA Weight Loss Centers or by joining online. Like the regular plan, it uses one-on-one counseling to design a personalized weight-loss strategy and allows dieters to eat at restaurants and prepare meals using foods available at the supermarket.

Legal troubles

LA Weight Loss Centers, Inc. has been involved in several legal disputes. In 2002, New York State Attorney General Eliot Spitzer reached a settlement with the company over allegations that they made false claims about the cost of their weight-loss program, were slow to issue refunds, and had not posted the bond required from health club service providers. The company was ordered to pay a civil penalty of $100,000, issue refunds to New York State customers who did not receive them, post a $275,000 bond, and cease misrepresenting the true cost of the program. In 2005, Washington State Attorney General Rob McKenna reached a settlement with the company over similar allegations. In that case, LA Weight Loss Centers were required to pay up to $800,000 in reimbursements to Washington customers, as well as a separate fine to be used for consumer education. In neither case did the company admit any wrong doing.

Function

LA Weight Loss Centers are intended to provide a source of support and guidance to those who want to lose weight and maintain good health. They are designed to provide one-on-one support for dieters, as well as help dieters design diet and exercise plans tailored to their specific needs and lifestyles.

Benefits

There are many benefits to losing weight, being healthy, and getting fit. The benefits of weight loss can be very significant, as many diseases and disorders, such as diabetes, are associated with being obese. The more overweight a person is, generally the greater their risk is for getting these diseases. Weight loss, if achieved at a moderate pace through a healthy diet and regular exercise, can reduce the risk of these and other obesity-related diseases. Increased exercise can also reduce the risk of cardiovascular diseases and improve overall health.

The LA Weight Loss Center's program may have additional benefits for some people. Because the program is designed around the dieter meeting one-on-one

---

KEY TERMS

Dietary supplement—A product, such as a vitamin, mineral, herb, amino acid, or enzyme, that is intended to be consumed in addition to an individual's diet with the expectation that it will improve health.

Mineral—An inorganic substance found in the earth that is necessary in small quantities for the body to maintain health. Examples: zinc, copper, iron.

Vitamin—A nutrient that the body needs in small amounts to remain healthy but that the body cannot manufacture for itself and must acquire through diet.

---

with counselors, this may help some people stay on track to achieve their desired weight-loss goals. This also means that counselors may be able to help the dieter design diet and exercise plans that center around the dieter's favorite foods or activities, or are designed to be able to fit into the dieter's busy schedule.

Precautions

Anyone thinking of beginning a new diet or exercise program should consult a doctor or other medical practitioner. Requirements of **calories**, fat, and nutrients can differ from person to person, depending on gender, age, weight, and many other factors such as the presence of any diseases or conditions. Pregnant or **breastfeeding** women should be especially cautious because they may need increased amounts of **vitamins** and **minerals**, and deficiencies can be harmful for a baby. Exercising too strenuously or beginning a rigorous exercise program too suddenly can lead to an increased risk of injury. Dieters should be advised that consultants for LA Weight Loss are not required to have certifications in personal fitness or nutrition. This means that dieters may want to consult other sources in addition to their counselors.

Risks

With any diet and exercise plan there are some risks. It can be difficult for a dieter to get enough vitamins and minerals when eating a limited diet. Anyone beginning a diet may want to consult their physician about whether taking a vitamin or supplement might help them reduce this risk. Supplements have their own risks and possibilities of side effects. Following proper warm-up and cool-down procedures can

QUESTIONS TO ASK YOUR DOCTOR

- Is this diet the best diet to meet my goals?
- At what level of intensity is it appropriate for me to begin exercising?
- Does diet or exercise pose any special risk for me that I should be aware of?
- Would a multivitamin or other dietary supplement be appropriate for me if I were to begin this diet?
- Is this diet appropriate for my entire family?
- Is it safe for me to follow this diet over a long period of time?
- Are there any signs or symptoms that might indicate a problem while on this diet?

help to minimize the risk of injury during exercise. It may be recommended that a dieter begin with light or moderate exercise and slowly increase the intensity of the exercise over weeks or months.

Research and general acceptance

There have been no scientific studies of the methods promoted by LA Weight Loss Centers. Their food products have not been proven to help dieters lose weight or live a healthier lifestyle. Because each dieter's diet will be different, it is difficult to say if the LA Weight Loss program will provide what is generally recognized as a healthy, well-balanced diet. The U.S. Department of Agriculture provides food guidelines in its MyPlate, the replacement for the food guide pyramid. Generally, for healthy adults, any diet program that is healthy should follow these guidelines. They can be found online at ChooseMyPlate.gov.

The LA Weight Loss plan is generally expected to include some form of exercise plan. The Centers for Disease Control and Prevention recommends that healthy adults get at least 30 minutes a day of light to moderate exercise. Because each dieter will have a personalized plan, it is not possible to determine if this minimum recommendation will be met. Exercise is a very important part of a healthy lifestyle and has been shown to reduce the risk of cardiovascular disease. Studies have shown that weight loss is achieved more effectively through programs that combine diet and exercise than programs that focus on just one aspect alone.

Resources

BOOKS

Larsen, Laura, ed. *Diet and Nutrition Sourcebook.* Detroit, MI: Omnigraphics, 2011.

Willis, Alicia P., ed. *Diet Therapy Research Trends.* New York: Nova Science, 2007.

PERIODICALS

Tsai, Adam Gilden, and Thomas A. Wadden. "Systematic Review: An Evaluation of Major Commercial Weight Loss Programs in the United States." *Annals of Internal Medicine* 142 (January 4, 2005): 56–66.

WEBSITES

LA Weight Loss official website. http://www.laweightloss.com (accessed October 3, 2012).

Wender, Samantha. "Welcome to LA Weight Loss." *ABC 2020*, February 16, 2007. http://abcnews.go.com/2020/story?id=2877644&page=1#.UGxNGa7bT9Q (accessed October 3, 2012).

Helen Davidson

Lactose intolerance diet

Definition

Lactose intolerance is a condition caused by the inability to digest lactose, a **sugar** found in milk. The lactose intolerance diet is a diet designed to treat the uncomfortable symptoms that can result from undigested lactose.

Origins

No single person originated the lactose intolerance diet. Physicians treating symptoms of lactose intolerance developed diet recommendations through observation and trial and error by their patients.

Description

Lactose is the main sugar in milk. When lactose reaches the small intestine, it is broken down into simpler sugars by the enzyme lactase. These simpler sugars are absorbed into the bloodstream and eventually are used as fuel for the body. Lactase is made in the cells that line the small intestine. In some people, however, these cells do not make enough lactase, and in a few people, they do not make any at all. When the body does not make enough lactase, it cannot properly digest lactose from food. Lactose that is not broken down cannot be absorbed into the blood and instead remains in the large

Calcium and lactose in common foods

Foods	Calcium content (mg)	Lactose content(g)
Soymilk, fortified, 1 cup	200–300	0
Sardines, with edible bones, 3 oz.	270	0
Salmon, canned, with edible bones, 3 oz.	205	0
Broccoli, raw, 1 cup	90	0
Orange, 1 medium	50	0
Pinto beans, ½ cup	40	0
Tuna, canned, 3 oz.	10	0
Lettuce greens, ½ cup	10	0
Dairy products		
Yogurt, plain, low-fat, 1 cup	415	5
Milk, reduced fat, 1 cup	295	11
Swiss cheese, 1 oz.	270	1
Ice cream, ½ cup	85	6
Cottage cheese, ½ cup	75	2–3

SOURCE: National Institute of Diabetes and Digestive and Kidney Diseases, National Institutes of Health, U.S. Department of Health and Human Services

(Table by GGS Information Services. © 2013 Cengage Learning.)

intestine (colon) where bacteria convert it into lactic acid. Lactic acid is a laxative and an irritant to the colon.

Symptoms of lactose intolerance include nausea, bloating, abdominal pain or cramps, abundant gas, and diarrhea. These symptoms usually begin anywhere from 30 minutes to 2 hours after eating a food that contains lactose. Symptoms of lactose intolerance can be uncomfortable and may temporarily interfere with daily activities. However, they do not harm the digestive system, and lactose intolerance does not progress to any other disease or disorder.

Lactose intolerance is an extremely common condition. It rarely develops before age six and is caused by a genetically programmed decline in lactase. This decline begins around age two, the age when most infants have finished the transition from breast milk to solid food. In some people this decline continues to the point where they develop lactose intolerance symptoms, usually by late childhood or early adulthood. Lactose intolerance is strongly linked to race and ethnicity. People of Northern European ancestry have the lowest rate of lactose intolerance, about 5%. In Hispanic, Jewish, and Southern European populations, the rate is about 70%, and it is thought to be 90% or more in Asian and African populations. Worldwide, the inability to digest lactose is much more common than the ability to digest it. Although the symptoms are similar, lactose intolerance is not the same as cow's milk intolerance. Cow's milk intolerance is a food allergy that produces an allergic reaction. Only about 3.4% of Americans have cow's milk intolerance.

The degree to which people are lactose intolerant varies widely. Some people can drink a glass of milk daily without developing unpleasant symptoms. Others can drink only small amounts of milk at a time and have fewer symptoms if milk is mixed with food. Some people can eat cheese, ice cream, or yogurt but cannot drink milk. A few people are 100% lactose intolerant, and even the smallest amount of lactose will produce unpleasant symptoms.

Although the greatest quantities of lactose are found in milk and dairy products, milk is used in the preparation of many processed foods such as chocolate bars, puddings, and soups. Food labels must list all of the ingredients in processed foods. Lactose intolerant individuals should look for words on the label that indicate the presence of lactose, such as milk, condensed milk, whey, curds, milk byproducts, or dry milk solids.

Besides dairy products, lactose is found in other unlikely places such as:

- bread, baked goods, and biscuit, pancake, and cookie mixes
- processed breakfast cereals and breakfast drinks
- instant mashed potatoes
- lunch meats (except kosher meats, which are lactose-free)
- salad dressings
- all chocolate, caramel, and butterscotch candies, as well as many others
- medications—as many as 6% of prescription and over-the-counter drugs contain lactose, used as filler

The amount of lactose found in these hidden sources is not enough to affect most people, but for the severely lactose intolerant, it can be enough to cause symptoms.

Many individuals diagnose themselves as lactose intolerant using an elimination diet. However, people who think they may be lactose intolerant should see their physician. Symptoms of lactose intolerance can be quite similar to other more serious and sometimes progressive diseases such as **celiac disease** (a gluten intolerance), **Crohn's disease**, giardia (a parasitic infection of the bowel), and **inflammatory bowel disease**. Lactose intolerance can be diagnosed by giving an individual lactose and then measuring changes in the sugar (glucose) level in their blood. In lactose intolerant individuals, lactose is not broken down into the sugars that can be absorbed from the intestine. Therefore, the level of glucose in the blood will be lower than expected. Lactose can also be diagnosed by a hydrogen breath test.

Lactose and diet

Lactose intolerance is treated by eliminating lactose from the diet beyond the level where it produces symptoms. Alternately, enzymes such as LACTAID or Dairy Ease can be added to milk 24 hours before drinking. These enzymes pre-digest lactose and can eliminate 70%–99% of lactose from milk and dairy drinks. Lactose-reduced milk is available at many supermarkets—all LACTAID and Dairy Ease milk is 70% lactose-free except for non-fat LACTAID, which contains no lactose. When eating other foods that contain lactose, LACTAID and Dairy Ease capsules are available that can be taken at the same time that an individual begins eating. These capsules contain enzymes to help digest lactose.

Since dairy products are a primary source of **calcium**, people who eliminate milk, cheese, yogurt, and other dairy products must adjust their diet to get enough calcium. Calcium is critical to building and maintaining strong bones and teeth and is needed for metabolic processes such as muscle contraction and nerve impulse transmission.

The U.S. Institute of Medicine (IOM) of the National Academy of Sciences developed recommended dietary allowances (RDA) for calcium based on the average daily amount of the nutrient needed to meet the health needs of 97%–98% of the population. The values were raised in 2010 after concerns that the previous recommendations were too low. The revised RDAs for calcium are:

- infants 0–6 months: 200 mg (adequate intake only; no RDA set)
- children 7–12 months: 260 mg (adequate intake only; no RDA set)
- children 1–3 years: 700 mg
- children 4–8 years: 1,000 mg
- children 9–13 years: 1,300 mg
- adolescents 14–18 years: 1,300 mg
- adult males 19–70 years: 1,000 mg
- adult females 19–50 years: 1,000 mg
- adult females 51–70 years: 1,200 mg
- adults over age 70: 1,200 mg
- pregnant or breastfeeding women 18 years and younger: 1,300 mg
- pregnant or breastfeeding women over age 18: 1,000 mg

Some good sources of calcium that do not contain lactose are:

- sardines with bones, canned in oil, 3 ounces: 270–325 mg

- salmon with bones, canned, 3 ounces: 180–205 mg
- soymilk, 1 cup: 200–300 mg
- orange juice, fortified with calcium, 6 ounces: 200–260 mg
- tofu, firm, made with calcium sulfate added, 1/2 cup: 204 mg
- white beans, cooked, 1/2 cup: 113 mg
- bok choy, cooked, 1/2 cup: 61 mg
- pinto or red beans, cooked, 1/2 cup: 43 mg
- bread, whole wheat, 1 slice: 20 mg

A registered dietitian can help people with lactose intolerance develop meal plans that will meet their dietary needs for calcium. Some people may also benefit from taking a calcium supplement. Calcium supplements are available over-the-counter at pharmacies and supermarkets.

Function

Lactose intolerance cannot be cured. The purpose of the lactose intolerance diet is to help people find alternatives to dairy and relieve symptoms of lactose intolerance so that they do not disrupt daily life.

Benefits

Following a lactose intolerance diet will help control the uncomfortable symptoms of bloating, nausea, stomach cramps, and diarrhea characteristic of lactose intolerance.

Precautions

Lactose intolerance diets are variable. Individuals must work out through trial and error how much and which lactose-containing foods they can eat without experiencing symptoms. It may take a little while for people to figure out what works best for them.

Risks

The greatest risk of lactose intolerance is that an individual will not get enough calcium. With careful planning, however, people with lactose intolerance can obtain enough calcium without consuming dairy products.

QUESTIONS TO ASK YOUR DOCTOR

- Do I have lactose intolerance, or are my symptoms being caused by another gastrointestinal disorder?

- Do you recommend using lactose-reduced milk or enzyme pre-treatment of milk, or is it better to simply eliminate milk from my diet?

- Should I take a calcium supplement? If so, how much and how often?

- Can my children inherit this condition?

Research and general acceptance

The lactose intolerance diet is accepted by medical professionals as a standard treatment for this condition. The diet has existed for many years and is not controversial.

Resources

BOOKS

Fleming, Alisa Marie. *Go Dairy Free: The Guide and Cookbook for Milk Allergies, Lactose Intolerance, and Casein-Free Living.* Henderson, NV: Fleming Ink, 2008.

Kafka, Barbara. *The Intolerant Gourmet: Glorious Food without Gluten and Lactose.* New York: Artisan, 2011.

Rockwell, Sally. *Calcium Rich & Dairy Free: How to Get Calcium Without the Cow.* Pomeroy, WA: Health Research Books, 2005.

Shreffler, Wayne, Qian Yuan, and Karen Asp. *Understanding Your Food Allergies and Intolerances: A Guide to Management and Treatment.* New York: St. Martin's Griffin, 2012.

PERIODICALS

Mattar, R., D.F. de Campos Mazo, and F.J. Carrilho. "Lactose Intolerance: Diagnosis, Genetic, and Clinical Factors." *Clinical and Experimental Gastroenterology* 5 (July 2012): 113–121. http://dx.doi.org/10.2147/CEG.S32368 (accessed August 16, 2012).

OTHER

Committee to Review Dietary Reference Intakes for Vitamin D and Calcium, Institute of Medicine. *Dietary Reference Intakes for Calcium and Vitamin D.* Washington, DC: The National Academies Press, 2011. http://www.iom.edu/Reports/2010/Dietary-Reference-Intakes-for-Calcium-and-Vitamin-D.aspx (accessed August 16, 2012).

WEBSITES

MedlinePlus. "Lactose Intolerance." U. S. National Library of Medicine, National Institutes of Health. http://www.nlm.nih.gov/medlineplus/lactoseintolerance.html (accessed August 16, 2012).

National Digestive Diseases Information Clearinghouse (NDDIC). "What I Need to Know about Lactose Intolerance." National Institute of Diabetes and Digestive and Kidney Diseases, U.S. National Institutes of Health. http://digestive.niddk.nih.gov/ddiseases/pubs/lactoseintolerance_ez/index.aspx (accessed August 16, 2012).

Nemours Foundation. "Lactose Intolerance." Teens Health.org. http://www.teenshealth.org/teen/food_fitness/nutrition/lactose_intolerance.html (accessed August 16, 2012).

Office of Dietary Supplements. "Dietary Supplement Fact Sheet: Calcium." U.S. National Institutes of Health. http://ods.od.nih.gov/factsheets/Calcium-HealthProfessional (accessed August 16, 2012).

ORGANIZATIONS

American Gastroenterological Association, 4930 Del Ray Ave., Bethesda, MD 20814, (301) 654-2055, Fax: (301) 654-5920, member@gastro.org, http://www.gastro.org.

International Foundation for Functional Gastrointestinal Disorders, PO Box 170864, Milwaukee, WI 53217, (414) 964-1799, (888) 964-2001, Fax: (414) 964-7176, iffgd@iffgd.org, http://www.iffgd.org.

National Digestive Diseases Information Clearinghouse, 2 Information Way, Bethesda, MD 20892–3570, (800) 891–5389, TTY: (866) 569–1162, Fax: (703) 738–4929, nddic@info.niddk.nih.gov, http://www.digestive.niddk.nih.gov.

Tish Davidson, AM

Lacto-vegetarianism

Definition

Vegetarian diets exclude animal products and are practiced with differing degrees of restriction. When most people think of a vegetarian diet, they are referring to an ovo-lacto-vegetarian diet, which excludes meat. Vegan diets exclude all animal products, including dairy, honey, and eggs. Lacto-vegetarian diets include dairy but exclude meat and eggs.

Origins

Vegetarianism has been practiced throughout history for a variety of religious, cultural, philosophical, social, and economic reasons. Similarly, people have expressed concerns about animal welfare and the environmental, ethical, and proposed health benefits associated with the consumption of animals and animal-based products. Many individuals over the years have chosen to either exclude or reduce their consumption of animal meats and associated products. Many followers of certain religious faiths have similarly adopted differing degrees of vegetarian-type eating patterns, including Buddhism, Jainism, and Hinduism.

Vegetarian eating patterns date back over hundreds of years. Famous vegetarians include Plato, Socrates, and Pythagoras. In the earlier stages of the vegetarian movement, there was a scarcity of evidence and knowledge to help support people in making the decision to adopt a vegetarian diet. Over the years, however, a wealth of evidence-based research has provided the public with information about how to ensure that dietary intake is balanced despite the exclusion of animal products. Research has also suggested health benefits associated with vegetarianism, such as reduced risk of disease.

Description

As with any pattern of eating, it is difficult to make generalizations about the pros and cons of vegetarianism, as the diet adopted by each individual will vary considerably depending on his or her reasons for adopting vegetarianism and the specific restrictions practiced. Whether or not a vegetarian diet is nutritionally balanced is dependent on the range and amounts of foods selected. As with all diets, care needs to be taken to ensure that enough different foods are selected to provide a nutritionally balanced mix. A varied lacto-vegetarian diet aims to provide all of the essential nutrients that the body requires in suitable amounts to help minimize the risk of vitamin or mineral deficiencies.

In 2011, the U.S. Department of Agriculture released a new form of its dietary recommendations—MyPlate—which replaced the food pyramid. **MyPlate** recommendations are illustrated in the form of a dinner plate separated into four sections: fruits, vegetables, grains, and **protein**, with a side dish for dairy. The MyPlate recommendations can be adapted to reflect the dietary needs of lacto-vegetarians. Ensuring that substitute foods of similar nutritional value to meat and eggs are introduced will help achieve an adequate protein intake.

Grains

The grains section contains starchy **carbohydrates** and is relatively similar for both meat eaters and lacto-vegetarians. Foods include bread, cereals, rice, potatoes, yams, oats, corn, rye, millet, barley, quinoa, buckwheat, and cous cous. Egg-free pasta is available as a noodle or pasta substitute. Quinoa is a particularly good grain for lacto- and other types of vegetarians, because it is one of the few plant-based complete proteins. Complete proteins provide the body with all of the essential amino acids that it needs and are usually meat products.

Grains are usually low in fat and are good sources of energy, and **whole grains** are typically high in **fiber**. Fiber helps people feel full quickly and for longer, reducing the risk of snacking throughout the day. Fiber-containing foods also help to regulate bowel movements and reduce the risk of **constipation**. For optimum benefits, food from this food group should be included at each mealtime.

Fruits and vegetables

Fruits and vegetables are important to vegetarian diets. These foods provide essential **vitamins** and minerals—including vitamins A and C, **folate**, and fiber—that can help reduce the risk of **cancer**, stroke, and heart disease and contribute to the maintenance of general good health. The worldwide recommendations for fruit and vegetables vary somewhat, but most sources encourage a minimum of five portions of fruit and vegetables per day.

Protein

Foods in the protein section that are appropriate for lacto-vegetarian diets include pulses, lentils, vegetarian cheese, nuts, textured vegetable protein, meat substitutes, seeds, **soy**, and peas (including chickpeas). Protein is a very important nutrient because it makes up part of the structure of every cell in the body. There is a constant turnover of cells in the body, so an adequate supply of protein is essential for good health. Protein foods should not be the main source of fuel for the body; this should come from starchy carbohydrates. Someone consuming large intakes of protein and only small amounts of starchy carbohydrates will end up using protein as their main energy source, which will leave insufficient amounts to meet the daily protein needs of the body. People following a lacto-vegetarian diet should consult with a qualified doctor or registered dietitian if they are concerned about consuming too much protein.

Dairy

Dairy products include milk, cheese, yogurt, fromage frais, and soy products. Even though lacto-vegetarian diets permit dairy products, some lacto-vegetarians may still choose to include some dairy-free options (such as soy-based products) as part of their dietary intake. It is important to note that soy-based products are typically low in **calcium** as compared to dairy foods, and individuals are encouraged to opt for

KEY TERMS

Amino acids—These compounds are the building blocks of protein. Some amino acids can be synthesized by the body but some cannot. The latter are referred to as essential amino acids and therefore must be obtained from protein in the diet.

Anemia—Anemia refers to a reduction in the quantity of the oxygen-carrying pigment hemoglobin in the blood. The main symptoms of anemia are excessive tiredness and fatigue, breathlessness on exertion, pallor, and poor resistance to infection.

Calcium—Calcium is a mineral present in large quantities in the body, mainly in the bones and teeth. A deficiency of calcium in the diet can increase risk of osteoporosis. Rich sources of calcium include milk, cheese, yogurt, and tofu.

Carbohydrates—Carbohydrates are a major source of energy. Carbohydrates in the diet are principally made up of starches, sugars, and dietary fiber.

Fats—Fat is a concentrated source of energy. Foods that are high in fat provide a lot of energy and are good sources of vitamins A, D, E, and K and provide essential fatty acids.

Fiber—Dietary fiber is a non-specific term for that fraction of dietary carbohydrate that cannot be digested in the human small intestine. An adequate intake of dietary fiber is required to maintain bowel function. Some types of fiber can help lower cholesterol.

Minerals—These are elements that are essential for the body's normal function including calcium, iron, phosphorous, magnesium, sodium, chloride, iodine, manganese, copper, and zinc.

Proteins—These are large molecules that are made up of thousands of amino acids. The primary function of protein is growth and repair of body tissues.

Vitamin B_1 (thiamin)—A vitamin that plays an important role in carbohydrate metabolism. A deficiency can lead to a disorder called Beri Beri, which results in widespread nerve degeneration that can damage the brain, spinal cord, and heart. Good sources of this vitamin for lacto-vegetarians include cereals, beans, potatoes, and nuts.

Vitamin B_2 (riboflavin)—A vitamin or coenzyme that functions by helping the enzymes in the body function correctly. A good source of this vitamin for lacto-vegetarians is milk.

Vitamins—These are compounds required by the body in small amounts to assist in energy production and in cell growth and maintenance. They are essential for life and, with the exception of vitamin D, cannot be made in the body. They should ideally be consumed from food. However, individuals who struggle to eat can obtain their vitamin requirements from dietary supplements.

brands that are fortified with calcium. Calcium is a mineral essential for healthy bones and teeth. Dairy foods are also a rich source of protein, energy, vitamin B_2 (**riboflavin**), **vitamin A**, and **vitamin B_{12}**.

Benefits

A lacto-vegetarian diet is generally lower in fat and higher in both fiber and **antioxidants** than a meat-based diet. Much research suggests that individuals who adopt vegetarian eating patterns are less likely to suffer from **obesity**, **coronary heart disease** (CHD), high blood pressure, type 2 diabetes, certain nutrition-related cancers, and constipation. People who choose vegetarian diets tend to lead healthier lifestyles.

Precautions

People wishing to adopt lacto-vegetarian eating habits need to know how to go about it safely. It is essential to ensure that foods excluded from the diet are replaced with suitable nutritional equivalents. Important nutrients such as **iron** are found primarily in meat and animal products, so vegetarians may risk vitamin and mineral deficiencies if they do not take steps to ensure that these needs are met.

Iron

Iron is essential for the formation of red blood cells, which carry oxygen to all parts of the body. A low body iron level can result in anemia. Iron from non-meat sources is referred to as nonheme iron, whereas iron from meat sources is heme iron. The body is able to absorb heme iron better than nonheme iron. Sources of nonheme iron include green leafy vegetables, pulses, wholemeal bread, fortified cereals, dried fruit, and nuts and seeds, including sesame, pumpkin, and sunflower seeds. Consuming **vitamin C** (such as in a glass of orange juice) with nonheme iron helps enhance the absorption of iron in the body.

Vitamin B$_{12}$

Vitamin B$_{12}$ is essential for healthy blood and nerve cells. This vitamin is not naturally found in plant foods, and the main sources of this vitamin are animal-based foods. Alternative sources for lacto-vegetarians include dairy products, yeast extracts, some vegetable stocks, soymilk, fortified breakfast cereals, and textured vegetable protein.

Fatty acids

The omega-3 essential fatty acids found in oily fish are found in vegetarian foods such as rapeseed (canola) oil, flaxseeds, and walnuts. **Omega-3 fatty acids** are thought to support heart health and also play an important role in the development of a baby's brain while in the womb, so pregnant women especially should aim to include plant-based sources of omega-3 in their diet.

Calcium

Calcium is essential for the formation of strong bones and teeth. During childhood, bones develop and become more dense until the mid-thirties. The combination of adequate dietary calcium intake and **vitamin D** levels in conjunction with regular exercise is essential to the development of bone mineral density and to helping safeguard against the development of osteoporosis (brittle bones) in later life.

Lacto-vegetarians typically receive most of their calcium intake from dairy products. Other sources of calcium include tofu, dried figs, pulses, tahini, sesame seeds, and some green vegetables (such as kale). Soy-based dairy products are typically low in calcium. Individuals are encouraged to either opt for brands that are fortified with calcium or ensure that calcium intake from other foods is sufficient.

Zinc

Zinc is an essential nutrient for health, growth, male fertility, and wound healing. Vegetarian diets in general may not always provide adequate intake, so it is important for lacto-vegetarians to be aware of zinc-rich foods. These include cheese, pulses, nuts, seeds, and whole-grain cereals.

Risks

Risks associated with lacto-vegetarian eating patterns are minimal as long as steps are taken to ensure adequate consumption of required nutrients. If a vegetarian diet is too restrictive, it may lead to **malnutrition** and vitamin and mineral deficiencies, adversely affecting overall health.

Research and general acceptance

According to the **Academy of Nutrition and Dietetics** (formerly the American Dietetic Association), vegetarian diets have been associated with a reduced risk of heart disease, high cholesterol, **hypertension** (high blood pressure), type 2 diabetes, and cancer. Vegetarians also tend to be leaner and are less likely to be obese than people who regularly eat meat. It is important to note, however, that risks of these illnesses in meat eaters are also reduced if dietary intake is based on the U.S. **dietary guidelines**.

Resources

BOOKS

Gelles, Carol. *AARP 1,000 Vegetarian Recipes*. Hoboken, NJ: John Wiley & Sons, 2011.

Polenz, Kathy. *Vegetarian Cooking*. Hoboken, NJ: Wiley, 2012.

Sutton, Jeanette. *Cooking for One or Two: Down to Earth Food for Vegan and Lacto-vegetarians*. Katikati, New Zealand: J. Sutton, 2010.

PERIODICALS

Craig, W.J., A.R. Mangels, and the Academy of Nutrition and Dietetics. "Position of the American Dietetic Association: Vegetarian Diets." *Journal of the American Dietetic Association* 109, no. 7 (2009): 1266–82.

OTHER

Kaiser Permamente. *Vegetarian Meal Planning: A Guide for Healthy Eating*. Permanente Medical Group, 2006. http://www.permanente.net/homepage/kaiser/pdf/6151.pdf (accessed on September 16, 2012).

WEBSITES

Bellows, L. "Vegetarian Diets." Colorado State University Extension. http://www.ext.colostate.edu/pubs/foodnut/09324.html (accessed September 16, 2012).

Mayo Clinic staff. "Vegetarian Diet: How to Get the Best Nutrition." MayoClinic.com. http://www.mayoclinic.com/health/vegetarian-diet/HQ01596 (accessed on September 16, 2012).

ORGANIZATIONS

Academy of Nutrition and Dietetics, 120 South Riverside Plz., Ste. 2000, Chicago, IL 60605, (312) 899-0400, (800) 877-1600, amacmunn@eatright.org, http://www.eatright.org.

Vegetarian Resource Group, PO Box 1463, Baltimore, MD 21203, (410) 366-8343, vrg@vrg.org, http://www.vrg.org.

Annette L. Dunne, BSc (Hons) MSc RD
David Newton

Latino diet *see* **Hispanic and Latino diet**

Liquid diets

Definition

Liquid diets is a term that encompasses a wide range of diets that serve a variety of functions. It can mean either partial or full meal replacement by either clear or non-clear fluids. Doctors often prescribe a liquid diet for before or after certain surgeries, or for patients who are medically obese. People also use them for fasting or weight loss.

Origins

The first uses of liquid diets date back centuries. Ancient religious ceremonies often involved fasting, and many cultures served only broth to sick patients. Doctors have been prescribing liquid diets to patients before they undergo surgery for decades. Only in the past few decades have several medically monitored weight-loss programs, such as **Optifast**, and commercially available weight-loss programs, such as **Slim-Fast**, become available.

Description

Liquid diets refer to a broad category of diets that can be used for a number of different reasons. In essence, a liquid diet is any diet that replaces regular meals of solid foods with fluid drinks. For many medical procedures it is helpful, or even necessary, if patients consume only liquids before or after the operation. People might also consume only liquids during periods of fasting. When a person is diagnosed as seriously obese, a physician may decide that he or she should undergo a medically observed weight-loss program, such as Optifast. There are also several programs, like Slim-Fast, that mimic the medically observed programs, but in a less severe way that can be followed without supervision.

Liquid diets for medical procedures

Before patients undergo certain medical procedures, their physicians may recommend a liquid diet. This is done to clear out the digestive system and decrease the strain on the digestive organs. It allows a patient to acquire the necessary **calories**, nutrients, and fluids, while minimizing the digestive impact. Tests that might require this include sigmoidoscopy, colonoscopy, magnetic resonance imaging (MRI), and certain x rays. Surgical procedures that can require a liquid diet include most types of serious oral surgery as well as almost any stomach or bowel surgery. Many surgical procedures, such as **bariatric surgery**, may also require that a patient follow a liquid diet after the operation while they regain the ability to digest solid foods.

Though guidelines will differ depending upon the procedure, following a liquid diet in preparation for a medical procedure will generally mean drinking only clear (translucent) liquids. Water, juice, broth, ice, and gelatin are usually acceptable. Soups that contain vegetables, noodles, meat, or rice are generally not allowed. While milk is usually acceptable, yogurt is usually restricted. When a physician prescribes a liquid diet, he or she will tell the patient the specific guidelines, including a time period during which the diet must be followed, and often provide literature that will describe the types of fluids that are allowed.

Fasting

Many people carry out periods of fasting for a variety of reasons. While some fasts require the faster to only drink water, or to consume no liquid at all, fasting typically means to refrain from eating food, but not from drinking liquids. Most of the world's popular religions call for periods of fasting at certain times for tradition, for reasons of atonement, to clear the mind, as a way of mourning, for purification, or for other spiritual reasons. Jewish tradition says that fasting should be done during Yom Kippur. Many Christians fast during Lent. Muslims traditionally fast during the days of Ramadan. Many ascetic Buddhists and Hindus practice periodic fasting. Many people also fast for health-related reasons, because they believe that it can cleanse the body of toxins and some even believe it can cure disease. Historically, fasting has also been used for political reasons as a form of protest, like those carried out by Mohandas Gandhi in the 1920s and 1930s.

For whatever reason it is done, fasting should never be used for weight loss. Medical professionals disagree about whether fasting should be used for other reasons, but it is overwhelmingly accepted that fasting is not an effective way to lose weight and that it can be very dangerous. Not only does fasting slow down the metabolic processes, meaning that it can actually result in overall weight gain, it also weakens the immune system and can make people vulnerable to many serious diseases and conditions, including liver and kidney failure. People considering a fast should always consult with their doctor to make sure that they will not be posing any risks to their health.

Liquid diets for medical weight loss

When a person is extremely obese, a physician may prescribe a medically monitored weight-loss program that involves replacing solid foods with a liquid substitute. The liquid substitute will usually supply between 500 and 800 calories each day, which means that it qualifies as a very low-calorie diet. The liquid substitute will also supply all of the necessary **vitamins** and

minerals that would normally be provided by solid food. Typically the liquid substitute comes in the form of a shake. Patients are told to drink a certain number of shakes every day, rather than eating, and to use that time period to break old eating habits. After a number of weeks of rapid weight loss and frequent meetings with the monitoring physician, solid foods may be slowly reintroduced. The entire process is difficult and risky. It should only be undertaken when prescribed by a physician and it must be monitored by a medical professional. Usually, this sort of liquid diet is only prescribed when serious health risks, caused by **obesity**, outweigh any risks from the program.

One popular medically observed liquid diet is called Optifast. It is produced by the Swiss company Nestlé Health Science, which is also known for making Gerber baby food. The company reported that, in a study of 20,000 people who used the Optifast program for 22 weeks, the average person lost 52 pounds and decreased their blood pressure by 10%. The Optifast system is extremely expensive and is not intended for the typical dieter.

Commercially available liquid diets

Possibly because of the reputation for rapid weight loss in seriously obese patients, several less expensive liquid meal replacements have become commercially available for weight loss without medical supervision. These products are not usually intended to replace every meal or all solid foods. These products are intended to help dieters lose weight quickly, though they often do little to affect long-term lifestyle changes.

One of the more popular commercially available liquid meal replacement diets is called Slim-Fast. The Slim-Fast plan says dieters should eat one regular meal during the day and replace the rest with low-calorie shakes. The shakes each provide one-third of the daily recommendations for a healthy diet. Slim-Fast is one of the few liquid replacement diets that defends its plan with controlled clinical studies. In a study done at the University of California, Los Angeles School of Medicine, 300 patients followed the Slim-Fast diet for 12 weeks. They lost an average of 15 pounds, and 76% were able to keep at least 80% of the weight off by one year later. However, most dietitians still maintain that a liquid replacement diet is not an appropriate substitute for a healthy lifestyle.

Function

Different liquid diets are intended for different functions. Many patients must follow a liquid diet before or after a medical procedure to clear out their digestive

system. Fasting is done for religious, medical, and even political reasons. Physicians prescribe medically supervised liquid diets to seriously obese patients to lower their risk of medical consequences of obesity. Many people also purchase similar, but commercially available, meal-replacement diets to lose weight.

Benefits

The possible benefits to a liquid diet depend upon which sort of liquid diet a person is considering. A patient that is told by a physician to refrain from eating solid foods can prevent everything from vomiting during surgery to an ineffective test. Some people believe that fasting can have spiritual benefits or can help to remove toxins from the body.

The greatest health benefits of a liquid diet, however, are probably experienced by extremely obese patients who lose weight on a medically supervised meal replacement liquid diet. Obesity has been linked with many serious diseases such as diabetes, heart disease, kidney failure, liver failure, and **cancer**. Obese individuals who lose weight can drastically reduce their risk of getting these diseases and even reduce the severity of their symptoms if they already suffer from them. Health benefits can also be gained by people who lose weight using a commercially available meal replacement liquid diet.

Precautions

Anyone who has been prescribed a liquid diet because of a medical procedure should get as much information as possible about the specific guidelines and follow those guidelines precisely. Doing so will give the procedure its greatest chance of success. Anyone considering a fast should consult their physician and describe the nature of the fast to him or her so that it can be determined if the fast will carry serious risks. People with health problems should not engage in prolonged fasting.

Very low-calorie liquid diets should not be undertaken without close medical supervision. These are only intended for people who have large amounts of weight to lose, generally over 50 pounds, and are experiencing health risks because of their obesity. People considering any kind of meal replacement liquid diet should consult their physician to be sure the diet is safe for them.

Risks

Short-term liquid diets for use before or after a medical procedure carry few risks and are generally considered safe if the patient follows the prescribed guidelines and is sure to get enough caloric intake through juice, broth, or other clear liquids. Longer fasting carries many risks including possible damage to the intestinal tract, impaired liver or kidney function, and hypoglycemia. Fasting also impairs the body's immune system, which makes the body more vulnerable to communicable diseases such as influenza or streptococcus. Gaining fat is also a common risk of fasting, because although the body may use stores of fat during the fast, once the fast is over the body usually rebuilds these stores quickly and often rebuilds more than was originally available.

Medically supervised meal-replacement diets can carry their own risks, though these are usually outweighed by the benefits of weight loss for the extremely obese. Side effects can include gallstone formation, nausea, fatigue, **constipation**, and diarrhea. Commercially available liquid diets also have many risks, depending on the brand. Some are considered very low-calorie diets that can result in **malnutrition**. Many do not adequately replace the vitamins and minerals that would usually be supplied by solid foods. This can result in deficiencies that can cause problems—for example, if the body does not get enough **calcium**, the risk of osteoporosis and rickets increases.

Research and general acceptance

For certain medical procedures, it is generally accepted that patients must refrain from eating solid foods for at least 24 hours before the procedure. Most hospitals have prepared patient literature about the precise guidelines that should be followed for these procedures.

QUESTIONS TO ASK YOUR DOCTOR

- What are the risks and benefits of a liquid diet?
- Is this diet safe for me?
- What sort of liquids should I drink on this diet?
- How long before I can eat solid foods?
- Is this the best diet to help me meet my weight loss goals?
- Will I get proper nutrition from my liquid diet?
- What symptoms or adverse effects are important enough that I should seek immediate treatment?

Doctors disagree about whether fasting can have health benefits, though most agree that it must be undertaken carefully and carries many risks. Most also agree that toxins do build up in the body when a person eats a diet that is high in processed foods and low in nutrients. However, the question of whether fasting can remove these toxins has yet to be conclusively answered. It is accepted that fasting is not a safe or effective method of weight loss.

Most medically supervised meal-replacement liquid diets are generally accepted. Some doctors question whether more traditional weight loss methods are better in cases of less extreme obesity, but it is generally believed that the risks and side effects of these programs are outweighed by the benefits for severely obese patients.

There are many commercially available liquid diets for weight loss, and their acceptance depends upon the brand and its program. Brands that include regular food, at least 1,200 calories each day, and some kind of exercise recommendations, like Slim-Fast, are more accepted than programs that are very low in calories and do not include exercise, such as the Hollywood Celebrity Miracle Diet.

Resources

BOOKS

Larsen, Laura, ed. *Diet and Nutrition Sourcebook*. 4th ed. Detroit, MI: Omnigraphics Inc, 2011.

Montgomery, Lisa. *Liquid Raw*. Hobart, NY: Hatherleigh Press, 2011.

Willis, Alicia P. ed. *Diet Therapy Research Trends*. New York: Nova Science, 2007.

PERIODICALS

Hemmingsson, Erik, et al. "Weight Loss and Dropout During a Commercial Weight-Loss Program Including a

Very-Low-Calorie Diet, a Low-Calorie Diet, or Restricted Normal Food: Observational Cohort Study." *American Journal of Clinical Nutrition* (September 18, 2012): e-pub ahead of print. http://dx.doi.org/10.3945/ajcn.112.038265 (accessed September 21, 2012).

WEBSITES

Mayo Clinic staff. "Clear Liquid Diet." MayoClinic.com. http://www.mayoclinic.com/health/clear-liquid-diet/MY00742 (accessed September 21, 2012).

Helen Davidson
Laura Jean Cataldo, RN, EdD

Local diet

Definition

A local diet is comprised of food produced as close as possible to a consumer's locale. The food may come from community-supported agriculture (CSA), also called family vegetable shares, community farms, or buying clubs; from individual or community gardens; or from local farms, either directly or via farmers' markets. People who follow a local diet are called locavores. First Lady Michelle Obama planted the White House Kitchen Garden in the spring of 2009, sparking a resurgence in vegetable gardening throughout the United States.

Origins

In the past most diets were primarily local. During World War II, urban gardens produced 40% of Britain's food supply, and Americans across the country planted "victory gardens." However, the second half of the twentieth century was marked by the industrialization of agriculture, which replaced family farms. Each food item in a typical American meal now travels an average of 1,500 miles from farm to table.

The current local diet phenomenon has several sources. The community garden movement originated in European cities and spread to the United States. In 1976, the Farmer-to-Consumer Direct Marketing Act led to a resurgence of farmers' markets—from about

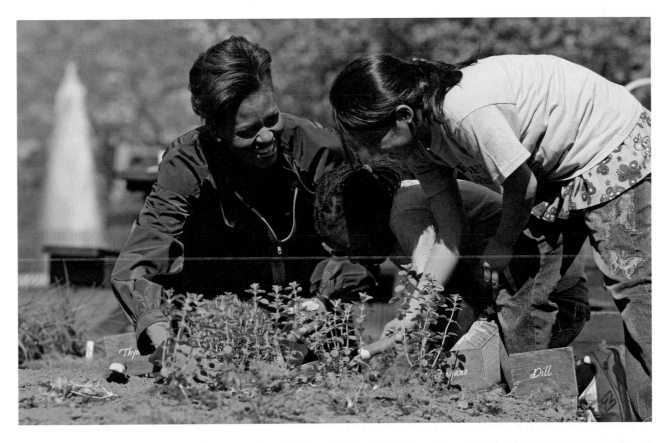

First Lady Michelle Obama works in the White House Kitchen Garden with children from a local elementary school. *(AP Photo/Charles Dharapak)*

350 to almost 4,800 in 2009—making it easier for consumers to buy locally grown food.

Robyn Van En introduced CSAs to North America in 1985. As of 2008, there were an estimated 1,700–2,000 CSAs operating in North America. In 1986, Slow Food International was founded in Italy "to protect the pleasures of the table from the homogenization of modern fast food and life." As of 2012, the organization had more than 100,000 members across the world devoted to promoting agricultural biodiversity and local, seasonal, and traditional foods.

Many restaurateurs and cookbook authors, such as Alice Waters, Rick Bayless, and Deborah Madson, promote the use of local, seasonal foods. Alice Waters's Edible Schoolyard brought organic gardening to inner-city schools, and similar programs appeared nationwide. In 2004, an amendment to the National School Lunch Act established the Farm-to-Cafeteria program to provide local meat and produce for school cafeterias and fund school garden projects In 2008, the National Cooperative Grocers Association launched their "Eat Local America" campaign, urging people to consume 80% local food during the summer months.

Description

"Local" generally refers to food that has been grown, raised, and processed within 50–100 miles. In non-food-producing regions, however, such as the Southwest desert of the United States, "local" may mean within a 250-mile radius. A local diet can involve:

- buying fresh food directly from a farm, roadside stand, or U-pick farm; through a CSA or buying club; or at a farmers' market
- finding local foods at a supermarket, independent grocery, or food co-op
- growing food in a yard, rooftop, windowsill, or community garden
- consuming foods that are in season
- storing, freezing, canning, and/or drying seasonal foods for the winter months
- home cooking
- eating local food in restaurants
- promoting farm-to-school programs
- giving local food to schools and food banks and as gifts

CSAs are programs where subscribers pay producers in the early spring and receive weekly supplies of produce throughout the season or year. Many CSAs allow or even require subscribers to work on the farms and some offer work-for-food arrangements. CSAs are generally small, but some are very large multi-farm operations and others are devoted solely to stocking food banks. Though most CSAs center on produce, some CSAs and buying clubs specialize in products such as milk or meat or in supplying restaurants.

In community gardens, neighbors work small plots and may share water, tools, and seeds. Some garden plots are rented and others are free. Some community gardens exist to supply local schools or specific at-need populations.

Local foods are often—but not always—from small and medium-sized farms. Some local farmers use cold frames and other devices to extend seasons, or heated greenhouses to provide fresh local produce year-round. Many small farmers maintain self-sufficiency by trading with other local farmers who grow or raise different foods.

The local food movement has led to the resurgence of smaller local processors, such as grain mills, slaughterhouses (including mobile units that travel to farms), smokehouses, dairies and creameries, and bakeries. Pastas, cereals, beer, wine, and bottled water are increasingly produced locally. Although locally grown coffee is impossible in the continental United States, local coffee roasting is a fast-growing business.

Farmers' market rules usually guarantee that products are both fresh and local. Some farmers' markets are producer-only, meaning that the vendors must grow their own wares, whereas others permit vendors who buy from wholesale distributors. Most farmers' market products are from small farms and connect consumers directly with farmers. Produce is likely to be organically grown, regardless of whether it is labeled as such. Some farmers sell directly to the public before and after market seasons.

First Lady Michelle Obama is a strong advocate of nutrition and home gardening. Hers was the first vegetable garden on the White House grounds since Eleanor Roosevelt's World War II victory garden. Local fifth-graders helped Obama plant and harvest annual and perennial herbs, a variety of vegetables, and raspberries and strawberries. The 1,100-square-foot year-round garden features heirloom varieties, honey bees for pollination, organic fertilizers, and biological insect control. In its first year, the garden yielded hundreds of pounds of vegetables for the White House kitchen and for Miriam's Kitchen, which serves Washington's homeless. The cost of seeds and soil amendments was about $200.

Popularity of local diets

In developing nations, gardening and farming is an essential part of life, but home gardens are increasing in developed countries. Shanghai, China, has over 600,000 acres of gardens. More than 80% of the produce in Havana, Cuba, comes from urban gardens. Even in the United States, it is estimated that 25% of households grow some of their own produce and that number is on the rise. More people are growing winter gardens, and as of 2009 there were more than one million community gardens in the United States, many of them in impoverished urban areas. An estimated 30,000-plus American farmers sell about $1 billion worth of food at farmers' markets to at least three million customers annually. Between 50% and 70% of Americans live within easy reach of a farmers' market, some of which are open all year. Diversified farming on the outskirts of cities is the fastest-growing sector of American agriculture, and many states have farm-to-school programs, with farm-to-college programs proliferating.

Many natural-food chain stores, food cooperatives (co-ops), and specialized markets promote local food. As a result of consumer demand, conventional grocery stores—especially locally owned stores—are carrying more local products. Even some chain supermarkets and box stores are beginning to specify the state or country of origin for their produce and are highlighting local produce. Some food processors, distributors, and cooperatives specialize in marketing locally produced food to supermarkets, and even some caterers, restaurants, and food-service corporations emphasize a local diet.

Local diets appeal to people across the socioeconomic spectrum. The nutritional assistance program coupons for women with infants and children (WIC) are redeemable at farmers' markets, and the Seniors Farmers Market Nutrition Program (SFMNP) helps low-income seniors buy fresh local produce. An increasing number of farmers' markets accept electronic benefits transfers (EBTs) from the Supplemental Nutrition Assistance Program (SNAP, formerly food stamps). Programs throughout the country link local farm produce with school cafeterias and food banks for the poor and homeless. Many communities have programs for diverting unsold produce from CSAs, farmers' markets, and even home gardeners to food banks.

Function

In addition to providing fresher, healthier foods, the local food movement encompasses broader issues, including environmental concerns, agricultural sustainability, and fair wages for labor. Smaller farms tend to be more sustainable over time because they use fewer chemicals, cause less soil erosion, and maintain more wildlife habitats. By limiting transportation, local diets may reduce oil consumption; per capita, a

conventional American diet consumes almost as much oil as Americans' automobiles. About 17% of America's energy usage is agricultural, with 80% of that going to processing, packaging, warehousing, refrigeration, and transport.

Local diets support family farms. These are more profitable per acre than corporate farms. Sometimes conventional farmers convert just a few of their acres to "high-value crops"—vegetables for the local market. A local diet provides small farmers with markets and allows them to keep more of their profits by selling directly to consumers.

Benefits

Prominent benefits of a local diet include the quality, nutritional value, and flavor of foods. Local foods are usually fresher and more flavorful. Small farms also tend to grow varieties of fruits and vegetables that are otherwise unavailable. Over their history, humans have consumed some 80,000 plant species, but over the past century—and especially since World War II—93% of North American crop varieties have disappeared from cultivation. Today, 75% of all human food is derived from just eight species—primarily genetically modified (GM) corn, **soy**, and canola. Local foods are more likely to include less common varieties that have not been selected for characteristics such as ease of transport.

Local foods are more likely to be organically grown, making them free of residues from petroleum-based fertilizers, herbicides, and pesticides. They are also less likely to be genetically modified. Local meat, eggs, and dairy products are more likely to come from humanely raised animals that have not been fed antibiotics and growth hormones. Pasture-raised meat has less saturated fat and more "good" cholesterol than meat from confined animal feeding operations (CAFOs). CSA members or consumers who buy directly from farmers can observe exactly how their food is produced.

Financially, a local diet returns more food money to the farmer, keeping it within the local economy. In contrast, 80–85 cents of every industrial food dollar goes not to the farmer but to processors, packagers, transporters, distributors, marketers, slotting fees for product placement, and waste management. The local diet movement has been a boon for economically depressed regions and for rural farmers who previously grew tobacco.

Precautions

A local diet may be difficult for some people to follow. Food grown locally on small farms tends to be more expensive than mass-produced supermarket produce. It may force people to become more creative in their shopping and cooking, planning meals around seasonal foods and learning new ways to prepare vegetables. For many people, this requires a major change in dietary habits and a commitment of time and energy. It may also require restraint and sacrificing some favorite foods and treats made from non-local ingredients.

Risks

There can be certain risks to a local diet:

- CSA members must organize their meals around the produce they receive each week and may not be able to use some of their produce.
- CSA members share in the risk that a harvest may fail.
- Certain local foods, especially raw milk, may be subject to bacterial contamination.
- Garden soil, especially in older urban neighborhoods, should be tested for toxins. For example, the soil in Michelle Obama's garden was found to contain 93 parts per million (ppm) of lead. Although this is well below the level considered harmful to humans, the U.S. Environmental Protection Agency (EPA) advises against growing food in soil with lead at 100 ppm or higher. The lead is believed to have come from sewage sludge used to fertilize the White House lawn during the 1990s.

QUESTIONS TO ASK YOUR DOCTOR

- Should I buy organic produce?
- If I follow a local diet, how can I ensure that my family gets all the required nutrients during the winter months?

Research and general acceptance

Local diets are becoming increasingly popular in the United States and other parts of the world; however, relatively few people are able to follow a completely local diet, at least for long periods of time. Several popular accounts written by locavores have contributed to the increased interest in eating local foods.

Resources

BOOKS

Cotler, Amy. *The Locavore Way: Discover and Enjoy the Pleasures of Locally Grown Food.* North Adams, MA: Storey Publishing, 2009.

Henderson, Elizabeth, with Robyn Van En. *Sharing the Harvest: A Citizen's Guide to Community Supported Agriculture.* Rev. ed. White River Junction, VT: Chelsea Green, 2007.

Kingsolver, Barbara, with Steven L. Hopp and Camille Kingsolver. *Animal, Vegetable, Miracle: A Year of Food Life.* New York: HarperCollins, 2007.

Smith, Alisa, and J. B. Mackinnon. *Plenty: One Man, One Woman, and a Raucous Year of Eating Locally.* New York: Harmony, 2007.

PERIODICALS

Roberts, Paul. "Spoiled." *Mother Jones* 34, no. 2 (March/April 2009): 28.

Walsh, Bryan. "America's Food Crisis and How to Fix It." *Time* 174, no. 8 (August 31, 2009): 30.

WEBSITES

Biodynamic Farming and Gardening Association. "Community Supported Agriculture: An Introduction to CSA." http://www.biodynamics.com/csa.html (accessed October 3, 2012).

Brandon, Katherine. "A Healthy Harvest." *The White House Blog,* June 17, 2009. http://www.whitehouse.gov/blog/A-Healthy-Harvest (accessed October 3, 2012).

Larsen, Steph. "It Takes a Community to Sustain a Small Farm." *Grist,* January 6, 2010. http://www.grist.org/article/2010-01-05-it-takes-a-community-to-sustain-a-small-farm (accessed October 3, 2012).

McFadden, Steven. "Community Farms in the 21st Century: Poised for Another Wave of Growth?" *The History of Community Supported Agriculture, Part I,* Rodale

Institute. http://newfarm.rodaleinstitute.org/features/
0104/csa-history/part1.shtml (accessed October 3, 2012).

Rodale Institute. "Farm Locator." http://
www.rodaleinstitute.org/farm_locator (accessed
October 3, 2012).

U.S. Department of Agriculture, Agricultural Marketing
Service. "Farmers Markets and Local Food Marketing."
http://www.ams.usda.gov/AMSv1.0/farmersmarkets
(accessed October 3, 2012).

U.S. Department of Agriculture, National Agricultural
Library. "Community Supported Agriculture."
Alternative Farming Systems Information Center.
http://www.nal.usda.gov/afsic/pubs/csa/csa.shtml
(accessed October 3, 2012).

"Why Buy Local?" FoodRoutes.org. http://www.
foodroutes.org/whycare.jsp (accessed October 3,
2012).

ORGANIZATIONS

American Community Garden Association, 1777 East
Broad St., Columbus, OH 43203-2040, info@community
garden.org, http://www.communitygarden.org.

Biodynamic Farming and Gardening Association, 25844
Butler Rd., Junction City, OR 97448, (888) 516-7797,
Fax: (541) 998-0106, info@biodynamics.com, http://
www.biodynamics.com.

City Farmer—Canada's Office of Urban Agriculture, Box
74567, Kitsilano RPO, Vancouver, BC, Canada V6K
4P4, (604) 685-5832, cityfarm@interchange.ubc.ca,
http://www.cityfarmer.org.

Community Food Security Coalition, 3830 SE Division St.,
Portland, OR 97202, (503) 954-2970, Fax: (503) 954-2959,
aleta@foodsecurity.org, http://www.foodsecurity.org.

Farmers Market Coalition, PO Box 504, Charlottesville, VA
22902, http://farmersmarketcoalition.org.

LocalHarvest, 220 21st Ave., Santa Cruz, CA 95062, (831)
515-5602, Fax: (831) 401-2418, http://
www.localharvest.org.

National Family Farm Coalition, 110 Maryland Ave. NE,
Ste. 307, Washington, DC 20002, (202) 543-5675,
Fax: (202) 543-0978, nffc@nffc.net, http://www.nffc.net.

Robyn Van En Center, Fulton Center for Sustainable Living,
Wilson College, 1015 Philadelphia Ave., Chambersburg,
PA 17201-9979, (717) 264-4141, ext. 3352, Fax: (717)
264-1578, csacenter@wilson.edu, http://www.wilson.edu/
wilson/asp/content.asp?id=804.

Slow Food International, Piazza XX Settembre, 5, 12042
Bra (Cuneo), Italy, +39 0172 419611, Fax: +39 0172
421293, international@slowfood.com, http://www.
slowfood.com.

U.S. Department of Agriculture, 1400 Independence Ave.
SW, Washington, DC 20250, (202) 720-2791, http://
www.usda.gov/wps/portal/usdahome.

Margaret Alic, PhD

Low-carb diets *see* **High-fat, low-carb diets**

Low-cholesterol diet

Definition

A low-cholesterol diet is a diet designed to reduce
the amount of cholesterol circulating in the blood.

Origins

No single person originated the low-cholesterol
diet. However, the American Heart Association has
been a major developer of this diet. The National
Cholesterol Education Program organized by the
National Heart, Lung, and Blood Institute monitors
research and new developments in cholesterol control,
including new approaches to low-cholesterol dieting.

Description

The low-cholesterol diet is designed to lower an
individual's cholesterol level. Cholesterol is a waxy
substance made by the liver and also acquired through
diet. Cholesterol does not dissolve in blood. Instead, it
moves through the circulatory system in combination
with carrier substances called lipoproteins. There are
two types of carrier-cholesterol combinations, low-
density lipoprotein (LDL) or "bad" cholesterol and
high-density lipoprotein or "good" cholesterol.

LDL picks up cholesterol in the liver and carries it
through the circulatory system. Most of the cholesterol in the body is LDL cholesterol. When too much
LDL cholesterol is present, it begins to drop out of the
blood and stick to the walls of the arteries. The arteries
are blood vessels carrying blood away from the heart

Cholesterol levels

Total Cholesterol	
Desirable	200
Borderline high	200–239
High	240
LDL Cholesterol (bad)	
Optimal	100
Near/above optimal	100–129
Borderline high	130–159
High	160–189
Very high	190
HDL Cholesterol (good)	
Low	40
High	60

SOURCE: National Heart, Lung and Blood Institute, National
Institutes of Health, U.S. Department of Health and Human
Services

(Table by GGS Information Services. © 2013 Cengage Learning.)

to other organs in the body. The coronary arteries are special arteries that supply blood to the heart. The sticky material on the artery walls is called cholesterol plaque. (It is different from dental plaque that accumulates on teeth.) Plaque can reduce the amount of blood flowing through the arteries and encourage blood clots to form. A heart attack occurs if the coronary arteries are blocked. A stroke occurs if arteries carrying blood to the brain are blocked.

Researchers believe that HDL works opposite LDL. HDL picks up cholesterol off the walls of the arteries and takes it back to the liver where it can be broken down and removed. This helps to keep the blood vessels open. Cholesterol can be measured by a simple blood test. To reduce the risk of cardiovascular disease, adults should keep their LDL cholesterol below 160 mg/dL and their HDL cholesterol above 40 mg/dL (on average).

Cholesterol is a necessary and important part of cell membranes. It also is converted into some types of steroid (sex) hormones. Cholesterol comes from two sources. The liver makes all the cholesterol the body needs from other nutrients. However, other animals also make cholesterol. When humans eat animal products, they take in more cholesterol. Cholesterol is found only in foods from animals, never in plant foods. The foods highest in cholesterol are organ meats such as liver, egg yolk (but not egg whites), whole-fat dairy products (butter, ice cream, whole milk), and marbled red meat. To reduce the risk of cardiovascular disease, adults should keep their consumption of cholesterol below 300 mg daily.

Cholesterol and fats

There are three types of **fats** in food. Saturated fats are animal fats such as butter, the fats in milk and cream, bacon fat, the fat under the skin of chickens, lard, or the fat on a piece of prime rib of beef. These fats are usually solid at room temperature, and they are considered "bad" fats because they raise LDL cholesterol.

Unsaturated fats can be monounsaturated or polyunsaturated. These fats are considered healthy fats and may help lower cholesterol levels. Olive oil, canola oil, and peanut oil are high in monounsaturated fats. Corn oil, soybean oil, safflower oil, and sunflower oil are high in polyunsaturated fats. Fish oils that are high in **omega-3 fatty acids** are polyunsaturated and may be beneficial in preventing heart disease.

Trans fat is made by a manufacturing process that creates hydrogenated or partially hydrogenated vegetable oils. *Trans* fat acts like saturated fat, raising the level of LDL cholesterol. It is found in some

margarines and in many commercially baked and fried foods. The U.S. Department of Agriculture's (USDA) *Dietary Guidelines for Americans* 2010 recommends that no more than 35% of an individual's daily **calories** come from fat, that no more than 10% of calories should come from saturated fat, and that people should consume as little *trans* fat as possible.

Managing a low-cholesterol diet

People who need to reduce their cholesterol levels can get help by reading food labels. Food labels are required to list in the nutrition information panel nutrition facts that include calories, calories from fat, total fat, saturated fat, *trans* fat, cholesterol, **sodium**, total **carbohydrates**, dietary **fiber**, sugars, **protein**, **vitamin A**, **vitamin C**, **calcium**, and **iron**. In addition, the following words have specific legal meanings on food labels:

- Cholesterol-free: Fewer than 2 mg of cholesterol and 2 g of saturated fat per serving.
- Low cholesterol: No more than 20 mg of cholesterol and 2 grams of saturated fat per serving.

When cooking, people can reduce cholesterol in the diet in the following ways:

- Choose lean cuts of meat. Select USDA graded cuts of beef and lamb marked Choice and Select. These cuts are leaner and less expensive than Prime.
- Bake or broil meats on a rack set in a pan, so that the fat can drip off.
- Refrigerate homemade soups and stews, then skim the solidified fat off the top before serving.
- If using canned soup or broth that contains fat, put the can in the refrigerator for a few hours, and skim the solid fat off the top before heating.
- Try cooking with olive or canola oil rather than corn oil.

To reduce cholesterol in meals when eating out:

- Order menu items that have the Heart Healthy stamp (may not be available in all restaurants).
- Choose items that are broiled, roasted, or baked and avoid fried foods.
- Select fish or chicken instead of beef or pork.
- Use margarine instead of butter on food.
- Ask for salad dressing, sauces, and gravy on the side.
- Order non-fat or 1% milk.

In addition to reducing fats, increasing soluble dietary fiber that is found in **whole grains** also helps lower cholesterol. Soluble fiber is found dissolved in water inside plant cells. In the body, it lowers LDL cholesterol. Good sources of soluble fiber include:

- oatmeal and oat bran
- kidney beans
- Brussels sprouts
- apples
- pears
- prunes

Walnuts and almonds are good sources of polyunsaturated fatty acids that help reduce blood cholesterol levels. Fish such as mackerel herring, sardines, lake trout, albacore tuna, and salmon, as well as walnuts, **flaxseed**, canola, and soybean oil are all rich in omega-3 fatty acids. These fatty acids help control fats in the blood and reduce blood clotting. Cholesterol-lowering drugs are available if changes in diet fail to control cholesterol levels. However, it is most desirable to control cholesterol through diet rather than medicine, as these drugs potentially have unwanted side effects.

Function

Low-cholesterol diets are healthy diets that are most effective if they become lifetime habits. Low-cholesterol diets work by reducing the amount of saturated (animal) fat to drive down LDL cholesterol and using more monounsaturated fats (olive oil, canola oil) and soluble fiber to drive up HDL cholesterol. By controlling fats in the diet, individuals may also lose weight.

Benefits

Low-cholesterol diets have the following benefits:
- decreased intake of dietary cholesterol
- decreased intake of saturated fats
- increased soluble fiber in diet
- decreased risk of developing cardiovascular disease

Precautions

Anyone over age two can safely follow a low-cholesterol diet. Children under age two need certain fats for the normal development of the nervous system and should be given whole-milk and whole-milk products.

Risks

There are no known risks to following a low-cholesterol diet.

Research and general acceptance

The relationship between cholesterol, saturated fat intake, and heart health has been documented in

---

KEY TERMS

Coronary arteries—The main arteries that provide blood to the heart. The coronary arteries surround the heart like a crown, coming out of the aorta, arching down over the top of the heart, and dividing into two branches. These are the arteries in which coronary artery disease occurs.

Dietary fiber—Also known as roughage or bulk. Insoluble fiber moves through the digestive system almost undigested and gives bulk to stools. Soluble fiber dissolves in water and helps keep stools soft.

Fatty acids—Complex molecules found in fats and oils. Essential fatty acids are fatty acids that the body needs but cannot synthesize. Essential fatty acids are made by plants and must be present in the diet to maintain health.

HDL cholesterol—High-density lipoprotein cholesterol is a component of cholesterol that helps protect against heart disease. HDL is nicknamed "good" cholesterol.

Hormone—A chemical messenger produced by the body that is involved in regulating specific bodily functions such as growth, development, reproduction, metabolism, and mood.

LDL cholesterol—Low-density lipoprotein cholesterol is the primary cholesterol molecule. High levels of LDL increase the risk of coronary heart disease. LDL is nicknamed "bad" cholesterol.

Plaque—A deposit of fatty and other substances that accumulate in the lining of the artery wall.

Steroid—A family of compounds that share a similar chemical structure. This family includes the hormones estrogen and testosterone, vitamin D, cholesterol, and the drugs cortisone and prednisone.

---

many studies. However, in a study of 49,000 women between the ages of 50 and 79 that was published in February 2007 in the *Journal of the American Medical Association*, women were divided randomly into a group that ate a **low-fat diet** and another group that had no restrictions and ate the average America diet. Researchers found no significant difference in the rates of heart attack or stroke between the two groups. They concluded that there was no justification in recommending a low-fat diet to the public as protection against heart disease. This study is particularly important because it was large, well-designed, and independent (it was funded by the federal government), and it followed the women for eight years.

QUESTIONS TO ASK YOUR DOCTOR

- What are the indications that I may need to begin or adhere to a low-cholesterol diet?
- What diagnostic tests are needed for a thorough assessment?
- What are my current cholesterol numbers?
- What are my current risk factors for cardiovascular disease?
- Should I see a specialist? If so, what kind of specialist should I contact?
- Does having high cholesterol put me at risk for other health conditions?
- Can my whole family go on this diet?
- Do I have any special health concerns that might affect this diet?

The American Heart Association has questioned these findings and continues to recommend a diet low in fat (especially animal fats) and low in cholesterol for the prevention of heart disease.

Critics of this study claim that the low-fat group did not reduce their fat significantly enough to make a difference in health and that the study did not cover enough time. Others said that eating unsaturated fat (a **Mediterranean diet**) was heart healthy and that this study did not distinguish between saturated and unsaturated fat intake. Supporters of the study have said that it shows that how much people eat and how much they exercise (their calorie balance) are more important than what they eat. This study is likely to stimulate more research into low-fat diets and the health differences between unsaturated and saturated fats.

More recently, in a May 2009 article about risk factors for heart disease, the *Journal of the American Medical Association* recommended that individuals "Check food labels and avoid saturated (usually from animals) fats and foods made with **trans fats** or hydrogenated fats."

Resources

BOOKS

American Heart Association. *American Heart Association Low-Fat, Low-Cholesterol Cookbook: Delicious Recipes to Help Lower Your Cholesterol.* 4th ed. New York: Clarkson Potter, 2010.

Gillinov, Marc, and Steven Nissen. *Heart 411: The Only Guide to Heart Health You'll Ever Need.* New York: Three Rivers Press, 2012.

Kowalski, Robert. *The New 8-Week Cholesterol Cure.* New York: HarperCollins, 2009.

Lipsky, Martin S, et al. *American Medical Association Guide to Preventing and Treating Heart Disease: Essential Information You and Your Family Need to Know About Having a Healthy Heart.* Hoboken, NJ: Wiley, 2008.

Mayo Clinic. *Mayo Clinic Healthy Heart for Life!* New York: Oxmoor House, 2012.

PERIODICALS

Hildreth, Carolyn J., Alison E. Burke, and Richard M. Glass. "Risk Factors for Heart Disease." *JAMA* 301, no. 20 (2009): 2176.

OTHER

National Heart, Lung, and Blood Institute. *Your Guide to Lowering your Cholesterol with TLC (Therapeutic Lifestyle Changes).* U.S. Department of Health and Human Services and National Institutes of Health, 2005. http://www.nhlbi.nih.gov/health/public/heart/chol/chol_tlc.pdf (accessed September 21, 2012).

WEBSITES

American Heart Association. "What Your Cholesterol Levels Mean." http://www.heart.org/HEARTORG/Conditions/Cholesterol/AboutCholesterol/What-Your-Cholesterol-Levels-Mean_UCM_305562_Article.jsp (accessed September 21, 2012).

Mayo Clinic staff. "Cholesterol: Top 5 Foods to Lower Your Numbers." MayoClinic.com. http://www.mayoclinic.com/health/cholesterol/CL00002 (accessed September 21, 2012).

ORGANIZATIONS

Academy of Nutrition and Dietetics, 120 South Riverside Plz., Ste. 2000, Chicago, IL 60606-6995, (312) 899-0040, (800) 877-1600, amacmunn@eatright.org, http://www.eatright.org.

American Heart Association, 7272 Greenville Ave., Dallas, TX 75231, (800) 242-8721, http://www.americanheart.org.

Centers for Disease Control and Prevention, Division for Heart Disease and Stroke Prevention, 4770 Buford Hwy NE, Mail Stop F-72, Atlanta, GA 30341-3717, (800) CDC-INFO (232-4636), TTY: (800) 232-6348, Fax: (770) 488-8151, cdcinfo@cdc.gov, http://www.cdc.gov/dhdsp.

National Heart, Lung, and Blood Institute, PO Box 30105, Bethesda, MD 20824-0105, (301) 592-8573, (240) 629-3255, Fax: (240) 629-3246, nhlbiinfo@nhlbi.nih.gov, http://www.nhlbi.nih.gov.

Tish Davidson, AM
Laura Jean Cataldo, RN, EdD

Low-fat diet

Definition

Different medical organizations, governments, and diet plans define "low fat" in slightly different ways. In general, a low-fat diet is one where 30% or less of the total daily **calories** come from **fats**. A very low-fat diet is one where 15% or less of the total daily calories come from fat. By comparison, in the average American diet about 35%–37% of calories come from fat.

Origins

When metabolized in the body, fats provide 9 calories per gram compared to 4 calories per gram from proteins and **carbohydrates**. Because of this, diet plans repeatedly target reduction in fats as a good way to lose weight. Examples of low-fat diets include the **Pritikin diet** and **Scarsdale diet**, both popular in the 1970s, Rosemary Conley's Hip and Thigh Diet (late 1980s), and the Dr. Dean Ornish Diet (2000s). Research into preventing cardiovascular disease also stimulated interest in low-fat diets as a preventative health measure.

Description

Fats are described as either saturated or unsaturated based on their chemical structure. Saturated fats are found in animal fats such as butter, the fats in milk and cream, bacon fat, the fat under the skin of chickens, lard, or the fat on a piece of prime rib of beef. These fats are usually solid at room temperature. Exceptions are palm oil and coconut oil, which are both liquid saturated fats. Saturated fats are often referred to as the "bad" fats. When consumed in high amounts, they raise the level of LDL cholesterol ("bad" cholesterol) in the blood. High LDL

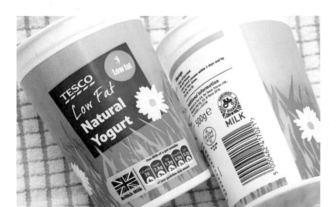

Low-fat yogurt. (© Libby Welch/Alamy)

cholesterol levels are associated with an increased risk of heart disease.

Unsaturated fats have a slightly different chemical structure that makes them liquid at room temperature. Unsaturated fats, especially monounsaturated fats, are considered "good" fats that can help lower cholesterol levels. Olive oil, canola oil, and peanut oil are high in monounsaturated fats. Corn oil, soybean oil, safflower oil, and sunflower oil are high in polyunsaturated fats. Fish oils are a rich source of two particular polyunsaturated fats termed long-chain omega-3 fatty acids, which have beneficial health effects.

Another type of fat, *trans* fat, is the by-product of a manufacturing process that hydrogenates or partially hydrogenates vegetable oils to make them more solid at room temperature. **Trans fats** also raise LDL cholesterol levels. They are found in some margarines and in many commercially baked and fried foods. During the past ten years, much work has been done to reduce *trans* fats in foods. A number of cities—including New York City—have passed full or partial bans on the use of *trans* fats in restaurants, and in 2008, California became the first state to enact a statewide ban (effective 2010).

The federal *Dietary Guidelines for Americans* 2010 recommend that 20%–35% of an adult's daily calories come from fat. Of that, no more than 10% of calories should come from saturated fat, and people should consume as little *trans* fat as possible. The American Heart Association's Nutrition Committee joined with the American Cancer Society, the American Academy of Pediatrics, and the National Institutes of Health to endorse these guidelines as part of a healthy diet. However, some experts believe that for heart health the amount of fats consumed should be much lower.

Nathan Pritikin, originator of the Pritikin Diet Plan, developed a very low-fat diet for heart health. The Pritikin Plan calls for less than 10% of calories to come from fat. The diet is also low in **protein** and high in whole-grain carbohydrates. Respected independent research shows that this diet does cause weight loss and lower risk factors for heart disease such as cholesterol and blood **triglycerides**. Critics of the diet say that it is too difficult to stay on and that the low-fat component of the diet does not allow people to get enough beneficial fats such as **omega-3 fatty acids**.

The Ornish diet is another very low-fat diet where only about 15% of calories come from fat. The Ornish diet is an almost-vegetarian diet. It too is designed to promote heart health, and again critics claim that it does not provide enough essential fatty acids.

Other low-fat diets are designed for people who have digestive disorders. People who have **gallstones** or gallbladder disease often benefit from reducing the amount of fats they eat. Bile, a digestive fluid made in the gallbladder, helps break down fats. When the gallbladder is not functioning well, a low-fat diet can improve digestion. Symptoms of other gastrointestinal problems, such as diarrhea, irritable bowel disorder, various malabsorptive disorders, and fatty liver, often improve on a low-fat diet. People who have had weight-loss surgery usually have fewer digestive problems if they eat a low-fat diet.

Managing a low-fat diet

People on low-fat diets need to avoid certain foods. High-fat foods include whole milk and whole-milk products such as ice cream or cream cheese, fried foods, marbled beef, chicken skin, spare ribs or any meat with visible fat, tuna packed in oil, regular salad dressing, potato chips and fried snack foods, and many baked goods—cookies, cakes, pies, and doughnuts.

People wishing to reduce the fat in their diet must read food labels. Food labels are required to list in the nutrition information panel nutrition facts that include calories, calories from fat, total fat, saturated fat, *trans* fat, cholesterol, **sodium**, total carbohydrates, dietary **fiber**, sugars, protein, **vitamin A**, **vitamin C**, **calcium**, and **iron**. In addition, the following words have specific legal meanings on food labels:

- Fat-free: Less than 0.5 grams of fat per serving.
- Low fat: No more than 3 grams or less of fat per serving.
- Less fat: A minimum of 25% less fat than the comparison food.
- Light (fat): A minimum of 50% less fat than the comparison food.

When cooking at home, people can reduce fat in the diet in the following ways:

- Remove all visible fat from meat and skin from poultry before cooking.
- Bake or broil meats on a rack set in a pan, so that the fat can drip off.
- Refrigerate homemade soups and stews, then skim the solidified fat off the top before serving.
- If using canned soup or broth that contains fat, put the can in the refrigerator for a few hours, and skim the solid fat off the top before heating.
- Use low-fat yogurt and herbs on baked potatoes in place of butter or sour cream.
- Top pasta with vegetables instead of oil, butter, or cheese.

To reduce fat in meals when eating out:

- Choose items that are broiled, roasted, or baked. Avoid fried foods.
- Select fish or chicken instead of beef or pork.
- Ask for salad dressing, butter, and gravy on the side.
- Fill up on salad with non-fat dressing at the salad bar.

Function

Low-fat diets work as weight-loss diets because they reduce caloric intake. The difficulty with low-fat and very low-fat diets is that they are difficult to maintain. Often when people go off these diets they gain weight back, then diet again, then gain weight back in a pattern of **weight cycling**. This happens with many diets, but some research shows that people who go off low-fat diets tend to binge or overeat more than people who go off more moderate diets.

In the 1990s and early 2000s, the public was encouraged to eat a low-fat diet not just to lose weight, but also to lower cholesterol and triglyceride levels. This, the public was told, would protect heart health and help prevent cardiovascular disease. This blanket statement is now in dispute.

Low-fat diets are effective in improving certain digestive symptoms. A general low-fat diet is usually prescribed first, and then fine-tuned with the aid of a physician to best treat the individual's digestive problems.

Benefits

People who go on low-fat diets can benefit in these ways:

- They lose weight.
- Their health usually improves.
- Their risk of developing cardiovascular disease may decrease.
- They get relief from unpleasant gastrointestinal symptoms.

Precautions

Young children, pregnant women, **breastfeeding** women, and the elderly have higher fat requirements and should not undergo low-fat diets unless advised to do so by a physician. Fat plays a key role in infant growth and development, and omega-3 fatty acids in particular may play a significant role in brain function and development.

Low-fat diets are difficult to maintain for long periods. They may increase the risk of yo-yo dieting or weight cycling.

Risks

Although many low-fat diets have been shown to be healthy, individual diets vary, and some low-fat diets are not nutritionally balanced.

Research and general acceptance

Many health claims have been made for low-fat diets. One is that they help people lose weight better than other diets. However, studies have shown that low-fat diets are no better at helping people lose weight and keep that weight off than regular low-calorie diets. The total amount of calories has more effect on weight loss than the particular foods those calories come from.

For many years, the public was told that low-fat diets helped protect against breast cancer, colon cancer, and heart disease. In a landmark study of 49,000 postmenopausal women, published in February 2006 in the *Journal of the American Medical Association*, researchers studied the effect of a low-fat diet on cancer risk. The women were divided randomly into a group that ate a low-fat diet and another group that had no restrictions and ate the average American diet. Researchers found no significant difference in the

rates of breast cancer, colon cancer, or heart attack and stroke between the two groups. They concluded that there was no justification in recommending a low-fat diet to the public as protection against these diseases. This study is particularly important because it was large, well-designed, and independent (it was funded by the federal government), and it followed women for 8 years. The American Heart Association has questioned these findings and continues to recommend a diet low in fat (especially animal fats) and low in cholesterol for the prevention of heart disease.

Critics of this study claim that the low-fat group did not reduce their fat significantly enough to make a difference in health and that the study did not cover enough time. Others said that eating unsaturated fat (a **Mediterranean diet**) was heart healthy and that this study did not distinguish between saturated and unsaturated fat intake. Supporters of the study have said that it shows that how much people eat and how much they exercise (their calorie balance) are more important than what they eat. This study is likely to stimulate more research into low-fat diets and the health differences between unsaturated and saturated fats.

Resources

BOOKS

American Heart Association. *American Heart Association Low-Fat, Low-Cholesterol Cookbook: Delicious Recipes to Help Lower Your Cholesterol.* 4th ed. New York: Clarkson Potter, 2010.

Gillinov, Marc, and Steven Nissen. *Heart 411: The Only Guide to Heart Health You'll Ever Need.* New York: Three Rivers Press, 2012.

Lipsky, Martin S., et al. *American Medical Association Guide to Preventing and Treating Heart Disease: Essential Information You and Your Family Need to Know About Having a Healthy Heart.* Hoboken, NJ: Wiley, 2008.

Mayo Clinic. *Mayo Clinic Healthy Heart for Life!* New York: Oxmoor House, 2012.

PERIODICALS

Hildreth, Carolyn J. "Risk Factors for Heart Disease." *JAMA* 301, no. 20 (2009): 2176. http://dx.doi.org/10.1001/jama.301.20.2176 (accessed September 25, 2012).

Prentice, Ross, et al. "Low-Fat Dietary Pattern and Risk of Invasive Breast Cancer: The Women's Health Initiative Randomized Controlled Dietary Modification Trial." *JAMA* 295, no. 6 (2006): 629–42. http://dx.doi.org/10.1001/jama.295.6.629 (accessed September 25, 2012).

WEBSITES

American Heart Association. "Fats & Oils." http://www.heart.org/HEARTORG/GettingHealthy/FatsAndOils/Fats-Oils_UCM_001084_SubHomePage.jsp (accessed September 25, 2012).

Centers for Disease and Prevention. "Dietary Fat." http://www.cdc.gov/nutrition/everyone/basics/fat/index.html (accessed September 25, 2012).

Hassink, Sandra. "Low Fat Diets for Babies." American Academy of Pediatrics, HealthyChildren.org. http://www.healthychildren.org/English/ages-stages/baby/feeding-nutrition/pages/Low-Fat-Diets-For-Babies.aspx? (accessed September 25, 2012).

McGreevy, Patrick. "State Bans Trans Fats." *Los Angeles Times*, July 26, 2008. http://articles.latimes.com/2008/jul/26/local/me-transfat26 (accessed September 25, 2012).

National Heart, Lung, and Blood Institute. "Low-Calorie, Lower Fat Alternative Foods." National Institutes of Health. http://www.nhlbi.nih.gov/health/public/heart/obesity/lose_wt/lcal_fat.htm (accessed September 25, 2012).

ORGANIZATIONS

Academy of Nutrition and Dietetics, 120 South Riverside Plz., Ste. 2000, Chicago, IL 60606-6995, (312) 899-0040, (800) 877-1600, amacmunn@eatright.org, http://www.eatright.org.

American Heart Association, 7272 Greenville Ave., Dallas, TX 75231, (800) 242-8721, http://www.americanheart.org.

Centers for Disease Control and Prevention, Division for Heart Disease and Stroke Prevention, 4770 Buford Hwy NE, Mail Stop F-72, Atlanta, GA 30341-3717, (800) CDC-INFO (232-4636), TTY: (800) 232-6348, Fax: (770) 488-8151, cdcinfo@cdc.gov, http://www.cdc.gov/dhdsp.

National Heart, Lung, and Blood Institute, PO Box 30105, Bethesda, MD 20824-0105, (301) 592-8573, (240) 629-3255, Fax: (240) 629-3246, nhlbiinfo@nhlbi.nih.gov, http://www.nhlbi.nih.gov.

Tish Davidson, A.M.
Laura Jean Cataldo, RN, EdD

Low-protein diet

Definition

A low-protein diet, a diet in which people are required to reduce their intake of **protein**, is used by people with abnormal kidney or liver function to prevent worsening of their disease.

Origins

The low-protein diet was developed by dietitians and nutritionists in response to adverse effects that protein can have on people with kidney or liver disease. Proteins are required for growth, upkeep, and repair of body tissues. They also help the body fight infections and heal wounds. Protein contains 16% nitrogen, which the body eliminates in the urine as urea. In cases where liver or kidney function is impaired, urea, ammonia, or other toxic nitrogen metabolites may build up in the blood. The low-protein diet is designed to reduce these nitrogen metabolites and ammonia in individuals with liver disease or kidney failure and to reduce the workload on the kidney or liver. If the kidneys, which are responsible for excretion of urea, are not functioning properly (renal failure), or if high levels of protein are continually present in the diet, urea and other toxic nitrogen compounds build up in the bloodstream, causing loss of appetite, nausea, headaches, bad taste in the mouth, and fatigue, as well as possibly further adversely affecting the kidney or liver.

Other conditions that require low-protein diets include tyrosinemia, phenylketonuria (PKU), and **maple syrup urine disease** (MSUD). In this conditions, the body cannot breakdown certain amino acids properly, causing them to accumulate in the body. These conditions can have serious consequences if left untreated.

Description

The low-protein diet focuses on obtaining most of a person's daily **calories** from complex **carbohydrates** rather than from proteins. There are two main sources of protein in the diet: higher levels are found in animal products, including fish, poultry, eggs, meat, and dairy products, while lower levels are found in vegetable products such as breads, cereals, rice, pasta, and dried beans. Generally foods in the high-protein group contain about 8 grams of protein per serving. Cereals and grains have about 2 grams of protein in 1/2 cup or 1 slice. Vegetables have about 1 gram of protein in 1/2 cup, while fruits have only a trace amount of protein in

1/2 cup. To control protein intake, foods such as starches, sugars, grains, fruits, vegetables, **fats**, and oils should be eaten at levels sufficient to meet daily energy needs. If a person has diabetes, the diet must also be designed to control blood sugar.

Protein should never be completely eliminated from the diet. The amount of protein that can be included in the diet depends on the degree of kidney or liver damage and the amount of protein needed for an individual to maintain good health. Laboratory tests are used to determine the amount of protein and protein waste breakdown products in the blood. A suggested acceptable level of protein in a low-protein diet is about 0.6 g/kg of body weight per day, or about 40 to 50 grams per day. A person suffering from a kidney disease such as nephrotic syndrome, where large amounts of protein are lost in the urine, should ingest moderate levels of protein (0.8 kg per kg of body weight per day).

A sample menu for one day might include:

- Breakfast: 1 orange, 1 egg or egg substitute, 1/2 cup rice or creamed cereal, 1 slice whole wheat bread (toasted), 1/2 tablespoon margarine or butter, 1/2 cup whole milk, hot non-caloric beverage, 1 tablespoon sugar (optional)
- Lunch: 1 ounce sliced turkey breast, 1/2 cup steamed broccoli, 1 slice whole wheat bread, 1/2 tablespoon margarine or butter, 1 apple, 1/2 cup gelatin dessert, 1 cup grape juice, hot non-caloric beverage, 1 tablespoon sugar (optional)
- Mid-Afternoon Snack: 6 squares salt-free soda crackers, 1/2 tablespoon margarine or butter, 1 to 2 tablespoons jelly, 1/2 cup apple juice
- Dinner: 1/2 cup tomato juice, 1 ounce beef, 1 baked potato, 1 teaspoon margarine or butter (optional), 1/2 cup steamed spinach, 1 slice whole wheat bread, 1/3 cup sherbet, 4 apricot halves, hot non-caloric beverage
- Evening Snack: 1 banana

This sample menu contains about 1850 calories, with a protein content of 8%.

Special, low-protein products, especially breads and pastas, are available from various food manufacturers for people who need to follow a low-protein diet. Specific information on the protein content of foods can be found on food labels. Books that list protein contents of various foods as well as low-protein cookbooks are also available.

In addition, it is recommended that fat calories be obtained from monounsaturated and polyunsaturated fats. Some people may also be required to reduce their **sodium** and potassium ingestion in foods. Sodium restriction improves the ability to control blood pressure and body fluid build-up as well as to avoid congestive heart failure. Foods with high sodium contents, such as processed, convenience and fast foods, salty snacks, and salty seasonings, should be avoided. Potassium is necessary for nerve and muscle health. Dietary potassium restriction is required if potassium is not excreted and builds to high levels in the blood, which may result in dangerous heart rhythms. At very high levels, potassium can even cause the heart to stop beating.

As kidney function decreases, the kidneys may reduce their production of urine, and the body can become overloaded with fluids. This fluid accumulation can result in swelling of the legs, hands, and face; high blood pressure; and shortness of breath. To relieve these symptoms, restriction of fluids, including water, soup, juice, milk, popsicles, and gelatin, should be incorporated into the low-protein diet. Liver disease may also require dietary fluid restrictions.

Function

The purpose of a low-protein diet is to prevent worsening of kidney or liver disease. The diet is effective because it decreases the stress on the kidney or liver.

Benefits

Protein restriction lessens the protein load on the kidney or liver, which slows down the continued development of disease.

Precautions

A person requiring a low-protein diet should consult a dietitian familiar with liver or kidney disease to provide guidance on developing an appropriate diet as well as to learn how to follow the diet effectively. The diet must meet the person's nutritional needs, cut down the work load on the kidneys or liver, help maintain the kidney or liver function that is left, control the build-up of waste products, and reduce symptoms of the kidney or liver disease. Strict adherence to the diet can be difficult, especially for children. Small amounts of protein-containing food combined with larger amounts of low or no-protein foods can be used to make the diet more acceptable. Some people eliminate meat, eggs, and cheese from their diets rather than measure the amounts of protein from these foods. However, care must be taken to make sure that some protein is included in a vegetarian diet to provide for growth and development, including building muscles and repairing wounds. Another approach, since it is difficult to manage portion sizes of foods other than milk, is to omit meats, fish, and chicken from the diet and use milk as the primary source of protein.

A person with both kidney disease and diabetes must be careful to eat only low-to-moderate amounts of carbohydrates along with monounsaturated and polyunsaturated fats.

The human body reacts to protein deficiency by taking amino acids (the building blocks of proteins) away from muscle tissue and other areas of the body. The process, in which the body basically metabolizes itself, is called catabolism and leads to muscle loss and weakness. The use of exercise and strength training is recommended to counter the effects of muscle loss.

Risks

The levels of **calcium** and phosphorus must be monitored closely, for in people with kidney disease, phosphorus levels can become too high, while levels of calcium can become too low. Monitoring of these two **minerals** may require an adjustment in dietary intakes of these minerals. Phosphorus is a mineral that helps to keep bones strong. Too much phosphorus, however, may cause itchy skin or painful joints. Calcium is required to maintain bone density and **vitamin D** is necessary to control the balance of calcium and phosphorus. If changes to add these nutrients to the diet are not adequate, then supplements and medications may be required. If phosphorus levels are too high, a person may have to take phosphorus binders that reduce the amount of phosphorus that enters the bloodstream from the intestine. Dairy products as well as seeds, nuts, dried peas, beans, and processed bran cereals, are high in phosphorus, so the use of these food sources may need to be limited.

A low-protein diet may also be deficient in some essential amino acids (which are the building blocks of protein); the **vitamins niacin**, thiamin, and **riboflavin**; and the mineral **iron** (most people with advanced kidney disease have severe anemia). Vitamin supplementation is dependent on the amount of protein restriction, the extent of kidney damage, and the vitamin content of food that is eaten. A person with kidney failure may have decreased urine output. The amount of fluids a person needs to drink is based on the amount of urine produced daily, the amount of fluid being retained, the amount of sodium in the diet, the use of diuretics, and whether the person has congestive heart failure.

In people with advanced kidney disease, a low-protein diet may lead to **malnutrition**. The person may lose muscle and weight, lack energy, and have difficulty fighting infections. Daily calorie intake is dependent on

---

KEY TERMS

Amino acids—These compounds are the building blocks of protein. Some amino acids can be synthesized by the body but some cannot. The latter are referred to as essential amino acids and must be obtained from protein in the diet.

Protein—A nutrient found in foods like meat, fish, poultry, eggs, dairy products, beans, nuts, and tofu. Protein molecules are comprised of thousands of amino acids. The primary function of protein is growth and repair of body tissues.

Uric acid—An acid found in urine and blood that is produced by the body's breakdown of nitrogen wastes.

---

the amount needed to prevent breakdown of body tissues. Body weight and protein status should be monitored periodically, which in some cases may be daily. Extra calories can be added to the diet by increasing the use of heart-healthy fats and eating candy or other sweet foods, such as canned or frozen fruits in heavy syrup.

Research and general acceptance

Very low-protein diets coupled with amino acid supplements have been shown to slow down the progression of and even cure certain types of kidney disease in people in early stages of the disease. In adults with moderate-to-severe chronic renal failure, reduced protein intake has also been shown to decrease the risk of end-stage renal disease, based on a systematic review of eight randomized trials with 1,524 patients who were followed for at least one year. Renal death was defined as initiation of dialysis, kidney transplant, or patient death. The incidence of renal death was 13.5% in patients following the low-protein diet compared with 19.4% in patients receiving the higher-protein diet. However, there was insufficient evidence to determine the optimal level of protein intake.

Although the low-protein diet may help those with chronic kidney or liver disease, it is known to lead to muscle loss. In 2004, researchers in the Nutrition, Exercise Physiology, and Sarcopenia Laboratory of the Jean Mayer USDA Human Nutrition Research Center on Aging at Tufts University (HNRCA) in Boston, Massachusetts, reported on a study involving a group of volunteers with chronic kidney disease who consumed a low-protein diet. About half the group engaged in resistance training, while the other half served as a control group. Among the strength-training participants who exercised for 45 minutes (including warm up and cool-down) three times per week for 12 weeks, measurements showed that, on average, total muscle **fiber** increased by 32%, and muscle strength increased by 30%. Those who did not exercise lost on average about 3% of their body weight, or about 9 pounds.

Researchers studying a group of vegetarians who had maintained a diet relatively low in protein and calories found that they had lower blood levels of several hormones and other substances that have been tied to certain cancers. Additionally, it has been shown that a low-protein diet protects against gout, which is caused by too much uric acid in the blood. The excess uric acid forms crystal deposits in joints, particularly in the big toe, feet, and ankles, resulting in episodes of pain.

A low-protein diet has also been shown to help people with Parkinson's disease. In this disease, dopamine-secreting neurons in the brain die off, leading to tremors, slowness, and rigidity. The most common treatment is a dopamine precursor called levodopa. However, the effects of this drug can decrease over time, resulting in "on" periods when the person exhibits few symptoms and other "off" periods when the person suffers from high and often debilitating symptoms. A research team in Italy showed that lowering the protein content of the diet can improve levodopa therapy and reduce the number and length of the "off periods." Additional studies are needed to confirm these results.

Resources

BOOKS

Erdman, John W., Jr., Ian A. MacDonald., and Steven H. Zeisel, eds. *Present Knowledge in Nutrition.* 10th ed. New York: Wiley-Blackwell, 2012.

Kang, Mandip S. *Doctors Kidney Diet: A Nutritional Guide to Manage, Slow Down and Halt the Progression of Kidney Disease.* Garden City Park, NY: Square One Publishers, 2012.

Thomas, Lynn K., and Jennifer Bohnstadt Othersen, eds. *Nutrition Therapy for Chronic Kidney Disease.* Boca Raton, FL: CRC Press, 2012.

WEBSITES

Adams, Maria. "Low-Protein Diet." Tufts Medical Center. http://www.tufts-nemc.org/apps/HealthGate/ Article.aspx?chunkiid = 197991 (accessed September 25, 2012).

National Kidney Foundation. "Enjoy Your Own Recipes Using Less Protein." http://www.kidney.org/atoz/ content/enjoy.cfm (accessed September 25, 2012).

ORGANIZATIONS

American Association of Kidney Patients, 2701 N. Rocky Point Dr., Ste. 150, Tampa, FL 33607, (800) 749-2257, Fax: (813) 636-8122, info@aakp.org, http://www. aakp.org.

American Diabetes Association, 1701 North Beauregard St., Alexandria, VA 22311, (800) DIABETES (342-2383), askADA@diabetes.org, http://www.diabetes.org.

American Liver Foundation, 39 Broadway, Ste. 2700, New York, NY 10006, (212) 668-1000, Fax: (212) 483-8179, (800) GO-LIVER (465-4837), http://www.liver foundation.org.

National Institute of Diabetes and Digestive and Kidney Diseases, 31 Center Dr., MSC 2560, Bldg 31, Rm 9A06, Bethesda, MD 20892, (301) 496-3583, http://www2. niddk.nih.gov.

National Kidney Foundation, 30 East 33rd St., New York, NY 10016, (212) 889-2210, Fax: (212) 689-9261, (800) 622-9010, http://www.kidney.org.

Tish Davidson, A.M.
Laura Jean Cataldo, RN, EdD

Low-sodium diet

Definition

A low-**sodium** diet is a diet that is low in salt, usually allowing less than 1 teaspoon per day. Many diseases, including kidney disease, heart disease, and diabetes, require patients to follow a low-sodium diet.

Origins

There is no single origin for the idea behind low-sodium diets. Many hospitals and health centers have long recommended that people with diseases that are affected by sodium intake lower the amount of salt in their diet.

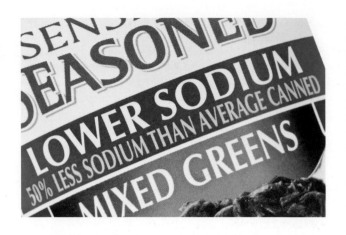

Low-sodium canned good. *(© Istockphoto.com/WendellandCarolyn)*

Description

The role of sodium

The majority of sodium consumed comes from sodium chloride (NaCl), better known as salt. Salt has many useful properties, both in food preservation and for the body. It helps to prevent spoilage by drawing the moisture out of foods. This helps to keep bacteria from growing in the food. It can also kill bacteria that are already growing on the surface of foods. Before refrigeration technology was developed, salting was one of the few methods available for preserving foods, such as meat, through the winter. Salt also dissolves into the **electrolytes** Na+ and Cl1, which help maintain the right balance of fluids in the body, transmit signals through the nervous system, and cause muscles to contract and relax.

The kidneys are responsible for regulating the amount of sodium in the body. When the body has too much sodium, the kidneys filter some out and the excess amounts are excreted from the body in the urine. When the body does not have enough sodium, the kidneys help to conserve sodium and return the needed amount into the bloodstream. When a person eats too much salt, however, and the kidneys are not able to filter enough out, sodium begins to build up in the blood. In the same way that salt pulls water out of foods, sodium in the blood pulls out and holds water from cells in the body. This increases the volume of the blood and puts strain on the heart and circulatory system.

Ways to reduce salt intake

According to a study done by the Mayo Clinic, the average American gets only 6% of their total salt intake from salt that is added at the table. Only 5% comes from salt that is added during cooking, and natural sources in food make up only another 11%. The remaining 77% comes from processed or prepared foods. Many packaged meats, as well as canned and frozen foods, contain a surprising amount of salt. Salt is used heavily by manufacturers because it acts as a preservative, adds flavor to foods, helps to keep foods from drying out, and can even increase the sweetness in desserts. Soups are often especially high in salt because salt helps to disguise chemical or metallic aftertastes.

One of the best ways to reduce salt intake is to cut back on heavily processed and prepared foods. Hot dogs, sausages, ham, and prepackaged deli meats usually contain much more salt than freshly sliced lean meats, such as chicken or fish. Most canned vegetables also have a much higher salt content than the same vegetable found in the fresh produce section. Frozen prepared meals should be avoided for the same reason, and canned soups usually contain much more salt than soups made at home. By reading the nutrition facts label on the side of commercially manufactured foods, consumers can determine how much sodium is in the food they are considering.

When choosing canned or frozen foods, people who wish to reduce their salt intake can often find a "low sodium" option. The U.S. Food and Drug Administration (FDA) sets legal standards for how much sodium can be contained in a product that is labeled "low sodium." Products labeled as such may not contain more than 140 milligrams of sodium per serving, while products labeled as "reduced sodium" only need to contain 25% less sodium than the usual amounts found in those products.

Meals served in restaurants are also often high in salt. Most restaurant kitchens use a great deal of processed foods. They then often add more salt because it is an inexpensive way to improve the taste. Recently, some chain restaurants have begun providing dietary information about their meals. Usually this is printed in a pamphlet that is separate from the menu, so customers may need to ask for it. Some restaurant chains even provide this information on their websites so that customers can decide on a low-sodium meal before they visit the restaurant. If this information is not available, dieters can use the same ideas for avoiding salt at the restaurant that they do at the supermarket. Salads and other foods made with fresh vegetables will usually have less salt than soups. Appetizers and meals with sauces should generally be avoided.

Another time that salt can be eliminated from the diet is when cooking or preparing meals at home. With the exception of baked goods, many recipes that call for salt do so only for taste, and it can be left out. By substituting herbs and spices for salt, the cook can avoid making bland food while still avoiding salt. When choosing an herb or spice mixture, it is important to select one that is not itself high in sodium. Using the zest of a lemon or lime is another a good way to add flavor without adding salt. There are also artificial salt substitutes available, although kidney patients should avoid these as they are usually high in potassium, another mineral that is regulated by the kidneys.

The most obvious way to reduce salt intake is to cut back on the amount of salt added at the table. Since salt is an acquired taste, many doctors recommend simply removing the salt shaker from the table altogether. Most condiments like ketchup, mustard, and pickle relish are high in salt. Eliminating these can be a significant help. Many commercially available sauces, dips, and salad dressings also contain a lot of salt. By checking the labels on these condiments before purchasing, consumers can often find options with less sodium.

Sodium content of popular foods

Many people are unaware of just how much sodium is in some of the most popular foods. A low-sodium diet generally consists of 1,500 to 2,400 milligrams of sodium each day. Some foods contain almost half of this in a single serving. The following is a list of foods and the approximate amount of sodium in one serving of each of them.

- 1 large cheeseburger: 1,220 mg
- 1 cup canned soup: 800 mg
- 1 hot dog: 650 mg
- 12-ounce can of soda: 25 mg
- 1/2 cup cottage cheese: 425 mg
- 1 Tablespoon soy sauce: 800 mg
- 1 bean burrito: 920 mg
- 1 Saltine cracker: 70 mg
- 1 frozen enchilada: 680 mg

Function

The low-sodium diet is designed to lower the amount of sodium that a person consumes. While this is generally considered healthy for most Americans, a low-sodium diet is particularly important for people suffering from certain conditions and diseases.

For kidney patients, reducing sodium is important because the kidneys are no longer capable of effectively filtering sodium out of the body. If these patients do not reduce their sodium intake, the buildup of sodium will cause fluid retention, which

---

KEY TERMS

Electrolyte—Ions in the body that participate in metabolic reactions. The major human electrolytes are sodium (Na+), potassium (K+), calcium (Ca 2+), magnesium (Mg2+), chloride (Cl-), phosphate (HPO4 2-), bicarbonate (HCO3-), and sulfate (SO4 2-).

Hyponatremia—An abnormally low concentration of sodium in the blood.

Mineral—An inorganic substance found in the earth that is necessary in small quantities for the body to maintain health. Examples: zinc, copper, iron.

---

can cause swelling in the lower extremities. A low-sodium diet will help to prevent this problem. For heart patients, a low-sodium diet is important to help reduce strain on the heart. Excess sodium in the bloodstream means that excess fluid is kept suspended, which increases the volume that the heart must pump.

Benefits

There are benefits of a low-sodium diet for people suffering from many different diseases and even for those who are not. A diet that is low in sodium can help to reduce blood pressure and the risk of heart disease and stroke. People who have a family history of heart problems, people of African decent, smokers, those who frequently drink alcohol, people who are overweight or do not exercise regularly, and people who live with a lot of unmanaged stress are all at higher risk for increased blood pressure and should consider a low-sodium diet. For heart disease patients, a low-sodium diet can be part of a plan to reduce their blood pressure and reduce the strain on their heart in order to slow the progress of current conditions and prevent future problems. For kidney patients, a low-sodium diet is necessary to prevent fluid retention.

Precautions

Anyone thinking of significantly altering their regular diet should talk to their physician. Each person has different dietary needs, which should be considered. In general, moderately lowering sodium intake is considered safe for most people. Dieters should be careful to not severely and abruptly increase their level of exercise and fluid intake while severely and abruptly lowering their sodium intake to avoid hyponatremia.

Risks

The risks of following a low-sodium diet are very low. Many experts believe that most Americans could benefit from following a low-sodium diet, even if they do not yet suffer from any of the conditions that might require them to do so. Most Americans consume between 3,000 and 5,000 milligrams of sodium per day, and a low-sodium diet reduces this to a healthier level of between 1,500 and 2,400 milligrams per day. Since the physiological requirement for sodium for adults is only 500 milligrams daily, there is little danger that a person following a low-sodium diet will consume so little sodium that it will endanger their health.

Some athletes and others who exercise frequently and ingest very little sodium yet drink a lot of water may be at risk of hyponatremia, a condition that occurs when the body does not have enough sodium. Though rare, low sodium levels can cause headache, nausea, lethargy, confusion, muscle twitching, and convulsions.

Research and general acceptance

Low-sodium diets are generally accepted as part of many programs that are aimed at lowering the serious risks posed by certain diseases, such as kidney and heart disease. Most health professionals agree that a low-sodium diet is not only necessary for patients suffering from these diseases, but would also be healthy and beneficial for most Americans. There is a great deal of scientific research that supports a direct link between salt intake and blood pressure.

Resources

BOOKS

American Heart Association. *American Heart Association Low-Salt Cookbook*. New York: Clarkson Potter, 2006.

Gazzaniga, Donald A., and Maureen A. Gazzaniga. *The No-Salt, Lowest Sodium Light Meals Book*. New York: Thomas Dunne Books, 2005.

Larsen, Laura, ed. *Diet and Nutrition Sourcebook*. Detroit, MI: Omnigraphics, 2011.

Willis, Alicia P., ed. *Diet Therapy Research Trends*. New York: Nova Science, 2007.

PERIODICALS

Graudal, N.A., T. Hubeck-Graudal, and G. Jürgens. "Effects of Low-Sodium Diet vs. High-Sodium Diet on Blood Pressure, Renin, Aldosterone, Catecholamines, Cholesterol, and Triglyceride (Cochrane Review)." *American Journal of Hypertension* 25, no. 1 (2012): 1–15.

WEBSITES

American Heart Association. "Sodium (Salt or Sodium Chloride)." http://www.heart.org/HEARTORG/ GettingHealthy/NutritionCenter/HealthyDietGoals/ Sodium-Salt-or-Sodium-Chloride_UCM_303290_ Article.jsp (accessed October 3, 2012).

Cleveland Clinic. "Low-Sodium Diet Guidelines." http:// my.clevelandclinic.org/healthy_living/Nutrition/ hic_Low-Sodium_Diet_Guidelines.aspx (accessed October 3, 2012).

MedlinePlus. "Dietary Sodium." U.S. National Library of Medicine, National Institutes of Health. http://www. nlm.nih.gov/medlineplus/dietarysodium.html (accessed October 3, 2012).

University of California San Francisco (UCSF) Medical Center. "Guidelines for a Low-Sodium Diet." http:// www.ucsfhealth.org/education/guidelines_for_a_ low_sodium_diet/index.html (accessed October 3, 2012).

Zeratsky, Katherine. "Low-Sodium Diet: Why is Processed Food So Salty?" MayoClinic.com. http:// www.mayoclinic.com/health/food-and-nutrition/ AN00350 (accessed October 3, 2012).

ORGANIZATIONS

Academy of Nutrition and Dietetics, 120 South Riverside Plz., Ste. 2000, Chicago, IL 60606-6995, (312) 899-0040, (800) 877-1600, amacmunn@eatright.org, http:// www.eatright.org.

American Heart Association, 7272 Greenville Ave., Dallas, TX 75231, (800) 242-8721, http://www.american heart.org.

British Nutrition Foundation, High Holborn House, 52-54 High Holborn, London, United Kingdom WC1V 6RQ, +44 20 7404 6504, Fax: +44 20 7404 6747, postbox@ nutrition.org.uk, http://www.nutrition.org.uk.

International Food Information Council Foundation, 1100 Connecticut Ave. NW, Ste. 430, Washington, DC 20036, (202) 296-6540, info@foodinsight.org, http:// www.foodinsight.org.

Tish Davidson, M.A.

Low-sugar diet

Definition

Low-sugar diets are weight-loss diets or eating plans focused on reducing or eliminating the amount of **sugar** that a person consumes. Sugars, which are a form of **carbohydrates**, occur naturally or are added to foods and beverages. Low-sugar diets include specialized eating plans to manage diets and weight-loss plans like Sugar Busters and the "nothing white" diets. In addition, many Americans in the twenty-first century consume so much sugar that organizations including the American Heart Association (AHA) issued recommendations to reduce that consumption and prevent health problems, including **obesity** and high blood pressure.

Origins

Low-sugar diets are a specialized form of low-carbohydrate diets for diabetes management or weight loss. Some are derived from general guidelines drawn up by such organizations as the AHA and the **American Diabetes Association** (ADA). Others, like Sugar Busters and "nothing white" diets, are weight-loss plans published by individuals or groups for the general public. Some low-sugar diets are based on reducing the total amount of sugar obtained in the diet from fruits, starches, and other foods, not just from table sugar and such other sweeteners as honey, molasses, or corn syrup. Other plans take the form of nutritional guidelines for the general public; recommendations include reducing the intake of added sugars that are found in products like sugar-sweetened beverages and baked goods.

During the 1920s and 1930s, there was much public interest in diets that promised quick weight loss. These **fad diets** included weight-loss plans where people ate a grapefruit with every meal, or ate meat but avoided certain food groups like vegetables. Some of these diets evolved into low-carbohydrate eating plans, which have been popular since the 1960s. Low-sugar diets, however, did not gain much attention from the general public until the 1990s. The concept of the glycemic index was introduced by David Jenkins, a Canadian physician, in 1981. The index is a classification of foods according to the speed at which the body converts carbohydrates to glucose (sugar). Glucose itself is assigned a value of 100 on the glycemic index and other foods are measured against it. Any food below 55 is considered to have a low GI. The first version of the Sugar Busters diet, based on the glycemic index, was published in New Orleans in 1998, with a revised version following in 2003.

Description

Sugars are sweet, water-soluble carbohydrates that occur naturally in some foods and are added to others. Fructose occurs naturally in fruit, and lactose occurs naturally in milk. Specific types of dietary sugars include:

- Simple sugars include monosaccharides (glucose, galactose, and fructose) and disaccharides (sucrose [glucose plus fructose], found in sugar cane, sugar beets, honey, and corn syrup; lactose [glucose plus galactose], found in milk products; and maltose [glucose plus glucose], found in malt).
- Complex carbohydrates (starches) contain glucose.
- Naturally occurring or intrinsic sugars are sugars that occur naturally in whole fruit, vegetable, and milk products.
- Added or extrinsic sugars are added during food processing or at the table.
- Total sugars refers to the sum total of naturally occurring and added sugars in a specific food.
- High-fructose corn syrup is a sweetener that is produced from corn syrup that undergoes enzymatic processing to increase its fructose content and is then mixed with glucose.

Added sugars

According to the AHA, the average American consumes 355 **calories** per day (22.5 tsp. or 122.5 g) in the form of sugars added to foods. The major sources of added sugars are:

- regular soft drinks
- sugars, candy, cakes, cookies, and pies
- fruit drinks
- dairy desserts and milk products including ice cream, sweetened yogurt, and sweetened milk
- sweetened grains, such as cinnamon toast and honey-nut waffles

Sugars are also added to many condiments and canned foods, including ketchup, tomato sauce, and soup.

A 12 oz. (0.35 L) can of sugar-sweetened soda contains 8 tsp. (40 g) of sugar, which represents 130 calories and is near the daily limit of sugar recommended by the association. The AHA recommends that women consume no more than 6 tsp. (30 g) of sugar daily, equal to about 100 calories from added sugar. For men, the limit is about 9 tsp. (0.43 kg), or about 150 calories. The recommended limits for children vary based on stage of development but average around 3–4 tsp. (15–20 g) daily, or 130–170 calories.

General low-sugar diets

Most **diabetic diet** plans are based on some form of carbohydrate counting or carbohydrate measurement, because carbohydrates are the nutrients with the greatest impact on blood glucose levels. Some low-sugar diets are based on the glycemic index, an approach to carbohydrate counting based on the knowledge that the body does not convert all carbohydrates in food to glucose with the same speed or efficiency.

Diabetes management

The American Diabetes Association provides numerous resources to help people customize plans that work for them. People could refer to the "What Do I Eat Now Section" of the ADA website for information about how foods fit into plans where carbohydrates or the glycemic index are tracked. For example, one cup (0.237 L) of milk or yogurt is equal to one small piece of fruit for carb counters or one slice of bread for those who use the glycemic index.

Sugar Busters diet

The Sugar Busters diet is a popularized version of a low-GI diet. There is a child's version of the diet available as well as a book for adults, written by a team of three doctors and the CEO of a Fortune 500 energy company (who is listed as the first author).

The Sugar Busters diet is essentially a diet that eliminates sources of sugar and other high-GI carbohydrates in order to lower blood **insulin** levels. It requires the dieter to eliminate all refined sugar, honey, and molasses; white flour and products made with it (white bread, cake, bagels, crackers, tortillas); potatoes; most forms of white rice; corn flour; sugared soft drinks; beer; and other foods that are high on the glycemic index. The general rule is that any permissible food must contain 3 g (0.10 oz) of sugar or less per serving. The published book contains little information on tailoring the diet to individual needs; a common criticism of it is that it is a one-size-fits-all approach to carbohydrate counting.

Nothing white diets

Nothing white diets, also known as "no white food" diets, are based on the elimination of white foods, including breads, potatoes, refined sugars, and salts. Processed foods containing these ingredients are also avoided. The diets have elements of low-glycemic diets and low– or no–refined sugar plans. Some versions of the diet allow people to drink milk. Measured portions and exercise are not required. Among the

---

promoters of this plan is Paul Array, author of the 2007 book *No White Diet*.

American Heart Association recommendations

The AHA recommendations for reducing sugar intake are targeted at helping people lose weight and improve or maintain good health. Instead of rules about portions and prohibited foods, the AHA wants people to be aware of how much sugar is in the food and beverage products they consume. Once they have this awareness, people can adjust their eating plans so that their consumption of sugar is within the daily limit that the AHA recommends.

Function

Low-sugar diets generally result in weight loss because fewer calories are consumed. According to the American Heart Association, the body does not need sugar to function properly. While calories from food provide energy for the body, a physically inactive person does not burn off excess calories. The AHA cautioned that products with added sugar have many added calories and zero nutrients. This could lead to weight gain and possibly obesity. The purpose of low-sugar diets is to assist in the long-term management of

---

diabetes mellitus, to enable weight loss or weight management, or both.

Benefits

The results of a properly designed low-sugar diabetic diet include improved stability in blood glucose levels, weight loss (if needed), lowered risk of the complications of diabetes, and patient satisfaction with the food choices and dishes allowed on the diet.

Some elements of low-sugar diets coincide with recommendations in the 2010 *Dietary Guidelines for Americans* and organizations including the AHA and the **Academy of Nutrition and Dietetics**, formerly known as the American Dietetic Association. The emphasis is on reducing the intake of sugar and salt and choosing whole-grain foods, lean meats, fruits, and vegetables. However, these organizations do recognize that there is nothing wrong with the occasional sweet treat, so long as these foods are consumed in moderation.

Precautions

Anyone interested in using a low-sugar or any other diet plan for weight loss should first consult their primary care physician. Preparation for following a low-sugar or any other diabetic diet may involve meeting with a dietitian or diabetes counselor as well as a doctor in order to plan a diet that will work well with the patient's food preferences and lifestyle. Children and adolescents, athletes, and people with type 1 diabetes need to take particular care regarding the timing of their meals as well as the total calories and specific foods included in the diet.

Consulting with a healthcare or nutrition professional is especially important because low-carbohydrate diets that allow unlimited consumption of foods ignore the calorie content and the nutritional value of these foods. While it may seem like sound advice to give up eating a starchy potato, replacing that vegetable with large portions of meat could result in weight gain. Furthermore, the Mayo Clinic cautioned that the glycemic index did not factor in the nutritional value of a food. The clinic noted that ice cream and potato chips have a lower GI than a baked potato.

In addition, people wishing to try the Sugar Busters diet should read the introduction to the book first and understand the theory underlying this diet before making food purchases and meal plans based on the diet.

The most important precautions for low-sugar diets, as for any other diet intended for weight control or diabetes management, are making sure that the diet is based on accurate medical information and sound nutritional advice, and that it includes foods and recipes that the individual enjoys for the sake of long-term compliance.

The major problem with low-sugar diets, as well as low-carbohydrate diets in general, is the difficulty most patients have in sticking with them over the long term because of the many restrictions. Researchers at the Mayo Clinic have noted that the dropout rate for these diets is the same as that for low-fat diets and other restrictive diet plans.

Risks

There are no risks in following the AHA's and other organizations' recommendations for sugar intake. Diets like the "nothing white" diet are not realistic and may be difficult to follow in the long term.

One group of people who should be particularly careful in trying a low-sugar diet is athletes, particularly long-distance or marathon runners. Athletes (or people who exercise vigorously for long periods of time) require more high–glycemic index foods in the diet that supply large quantities of glucose quickly to meet the body's needs for energy.

In addition, people with diabetes are at risk of complications from their disease if they try extreme fad diets for rapid weight loss or if they fail to stay within their individual **dietary guidelines**.

Research & general acceptance

The U.S. Department of Health and Human Services and organizations including the American Heart Association recognize the need for Americans to reduce their daily intake of sugar. The recommendations of these groups include foods that are allowed on low-sugar diets, like Sugar Busters and the Nothing White diet. However, those diets do not take into account the nutritional value of foods and are considered fad diets.

QUESTIONS TO ASK YOUR DOCTOR

- Should I reduce my sugar intake?
- How many calories from added sugar can I consume each day?
- Are there safe substitutes I can use in place of sugar?

In the Mayo Clinic evaluation of **glycemic index diets**, the clinic noted that the index could help guide a person to healthier food choices. However, results from studies were mixed about the effectiveness of glycemic index diets. Some research showed little difference in the sensation of hunger after subjects consumed a high-GI food or a low-index eating plan. Other research indicated that a person was more likely to lose weight on a glycemic index diet than on a traditional weight-loss plan, according to the clinic.

Resources

BOOKS

Array, Paul. *No White Diet*. Charleston, SC: 2007.
Dufty, William. *Sugar Blues*. New York: Warner Books, 1993.
Maccaro, Janet. *Change Your Food, Change Your Mood*. Lake Mary, FL: Siloam, 2008.
Steward, Leighton H., et al. *The New Sugar Busters! Cut Sugar to Trim Fat*. New York: Ballantine Books, 2003.

PERIODICALS

American Diabetes Association (ADA). "Position Statement: Nutrition Recommendations and Interventions for Diabetes." *Diabetes Care* 31 (January 2008), Suppl. 1, 561–578. http://dx.doi.org/10.2337/dc08-S061 (accessed September 19, 2012).
Gellar, L.A., et al. "Healthy Eating Practices: Perceptions, Facilitators, and Barriers among Youth with Diabetes." *Diabetes Educator* 33 (Jul–Aug 2007): 671–79.
Johnson, R.K., et al. "Dietary Sugars Intake and Cardiovascular Health: A Scientific Statement from the American Heart Association." *Circulation* 120 (September 15, 2009): 1011–20. http://dx.doi.org/10.1056/NEJMoa1203039 (accessed September 25, 2012).
Qi, Q., et al. "Sugar-Sweetened Beverages and Genetic Risk of Obesity." *New England Journal of Medicine* (September 21, 2012): e-pub ahead of print. http://circ.ahajournals.org/content/120/11/1011.full.pdf (accessed September 19, 2012).
Vega-Lopez, S., and S.N. Mayol-Kreiser. "Use of the Glycemic Index for Weight Loss and Glycemic Control: A Review of Recent Evidence." *Current Diabetes Reports* 9 (October 2009): 379–88.
Ventura, E., et al. "Reduction in Risk Factors for Type 2 Diabetes Mellitus in Response to a Low-Sugar, High-Fiber Dietary Intervention in Overweight Latino Adolescents." *Archives of Pediatric and Adolescent Medicine* 163 (April 2009): 320–27.

WEBSITES

Academy of Nutrition and Dietetics. "Is Your Diet Heart-Healthy?" Academy of Nutrition and Dietetics (January 13, 2012). http://www.eatright.org/Public/content.aspx?id=6442463087&terms=low-sugar+diet (accessed September 19, 2012).
American Diabetes Association. "What Can I Eat?" http://www.diabetes.org/food-and-fitness/food/what-can-i-eat (accessed September 19, 2012).
American Heart Association. "Sugars and Carbohydrates." http://www.heart.org/HEARTORG/GettingHealthy/NutritionCenter/HealthyDietGoals/Sugars-and-Carbohydrates_UCM_303296_Article.jsp (accessed September 25, 2012).
Joslin Diabetes Center. "The Glycemic Index and Diabetes." http://www.joslin.org/info/the_glycemic_index_and_diabetes.html (accessed September 19, 2012).
Mayo Clinic staff. "Glycemic Index Diet: What's Behind the Claims." MayoClinic.com. http://www.mayoclinic.com/health/glycemic-index-diet/MY00770 (accessed July 5, 2012).
Rodale, Maya. "The 'Nothing White Diet.'" *Prevention*, April 20, 2012. Available online at: http://www.foxnews.com/health/2012/04/18/nothing-white-diet (accessed July 5, 2012).
U.S. Department of Agriculture and U.S. Department of Health and Human Services. *Dietary Guidelines for Americans, 2010*. 7th ed. Washington, DC: U.S. Government Printing Office, December 2010. http://health.gov/dietaryguidelines (accessed February 22, 2012).

ORGANIZATIONS

Academy of Nutrition and Dietetics, 120 South Riverside Plz., Ste. 2000, Chicago, IL 60606-6995, (312) 899-0040, (800) 877-1600, amacmunn@eatright.org, http://www.eatright.org.
American Diabetes Association, 1701 North Beauregard St., Alexandria, VA 22311, (800) DIABETES (342-2383), askADA@diabetes.org, http://www.diabetes.org.
American Heart Association, 7272 Greenville Ave., Dallas, TX 75231, (800) 242-8721, http://www.americanheart.org..

Rebecca J. Frey, PhD
Liz Swain